S A U N D E R S

# PHARMACEUTICAL

# WORD BOOK

## 2005

ELLEN DRAKE, CMT
RANDY DRAKE, MS

SAUNDERS

PHARMACEUTICAL

WORD BOOK

2005

ELSEVIER
SAUNDERS

**ELSEVIER
SAUNDERS**

11830 Westline Industrial Drive
St. Louis, Missouri 63146

SAUNDERS PHARMACEUTICAL WORD BOOK 2005          1-4160-0294-4
Copyright © 2005, Elsevier Inc.

---

### NOTICE

Pharmacology is an ever-changing field. Standard safety precautions must be followed,
but as new research and clinical experience broaden our knowledge, changes in treatment and drug therapy may become necessary or appropriate. Readers are advised to
check the most current product information provided by the manufacturer of each drug
to be administered to verify the recommended dose, the method and duration of administration, and contraindications. It is the responsibility of the licensed prescriber, relying
on experience and knowledge of the patient, to determine dosages and the best treatment for each individual patient. Neither the publisher nor the author assumes any lia-
bility for any injury and/or damage to persons or property arising from this publication.

---

Previous editions copyrighted 2004, 2003, 2002, 2001, 2000, 1999, 1998, 1997, 1996, 1995,
1994, 1992

**International Standard Series Number 1072-7779**
**International Standard Book Number 1-4160-0294-4**

Printed in the United States of America

Last digit is the print number:    9   8   7   6   5   4   3   2   1

# Contents

Preface . . . . . . . . . . . . . . . . . . . . . . . . . . . . . . . . . . . . . . . . . . . . . . . . . . . ix

Notes on Using the Text . . . . . . . . . . . . . . . . . . . . . . . . . . . . . . . . . . . . xi
    How the Book Is Arranged
    Experimental, Investigational, and Orphan Drugs
    A Brief Note on the Transcription of Drugs

Pharmaceutical List . . . . . . . . . . . . . . . . . . . . . . . . . . . . . . . . . . . . . . . . . 1
    27,156 Total Entries, including:
        518 New Entries (not in the 2004 edition)
        805 Modified Entries (changes from the 2004 edition)
      3670 Official USAN Generic Drugs
      9156 Brand Name Drugs
      1570 Experimental and Investigational Drugs
      1118 FDA-Designated Orphan Drugs
      1642 Chemotherapy Drugs and Protocols
      1926 Medicinal Herbs and Natural Remedies
      1430 Recently Discontinued Brands (2000 to date)

Appendix A: Sound-Alikes . . . . . . . . . . . . . . . . . . . . . . . . . . . . . . . . . . . 739
    677 Drugs with One or More Similarly Sounding Names

Appendix B: Abbreviations Used with Medications and Dosages . . . . . . . . . 753

Appendix C: Therapeutic Drug Levels . . . . . . . . . . . . . . . . . . . . . . . . . . . . 755

Appendix D: The Most Prescribed Drugs . . . . . . . . . . . . . . . . . . . . . . . . . . 757

# Preface

*Saunders Pharmaceutical Word Book* has been compiled primarily with the medical transcriptionist in mind, although it will certinly appeal to coders, quality assurance personnel, nurses, ward clerks, students of all allied health professions—anyone who has a need for a quick, easy-to-use drug reference that gives more information than just the spelling. Even physicians may find it useful to get quick information on medications their patients may be using for conditions outside their specialty. The "Note on Using the Text" will explain the variety of information this book contains as well as how to find that information.

We think you will find this twelfth edition more complete and more valuable than ever; however, no book is ever perfect. We plan to keep our database current by adding new entries as the information becomes available. Although we have diligently tried to be as accurate and comprehensive as possible, we will certainly welcome your comments regarding additions, inconsistencies, or inaccuracies. Please send them to us via e-mail at the address below, or via regular mail to Elsevier Saunders, 11830 Westline Industrial Drive, St. Louis, MO 63146-3313. We welcome your suggestions.

Authors' e-mail address:
  spwb@saunders.net
Authors' web site:
  spwb.saunders.net

ELLEN DRAKE, CMT
RANDY DRAKE, MS
Atlanta, Georgia

# Notes on Using the Text

The purpose of the *Saunders Pharmaceutical Word Book* is to provide the medical transcriptionist (as well as medical record administrators and technicians, coders, nurses, ward clerks, court reporters, legal secretaries, medical assistants, allied health students, physicians, and even pharmacists) a quick, easy-to-use reference that gives not only the correct spellings and capitalizations of drugs, but the designated uses of those drugs, the cross-referencing of brand names to generics, and the usual methods of administration (e.g., capsule, IV, cream). The indication of the preferred nonproprietary (generic) names and the agencies adopting these names (e.g., USAN, USP) should be particularly useful to those writing for publication. The reader will also find various trademarked or proprietary names (e.g., Spansule, Dosepak) that are not drugs but are closely associated with the packaging or administration of drugs.

There are four different ways to refer to drugs. One of these ways is not the name of the drug itself but the class to which it belongs—aminoglycosides, for example. Inexperienced transcriptionists sometimes confuse these classes with the names of drugs. We have included some 200 drug classes in the main list, with a brief description of the therapeutic use and/or method of action common to drugs in the class. Beyond a class description, each drug has three names. The first is the *chemical name*, which describes its chemical composition and how the molecules are arranged. It is often long and complex, sometimes containing numbers, Greek letters, italicized letters, and hyphens between elements. This name is rarely used in dictation except in research hospitals and sometimes in the laboratory section when the blood or urine is examined for traces of the drug. The second name for a drug is the *nonproprietary* or *generic name*. This is a name chosen by the discovering manufacturer or agency and submitted to a nomenclature committee (the United States Adopted Names Council, for example). The name is simpler than the chemical name but often reflects the chemical entity. It is arrived at by using guidelines provided by the nomenclature committee—beta-blockers must end in "olol," for example—and must be unique. There is increasing emphasis on the adoption of the same nonproprietary name by various nomenclature committees worldwide (see the list on page xiii). The third name for a drug is the *trade* or *brand name*. There may be several trade names for the same generic drug, each marketed by a different company. These are the ones that are highly advertised, and sometimes have unusual capitalization. An interesting article on the naming of drugs is "Pharmaceutical Nomenclature: The Lawless Language" in *Perspectives on the Medical Transcription Profession.*[1] *Understanding Pharmacology*[2] also discusses the naming of drugs.

We have included many foreign names of drugs for our Canadian friends, and also because we have so many visitors to the United States from other countries (and they get sick, too). The international and British spellings of generic drugs are cross-referenced to the American spellings, and vice versa. Occasionally there will be three different spellings—one American, one international, and another British—which are all cross-referenced to each other. Other special features that may be useful, especially for students, are the commonly used prescribing abbreviations and the sound-alike lists that are found in the appendices. The Therapeutic Drug Levels and Most Prescribed Drugs appendices will be useful as well.

This information was compiled using a variety of sources including direct communication with over 500 drug companies. The orphan entries are taken directly from the latest list issued by the FDA. When sources differed, we ranked our sources as to reliability and went with what we thought was the most reliable source. We recognize that there may be several published ways in which to type a single drug, but we have chosen to use only one of those ways. In the instance of internal capitalization (e.g., pHisoHex), it should be recognized that in most instances it is acceptable to type such words with initial capitalization only (Phisohex).

## How the Book Is Arranged

While other pharmaceutical references have separate listings for brand names and generics, or put entries into separate sections by body system or therapeutic use, we have chosen to list all entries in one comprehensive alphabetical listing. Therefore, it is not necessary to know if the term sought is a brand name, a generic, a drug class, a chemotherapy protocol, approved or investigational, or slang; what it's used for; or which body system it affects. If it's given to a patient, it's in "the list." In addition to strict pharmaceuticals, we have included other "consumable" products, such as in vitro testing kits, radiographic contrast and other imaging agents, wound dressings, etc.

All entries are in alphabetical order by word. Initial numbers, chemical prefixes (N-, p-, L-, D-, etc.), and punctuation (prime, ampersands, etc.) are ignored. For example, L-dopa would be alphabetized under "dopa," but levodopa under "levo."

We have indicated brand names with initial capital letters unless an unusual combination of capitals and lowercase has been designated by the manufacturer (e.g., pHisoHex, ALternaGEL). Generic names are rendered in lowercase. Where the same name can be either generic or brand, both have been included.

**The general format of a *generic* entry is:**

**entry** council(s) *designated use* [other references] dosages 🕮 sound-alike(s)

| #1 | | #2 | | #3 | | #4 | | #5 | | #6 |

1. The name of the drug (in bold).
2. The various agencies that have approved the name, shown in small caps, which may be any or all of the following (listed according to appearance in the book):

   USAN      United States Adopted Name Council

   USP       United States Pharmacopeial Convention

   NF         National Formulary

   FDA       U.S. Food and Drug Administration

   INN        International Nonproprietary Name (a project of the World Health Organization)

   BAN      British Approved Name

   JAN       Japanese Accepted Name

   DCF      Dénomination Commune Française (French)
3. The indications, sometimes referred to as the drug's "designated use," "approved use," or "therapeutic action." This is provided only for official FDA-approved names or other names for the same substance (e.g., the British name of an official U.S. generic). This entry is always in italic.
4. The entry in brackets is one of four cross-references:

   see:        refers the reader to the "official" name(s).

   now:      for an older generic name no longer used, refers reader to the current official name(s).

   also:      a substance that has two or more different names, each officially recognized by one of the above groups, will cross-reference the other name(s).

   q.v.        Latin for quod vide; which see. Used exclusively for abbreviations, it invites the reader to turn to the reference in parentheses.

   If there is more than one cross reference, alternate names will follow the order of the above agency list; i.e., U.S. names, then international names, then British, Japanese, and French names. The first cross-reference will always be to the approved U.S. name, unless the entry itself is the U.S. name.
5. Dosage information, including the delivery form(s), is given for medications that may be dispensed generically. No dosage information appears for drugs dispensed only under the brand name, or for those containing multiple ingredients. Some drugs may be available in more than one strength, indicated by a comma in the dosage field:

   > **erythromycin stearate** USP, BAN *macrolide antibiotic* 250, 500 mg oral

   A semicolon in the dosage field separates different delivery forms, such as:

   > **nitroglycerin** USP *coronary vasodilator; antianginal; antihypertensive* [also: glyceryl trinitrate] 0.3, 0.4, 0.6 mg sublingual; 2.5, 6.5, 9 mg oral; 5 mg/mL injection; 0.2, 0.4, 0.6 mg/hr. transdermal; 2% topical

   (Note that some delivery forms come in multiple strengths.)
6. Sound-alike drugs follow the "ear" icon.

**The general format for a *brand name* entry is:**

**Entry** Ⓒᴬᴺ form(s)  ℞/OTC *designated use* [generics] dosages ② sound-alike(s)

| #1 | #2 | #3 | #4 | #5 | #6 | #7 | #8 |

1. The drug name (in bold), which almost always starts with a capital letter.
2. If a brand is not marketed in the U.S., an icon designates the country where it is available. Canadian brands are designated by Ⓒᴬᴺ.
3. The form of administration; e.g., tablets, capsules, syrup. (Sometimes these words are slurred by the dictator, causing confusion regarding the name.)
4. The ℞ or OTC status. A few drugs may be either ℞ or OTC depending on strength or various state laws.
5. The designated use in italics as for generics. These are more complete or less complete as supplied by the individual drug companies.
6. The brackets that follow contain the generic names of the active ingredients to which the reader may refer for further information.
7. Dosage information follows the generics. For multi-ingredient drugs, a bullet separates the dosages of each ingredient, listed in the same order as the generics. For example,

    **Ser-Ap-Es** tablets ℞ *antihypertensive; vasodilator; diuretic* [hydrochlorothiazide; reserpine; hydralazine HCl] 15•0.1•25 mg

    shows a three-ingredient product containing 15 mg hydrochlorothiazide, 0.1 mg reserpine, and 25 mg hydralazine HCl.

    Some drugs may have more than one strength, indicated by a comma in the dosage field:

    **Norpace** capsules ℞ *antiarrhythmic* [disopyramide phosphate] 100, 150 mg

    A semicolon in the dosage field separates either different products listed together, such as:

    **Pred Mild; Pred Forte** eye drop suspension ℞ *corticosteroidal anti-inflammatory* [prednisolone acetate] 0.12%; 1%

    Or different delivery forms:

    **Phenergan** tablets, suppositories, injection ℞ *antihistamine; sedative; antiemetic; motion sickness relief* [promethazine HCl] 12.5, 25, 50 mg; 12.5, 25, 50 mg; 25, 50 mg/mL

    (Note that all three delivery forms of Phenergan come in multiple strengths.)

    Liquid delivery forms show the strength per usual dose where appropriate. Thus injectables and drops are usually shown per milliliter (mL), with oral liquids and syrups shown per 5 mL or 15 mL.

    The ② symbol indicates that dosage information has not been supplied by the manufacturer for one or more ingredients.

    The ② symbol is used when a value *cannot* be given because the generic entry refers to multiple ingredients.
8. Sound-alike drugs follow the "ear" icon.

# Experimental, Investigational, and Orphan Drugs

Before a drug can be advertised or sold in the United States, it must first be approved for marketing by the U.S. Food and Drug Administration. With a few exceptions, FDA approval is contingent solely upon the manufacturer demonstrating that the proposed drug is both safe and effective.

To provide such proof, the manufacturer undertakes a series of tests. Preclinical (before human) research is done through computer simulation, then *in vitro* (L. "in glass," meaning laboratory) tests, then in animals. In most cases neither the public nor the general medical community hears about "experimental drugs" in this stage of testing. Neither are they listed in this reference.

If safety and efficacy are successfully demonstrated during the preclinical stage, an Investigational New Drug (IND) application is filed with the FDA. There are three phases of clinical trials, designated Phase I, Phase II, and Phase III. After each phase, the FDA will review the findings and approve or deny further testing.

Phase I trials involve 20 to 100 patients, primarily to establish safety. Phase II trials may involve several hundred patients for up to two years. The goal in this phase is to determine the drug's effectiveness for the proposed indication. Phase III trials, which routinely last up to four years and involve several thousand patients, determine the optimum effective, but safe, dosage. The manufacturer will then file a New Drug Application (NDA) with the FDA, requesting final marketing approval. Only 20% of drugs entering Phase I trials will ultimately be approved for marketing, at an average cost of $359 million and 8½ years in testing.[3]

An orphan drug is a drug or biological product for the diagnosis, treatment, or prevention of a rare disease or condition. A rare disease is one that affects less than 200,000 persons or for which there is no reasonable expectation that the cost of development and testing will be recovered through U.S. sales of the product. Federal subsidies are provided to the manufacturer or sponsor for the development of orphan drugs. Applications for orphan status are made through the FDA, and may be made during drug development or after marketing approval.

# A Brief Note on the Transcription of Drugs

Many references are available describing several acceptable ways to transcribe drug information when dictated. We offer the following only as brief guidelines.

Although some institutions favor capitalizing every drug, others promote not capitalizing any drug, and yet others put drugs in all capital letters, the generally accepted style today for the transcription of medical reports for hospital and doctors' office charts (see the American Medical Association *Manual of Style*[4] for publications) is to capitalize the initial letter of brand name drugs and lowercase generic name drugs. The institution may also designate that brand name drugs with unusual capitalization may be typed with initial capital letter only, or typed using the manufacturer's scheme.

In general, commas are omitted between the drug name, the dosage, and the instructions for purposes of simplification. Items in a series may be separated by either commas (if no internal commas are used) or semicolons. A simple series might be typed thus:

Procardia, nitroglycerin sublingual, and Tolinase

or

Procardia 10 mg three times a day, nitroglycerin 1/150 p.r.n., and Tolinase 100 mg twice a day.

or

Procardia 10 mg t.i.d., nitroglycerin 1/150 p.r.n., and Tolinase 100 mg b.i.d.

A more complex or lengthy list of medications, or a list with internal commas, may require the use of semicolons to separate the items in a series. For example,

Procardia 10 mg, one t.i.d.; nitroglycerin 1/150 p.r.n., to take one with onset of pain, a second in five minutes, and a third five minutes later, if no relief to go immediately to the ER; Tolinase 100 mg, one b.i.d.; and Coumadin 2.5 mg on Mondays, Wednesdays, and Fridays, and 5 mg on Tuesdays, Thursdays, and Saturdays...

Note that the "one" following Procardia 10 mg and Tolinase 100 mg is not necessary, but many doctors dictate something like this; when they do, it is acceptable to place a comma after the dosage. In addition, when two numbers are adjacent to each other, write out one number and use a numeral for the other.

The typing of chemicals with superscripts or subscripts, italics, small capitals, and Greek letters often presents a problem to the medical transcriptionist. In general, Greek letters are written out (alpha-, beta-, gamma-, etc.). Italics and small capitals are written as standard letters followed by a hyphen (dl-alpha-tocopherol, L-dopa).

When typing nonproprietary (generic) isotope names, element symbols should be included with the name. It may appear to be redundant, but it is the correct form. Therefore, we would type sodium pertechnetate Tc 99m, iodohippurate sodium I 131, or sodium iodide I 125. Occasionally the physician may simply dictate isotopes such as Tc 99m, iodine 131 or I 131, or sodium iodide I 125, and unless he is indicating a trademarked name, it should be typed with a space, no hyphen, and no superscript. This reference indicates proper capitalization, spacing, and hyphenation of isotope entries.

Other combinations of letters and numbers are usually written without spaces or hyphens (OKT1, OKT3, T101, SC1), but this is a complex subject and is dealt with extensively in the AMA *Manual of Style*.

---

[1] Dirckx, John, M.D.: "Pharmaceutical Nomenclature: The Lawless Language," *Perspectives on the Medical Transcription Profession*, Vol. 1, No. 4. Modesto: Health Professions Institute, 1991, p. 9.

[2] Turley, Susan M.: *Understanding Pharmacology for Health Professionals*–2nd ed.. Upper Saddle River, NJ: Prentice-Hall, 1999.

[3] *FDA Consumer*, January, 1995. www.fda.gov/fdac/special/newdrug/ndd_toc.html

[4] American Medical Association: *Manual of Style*, 9th ed. Baltimore: Williams & Wilkins, 1997.

SAUNDERS

# PHARMACEUTICAL WORD BOOK

## 2005

**a-(3-aminophthalimido) glutaramide** *investigational (orphan) agent for lupus nephritis*

**A (vitamin A)** [q.v.]

**A and D** ointment OTC *moisturizer; emollient* [fish liver oil (vitamins A and D); cholecalciferol; lanolin]

**A and D Medicated** ointment OTC *diaper rash treatment* [zinc oxide; vitamins A and D]

**A + D (ara-C, daunorubicin)** *chemotherapy protocol*

**A1cNOW** fingerstick test kit for home use ℞ *in vitro diagnostic aid for glycosylated hemoglobin levels*

**A-200** shampoo concentrate OTC *pediculicide for lice* [pyrethrins; piperonyl butoxide] 0.33%•4%

**AA (ara-C, Adriamycin)** *chemotherapy protocol*

**AA (arachadonic acid)** [q.v.]

**AA-HC Otic** ear drops (discontinued 2000) ℞ *corticosteroidal anti-inflammatory; antibacterial; antifungal* [hydrocortisone; acetic acid] 1%•2%

**abacavir succinate** USAN *antiviral nucleoside reverse transcriptase inhibitor for HIV infection*

**abacavir sulfate** USAN *antiviral nucleoside reverse transcriptase inhibitor for HIV infection*

**abacavir sulfate & amprenavir** *investigational (Phase III) nucleoside analogue and protease inhibitor combination for HIV and AIDS*

**abafilcon A** USAN *hydrophilic contact lens material*

**abamectin** USAN, INN *antiparasitic*

**abanoquil** INN, BAN

**abarelix** USAN *GnRH antagonist to suppress LH and FSH, leading to the cessation of testosterone production (medical castration, androgen ablation); treatment for prostate cancer; investigational for uterine fibroids, endometriosis, and precocious puberty*

**Abarelix-Depot-M** (name changed to Plenaxis upon marketing release in 2004)

**abavca & perthon** *investigational (Phase I/II) plant derivative combination for HIV and AIDS*

**Abbokinase** powder for IV or intra-coronary artery infusion ℞ *thrombolytic enzymes for pulmonary embolism or coronary artery thrombosis* [urokinase] 250 000 IU/vial

**Abbokinase Open-Cath** powder for catheter clearance (discontinued 2003) ℞ *thrombolytic enzymes* [urokinase] 5000 IU/mL

**Abbo-Pac** (trademarked packaging form) *unit dose package*

**Abbott TestPack Plus hCG-Urine Plus** test kit for professional use *in vitro diagnostic aid; urine pregnancy test* [monoclonal antibody-based enzyme immunoassay]

**ABC (Adriamycin, BCNU, cyclophosphamide)** *chemotherapy protocol*

**ABC to Z** tablets OTC *vitamin/mineral/iron supplement* [multiple vitamins & minerals; ferrous fumarate; folic acid; biotin] ±•18 mg•0.4 mg•30 μg

**abciximab** USAN, INN *glycoprotein (GP) IIb/IIIa receptor antagonist; antithrombotic monoclonal antibody; antiplatelet agent for PTCA and acute arterial occlusive disorders*

**ABCM (Adriamycin, bleomycin, cyclophosphamide, mitomycin)** *chemotherapy protocol*

**ABD (Adriamycin, bleomycin, DTIC)** *chemotherapy protocol*

**ABDIC (Adriamycin, bleomycin, DIC, [CCNU, prednisone])** *chemotherapy protocol*

**ABDV (Adriamycin, bleomycin, DTIC, vinblastine)** *chemotherapy protocol*

**ABE (antitoxin botulism equine)** [see: botulism equine antitoxin, trivalent]

**abecarnil** INN *investigational anxiolytic*

**Abelcet** suspension for IV infusion ℞ *systemic polyene antifungal for aspergillosis and other resistant fungal infections (orphan)* [amphotericin B lipid complex (ABLC)] 100 mg/20 mL

*Abelmoschus moschatus* medicinal herb [see: ambrette]

**Abenol** ⊛ suppositories OTC *analgesic; antipyretic* [acetaminophen] 120, 325, 650 mg

**abetimus sodium** USAN *investigational (NDA filed, orphan) oligonucleotide immunosuppressant for systemic lupus erythematosus–associated nephritis*

**Abilify** tablets ℞ *antipsychotic for schizophrenia* [aripiprazole] 5, 10, 15, 20, 30 mg

**Abilitat** (name changed to Abilify upon marketing release in 2002)

**ABLC** [see: TLC ABLC]

**ABLC (amphotericin B lipid complex)** [q.v.]

**ablukast** USAN, INN *antiasthmatic; leukotriene antagonist*

**ablukast sodium** USAN *antiasthmatic; leukotriene antagonist*

**Abolic** *a veterinary steroid abused as a street drug*

**abortifacients** *a class of agents that stimulate uterine contractions sufficient to produce uterine evacuation*

**ABP (Adriamycin, bleomycin, prednisone)** *chemotherapy protocol*

**ABPP (aminobromophenylpyrimidinone)** [see: bropirimine]

**Abreva** cream OTC *antiviral for cold sores and fever blisters* [docosanol] 10%

**abrineurin** USAN *treatment for amyotrophic lateral sclerosis (ALS)*

*Abrus precatorius* medicinal herb [see: precatory bean]

**absinthe; absinthites; absinthium** medicinal herb [see: wormwood]

**absorbable cellulose cotton** [see: cellulose, oxidized]

**absorbable collagen sponge** [see: collagen sponge, absorbable]

**absorbable dusting powder** [see: dusting powder, absorbable]

**absorbable gelatin film** [see: gelatin film, absorbable]

**absorbable gelatin powder** [see: gelatin powder, absorbable]

**absorbable gelatin sponge** [see: gelatin sponge, absorbable]

**absorbable surgical suture** [see: suture, absorbable surgical]

**Absorbase** OTC *ointment base* [water-in-oil emulsion of cholesterolized petrolatum and purified water]

**absorbent gauze** [see: gauze, absorbent]

**Absorbine Antifungal Foot** aerosol powder OTC *antifungal* [miconazole nitrate; alcohol 10%] 2%

**Absorbine Arthritis Strength Liquid with Capsaicin** topical liquid OTC *analgesic; counterirritant* [menthol; capsaicin] 4%•0.025%

**Absorbine Athlete's Foot** cream OTC *antifungal* [tolnaftate] 1%

**Absorbine Footcare** spray liquid OTC *antifungal* [tolnaftate] 1%

**Absorbine Jr.** liniment OTC *analgesic; counterirritant* [menthol] 1.27%, 4%

**Absorbine Jr. Extra Strength** topical liquid OTC *analgesic; counterirritant* [menthol] 4%

**abunidazole** INN

**ABV (actimomycin D, bleomycin, vincristine)** *chemotherapy protocol*

**ABV (Adriamycin, bleomycin, vinblastine)** *chemotherapy protocol for Kaposi sarcoma*

**ABV (Adriamycin, bleomycin, vincristine)** *chemotherapy protocol for Kaposi sarcoma*

**ABVD (Adriamycin, bleomycin, vinblastine, dacarbazine)** *chemotherapy protocol for Hodgkin lymphoma*

**ABVD/MOPP (alternating cycles of ABVD and MOPP)** *chemotherapy protocol*

**9-AC (9-aminocamptothecin)** [q.v.]

**AC (Adriamycin, carmustine)** *chemotherapy protocol*

**AC (Adriamycin, CCNU)** *chemotherapy protocol*

**AC (Adriamycin, cisplatin)** *chemotherapy protocol for bone sarcoma*

**AC; A-C (Adriamycin, cyclophos-phamide)** *chemotherapy protocol for breast cancer and pediatric neuroblas-toma*

**AC/paclitaxel, sequential (Adria-mycin, cyclophosphamide; pacli-taxel)** *chemotherapy protocol for breast cancer*

**ACA125** *investigational (orphan) agent for epithelial ovarian cancer*

**acacia** NF, JAN *suspending agent; emol-lient; demulcent*

**acacia (Acacia senegal; A. verek)** gum *medicinal herb for colds, cough, periodontal disease, and wound healing*

**acadesine** USAN, INN, BAN *platelet aggregation inhibitor*

**acamprosate** INN

**acamprosate calcium** *agent for the treatment of alcoholism*

**acamylophenine** [see: camylofin]

*Acanthopanax senticosus medicinal herb* [see: Siberian ginseng]

**acaprazine** INN

**acarbose** USAN, INN, BAN *antidiabetic agent for type 2 diabetes; alpha-glucosi-dase inhibitor that delays the digestion of dietary carbohydrates*

**ACAT (acylCoA transferase) inhib-itors** *a class of antihyperlipidemics that lower serum cholesterol levels*

**Accolate** film-coated tablets ℞ *leuko-triene receptor antagonist (LTRA) for prevention and chronic treatment of asthma* [zafirlukast] 10, 20 mg

**Accu-Chek Advantage** reagent strips for home use *in vitro diagnostic aid for blood glucose*

**AccuHist DM Pediatric** oral drops OTC *decongestant; antihistamine; anti-tussive* [pseudoephedrine HCl; brom-pheniramine maleate; dextromethor-phan hydrobromide] 15•1•4 mg/mL

**AccuHist DM Pediatric** syrup OTC *decongestant; antihistamine; antitus-sive; expectorant* [pseudoephedrine HCl; brompheniramine maleate; dextromethorphan hydrobromide; guaifenesin] 30•2•5•50 mg/5 mL

**AccuHist LA** sustained-release cap-lets ℞ *decongestant; antihistamine; anticholinergic* [phenylephrine HCl; chlorpheniramine maleate; hyoscy-amine sulfate; atropine sulfate; sco-polamine hydrobromide] 20•8•0.19•0.04•0.01 mg

**AccuHist PDX** oral drops ℞ *decon-gestant; antihistamine; antitussive* [pseudoephedrine HCl; brompheni-ramine maleate; dextromethorphan hydrobromide] 12.5•1•3 mg/mL

**AccuHist PDX** syrup ℞ *decongestant; antihistamine; antitussive; expectorant* [phenylephrine HCl; brompheni-ramine maleate; dextromethorphan hydrobromide; guaifenesin] 5•2•5•50 mg/5 mL

**AccuHist Pediatric** oral drops (discon-tinued 2004) OTC *decongestant; antihis-tamine* [pseudoephedrine HCl; brom-pheniramine maleate] 12.5•1 mg/mL

**AccuNeb** solution for inhalation ℞ *sympathomimetic bronchodilator for children 2–12 years* [albuterol sulfate] 0.63, 1.25 mg/3 mL

**Accu-Pak** (trademarked packaging form) *unit dose blister pack*

**Accupep HPF** powder OTC *enteral nutritional therapy for GI impairment*

**Accupril** film-coated tablets ℞ *antihy-pertensive; angiotensin-converting enzyme (ACE) inhibitor; adjunctive treatment for CHF* [quinapril HCl] 5, 10, 20, 40 mg

**Accurbron** syrup ℞ *antiasthmatic; bronchodilator* [theophylline; alcohol 7.5%] 150 mg/15 mL ⊡ Accutane

**Accuretic** film-coated tablets ℞ *anti-hypertensive; angiotensin-converting enzyme (ACE) inhibitor; diuretic* [quinapril HCl; hydrochlorothiazide] 10•12.5, 20•12.5, 20•25 mg

**Accutane** capsules ℞ *keratolytic for severe recalcitrant cystic acne; investi-gational (Phase III) for neuroblastoma* [isotretinoin] 10, 20, 40 mg ⊡ Accurbron

**Accuzyme** ointment ℞ *enzyme for wound debridement; vulnerary* [papain; urea] 830 000 IU/g•10%

**ACD solution (acid citrate dextrose; anticoagulant citrate dextrose)** [see: anticoagulant citrate dextrose solution]

**ACD whole blood** [see: blood, whole]

**ACe (Adriamycin, cyclophosphamide)** *chemotherapy protocol for breast cancer*

**ACE (Adriamycin, cyclophosphamide, etoposide)** *chemotherapy protocol for small cell lung cancer (SCLC)* [also: CAE]

**ACE inhibitors (angiotensin-converting enzyme inhibitors)** [q.v.]

**acebrochol** INN, DCF

**aceburic acid** INN, DCF

**acebutolol** USAN, INN, BAN *antihypertensive; antianginal; antiarrhythmic; antiadrenergic (β-receptor)* [also: acebutolol HCl]

**acebutolol HCl** JAN *antihypertensive; antianginal; antiarrhythmic; antiadrenergic (β-receptor)* [also: acebutolol] 200, 400 mg oral

**acecainide** INN *antiarrhythmic* [also: acecainide HCl]

**acecainide HCl** USAN *antiarrhythmic* [also: acecainide]

**acecarbromal** INN *CNS depressant; sedative; hypnotic*

**aceclidine** USAN, INN *cholinergic*

**aceclofenac** INN, BAN

**acedapsone** USAN, INN, BAN *antimalarial; antibacterial; leprostatic*

**acediasulfone sodium** INN, DCF

**acedoben** INN

**acefluranol** INN, BAN

**acefurtiamine** INN

**acefylline clofibrol** INN

**acefylline piperazine** INN, DCF [also: acepifylline]

**aceglaton** JAN [also: aceglatone]

**aceglatone** INN [also: aceglaton]

**aceglutamide** INN *antiulcerative* [also: aceglutamide aluminum]

**aceglutamide aluminum** USAN, JAN *antiulcerative* [also: aceglutamide]

**ACEIs (angiotensin-converting enzyme inhibitors)** [q.v.]

**Acel-Imune** IM injection (discontinued 2001) ℞ *immunization against diphtheria, tetanus and pertussis* [diphtheria & tetanus toxoids & acellular pertussis (DTaP) vaccine] 7.5 LfU•5 LfU•300 HAU per 0.5 mL

**acellular pertussis vaccine** [see: diphtheria & tetanus toxoids & acellular pertussis (DTaP) vaccine, adsorbed]

**Acel-P** ⓒᴬᴺ suspension for IM injection (discontinued 2001) ℞ *active immunization against pertussis* [pertussis vaccine, acellular adsorbed] 300 HAU/0.5 mL

**acemannan** USAN, INN *hydrogel wound dressing*

**acemetacin** INN, BAN, JAN

**acemethadone** [see: methadyl acetate]

**aceneuramic acid** INN

**acenocoumarin** [see: acenocoumarol]

**acenocoumarol** NF, INN [also: nicoumalone]

**Aceon** tablets ℞ *antihypertensive; angiotensin-converting enzyme (ACE) inhibitor* [perindopril erbumine] 2, 4, 8 mg

**aceperone** INN

**Acephen** suppositories OTC *analgesic; antipyretic* [acetaminophen] 120, 325, 650 mg

**acephenazine dimaleate** [see: acetophenazine maleate]

**acepifylline** BAN [also: acefylline piperazine]

**acepromazine** INN, BAN *veterinary sedative* [also: acepromazine maleate]

**acepromazine maleate** USAN *veterinary sedative* [also: acepromazine]

**aceprometazine** INN, DCF

**acequinoline** INN, DCF

**acerola (Malpighia glabra; M. punicifolia)** fruit *natural dietary source of vitamin C*

**acesulfame** INN, BAN

**Aceta** tablets, elixir OTC *analgesic; antipyretic* [acetaminophen] 325, 500 mg; 120 mg/5 mL

**Aceta with Codeine** tablets ℞ *narcotic analgesic; antitussive* [codeine phosphate; acetaminophen] 30•300 mg

**Acetadote** IV injection ℞ *antidote to severe acetaminophen overdose (orphan)* [acetylcysteine] 20% in 30 mL single-dose vials

**Aceta-Gesic** tablets OTC *analgesic; antihistaminic sleep aid* [acetaminophen; phenyltoloxamine citrate] 325•30 mg

*p*-**acetamidobenzoic acid** [see: acedoben]

**6-acetamidohexanoic acid** [see: acexamic acid]

**4-acetamidophenyl acetate** [see: diacetamate]

**acetaminocaproic acid** [see: acexamic acid]

**acetaminophen** USP *analgesic; antipyretic* [also: paracetamol] 80, 325, 500, 650 mg, 100 mg/mL, 120, 160 mg/5 mL, 500/15 mL oral; 120, 300, 325, 650 mg suppository

**acetaminophen & butalbital & caffeine** *analgesic; barbiturate sedative* 325•50•40, 500•50•40 mg oral

**acetaminophen & codeine** *narcotic analgesic* 300•15, 300•30, 300•60 mg oral; 30•12 mg/5 mL oral

**acetaminophen & hydrocodone bitartrate** *analgesic; narcotic antitussive* 325•5, 325•10, 500•10, 650•7.5, 650•10, 750•7.5, 750•10 mg oral; 167•2.5 mg/5 mL oral

**acetaminophen & isometheptene mucate & dichloralphenazone** *cerebral vasoconstrictor and analgesic for vascular and tension headaches; "possibly effective" for migraine headaches* 325•65•100 mg oral

**acetaminophen & pentazocine HCl** *narcotic analgesic* 650•25 mg oral

**acetaminophenol** [see: acetaminophen]

**acetaminosalol** INN, DCF

**acetanilid (or acetanilide)** NF

**acetannin** [see: acetyltannic acid]

**acetarsol** INN, BAN, DCF [also: acetarsone]

**acetarsone** NF [also: acetarsol]

**acetarsone salt of arecoline** [see: drocarbil]

**Acetasol** ear drops ℞ *antibacterial; antifungal* [acetic acid] 2%

**Acetasol HC** ear drops ℞ *corticosteroidal anti-inflammatory; antibacterial; antifungal* [hydrocortisone; acetic acid] 1%•2%

**acetazolamide** USP, INN, BAN, JAN *carbonic anhydrase inhibitor; diuretic; anticonvulsant; antiglaucoma; treatment for acute mountain sickness* 125, 250 mg oral; 500 mg injection

**acetazolamide sodium** USP, JAN *carbonic anhydrase inhibitor; diuretic; anticonvulsant; antiglaucoma; treatment for acute mountain sickness*

**acetcarbromal** [see: acecarbromal]

**acet-dia-mer-sulfonamide (sulfacetamide, sulfadiazine & sulfamerazine)** [q.v.]

**acetergamine** INN

**Acetest** reagent tablets for professional use *in vitro diagnostic aid for acetone (ketones) in the urine or blood*

**acetiamine** INN

**acetic acid** NF, JAN *acidifying agent* 0.25%

**acetic acid, aluminum salt** [see: aluminum acetate]

**acetic acid, calcium salt** [see: calcium acetate]

**acetic acid, diluted** NF *bladder irrigant*

**acetic acid, ethyl ester** [see: ethyl acetate]

**acetic acid, glacial** USP, INN *acidifying agent*

**acetic acid, potassium salt** [see: potassium acetate]

**acetic acid, sodium salt trihydrate** [see: sodium acetate]

**acetic acid, zinc salt dihydrate** [see: zinc acetate]

**acetic acid 5-nitrofurfurylidenehydrazide** [see: nihydrazone]

**aceticyl** [see: aspirin]

**acetilum acidulatum** [see: aspirin]

**acetiromate** INN

**acetohexamide** USAN, USP, INN, BAN, JAN *sulfonylurea antidiabetic* 250, 500 mg oral

**acetohydroxamic acid (AHA)** USAN, USP, INN *urease enzyme inhibitor for chronic urea-splitting urinary infections*

**acetol** [see: aspirin]

**acetomenaphthone** BAN

**acetomeroctol**

**acetone** NF *solvent; antiseptic*

**acetophen** [see: aspirin]

**acetophenazine** INN *antipsychotic* [also: acetophenazine maleate]

**acetophenazine maleate** USAN, USP *antipsychotic* [also: acetophenazine]

**p-acetophenetidide** (*withdrawn from market*) [see: phenacetin]

**acetophenetidin** (*withdrawn from market*) [now: phenacetin]

**acetorphan** *investigational enkephalinase inhibitor for acute diarrhea*

**acetorphine** INN, BAN *enkephalinase inhibitor for acute diarrhea; investigational for opioid withdrawal and GERD*

**acetosal** [see: aspirin]

**acetosalic acid** [see: aspirin]

**acetosalin** [see: aspirin]

**acetosulfone sodium** USAN *antibacterial; leprostatic* [also: sulfadiasulfone sodium]

**acetoxyphenylmercury** [see: phenylmercuric acetate]

**acetoxythymoxamine** [see: moxisylyte]

**acetphenarsine** [see: acetarsone]

**acetphenetidin** (*withdrawn from market*) [now: phenacetin]

**acetphenolisatin** [see: oxyphenisatin acetate]

**acetrizoate sodium** USP [also: sodium acetrizoate]

**acetrizoic acid** USP

**acetryptine** INN

**acetsalicylamide** [see: salacetamide]

**acet-theocin sodium** [see: theophylline sodium acetate]

**aceturate** USAN, INN *combining name for radicals or groups*

**acetyl adalin** [see: acetylcarbromal]

**N-acetyl cysteine (NAC)** *natural source of cysteine; promotes an increase in the endogenous antioxidant glutathione*

**acetyl sulfisoxazole** [see: sulfisoxazole acetyl]

**l-acetyl-α-methadol (LAAM)** [see: levomethadyl acetate]

**p-acetylaminobenzaldehyde thiosemicarbazone** [see: thioacetazone; thiacetazone]

**acetylaminobenzene** [see: acetanilid]

**N-acetyl-p-aminophenol (APAP; NAPA)** [see: acetaminophen]

**acetylaniline** [see: acetanilid]

**acetylated polyvinyl alcohol** *viscosity-increasing agent*

**acetyl-bromo-diethylacetylcarbamide** [see: acecarbromal]

**acetylcarbromal** [see: acecarbromal]

**acetylcholine chloride** USP, INN, BAN, JAN *cardiac depressant; cholinergic; miotic; peripheral vasodilator*

**acetylcholinesterase (AChE) inhibitors** *a class of drugs that alter acetylcholine neurotransmitters, used as a cognition adjuvant in Alzheimer dementia* [also called: cholinesterase inhibitors]

**acetylcysteine (N-acetylcysteine)** USAN, USP, INN, BAN *mucolytic inhaler; antidote to severe acetaminophen overdose (orphan)* [also: N-acetyl-L-cysteine; NAC] 10%, 20% oral

**acetylcysteine sodium** *mucolytic inhaler* 10%, 20% inhalation

**acetyldigitoxin (α-acetyldigitoxin)** NF, INN

**acetyldihydrocodeinone** [see: thebacon]

**N-acetyl-DL-leucine** [see: acetylleucine]

**acetylhydrolase** *investigational (Phase II/III) platelet-activating factor for acute respiratory distress syndrome*

**acetylin** [see: aspirin]

**acetylkitasamycin** JAN *antibacterial* [also: kitasamycin; kitasamycin tartrate]

**acetyl-L-carnitine (ALC; ALCAR)** *natural protector of neurologic and cardiac function; biologically active amino acid that transports fatty acids into the* cellular mitochondria for increased energy output; acetylated form of L-carnitine

**N-acetyl-L-cysteine** JAN *mucolytic inhaler* [also: acetylcysteine]

**N-acetyl-L-cysteine salicylate** [see: salnacedin]

**acetylleucine (N-acetyl-DL-leucine)** INN

**acetylmethadol** INN, DCF *narcotic analgesic* [also: methadyl acetate]

**acetyloleandomycin** [see: troleandomycin]

**2-acetyloxybenzoic acid** [see: aspirin]

**acetylpheneturide** JAN [also: pheneturide]

**acetylphenylisatin** [see: oxyphenisatin acetate]

**N-acetyl-procainamide (NAPA)** [see: acecainide HCl]

**acetylpropylorvinol** [see: acetorphine]

**acetylresorcinol** [see: resorcinol monoacetate]

**acetylsal** [see: aspirin]

**N-acetylsalicylamide** [see: salacetamide]

**acetylsalicylate aluminum** [see: aspirin aluminum]

**acetylsalicylic acid (ASA)** [now: aspirin]

**acetylsalicylic acid, phenacetin & caffeine** [see: APC]

**acetylspiramycin** JAN *macrolide antibiotic* [also: spiramycin]

**acetylsulfamethoxazole** JAN *broad-spectrum sulfonamide bacteriostatic* [also: sulfamethoxazole; sulphamethoxazole; sulfamethoxazole sodium]

**N¹-acetylsulfanilamide** [see: sulfacetamide]

**acetyltannic acid** USP

**acetyltannin** [see: acetyltannic acid]

**acevaltrate** INN

**acexamic acid** INN, DCF

**ACFUCY (actinomycin D, fluorouracil, cyclophosphamide)** *chemotherapy protocol*

**AChE (acetylcholinesterase) inhibitors** [q.v.]

*Achillea millefolium medicinal herb* [see: yarrow]

**aciclovir** INN, JAN *antiviral* [also: acyclovir]

**acid acriflavine** [see: acriflavine HCl]

**acid alpha-glucosidase, human** [see: human acid alpha-glucosidase]

**acid citrate dextrose (ACD)** [see: anticoagulant citrate dextrose solution]

**acid histamine phosphate** [see: histamine phosphate]

**Acid Mantle** OTC *cream base*

**acid sphingomyelinase** *investigational (orphan) agent for Niemann-Pick disease type B*

**acid trypaflavine** [see: acriflavine HCl]

**acidogen** [see: glutamic acid HCl]

**acidol HCl** [see: betaine HCl]

**acidophilus (*Lactobacillus acidophilus*)** *natural bacteria for replenishment of normal flora in the gastrointestinal tract and vagina; not generally regarded as safe and effective as an antidiarrheal*

**acidulated phosphate fluoride (sodium fluoride & hydrofluoric acid)** *dental caries prophylactic*

**acidum acetylsalicylicum** [see: aspirin]

**Acid-X** tablets OTC *analgesic; antipyretic; antacid* [acetaminophen; calcium carbonate] 500•250 mg

**acifran** USAN, INN *antihyperlipoproteinemic*

**aciglumin** [see: glutamic acid HCl]

**Aci-jel** vaginal jelly OTC *antibacterial; acidity modifier* [acetic acid; oxyquinoline sulfate; ricinoleic acid; glycerin] 0.921%•0.025%•0.7%•5%

**acinitrazole** BAN *veterinary antibacterial* [also: nithiamide; aminitrozole]

**Aciphex** enteric-coated delayed-release tablets ℞ *proton pump inhibitor for duodenal ulcers, erosive or ulcerative gastroesophageal reflux disease (GERD), H. pylori infection, and other gastroesophageal disorders* [rabeprazole sodium] 20 mg ⧄ AcuTect

**acipimox** INN, BAN

**acistrate** INN *combining name for radicals or groups*

**acitemate** INN

**acitretin** USAN, INN, BAN *systemic anti-psoriatic; retinoic acid analogue*

**acivicin** USAN, INN *antineoplastic*

**ackee *(Blighia sapida)*** fruit *medicinal herb for colds, fever, edema, and epilepsy; not generally regarded as safe and effective as seeds and unripened fruit are highly toxic*

**aclacinomycin A** [now: aclarubicin]

**aclantate** INN

**Aclaro** emulsion Ŗ *hyperpigmentation bleaching agent* [hydroquinone] 4%

**aclarubicin** USAN, INN, BAN *antibiotic antineoplastic* [also: aclarubicin HCl]

**aclarubicin HCl** JAN *antibiotic antineoplastic* [also: aclarubicin]

**aclatonium napadisilate** INN, BAN, JAN

**Aclophen** long-acting tablets (discontinued 2002) Ŗ *decongestant; antihistamine; analgesic* [phenylephrine HCl; chlorpheniramine maleate; acetaminophen] 40•8•500 mg

**Aclovate** ointment, cream Ŗ *corticosteroidal anti-inflammatory* [alclometasone dipropionate] 0.05%

**ACM (Adriamycin, cyclophosphamide, methotrexate)** *chemotherapy protocol*

**A.C.N.** tablets OTC *vitamin supplement* [vitamins A, B₃, and C] 25 000 IU• 25 mg•250 mg

**Acne Lotion 10** OTC *antibacterial and exfoliant for acne* [colloidal sulfur] 10%

**Acne-5** lotion, mask (discontinued 2003) OTC *keratolytic for acne* [benzoyl peroxide] 5%

**Acne-10** lotion (discontinued 2003) OTC *keratolytic for acne* [benzoyl peroxide] 10%

**Acno** lotion OTC *acne treatment* [sulfur] 3%

**Acno Cleanser** topical liquid OTC *cleanser for acne* [isopropyl alcohol] 60%

**Acnomel; Adult Acnomel** cream OTC *acne treatment* [sulfur; resorcinol; alcohol] 8%•2%•11%

**Acnotex** lotion OTC *acne treatment* [sulfur; resorcinol; isopropyl alcohol] 8%•2%•20%

**ACNU (1-(4-amino-2-methyl-5-pyrimidnyl)-methyl-3-(2-chloro-ethyl)-3-nitrosourea)** [see: nimustin]

**acodazole** INN *antineoplastic* [also: acodazole HCl]

**acodazole HCl** USAN *antineoplastic* [also: acodazole]

**Acomplia** Ŗ *investigational (Phase III) selective cannabinoid CB-1 blocker for smoking cessation, weight loss, increasing HDL, increasing insulin sensitivity, and decreasing C-reactive protein (CRP) levels* [rimonabant]

**aconiazide** INN *investigational (orphan) agent for tuberculosis*

**aconite *(Aconitum napellus)*** plant and root *medicinal herb for fever, hypertension, and neuralgia; not generally regarded as safe and effective as it is highly toxic*

**aconitine** USP

**ACOP (Adriamycin, cyclophosphamide, Oncovin, prednisone)** *chemotherapy protocol*

**ACOPP; A-COPP (Adriamycin, cyclophosphamide, Oncovin, procarbazine, prednisone)** *chemotherapy protocol*

**acortan** [see: corticotropin]

***Acorus calamus*** *medicinal herb* [see: calamus]

**Acova** IV infusion Ŗ *anticoagulant for thrombosis due to heparin-induced thrombocytopenia (HIT); investigational (Phase II) for myocardial infarction* [argatroban] 1 mg/mL

**acoxatrine** INN

**9-acridinamine monohydrochloride** [see: aminacrine HCl]

**acridinyl anisidide** [see: amsacrine]

**acridinylamine methanesulfon anisidide (AMSA)** [see: amsacrine]

**acridorex** INN

**acrids** *a class of agents that have a pungent taste or cause heat and irritation when applied to the skin*

**acriflavine** NF

**acriflavine HCl** NF [also: acriflavinium chloride]

**acriflavinium chloride** INN [also: acriflavine HCl]

**acrihellin** INN

**acrinol** JAN [also: ethacridine lactate; ethacridine]

**acrisorcin** USAN, USP, INN *antifungal*

**acrivastine** USAN, INN, BAN *antihistamine*

**acrocinonide** INN, DCF

**acronine** USAN, INN *antineoplastic*

**acrosoxacin** BAN *antibacterial* [also: rosoxacin]

**AcryDerm Strands** wound dressing *high-exudate absorbent dressing for cavitated wounds*

**ACT** oral rinse OTC *dental caries preventative* [sodium fluoride; alcohol 7%] 0.05%

**ACT (activated cellular therapy)** [q.v.]

*Actaea alba; A. pachypoda; A. rubra medicinal herb* [see: white cohosh]

*Actaea racemosa medicinal herb* [see: black cohosh]

**actagardin** INN

**Actagen** tablets, syrup (discontinued 2002) OTC *decongestant; antihistamine* [pseudoephedrine HCl; triprolidine HCl] 60•2.5 mg; 30•1.25 mg/5 mL

**Actagen-C Cough** syrup (discontinued 2002) ℞ *narcotic antitussive; decongestant; antihistamine* [codeine phosphate; pseudoephedrine HCl; triprolidine HCl] 10•30•2 mg/5 mL

**actaplanin** USAN, INN, BAN *veterinary growth stimulant*

**actarit** INN

**ACTH** powder for IM or subcu injection (discontinued 2002) ℞ *corticosteroid; anti-inflammatory* [corticotropin] 40 U/vial

**ACTH (adrenocorticotropic hormone)** [see: corticotropin]

**ACTH-80** subcu or IM injection (discontinued 2002) ℞ *corticosteroid; anti-inflammatory* [corticotropin repository] 80 U/mL

**Acthar** powder for IM or subcu injection (discontinued 2002) ℞ *corticosteroid; anti-inflammatory* [corticotropin] 25, 40 U/vial

**Acthar Gel** [see: H.P. Acthar Gel]

**ActHIB** powder for injection ℞ *infant (2–18 months) vaccine for Haemophilus influenzae type b (HIB) and invasive diseases (15–18 months) caused by HIB* [Hemophilus b conjugate vaccine; tetanus toxoid] 10•24 μg/0.5 mL

**ActHIB/Tripedia** IM injection ℞ *pediatric vaccine for children younger than 5 months old* [Hemophilus b conjugate vaccine; diphtheria & tetanus toxoids & acellular pertussis (DTaP) vaccine] 10 μg•6.7 LfU•5 LfU•46.8 μg per 0.5 mL

**Acthrel** IV infusion ℞ *diagnostic aid for adrenocorticotropic hormone (ACTH)-dependent Cushing syndrome (orphan)* [corticorelin ovine triflutate] 100 μg

**ActiBath** effervescent tablets OTC *moisturizer; emollient* [colloidal oatmeal] 20%

**Actical Plus** ⊛ tablets OTC *dietary supplement* [calcium citrate; multiple minerals; vitamin D₃] 135 mg• ± •40 IU

**Acticin** cream ℞ *pediculicide for lice; scabicide* [permethrin] 5%

**Acticort 100** lotion ℞ *corticosteroidal anti-inflammatory* [hydrocortisone] 1%

**Actidose with Sorbitol** oral suspension OTC *adsorbent antidote for poisoning; reduces intestinal transit time* [activated charcoal; sorbitol] 25• ≟ g/120 mL; 50• ≟ g/240 mL

**Actidose-Aqua** oral suspension OTC *adsorbent antidote for poisoning* [activated charcoal] 25 g/120 mL, 50 g/240 mL

**Actifed Allergy** daytime caplets + nighttime caplets (discontinued 2002) OTC *decongestant; (antihistamine/sleep aid added at night)* [pseudoephedrine HCl; (diphenhydramine HCl added at night)] 30 mg; 30•25 mg ⊠ Actidil

**Actifed Cold & Allergy** tablets OTC *decongestant; antihistamine* [pseudoephedrine HCl; triprolidine HCl] 60•2.5 mg ⊠ Actidil

**Actifed Cold & Sinus** caplets OTC
*decongestant; antihistamine; analgesic*
[pseudoephedrine HCl; chlorpheniramine maleate; acetaminophen] 30•
2•500 mg

**Actifed Plus** caplets, tablets (discontinued 2002) OTC *decongestant; antihistamine; analgesic* [pseudoephedrine
HCl; triprolidine HCl; acetamino-
phen] 30•1.25•500 mg ② Actidil

**Actifed Sinus** daytime caplets +
nighttime caplets (discontinued
2002) OTC *decongestant; analgesic;
(antihistamine/sleep aid added at night)*
[pseudoephedrine HCl; acetaminophen; (diphenhydramine HCl added
at night)] 30•325 mg; 30•500•25
mg ② Actidil

**Actigall** capsules ℞ *gallstone dissolving
agent; also for primary biliary cirrhosis
(orphan)* [ursodiol] 300 mg

**Actimid** ℞ *investigational (orphan)
agent for lupus nephritis* [a-(3-amino-
phthalimido) glutaramide]

**Actimmune** subcu injection ℞ *immunoregulator for chronic granulomatous
disease (orphan) and severe congenital
osteopetrosis (orphan); investigational
(orphan) for renal cell carcinoma;
investigational (Phase III) for multidrug-resistant pulmonary tuberculosis*
[interferon gamma-1b] 100 μg (2
million IU) per 0.5 mL

**actinium** *element (Ac)*

**actinomycin C** BAN *antibiotic antineoplastic* [also: cactinomycin] ② Achro-
mycin; Aureomycin

**actinomycin D** JAN *antibiotic antineoplastic* [also: dactinomycin] ② Ach-
romycin; Aureomycin

**actinoquinol** INN *ultraviolet screen*
[also: actinoquinol sodium]

**actinoquinol sodium** USAN *ultraviolet
screen* [also: actinoquinol]

**actinospectocin** [see: spectinomycin]

**Actiq** "lollipops" ℞ *oral transmucosal
narcotic analgesic for breakthrough pain
in cancer patients* [fentanyl citrate]
200, 400, 600, 800, 1200, 1600 μg

**Actisite** periodontal fiber (discontinued 2004) ℞ *oral antibiotic for periodontitis* [tetracycline] 12.7 mg/23 cm

**actisomide** USAN, INN *antiarrhythmic*

**Activase** powder for IV infusion ℞ *tissue plasminogen activator (tPA) for
acute myocardial infarction, acute
ischemic stroke, or pulmonary embolism;
investigational (orphan) for intraventricular hemorrhage with intracerebral
hemorrhage* [alteplase] 50, 100 mg/
vial (29, 58 million IU/vial)

**Activase Cathflo** [see: Cathflo Acti-
vase]

**activated attapulgite** [see: attapulgite,
activated]

**activated carbon**

**activated cellular therapy (ACT)**
*investigational (Phase II) agent for AIDS*

**activated charcoal** [see: charcoal,
activated]

**activated 7-dehydrocholesterol** [see:
cholecalciferol]

**activated ergosterol** [see: ergocalciferol]

**activated prothrombin complex** BAN

**Activella** tablets (in packs of 28) ℞
*hormone replacement therapy for post-
menopausal symptoms* [estradiol; norethindrone acetate] 1•0.5 mg

**actodigin** USAN, INN *cardiotonic*

**Actonel** film-coated tablets ℞ *bisphosphonate bone resorption inhibitor for
osteoporosis and Paget disease* [risedro-
nate sodium] 5, 30, 35 mg

**Actos** tablets ℞ *thiazolidinedione antidiabetic; increases cellular response to
insulin without increasing insulin secretion* [pioglitazone HCl] 15, 30, 45 mg

**Act-O-Vial** (trademarked packaging
form) *vial system*

**Actron** tablets (discontinued 2000)
OTC *analgesic; antiarthritic; nonste-
roidal anti-inflammatory drug
(NSAID)* [ketoprofen] 12.5 mg

**ACU-dyne** ointment, perineal wash
concentrate, prep solution, skin
cleanser, prep swabs, swabsticks OTC
*broad-spectrum antimicrobial* [povi-
done-iodine]

**ACU-dyne Douche** concentrate OTC *antiseptic/germicidal; vaginal cleanser and deodorizer* [povidone-iodine]

**Acular; Acular LS** eye drops ℞ *nonsteroidal anti-inflammatory drug (NSAID) for allergic conjunctivitis or cataract extraction* [ketorolac tromethamine] 0.5%; 0.4%

**Acular PF** eye drops (discontinued 2004) ℞ *nonsteroidal anti-inflammatory drug (NSAID) for allergic conjunctivitis or cataract extraction* [ketorolac tromethamine] 0.5%

**AcuTect** ℞ *radiopharmaceutical diagnostic aid for acute venous thrombosis* [technetium Tc 99m apcitide] ⑨ Aciphex

**Acutrim 16 Hour; Acutrim Late Day; Acutrim II** precision-release tablets (discontinued 2001) OTC *diet aid* [phenylpropanolamine HCl] 75 mg

**AcuTrim Diet** chewing gum (discontinued 2001) OTC *diet aid* [phenylpropanolamine HCl] 75 mg

**acycloguanosine** [see: acyclovir]

**acyclovir** USAN, USP, BAN *oral antiviral for herpes simplex virus type 2 (HSV-2, genital herpes), herpes zoster (shingles), and adult-onset varicella (chickenpox); prophylaxis of viral infections in immunocompromised patients* [also: aciclovir] 200, 400, 800 mg oral; 200/5 mL oral

**acyclovir redox** [see: redox-acyclovir]

**acyclovir sodium** USAN *parenteral antiviral for herpes simplex virus types 1 and 2 (HSV-1 and HSV-2), herpes simplex encephalitis, and neonatal HSV infections; prophylaxis of viral infections in immunocompromised patients* 50 mg/mL injection

**acylCoA transferase (ACAT) inhibitors** *a class of antihyperlipidemics that lower serum cholesterol levels*

**acylpyrin** [see: aspirin]

**AD (Adriamycin, dacarbazine)** *chemotherapy protocol for soft tissue sarcoma*

**ad5CMV-p53** [see: adenoviral p53 gene]

**ADA (adenosine deaminase)** [see: pegademase bovine; pegademase]

**Adacel** ⓒ IM injection ℞ *active immunizing agent for diphtheria, tetanus and pertussis* [diphtheria & tetanus toxoids & acellular pertussis (DTaP) vaccine, adsorbed] 2 LfU•5 LfU•2.5 μg per 0.5 mL dose

**adafenoxate** INN

**Adagen** IM injection ℞ *adenosine deaminase (ADA) enzyme replacement for severe combined immunodeficiency disease (orphan)* [pegademase bovine] 250 U/mL

**Adalat** capsules ℞ *antianginal; antihypertensive; calcium channel blocker* [nifedipine] 10, 20 mg

**Adalat CC** film-coated sustained-release tablets ℞ *antianginal; antihypertensive; calcium channel blocker* [nifedipine] 30, 60, 90 mg

**Adalat XL** ⓒ extended-release tablets ℞ *antianginal; antihypertensive; calcium channel blocker* [nifedipine] 20, 30, 60 mg

**adalimumab** *recombinant human immunoglobulin G1 (IgG1); tumor necrosis factor-α (TNF-α) blocker; disease-modifying antirheumatic drug (DMARD) for moderate to severe rheumatoid arthritis*

**adamantanamine** [see: amantadine]

**adamantanamine HCl** [see: amantadine HCl]

**adamexine** INN

**adapalene** USAN, INN, BAN *synthetic retinoid analogue for topical treatment of acne*

**Adapettes** solution OTC *rewetting solution for hard contact lenses*

**Adapettes Especially for Sensitive Eyes** solution OTC *rewetting solution for soft contact lenses*

**adaprolol maleate** USAN *ophthalmic antihypertensive (β-blocker)*

**adatanserin** INN *anxiolytic; antidepressant* [also: adatanserin HCl]

**adatanserin HCl** USAN *anxiolytic; antidepressant* [also: adatanserin]

**AdatoSil 5000** intraocular injection ℞ *retinal tamponade for retinal detachment* [polydimethylsiloxane] 10, 15 mL

**Adavite** tablets OTC *vitamin supplement* [multiple vitamins; folic acid; biotin] ± •400•35 µg

**Adavite-M** tablets OTC *vitamin/mineral/iron supplement* [multiple vitamins & minerals; iron; folic acid; biotin] ± •27 mg•0.4 mg•30 µg

**ADBC (Adriamycin, DTIC, bleomycin, CCNU)** *chemotherapy protocol*

**ADC with Fluoride** pediatric oral drops ℞ *vitamin supplement; dental caries preventative* [vitamins A, C, and D; fluoride] 1500 IU•35 mg•400 IU•0.5 mg per mL

**Adcon-L** gel ℞ *investigational (NDA filed) postsurgical adhesion barrier to inhibit the formation of scars and adhesions following lumbar discectomy and breast augmentation surgery* [carbohydrate polymer gel]

**Adcon-P** ℞ *investigational (NDA filed) postsurgical adhesion control barrier to inhibit the formation of scars and adhesions in the peritoneal cavity*

**Adderall** tablets ℞ *CNS stimulant for attention-deficit hyperactivity disorder (ADHD), narcolepsy, and obesity* [amphetamine aspartate; amphetamine sulfate; dextroamphetamine sulfate; dextroamphetamine saccharate] 5, 7.5, 10, 12.5, 15, 20, 30 mg total amphetamines (25% of each)

**Adderall XR** capsules containing extended-release spheres ℞ *CNS stimulant for attention-deficit hyperactivity disorder (ADHD); once-daily doseform* [amphetamine aspartate; amphetamine sulfate; dextroamphetamine sulfate; dextroamphetamine saccharate] 5, 10, 15, 20, 25, 30 mg total amphetamines (25% of each)

**adder's mouth** *medicinal herb* [see: chickweed]

**adder's tongue (Erythronium americanum)** bulb and leaves *medicinal herb used as an emetic, antiscrofulous agent, and emollient*

**ADD-Vantage** (trademarked delivery system) *intravenous drug admixture system*

**ADE (ara-C, daunorubicin, etoposide)** *chemotherapy protocol*

**Adeflor M** tablets (discontinued 2004) ℞ *pediatric vitamin deficiency and dental caries prevention* [multiple vitamins; fluoride; calcium; iron] ± •1•250•30 mg

**adefovir dipivoxil** USAN *nucleotide analogue reverse transcriptase inhibitor for chronic hepatitis B virus (HBV) infection*

**ADEKs** chewable tablets OTC *vitamin/mineral supplement* [multiple vitamins & minerals; folic acid; biotin] ± •200•50 µg

**ADEKs** pediatric drops OTC *vitamin/mineral supplement* [multiple vitamins & minerals; biotin] ± •15 µg

**adelmidol** INN

**ademetionine** INN

**adenazole** [see: tocladesine]

**adenine** USP, JAN *amino acid*

**adenine arabinoside (ara-A)** [see: vidarabine]

**adeno-associated viral vector containing the gene for human coagulation Factor IX** *investigational (orphan) agent for moderate to severe hemophilia*

**adeno-associated viral-based vector cystic fibrosis gene therapy** *investigational (orphan) for cystic fibrosis*

**Adenocard** IV injection ℞ *antiarrhythmic* [adenosine] 3 mg/mL

**Adenoscan** IV infusion ℞ *cardiac diagnostic aid; cardiac stressor; adjunct to thallium 201 myocardial perfusion scintigraphy* [adenosine] 3 mg/mL

**adenosine** USAN, BAN *antiarrhythmic for paroxysmal supraventricular tachycardia; diagnostic aid; investigational (orphan) for brain tumors* 3 mg/mL injection

**adenosine deaminase (ADA)** [see: pegademase bovine; pegademase]

**adenosine monophosphate (AMP)** [see: adenosine phosphate]

**adenosine phosphate** USAN, INN, BAN *nutrient; treatment for varicose veins and herpes infections* 25 mg/mL IM injection

**adenosine triphosphate (ATP) disodium** JAN

**S-adenosyl-L-methionine (SAMe)** *natural amino acid derivative used to treat depression and protect the liver from toxic overload; regenerates liver function and restores hepatic glutathione levels when taken with vitamins $B_6$, $B_{12}$, and folic acid*

**adenoviral p53 gene** *investigational (Phase III) gene therapy for head and neck cancer* [also: p53 adenoviral gene]

**adenovirus-based vector Factor VIII complementary DNA to somatic cells** *investigational (orphan) agent for hemophilia A*

**adenovirus-mediated herpes simplex virus-thymidine kinase gene** *investigational (orphan) agent for malignant glioma*

**5'-adenylic acid** [see: adenosine phosphate]

**adepsine oil** [see: mineral oil]

**adhesive bandage** [see: bandage, adhesive]

**adhesive tape** [see: tape, adhesive]

**adibendan** INN

**A-DIC (Adriamycin, dacarbazine)** *chemotherapy protocol*

**adicillin** INN, BAN

**adimolol** INN

**adinazolam** USAN, INN, BAN *antidepressant; sedative*

**adinazolam mesylate** USAN *antidepressant*

**Adipex-P** capsules, tablets ℞ *anorexiant; CNS stimulant* [phentermine HCl] 37.5 mg

**adiphenine** INN *smooth muscle relaxant* [also: adiphenine HCl]

**adiphenine HCl** USAN *smooth muscle relaxant* [also: adiphenine]

**adipiodone** INN, JAN *parenteral radiopaque contrast medium* [also: iodipamide]

**adipiodone meglumine** JAN *parenteral radiopaque contrast medium (49.42% iodine)* [also: iodipamide meglumine]

**Adipost** slow-release capsules (discontinued 2001) ℞ *anorexiant; CNS stimulant* [phendimetrazine tartrate] 105 mg

**aditeren** INN

**aditoprim** INN

**Adlone** injection ℞ *corticosteroid; anti-inflammatory* [methylprednisolone acetate] 40, 80 mg/mL

**adnephrine** [see: epinephrine]

**ADOAP (Adriamycin, Oncovin, ara-C, prednisone)** *chemotherapy protocol*

**Adolph's Salt Substitute** OTC *salt substitute* [potassium chloride] 64 mEq K/5 g; 35 mEq K/5 g

**ADOP (Adriamycin, Oncovin, prednisone)** *chemotherapy protocol*

**adosopine** INN

**Adoxa** film-coated tablets ℞ *tetracycline antibiotic* [doxycycline monohydrate] 50, 75, 100 mg

**adozelesin** USAN, INN *antineoplastic*

**Adprin-B** coated tablets OTC *analgesic; antipyretic; anti-inflammatory; antirheumatic* [aspirin (buffered with calcium carbonate, magnesium oxide, and magnesium carbonate)] 325, 500 mg

**ADR (Adriamycin)** [see: Adriamycin; doxorubicin HCl]

**adrafinil** INN

**adrenal** [see: epinephrine]

**adrenal cortical steroids** *a class of steroid hormones that stimulate the adrenal cortex*

**Adrenalin Chloride** nose drops, nasal spray ℞ *nasal decongestant* [epinephrine HCl] 0.1%

**Adrenalin Chloride** solution for inhalation ℞ *sympathomimetic bronchodilator* [epinephrine HCl] 1:100, 1:1000

**Adrenalin Chloride** subcu, IV, IM or intracardiac injection ℞ *sympathomimetic bronchodilator for bronchial asthma, bronchospasm, and COPD;*

*vasopressor for shock* [epinephrine HCl] 1:1000 (1 mg/mL)

**adrenaline** BAN *vasoconstrictor; sympathomimetic bronchodilator; topical antiglaucoma agent; vasopressor for shock* [also: epinephrine] ② adrenalone

**adrenaline bitartrate** [see: epinephrine bitartrate]

**adrenaline HCl** [see: epinephrine HCl]

**adrenalone** USAN, INN *ophthalmic adrenergic* ② adrenaline

**adrenamine** [see: epinephrine]

**adrenergic agonists** *a class of bronchodilators that relax the bronchial muscles, reducing bronchospasm; a class of cardiac agents that increase myocardial contractility, causing a vasopressor effect to counteract shock (inadequate tissue perfusion)* [also called: sympathomimetics]

**adrenine** [see: epinephrine]

**adrenochromazone** [see: carbazochrome salicylate]

**adrenochrome** [see: carbazochrome salicylate]

**adrenochrome guanylhydrazone mesilate** JAN

**adrenochrome monoaminoguanidine sodium methylsulfonate** [see: adrenochrome guanylhydrazone mesilate]

**adrenochrome monosemicarbazone sodium salicylate** [see: carbazochrome salicylate]

**adrenocorticotrophin** [see: corticotropin]

**adrenocorticotropic hormone (ACTH)** [see: corticotropin]

**adrenone** [see: adrenalone]

**Adria + BCNU (Adriamycin, BCNU)** *chemotherapy protocol*

**Adria-L-PAM (Adriamycin, L-phenylalanine mustard)** *chemotherapy protocol*

**Adriamycin PFS** (preservative-free solution) IV injection ℞ *anthracycline antibiotic antineoplastic* [doxorubicin HCl] 2 mg/mL

**Adriamycin RDF** (rapid dissolution formula) powder for IV injection ℞ *anthracycline antibiotic antineoplastic*

[doxorubicin HCl] 10, 20, 50, 150 mg/vial

**Adria-Oncoline Chemo-Pin** (trademarked delivery system)

**adrogolide HCl** USAN *dopamine $D_1$ receptor agonist for Parkinson disease*

**Adrucil** IV injection ℞ *antimetabolite antineoplastic for colorectal (orphan), esophageal (orphan), breast, stomach, and pancreatic cancers; investigational (orphan) for glioblastoma multiforme* [fluorouracil] 50 mg/mL

**ADS (azodisal sodium)** [now: olsalazine sodium]

**adsorbed diphtheria toxoid** [see: diphtheria toxoid, adsorbed]

**Adsorbocarpine** eye drops ℞ *antiglaucoma agent; direct-acting miotic* [pilocarpine HCl] 1%, 2%, 4%

**Adsorbonac** eye drops OTC *corneal edema-reducing agent* [sodium chloride (hypertonic saline solution)] 2%, 5%

**ADT** (trademarked dosage form) *alternate-day therapy*

**Adult Acnomel** [see: Acnomel]

**Advair** Diskus (powder for inhalation) ℞ *bronchodilator and corticosteroidal anti-inflammatory combination for asthma and chronic obstructive pulmonary disease (COPD)* [salmeterol xinafoate; fluticasone propionate] 50•100, 50•250, 50•500 µg

**Advance** test stick for home use *in vitro diagnostic aid; urine pregnancy test*

**Advanced Care Cholesterol Test** kit for home use *in vitro diagnostic aid for cholesterol in the blood*

**"Advanced Formula"** products [see under product name]

**Advanced-RF Natal Care** tablets ℞ *vitamin/mineral/calcium/iron supplement; stool softener* [multiple vitamins & minerals; calcium; iron; folic acid; docusate sodium] ±•200•90•1•50 mg

**Advantage 24** vaginal gel OTC *spermicidal contraceptive (for use with a diaphragm)* [nonoxynol 9] 3.5%

**Advate** powder for injection ℞ *antihemophilic for the prevention and control*

of bleeding in hemophilia A [antihemophilic factor VIII, recombinant (rAHF; rFVIII)] 250, 500, 1000, 1500 U/vial

**Advera** oral liquid OTC *enteral nutritional therapy for HIV and AIDS patients* [lactose-free formula] 240 mL

**Advexin** R *investigational (Phase III) gene therapy for head and neck cancer* [p53 adenoviral gene]

**Advicor** caplets R *combination antihyperlipidemic for hypercholesterolemia and hypertriglyceridemia* [lovastatin; extended-release niacin] 20•500, 20•750, 20•1000 mg

**Advil** tablets, Liqui-Gels (soft liquid-filled gelatin capsules) OTC *analgesic; antiarthritic; antipyretic; nonsteroidal anti-inflammatory drug (NSAID)* [ibuprofen] 200 mg ⧉ Avail

**Advil, Children's** chewable tablets, oral suspension OTC *analgesic; antipyretic; nonsteroidal anti-inflammatory drug (NSAID)* [ibuprofen] 50 mg; 100 mg/5 mL

**Advil, Junior Strength** chewable tablets OTC *analgesic; antiarthritic; antipyretic; nonsteroidal anti-inflammatory drug (NSAID)* [ibuprofen] 100 mg

**Advil Allergy Sinus** tablets OTC *decongestant; antihistamine; analgesic; antipyretic* [pseudoephedrine HCl; chlorpheniramine maleate; ibuprofen] 30•2•200 mg

**Advil Cold, Children's** oral suspension OTC *pediatric decongestant, analgesic, and antipyretic* [pseudoephedrine HCl; ibuprofen] 15•100 mg/5 mL

**Advil Cold & Sinus** Liqui-gels (liquid-filled gelcaps), caplets OTC *decongestant; analgesic; antipyretic* [pseudoephedrine HCl; ibuprofen] 30•200 mg

**Advil Flu & Body Ache** caplets OTC *decongestant; analgesic; antipyretic* [pseudoephedrine HCl; ibuprofen] 30•200 mg

**Advil Migraine** liquid-filled capsules OTC *analgesic; antipyretic; nonsteroidal anti-inflammatory drug (NSAID)* [ibuprofen] 200 mg

**Advil Pediatric Drops** oral suspension OTC *analgesic; antipyretic; nonsteroidal anti-inflammatory drug (NSAID)* [ibuprofen] 100 mg/2.5 mL

**AE-941** *investigational (Phase III) shark cartilage–based angiogenesis inhibitor for osteoarthritis, rheumatoid arthritis, and various cancers; investigational (orphan) for renal cell carcinoma*

**AEDs (anti-epileptic drugs)** [see: anticonvulsants]

**A-E-R** pads OTC *astringent* [hamamelis water] 50%

**Aerius** ⒸⒶⓃ tablets R *nonsedating antihistamine for allergic rhinitis* [desloratadine] 5 mg

**Aeroaid** spray OTC *antiseptic; antibacterial; antifungal* [thimerosal; alcohol 72%] 1:1000

**AeroBid; AeroBid-M** oral inhalation aerosol R *corticosteroidal anti-inflammatory for chronic asthma* [flunisolide] 250 μg/dose

**AeroCaine** aerosol solution OTC *local anesthetic* [benzocaine; benzethonium chloride] 13.6%•0.5%

**AeroChamber** (trademarked form) *aerosol holding chamber*

**Aerodine** aerosol (discontinued 2004) OTC *broad-spectrum antimicrobial* [povidone-iodine]

**AeroDose** (trademarked delivery system) R *investigational (Phase I) inhaler*

**Aerofreeze** spray OTC *vapo-coolant anesthetic* [trichloromonofluoromethane; dichlorodifluoromethane]

**AeroHist Plus** extended-release caplets R *decongestant; antihistamine; anticholinergic to dry mucosal secretions* [phenylephrine HCl; chlorpheniramine maleate; methscopolamine nitrate] 20•8•2.5 mg

**AeroKid** syrup R *decongestant; antihistamine; anticholinergic to dry mucosal secretions* [phenylephrine HCl; chlorpheniramine maleate; methscopolamine nitrate] 10•4•125 mg/5 mL

**Aerolate Sr.; Aerolate Jr.; Aerolate III** timed-action capsules ℞ *antiasthmatic; bronchodilator* [theophylline] 260 mg; 130 mg; 65 mg

**Aerolizer** (trademarked delivery system) *oral inhaler for encapsulated dry powder*

**Aeropin** *investigational (orphan) for cystic fibrosis* [heparin, 2-0-desulfated]

**Aeroseb-Dex** aerosol spray ℞ *corticosteroidal anti-inflammatory* [dexamethasone] 0.01%

**aerosol OT** [see: docusate sodium]

**aerosolized pooled immune globulin** [see: globulin, aerosolized pooled immune]

**AeroTherm** aerosol solution (discontinued 2004) OTC *local anesthetic* [benzocaine; benzethonium chloride] 13.6%•0.5%

**Aerotrol** (trademarked form) *inhalation aerosol*

**AeroZoin** spray OTC *skin protectant* [benzoin; isopropyl alcohol 44.8%] 30%

**AERx** ℞ *investigational (Phase III) insulin inhalation system for diabetes management* [morphine sulfate]

*Aesculus hippocastanum; A. californica; A. glabra medicinal herb* [see: horse chestnut]

*Aethusa cynapium medicinal herb* [see: dog poison]

**aethylis chloridum** [see: ethyl chloride]

**afalanine** INN

**Afeditab CR** extended-release tablets ℞ *antianginal; antihypertensive; calcium channel blocker* [nifedipine] 30, 60 mg

**Affinitac** ℞ *investigational (Phase III) antisense agent for lung cancer*

**afloqualone** INN, JAN

**AFM (Adriamycin, fluorouracil, methotrexate [with leucovorin rescue])** *chemotherapy protocol*

**afovirsen** INN *antisense antiviral*

**afovirsen sodium** USAN *antisense antiviral; investigational for genital warts*

**African ginger** *medicinal herb* [see: ginger]

**African pepper; African red pepper** *medicinal herb* [see: cayenne]

**Afrin** extended-release tablets (discontinued 2002) OTC *nasal decongestant* [pseudoephedrine sulfate] 120 mg ☒ aspirin

**Afrin 12-Hour Original** nasal spray, pump spray OTC *nasal decongestant* [oxymetazoline HCl] 0.05% ☒ aspirin

**Afrin Children's Nose Drops** (discontinued 2002) OTC *pediatric nasal decongestant* [oxymetazoline HCl] 0.025% ☒ aspirin

**Afrin Children's Pump Mist** nasal spray OTC *nasal decongestant* [phenylephrine HCl] 0.25%

**Afrin Moisturizing Saline Mist** solution OTC *nasal moisturizer* [sodium chloride (saline solution)] 0.64% ☒ aspirin

**Afrin No-Drip 12-Hour; Afrin No-Drip 12-Hour Extra Moisturizing; Afrin No-Drip 12-Hour Severe Congestion with Menthol** nasal spray OTC *nasal decongestant* [oxymetazoline HCl] 0.05%

**Afrin Severe Congestion with Menthol** nasal spray OTC *nasal decongestant* [oxymetazoline HCl] 0.05%

**Afrin Sinus** nasal spray OTC *nasal decongestant* [oxymetazoline HCl] 0.05% ☒ aspirin

**Afrin Sinus with Vapornase; Afrin No-Drip Sinus with Vapornase** nasal spray OTC *nasal decongestant* [oxymetazoline HCl] 0.05%

**Aftate for Athlete's Foot** spray powder, spray liquid OTC *antifungal* [tolnaftate] 1%

**Aftate for Jock Itch** spray powder OTC *topical antifungal* [tolnaftate] 1%

**afurolol** INN

**A/G Pro** tablets OTC *dietary supplement* [protein hydrolysate; multiple vitamins & minerals; multiple amino acids] 542•≛ mg

**AG-1549** *investigational (Phase II) nonnucleoside reverse transcriptase inhibitor (NNRTI) for HIV and AIDS*

**agalsidase alfa** *investigational (NDA filed, orphan) enzyme replacement therapy for Fabry disease*

**agalsidase beta** *enzyme replacement therapy for Fabry disease (orphan)*

**aganodine** INN

**agar** NF, JAN *suspending agent*

**agar-agar** [see: agar]

*Agathosma betulina medicinal herb* [see: buchu]

**agave (Agave americana)** *plant medicinal herb used as an antiseptic, diuretic, and laxative and for jaundice and liver disease, pulmonary tuberculosis, and syphilis; also used to combat putrefactive bacteria in the stomach and intestines*

**age cross-link breakers** *a class of investigational antiaging compounds that break age-mediated bonds between proteins*

**Agenerase** capsules, oral solution ℞ *protease inhibitor antiviral for HIV infection* [amprenavir; vitamin E] 50 mg•36 IU, 150 mg•109 IU; 15 mg•46 IU per mL

**Aggrastat** IV infusion ℞ *GP IIb/IIIa platelet aggregation inhibitor for acute coronary syndrome, unstable angina, myocardial infarction, and cardiac surgery* [tirofiban HCl] 50, 250 μg/mL

**aggregated albumin** [see: albumin, aggregated]

**aggregated radio-iodinated I 131 serum albumin** [see: albumin, aggregated iodinated I 131 serum]

**Aggrenox** combination-release capsules ℞ *platelet aggregation inhibitor for stroke* [dipyridamole (extended release); aspirin (immediate release)] 200•25 mg

**Agilect** ℞ *investigational (NDA filed) once-daily monoamine oxidase B (MAO-B) inhibitor for Parkinson disease* [rasagiline mesylate]

**aglepristone** INN

**AGN-191024** *investigational (Phase III) agent for glaucoma*

**agofollin** [see: estradiol]

**Agoral** oral liquid OTC *stimulant laxative* [sennosides] 25 mg/15 mL ⊠ Argyrol

**agrimony (Agrimonia eupatoria)** plant *medicinal herb for diarrhea, gastroenteritis, jaundice, kidney stones,* liver disorders, mucous membrane inflammation with discharge; also used topically as an astringent and antiseptic

**agrimony, hemp** *medicinal herb* [see: hemp agrimony]

*Agropyron repens medicinal herb* [see: couch grass]

**Agrylin** capsules ℞ *thrombolytic and antiplatelet agent for essential thrombocytopenia (orphan); investigational (orphan) for thrombocytosis and polycythemia vera* [anagrelide HCl] 0.5, 1 mg

**ague tree** *medicinal herb* [see: sassafras]

**agurin** [see: theobromine sodium acetate]

**AHA (acetohydroxamic acid)** [q.v.]

**AHA (alpha hydroxy acids)** [see: glycolic acid]

**AH-chew** chewable tablets ℞ *decongestant; antihistamine; anticholinergic to dry mucosal secretions* [phenylephrine HCl; chlorpheniramine maleate; methscopolamine nitrate] 10•2•1.25 mg

**AH-chew D** chewable tablets ℞ *nasal decongestant* [phenylephrine HCl] 10 mg

**AHF (antihemophilic factor)** [q.v.]

**AHG (antihemophilic globulin)** [see: antihemophilic factor]

**A-Hydrocort** IV or IM injection ℞ *corticosteroid; anti-inflammatory* [hydrocortisone sodium succinate] 100, 250, 500, 1000 mg/vial

**AIDS vaccine** (several different compounds are included in this general category; e.g., gp120, rgp160, rgp160 MN, rp24) *investigational (Phase I–III) antiviral for HIV and AIDS treatment and prophylaxis* [also: gp120; rgp160; rp24]

**AIDSVax** ℞ *investigational (Phase III) bivalent HIV vaccine* [gp120 antigens]

**AIIRAs (angiotensin II receptor antagonists)** [q.v.]

**air, compressed** [see: air, medical]

**air, medical** USP *medicinal gas*

**Airet** solution for inhalation ℞ *sympathomimetic bronchodilator* [albuterol sulfate] 0.083%

**Airomir** ⓒ CFC-free pMDI (pressurized metered-dose inhaler) *sympathomimetic bronchodilator* [salbutamol sulfate] 100 µg/dose

**Airozin** ℞ *investigational leukotriene synthesis inhibitor for asthma*

**AI-RSA** *investigational (orphan) agent for autoimmune uveitis*

**ajmaline** JAN

**Akarpine** eye drops ℞ *antiglaucoma agent; direct-acting miotic* [pilocarpine HCl] 1%, 2%, 4%

**AKBeta** eye drops ℞ *antiglaucoma agent (β-blocker)* [levobunolol HCl] 0.25%, 0.5%

**AK-Chlor** eye drops, ophthalmic ointment ℞ *antibiotic* [chloramphenicol] 5 mg/mL; 10 mg/g

**AK-Cide** eye drop suspension, ophthalmic ointment (discontinued 2004) ℞ *corticosteroidal anti-inflammatory; antibiotic* [prednisolone acetate; sulfacetamide sodium] 0.5%•10%

**AK-Con** eye drops ℞ *decongestant; vasoconstrictor* [naphazoline HCl] 0.1%

**AK-Dex** eye drops (discontinued 2004) ℞ *corticosteroidal anti-inflammatory* [dexamethasone sodium phosphate] 0.1%

**AK-Dilate** eye drops ℞ *decongestant; vasoconstrictor; mydriatic* [phenylephrine HCl] 2.5%, 10%

**AK-Fluor** antecubital venous injection ℞ *ophthalmic diagnostic agent* [fluorescein] 10%, 25%

**Akineton** IV or IM injection ℞ *anticholinergic; antiparkinsonian* [biperiden lactate] 5 mg/mL

**Akineton** tablets ℞ *anticholinergic; antiparkinsonian* [biperiden HCl] 2 mg

**aklomide** USAN, INN, BAN *coccidiostat for poultry*

**AK-NaCl** eye drops, ophthalmic ointment OTC *corneal edema-reducing agent* [sodium chloride (hypertonic saline solution)] 5%

**AK-Nefrin** eye drops (discontinued 2003) OTC *ophthalmic decongestant* [phenylephrine HCl] 0.12%

**Akne-Mycin** ointment ℞ *antibiotic for acne* [erythromycin] 2% ⓢ Ak-Mycin

**Akne-Mycin** topical solution (discontinued 2003) ℞ *antibiotic for acne* [erythromycin] 2% ⓢ Ak-Mycin

**AK-Neo-Dex** eye drops (discontinued 2000) ℞ *corticosteroidal anti-inflammatory; antibiotic* [dexamethasone sodium phosphate; neomycin sulfate] 0.1%•0.35%

**AK-Pentolate** eye drops ℞ *mydriatic; cycloplegic* [cyclopentolate HCl] 1%

**AK-Poly-Bac** ophthalmic ointment ℞ *antibiotic* [polymyxin B sulfate; bacitracin zinc] 10 000•500 U/g

**AK-Pred** eye drops ℞ *corticosteroidal anti-inflammatory* [prednisolone sodium phosphate] 0.125%, 1%

**AKPro** eye drops ℞ *antiglaucoma agent* [dipivefrin HCl] 0.1%

**AK-Rinse** ophthalmic solution OTC *extraocular irrigating solution* [sterile isotonic solution]

**AK-Spore** eye drops ℞ *antibiotic* [polymyxin B sulfate; neomycin sulfate; gramicidin] 10 000 U•1.75 mg•0.025 mg per mL

**AK-Spore** ophthalmic ointment ℞ *antibiotic* [polymyxin B sulfate; neomycin sulfate; bacitracin zinc] 10 000 U•5 mg•400 U per g

**AK-Spore H.C.** ear drops, otic suspension (discontinued 2004) ℞ *corticosteroidal anti-inflammatory; antibiotic* [hydrocortisone; neomycin sulfate; polymyxin B sulfate] 1%•5 mg•10 000 U per mL

**AK-Spore H.C.** eye drop suspension (discontinued 2000) ℞ *corticosteroidal anti-inflammatory; antibiotic* [hydrocortisone; neomycin sulfate; polymyxin B sulfate] 1%•0.35%•10 000 U per mL

**AK-Spore H.C.** ophthalmic ointment ℞ *corticosteroidal anti-inflammatory; antibiotic* [hydrocortisone; neomycin sulfate; bacitracin zinc; polymyxin B sulfate] 1%•0.35%•400 U/g•10 000 U/g

**AK-Sulf** eye drops, ophthalmic ointment ℞ *antibiotic* [sulfacetamide sodium] 10%

**AKTob** eye drops ℞ *antibiotic* [tobramycin] 0.3%

**AK-Tracin** ophthalmic ointment ℞ *antibiotic* [bacitracin] 500 U/g

**AK-Trol** eye drop suspension (discontinued 2004) ℞ *corticosteroidal anti-inflammatory; antibiotic* [dexamethasone; neomycin sulfate; polymyxin B sulfate] 0.1%•0.35%•10 000 U/mL

**AK-Trol** ophthalmic ointment ℞ *corticosteroidal anti-inflammatory; antibiotic* [dexamethasone; neomycin sulfate; polymyxin B sulfate] 0.1%•0.35%•10 000 U/g

**Akwa Tears** eye drops OTC *moisturizer/lubricant* [polyvinyl alcohol] 1.4%

**Akwa Tears** ophthalmic ointment OTC *moisturizer/lubricant* [white petrolatum; mineral oil]

**ALA (alpha lipoic acid)** *natural antioxidant* [q.v.]

**ALA; 5-ALA HCl** [see: aminolevulinic acid HCl]

**alacepril** INN, JAN

**Alacol DM** syrup ℞ *pediatric decongestant, antihistamine, and expectorant* [phenylephrine HCl; brompheniramine maleate; dextromethorphan hydrobromide] 5•2•10 mg/5 mL

**Ala-Cort** cream, lotion ℞ *topical corticosteroidal anti-inflammatory* [hydrocortisone] 1%

**Alacramyn** ℞ *investigational (orphan) antitoxin for scorpion stings* [centruroides immune Fab 2]

**alafosfalin** INN, BAN

**Alamag** oral suspension OTC *antacid* [aluminum hydroxide; magnesium hydroxide] 225•200 mg/5 mL ⃝ Alma-Mag

**Alamag Plus** oral suspension OTC *antacid; antiflatulent* [aluminum hydroxide; magnesium hydroxide; simethicone] 225•200•25 mg/5 mL

**Alamast** eye drops ℞ *mast cell stabilizer for allergic conjunctivitis* [pemirolast potassium] 0.1%

**alamecin** USAN *antibacterial*

**alanine (L-alanine)** USAN, USP, INN *nonessential amino acid; symbols: Ala, A*

**alanine nitrogen mustard** [see: melphalan]

**alanosine** INN

**alaproclate** USAN, INN *antidepressant*

**Ala-Quin** cream ℞ *corticosteroidal anti-inflammatory; antifungal; antibacterial* [hydrocortisone; clioquinol] 0.5%•3%

**Ala-Scalp** lotion ℞ *corticosteroidal anti-inflammatory* [hydrocortisone] 2%

**AlaSTAT** lab test for professional use *test for allergic reaction to latex*

**Alasulf** vaginal cream ℞ *broad-spectrum antibiotic; antiseptic; vulnerary* [sulfanilamide; aminacrine HCl; allantoin] 15%•0.2%•2%

**alatrofloxacin mesylate** USAN *broad-spectrum fluoroquinolone antibiotic*

**Alavert** orally disintegrating tablets OTC *nonsedating antihistamine for allergic rhinitis and chronic idiopathic urticaria* [loratadine] 10 mg

**Alavert D-12 Hour, Allergy & Sinus** extended-release tablets OTC *nonsedating antihistamine; decongestant* [loratadine; pseudoephedine HCl] 5•120 mg

**alazanine triclofenate** INN

**Albalon** eye drops ℞ *topical ophthalmic decongestant and vasoconstrictor and lubricant* [naphazoline HCl; polyvinyl alcohol] 0.1%•1.4%

**Albamycin** capsules (discontinued 2004) ℞ *bacteriostatic antibiotic* [novobiocin sodium] 250 mg

**Albay** subcu or IM injection ℞ *venom sensitivity testing (subcu); venom desensitization therapy (IM)* [extracts of honeybee, yellow jacket, yellow hornet, white-faced hornet, mixed vespid, and wasp venom]

**albendazole** USAN, INN, BAN *anthelmintic for neurocysticercosis (tapeworm) and cestode-induced hydatid cyst disease (orphan)*

**albendazole oxide** INN, BAN

**Albenza** Tiltab (film-coated tablets) ℞ *anthelmintic for neurocysticercosis (tapeworm) and cestode-induced hydatid cyst disease (orphan)* [albendazole]

**Alberta Lens, The** ℞ *contact lens* [sulfocon B]

**Albright solution (sodium citrate and citric acid)** *urine alkalizer; compounding agent*

**albucid** [see: sulfacetamide]

**albumin, aggregated** USAN *lung imaging aid (with technetium Tc 99m)*

**albumin, aggregated iodinated I 131 serum** USAN, USP *radioactive agent*

**albumin, chromated Cr 51 serum** USAN *radioactive agent*

**albumin, human** USP *blood volume supporter* 5%, 25% injection

**albumin, iodinated ($^{125}$I) human serum** INN *radioactive agent; blood volume test* [also: albumin, iodinated I 125 serum]

**albumin, iodinated ($^{131}$I) human serum** INN, JAN *radioactive agent; intrathecal imaging agent; blood volume test* [also: albumin, iodinated I 131 serum]

**albumin, iodinated I 125** USP *radioactive agent; blood volume test*

**albumin, iodinated I 125 serum** USAN, USP *radioactive agent; blood volume test* [also: iodinated ($^{125}$I) human serum albumin]

**albumin, iodinated I 131** USP *radioactive agent; intrathecal imaging agent; blood volume test*

**albumin, iodinated I 131 serum** USAN, USP *radioactive agent; intrathecal imaging agent; blood volume test* [also: iodinated ($^{131}$I) human serum albumin]

**albumin, normal human serum** [now: albumin, human]

**Albuminar-5; Albuminar-25** IV infusion ℞ *blood volume expander for shock, burns, and hypoproteinemia* [human albumin] 5%; 25%

**Albunex** injection ℞ *ultrasound heart imaging agent; investigational (Phase III) diagnostic aid for infertility due to obstructed fallopian tubes* [human albumin, sonicated] 5%

**Albustix** reagent strips for professional use *in vitro diagnostic aid for albumin (protein) in the urine*

**Albutein 5%; Albutein 25%** IV infusion ℞ *blood volume expander for shock, burns, and hypoproteinemia* [human albumin] 5%; 25%

**albuterol** USAN, USP *sympathomimetic bronchodilator; investigational (orphan) to prevent paralysis cased by spinal cord injury* [also: salbutamol] 90 μg inhalation

**albuterol sulfate** USAN, USP *sympathomimetic bronchodilator* [also: salbutamol sulfate] 2, 4 mg oral; 2 mg/5 mL oral; 0.083%, 0.5% inhalation

**albutoin** USAN, INN *anticonvulsant*

**ALC (acetyl-L-carnitine)** [q.v.]

**Alcaine** Drop-Tainers (eye drops) ℞ *topical ophthalmic anesthetic* [proparacaine HCl] 0.5%

**alcanna** *medicinal herb* [see: henna (Alkanna)]

**Alcar** ℞ *investigational (Phase III) treatment for Alzheimer disease* [levacecarnine]

**ALCAR (acetyl-L-carnitine)** [q.v.]

**Alcare** foam OTC *topical antiseptic* [ethyl alcohol] 62%

**Alchemilla xanthochlora; A. vulgaris** *medicinal herb* [see: lady's mantle]

**alclofenac** USAN, INN, BAN, JAN *anti-inflammatory*

**alclometasone** INN, BAN *topical corticosteroidal anti-inflammatory* [also: alclometasone dipropionate]

**alclometasone dipropionate** USAN, USP, JAN *topical corticosteroidal anti-inflammatory* [also: alclometasone]

**alcloxa** USAN, INN *astringent; keratolytic* [also: aluminum chlorohydroxy allantoinate]

**Alco-Gel** OTC *topical antiseptic for instant sanitation of hands* [ethyl alcohol] 60% ⍰ aloe gel

**alcohol** USP *topical anti-infective/antiseptic; astringent; solvent; a widely* abused "*legal street drug*" *used to produce euphoria* [also: ethanol]

**alcohol, dehydrated** USP *antidote* [also: ethanol, dehydrated]

**alcohol, diluted** NF *solvent*

**alcohol, rubbing** USP, INN *rubefacient*

**5% Alcohol and 5% Dextrose in Water; 10% Alcohol and 5% Dextrose in Water** IV infusion ℞ *for caloric replacement and rehydration* [dextrose; alcohol] 5%•5%; 10%•5%

**Alcon Saline Especially for Sensitive Eyes** solution OTC *rinsing/storage solution for soft contact lenses* [sodium chloride (preserved saline solution)]

**Alconefrin** nose drops, nasal spray (discontinued 2002) OTC *nasal decongestant* [phenylephrine HCl] 0.25%, 0.5%

**Alconefrin 12** nose drops (discontinued 2002) OTC *nasal decongestant* [phenylephrine HCl] 0.16%

**Alcortin** gel ℞ *corticosteroidal antiinflammatory* [hydrocortisone] 2%

**alcuronium chloride** USAN, INN, BAN, JAN *skeletal muscle relaxant*

**Aldactazide** tablets ℞ *antihypertensive; diuretic* [spironolactone; hydrochlorothiazide] 25•25, 50•50 mg ⊡ Aldactone

**Aldactone** tablets ℞ *antihypertensive; potassium-sparing diuretic* [spironolactone] 25, 50, 100 mg ⊡ Aldactazide

**Aldara** cream ℞ *immunomodulator for external genital warts, perianal warts, actinic keratoses, and superficial basal cell carcinoma* [imiquimod] 5% in 250 mg single-use packets

**alder, spotted** *medicinal herb* [see: witch hazel]

**alder, striped** *medicinal herb* [see: winterberry; witch hazel]

**alder buckthorn; European black alder** *medicinal herb* [see: buckthorn]

**alderlin** [see: pronethalol]

**aldesleukin** USAN, INN, BAN *immunostimulant; biological response modifier; antineoplastic for metastatic melanoma and renal cell carcinoma (orphan); investigational (Phase III, orphan) for* immunodeficiency diseases and acute myelogenous leukemia (AML); investigational (Phase II) for non-Hodgkin lymphoma

**aldesulfone sodium** INN, DCF *antibacterial; leprostatic* [also: sulfoxone sodium]

**aldioxa** USAN, INN, JAN *astringent; keratolytic*

**Aldoclor-150; Aldoclor-250** film-coated tablets ℞ *antihypertensive* [chlorothiazide; methyldopa] 150•250 mg; 250•250 mg

**aldocorten** [see: aldosterone]

**Aldomet** film-coated tablets, oral suspension (discontinued 2002) ℞ *antihypertensive* [methyldopa] 125, 250, 500 mg; 250 mg/5 mL

**Aldomet; Aldomet Ester HCl** IV injection ℞ *antihypertensive* [methyldopate HCl] 50 mg/mL

**Aldoril 15; Aldoril 25; Aldoril D30; Aldoril D50** film-coated tablets ℞ *antihypertensive; diuretic* [hydrochlorothiazide; methyldopa] 15•250 mg; 25•250 mg; 30•500 mg; 50•500 mg ⊡ Elavil; Eldepryl; Enovil; Equanil; Mellaril

**aldosterone** INN, BAN, DCF

**Aldurazyme** powder for IV infusion ℞ *enzyme replacement therapy for mucopolysaccharidosis I (MPS I) (orphan)* [laronidase] 2.9 mg/vial

**Alec** ℞ *investigational (orphan) agent to prevent or treat neonatal respiratory distress syndrome* [colfosceril palmitate; phosphatidylglycerol]

**alefacept** USAN *immunosuppressant; recombinant human LFA-3/IgG1 (leukocyte function–associated antigen, type 3/immunoglobulin G1) fusion protein for chronic plaque psoriasis*

**alemcinal** USAN *motilin agonist to stimulate gastrointestinal peristaltic action*

**alemtuzumab** *humanized monoclonal antibody (huMAb) immunosuppressant for chronic lymphocytic leukemia (orphan); investigational (Phase II) for non-Hodgkin lymphoma, organ transplants, and multiple sclerosis*

**alendronate sodium** USAN *bisphosphonate bone resorption inhibitor for Paget disease and corticosteroid-induced or age-related osteoporosis in men and women; investigational (orphan) for bone manifestations of Gaucher disease and pediatric osteogenesis imperfecta*

**alendronic acid** INN, BAN

**Alenic Alka** chewable tablets OTC *antacid* [aluminum hydroxide; magnesium trisilicate] 80•20 mg

**Alenic Alka** oral liquid OTC *antacid* [aluminum hydroxide; magnesium carbonate] 31.7•137.3 mg/5 mL

**Alenic Alka, Extra Strength** chewable tablets OTC *antacid* [aluminum hydroxide; magnesium carbonate] 160•105 mg

**alentemol** INN *antipsychotic; dopamine agonist* [also: alentemol hydrobromide]

**alentemol hydrobromide** USAN *antipsychotic; dopamine agonist* [also: alentemol]

**alepride** INN

**Alertec** ⒸⒶⓃ tablets Ŗ *analeptic for excessive daytime sleepiness of narcolepsy* [modafinil] 100 mg

**Alesse** tablets (in packs of 28) Ŗ *monophasic oral contraceptive* [levonorgestrel; ethinyl estradiol] 0.1 mg•20 µg

**alestramustine** INN

**aletamine HCl** USAN *antidepressant* [also: alfetamine]

*Aletris farinosa medicinal herb* [see: star grass]

*Aleurites moluccana; A. cordata medicinal herb* [see: tung seed]

**Aleve** tablets, capsules, gelcaps OTC *analgesic; antiarthritic; antipyretic; nonsteroidal anti-inflammatory drug (NSAID)* [naproxen sodium] 220 mg (=200 mg base)

**Aleve Cold & Sinus; Aleve Sinus & Headache** extended-release caplets OTC *decongestant; analgesic; antipyretic* [pseudoephedrine HCl; naproxen sodium] 120•220 mg

**alexidine** USAN, INN *antibacterial*

**alexitol sodium** INN, BAN

**alexomycin** USAN *veterinary growth promoter for poultry and swine*

**alfacalcidol (1α-hydroxycholecalciferol; 1α-hydroxyvitamin D₃)** INN, BAN, JAN *vitamin D precursor (converted to calcifediol in the body); calcium regulator for treatment of hypocalcemia and osteodystrophy from chronic renal dialysis*

**alfadex** INN

**alfadolone** INN, DCF [also: alphadolone]

**alfalfa (Medicago sativa)** leaves and flowers *medicinal herb for anemia, appetite stimulation, arthritis, atherosclerosis, blood cleansing, diabetes, hemorrhages, kidney cleansing, lowering cholesterol levels, nausea, pituitary disorders, and peptic ulcers*

**alfaprostol** USAN, INN, BAN *veterinary prostaglandin*

**alfaxalone** INN, JAN, DCF [also: alphaxalone]

**Alfenta** IV or IM injection Ŗ *narcotic analgesic; anesthetic* [alfentanil HCl] 500 µg/mL

**alfentanil** INN, BAN *narcotic analgesic* [also: alfentanil HCl]

**alfentanil HCl** USAN *narcotic analgesic* [also: alfentanil]

**Alferon LDO** (low dose oral) Ŗ *investigational (Phase I/II) cytokine for HIV, AIDS, and ARC* [interferon alfa-n3]

**Alferon N** intralesional injection Ŗ *immunomodulator and antiviral for condyloma acuminata; investigational (Phase III) cytokine for HIV, AIDS, ARC, and hepatitis C* [interferon alfa-n3] 5 million IU/mL

**alfetamine** INN *antidepressant* [also: aletamine HCl]

**alfetamine HCl** [see: aletamine HCl]

**alfuzosin** INN, BAN *alpha₁-adrenergic blocker for hypertension and benign prostatic hyperplasia (BPH)* [also: alfuzosin HCl]

**Alfuzosin** tablets Ŗ *anti-inflammatory for benign prostatic hyperplasia (BPH)* [leflunomide]

**alfuzosin HCl** USAN *alpha₁-adrenergic blocker for hypertension and benign prostatic hyperplasia (BPH)* [also: alfuzosin]

**algeldrate** USAN, INN *antacid*

**algestone** INN *anti-inflammatory* [also: algestone acetonide]

**algestone acetonide** USAN, BAN *anti-inflammatory* [also: algestone]

**algestone acetophenide** USAN *progestin*

**algin** [see: sodium alginate]

**alginic acid** NF, BAN *tablet binder and emulsifying agent*

**alginic acid, sodium salt** [see: sodium alginate]

**alglucerase** USAN, INN, BAN *glucocerebrosidase enzyme replacement for Gaucher disease type I (orphan); investigational (orphan) for types II and III*

**alibendol** INN, DCF

**Alibra** ℞ *investigational (NDA filed) treatment for erectile dysfunction*

**alicaforsen sodium** USAN, INN *anti-inflammatory; antisense inhibitor of intercellular adhesion molecule 1 (ICAM-1); investigational (Phase III) injection for Crohn disease; investigational (Phase II) suppository for ulcerative colitis; investigational (Phase II) topical treatment of psoriasis*

**aliconazole** INN

**alidine dihydrochloride** [see: anileridine]

**alidine phosphate** [see: anileridine]

**alifedrine** INN

**aliflurane** USAN, INN *inhalation anesthetic*

**alimadol** INN

**alimemazine** INN *phenothiazine antihistamine; antipruritic* [also: trimeprazine tartrate; trimeprazine; alimemazine tartrate]

**alimemazine tartrate** JAN *phenothiazine antihistamine; antipruritic* [also: trimeprazine tartrate; alimemazine; trimeprazine]

**Alimentum** ready-to-use oral liquid OTC *hypoallergenic infant food* [casein protein formula]

**Alimentum Advance** ready-to-use oral liquid OTC *hypoallergenic infant food with omega-3 and omega-6 fatty acids* [casein protein formula; iron; docosahexaenoic acid (DHA); arachidonic acid (AA)]

**Alimta** powder for IV infusion ℞ *antineoplastic for malignant pleural mesothelioma (MPM)* [pemetrexed disodium] 500 mg/vial

**Alinia** powder for oral suspension ℞ *antiprotozoal for pediatric diarrhea due to* Cryptosporidium parvum *and* Giardia lamblia *infections* [nitazoxanide] 100 mg/5 mL

**alinidine** INN, BAN

**alipamide** USAN, INN, BAN *diuretic; antihypertensive*

**alisactide** [see: alsactide]

**alisobumal** [see: butalbital]

**Alista** cream ℞ *investigational (Phase II/III) treatment for female sexual arousal disorder* [alprostadil]

**alitame** USAN *sweetener*

**alitretinoin** USAN *retinoic acid for topical treatment of cutaneous lesions of AIDS-related Kaposi sarcoma (orphan); investigational (Phase III, orphan) oral treatment for Kaposi sarcoma and acute promyelocytic leukemia (APL)*

**alitretinoin & interferon** *investigational (Phase I/II) combination treatment for AIDS-related Kaposi sarcoma*

**alizapride** INN

**Alka-Mints** chewable tablets OTC *antacid* [calcium carbonate] 850 mg

*Alkanna tinctoria* medicinal herb [see: henna]

**Alka-Seltzer** effervescent tablets OTC *antacid; analgesic* [sodium bicarbonate; citric acid; aspirin; phenylalanine] 1700•1000•325•9 mg

**Alka-Seltzer, Extra Strength** effervescent tablets OTC *antacid; analgesic* [sodium bicarbonate; citric acid; aspirin] 1985•1000•500 mg

**Alka-Seltzer, Gold** effervescent tablets OTC *antacid* [sodium bicarbonate; citric acid; potassium bicarbonate] 958•832•312 mg

**Alka-Seltzer, Original** effervescent tablets OTC *antacid; analgesic* [sodium bicarbonate; citric acid; aspirin] 1916•1000•325 mg

**Alka-Seltzer Plus Allergy** Liqui-Gels (liquid-filled gelcaps) (discontinued 2002) OTC *decongestant; antihistamine; analgesic* [pseudoephedrine HCl; chlorpheniramine maleate; acetaminophen] 30•2•250 mg

**Alka-Seltzer Plus Children's Cold** effervescent tablets (discontinued 2002) OTC *antitussive; decongestant; antihistamine* [dextromethorphan hydrobromide; phenylpropanolamine bitartrate; chlorpheniramine maleate] 5•10•1 mg

**Alka-Seltzer Plus Cold & Cough** Liqui-Gels (liquid-filled gelcaps) OTC *antitussive; decongestant; antihistamine; analgesic* [dextromethorphan hydrobromide; pseudoephedrine HCl; chlorpheniramine maleate; acetaminophen] 10•30•2•325 mg

**Alka-Seltzer Plus Cold & Cough Medicine** effervescent tablets OTC *antitussive; decongestant; antihistamine* [dextromethorphan hydrobromide; phenylephrine HCl; chlorpheniramine maleate] 10•5•2 mg

**Alka-Seltzer Plus Cold Medicine** effervescent tablets OTC *decongestant; antihistamine; analgesic* [phenylephrine HCl; chlorpheniramine maleate; acetaminophen] 5•2•250 mg

**Alka-Seltzer Plus Cold Medicine** Liqui-Gels (liquid-filled gelcaps) OTC *decongestant; antihistamine; analgesic* [pseudoephedrine HCl; chlorpheniramine maleate; acetaminophen] 30•2•325 mg

**Alka-Seltzer Plus Cold Medicine; Alka-Seltzer Plus Cold Tablets** for oral solution (discontinued 2001) OTC *decongestant; antihistamine; analgesic; antipyretic* [phenylpropanolamine bitartrate; brompheniramine maleate; aspirin] 20•2•325 mg; 24.08•2•325 mg

**Alka-Seltzer Plus Cold & Sinus** effervescent tablets OTC *decongestant;*

*analgesic; antipyretic* [phenylephrine HCl; aspirin] 5•250 mg

**Alka-Seltzer Plus Cold & Sinus** Liqui-Gels (liquid-filled gelcaps) OTC *decongestant; analgesic* [pseudoephedrine HCl; acetaminophen] 30•325 mg

**Alka-Seltzer Plus Flu & Body Aches Non-Drowsy** Liqui-Gels (name changed to Alka-Seltzer Plus Flu Medicine in 2002)

**Alka-Seltzer Plus Flu Medicine** effervescent tablets OTC *antitussive; antihistamine; analgesic* [dextromethorphan hydrobromide; chlorpheniramine maleate; aspirin] 15•2•500 mg

**Alka-Seltzer Plus Flu Medicine** Liqui-Gels (liquid-filled gelcaps) OTC *antitussive; decongestant; analgesic* [dextromethorphan hydrobromide; pseudoephedrine HCl; acetaminophen] 10•30•325 mg

**Alka-Seltzer Plus Night-Time Cold** Liqi-Gels (liquid-filled gelcaps) OTC *antitussive; decongestant; antihistamine; analgesic* [dextromethorphan hydrobromide; pseudoephedrine HCl; doxylamine succinate; acetaminophen] 10•30•6.25•250 mg

**Alka-Seltzer Plus Night-Time Cold** tablets (discontinued 2002) OTC *antitussive; decongestant; antihistamine; analgesic; antipyretic* [dextromethorphan hydrobromide; phenylpropanolamine bitartrate; doxylamine succinate; aspirin] 10•20•6.25•500 mg

**Alka-Seltzer Plus Night-Time Cold Medicine** effervescent tablets OTC *antitussive; decongestant; antihistamine* [dextromethorphan hydrobromide; phenylephrine HCl; doxylamine succinate] 10•5•6.25 mg

**Alka-Seltzer Plus Nose & Throat** effervescent tablets OTC *antitussive; antihistamine; analgesic* [dextromethorphan hydrobromide; chlorpheniramine maleate; acetaminophen] 10•2•250 mg

**Alka-Seltzer Plus Sinus** tablets (discontinued 2002) OTC *decongestant;*

analgesic; antipyretic [phenylpropanol-
amine bitartrate; aspirin] 20•325 mg

**Alka-Seltzer with Aspirin** effervescent tablets OTC antacid; analgesic
[sodium bicarbonate; citric acid;
aspirin] 1900•1000•325, 1900•
1000•500 mg

**alkavervir (Veratrum viride alka-
loids)**

**Alkavite** extended-release tablets OTC
vitamin/mineral supplement for alcohol-
related deficiencies [multiple vitamins
& minerals; calcium carbonate; iron
sulfate; folic acid; biotin] ≛•68.5•
60•1•0.03 mg

**Alkeran** film-coated tablets, powder
for IV infusion Ṛ nitrogen mustard-
type alkylating antineoplastic for multiple myeloma (orphan) and ovarian
cancer; investigational (orphan) for
metastatic melanoma [melphalan] 2
mg; 50 mg

**Alkets** chewable tablets OTC antacid
[calcium carbonate] 500, 750 mg

**alkyl aryl sulfonate** surfactant/wetting
agent

**alkylade** investigational (Phase III)
AGT inhibitor for brain cancer

**alkylamines** a class of antihistamines

**alkylbenzyldimethylammonium
chloride** [see: benzalkonium chloride]

**alkyldimethylbenzylammonium
chloride** [see: benzalkonium chloride]

**alkylpolyaminoethylglycine** JAN

**alkylpolyaminoethylglycine HCl** JAN

**All Clear; All Clear AR** eye drops
OTC decongestant; vasoconstrictor
[naphazoline HCl] 0.012%; 0.03%

**allantoin** USAN, BAN topical vulnerary;
investigational (orphan) for skin blistering and erosions associated with inherited epidermolysis bullosa

**Allbee C-800** film-coated tablets OTC
vitamin supplement [multiple B vitamins; vitamins C and E] ≛•800•45
mg

**Allbee C-800 plus Iron** film-coated
tablets OTC vitamin/iron supplement
[ferrous fumarate; multiple B vita-

mins; vitamins C and E; folic acid]
27 mg•≛•800 mg•45 IU•0.4 mg

**Allbee with C** caplets OTC vitamin
supplement [multiple B vitamins;
vitamin C] ≛•300 mg

**Allbee-T** tablets OTC vitamin supplement [multiple B vitamins; vitamin
C] ≛•500 mg

**Allegra** film-coated tablets, capsules Ṛ
nonsedating antihistamine for allergic
rhinitis and chronic idiopathic urticaria
[fexofenadine HCl] 30, 60, 180 mg;
60 mg

**Allegra 24 Hour** ⓒⒶⓃ extended-release
tablets OTC nonsedating antihistamine
for allergic rhinitis [fexofenadine HCl]
120 mg

**Allegra-D** extended-release film-coated
tablets Ṛ decongestant; nonsedating
antihistamine [pseudoephedrine HCl;
fexofenadine HCl] 120•60 mg

**allegron** [see: nortriptyline]

**Allent** sustained-release capsules Ṛ
decongestant; antihistamine [pseudo-
ephedrine HCl; brompheniramine
maleate] 120•12 mg

**Aller-Chlor** tablets, syrup OTC antihistamine [chlorpheniramine maleate] 4
mg; 2 mg/5 mL

**Allercon** tablets (discontinued 2002)
OTC decongestant; antihistamine [pseu-
doephedrine HCl; triprolidine HCl]
60•2.5 mg

**Allercreme Skin** lotion (discontinued
2004) OTC moisturizer; emollient

**Allercreme Ultra Emollient** cream
(discontinued 2004) OTC moisturizer;
emollient

**Allerest** eye drops OTC topical ophthalmic decongestant and vasoconstrictor
[naphazoline HCl] 0.012%

**Allerest** tablets OTC decongestant; antihistamine [pseudoephedrine HCl;
chlorpheniramine maleate] 30•2 mg

**Allerest, Children's** chewable tablets
(discontinued 2001) OTC pediatric
decongestant and antihistamine [phen-
ylpropanolamine HCl; chlorpheniramine maleate] 9.4•1 mg

**Allerest 12 Hour** nasal spray (discontinued 2002) OTC *nasal decongestant* [oxymetazoline HCl] 0.05%

**Allerest 12 Hour** sustained-release caplets (discontinued 2001) OTC *decongestant; antihistamine* [phenylpropanolamine HCl; chlorpheniramine maleate] 75•12 mg

**Allerest Allergy & Sinus Relief** tablets OTC *decongestant; analgesic* [pseudoephedrine HCl; acetaminophen] 30•325 mg

**Allerest Headache; Allerest Sinus Pain Formula** tablets (discontinued 2002) OTC *decongestant; antihistamine; analgesic* [pseudoephedrine HCl; chlorpheniramine maleate; acetaminophen] 30•2•325 mg; 30•2•500 mg

**Allerest No Drowsiness** tablets, caplets (discontinued 2002) OTC *decongestant; analgesic* [pseudoephedrine HCl; acetaminophen] 30•500 mg; 30•325 mg

**Allerfrim** film-coated tablets, syrup OTC *decongestant; antihistamine* [pseudoephedrine HCl; triprolidine HCl] 60•2.5 mg; 60•2.5 mg/10 mL

**Allerfrim with Codeine** syrup (discontinued 2002) ℞ *narcotic antitussive; decongestant; antihistamine* [codeine phosphate; pseudoephedrine HCl; triprolidine HCl] 10•30•1.25 mg/5 mL

**Allergan Enzymatic** tablets OTC *enzymatic cleaner for soft contact lenses* [papain] ☒ allergen; Auralgan

**Allergan Hydrocare** [see: Hydrocare]

**Allergen Ear Drops** ℞ *topical local anesthetic; analgesic* [benzocaine; antipyrine] 1.4%•5.4%

**allergenic extracts** *a class of agents derived from various biological sources containing antigens that possess immunologic activity*

**allergenic extracts (aqueous, glycerinated, or alum-precipitated)** *over 900 allergens available for diagnosis of and desensitization to specific allergies*

**Allergy** tablets OTC *antihistamine* [chlorpheniramine maleate] 4 mg

**Allergy Drops** eye drops OTC *topical ophthalmic decongestant and vasoconstrictor* [naphazoline HCl] 0.012%; 0.03%

**Allergy Relief** tablets OTC *antihistamine* [chlorpheniramine maleate] 4 mg

**AllerMax** caplets, oral liquid OTC *antihistamine; sleep aid* [diphenhydramine HCl] 50 mg; 12.5 mg/5 mL

**AllerMax Allergy & Cough Formula** oral liquid (discontinued 2002) OTC *antihistamine* [diphenhydramine HCl] 6.25 mg/5 mL

**Allermed** capsules (discontinued 2002) OTC *nasal decongestant* [pseudoephedrine HCl] 60 mg

**Allerphed** syrup (discontinued 2002) OTC *decongestant; antihistamine* [pseudoephedrine HCl; triprolidine HCl] 30•1.25 mg/5 mL

**AlleRx** pediatric oral suspension ℞ *decongestant; antihistamine* [phenylephrine tannate; chlorpheniramine tannate; pyrilamine tannate] 5•2•12.5 mg/5 mL

**AlleRx Dose Pack** controlled-release tablets (AM and PM) ℞ AM: *decongestant, anticholinergic;* PM: *antihistamine, anticholinergic* [AM: pseudoephedrine HCl, methscopolamine nitrate; PM: chlorpheniramine maleate, methscopolamine nitrate] AM: 120•2.5 mg; PM: 8•2.5 mg

**AlleRx-D** controlled-release caplets ℞ *decongestant; anticholinergic to dry mucosal secretions* [pseudoephedrine HCl; methscopolamine nitrate] 120•2.5 mg

**alletorphine** BAN, INN

**Allfen** sustained-release tablets (discontinued 2004) ℞ *expectorant* [guaifenesin] 1000 mg

**Allfen Jr.** tablets ℞ *expectorant* [guaifenesin] 400 mg

**Allfen-DM** sustained-release tablets ℞ *antitussive; expectorant* [dextromethorphan hydrobromide; guaifenesin] 55•1000 mg

**all-heal** *medicinal herb* [see: mistletoe; valerian]

*Allium cepa medicinal herb* [see: onion]

*Allium porrum medicinal herb* [see: leek]

*Allium sativum medicinal herb* [see: garlic]

**All-Nite Children's Cold/Cough Relief** oral liquid OTC *antitussive; decongestant; antihistamine* [dextromethorphan hydrobromide; pseudoephedrine HCl; chlorpheniramine maleate] 15•30•2 mg/15 mL

**All-Nite Cold Formula** oral liquid (name changed to All-Nite Liquid in 2002)

**All-Nite Liquid** OTC *antitussive; decongestant; antihistamine; analgesic* [dextromethorphan hydrobromide; pseudoephedrine HCl; doxylamine succinate; acetaminophen; alcohol 10%] 30•60•12.5•1000 mg/30 mL

**allobarbital** USAN, INN *hypnotic*

**allobarbitone** [see: allobarbital]

**alloclamide** INN, DCF

**allocupreide sodium** INN, DCF

**allomethadione** INN, DCF [also: aloxidone]

**allopurinol** USAN, USP, INN, BAN, JAN *xanthine oxidase inhibitor for gout and hyperuricemia; antineoplastic adjunct for reducing uric acid levels following chemotherapy for leukemia, lymphoma, and solid tumor malignancies (orphan)* 100, 300 mg oral

**allopurinol riboside** *investigational (orphan) agent for Chagas disease and for cutaneous and visceral leishmaniasis*

**allopurinol sodium** *antineoplastic adjunct for reducing uric acid levels following chemotherapy for leukemia, lymphoma, and solid tumor malignancies (orphan); investigational (orphan) for ex vivo preservation of organs for transplant*

**Allovectin-7** ℞ *investigational (Phase II) treatment for head and neck cancer; investigational (Phase II/III, orphan) for invasive and metastatic melanoma*

**Allpyral** subcu or IM injection ℞ *allergenic sensitivity testing (subcu); allergenic desensitization therapy (IM)* [allergenic extracts, alum-precipitated]

**allspice (*Eugenia pimenta; Pimenta dioica; P. officinalis*)** unripe fruit and leaves *medicinal herb for diarrhea and gas; also used as a purgative and tonic*

**all-*trans*-retinoic acid** [see: tretinoin]

**allyl isothiocyanate** USAN, USP

**allylamines** *a class of antifungals*

**allylbarbituric acid** [now: butalbital]

**allylestrenol** INN, JAN [also: allyloestrenol]

**allyl-isobutylbarbituric acid** [see: butalbital]

**allylisopropylmalonylurea** [see: aprobarbital]

**4-allyl-2-methoxyphenol** [see: eugenol]

**N-allylnoretorphine** [see: alletorphine]

**N-allylnoroxymorphone HCl** [see: naloxone HCl]

**allyloestrenol** BAN [also: allylestrenol]

**allylprodine** INN, BAN, DCF

**5-allyl-5-*sec*-butylbarbituric acid** [see: talbutal]

**allylthiourea** INN

**allypropymal** [see: aprobarbital]

**Almacone** chewable tablets, oral liquid OTC *antacid; antiflatulent* [aluminum hydroxide; magnesium hydroxide; simethicone] 200•200•20 mg; 200•200•20 mg/5 mL

**Almacone II** oral liquid OTC *antacid; antiflatulent* [aluminum hydroxide; magnesium hydroxide; simethicone] 400•400•40 mg/5 mL

**almadrate sulfate** USAN, INN *antacid*

**almagate** USAN, INN *antacid*

**almagodrate** INN

**almasilate** INN, BAN

**Almebex Plus B$_{12}$** oral liquid OTC *vitamin supplement* [multiple B vitamins]

**almecillin** INN

**almestrone** INN

**alminoprofen** INN, JAN

**almitrine** INN, BAN

**almokalant** INN *investigational antiarrhythmic*

**almond** *(Prunus amygdalus)* kernels *medicinal herb used as a demulcent, emollient, and pectoral*

**almond oil** NF *emollient and perfume; oleaginous vehicle*

**Almora** tablets OTC *magnesium supplement* [magnesium gluconate dihydride] 500 mg (27 mg Mg)

**almotriptan** USAN, INN *vascular serotonin 5-HT$_{1B/1D/1F}$ receptor agonist for the acute treatment of migraine*

**almotriptan malate** USAN *vascular serotonin 5-HT$_{1B/1D/1F}$ receptor agonist for the acute treatment of migraine*

**almoxatone** INN

**alnespirone** INN

**alniditan dihydrochloride** USAN *serotonin 5-HT$_{1D}$ agonist for migraine*

***Alnus glutinosa*** *medicinal herb* [see: black alder]

**Alocril** eye drops ℞ *mast cell stabilizer for allergic conjunctivitis* [nedocromil sodium] 2%

**aloe** USP ② Alco-Gel

**aloe (*Aloe vera* and over 500 other species)** leaves and juice *medicinal herb for burns, hemorrhoids, insect bites, and scalds; also used as a deodorant and to aid digestion and limit scarring; not generally regarded as safe and effective as a cathartic*

**Aloe Grande** lotion OTC *moisturizer; emollient; skin protectant* [vitamins A and E; aloe] 3333.3•50•⸛ U/g

**Aloe Vesta** lotion OTC *emollient/protectant* [dimethicone; aloe vera gel] 3%•⸛

**Aloe Vesta Perineal** solution OTC *emollient/protectant* [propylene glycol; aloe vera gel]

**alofilcon A** USAN *hydrophilic contact lens material*

**aloin** BAN

**ALOMAD (Adriamycin, Leukeran, Oncovin, methotrexate, actinomycin D, dacarbazine)** *chemotherapy protocol* ② Alomide

**Alomide** Drop-Tainers (eye drops) ℞ *topical antiallergic for vernal keratoconjunctivitis (orphan)* [lodoxamide tromethamine] 0.1% ② ALOMAD

**alonacic** INN

**alonimid** USAN, INN *sedative; hypnotic*

**Alophen** enteric-coated tablets OTC *stimulant laxative* [bisacodyl] 5 mg

**Aloprim** powder for IV infusion ℞ *antineoplastic adjunct for reducing uric acid levels following chemotherapy for leukemia, lymphoma, and solid-tumor malignancies (orphan); investigational (orphan) for ex vivo preservation of organs for transplant* [allopurinol sodium] 500 mg

**Alor 5/500** tablets ℞ *narcotic analgesic* [hydrocodone bitartrate; aspirin] 5• 500 mg

**Alora** transdermal patch ℞ *estrogen replacement therapy for the treatment of postmenopausal symptoms and prevention of postmenopausal osteoporosis* [estradiol] 25, 50, 75, 100 µg/day

**aloracetam** INN

**alosetron** INN, BAN *antiemetic; 5-HT$_3$ receptor antagonist for irritable bowel syndrome* [also: alosetron HCl]

**alosetron HCl** USAN *antiemetic; 5-HT$_3$ receptor antagonist for irritable bowel syndrome (IBS)* (base=89%) [also: alosetron]

**alovudine** USAN, INN *antiviral*

**Aloxi** IV injection ℞ *antiemetic for chemotherapy-induced nausea and vomiting (CINV)* [palonosetron HCl] 0.25 mg/5 mL

**aloxidone** BAN [also: allomethadione]

**aloxiprin** INN, BAN, DCF

**aloxistatin** INN

***Aloysiatriphylla* spp.** *medicinal herb* [see: lemon verbena]

**alozafone** INN

**alpertine** USAN, INN *antipsychotic*

**alpha amylase (α-amylase)** USAN *anti-inflammatory*

**alpha hydroxy acids (AHA)** [see: glycolic acid]

**alpha interferon-2A** [see: interferon alfa-2A]

**alpha interferon-2B** [see: interferon alfa-2B]

**alpha interferon-N1** [see: interferon alfa-N1]

**alpha interferon-N3** [see: interferon alfa-N3]

**Alpha Keri Moisturizing Soap** bar (discontinued 2004) oTc *therapeutic skin cleanser*

**Alpha Keri Spray** (discontinued 2004) oTc *bath emollient*

**Alpha Keri Therapeutic Bath Oil** oTc *bath emollient*

**alpha lipoic acid (ALA)** *natural antioxidant that is both fat- and water-soluble and readily crosses cell membranes; used in the treatment of AIDS, diabetes, liver ailments, oxidative stress injuries, and various cancers*

**d-alpha tocopherol** *(relative potency: 100%)* [see: vitamin E]

**dl-alpha tocopherol** *(relative potency: 74%)* [see: vitamin E]

**d-alpha tocopheryl acetate** *(relative potency: 91%)* [see: vitamin E]

**dl-alpha tocopheryl acetate** *(relative potency: 67%)* [see: vitamin E]

**d-alpha tocopheryl acid succinate** *(relative potency: 81%)* [see: vitamin E]

**dl-alpha tocopheryl acid succinate** *(relative potency: 60%)* [see: vitamin E]

**alpha$_1$ PI (alpha$_1$-proteinase inhibitor)** [q.v.]

**alpha$_1$-adrenergic blockers** *a class of agents that block the alpha$_1$ adrenergic receptors, used for the treatment of hypertension and benign prostatic hyperplasia (BPH) also called: antiadrenergics*

**alpha$_1$-antitrypsin (AAT), recombinant** *investigational (orphan) for alpha$_1$-antitrypsin deficiency in the ZZ phenotype population*

**alpha$_1$-antitrypsin, transgenic human** *investigational (Phase II, orphan) for cystic fibrosis*

**alpha$_1$-proteinase inhibitor (alpha$_1$ PI)** *enzyme replacement therapy for hereditary alpha$_1$ PI deficiency, which leads to progressive panacinar emphysema (orphan)*

**alphacemethadone** [see: alphacetylmethadol]

**alphacetylmethadol** BAN, INN, DCF

**alpha-chymotrypsin** [see: chymotrypsin]

**alpha-cypermethrin** BAN

**α-D-galactopyranose** [see: galactose]

**alpha-D-galactosidase** *digestive enzyme*

**alphadolone** BAN [also: alfadolone]

**alpha-estradiol** [see: estradiol]

**alpha-estradiol benzoate** [see: estradiol benzoate]

**alpha-ethyltryptamine (alpha-EtT)** *a hallucinogenic street drug chemically related to MDMA* [see also: MDMA; alpha-methyltryptamine]

**alphafilcon A** USAN *hydrophilic contact lens material*

**alpha-galactosidase A** [see: agalsidase alfa; agalsidase beta]

**agalsidase beta & ceramide trihexosidase (CTH)** *investigational (orphan) enzyme replacement therapy for Fabry disease*

**Alphagan; Alphagan P** eye drops ℞ *selective α$_2$ agonist for open-angle glaucoma and ocular hypertension; investigational (orphan) for anterior ischemic optic neuropathy* [brimonidine tartrate] 0.2%; 0.15%

**alpha-glucosidase, human acid** [see: human acid alpha-glucosidase]

**alpha-hypophamine** [see: oxytocin]

**alpha-L-iduronidase** [now: laronidase]

**alpha-melanocyte stimulating hormone** *investigational (orphan) agent for the prevention and treatment of acute renal failure due to ischemia*

**alphameprodine** INN, BAN, DCF

**alphamethadol** INN, BAN, DCF

**alpha-methyldopa** [now: methyldopa]

**alpha-methyltryptamine (alpha-MeT)** *a hallucinogenic street drug chemically related to MDMA* [see also: MDMA; alpha-ethyltryptamine]

**Alphanate** powder for IV injection ℞ *antihemophilic; investigational (orphan) for von Willebrand disease* [antihemophilic factor concentrate, solvent/detergent treated]

**AlphaNine SD** powder for IV injection ℞ *antihemophilic for factor IX deficiency (hemophilia B; Christmas disease) (orphan)* [factor IX, solvent/detergent treated]

**alpha-phenoxyethyl penicillin, potassium** [see: phenethicillin potassium]

**alphaprodine** INN, BAN [also: alphaprodine HCl]

**alphaprodine HCl** USP [also: alphaprodine]

**alphasone acetophenide** [now: algestone acetonide]

**Alphatrex** cream ℞ *corticosteroidal anti-inflammatory* [betamethasone dipropionate] 0.05%

**Alphatrex** ointment, lotion (discontinued 2003) ℞ *corticosteroidal anti-inflammatory* [betamethasone dipropionate] 0.05%

**alphaxalone** BAN [also: alfaxalone]

**alpidem** USAN, INN, BAN *anxiolytic*

*Alpinia officinarum; A. galanga* medicinal herb [see: galangal]

*Alpinia oxyphylla; A. fructus* medicinal herb [see: bitter cardamom]

*Alpinia speciosa* medicinal herb for edema, fungal infections, hypertension, and thrombosis

**alpiropride** INN

**alprafenone** INN

**alprazolam** USAN, USP, INN, BAN, JAN *benzodiazepine anxiolytic; sedative; treatment for panic disorders and agoraphobia* 0.25, 0.5, 1, 2 mg oral

**Alprazolam Intensol** oral drops ℞ *benzodiazepine anxiolytic; sedative* [alprazolam] 1 mg/mL

**alprenolol** INN, BAN *antiadrenergic (β-receptor)* [also: alprenolol HCl]

**alprenolol HCl** USAN, JAN *antiadrenergic (β-receptor)* [also: alprenolol]

**alprenoxime HCl** USAN *antiglaucoma agent*

**alprostadil** USAN, USP, INN, BAN, JAN *vasodilator for erectile dysfunction; platelet aggregation inhibitor; investigational (orphan) for peripheral arterial occlusive disease; investigational (Phase II/III) topical treatment for female sexual arousal disorder*

**alprostadil, liposomal** *investigational (Phase III) for erectile dysfunction; investigational (orphan) for acute respiratory distress and ischemic ulcerations due to peripheral artery disease*

**alprostadil alfadex** BAN

**Alredase** ℞ *investigational (NDA filed) aldose reductase inhibitor for diabetic neuropathy* [tolrestat]

**alrestatin** INN *aldose reductase enzyme inhibitor* [also: alrestatin sodium]

**alrestatin sodium** USAN *aldose reductase enzyme inhibitor* [also: alrestatin]

**Alrex** eye drop suspension ℞ *corticosteroidal anti-inflammatory* [loteprednol etabonate] 0.2%

**alsactide** INN

**alseroxylon** JAN *antihypertensive; rauwolfia derivative*

**ALT-711** *investigational (Phase II) anti-aging compound; reverses collagen cross-linkage formed by advanced glycation end-products (AGE)*

**Altace** capsules ℞ *angiotensin-converting enzyme (ACE) inhibitor for hypertension, myocardial infarction, CHF, and stroke* [ramipril] 1.25, 2.5, 5, 10 mg

**altanserin** INN *serotonin antagonist* [also: altanserin tartrate]

**altanserin tartrate** USAN *serotonin antagonist* [also: altanserin]

**altapizone** INN

**Altarussin** syrup OTC *expectorant* [guaifenesin] 100 mg/5 mL

**alteconazole** INN

**alteplase** USAN, INN, BAN, JAN *tissue plasminogen activator (tPA) for acute myocardial infarction, acute ischemic stroke, or pulmonary embolism; investigational (orphan) for intraventricular hemorrhage with intracerebral hemorrhage*

**alteratives** *a class of agents that produce gradual beneficial changes in the body, usually by improving nutrition, without having any marked specific effect*

**ALternaGEL** oral liquid OTC *antacid* [aluminum hydroxide gel] 600 mg/ 5 mL

*Althaea officinalis medicinal herb* [see: marsh mallow]

**althiazide** USAN *antihypertensive* [also: altizide]

**Alti-Amiodarone** 🇨🇦 tablets ℞ *antiarrhythmic* [amiodarone HCl] 200 mg

**Alti-Amoxi Clav** 🇨🇦 tablets ℞ *aminopenicillin antibiotic* [amoxicillin; clavulanic acid] 250•125, 500•125 mg

**Alti-Clindamycin** 🇨🇦 capsules ℞ *lincosamide antibiotic* [clindamycin HCl] 150, 300 mg

**Alti-Clobazam** 🇨🇦 tablets ℞ *minor tranquilizer and anxiolytic; adjunct to anticonvulsant therapy* [clobazam] 10 mg

**Alti-Dexamethasone** 🇨🇦 tablets ℞ *corticosteroid; anti-inflammatory* [dexamethasone] 0.5, 0.75, 4 mg

**Alti-Doxazosin** 🇨🇦 tablets ℞ *antihypertensive (α-blocker)* [doxazosin mesylate] 1, 2, 4 mg

**Alti-Famotidine** 🇨🇦 film-coated tablets ℞ *histamine $H_2$ antagonist for gastric and duodenal ulcers* [famotidine] 20, 40 mg

**Alti-Flunisolide** 🇨🇦 nasal spray ℞ *corticosteroidal anti-inflammatory for chronic asthma and rhinitis* [flunisolide] 0.025% (25 μg/metered dose)

**Alti-Fluoxetine** 🇨🇦 capsules ℞ *selective serotonin reuptake inhibitor (SSRI) for depression, obsessive-compulsive disorder (OCD), and bulimia nervosa* [fluoxetine HCl] 10, 20 mg

**Alti-Ipratropium** 🇨🇦 nasal spray, solution for inhalation ℞ *anticholinergic bronchodilator for bronchospasm; antisecretory for rhinorrhea* [ipratropium bromide] 0.03%; 0.0125%, 0.025%

**Alti-Metformin HCl** 🇨🇦 film-coated tablets ℞ *biguanide antidiabetic* [metformin HCl] 500, 850 mg

**Alti-MPA** 🇨🇦 tablets ℞ *progestin for secondary amenorrhea, abnormal uterine bleeding, and endometrial hyperplasia* [medroxyprogesterone acetate] 2.5, 5, 10 mg

**Altinac** cream (discontinued 2004) ℞ *keratolytic for acne* [tretinoin] 0.025%, 0.05%, 0.1%

**altinicline maleate** USAN *investigational (Phase II) nicotinic acetylcholine receptor agonist for Parkinson disease*

**Alti-Nortriptylene Hydrochloride** 🇨🇦 capsules ℞ *tricyclic antidepressant* [nortriptyline HCl] 10, 25 mg

**Alti-Ticlopidine** 🇨🇦 film-coated tablets ℞ *platelet aggregation inhibitor for stroke* [ticlopidine HCl] 250 mg

**Alti-Timolol** 🇨🇦 eye drops ℞ *topical antiglaucoma agent (β-blocker)* [timolol maleate] 0.25%, 0.5%

**altizide** INN, DCF *antihypertensive* [also: althiazide]

**Alti-Zopiclone** 🇨🇦 tablets ℞ *sedative; hypnotic* [zopiclone] 7.5 mg

**Altocor** (name changed to Altoprev in 2004)

**Altoprev** extended-release tablets ℞ *HMG-CoA reductase inhibitor for hyperlipidemia and atherosclerosis; also for primary prevention of coronary heart disease* [lovastatin] 10, 20, 40, 60 mg

**altoqualine** INN

**Altracin** *investigational (orphan) antibiotic for pseudomembranous enterocolitis* [bacitracin]

**altrenogest** USAN, INN, BAN *veterinary progestin*

**altretamine** USAN, INN, BAN *antineoplastic for advanced ovarian adenocarcinoma (orphan)*

**Altropane** *investigational (Phase III) single photon emission tomography imaging agent for Parkinson disease; investigational (Phase II) radioimaging agent for attention-deficit hyperactivity disorder (ADHD)*

**altumomab** USAN, INN *radiodiagnostic monoclonal antibody for colorectal carcinoma; anticarcinoembryonic antigen (anti-CEA)* [also: indium In 111 altumomab pentetate]

**altumomab pentetate** USAN *monoclonal antibody conjugate* [also: indium In 111 altumomab pentetate]

**Alu-Cap** capsules OTC *antacid* [aluminum hydroxide gel] 400 mg

**Aludrox** oral suspension OTC *antacid; antiflatulent* [aluminum hydroxide; magnesium hydroxide; simethicone] 307•103• ± mg/5 mL

**alukalin** [see: kaolin]

**alum, ammonium** USP *topical astringent*

**alum, potassium** USP *topical astringent* [also: aluminum potassium sulfate]

**alum root (*Geranium maculatum*)** *medicinal herb used as an astringent, hemostatic, and antiseptic*

**Alumadrine** tablets (discontinued 2001) ℞ *decongestant; antihistamine; analgesic* [phenylpropanolamine HCl; chlorpheniramine maleate; acetaminophen] 25•4•500 mg

**alumina & magnesia** USP *antacid*

**aluminopara-aminosalicylate calcium (alumino *p*-aminosalicylate calcium)** JAN

**aluminosilicic acid, magnesium salt hydrate** [see: silodrate]

**aluminum** *element (Al)*

**aluminum, micronized** *astringent*

**aluminum acetate** USP *topical astringent; Burow solution*

**aluminum aminoacetate** [see: dihydroxyaluminum aminoacetate]

**aluminum ammonium sulfate dodecahydrate** [see: alum, ammonium]

**aluminum bismuth oxide** [see: bismuth aluminate]

**aluminum carbonate, basic** USAN, USP *antacid*

**aluminum chlorhydroxide** [now: aluminum chlorohydrate]

**aluminum chlorhydroxide alcohol soluble complex** [now: aluminum chlorohydrex]

**aluminum chloride** USP *topical astringent for hyperhidrosis* 20% topical

**aluminum chloride, basic** [see: aluminum sesquichlorohydrate]

**aluminum chloride hexahydrate** [see: aluminum chloride]

**aluminum chloride hydroxide hydrate** [see: aluminum chlorohydrate]

**aluminum chlorohydrate** USAN *anhidrotic*

**aluminum chlorohydrex** USAN *topical astringent*

**aluminum chlorohydrol propylene glycol complex** [now: aluminum chlorohydrex]

**aluminum chlorohydroxy allantoinate** JAN *astringent; keratolytic* [also: alcloxa]

**aluminum clofibrate** INN, BAN, JAN

**aluminum dihydroxyaminoacetate** [see: dihydroxyaluminum aminoacetate]

**aluminum flufenamate** JAN

**aluminum glycinate, basic** [see: dihydroxyaluminum aminoacetate]

**aluminum hydroxide gel** USP *antacid* 320, 450, 600 mg/5 mL oral

**aluminum hydroxide gel, dried** USP, JAN *antacid*

**aluminum hydroxide glycine** [see: dihydroxyaluminum aminoacetate]

**aluminum hydroxide hydrate** [see: algeldrate]

**aluminum hydroxychloride** [now: aluminum chlorohydrate]

**aluminum magnesium carbonate hydroxide dihydrate** [see: almagate]

**aluminum magnesium hydroxide carbonate hydrate** [see: hydrotalcite]

**aluminum magnesium hydroxide oxide sulfate** [see: almadrate sulfate]

**aluminum magnesium hydroxide oxide sulfate hydrate** [see: almadrate sulfate]

**aluminum magnesium hydroxide sulfate** [see: magaldrate]

**aluminum magnesium hydroxide sulfate hydrate** [see: magaldrate]

**aluminum monostearate** NF, JAN

**aluminum oxide**

**Aluminum Paste** ointment OTC *occlusive skin protectant* [metallic aluminum] 10%

**aluminum phosphate gel** USP *antacid (disapproved for use as an antacid in 1989)*

**aluminum potassium sulfate** JAN *topical astringent* [also: alum, potassium]

**aluminum potassium sulfate dodecahydrate** [see: alum, potassium]

**aluminum sesquichlorohydrate** USAN *anhidrotic*

**aluminum silicate, natural** JAN

**aluminum silicate, synthetic** JAN

**aluminum sodium carbonate hydroxide** [see: dihydroxyaluminum sodium carbonate]

**aluminum subacetate** USP *topical astringent*

**aluminum sulfate** USP *anhidrotic*

**aluminum sulfate hydrate** [see: aluminum sulfate]

**aluminum zirconium glycine tetrachloro hydrate complex** [see: aluminum zirconium tetrachlorohydrex gly]

**aluminum zirconium glycine trichloro hydrate complex** [see: aluminum zirconium trichlorohydrex gly]

**aluminum zirconium octachlorohydrate** USP *anhidrotic*

**aluminum zirconium octachlorohydrex gly** USP *anhidrotic*

**aluminum zirconium pentachlorohydrate** USP *anhidrotic*

**aluminum zirconium pentachlorohydrex gly** USP *anhidrotic*

**aluminum zirconium tetrachlorohydrate** USP *anhidrotic*

**aluminum zirconium tetrachlorohydrex gly** USAN, USP *anhidrotic*

**aluminum zirconium trichlorohydrate** USP *anhidrotic*

**aluminum zirconium trichlorohydrex gly** USAN, USP *anhidrotic*

**Alupent** inhalation aerosol powder, solution for inhalation ℞ *sympathomimetic bronchodilator* [metaproterenol sulfate] 0.65 mg/dose; 0.4%, 0.6%, 5%

**Alupent** syrup (discontinued 2001) ℞ *sympathomimetic bronchodilator* [metaproterenol sulfate] 10 mg/5 mL

**Alurate** elixir (discontinued 2004) ℞ *sedative; hypnotic* [aprobarbital] 40 mg/5 mL

**Alustra** cream ℞ *hyperpigmentation bleaching agent* [hydroquinone; tretinoin (in a base containing glycolic acid and vitamins C and E)] 4% • 0.1% ☒ Lustra

**alusulf** INN

**Alu-Tab** film-coated tablets OTC *antacid* [aluminum hydroxide gel] 500 mg

**ALVAC-120TMG** *investigational (Phase II) vaccine for HIV* [also: VCP 205]

**alverine** INN, BAN *anticholinergic* [also: alverine citrate]

**alverine citrate** USAN, NF *anticholinergic* [also: alverine]

**Alvesco** (approved in Europe) ℞ *investigational (NDA filed) inhaled corticosteroid for asthma* [ciclesonide]

**alvimopan** *investigational (NDA filed) narcotic analgesic; opioid receptor antagonist*

**alvircept sudotox** USAN, INN *antiviral; investigational (Phase II) for AIDS*

**Alwextin** ℞ *investigational (orphan) topical vulnerary for skin blistering and erosions associated with inherited epidermolysis bullosa* [allantoin]

**ALX-0600** *investigational (Phase II, orphan) glucagon analogue for short bowel syndrome*

**Alzhemed** ℞ *investigational (Phase III) amyloid protein–binding agent for Alzheimer disease*

**AM Caps** ⓒⒶⓃ OTC *vitamin supplement* [multiple vitamins; folic acid; biotin] ≛ • 0.2 • 0.15 mg

**amabevan** [see: carbarsone]

**amacetam HCl** [now: pramiracetam HCl]

**amacetam sulfate** [now: pramiracetam sulfate]

**amadinone** INN *progestin* [also: amadinone acetate]

**amadinone acetate** USAN *progestin* [also: amadinone]

**amafolone** INN, BAN

**amalgucin**

**Amanita muscaria** **mushrooms** *a species that produces muscarine and ibotenic acid, a psychotropic substance ingested as a street drug*

**amanozine** INN

**amantadine** INN, BAN *antiviral for influenza A virus; dopaminergic antiparkinson agent* [also: amantadine HCl]

**amantadine HCl** USAN, USP, JAN *antiviral for influenza A infections; dopaminergic antiparkinson agent* [also: amantadine] 100 mg oral; 50 mg/5 mL oral

**amantanium bromide** INN

**amantocillin** INN

**Amaphen** capsules (discontinued 2000) ℞ *analgesic; barbiturate sedative* [acetaminophen; caffeine; butalbital] 325•40•50 mg

**amara; amargo** *medicinal herb* [see: quassia]

**amaranth (*Amnaranthus* spp.)** leaves and flowers *medicinal herb for diarrhea, dysentery, excessive menstruation, and nosebleeds*

**amaranth (FD&C Red No. 2)** USP

**amargo; amara** *medicinal herb* [see: quassia]

**amarsan** [see: acetarsone]

**Amaryl** tablets ℞ *once-daily sulfonylurea antidiabetic* [glimepiride] 1, 2, 4 mg

**ambamustine** INN

**ambasilide** INN *investigational antiarrhythmic*

**ambazone** INN, BAN, DCF

**ambenonium chloride** USP, INN, BAN, JAN *anticholinesterase muscle stimulant*

**ambenoxan** INN, BAN

**Ambenyl Cough** syrup (discontinued 2002) ℞ *narcotic antitussive; antihistamine* [codeine phosphate; bromodiphenhydramine HCl; alcohol 5%] 10•12.5 mg/5 mL ⬚ Aventyl

**Ambenyl-D** oral liquid (discontinued 2002) OTC *antitussive; decongestant; expectorant* [dextromethorphan hydrobromide; pseudoephedrine HCl; guaifenesin; alcohol 9.5%] 10•30•100 mg/5 mL

**amber; amber touch-and-heal** *medicinal herb* [see: St. John wort]

**Ambi 10** bar OTC *therapeutic skin cleanser*

**Ambi 10** cream (discontinued 2003) OTC *keratolytic for acne* [benzoyl peroxide] 10%

**Ambi 60/580** caplets ℞ *decongestant; expectorant* [pseudoephedrine HCl; guaifenesin] 60•580 mg

**Ambi 60/580/30** extended-release caplets ℞ *decongestant; expectorant; antitussive* [pseudoephedrine HCl; guaifenesin; dextromethorphan hydrobromide] 60•580•30 mg

**Ambi 600; Ambi 800; Ambi 1000; Ambi 1200** sustained-release caplets (discontinued 2004) ℞ *expectorant* [guaifenesin] 600 mg; 800 mg; 1000 mg; 1200 mg

**Ambi 1000/55** extended-release tablets ℞ *expectorant; antitussive* [guaifenesin; dextromethorphan hydrobromide] 1000•55 mg

**Ambi Skin Tone** cream (discontinued 2003) OTC *hyperpigmentation bleaching agent* [hydroquinone (in a sunscreen base)]

**ambicromil** INN, BAN *prophylactic antiallergic* [also: probicromil calcium]

**ambicromil calcium** [see: probicromil calcium]

**Ambien** film-coated tablets ℞ *imidazopyridine sedative and hypnotic* [zolpidem tartrate] 5, 10 mg

**AmBisome** powder for IV infusion ℞ *systemic polyene antifungal for cryptococcal meningitis, visceral leishmaniasis, and histoplasmosis* (orphan) [amphotericin B lipid complex (ABLC)] 50 mg/vial

**ambomycin** USAN, INN *antineoplastic*

**ambrette (*Abelmoschus moschatus*)** seeds and oil *medicinal herb for gastric cancer, gonorrhea, hysteria, and respiratory disorders; also used as a fragrance in cosmetics and a flavoring in alcoholic beverages, bitters, and coffees; not generally regarded as safe and effective for medicinal uses*

**ambroxol** INN [also: ambroxol HCl]
**ambroxol HCl** JAN [also: ambroxol]
**ambruticin** USAN, INN *antifungal*
**ambucaine** INN, DCF
**ambucetamide** INN, BAN
**ambuphylline** USAN *diuretic; smooth muscle relaxant* [also: bufylline]
**ambuside** USAN, INN, BAN *diuretic*
**ambuterol** [see: mabuterol]
**ambutonium bromide** BAN
**ambutoxate** [see: ambucaine]
**amcinafal** USAN, INN *anti-inflammatory*
**amcinafide** USAN, INN *anti-inflammatory*
**amcinonide** USAN, USP, INN, BAN, JAN *topical corticosteroidal anti-inflammatory* 0.1% topical
**Amcort** IM injection ℞ *corticosteroid; anti-inflammatory* [triamcinolone diacetate] 40 mg/mL
**AMD-3100** *investigational (Phase II) for HIV infection*
**amdinocillin** USAN, USP *aminopenicillin antibiotic* [also: mecillinam]
**amdinocillin pivoxil** USAN *antibacterial* [also: pivmecillinam; pivmecillinam HCl]
**amdoxovir** USAN *antiviral for HIV-1 and hepatitis B infections*
**Amdray** IV infusion, oral solution, capsules ℞ *investigational (Phase III) P-glycoprotein (P-gp) inhibitor for multi-drug–resistant (MDR) cancers, including acute myelogenous leukemia (AML), multiple myeloma, and ovarian cancer* [valspodar]
**ameban** [see: carbarsone]
**amebarsone** [see: carbarsone]
**amebicides** *a class of drugs that kill amoebae*
**amebucort** INN
**amechol** [see: methacholine chloride]
**amedalin** INN *antidepressant* [also: amedalin HCl]
**amedalin HCl** USAN *antidepressant* [also: amedalin]
**ameltolide** USAN, INN, BAN *anticonvulsant*
**Amen** tablets (discontinued 2004) ℞ *synthetic progestin for secondary amenorrhea, abnormal uterine bleeding, and* endometrial hyperplasia [medroxyprogesterone acetate] 10 mg
**amenozine** [see: amanozine]
**Amerge** film-coated tablets ℞ *vascular serotonin 5-HT$_{1D}$ receptor agonist for the acute treatment of migraine* [naratriptan HCl] 1, 2.5 mg
**Americaine** ointment, anorectal ointment, aerosol spray OTC *topical local anesthetic* [benzocaine] 20%
**Americaine Anesthetic Lubricant** gel ℞ *anesthetic lubricant for upper GI procedures* [benzocaine] 20%
**Americaine First Aid** ointment OTC *topical local anesthetic* [benzocaine] 20%
**Americaine Otic** ear drops (discontinued 2004) ℞ *local anesthetic* [benzocaine] 20%
**American angelica** *medicinal herb* [see: angelica]
**American aspen** *medicinal herb* [see: poplar]
**American centaury (Sabatia angularis)** plant *medicinal herb used as a bitter tonic, emmenagogue, febrifuge, and vermifuge*
**American elder** *medicinal herb* [see: elderberry]
**American elm** *medicinal herb* [see: slippery elm]
**American foxglove** *medicinal herb* [see: feverweed]
**American ginseng (Panax quinquefolia)** *medicinal herb* [see: ginseng]
**American hellebore (Veratrum viride)** [see: hellebore]
**American ivy (Parthenocissus quinquefolia)** bark and twigs *medicinal herb used as an alterative, astringent, and expectorant*
**American nightshade** *medicinal herb* [see: pokeweed]
**American pepper; American red pepper** *medicinal herb* [see: cayenne]
**American saffron** *medicinal herb* [see: safflower]
**American valerian** *medicinal herb* [see: lady's slipper]

**American vegetable tallow tree; American vegetable wax** *medicinal herb* [see: bayberry]

**American woodbine** *medicinal herb* [see: American ivy]

**Americet** tablets ℞ *analgesic; barbiturate sedative* [aspirin; caffeine; butalbital] 325•40•50 mg

**americium** *element (Am)*

**Amerifed** oral liquid OTC *pediatric decongestant and antihistamine* [pseudoephedrine HCl; chlorpheniramine maleate] 80•4 mg/5 mL

**Amerigel** lotion, ointment OTC *emollient; diaper rash treatment*

**Amerituss AD** oral liquid ℞ *pediatric decongestant, antihistamine, and expectorant* [phenylephrine HCl; chlorpheniramine maleate; dextromethorphan hydrobromide] 10•3•15 mg/5 mL

**amesergide** USAN, INN *serotonin antagonist; investigational antidepressant*

**ametantrone** INN *antineoplastic* [also: ametantrone acetate]

**ametantrone acetate** USAN *antineoplastic* [also: ametantrone]

**ametazole** BAN [also: betazole HCl; betazole]

**A-Methapred** powder for injection ℞ *corticosteroid; anti-inflammatory; immunosuppressant* [methylprednisolone sodium succinate] 40, 125, 500, 1000 mg/vial

**amethocaine** BAN *topical anesthetic* [also: tetracaine]

**amethocaine HCl** BAN *local anesthetic* [also: tetracaine HCl]

**amethopterin** [now: methotrexate]

**Amevive** powder for IV or IM injection ℞ *immunosuppressant for chronic plaque psoriasis* [alefacept] 7.5 mg/dose IV, 15 mg/dose IM

**amezepine** INN

**amezinium metilsulfate** INN, JAN

**amfebutamone** INN *aminoketone antidepressant; non-nicotine aid to smoking cessation* [also: bupropion HCl; bupropion]

**amfebutamone HCl** [see: bupropion HCl]

**amfecloral** INN, BAN *anorectic* [also: amphecloral]

**amfenac** INN, BAN *anti-inflammatory* [also: amfenac sodium]

**amfenac sodium** USAN, JAN *anti-inflammatory* [also: amfenac]

**amfepentorex** INN, DCF

**amfepramone** INN, DCF *anorexiant* [also: diethylpropion HCl; diethylpropion]

**amfepramone HCl** *anorexiant* [see: diethylpropion HCl]

**amfetamine** INN *CNS stimulant* [also: amphetamine sulfate; amphetamine]

**amfetaminil** INN

**amfilcon A** USAN *hydrophilic contact lens material*

**amflutizole** USAN, INN *gout suppressant*

**amfodyne** [see: imidecyl iodine]

**amfomycin** INN, DCF *antibacterial* [also: amphomycin]

**amfonelic acid** USAN, INN, BAN *CNS stimulant*

**AMG 531** *investigational (orphan) agent for immune thrombocytopenic purpura*

**Amgenal Cough** syrup (discontinued 2002) ℞ *narcotic antitussive; antihistamine* [codeine phosphate; bromodiphenhydramine HCl] 10•12.5 mg/5 mL

**AMI-7228** *investigational magnetic resonance angiography contrast agent*

**amibiarson** [see: carbarsone]

**Amicar** tablets, syrup, IV infusion ℞ *systemic hemostatic to control excessive bleeding* [aminocaproic acid] 500, 1000 mg; 250 mg/mL; 250 mg/mL ⧉ Amikin

**amicarbalide** INN, BAN

**amicibone** INN

**amicloral** USAN *veterinary food additive*

**amicycline** USAN, INN *antibacterial*

**amidantel** INN, BAN

**amidapsone** USAN, INN *antiviral for poultry*

**Amidate** IV injection ℞ *rapid-acting nonbarbiturate general anesthetic* [etomidate] 2 mg/mL amidefrine mesilate INN *adrenergic* [also: amidephrine mesylate; amidephrine]

amidephrine BAN *adrenergic* [also: amidephrine mesylate; amidefrine mesilate]

amidephrine mesylate USAN *adrenergic* [also: amidefrine mesilate; amidephrine]

amidofebrin [see: aminopyrine]

amidol [see: dimepheptanol]

amidone HCl [see: methadone HCl]

amidopyrazoline [see: aminopyrine]

amidopyrine [now: aminopyrine]

amidotrizoate sodium [see: diatrizoate sodium]

amidotrizoic acid JAN *radiopaque contrast medium* [also: diatrizoic acid]

amiflamine INN

amifloverine INN, DCF

amifloxacin USAN, INN, BAN *broad-spectrum fluoroquinolone antibiotic*

amifloxacin mesylate USAN *broad-spectrum fluoroquinolone antibiotic*

amifostine USAN, INN, BAN *chemoprotective agent for cisplatin and paclitaxel chemotherapy (orphan); investigational (orphan) for cyclophosphamide; treatment for moderate to severe xerostomia following postoperative radiation therapy (orphan)*

Amigesic *film-coated tablets, film-coated caplets, capsules* ℞ *analgesic; antipyretic; anti-inflammatory; antirheumatic* [salsalate] 500 mg; 750 mg; 500 mg

amikacin USP, INN, BAN *aminoglycoside antibiotic; investigational (Phase II) liposomal formulation for complicated urinary tract infections and AIDS-related Mycobacterial infection*

amikacin sulfate USAN, USP, JAN *aminoglycoside antibiotic* 50, 250 mg/mL injection

amikhelline INN

Amikin *IV or IM injection, pediatric injection* ℞ *aminoglycoside antibiotic* [amikacin sulfate] 250 mg/mL; 50 mg/mL ⊘ Amicar

amilomer INN

amiloride INN, BAN *antihypertensive; potassium-sparing diuretic* [also: amiloride HCl]

amiloride HCl USAN, USP *antihypertensive; potassium-sparing diuretic; investigational (orphan) inhalant for cystic fibrosis* [also: amiloride]

amiloxate USAN *ultraviolet B sunscreen*

aminacrine BAN *topical anti-infective/antiseptic* [also: aminacrine HCl; aminoacridine]

aminacrine HCl USAN *vaginal antibacterial and antiseptic* [also: aminoacridine; aminacrine]

aminarsone [see: carbarsone]

amindocate INN

amine resin [see: polyamine-methylene resin]

amineptine INN

Aminess 5.2% *IV infusion* ℞ *nutritional therapy for renal failure* [multiple essential amino acids]

Aminess N *film-coated tablets* ℞ *nutritional therapy for dialysis patients* [multiple essential amino acids]

aminicotin [see: niacinamide]

aminitrozole INN *veterinary antibacterial* [also: nithiamide; acinitrazole]

2-amino-2-deoxyglucose [see: glucosamine]

aminoacetic acid JAN *nonessential amino acid; urologic irrigant; symbols: Gly, G* [also: glycine]

aminoacridine INN *topical anti-infective/antiseptic* [also: aminacrine HCl; aminacrine]

aminoacridine HCl [see: aminacrine HCl]

9-aminoacridine monohydrochloride [see: aminacrine HCl]

*p*-aminobenzenearsonic acid [see: arsanilic acid]

*p*-aminobenzenesulfonamide [see: sulfanilamide]

*p*-aminobenzene-sulfonylacetylimide [see: sulfacetamide]

aminobenzoate potassium USP *water-soluble vitamin; analgesic; "possibly effective" for scleroderma and other skin diseases and Peyronie disease* 500 mg oral

**aminobenzoate sodium** USP *analgesic*

*p*-**aminobenzoic acid** [see: aminobenzoic acid]

**aminobenzoic acid (4-aminobenzoic acid)** USP *water-soluble vitamin; ultraviolet screen*

**aminobenzylpenicillin** [see: ampicillin]

γ-**amino-β-hydroxybutyric acid** JAN

**aminobromophenylpyrimidinone (ABPP)** [see: bropirimine]

γ-**aminobutyric acid (GABA)** JAN *inhibitory neurotransmitter*

**9-aminocamptothecin (9-AC)** *topoisomerase I inhibitor; investigational (Phase I/II) anticancer agent; investigational (Phase II) for AIDS-related Kaposi sarcoma*

**aminocaproic acid** USAN, USP, INN, BAN *systemic hemostatic; investigational (orphan) topical treatment for traumatic hyphema of the eye* [also: ε-aminocaproic acid] 250 mg/mL injection; 250 mg/mL oral

ε-**aminocaproic acid** JAN *systemic hemostatic* [also: aminocaproic acid]

**aminocardol** [see: aminophylline]

**Amino-Cerv pH 5.5** vaginal cream ℞ *emollient; antifungal; anti-inflammatory* [urea; sodium propionate; methionine; cystine; inositol] 8.34%•0.5%•0.83%•0.35%•0.83%

**aminodeoxykanamycin** [see: bekanamycin]

**2-aminoethanethiol** [see: cysteamine]

**2-aminoethanethiol HCl** [see: cysteamine HCl]

**2-aminoethanol** [see: monoethanolamine]

**aminoethyl nitrate (2-aminoethyl nitrate)** INN, DCF

**amino-ethyl-propanol** [see: ambuphylline]

**aminoethylsulfonic acid** JAN [also: taurine]

**aminoform** [see: methenamine]

**2-aminoglutaramic acid** [see: glutamine]

**aminoglutethimide** USP, INN, BAN *adrenal steroid inhibitor; antisteroidal antineoplastic*

**aminoglycosides** *a class of bactericidal antibiotics effective against gram-negative organisms* [also called: "mycins"]

**aminoguanidine monohydrochloride** [see: pimagedine HCl]

**6-aminohexanoic acid** [see: aminocaproic acid]

**aminohippurate sodium** USP *diagnostic aid for renal function* [also: p-aminohippurate sodium] 20% injection

*p*-**aminohippurate sodium** JAN *renal function test* [also: aminohippurate sodium]

**aminohippuric acid (p-aminohippuric acid)** USP

**aminohydroxypropylidene diphosphonate (APD)** [see: pamidronate disodium]

**aminoisobutanol** [see: ambuphylline]

**3-(4'-aminoisoindoline-1'-one)-1-piperidine-2,6-dione** *investigational (orphan) for multiple myeloma*

**aminoisometradine** [see: methionine]

**aminoketones** *a class of oral antidepressants*

**5-aminolevulinic acid HCl (5-ALA HCl)** USAN *photosensitizer for photodynamic therapy of precancerous actinic keratoses of the face and scalp (for use with the BLU-U Blue Light Photodynamic Therapy Illuminator)*

**aminometradine** INN, BAN

**Amino-Min-D** capsules OTC *dietary supplement* [calcium carbonate; multiple minerals; vitamin D] 250 mg• ± •100 IU

**aminonat** [see: protein hydrolysate]

**Amino-Opti-C** sustained-release tablets OTC *vitamin C supplement with multiple bioflavonoids* [vitamin C; rose hips; lemon bioflavonoids; rutin; hesperidin] 1000• ± •250• ± • ± mg

**aminopenicillins** *a subclass of penicillins (q.v.)*

**aminopentamide sulfate** [see: dimevamide]

**aminophenazone** INN [also: aminopyrine]

**aminophenazone cyclamate** INN

**p-aminophenylarsonic acid** [see: arsanilic acid]

**aminophylline** USP, INN, BAN, JAN *smooth muscle relaxant; bronchodilator* 100, 200 mg oral; 105 mg/5 mL oral; 250 mg/10 mL injection; 250, 500 suppositories

**aminopromazine** INN, DCF [also: proquamezine]

**aminopterin sodium** INN, BAN, DCF *investigational (Phase II) antifolate for breast and ovarian cancer*

**4-aminopyridine** [see: fampridine]

**aminopyrine** NF, JAN [also: aminophenazone]

**aminoquin naphthoate** [see: pamaquine naphthoate]

**aminoquinol** INN

**aminoquinoline** [see: aminoquinol]

**4-aminoquinoline** [see: chloroquine phosphate]

**8-aminoquinoline** [see: primaquine phosphate]

**aminoquinuride** INN

**aminorex** USAN, INN, BAN *anorectic*

**aminosalicylate calcium** USP [also: calcium para-aminosalicylate]

**aminosalicylate potassium** USP

**aminosalicylate sodium (p-aminosalicylate sodium)** USP *bacteriostatic; tuberculosis retreatment agent; investigational (orphan) for Crohn disease*

**aminosalicylic acid (4-aminosalicylic acid)** USP *antibacterial; tuberculostatic (orphan); investigational (orphan) for ulcerative colitis*

**5-aminosalicylic acid (5-ASA)** [see: mesalamine]

**aminosalyle sodium** [see: aminosalicylate sodium]

**aminosidine** *investigational (orphan) agent for tuberculosis,* Mycobacterium avium *complex (MAC), and visceral leishmaniasis*

**aminosidine sulfate** [see: paromomycin sulfate]

**21-aminosteroids** *a class of potent antioxidants that can protect against oxygen radical–mediated lipid peroxidation and progressive neuronal degeneration following brain or spinal trauma, subarachnoid hemorrhage, or stroke* [also called: lazaroids]

**aminosuccinic acid** [see: aspartic acid]

**Aminosyn 3.5% (5%, 7%, 8.5%, 10%); Aminosyn (pH6) 10%; Aminosyn II 3.5% (5%, 7%, 8.5%, 10%, 15%); Aminosyn-PF 7% (10%)** IV infusion ℞ *total parenteral nutrition (except 3.5%); peripheral parenteral nutrition (all)* [multiple essential and nonessential amino acids]

**Aminosyn 3.5% M; Aminosyn II 3.5% M** IV infusion ℞ *peripheral parenteral nutrition* [multiple essential and nonessential amino acids; electrolytes]

**Aminosyn 7% (8.5%) with Electrolytes; Aminosyn II 7% (8.5%, 10%) with Electrolytes** IV infusion ℞ *total parenteral nutrition; peripheral parenteral nutrition* [multiple essential and nonessential amino acids; electrolytes]

**Aminosyn II 3.5% in 5% (25%) Dextrose; Aminosyn II 4.25% in 10% (20%, 25%) Dextrose; Aminosyn II 5% in 25% Dextrose** IV infusion ℞ *total parenteral nutrition (except 3.5% in 5%); peripheral parenteral nutrition (not 20% and 25%)* [multiple essential and nonessential amino acids; dextrose]

**Aminosyn II 3.5% M in 5% Dextrose; Aminosyn II 4.25% M in 10% Dextrose** IV infusion ℞ *total parenteral nutrition (4.25% in 10% only); peripheral parenteral nutrition (both)* [multiple essential and nonessential amino acids; electrolytes; dextrose]

**Aminosyn-HBC 7%** IV infusion ℞ *nutritional therapy for high metabolic stress* [multiple branched-chain essential and nonessential amino acids; electrolytes]

**Aminosyn-RF 5.2%** IV infusion ℞ *nutritional therapy for renal failure* [multiple essential amino acids]

**aminothiazole** INN

**aminotrate phosphate** [see: trolnitrate phosphate]

**aminoxaphen** [see: aminorex]

**Aminoxin** enteric-coated tablets OTC *vitamin B₆ supplement* [pyridoxal-5′-phosphate] 20 mg

**aminoxytriphene** INN

**aminoxytropine tropate HCl** [see: atropine oxide HCl]

**Amio-Aqueous** ℞ *investigational (orphan) antiarrhythmic for incessant ventricular tachycardia* [amiodarone]

**amiodarone** USAN, INN, BAN *investigational (orphan) ventricular antiarrhythmic for incessant ventricular tachycardia*

**amiodarone HCl** *ventricular antiarrhythmic for acute ventricular tachycardia and fibrillation (orphan)* 200 mg oral; 50 mg/mL injection

**amiperone** INN

**amiphenazole** INN, BAN

**amipizone** INN

**amipramidine** [see: amiloride HCl]

**amiprilose** INN *synthetic monosaccharide anti-inflammatory* [also: amiprilose HCl]

**amiprilose HCl** USAN *investigational (NDA filed) synthetic monosaccharide anti-inflammatory for rheumatoid arthritis* [also: amiprilose]

**amiquinsin** INN *antihypertensive* [also: amiquinsin HCl]

**amiquinsin HCl** USAN *antihypertensive* [also: amiquinsin]

**amisometradine** NF, INN, BAN

**amisulpride** INN

**amiterol** INN

**Ami-Tex LA** long-acting tablets (discontinued 2002) ℞ *decongestant; expectorant* [phenylpropanolamine HCl; guaifenesin] 75•400 mg

**amithiozone** [see: thioacetazone; thiacetazone]

**amitivir** USAN, INN *investigational influenza vaccine*

**Amitone** chewable tablets OTC *antacid* [calcium carbonate] 350 mg

**amitraz** USAN, INN, BAN *scabicide*

**amitriptyline (AMT)** INN, BAN *tricyclic antidepressant* [also: amitriptyline HCl] ⊠ nortriptyline

**amitriptyline HCl** USP, JAN *tricyclic antidepressant* [also: amitriptyline] 10, 25, 50, 75, 100, 150 mg oral

**amitriptylinoxide** INN

**amixetrine** INN, DCF

**AmLactin** cream, lotion OTC *moisturizer; emollient* [ammonium lactate] 12%

**AmLactin AP** cream OTC *local anesthetic; moisturizer; emollient* [pramoxine HCl; lactic acid] 1%•12%

**amlexanox** USAN, INN, JAN *antiallergic; anti-inflammatory for aphthous ulcers*

**amlintide** USAN *antidiabetic for type 1 diabetes*

**amlodipine** INN, BAN *antianginal; antihypertensive; calcium channel blocker* [also: amlodipine besylate]

**amlodipine besylate** USAN *antianginal; antihypertensive; calcium channel blocker* [also: amlodipine]

**amlodipine maleate** USAN *antianginal; antihypertensive*

**ammi (*Ammi majus; A. visnaga*)** dried ripe fruits *medicinal herb for angina, bronchial asthma, diabetes, diuresis, kidney and bladder stones, psoriasis, respiratory diseases, and vitiligo*

**ammoidin** [see: methoxsalen]

**[¹³N]ammonia** [see: ammonia N 13]

**ammonia** [see: ammonia spirit, aromatic]

**ammonia N 13** USAN, USP *radioactive diagnostic aid for cardiac and liver imaging*

**ammonia solution, strong** NF *solvent; source of ammonia* [also: ammonia water]

**ammonia spirit, aromatic** USP *respiratory stimulant*

**ammonia water** JAN *solvent; source of ammonia* [also: ammonia solution, strong]

**ammoniated mercury** [see: mercury, ammoniated]

**ammonio methacrylate copolymer** NF *coating agent*

**ammonium alum** [see: alum, ammonium]

**ammonium benzoate** USP

**ammonium carbonate** NF *source of ammonia*

**ammonium chloride** USP, JAN *urinary acidifier; diuretic; expectorant* 486, 500 mg oral; 5 mEq/mL (26.75%) injection

**ammonium 2-hydroxypropanoate** [see: ammonium lactate]

**ammonium ichthosulfonate** [see: ichthammol]

**ammonium lactate (lactic acid neutralized with ammonium hydroxide)** USAN *antipruritic; emollient for xerosis*

**ammonium mandelate** USP

**ammonium molybdate** USP *dietary molybdenum supplement* 25 μg/mL injection

**ammonium molybdate tetrahydrate** [see: ammonium molybdate]

**ammonium phosphate** NF *pharmaceutic aid*

**ammonium salicylate** NF

**ammonium tetrathiomolybdate** *investigational (orphan) for Wilson disease*

**ammonium valerate** NF

**Ammonul** ℞ *investigational (orphan) agent to prevent and treat hyperammonemia of urea cycle enzymopathy* [sodium benzoate; sodium phenylacetate]

**ammophyllin** [see: aminophylline]

*Amnaranthus spp.* *medicinal herb* [see: amaranth]

**Amnesteem** capsules ℞ *keratolytic for severe recalcitrant cystic acne* [isotretinoin] 10, 20, 40 mg

**AMO Endosol; AMO Endosol Extra** ophthalmic solution ℞ *intraocular irrigating solution* [sodium chloride (balanced saline solution)]

**AMO Vitrax** intraocular injection ℞ *viscoelastic agent for ophthalmic surgery* [hyaluronate sodium] 30 mg/mL

**amobarbital** USP, INN, JAN *sedative; hypnotic; anticonvulsant; also abused as a street drug* [also: amylobarbitone]

**amobarbital sodium** USP, JAN *hypnotic; sedative; anticonvulsant; also abused as a street drug*

**amocaine chloride** [see: amolanone HCl]

**amocarzine** INN

**amodiaquine** USP, INN, BAN *antiprotozoal*

**amodiaquine HCl** USP *antimalarial*

**amogastrin** INN, JAN

**amolanone** INN

**amolanone HCl** [see: amolanone]

**amonafide** INN *investigational antineoplastic*

**amoproxan** INN, DCF

**amopyroquine** INN

**amorolfine** USAN, INN, BAN *antimycotic*

*Amorphophallus konjac* *medicinal herb* [see: glucomannan]

**Amosan** powder OTC *oral antibacterial* [sodium peroxyborate monohydrate]

**amoscanate** INN

**amosulalol** INN [also: amosulalol HCl]

**amosulalol HCl** JAN [also: amosulalol]

**amotriphene** [see: aminoxytriphene]

**amoxapine** USAN, USP, INN, BAN, JAN *tricyclic antidepressant* 25, 50, 100, 150 mg oral ⍰ amoxicillin; Amoxil

**amoxecaine** INN

**amoxicillin** USAN, USP, JAN *aminopenicillin antibiotic* [also: amoxicilline; amoxycillin] 125, 200, 250, 400, 500, 875 mg oral; 125, 200, 250, 400 mg/5 mL oral ⍰ amoxapine

**amoxicillin & clavulanate potassium** *aminopenicillin antibiotic plus synergist* 200•28.5, 400•57, 500•125, 875•125 mg oral; 200•28.5, 400•57 mg/5 mL oral

**amoxicillin sodium** USAN *aminopenicillin antibiotic*

**amoxicillin trihydrate** [see: amoxicillin]

**amoxicilline** INN *aminopenicillin antibiotic* [also: amoxicillin; amoxycillin]

**Amoxil** capsules, film-coated caplets, chewable tablets, powder for oral suspension, pediatric drops ℞ *aminopenicillin antibiotic* [amoxicillin] 250, 500 mg; 500, 875 mg; 200, 400 mg; 125, 200, 250, 400 mg/5 mL; 50 mg/mL ② amoxapine

**amoxycillin** BAN *aminopenicillin antibiotic* [also: amoxicillin; amoxicilline]

**amoxydramine camsilate** INN [also: amoxydramine camsylate]

**amoxydramine camsylate** DCF [also: amoxydramine camsilate]

**AMP; A₅MP (adenosine monophosphate)** [see: adenosine phosphate]

**amperozide** INN, BAN *investigational antipsychotic for schizophrenia*

**amphecloral** USAN *anorectic* [also: amfecloral]

**amphenidone** INN

**amphetamine** BAN *CNS stimulant; widely abused as a street drug, which causes strong psychic dependence* [also: amphetamine sulfate; amfetamine]

*d*-**amphetamine** [see: dextroamphetamine]

(+)-**amphetamine** [see: dextroamphetamine]

*l*-**amphetamine** [see: levamphetamine]

(–)-**amphetamine** [see: levamphetamine]

**amphetamine aspartate** *CNS stimulant*

**amphetamine complex (resin complex of amphetamine & dextroamphetamine)** [q.v.]

**amphetamine phosphate, dextro** [see: dextroamphetamine phosphate]

**Amphetamine Salt Combo** tablets ℞ *CNS stimulant mixture for attention-deficit hyperactivity disorder (ADHD)* [amphetamine aspartate; amphetamine sulfate; dextroamphetamine sulfate; dextroamphetamine saccharate] 5, 10, 20, 30 mg total amphetamines (1.25, 2.5, 5, 7.5 mg of each)

**amphetamine succinate, levo** [see: levamphetamine succinate]

**amphetamine sulfate** USP *CNS stimulant; widely abused as a street drug, which causes strong psychic dependence* [also: amfetamine; amphetamine]

**amphetamine sulfate, dextro** [see: dextroamphetamine sulfate]

**amphetamines** *a class of CNS stimulants that includes amphetamine, dextroamphetamine, levamphetamine, methamphetamine, and their salts*

**amphetamines, mixed** (equal parts amphetamine aspartate, amphetamine sulfate, dextroamphetamine sulfate, and dextroamphetamine saccharate) *CNS stimulant for attention-deficit hyperactivity disorder (ADHD), narcolepsy, and obesity; also abused as a street drug, which causes strong psychic dependence* [5, 10, 20, 30 mg oral]

**Amphocin** powder for IV infusion ℞ *systemic polyene antifungal* [amphotericin B deoxycholate] 50 mg/vial

**amphocortrin** [see: amphomycin]

**Amphojel** oral suspension (discontinued 2004) OTC *antacid* [aluminum hydroxide gel] 320 mg/5 mL ② Amphocil

**Amphojel** tablets OTC *antacid* [aluminum hydroxide gel] 300, 600 mg ② Amphocil

**amphomycin** USAN, BAN *antibacterial* [also: amfomycin]

**amphotalide** INN, DCF

**Amphotec** powder for IV infusion ℞ *systemic polyene antifungal for invasive aspergillosis* [amphotericin B cholesteryl sulfate] 50, 100 mg/vial

**amphotericin B** USP, INN, BAN, JAN *polyene antifungal*

**amphotericin B cholesteryl** *systemic polyene antifungal for invasive aspergillosis*

**amphotericin B deoxycholate** *systemic polyene antifungal* 50 mg injection

**amphotericin B lipid complex (ABLC)** *systemic polyene antifungal for meningitis, leishmaniasis, histoplasmosis, and other invasive infections (orphan)*

**ampicillin** USAN, USP, INN, BAN, JAN *aminopenicillin antibiotic* 250, 500 mg oral

**ampicillin sodium** USAN, USP, JAN *aminopenicillin antibiotic* 250, 500 mg, 1, 2 g injection

**ampicillin sodium & sulbactam sodium** *aminopenicillin antibiotic plus synergist* 1•0.5, 2•1 g injection

**ampiroxicam** INN, BAN

**Amplicor Chlamydia** test kit for professional use *in vitro diagnostic aid for* Chlamydia trachomatis [DNA amplification test]

**Amplicor HIV-1 Monitor** test kit for professional use *in vitro diagnostic aid for HIV-1 in blood* [polymerase chain reaction (PCR) test]

**Amplicor MTB** test kit for professional use *in vitro diagnostic aid for* Mycobacterium *tuberculosis* [polymerase chain reaction (PCR) test]

**Ampligen** Ŗ *investigational (Phase III, orphan) RNA synthesis inhibitor and immunomodulator for HIV, renal cell carcinoma, metastatic melanoma, and chronic fatigue syndrome* [poly I: poly C12U]

**amprenavir** USAN *protease inhibitor antiviral for HIV infection*

**amprenavir & abacavir sulfate** *investigational (Phase III) protease inhibitor and nucleoside analogue combination for HIV and AIDS*

**amprenavir & indinavir sulfate** *investigational (Phase II) protease inhibitor combination for AIDS*

**amprenavir & lamivudine & zidovudine** *investigational (Phase III) second-generation protease inhibitor combination for AIDS*

**amprenavir & nelfinavir mesylate** *investigational (Phase II) protease inhibitor combination for AIDS*

**amprenavir & saquinavir** *investigational (Phase II) protease inhibitor combination for AIDS*

**amprocidum** [see: amprolium]

**amprolium** USP, INN, BAN *coccidiostat for poultry*

**amprotropine phosphate**

**ampyrimine** INN

**ampyzine** INN *CNS stimulant* [also: ampyzine sulfate]

**ampyzine sulfate** USAN *CNS stimulant* [also: ampyzine]

**amquinate** USAN, INN *antimalarial*

**amrinone** INN, BAN *cardiotonic* [also: inamrinone (USAN changed 2000)]

**amrinone lactate** [now: inamrinone lactate]

**amrubicin** INN

**AMSA; *m*-AMSA (acridinylamine methanesulfon anisidide)** [see: amsacrine]

**amsacrine** USAN, INN, BAN *investigational (NDA filed, orphan) antineoplastic for acute adult leukemias (AML, APL, and ALL) and lymphomas*

**Amsidyl** Ŗ *investigational (NDA filed, orphan) antineoplastic for acute adult leukemias (AML, APL, and ALL) and lymphomas* [amsacrine]

**amsonate** INN, BAN *combining name for radicals or groups*

**AMT (amitriptyline HCl)** [q.v.]

**amtolmetin guacil** INN

**Amvaz** tablets Ŗ *antianginal; antihypertensive; calcium channel blocker* [amlodipine] 2.5, 5, 10 mg

**Amvisc; Amvisc Plus** intraocular injection Ŗ *viscoelastic agent for ophthalmic surgery* [hyaluronate sodium] 12 mg/mL; 16 mg/mL

**amyl alcohol, tertiary** [see: amylene hydrate]

**amyl nitrite** USP, JAN *vasodilator; antianginal; also abused as a euphoric street drug and sexual stimulant* 0.3 mL inhalant

**amylase** *digestive enzyme* [100 IU/mg in pancrelipase; 25 IU/mg in pancreatin]

**amylase** [see: alpha amylase]

**amylene hydrate** NF *solvent*

**amylin** [see: amlintide]

**amylmetacresol** INN, BAN

**amylobarbitone** BAN *sedative; hypnotic; anticonvulsant* [also: amobarbital]

**amylocaine** BAN

**amylopectin sulfate, sodium salt**
[see: sodium amylosulfate]

**amylosulfate sodium** [see: sodium amylosulfate]

**Amytal Sodium** powder for injection R̞ *sedative; hypnotic; anxiolytic; anticonvulsant; also abused as a street drug* [amobarbital sodium]

**anabolic steroids** *a class of hormones derived from or closely related to testosterone that increase anabolic (tissue-building) and decrease catabolic (tissue-depleting) processes*

**Anacin** caplets, tablets OTC *analgesic; antipyretic; anti-inflammatory* [aspirin; caffeine] 400•32 mg; 400•32, 500•32 mg ⊠ Unisom; Unasyn

**Anacin Aspirin Free** tablets, caplets, gelcaps OTC *analgesic; antipyretic* [acetaminophen] 500 mg ⊠ Unisom; Unasyn

**Anacin P.M., Aspirin Free** film-coated caplets OTC *antihistaminic sleep aid; analgesic* [diphenhydramine HCl; acetaminophen] 25•500 mg ⊠ Unisom; Unasyn

**Anadrol-50** tablets R̞ *anabolic steroid for anemias; also abused as a street drug* [oxymetholone] 50 mg

**anafebrina** [see: aminopyrine]

**Anafranil** capsules R̞ *tricyclic antidepressant for obsessive-compulsive disorders* [clomipramine HCl] 25, 50, 75 mg ⊠ enalapril

**anagestone** INN *progestin* [also: anagestone acetate]

**anagestone acetate** USAN *progestin* [also: anagestone]

**anagrelide** INN *antithrombotic/antiplatelet agent* [also: anagrelide HCl]

**anagrelide HCl** USAN *antithrombotic/antiplatelet agent for essential thrombocythemia (orphan); investigational (orphan) for thrombocytosis and polycythemia vera* [also: anagrelide]

**Ana-Guard** subcu or IM injection (discontinued 2001) R̞ *sympathomimetic bronchodilator for emergency treatment of anaphylaxis; vasopressor for shock* [epinephrine] 1:1000

**anakinra** USAN, INN *interleukin-1 receptor antagonist (IL-1ra); nonsteroidal anti-inflammatory for inflammatory bowel disease and rheumatoid arthritis (RA); investigational (Phase II, orphan) for juvenile rheumatoid arthritis (JRA) and graft vs. host disease (GVHD)*

**Ana-Kit** (discontinued 2002) R̞ *emergency treatment of anaphylaxis* [epinephrine; chlorpheniramine maleate; alcohol; tourniquet] 1:100 000•2 mg

**analeptics** *a class of central nervous system stimulants used to maintain or improve alertness*

**Analgesia Creme** OTC *topical analgesic* [trolamine salicylate] 10%

**Analgesic Balm** OTC *analgesic; counterirritant* [methyl salicylate; menthol]

**analgesics** *a class of drugs that relieve pain or reduce sensitivity to pain without causing loss of consciousness*

**analgesine** [see: antipyrine]

**Analpram-HC** anorectal cream R̞ *corticosteroidal anti-inflammatory; local anesthetic* [hydrocortisone acetate; pramoxine] 1%•1%, 2.5%•1% ⊠ Analbalm

**AnaMantle HC** cream R̞ *corticosteroidal anti-inflammatory; local anesthetic* [hydrocortisone acetate; lidocaine] 0.5%•3%

**Anamine** syrup (discontinued 2002) R̞ *decongestant; antihistamine* [pseudoephedrine HCl; chlorpheniramine maleate] 30•2 mg/5 mL

**Anamine T.D.** sustained-release capsules (discontinued 2002) R̞ *decongestant; antihistamine* [pseudoephedrine HCl; chlorpheniramine maleate] 120•8 mg

***Anamirta cocculus; A. paniculata*** *medicinal herb* [see: levant berry]

**ananain** *investigational (orphan) proteolytic enzymes for debridement of severe burns*

***Ananas comosus*** *medicinal herb* [see: pineapple]

**Anandron** Ⓒᴬᴺ tablets (also available in Europe and Latin America) R̞ antiandrogen antineoplastic adjunct to surgical or chemical castration for metastatic prostate cancer [nilutamide] 50, 100 mg

**Anaphalis margaritacea; Gnaphalium polycephalum; G. uliginosum** medicinal herb [see: everlasting]

**anaphrodisiacs** a class of agents that reduce sexual desire or potency

**Anaplex** oral liquid (discontinued 2002) ℞ decongestant; antihistamine [pseudoephedrine HCl; chlorpheniramine maleate] 30•2 mg/5 mL

**Anaplex HD** oral liquid ℞ narcotic antitussive; decongestant; antihistamine [hydrocodone bitartrate; pseudoephedrine HCl; brompheniramine maleate] 3.4•60•4 mg/10 mL

**Anaplex-DM** oral liquid ℞ antitussive; decongestant; antihistamine [dextromethorphan hydrobromide; pseudoephedrine HCl; brompheniramine maleate] 30•60•4 mg/5 mL

**Anaprox; Anaprox DS** film-coated tablets ℞ analgesic; antiarthritic; nonsteroidal anti-inflammatory drug (NSAID) [naproxen sodium] 275 mg (=250 mg base); 550 mg (=500 mg base)

**anarel** [see: guanadrel sulfate]

**anaritide** INN, BAN antihypertensive; diuretic [also: anaritide acetate]

**anaritide acetate** USAN antihypertensive; diuretic; investigational (orphan) for acute renal failure and renal transplants

**Anaspaz** tablets ℞ GI/GU antispasmodic; antiparkinsonian; anticholinergic "drying agent" for allergic rhinitis and hyperhidrosis [hyoscyamine sulfate] 0.125 mg

**anastrozole** USAN, INN, BAN aromatase inhibitor; estrogen antagonist; antineoplastic for advanced breast cancer

**Anatrast** rectal paste ℞ radiopaque contrast medium for defecography [barium sulfate] 100%

**Anatrofin** brand name for stenbolone acetate, an anabolic steroid abused as a street drug

**Anatuss** film-coated tablets (discontinued 2002) ℞ antitussive; decongestant; expectorant; analgesic [dextromethorphan hydrobromide; phenylpropanolamine HCl; guaifenesin; acetaminophen] 15•25•100•325 mg

**Anatuss** syrup (discontinued 2002) OTC antitussive; decongestant; expectorant [dextromethorphan hydrobromide; phenylpropanolamine HCl; guaifenesin] 15•25•100 mg/5 mL

**Anatuss DM** tablets, syrup (discontinued 2002) OTC antitussive; decongestant; expectorant [dextromethorphan hydrobromide; pseudoephedrine HCl; guaifenesin] 20•60•400 mg; 10•30•100 mg/5 mL

**Anatuss LA** long-acting tablets (discontinued 2002) ℞ decongestant; expectorant [pseudoephedrine HCl; guaifenesin] 120•400 mg

**Anavar** brand name for oxandrolone, an anabolic steroid abused as a street drug

**anaxirone** INN

**anayodin** [see: chiniofon]

**anazocine** INN

**anazolene sodium** USAN, INN blood volume and cardiac output test [also: sodium anoxynaphthonate]

**Anbesol** topical liquid, gel OTC mucous membrane anesthetic; antipruritic/counterirritant; antiseptic [benzocaine; phenol; alcohol 70%] 6.3%•0.5%

**Anbesol, Baby** gel OTC topical oral anesthetic [benzocaine] 7.5%

**Anbesol, Maximum Strength** topical liquid, gel OTC mucous membrane anesthetic [benzocaine; alcohol 60%] 20%

**ancarolol** INN

**Ancef** powder or frozen premix for IV or IM injection ℞ cephalosporin antibiotic [cefazolin sodium] 0.5, 1, 5, 10 g

**ancestim** USAN recombinant-methionyl human stem cell factor (r-metHuSCF); hematopoietic growth factor; investigational (NDA filed, orphan) myelosuppressive and myeloablative therapy for non-Hodgkin lymphoma, breast and ovarian cancer, and multiple myeloma

**Ancet** topical liquid OTC soap-free therapeutic skin cleanser

**anchusa** *medicinal herb* [see: henna (Alkanna)]

**ancitabine** INN [also: ancitabine HCl]

**ancitabine HCl** JAN [also: ancitabine]

**Ancobon** capsules ℞ *systemic antifungal* [flucytosine] 250, 500 mg ⊡ Oncovin

**ancrod** USAN, INN, BAN *anticoagulant enzyme derived from the venom of the Malayan pit viper; investigational (orphan) for cardiopulmonary bypass in heparin-intolerant patients*

**Andehist** pediatric oral drops (discontinued 2004) ℞ *decongestant; antihistamine* [pseudoephedrine HCl; carbinoxamine maleate] 15•2 mg/mL

**Andehist** syrup (discontinued 2004) ℞ *decongestant; antihistamine* [pseudoephedrine HCl; brompheniramine maleate] 60•4 mg/5 mL

**Andehist DM NR** pediatric oral drops ℞ *antitussive; decongestant; antihistamine* [dextromethorphan hydrobromide; pseudoephedrine HCl; carbinoxamine maleate] 4•15•1 mg/mL

**Andehist-DM** syrup (discontinued 2004) ℞ *antitussive; decongestant; antihistamine* [dextromethorphan hydrobromide; pseudoephedrine HCl; brompheniramine maleate] 15•60•4 mg/5 mL

**andolast** INN

**andrachne** *(Andrachne aspera; A. cordifolia; A. phyllanthoides)* root *medicinal herb for eye inflammation; not generally regarded as safe and effective*

**Andro 100; Andro 200** [see: depAndro 100; depAndro 200]

**Andro L.A. 200** IM injection (discontinued 2001) ℞ *androgen replacement for delayed puberty or breast cancer* [testosterone enanthate] 200 mg/mL

**Androcur** *investigational (orphan) antiandrogen for severe hirsutism* [cyproterone acetate]

**Androderm** transdermal patch (for nonscrotal area) ℞ *hormone replacement therapy for male hypogonadism; investigational (Phase III) for AIDS-wasting syndrome* [testosterone] 2.5, 5 mg/day (12.2, 24.3 mg total)

**AndroGel** ℞ *hormone replacement for male hypogonadism; investigational (orphan) for AIDS-wasting syndrome* [testosterone; alcohol 67%] 1% (25, 50 mg/pkt.)

**Androgel-DHT** ℞ *investigational (Phase III) transdermal testosterone replacement in elderly men; investigational (Phase II, orphan) for AIDS-wasting syndrome* [dihydrotestosterone]

**androgens** *a class of sex hormones responsible for the development of the male sex organs and secondary sex characteristics*

**Androgyn** [see: depAndrogyn]

**Android** capsules ℞ *androgen for hypogonadism or testosterone deficiency in men, delayed puberty in boys, and metastatic breast cancer in women* [methyltestosterone] 10 mg

**Android-10; Android-25** tablets (discontinued 2001) ℞ *androgen for hypogonadism or testosterone deficiency in men, delayed puberty in boys, and metastatic breast cancer in women* [methyltestosterone] 10 mg; 25 mg

**Androlone-D 200** IM injection (discontinued 2000) ℞ *anabolic steroid for anemia of renal insufficiency* [nandrolone decanoate (in oil)] 200 mg/mL

**Andropogon citratus** *medicinal herb* [see: lemongrass]

**Andropository-200** IM injection (discontinued 2001) ℞ *androgen replacement for delayed puberty or breast cancer* [testosterone enanthate] 200 mg/mL

**androstanazole** [now: stanozolol]

**androstane** [see: androstanolone; stanolone]

**androstanolone** INN *investigational (orphan) for AIDS-wasting syndrome* [also: stanolone]

**androtest P** [see: testosterone propionate]

**Androvite** tablets OTC *vitamin/mineral/iron supplement* [multiple vitamins &

minerals; iron; folic acid; biotin] ± •
3•0.06• ⸧ mg

**anecortave acetate** USAN *angiostatic steroid for neovascularization of the eye*

**Anectine** IV or IM injection, Flo-Pack (powder for injection) ℞ *muscle relaxant; anesthesia adjunct* [succinylcholine chloride] 20 mg/mL; 500, 1000 mg

**Anemagen** gelcaps (discontinued 2004) ℞ *hematinic; vitamin/iron supplement* [multiple vitamins; ferrous fumarate] ± •200 mg

**Anemagen OB** gelcaps ℞ *vitamin/calcium/iron supplement* [multiple vitamins; calcium; ferrous fumarate; folic acid] ± •200•27•1 mg

*Anemone patens medicinal herb* [see: pasque flower]

**Anergan 50** IM injection (discontinued 2002) ℞ *antihistamine; sedative; antiemetic; motion sickness relief* [promethazine HCl] 50 mg/mL

**anertan** [see: testosterone propionate]

**Anestacon** jelly ℞ *mucous membrane anesthetic* [lidocaine HCl] 2%

**anesthesin** [see: benzocaine]

**anesthetics** *a class of agents that abolish the sensation of pain*

**anesthrone** [see: benzocaine]

**anethaine** [see: tetracaine HCl]

**anethole** NF *flavoring agent*

**anetholtrithion** JAN

*Anethum foeniculum medicinal herb* [see: fennel]

*Anethum graveolens medicinal herb* [see: dill]

**aneurine HCl** [see: thiamine HCl]

**Anexsia; Anexsia 5/500; Anexsia 7.5/650; Anexsia 10/660** tablets ℞ *narcotic analgesic* [hydrocodone bitartrate; acetaminophen] 5•325, 7.5• 325 mg; 5•500 mg; 7.5•650 mg; 10•660 mg

**angelica (*Angelica atropurpurea*)** root *medicinal herb for appetite stimulation, bronchial disorders, colds, colic, cough, exhaustion, gas, heartburn, and rheumatism; also used as a tonic*

*Angelica levisticum medicinal herb* [see: lovage]

*Angelica polymorpha; A. sinensis; A. dahurica medicinal herb* [see: dong quai]

**Angiomax** powder for IV injection ℞ *anticoagulant thrombin inhibitor for patients with unstable angina undergoing percutaneous transluminal coronary angioplasty (PTCA)* [bivalirudin] 250 mg/vial

**angiotensin 1-7** *investigational (orphan) agent for myelodysplastic syndrome and neutropenia due to bone marrow transplantation*

**angiotensin II** INN

**angiotensin II receptor antagonists (AIIRAs)** *a class of antihypertensives that reduce the vasoconstricting effects of angiotensin II by blocking the angiotensin II receptor sites in the vascular smooth muscles* [compare to: angiotensin-converting enzyme inhibitors]

**angiotensin amide** USAN, NF, BAN *vasoconstrictor* [also: angiotensinamide]

**angiotensinamide** INN *vasoconstrictor* [also: angiotensin amide]

**angiotensin-converting enzyme inhibitors (ACEIs)** *a class of antihypertensives that reduce the vasoconstricting effects of angiotensin II by blocking the enzyme (kininase II) that converts angiotensin I to angiotensin II* [compare to: angiotensin II receptor antagonists]

**anhidrotics** *a class of agents that reduce or suppress perspiration* [also called: anidrotics; antihydrotics]

**anhydrohydroxyprogesterone** [now: ethisterone]

**anhydrous lanolin** [see: lanolin, anhydrous]

**anidoxime** USAN, INN, BAN *analgesic*

**anidrotics** *a class of agents that reduce or suppress perspiration* [also called: anhidrotics; antihydrotics]

**anidulafungin** USAN *antifungal for* Candida, Aspergillus, *and* Pneumocystis *infections; investigational (Phase III) for esophageal candidiasis*

**anilamate** INN

**anileridine** USP, INN, BAN *narcotic analgesic*

**anileridine HCl** USP *narcotic analgesic*

**anilopam** INN *analgesic* [also: anilopam HCl]

**anilopam HCl** USAN *analgesic* [also: anilopam]

**Animal Shapes** chewable tablets OTC *vitamin supplement* [multiple vitamins; folic acid] ± • 0.3 mg

**Animal Shapes + Iron** chewable tablets OTC *vitamin/iron supplement* [multiple vitamins; iron; folic acid] ± • 15 • 0.3 mg

**anion exchange resin** [see: polyamine-methylene resin]

**anipamil** INN

**aniracetam** USAN, INN *mental performance enhancer*

**anirolac** USAN, INN *anti-inflammatory; analgesic*

**anisacril** INN

**anisatil** USAN *combining name for radicals or groups*

**anise (Pimpinella anisum)** oil and seeds *medicinal herb for colic, convulsions, cough, gas, intestinal cleansing, iron-deficiency anemia, mucous discharge, promoting expectoration, and psoriasis; also used as an antibacterial, antimicrobial, and antiseptic*

**anise oil** NF

**anise root; sweet anise** *medicinal herb* [see: sweet cicely]

**anisindione** NF, INN, BAN *indanedione-derivative anticoagulant*

**anisopirol** INN

**anisopyradamine** [see: pyrilamine maleate]

**anisotropine methylbromide** USAN, JAN *anticholinergic; peptic ulcer adjunct* [also: octatropine methylbromide] 50 mg oral

**anisoylated plasminogen streptokinase activator complex (APSAC)** [see: anistreplase]

**anistreplase** USAN, INN, BAN *fibrinolytic; thrombolytic enzyme for acute myocardial infarction*

**Anisum officinarum; A. vulgare** *medicinal herb* [see: anise]

**anitrazafen** USAN, INN *topical anti-inflammatory*

**anodynes** *a class of agents that lessen or relieve pain*

**anodynine** [see: antipyrine]

**anodynon** [see: ethyl chloride]

**Anogesic** ointment ℞ *investigational (Phase III) topical treatment for hemorrhoids and anal fissures* [nitroglycerin]

**Anoquan** capsules (discontinued 2000) ℞ *analgesic; barbiturate sedative* [acetaminophen; caffeine; butalbital] 325 • 40 • 50 mg

**anorectics** *a class of central nervous system stimulants that suppress the appetite* [also called: anorexiants; anorexigenics]

**anorexiants** *a class of central nervous system stimulants that suppress the appetite* [also called: anorectics; anorexigenics]

**anorexigenics** *a class of central nervous system stimulants that suppress the appetite* [also called: anorexiants; anorectics]

**anovlar** [see: norethindrone & ethinyl estradiol]

**anoxomer** USAN *antioxidant; food additive*

**anoxynaphthonate sodium** [see: anazolene sodium]

**anpirtoline** INN

**Ansaid** film-coated tablets ℞ *antiarthritic; nonsteroidal anti-inflammatory drug (NSAID)* [flurbiprofen] 50, 100 mg ☑ NSAID

**ansamycin** [see: rifabutin]

**ansoxetine** INN

**Answer One-Step; Answer Plus; Answer Quick & Simple** test kit for home use *in vitro diagnostic aid; urine pregnancy test*

**Answer Ovulation** test kit for home use *in vitro diagnostic aid to predict ovulation time*

**Antabuse** tablets ℞ *deterrent to alcohol consumption* [disulfiram] 250 mg

**Antacid** chewable tablets OTC *antacid* [calcium carbonate] 500, 750 mg

**Antacid** oral suspension OTC *antacid* [aluminum hydroxide; magnesium hydroxide] 225•200 mg/5 mL

**antacids** *a class of drugs that neutralize gastric acid*

**antafenite** INN

**Antagon** subcu injection ℞ *gonadotropin-releasing hormone (GnRH) antagonist for infertility* [ganirelix acetate] 250 µg/0.5 mL

**antastan** [see: antazoline HCl]

**antazoline** INN, BAN [also: antazoline HCl]

**antazoline HCl** USP [also: antazoline]

**antazoline phosphate** USP *antihistamine*

**antazoline phosphate & naphazoline HCl** *topical ocular antihistamine and decongestant* 0.5%•0.05%

**antazonite** INN

**Antegren** ℞ *investigational (NDA filed) humanized monoclonal antibody (huMAb) for treatment of multiple sclerosis and Crohn disease* [natalizumab]

**antelmycin** INN *anthelmintic* [also: anthelmycin]

**anterior pituitary**

**anthelmintics** *a class of drugs effective against parasitic infections* [also called: vermicides; vermifuges]

**anthelmycin** USAN *anthelmintic* [also: antelmycin]

*Anthemis nobilis* medicinal herb [see: chamomile]

**anthiolimine** INN

*Anthoxanthum odoratum* medicinal herb [see: sweet vernal grass]

**anthracyclines** *a class of antibiotic antineoplastics*

**Anthra-Derm** ointment ℞ *topical antipsoriatic* [anthralin] 0.1%, 0.25%, 0.5%, 1%

**anthralin** USP *topical antipsoriatic* [also: dithranol] 1% topical

**anthramycin** USAN *antineoplastic* [also: antramycin]

**anthraquinone of cascara** [see: cascara sagrada]

**anthrax test** [see: Rapid Anthrax Test]

**anthrax vaccine, adsorbed (AVA)** *active bacterin derived from an attenuated strain of* Bacillus anthracis

*Anthriscus cerefolium* medicinal herb [see: chervil]

**anti pan T lymphocyte monoclonal antibodies (MAb)** *investigational (orphan) agent for in vivo and ex vivo treatment of bone marrow transplants* [also: anti-T lymphocyte immunotoxin XMMLY-H65-RTA]

**anti-A blood grouping serum** USP *in vitro blood testing*

**antiadrenergics** *a class of agents that block the alpha₁ adrenergic receptors, used for the treatment of hypertension and benign prostatic hyperplasia (BPH)* also called: alpha₁-adrenergic blockers

**antiadrenergics** *a class of cardiovascular drugs that block the passage of impulses through the sympathetic nervous system* [also called: sympatholytics]

**antiandrogens** *a class of hormonal antineoplastics*

**antib** [see: thioacetazone; thiacetazone]

**anti-B blood grouping serum** USP *in vitro blood testing*

**antibason** [see: methylthiouracil]

**AntibiOtic** ear drops, otic suspension ℞ *topical corticosteroidal anti-inflammatory; antibiotic* [hydrocortisone; neomycin sulfate; polymyxin B sulfate] 1%•5 mg•10 000 U per mL

**Antibiotic Ear Solution** ℞ *topical corticosteroidal anti-inflammatory; antibiotic* [hydrocortisone; neomycin sulfate; polymyxin B sulfate] 1%•5 mg•10 000 U per mL

**Antibiotic Ear Suspension** ℞ *topical corticosteroidal anti-inflammatory; antibiotic* [hydrocortisone; neomycin sulfate; polymyxin B sulfate] 1%•5 mg•10 000 U per mL

**antibiotics** *a class of agents that destroy or arrest the growth of micro-organisms*

**antibromics** *a class of agents that mask undesirable or offensive odors* [also called: deodorants]

**anti-C blood grouping serum** [see: blood grouping serum, anti-C]

**anti-c blood grouping serum** [see: blood grouping serum, anti-c]

**anti-CD3** [see: muromonab-CD3]

**anti-CD23 kappa monoclonal antibodies (MAb) to immunoglobulin G1 (IgG1)** *investigational (orphan) agent for chronic lymphocytic leukemia*

**anti-CD45 monoclonal antibodies (MAb)** *investigational (orphan) agent to prevent acute graft rejection of human organ transplants*

**anti-CEA sheep-human chimeric monoclonal antibodies (MAb) radiolabeled with iodine I 131** *investigational (orphan) agent for pancreatic cancer*

**anticholinergics** *a class of agents that block parasympathetic nerve impulses, producing antiemetic, antinausea, and antispasmodic effects; also used to dry mucosal secretions*

**anticoagulant citrate dextrose (ACD) solution** USP *anticoagulant for storage of whole blood and during cardiac surgery*

**anticoagulant citrate phosphate dextrose adenine solution** USP *anticoagulant for storage of whole blood*

**anticoagulant citrate phosphate dextrose solution** USP *anticoagulant for storage of whole blood*

**anticoagulant heparin solution** USP *anticoagulant for storage of whole blood*

**anticoagulant sodium citrate solution** USP *anticoagulant for plasma and for blood for fractionation*

**anticoagulants** *a class of therapeutic agents that inhibit or inactivate blood clotting factors*

**anticonvulsants** *a class of drugs that prevent seizures by suppressing abnormal neuronal discharges in the central nervous system* [also called: anti-epileptic drugs (AEDs)]

**Anticort** ℞ *investigational anti-aging and anticancer agent; investigational (Phase II) for HIV infection* [procaine HCl]

**anticytomegalovirus monoclonal antibodies (MAb)** *investigational (orphan) agent to prevent or treat cytomegalovirus infections due to bone marrow transplants, organ transplants, or AIDS*

**anti-D antibodies** [see: Rh$_O$(D) immune globulin]

**antidopaminergics** *a class of antiemetic drugs*

**antidotes** *a class of drugs that counteract the effects of toxic doses of other drugs or toxic substances*

**anti-E blood grouping serum** [see: blood grouping serum, anti-E]

**anti-e blood grouping serum** [see: blood grouping serum, anti-e]

**antiemetics** *a class of agents that prevent or alleviate nausea and vomiting* [also called: antinauseants]

**antiendotoxin monoclonal antibodies (MAb) E5** [now: edobacomab]

**antienite** INN

**antiepilepsirine** [now: ilepcimide]

**anti-epileptic drugs (AEDs)** *a class of drugs that prevent seizures by suppressing abnormal neuronal discharges in the central nervous system* [also called: anticonvulsants]

**antiestrogen** [see: tamoxifen citrate]

**antiestrogens** *a class of hormonal antineoplastics*

**antifebriles** *a class of agents that relieve or reduce fever* [also called: antipyretics; antithermics; febricides; febrifuges]

**antifebrin** [see: acetanilide]

**antifolic acid** [see: methotrexate]

**antiformin, dental** JAN [also: sodium hypochlorite, diluted]

**antigen-presenting cells pulsed with tumor immunoglobulin idiotype** *investigational (orphan) agent for multiple myeloma*

**antihemophilic factor (AHF; FVIII)** USP *systemic hemostatic; antihemophilic for von Willebrand disease (orphan)*

**Antihemophilic Factor (Porcine) Hyate:C** powder for IV injection ℞ *antihemophilic to correct coagulation deficiency* [antihemophilic factor VIII:C] 400–700 porcine units/vial

**antihemophilic factor, human** [now: antihemophilic factor]

**antihemophilic factor, recombinant (rFVIII)** *antihemophilic for treatment of hemophilia A and presurgical prophylaxis for hemophiliacs (orphan)*

**antihemophilic factor A** [see: antihemophilic factor]

**antihemophilic factor B** [see: factor IX complex]

**antihemophilic globulin (AHG)** [see: antihemophilic factor]

**antihemophilic human plasma** [now: plasma, antihemophilic human]

**antihemophilic plasma, human** [now: plasma, antihemophilic human]

**antiheparin** [see: protamine sulfate]

**Antihist-1** tablets (discontinued 2002) OTC *antihistamine* [clemastine fumarate] 1.34 mg

**antihistamines** *a class of drugs that counteract the effect of histamine*

**Antihist-D** tablets (discontinued 2001) OTC *decongestant; antihistamine* [phenylpropanolamine HCl (extended release); clemastine fumarate (immediate release)] 75•1.34 mg

**antihydrotics** *a class of agents that reduce or suppress perspiration* [also called: anhidrotics; anidrotics]

**antihyperlipidemic agents** *a class of drugs that lower serum lipid levels* [also called: antilipemics]

**anti-inhibitor coagulant complex** *antihemophilic*

**anti-interferon-gamma Fab from goats** *investigational (orphan) immunologic for corneal allograft rejection*

**Anti-Itch** gel OTC *poison ivy treatment* [camphor; alcohol 37%] 0.45%

**antilipemics** *a class of drugs that lower serum lipid levels* [also called: antihyperlipidemics]

**Antilirium** IV or IM injection ℞ *cholinergic to reverse anticholinergic overdose; investigational (orphan) for Friedreich and other inherited ataxias* [physostigmine salicylate] 1 mg/mL

**antilithics** *a class of agents that prevent the formation of stone or calculus* [see also: litholytics]

**antilymphocyte immunoglobulin** BAN

**antimelanoma antibody XMMME-001-DTPA 111 indium** *investigational (orphan) imaging aid for systemic and nodal melanoma metastasis*

**antimelanoma antibody XMMME-001-RTA** *investigational (orphan) agent for melanoma*

**Antiminth** oral suspension (discontinued 2004) OTC *anthelmintic for ascariasis (roundworm) and enterobiasis (pinworm)* [pyrantel pamoate] 50 mg/mL

**antimony** *element (Sb)*

**antimony potassium tartrate** USP *antischistosomal*

**antimony sodium tartrate** USP, JAN *antischistosomal*

**antimony sodium thioglycollate** USP

**antimony sulfide** [see: antimony trisulfide colloid]

**antimony trisulfide colloid** USAN *pharmaceutic aid*

**antimonyl potassium tartrate** [see: antimony potassium tartrate]

**antimuscarinics** *a class of anticholinergic agents*

**antinauseants** *a class of agents that prevent or alleviate nausea and vomiting* [also called: antiemetics]

**antineoplastics** *a class of chemotherapeutic agents capable of selective action on neoplastic (abnormally proliferating) tissues*

**antineoplastons** *a class of naturally occurring peptides that suppress cancer oncogenes and stimulate the body's cancer suppressor genes*

**Antiox** capsules OTC *vitamin supplement* [vitamins C and E; beta carotene] 120 mg•100 IU•25 mg

**anti-pellagra vitamin** [see: niacin]

**antiperiodics** *a class of agents that prevent periodic or intermittent recurrence of symptoms, as in malaria*

**anti-pernicious anemia principle** [see: cyanocobalamin]

**antiphlogistics** *a class of agents that reduce inflammation and fever*

**antipyretics** *a class of agents that relieve or reduce fever* [also called: antifebriles; antithermics; febricides; febrifuges]

**antipyrine** USP, JAN *analgesic; investigational (orphan) diagnostic agent to determine hepatic drug metabolizing activity* [also: phenazone]

**N-antipyrinylnicotinamide** [see: nifenazone]

**antirabies serum (ARS)** USP *passive immunizing agent*

**anti-Rh antibodies** [see: $Rh_O(D)$ immune globulin]

**anti-Rh typing serums** [now: blood grouping serums]

**antiscorbutic vitamin** [see: ascorbic acid]

**antiscorbutics** *a class of agents that are sources of vitamin C and are effective in the prevention or relief of scurvy*

**antiscrofulous herbs** *a class of agents that counteract scrofuloderma (tuberculous cervical lymphadenitis)*

**antisense 20-mer phosphorothiolate oligonucleotide** *investigational (orphan) agent for renal cell carcinoma*

**antisense drugs** *a class of antiviral drugs that interfere with the replication of viral protein*

**antiseptics** *a class of agents that inhibit the growth and development of microorganisms, usually on a body surface, without necessarily killing them* [see also: disinfectants; germicides]

**Antispas** IM injection ℞ *GI antispasmodic* [dicyclomine HCl] 10 mg/mL

**Antispasmodic** elixir ℞ *GI antispasmodic; anticholinergic; sedative* [atropine sulfate; scopolamine hydrobromide; hyoscyamine sulfate; phenobarbital] 0.0194•0.0065•0.1037•16.2 mg/5 mL

**antispasmodics** *a class of agents that relieve spasms or cramps, usually of gastrointestinal tract or blood vessels*

**antisterility vitamin** [see: vitamin E]

**anti-T lymphocyte immunotoxin XMMLY-H65-RTA** *investigational (orphan) agent for in vivo and ex vivo treatment of bone marrow transplants* [also: anti pan T lymphocyte monoclonal antibody]

**anti-tac, humanized; SMART anti-tac** [now: dacliximab]

**anti-tap-72 immunotoxin** *investigational (orphan) for metastatic colorectal adenocarcinoma*

**antithermics** *a class of agents that relieve or reduce fever* [also called: antifebriles; antipyretics; febricides; febrifuges]

**antithrombin III (AT-III)** INN, BAN *agent for thrombosis and pulmonary emboli of congenital AT-III deficiency (orphan); investigational (Phase III, orphan) for heparin resistance in patients undergoing coronary artery bypass grafts and other surgical procedures*

**antithrombin III, human** [see: antithrombin III]

**antithrombin III, recombinant human (rhATIII)** [see: antithrombin III]

**antithrombin III concentrate IV** [see: antithrombin III]

**antithymocyte globulin (ATG)** *treatment for aplastic anemia; passive immunizing agent to prevent allograft rejection of renal transplants (orphan); investigational (orphan) for other solid organ and bone marrow transplants; investigational (orphan) for myelodysplastic syndrome (MDS)* [also: lymphocyte immune globulin (LIG)]

**antithymocyte serum** [see: antithymocyte globulin]

**anti-TNF (tumor necrosis factor) monoclonal antibodies (MAb)** [now: nerelimomab]

**antitoxin botulism equine (ABE)** [see: botulism equine antitoxin, trivalent]

**antitoxins** *a class of drugs used for passive immunization that consist of antibodies which combine with toxins to neutralize them*

**$\alpha_1$-antitrypsin** [see: alpha$_1$-antitrypsin]

**antituberculous agents** *a class of antibiotics, divided into primary and retreatment agents*

**Anti-Tuss** syrup (discontinued 2004) OTC *expectorant* [guaifenesin; alcohol 3.5%] 100 mg/5 mL

**antitussives** *a class of drugs that prevent or relieve cough*

**antivenin (Crotalidae) polyvalent** USP *passive immunizing agent for pit viper (rattlesnake, copperhead, and cottonmouth moccasin) bites*

**antivenin (Crotalidae) polyvalent immune Fab (equine)** *investigational (orphan) treatment for pit viper (rattlesnake, copperhead, and cottonmouth moccasin) bites*

**antivenin (Crotalidae) polyvalent immune Fab (ovine)** *treatment for pit viper (rattlesnake, copperhead, and cottonmouth moccasin) bites (orphan)*

**antivenin (Crotalidae) purified (avian)** *investigational (orphan) treatment for pit viper (rattlesnake, copperhead, and cottonmouth moccasin) bites*

**antivenin (*Latrodectus mactans*)** USP *passive immunizing agent for black widow spider bites* 6000 U/vial

**antivenin (*Micrurus fulvius*)** USP *passive immunizing agent for coral snake bites*

**antivenins** *a class of drugs used for passive immunization against or treatment for venomous bites and stings*

**Antivert; Antivert/25; Antivert/50** tablets ℞ *anticholinergic; antihistamine; antivertigo agent; motion sickness preventative* [meclizine HCl] 12.5 mg; 25 mg; 50 mg

**Antivipmyn** ℞ *investigational (orphan) treatment for pit viper (rattlesnake, copperhead, and cottonmouth moccasin) bites* [antivenin (Crotalidae) polyvalent immune Fab (equine)]

**antivirals** *a class of drugs effective against viral infections*

**antixerophthalmic vitamin** [see: vitamin A]

**Antizol** injection ℞ *alcohol dehydrogenase inhibitor for methanol or ethylene glycol poisoning (orphan)* [fomepizole] 1 g/mL

**antler (deer and elk)** *natural remedy for aging, energy, hormone balancing, impotence, infertility, and longevity*

**antrafenine** INN

**antramycin** INN *antineoplastic* [also: anthramycin]

**Antril** ℞ *nonsteroidal anti-inflammatory drug (NSAID) for inflammatory bowel disease; investigational (orphan) for juvenile rheumatoid arthritis and graft vs. host disease* [anakinra]

**Antrin** ℞ *investigational photodynamic therapy for peripheral vascular and cardiovascular atherosclerosis*

**Antrizine** tablets ℞ *anticholinergic; antihistamine; antivertigo agent; motion sickness preventative* [meclizine HCl] 12.5 mg

**Antrocol** elixir ℞ *GI anticholinergic; sedative* [atropine sulfate; phenobarbital] 0.195•16 mg/5 mL

**Antrypol** (available only from the Centers for Disease Control) ℞ *antiparasitic for African trypanosomiasis and onchocerciasis* [suramin sodium]

**antrypol** [see: suramin sodium]

**Anturane** tablets, capsules ℞ *uricosuric for gout* [sulfinpyrazone] 100 mg; 200 mg ⊡ Artane

**Anucort HC** rectal suppositories ℞ *corticosteroidal anti-inflammatory* [hydrocortisone acetate] 25 mg

**Anumed** rectal suppositories OTC *temporary relief of hemorrhoidal symptoms* [bismuth subgallate; bismuth resorcin compound; benzyl benzoate; zinc oxide; peruvian balsam] 2.25%•1.75%•1.2%•11%•1.8%

**Anumed HC** rectal suppositories ℞ *corticosteroidal anti-inflammatory* [hydrocortisone acetate] 10 mg

**Anusol** anorectal ointment OTC *local anesthetic; astringent* [pramoxine HCl; zinc oxide] 1%•12.5% ⊡ Aplisol

**Anusol** rectal suppositories OTC *emollient* [topical starch] 51%

**Anusol-HC** anorectal cream ℞ *topical corticosteroidal anti-inflammatory* [hydrocortisone] 2.5%

**Anusol-HC** rectal suppositories ℞ *corticosteroidal anti-inflammatory* [hydrocortisone acetate] 25 mg

**Anusol-HC 1** ointment ℞ *topical corticosteroidal anti-inflammatory* [hydrocortisone acetate] 1%

**Anuzinc** ⓒᴬᴺ anorectal ointment, suppositories ℞ *topical astringent* [zinc sulfate] 0.5%; 10 mg

**Anzemet** film-coated tablets, IV injection ℞ *serotonin 5-HT₃ receptor antagonist; antiemetic for nausea following chemotherapy, radiation, or surgery* [dolasetron mesylate] 50, 100 mg; 20 mg/mL

**AOPA (ara-C, Oncovin, prednisone, asparaginase)** *chemotherapy protocol*

**AOPE (Adriamycin, Oncovin, prednisone, etoposide)** *chemotherapy protocol*

**Aosept + Aodisc** solution + tablet OTC *two-step chemical disinfecting system for soft contact lenses* [hydrogen peroxide based] 3%

**AP (Adriamycin, Platinol)** *chemotherapy protocol for ovarian and endometrial cancer*

**AP-1903** *investigational (orphan) agent for graft-versus-host disease*

**Apacet** chewable tablets, drops OTC *analgesic; antipyretic* [acetaminophen] 80 mg; 100 mg/mL

**apafant** USAN, INN *platelet activating factor antagonist for allergies, asthma, and acute pancreatitis*

**apalcillin sodium** USAN, INN *antibacterial*

**APAP (N-acetyl-p-aminophenol)** [see: acetaminophen]

**APAP Plus** tablets OTC *analgesic; antipyretic* [acetaminophen; caffeine] 500•65 mg

**Apatate** chewable tablets, oral liquid (discontinued 2004) OTC *vitamin supplement* [vitamins B₁, B₆, and B₁₂] 15•0.5•0.025 mg; 15•0.5•0.025 mg/5 mL

**Apatate with Fluoride** oral liquid ℞ *pediatric vitamin supplement and dental caries preventative* [vitamins B₁, B₆, and B₁₂; fluoride] 15•0.5•0.025•0.5 mg/5 mL

**apaxifylline** USAN, INN *selective adenosine A₁ antagonist for cognitive deficits*

**apazone** USAN *anti-inflammatory* [also: azapropazone]

**APC (AMSA, prednisone, chlorambucil)** *chemotherapy protocol*

**APC (aspirin, phenacetin & caffeine)** [q.v.]

**apcitide** [see: technetium Tc 99m apcitide]

**APD (aminohydroxypropylidene diphosphonate)** [see: pamidronate disodium]

**APE (Adriamycin, Platinol, etoposide)** *chemotherapy protocol*

**APE (aminophylline, phenobarbital, ephedrine)**

**APE (ara-C, Platinol, etoposide)** *chemotherapy protocol*

**aperients** *a class of agents that have a mild purgative or laxative effect* [see also: aperitives]

**aperitives** *a class of agents that stimulate the appetite or have a mild purgative or laxative effect* [see also: aperients]

**Apetil** oral liquid OTC *vitamin/mineral supplement* [multiple B vitamins; multiple minerals]

**ApexiCon** ointment ℞ *corticosteroidal anti-inflammatory* [diflorasone diacetate] 0.05%

**ApexiCon E** cream ℞ *corticosteroidal anti-inflammatory; emollient* [diflorasone diacetate] 0.05%

**aphrodisiacs** *a class of agents that arouse or increase sexual desire or potency*

**Aphrodyne** tablets ℞ *alpha₂-adrenergic blocker for impotence and orthostatic hypotension; sympatholytic; mydriatic; may have aphrodisiac activity; no FDA-sanctioned indications* [yohimbine HCl] 5.4 mg

**Aphthasol** oral paste ℞ *anti-inflammatory for aphthous ulcers* [amlexanox] 5%

**apicillin** [see: ampicillin]

**apicycline** INN

**Apidra** subcu injection ℞ *human insulin analogue; rapid-onset, short-acting antidiabetic* [insulin glulisine (rDNA)] 100 IU/mL

**apiquel fumarate** [see: aminorex]

*Apium graveolens* medicinal herb [see: celery]

**A.P.L.** powder for IM injection (discontinued 2004) ℞ *hormone for prepubertal cryptorchidism and hypogonadism; ovulation stimulant* [chorionic gonadotropin] 500, 1000, 2000 U/mL

**APL 400-020 V-Beta DNA vaccine** *investigational (orphan) agent for cutaneous T-cell lymphoma*

**Apligraf** ℞ *living skin construct for diabetic foot ulcers and pressure sores* [graftskin]

**Aplisol** intradermal injection *tuberculosis skin test* [tuberculin purified protein derivative (PPD)] 5 U/0.1 mL ⊉ Anusol; Apresoline

**Aplitest** single-use intradermal puncture test device (discontinued 2002) *tuberculosis skin test* [tuberculin purified protein derivative (PPD)] 5 U

**aplonidine HCl** [see: apraclonidine HCl]

**APO (Adriamycin, prednisone, Oncovin)** *chemotherapy protocol*

**Apo-Acetaminophen** ⓒⒶⓃ tablets, film-coated caplets OTC *analgesic; antipyretic* [acetaminophen] 325, 500 mg

**Apo-Acyclovir** ⓒⒶⓃ tablets ℞ *antiviral for herpes infections* [acyclovir] 200, 400, 800 mg

**Apo-Amitriptyline** ⓒⒶⓃ film-coated tablets ℞ *tricyclic antidepressant* [amitriptyline HCl] 10, 25, 50, 75 mg

**Apo-Amoxi** ⓒⒶⓃ capsules, oral suspension ℞ *aminopenicillin antibiotic* [amoxicillin trihydrate] 250, 500 mg; 125, 250 mg/5 mL

**Apo-Atenolol** ⓒⒶⓃ tablets ℞ *antihypertensive; antianginal; antiadrenergic (β-blocker)* [atenolol] 50, 100 mg

**Apo-Beclomethasone** ⓒⒶⓃ nasal spray ℞ *corticosteroidal anti-inflammatory for chronic asthma and rhinitis* [beclomethasone dipropionate] 50 μg/spray

**Apo-Benzydamine** ⓒⒶⓃ oral rinse ℞ *topical analgesic and anti-inflammatory* [benzydamine HCl] 0.15%

**Apo-Butorphanol** ⓒⒶⓃ nasal spray ℞ *narcotic agonist-antagonist analgesic; antimigraine agent* [butorphanol tartrate] 10 mg/mL

**Apo-Carbamazepine CR** ⓒⒶⓃ controlled-release tablets ℞ *twice-daily anticonvulsant; antipsychotic* [carbamazepine] 100, 200, 400 mg

**Apo-Cefaclor** ⓒⒶⓃ capsules, oral suspension ℞ *cephalosporin antibiotic* [cefaclor] 250, 500 mg; 125, 250, 375 mg/5 mL

**Apo-Cefadroxil** ⓒⒶⓃ capsules ℞ *cephalosporin antibiotic* [cefadroxil] 500 mg

**Apo-Cetirizine** ⓒⒶⓃ tablets OTC *antihistamine* [cetirizine HCl] 10 mg

**Apo-Chlorhexidine** ⓒⒶⓃ oral rinse ℞ *antimicrobial; gingivitis treatment* [chlorhexidine gluconate] 0.12%

**Apo-Cimetidine** ⓒⒶⓃ film-coated tablets, oral liquid ℞ *histamine $H_2$ antagonist for gastric and duodenal ulcers and gastric hypersecretory conditions* [cimetidine] 200, 300, 400, 600, 800 mg; 300 mg/5 mL

**Apo-Clonazepam** ⓒⒶⓃ tablets ℞ *anticonvulsant* [clonazepam] 0.5, 2 mg

**Apo-Cromolyn** ⓒⒶⓃ nasal spray ℞ *anti-inflammatory/mast cell stabilizer for the prophylaxis of allergic rhinitis* [cromolyn sodium (sodium cromoglycate)] 2% (5.2 mg/dose)

**Apo-Cromolyn** ⓒⒶⓃ Sterules (solution for nebulization) ℞ *anti-inflammatory/mast cell stabilizer for the prophylaxis of asthma and bronchospasm* [cromolyn sodium (sodium cromoglycate)] 1% (20 mg/2 mL dose)

*Apocynum androsaemifolium* medicinal herb [see: dogbane]

**Apo-Desmopressin** ⓒⒶⓃ nasal spray ℞ *posterior pituitary hormone; antidi-*

uretic for nocturnal enuresis [desmo-pressin acetate] 10 μg/dose

**Apo-Diazepam** Ⓒ tablets ℞ *benzodi-azepine sedative; anxiolytic; anticon-vulsant; skeletal muscle relaxant* [diazepam] 2, 5, 10 mg

**Apo-Diclo Rapide** Ⓒ tablets ℞ *anal-gesic; antiarthritic; nonsteroidal anti-inflammatory drug (NSAID)* [diclo-fenac potassium] 50 mg

**Apo-Diltiaz** Ⓒ IV injection ℞ *calcium channel blocker for atrial fibrillation or paroxysmal supraventricular tachycar-dia (PSVT)* [diltiazem HCl] 5 mg/mL

**Apo-Diltiaz** Ⓒ tablets ℞ *antianginal; antihypertensive; antiarrhythmic; cal-cium channel blocker* [diltiazem HCl] 30, 60 mg

**Apo-Diltiaz CD** Ⓒ (once daily) sus-tained-release capsules ℞ *antihyper-tensive; antianginal; antiarrhythmic; calcium channel blocker* [diltiazem HCl] 120, 180, 240, 300 mg

**Apo-Diltiaz SR** Ⓒ (twice daily) sus-tained-release capsules ℞ *antihyper-tensive; antianginal; antiarrhythmic; calcium channel blocker* [diltiazem HCl] 60, 90, 120 mg

**Apo-Dipivefrin** Ⓒ eye drops ℞ *topical antiglaucoma agent* [dipivefrin HCl] 0.1%

**Apo-Divalproex** Ⓒ enteric-coated tablets ℞ *anticonvulsant* [divalproex sodium] 125, 250, 500 mg

**apodol** [see: anileridine HCl]

**Apo-Domperidone** Ⓒ film-coated tablets ℞ *antiemetic for diabetic gas-troparesis and chronic gastritis* [dom-peridone maleate] 10 mg

**Apo-Doxazosin** Ⓒ tablets ℞ *antihy-pertensive (α-blocker); treatment for benign prostatic hyperplasia* [doxazosin mesylate] 1, 2, 4 mg

**Apo-Etodolac** Ⓒ capsules ℞ *nonste-roidal anti-inflammatory drug; analgesic; antiarthritic* [etodolac] 200, 300 mg

**Apo-Fluconazole** Ⓒ tablets ℞ *broad-spectrum antifungal* [fluconazole] 50, 100, 200 mg

**Apo-Flunisolide** Ⓒ metered dose nasal spray ℞ *corticosteroidal anti-inflammatory for seasonal or perennial rhinitis* [flunisolide] 25 μg/dose

**Apo-Fluphenazine** Ⓒ tablets ℞ *con-ventional (typical) antipsychotic* [flu-phenazine HCl] 1, 2, 5 mg

**Apo-Fluphenazine Decanoate** Ⓒ injection ℞ *conventional (typical) antipsychotic* [fluphenazine decano-ate] 25 mg/mL

**Apo-Flutamide** Ⓒ tablets ℞ *antiandro-gen antineoplastic* [flutamide] 250 mg

**Apo-Furosemide** Ⓒ tablets ℞ *antihy-pertensive; loop diuretic* [furosemide] 20, 40, 80 mg

**Apo-Gemfibrozil** Ⓒ capsules, tablets ℞ *antihyperlipidemic for hypertriglycer-idemia and coronary heart disease* [gemfibrozil] 300 mg; 600 mg

**Apo-Glyburide** Ⓒ tablets ℞ *sulfonyl-urea antidiabetic* [glyburide] 2.5, 5 mg

**Apo-Haloperidol LA** Ⓒ long-acting IM injection ℞ *conventional (typical) antipsychotic* [haloperidol decanoate] 50, 100 mg/mL

**Apo-Hydro** Ⓒ tablets ℞ *antihyperten-sive; diuretic* [hydrochlorothiazide] 25, 50, 100 mg

**Apo-Ipravent** Ⓒ Sterules (solution for nebulization), solution for inhalation ℞ *anticholinergic bronchodilator for bronchospasm; antisecretory for rhinor-rhea* [ipratropium bromide] 250 μg/mL

**Apo-Ketoconazole** Ⓒ tablets ℞ *sys-temic antifungal* [ketoconazole] 200 mg

**Apo-Ketorolac** Ⓒ tablets, IM or IV injection ℞ *analgesic; nonsteroidal anti-inflammatory drug (NSAID)* [ketorolac tromethamine] 10 mg; 30 mg/mL

**Apokinon** (French name for U.S. product Apokyn)

**Apokyn** subcu injection ℞ *dopamine agonist for hypomobility episodes of late-stage Parkinson disease (orphan)* [apomorphine HCl] 10 mg/mL

**Apo-Lactulose** Ⓒ oral/rectal solution ℞ *hyperosmotic laxative* [lactulose] 10 g/15 mL

**Apo-Levobunolol** ⓒᴬᴺ eye drops ℞ *topical antiglaucoma agent (β-blocker)* [levobunolol HCl] 0.25%, 0.5%

**Apo-Lithium** ⓒᴬᴺ capsules ℞ *antipsychotic for manic episodes* [lithium carbonate] 150, 300 mg

**Apo-Lorazepam** ⓒᴬᴺ tablets ℞ *benzodiazepine anxiolytic* [lorazepam] 0.5, 1, 2 mg

**Apo-Loxapine** ⓒᴬᴺ film-coated tablets ℞ *conventional (typical) antipsychotic for schizophrenia* [loxapine succinate] 5, 10, 25, 50 mg

**Apo-Methoprazine** ⓒᴬᴺ tablets ℞ *CNS depressant; neuroleptic* [methotrimeprazine maleate] 2, 5, 25, 50 mg

**Apo-Metoprolol** ⓒᴬᴺ tablets ℞ *antihypertensive; antianginal; antiadrenergic (β-blocker)* [metoprolol tartrate] 50, 100 mg

**Apo-Metoprolol L** ⓒᴬᴺ film-coated caplets ℞ *antihypertensive; antianginal; antiadrenergic (β-blocker)* [metoprolol tartrate] 50, 100 mg

**Apo-Moclobemide** ⓒᴬᴺ film-coated tablets ℞ *antidepressant; MAO inhibitor* [moclobemide] 100, 150 mg

**apomorphine** BAN *dopamine $D_1$ agonist* [also: apomorphine HCl]

**apomorphine HCl** USP *dopamine $D_1$ agonist for hypomobility episodes of late-stage Parkinson disease (orphan); investigational (NDA filed) for erectile dysfunction* [also: apomorphine]

**Apo-Nabumetone** ⓒᴬᴺ tablets ℞ *antiarthritic; nonsteroidal anti-inflammatory drug (NSAID)* [nabumetone] 500 mg

**Apo-Naproxen** ⓒᴬᴺ tablets ℞ *analgesic; antiarthritic; nonsteroidal anti-inflammatory drug* [naproxen] 125, 250, 375, 500 mg

**Apo-Naproxen SR** ⓒᴬᴺ sustained-release tablets ℞ *analgesic; antiarthritic; nonsteroidal anti-inflammatory drug (NSAID)* [naproxen] 750 mg

**Apo-Nefazodone** ⓒᴬᴺ tablets ℞ *antidepressant* [nefazodone HCl] 50, 100, 150, 200 mg

**Apo-Norflox** ⓒᴬᴺ tablets ℞ *broad-spectrum fluoroquinolone antibiotic* [norfloxacin] 400 mg

**Apo-Oflox** ⓒᴬᴺ film-coated tablets ℞ *broad-spectrum fluoroquinolone antibiotic* [ofloxacin] 200, 300, 400 mg

**Apo-Orciprenaline** ⓒᴬᴺ syrup ℞ *sympathomimetic bronchodilator* [orciprenaline sulfate] 10 mg/5 mL

**Apo-Oxazepam** ⓒᴬᴺ tablets ℞ *benzodiazepine anxiolytic* [oxazepam] 10, 15, 30 mg

**Apo-Pen VK** ⓒᴬᴺ tablets, powder for oral solution ℞ *natural penicillin antibiotic* [penicillin V potassium] 300 mg; 125, 300 mg/5 mL

**Apo-Perphenazine** ⓒᴬᴺ film-coated tablets ℞ *conventional (typical) antipsychotic; antiemetic* [perphenazine] 4, 8, 16 mg

**Apo-Pravastatin** ⓒᴬᴺ tablets ℞ *HMG-CoA reductase inhibitor for hyperlipidemia and hypertriglyceridemia* [pravastatin sodium] 10, 20, 40 mg

**Apo-Prednisone** ⓒᴬᴺ tablets ℞ *corticosteroid; anti-inflammatory* [prednisone] 1, 5, 50 mg

**Apo-Prochlorazine** ⓒᴬᴺ tablets ℞ *conventional (typical) antipsychotic; antiemetic* [prochlorperazine maleate] 5, 10 mg

**Apo-Propafenone** ⓒᴬᴺ film-coated tablets ℞ *antiarrhythmic* [propafenone HCl] 150, 300 mg

**Apo-Ranitidine** ⓒᴬᴺ film-coated tablets OTC *histamine $H_2$ antagonist for episodic heartburn* [ranitidine HCl] 75 mg

**Apo-Ranitidine** ⓒᴬᴺ film-coated tablets ℞ *histamine $H_2$ antagonist for gastric and duodenal ulcers* [ranitidine HCl] 150, 300 mg

**Apo-Salvent** ⓒᴬᴺ inhaler ℞ *sympathomimetic bronchodilator* [salbutamol] 100 μg/dose

**Apo-Salvent** ⓒᴬᴺ tablets, solution for nebulization ℞ *sympathomimetic bronchodilator* [salbutamol sulfate] 2, 4 mg; 1, 2 mg/mL

**Apo-Sertraline** ⓒᴬᴺ capsules ℞ *selective serotonin reuptake inhibitor (SSRI) for*

*depression, obsessive-compulsive disorder (OCD), and panic disorder* [sertraline HCl] 25, 50, 100 mg

**Apo-Temazepam** ⒸⒶⓃ capsules ℞ *benzodiazepine sedative; hypnotic* [temazepam] 15, 30 mg

**Apo-Terazosin** ⒸⒶⓃ tablets ℞ *antihypertensive (α-blocker); treatment for benign prostatic hyperplasia (BPH)* [terazosin HCl] 1, 2, 5, 10 mg

**Apo-Terbinafine** ⒸⒶⓃ tablets ℞ *systemic allylamine antifungal* [terbinafine HCl] 250 mg

**Apo-Thioridazine** ⒸⒶⓃ film-coated tablets ℞ *conventional (typical) antipsychotic* [thioridazine HCl] 10, 25 mg

**Apo-Ticlopidine** ⒸⒶⓃ film-coated tablets ℞ *platelet aggregation inhibitor for stroke* [ticlopidine HCl] 250 mg

**Apo-Trifluoperazine** ⒸⒶⓃ film-coated tablets ℞ *conventional (typical) antipsychotic; anxiolytic* [trifluoperazine HCl] 1, 2, 5, 10, 20 mg

**Apo-Valproic** ⒸⒶⓃ capsules, syrup ℞ *anticonvulsant* [valproic acid] 250 mg; 250 mg/5 mL

**apovincamine** INN

**Apo-Warfarin** ⒸⒶⓃ tablets ℞ *coumarin-derivative anticoagulant* [warfarin sodium] 1, 2, 2.5, 4, 5, 10 mg

**Appedrine** tablets (discontinued 2001) OTC *nonprescription diet aid; vitamin/mineral supplement* [phenylpropanolamine HCl; multiple vitamins & minerals; folic acid] 25● ± ● 0.4 mg ⍰ aprindine; ephedrine

**appetizers** *a class of agents that stimulate the appetite* [see also: aperitives]

**APPG (aqueous penicillin G procaine)** [see: penicillin G procaine]

**apple (Pyrus malus)** fruit *medicinal herb for constipation and diarrhea, dysentery, fever, heart ailments, scurvy, and warts*

**apple, ground** *medicinal herb* [see: chamomile]

**apple, hog; Indian apple; May apple** *medicinal herb* [see: mandrake]

**Appli-Kit** (trademarked form) *ointment and adhesive dosage covers*

**Appli-Ruler** (trademarked name) OTC *dose-determining pads*

**Appli-Tape** (trademarked name) OTC *dosage covers*

**Apra** ℞ *investigational (Phase II, orphan) antineoplastic for soft tissue sarcomas and malignant mesothelioma* [CT-2584 mesylate (code name—generic name not yet assigned)]

**Apra** oral liquid OTC *analgesic; antipyretic* [acetaminophen] 160 mg/5 mL

**apraclonidine** INN, BAN *topical adrenergic for glaucoma* [also: apraclonidine HCl]

**apraclonidine HCl** USAN *topical adrenergic for glaucoma* [also: apraclonidine]

**apramycin** USAN, INN, BAN *antibacterial*

**aprepitant** USAN *neurokinin NK$_1$ receptor antagonist; antiemetic for chemotherapy*

**Apresazide 25/25; Apresazide 50/50; Apresazide 100/50** capsules ℞ *antihypertensive; vasodilator; diuretic* [hydralazine HCl; hydrochlorothiazide] 25●25 mg; 50●50 mg; 100●50 mg

**Apresoline** tablets ℞ *antihypertensive; vasodilator* [hydralazine HCl] 10, 25, 50, 100 mg

**Apri** tablets (in packs of 28) ℞ *monophasic oral contraceptive* [desogestrel; ethinyl estradiol] 0.15 mg●30 μg

**apricot (Prunus armeniaca)** fruit, seeds, and kernel oil *medicinal herb for asthma, constipation, cough, eye inflammation, hemorrhage, infertility, spasm, and vaginal infections; not generally regarded as safe and effective as apricot kernel ingestion causes cyanide poisoning*

**apricot kernel water** JAN

**aprikalim** INN *investigational antianginal*

**aprindine** USAN, INN, BAN *antiarrhythmic* ⍰ Appedrine; ephedrine

**aprindine HCl** USAN, JAN *antiarrhythmic*

**aprobarbital** NF, INN, DCF *sedative*

**Aprodine** tablets, syrup OTC *decongestant; antihistamine* [pseudoephedrine HCl; triprolidine HCl] 60●2.5 mg; 60●2.5 mg/10 mL

**Aprodine with Codeine** syrup (discontinued 2002) ℞ *narcotic antitussive; decongestant; antihistamine* [codeine phosphate; pseudoephedrine HCl; triprolidine HCl] 10•30•1.25 mg/5 mL

**aprofene** INN

**aprosulate sodium** INN

**aprotinin** USAN, INN, BAN, JAN *systemic hemostatic for coronary artery bypass graft (CABG) surgery (orphan); protease inhibitor*

**A.P.S. (aspirin, phenacetin & salicylamide)** [q.v.]

**APSAC (anisoylated plasminogen streptokinase activator complex)** [see: anistreplase]

**aptazapine** INN *antidepressant* [also: aptazapine maleate]

**aptazapine maleate** USAN *antidepressant* [also: aptazapine]

**aptiganel HCl** USAN *investigational (Phase III) NMDA ion channel blocker for stroke and traumatic brain injury*

**aptocaine** INN, BAN, DCF

**Aptosyn** ℞ *investigational (NDA filed, orphan) apoptosis modulator for adenomatous polyposis coli (APC); investigational (Phase III) for lung cancer* [exisulind]

**apyron** [see: magnesium salicylate]

**AquaBalm** cream OTC *moisturizer; emollient*

**Aqua-Ban** enteric-coated tablets OTC *diuretic* [ammonium chloride; caffeine] 325•100 mg

**Aqua-Ban, Maximum Strength** tablets OTC *diuretic* [pamabrom] 50 mg

**Aqua-Ban Plus** enteric-coated tablets OTC *diuretic; iron supplement* [ammonium chloride; caffeine; ferrous sulfate] 650•200•6 mg

**Aquabase** OTC *ointment base*

**Aquacare** cream, lotion OTC *moisturizer; emollient; keratolytic* [urea] 10%

**Aquachloral** Supprettes (suppositories) ℞ *sedative; hypnotic* [chloral hydrate] 324, 648 mg

**aquaday** [see: menadione]

**aquakay** [see: menadione]

**AquaMEPHYTON** IM or subcu injection ℞ *coagulant to correct anticoagulant-induced prothrombin deficiency; vitamin K supplement* [phytonadione] 2, 10 mg/mL

**Aquanil** lotion OTC *moisturizer; emollient*

**Aquanil Cleanser** lotion OTC *soap-free therapeutic skin cleanser*

**Aquaphilic** OTC *ointment base*

**Aquaphilic with Carbamide** OTC *ointment base* [urea] 10%, 20%

**Aquaphor** OTC *ointment base*

**Aquaphyllin** syrup (discontinued 2004) ℞ *antiasthmatic; bronchodilator* [theophylline] 80 mg/15 mL

**AquaSite** eye drops (discontinued 2004) OTC *ophthalmic moisturizer/lubricant* [polyethylene glycol 400] 0.2%

**Aquasol A** IM injection ℞ *vitamin deficiency therapy* [vitamin A] 50 000 IU/mL

**Aquatab C** extended-release tablets ℞ *antitussive; decongestant; expectorant* [dextromethorphan hydrobromide; pseudoephedrine HCl; guaifenesin] 60•60•1200 mg

**Aquatab D** extended-release tablets ℞ *decongestant; expectorant* [pseudoephedrine HCl; guaifenesin] 75•1200 mg

**Aquatab D Dose Pack** sustained-release tablets ℞ *decongestant; expectorant* [pseudoephedrine HCl; guaifenesin] 60•600 mg

**Aquatab DM** tablets, syrup ℞ *antitussive; expectorant* [dextromethorphan hydrobromide; guaifenesin] 60•1200 mg; 10•200 mg/5 mL

**AquaTar** gel (discontinued 2003) OTC *antipsoriatic; antiseborrheic* [coal tar extract] 2.5%

**Aquatensen** tablets ℞ *diuretic; antihypertensive* [methyclothiazide] 5 mg

**Aquavit-E** drops ℞ *vitamin supplement* [vitamin E (as *dl*-alpha tocopheryl acetate)] 15 IU/0.3 mL

**aqueous penicillin G procaine (APPG)** [see: penicillin G procaine]

*Aquilegia vulgaris* *medicinal herb* [see: columbine]

**aquinone** [see: menadione]

**AR-177** *investigational (Phase I/II) antiviral/oligonucleotide/integrase inhibitor for HIV infection*

**ara-A (adenine arabinoside)** [see: vidarabine]

**ara-AC (azacytosine arabinoside)** [see: fazarabine]

**arabinofuranosylcytosine** [see: cytarabine]

**arabinogalactans** *a class of dietary fiber used as an immune booster; stimulates macrophages, increases levels of natural killer (NK) cells, interferon-gamma (IFN-γ), tumor necrosis factor-alpha (TNF-α), and interleukin-1 beta (IL-1 β)* [see also: larch]

**arabinoluranosylcytosine HCl** [see: cytarabine HCl]

**arabinosyl cytosine** [see: cytarabine]

**ara-C (cytosine arabinoside)** [see: cytarabine] ☒ ERYC

**ara-C + 6-TG (ara-C, thioguanine)** *chemotherapy protocol*

**ara-C + ADR (ara-C, Adriamycin)** *chemotherapy protocol*

**ara-C + DNR + PRED + MP (ara-C, daunorubicin, prednisolone, mercaptopurine)** *chemotherapy protocol*

**ARAC-DNR (ara-C, daunorubicin)** *chemotherapy protocol for acute myelocytic leukemia (AML)*

**arachadonic acid (AA)** *natural omega-6 fatty acid*

**arachis oil** [see: peanut oil]

**ara-C-HU (ara-C, hydroxyurea)** *chemotherapy protocol*

**ara-cytidine** [see: cytarabine]

**Aralast** powder for IV infusion ℞ *enzyme replacement therapy for hereditary alpha₁-proteinase inhibitor deficiency, which leads to progressive panacinar emphysema* [alpha₁-proteinase inhibitor] ≥ 16 mg/mL (400, 800 mg/vial)

**Aralen HCl** IM injection ℞ *antimalarial; amebicide* [chloroquine HCl] 50 mg/mL ☒ Arlidin

**Aralen Phosphate** film-coated tablets ℞ *antimalarial; amebicide* [chloroquine phosphate] 500 mg

*Aralia racemosa* *medicinal herb* [see: spikenard]

*Aralia* **spp.** *medicinal herb* [see: ginseng]

**Aramine** IV, subcu or IM injection ℞ *vasopressor for acute hypotensive shock, anaphylaxis, or traumatic shock* [metaraminol bitartrate] 10 mg/mL

**Aranesp** IV or subcu injection, prefilled syringes ℞ *hematopoietic; recombinant erythropoietin analogue for anemia associated with chronic renal failure* [darbepoetin alfa] 25, 40, 60, 100, 200, 300, 500 μg/mL; 25, 40, 60, 100, 150, 200, 300, 500 μg/dose

**aranidipine** INN

**aranotin** USAN, INN *antiviral*

**araprofen** INN

**Arava** film-coated tablets ℞ *anti-inflammatory for rheumatoid arthritis (RA)* [leflunomide] 10, 20, 100 mg

**ARBs (angiotensin II receptor blockers)** [see: angiotensin II receptor antagonists]

**arbaprostil** USAN, INN *gastric antisecretory*

**arbekacin** INN

**arberry** *medicinal herb* [see: uva ursi]

**arbutamine** INN, BAN *cardiac stressor for diagnosis of coronary artery disease* [also: arbutamine HCl]

**arbutamine HCl** USAN *cardiac stressor for diagnosis of coronary artery disease* [also: arbutamine]

*Arbutus uva ursi* *medicinal herb* [see: uva ursi]

**archangel** *medicinal herb* [see: angelica]

**arcitumomab** USAN *investigational (orphan) imaging agent for detection of recurrent or metastatic thyroid cancers; investigational (Phase III) for lung cancer*

**arclofenin** USAN, INN *hepatic function test*

**Arcobee with C** caplets OTC *vitamin supplement* [multiple B vitamins; vitamin C] ≜•300 mg

**Arco-Lase** chewable tablets (discontinued 2002) OTC *digestive enzymes*

[amylase; protease; lipase; cellulase] 30•6•25•2 mg

**Arco-Lase Plus** tablets (discontinued 2002) ℞ *digestive enzymes; GI antispasmodic; sedative* [amylase; protease; lipase; cellulase; hyoscyamine sulfate; atropine sulfate; phenobarbital] 30•6•25•2•0.1•0.02•7.5 mg

**Arcoxia** tablets *investigational (NDA filed) COX-2 inhibitor for osteoarthritis, rheumatoid arthritis, musculoskeletal pain, and gout* [etoricoxib] 60, 90, 10 mg

**Arctium lappa; A. majus; A. minus** *medicinal herb* [see: burdock]

**Arctostaphylos uva ursi** *medicinal herb* [see: uva ursi]

**ardacin** INN

**ardeparin sodium** USAN, INN *a low molecular weight heparin–type anticoagulant and antithrombotic for the prevention of deep vein thrombosis (DVT) following knee replacement surgery*

**Arduan** powder for IV injection ℞ *nondepolarizing neuromuscular blocking agent; muscle relaxant; adjunct to general anesthesia* [pipecuronium bromide] 10 mg/vial

**arecoline acetarsone salt** [see: drocarbil]

**arecoline hydrobromide** NF

**Aredia** powder for IV infusion ℞ *bisphosphonate bone resorption inhibitor for Paget disease, hypercalcemia of malignancy, breast cancer, and multiple myeloma* [pamidronate disodium] 30, 90 mg

**Arestin** sustained-release microspheres for subgingival injection ℞ *antibiotic for periodontitis* [minocycline HCl] 1 mg

**arfalasin** INN

**arfendazam** INN

**argatroban** USAN, INN, JAN *anticoagulant for heparin-induced thrombocytopenia (HIT) and thrombosis syndrome (HITTS); prevention of HIT or HITTS in percutaneous coronary intervention (PCI)* 1 mg/mL injection

**Argesic** cream OTC *analgesic; counterirritant* [methyl salicylate; trolamine]

**Argesic-SA** tablets ℞ *analgesic; antiinflammatory* [salsalate] 500 mg

**argimesna** INN

**Arginaid Extra** oral liquid OTC *enteral nutritional treatment for wound healing* [whey protein–based]

**L-argininamide** [see: iseganan HCl]

**arginine (L-arginine)** USP, INN *nonessential amino acid; ammonia detoxicant; diagnostic aid for pituitary function; symbols: Arg, R*

**arginine butanoate** [see: arginine butyrate]

**arginine butyrate (L-arginine butyrate)** USAN *investigational (orphan) for beta-hemoglobinopathies, beta-thalassemia, and sickle cell disease*

**arginine glutamate (L-arginine L-glutamate)** USAN, BAN, JAN *ammonia detoxicant*

**arginine HCl** USAN, USP, JAN *ammonia detoxicant; pituitary (growth hormone) function diagnostic aid*

**L-arginine monohydrochloride** [see: arginine HCl]

**8-L-arginine vasopressin** [see: vasopressin]

**8-arginineoxytocin** [see: argiprestocin]

**8-L-argininevasopressin tannate** [see: argipressin tannate]

**argipressin** INN, BAN *antidiuretic* [also: argipressin tannate]

**argipressin tannate** USAN *antidiuretic* [also: argipressin]

**argiprestocin** INN

**argon** *element (Ar)*

**argyn** [see: silver protein, mild]

**Aricept** tablets ℞ *reversible acetylcholinesterase (AChE) inhibitor; cognition adjuvant for Alzheimer dementia* [donepezil HCl] 5, 10 mg ⃞ Erycette

**Ariflo** tablets ℞ *investigational (NDA filed) pulmonary anti-inflammatory for COPD* [cilomilast] 15 mg

**arildone** USAN, INN *antiviral*

**Arilvax** ℞ *investigational (Phase III) single-dose, live attenuated yellow fever vaccine*

**Arimidex** film-coated tablets ℞ *aromatase inhibitor; estrogen antagonist; antineoplastic for breast cancer* [anastrozole] 1 mg

**aripiprazole** USAN *quinolinone antipsychotic; dopamine $D_2$ and serotonin 5-$HT_1$ and 5-$HT_2$ receptor agonist*

**Aristocort** ointment, cream ℞ *topical corticosteroidal anti-inflammatory* [triamcinolone acetonide] 0.1%, 0.5%; 0.025%, 0.1%, 0.5%

**Aristocort** tablets ℞ *corticosteroid; anti-inflammatory* [triamcinolone] 1, 2, 4, 8 mg

**Aristocort A** ointment, cream ℞ *topical corticosteroidal anti-inflammatory* [triamcinolone acetonide in a water-washable base] 0.1%; 0.025%, 0.1%, 0.5%

**Aristocort Forte** IM injection (discontinued 2004) ℞ *corticosteroid; anti-inflammatory* [triamcinolone diacetate] 40 mg/mL

**Aristocort Intralesional** injection ℞ *corticosteroid; anti-inflammatory* [triamcinolone diacetate] 25 mg/mL

*Aristolochia clematitis* medicinal herb [see: birthwort]

**Aristospan Intra-articular** injection ℞ *corticosteroid; anti-inflammatory* [triamcinolone hexacetonide] 20 mg/mL

**Aristospan Intralesional** injection ℞ *corticosteroid; anti-inflammatory* [triamcinolone hexacetonide] 5 mg/mL

**Arixtra** subcu injection in prefilled syringes ℞ *selective factor Xa inhibitor; antithrombotic for prevention of deep vein thrombosis (DVT) and acute pulmonary embolism following orthopedic surgery* [fondaparinux sodium] 2.5 mg/0.5 mL dose

**A.R.M. (Allergy Relief Medicine)** caplets (discontinued 2001) OTC *decongestant; antihistamine* [phenylpropanolamine HCl; chlorpheniramine maleate] 25•4 mg

**Arm-A-Med** (trademarked packaging form) *single-dose plastic vial*

**Arm-A-Vial** (trademarked packaging form) *single-dose plastic vial*

*Armoracia rusticana; A. lapathiofolia* medicinal herb [see: horseradish]

**Armour Thyroid** tablets ℞ *thyroid replacement therapy for hypothyroidism or thyroid cancer* [thyroid, desiccated (porcine)] 15, 30, 60, 90, 120, 180, 240, 300 mg

**arnica** *(Arnica montana; A. cordifolia; A. fulgens)* flowers *medicinal herb used as a topical counterirritant and vulnerary for acne, bruises, rashes, and other dermal lesions; not generally regarded as safe and effective taken internally as it is highly toxic*

**arnolol** INN

**arofylline** USAN *phosphodiesterase IV inhibitor for asthma*

**Aromasin** tablets ℞ *aromatase inhibitor; antihormonal antineoplastic for advanced breast cancer in postmenopausal women (orphan)* [exemestane] 25 mg

**aromatase inhibitors** *a class of antihormonal antineoplastics which block the conversion of androgens to estrogens, effectively depriving hormone-dependent tumors of estrogen in postmenopausal women*

**aromatic ammonia spirit** [see: ammonia spirit, aromatic]

**aromatic cascara fluidextract** [see: cascara fluidextract, aromatic]

**aromatic cascara sagrada** [see: cascara fluidextract, aromatic]

**aromatic elixir** NF *flavored and sweetened vehicle*

**aromatics** *a class of agents that have an agreeable odor and stimulating qualities; also, substances with a specific molecular structure in organic chemistry*

**aronixil** INN

**Aroplatin** ℞ *investigational (orphan) antineoplastic*

**arotinolol** INN [also: arotinolol HCl]

**arotinolol HCl** JAN [also: arotinolol]

**arprinocid** USAN, INN, BAN *coccidiostat*

**arpromidine** INN

**Arrestin** IM injection (discontinued 2000) ℞ *antiemetic; anticholinergic* [trimethobenzamide HCl] 100 mg/mL

**arrow wood; Indian arrow wood; Indian arrow** *medicinal herb* [see: wahoo]

**ARS (antirabies serum)** [q.v.]

**arsambide** [see: carbarsone]

**arsanilic acid** INN, BAN *investigational (Phase I/II, orphan) immunomodulator for AIDS*

**arseclor** [see: dichlorophenarsine HCl]

**arsenic** *element (As)*

**arsenic acid, sodium salt** [see: sodium arsenate]

**arsenic trioxide (AsO$_3$)** JAN *antineoplastic for acute promyelocytic leukemia (orphan); investigational (NDA filed) for renal cell carcinoma; investigational (orphan) for multiple myeloma and myelodysplastic syndromes*

**arsenobenzene** [see: arsphenamine]

**arsenobenzol** [see: arsphenamine]

**arsenphenolamine** [see: arsphenamine]

**Arsobal** (available only from the Centers for Disease Control) ℞ *investigational anti-infective for trypanosomiasis* [melarsoprol]

**arsphenamine** USP

**arsthinenol** DCF [also: arsthinol]

**arsthinol** INN [also: arsthinenol]

**Artane** tablets, elixir, Sequels (sustained-release capsules) (discontinued 2001) ℞ *anticholinergic; antiparkinsonian* [trihexyphenidyl HCl] 2, 5 mg; 2 mg/5 mL; 5 mg ⬚ Anturane

**arteflene** USAN, INN *antimalarial*

**artegraft** USAN *arterial prosthetic aid*

**artemether** INN

*Artemisia absinthium* *medicinal herb* [see: wormwood]

*Artemisia dracunculus* *medicinal herb* [see: tarragon]

*Artemisia vulgaris* *medicinal herb* [see: mugwort]

**artemisinin** INN *natural herbal drug for malaria*

**arterenol** [see: norepinephrine bitartrate]

**artesunate** INN *antimalarial; investigational (NDA filed, orphan) rectal suppositories for emergency treatment of malaria*

**Artha-G** tablets OTC *analgesic; anti-inflammatory* [salsalate] 750 mg

**ArthriCare, Double Ice** gel OTC *topical analgesic; counterirritant* [menthol; camphor] 4%•3.1%

**ArthriCare, Odor Free** rub OTC *topical analgesic; counterirritant* [menthol; methyl nicotinate; capsaicin] 1.25%•0.25%•0.025%

**ArthriCare Triple Medicated** gel OTC *analgesic; counterirritant* [methyl salicylate; menthol; methyl nicotinate] 30%•1.5%•0.7%

**Arthriten** tablets (discontinued 2000) OTC *analgesic; antipyretic* [acetaminophen; magnesium salicylate; caffeine (buffered with magnesium carbonate, magnesium oxide, and calcium carbonate)] 250•250•32.5 mg

**"Arthritis Formula"; "Arthritis Strength"** products [see under product name]

**Arthritis Hot Creme** OTC *analgesic; counterirritant* [methyl salicylate; menthol] 15%•10%

**Arthritis Pain Formula** caplets OTC *analgesic; antipyretic; anti-inflammatory; antirheumatic* [aspirin (buffered with magnesium hydroxide and aluminum hydroxide)] 500 mg

**Arthropan** IM injection ℞ *analgesic; antipyretic; anti-inflammatory; antirheumatic* [choline salicylate] 870 mg/5 mL

**Arthrotec** film-coated tablets ℞ *anti-arthritic NSAID with a coating to protect gastric mucosa* [diclofenac sodium (enteric-coated core); misoprostol (coating)] 50•0.2, 75•0.2 mg

**articaine** INN *amide local anesthetic for dentistry* [also: carticaine]

**articaine HCl** USAN *amide local anesthetic for dentistry* [also: articaine; carticaine]

**artichoke (Cynara scolymus)** flower heads *medicinal herb for albuminuria, bile stimulation, diabetes, diuresis, dyspepsia, jaundice, liver diseases, and postoperative anemia*

**Articoat** bandages OTC *antimicrobial dressings*

**Articulose L.A.** IM injection ℞ *corticosteroid; anti-inflammatory* [triamcinolone diacetate] 40 mg/mL

**Artificial Tears** eye drops OTC *ocular moisturizer/lubricant*

**Artificial Tears** ophthalmic ointment OTC *ocular moisturizer/lubricant* [white petrolatum; mineral oil; lanolin]

**Artificial Tears Plus** eye drops OTC *ophthalmic moisturizer/lubricant* [polyvinyl alcohol] 1.4%

**artilide** INN *antiarrhythmic* [also: artilide fumarate]

**artilide fumarate** USAN *antiarrhythmic* [also: artilide]

**arzoxifene HCl** USAN *selective estrogen receptor modulator (SERM) for breast cancer, uterine fibroids, endometriosis, and dysfunctional uterine bleeding*

[74]**As** [see: sodium arsenate As 74]

**5-ASA (5-aminosalicylic acid)** [see: mesalamine]

**ASA (acetylsalicylic acid)** [see: aspirin]

**Asacol** delayed-release tablets ℞ *anti-inflammatory for active ulcerative colitis, proctosigmoiditis, and proctitis* [mesalamine (5-aminosalicylic acid)] 400 mg

**asafetida; asafoetida** *(Ferula assafoetida; F. foetida; F. rubricaulis)* gum resin from dried roots and rhizomes *medicinal herb for abdominal tumors, amenorrhea, asthma, colic, convulsions, corns and calluses, edema; also used as an expectorant; not generally regarded as safe and effective in children as it may induce methemoglobinemia*

**asafoetida** *medicinal herb* [see: asafetida]

*Asarum canadense* *medicinal herb* [see: wild ginger]

*Asclepias geminata* *medicinal herb* [see: gymnema]

*Asclepias syriaca* *medicinal herb* [see: milkweed]

*Asclepias tuberosa* *medicinal herb* [see: pleurisy root]

**Ascocaps** capsules OTC *vitamin C supplement* [ascorbic acid] 500 mg

**Ascomp with Codeine** capsules ℞ *narcotic analgesic; barbiturate sedative* [codeine phosphate; aspirin; caffeine; butalbital] 30•325•40•50 mg

**Ascor L** injection ℞ *vitamin C supplement* [ascorbic acid] 500 mg/mL

**ascorbic acid (L-ascorbic acid; vitamin C)** USP, INN, BAN, JAN *water-soluble vitamin; antiscorbutic; urinary acidifier; topical sunscreen* 250, 500, 1000, 1500 mg oral; 240 mg/tsp. oral; 500 mg/5 mL oral; 500 mg/mL injection

**L-ascorbic acid, monosodium salt** [see: sodium ascorbate]

**L-ascorbic acid 6-palmitate** [see: ascorbyl palmitate]

**ascorbyl palmitate** NF *antioxidant*

**Ascriptin; Ascriptin A/D** coated tablets OTC *analgesic; antipyretic; anti-inflammatory; antirheumatic* [aspirin (buffered with magnesium hydroxide, aluminum hydroxide, and calcium carbonate)] 325, 500 mg; 325 mg

**Asendin** tablets ℞ *tricyclic antidepressant* [amoxapine] 25, 50, 100, 150 mg

**aseptichrome** [see: merbromin]

**Aseptone 1; Aseptone 2; Aseptone 5; Aseptone QUAT** (CAN) solution OTC *antiseptic; disinfectant; germicide*

**ash, bitter** *medicinal herb* [see: quassia; wahoo]

**ash, mountain; American mountain ash; European mountain ash** *medicinal herb* [see: mountain ash]

**ash, poison** *medicinal herb* [see: fringe tree]

**ASHAP; A-SHAP (Adriamycin, Solu-Medrol, high-dose ara-C, Platinol)** *chemotherapy protocol*

*Asimina triloba* *medicinal herb* [see: pawpaw]

**Aslera** ℞ *investigational (Phase III) treatment for systemic lupus erythematosus (SLE)* [prasterone]

**Asmalix** elixir ℞ *antiasthmatic; bronchodilator* [theophylline] 80 mg/15 mL

**AsO₃ (arsenic trioxide)** [q.v.]

**asobamast** INN, BAN

**asocainol** INN

*Aspalathus linearis; A. contaminata; Borbonia pinifolia* medicinal herb [see: red bush tea]

**asparaginase (L-asparaginase)** USAN, JAN *antineoplastic for acute lymphocytic leukemia* [also: colaspase]

**asparagine (L-asparagine)** *nonessential amino acid; symbols: Asn, N*

**L-asparagine amidohydrolase** [see: asparaginase]

**asparagus** *(Asparagus officinalis)* roots, seeds *medicinal herb for acne, constipation, contraception, edema, neuritis, parasites, rheumatism, stimulating hair growth, and toothache*

**aspartame** USAN, NF, INN, BAN *sweetener*

**L-aspartate potassium** JAN

**aspartic acid (L-aspartic acid)** USAN, INN *nonessential amino acid; symbols: Asp, D*

**L-aspartic acid insulin** [see: insulin aspart]

**aspartocin** USAN, INN *antibacterial*

**A-Spas S/L** sublingual tablets ℞ *GI/ GU antispasmodic; anticholinergic* [hyoscyamine sulfate] 0.125 mg

**aspen, European** *medicinal herb* [see: black poplar]

**aspen poplar; American aspen; quaking aspen** *medicinal herb* [see: poplar]

**Aspercreme** cream OTC *analgesic* [trolamine salicylate] 10%

**Aspercreme Rub** lotion OTC *analgesic* [trolamine salicylate] 10%

*Aspergillus oryase* proteinase [see: asperkinase]

**Aspergum** chewing gum tablets OTC *analgesic; antipyretic; anti-inflammatory; antirheumatic* [aspirin] 227.5 mg

**asperkinase**

**asperlin** USAN *antibacterial; antineoplastic*

*Asperula odorata* medicinal herb [see: sweet woodruff]

**aspidium** *(Dryopteris filix-mas)* plant *medicinal herb for bloody nose, menorrhagia, worm infections including tapeworm and ringworm, and wound healing; not generally regarded as safe and effective for internal use as it is highly toxic*

**aspidosperma** USP

**aspirin** USP, BAN, JAN *analgesic; antipyretic; anti-inflammatory; antirheumatic* 325, 500, 650, 975 mg oral; 120, 200, 300, 600 mg suppositories ⃝ Afrin

**aspirin, buffered** USP *analgesic; antipyretic; anti-inflammatory; antirheumatic* 325 mg oral

**aspirin aluminum** NF, JAN

**aspirin & butalbital & caffeine** *analgesic; barbiturate sedative* 325•50•40 mg oral

**aspirin & codeine phosphate** *antipyretic; analgesic; narcotic antitussive* 15•325 mg oral

**aspirin DL-lysine** JAN

**Aspirin Free Excedrin** caplets, geltabs OTC *analgesic; antipyretic* [acetaminophen; caffeine] 500•65 mg

**Aspirin with Codeine No. 2, No. 3, and No. 4** tablets ℞ *narcotic antitussive; analgesic* [codeine phosphate; aspirin] 15•325 mg; 30•325 mg; 60•325 mg

**ASPIRINcheck** urine test kit for professional use *in vitro diagnostic aid for antiplatelet metabolites of aspirin*

**Aspirin-Free Pain Relief** tablets, caplets OTC *analgesic; antipyretic* [acetaminophen] 325, 500 mg; 500 mg

**Aspirol** (trademarked delivery form) *crushable ampule for inhalation*

**aspogen** [see: dihydroxyaluminum aminoacetate]

**aspoxicillin** INN, JAN

**Asprimox; Asprimox Extra Protection for Arthritis Pain** tablets, caplets OTC *analgesic; antipyretic; anti-inflammatory; antirheumatic* [aspirin (buffered with aluminum hydroxide, magnesium hydroxide, and calcium carbonate)] 325 mg

**aspro** [see: aspirin]

**astatine** *element (At)*

**Astelin Ready-Spray** nasal spray in a metered-dose pump sprayer ℞ *peripherally selective phthalazinone antihistamine and mast cell stabilizer* for allergic and vasomotor rhinitis [azel-astine HCl] 137 µg/spray

**astemizole** USAN, INN, BAN antiallergic; second-generation piperidine antihistamine

**AsthmaHaler** inhalation aerosol (discontinued 2002) OTC sympathomimetic bronchodilator [epinephrine bitartrate] 0.35 mg/dose

**AsthmaNefrin** solution for inhalation (discontinued 2001) OTC sympathomimetic bronchodilator [racepinephrine HCl] 2.25%

**astifilcon A** USAN hydrophilic contact lens material

**Astracaine; Astracaine Forte** ⓒᴬᴺ intraoral injection R local anesthetic for dentistry [articaine HCl; epinephrine] 4%•1:200 000; 4%•1:100 000

**astragalus (Astragalus membranaceus)** root medicinal herb for cancer, chronic fatigue, and Epstein-Barr syndrome; also used to strengthen the immune system, especially after chemotherapy and HIV treatments

**Astramorph PF** (preservative free) IV, subcu or IM injection R narcotic analgesic [morphine sulfate] 0.5, 1 mg/mL

**astringents** a class of agents that contract tissue, reducing secretions or discharges [see also: hemostatics; styptics]

**Astroglide** vaginal gel OTC lubricant [glycerin; propylene glycol]

**astromicin** INN antibacterial [also: astromicin sulfate]

**astromicin sulfate** USAN, JAN antibacterial [also: astromicin]

**AT-III (antithrombin III)** [q.v.]

**Atacand** tablets R antihypertensive; angiotensin II receptor antagonist; investigational (Phase III) for the prevention of diabetic retinopathy [candesartan cilexetil] 4, 8, 16, 32 mg ◫ Ativan

**Atacand HCT 16-12.5; Atacand HCT 32-12.5** tablets R antihypertensive; angiotensin II receptor antagonist; diuretic [candesartan cilexetil; hydrochlorothiazide] 16•12.5; 32•12.5 mg

**Atacand Plus** ⓒᴬᴺ tablets R antihypertensive; angiotensin II receptor antago-

nist; diuretic [candesartan cilexetil; hydrochlorothiazide] 16•12.5 mg

**atamestane** INN investigational (Phase III) aromatase inhibitor for breast cancer

**ataprost** INN

**Atarax** tablets, syrup (discontinued 2004) R anxiolytic; minor tranquilizer [hydroxyzine HCl] 10, 25, 50, 100 mg; 10 mg/5 mL ◫ Marax

**Atarax 100** tablets (discontinued 2004) R anxiolytic; minor tranquilizer; antihistamine for allergic pruritus [hydroxyzine HCl] 100 mg ◫ Marax

**atarvet** [see: acepromazine]

**atazanavir sulfate** antiviral; azapeptide protease inhibitor for HIV-1 infection

**atenolol** USAN, INN, BAN, JAN antihypertensive; antiadrenergic (β-receptor) 25, 50, 100 mg oral ◫ timolol

**atevirdine** INN antiviral [also: atevirdine mesylate]

**atevirdine mesylate** USAN antiviral; investigational (Phase II/III) nonnucleoside reverse transcriptase inhibitor (NNRTI) for HIV and AIDS [also: atevirdine]

**ATG (antithymocyte globulin)** [q.v.]

**Atgam** IV infusion R treatment for aplastic anemia; immunizing agent to prevent allograft rejection of renal transplants; investigational (orphan) for organ and bone marrow transplants [antithymocyte globulin, equine] 50 mg/mL

**athyromazole** [see: carbimazole]

**atipamezole** USAN, INN, BAN $\alpha_2$-receptor antagonist

**atiprimod dihydrochloride** USAN immunomodulator; anti-inflammatory; antiarthritic

**atiprimod dimaleate** USAN immunomodulator; anti-inflammatory; antiarthritic

**atiprosin** INN antihypertensive [also: atiprosin maleate]

**atiprosin maleate** USAN antihypertensive [also: atiprosin]

**Ativan** IV or IM injection R benzodiazepine anxiolytic; preanesthetic sedative; anticonvulsant [lorazepam] 2, 4 mg/mL ◫ Atacand; Adapin; Avitene

**Ativan** tablets (discontinued 2003) ℞ benzodiazepine anxiolytic; sedative [lorazepam] 0.5, 1, 2 mg ▣ Adapin; Avitene

**atlafilcon A** USAN hydrophilic contact lens material

**ATnativ** ℞ investigational (orphan) agent for congenital AT-III deficiency in patients undergoing surgical or obstetrical procedures [antithrombin III]

**atolide** USAN, INN anticonvulsant

**Atolone** tablets ℞ corticosteroid; antiinflammatory [triamcinolone] 4 mg

**atomoxetine HCl** selective norepinephrine reuptake inhibitor for attention-deficit hyperactivity disorder (ADHD); investigational (orphan) for Tourette syndrome

**Atopik** ℞ investigational (Phase III) topical phosphodiesterase 4 ($PDE_4$) inhibitor for eczema

**atorvastatin calcium** USAN HMG-CoA reductase inhibitor for hypercholesterolemia, dysbetalipoproteinemia, and hypertriglyceridemia

**atosiban** USAN, INN oxytocin antagonist

**atovaquone** USAN, INN, BAN antimalarial; antiprotozoal for AIDS-related Pneumocystis carinii pneumonia (orphan); investigational (orphan) for AIDS-related Toxoplasma gondii encephalitis

**ATP (adenosine triphosphate)** [see: adenosine triphosphate disodium]

**ATPase (adenosine triphosphatase) inhibitors** a class of gastric antisecretory agents that inhibit the ATPase "proton pump" within the gastric parietal cell [also called: proton pump inhibitors; substituted benzimidazoles]

**atracurium besilate** INN skeletal muscle relaxant; nondepolarizing neuromuscular blocker; adjunct to anesthesia [also: atracurium besylate]

**atracurium besylate** USAN, BAN skeletal muscle relaxant; nondepolarizing neuromuscular blocker; adjunct to anesthesia [also: atracurium besilate]

**Atragen** ℞ investigational (NDA filed, orphan) antineoplastic for acute pro-myelocytic leukemia; investigational (orphan) for other leukemias and ophthalmic squamous metaplasia; investigational (Phase II) for relapsed or refractory non-Hodgkin lymphoma and AIDS-related Kaposi sarcoma [tretinoin]

**atrasentan HCl** USAN endothelin $ET_A$ receptor antagonist for bone pain due to metastatic prostate cancer

**atreleuton** USAN 5-lipoxygenase inhibitor for asthma

**Atretol** tablets (discontinued 2004) ℞ anticonvulsant; analgesic for trigeminal neuralgia; antipsychotic [carbamazepine] 200 mg

**Atridox** controlled-release gel for subgingival injection ℞ antibiotic for periodontal disease [doxycycline hyclate] 10%

**Atrigel** (trademarked delivery system) sustained-release delivery

**Atrigel Depot** (trademarked delivery system) sustained-release subcu injection

**atrimustine** INN

**atrinositol** INN

**Atrisone** gel ℞ investigational (Phase II) topical acne treatment

**Atrisorb FreeFlow GTR Barrier** ℞ investigational (NDA filed) guided tissue regeneration (GTR) therapy for severe periodontal disease

**Atrohist Pediatric** oral suspension (discontinued 2002) ℞ pediatric decongestant and antihistamine [phenylephrine tannate; chlorpheniramine tannate; pyrilamine tannate] 5•2•12.5 mg/5 mL

**Atrohist Pediatric** sustained-release capsules (discontinued 2002) ℞ pediatric decongestant and antihistamine [pseudoephedrine HCl; chlorpheniramine maleate] 60•4 mg

**Atrohist Plus** sustained-release tablets (discontinued 2001) ℞ decongestant; antihistamine; anticholinergic [phenylpropanolamine HCl; phenylephrine HCl; chlorpheniramine maleate; hyoscyamine sulfate; atropine sulfate; scopolamine hydrobromide] 50•25•8•0.19•0.04•0.01 mg

**atromepine** INN, DCF

**Atromid-S** capsules (discontinued 2002) ℞ *triglyceride-lowering antihyperlipidemic for primary dysbetalipoproteinemia (type III hyperlipidemia) and hypertriglyceridemia (types IV and V hyperlipidemia)* [clofibrate] 500 mg (1 g available in Canada)

*Atropa belladonna* medicinal herb [see: belladonna]

**AtroPen** auto-injector (automatic IM injection device) ℞ *antidote for organophosphorous or carbamate insecticides* [atropine sulfate] 0.5, 1, 2 mg/0.7 mL dose

**atropine** USP, BAN *anticholinergic*

**Atropine Care** eye drops (discontinued 2004) ℞ *mydriatic; cycloplegic* [atropine sulfate] 1%

**atropine methonitrate** INN, BAN *anticholinergic* [also: methylatropine nitrate]

**atropine methylnitrate** [see: methylatropine nitrate]

**atropine oxide** INN *anticholinergic* [also: atropine oxide HCl]

**atropine oxide HCl** USAN *anticholinergic* [also: atropine oxide]

**atropine propionate** [see: prampine]

**atropine sulfate** USP, JAN *GI/GU antispasmodic; antiparkinsonian; bronchodilator; cycloplegic; mydriatic; antidote to insecticide poisoning* [also: atropine sulphate] 0.4, 0.6 mg oral; 1%, 2% eye drops; 0.05, 0.1, 0.3, 0.4, 0.5, 0.8, 1 mg/mL injection

**atropine sulphate** BAN *GI/GU antispasmodic; antiparkinsonian; bronchodilator; cycloplegic; mydriatic* [also: atropine sulfate]

**Atropine-1** eye drops ℞ *mydriatic; cycloplegic* [atropine sulfate] 1%

**Atropisol** Dropperettes (eye drops) (discontinued 2003) ℞ *cycloplegic; mydriatic* [atropine sulfate] 1%

**Atrosept** sugar-coated tablets ℞ *urinary antibiotic; analgesic; antispasmodic; acidifier* [methenamine; phenyl salicylate; atropine sulfate; methylene blue; hyoscyamine sul-

fate; benzoic acid] 40.8•18.1•0.03•5.4•0.03•4.5 mg

**Atrovent** nasal spray, solution for inhalation, inhalation aerosol ℞ *anticholinergic bronchodilator for bronchospasm; antisecretory for rhinorrhea* [ipratropium bromide] 0.03%, 0.06%; 0.02%; 18 μg/dose ② Trovan

**A/T/S** topical solution, gel ℞ *antibiotic for acne* [erythromycin; alcohol 66%–92%] 2%

**Attain** oral liquid OTC *enteral nutritional therapy* [lactose-free formula]

**attapulgite, activated** USP *suspending agent; GI adsorbent*

**Attenuvax** powder for subcu injection ℞ *measles vaccine* [measles virus vaccine, live attenuated] 0.5 mL

**Atuss DM** syrup ℞ *antitussive; decongestant; antihistamine* [dextromethorphan hydrobromide; phenylephrine HCl; chlorpheniramine maleate] 30•20•4 mg/10 mL

**Atuss EX** syrup ℞ *narcotic antitussive; expectorant* [hydrocodone bitartrate; potassium guaiacolsulfonate] 5•240 mg/10 mL

**Atuss G** syrup ℞ *narcotic antitussive; decongestant; expectorant* [hydrocodone bitartrate; phenylephrine HCl; guaifenesin] 4•20•200 mg/10 mL

**Atuss HC; Atuss HD; Atuss MS** oral liquid ℞ *narcotic antitussive; decongestant; antihistamine* [hydrocodone bitartrate; phenylephrine HCl; chlorpheniramine maleate] 2.5•10•2 mg/5 mL; 2.5•10•4 mg/5 mL; 5•10•2 mg/5 mL

**Atuss-12 DM** extended-release oral suspension ℞ *antitussive; decongestant; antihistamine* [dextromethorphan polistirex; pseudoephedrine polistirex; chlorpheniramine polistirex] 30•30•6 mg/5 mL

**Atuss-12 DX** extended-release oral suspension ℞ *antitussive; expectorant* [dextromethorphan hydrobromide; guaifenesin] 30•200 mg/5 mL

**"atypical" antipsychotics** [see: novel antipsychotics]

**198Au** [see: gold Au 198]

**augmented betamethasone dipropi-onate** *topical corticosteroid*

**Augmentin** film-coated tablets, chew-able tablets, powder for oral suspen-sion ℞ *aminopenicillin antibiotic plus synergist* [amoxicillin; clavulanate potassium] 250•125, 500•125, 875•125 mg; 125•31.25, 200•28.5, 250•62.5, 400•57 mg; 125•31.25, 200•28.5, 250•62.5, 400•57 mg/5 mL

**Augmentin ES-600** powder for oral suspension ℞ *aminopenicillin antibi-otic plus synergist* [amoxicillin; clavu-lanate potassium] 600•43 mg/5 mL

**Augmentin XR** extended-release film-coated tablets ℞ *aminopenicillin anti-biotic plus synergist* [amoxicillin; clav-ulanate potassium] 1000•62.5 mg

**augmerosen** *investigational (NDA filed, orphan) antineoplastic for malig-nant melanoma; investigational (Phase III, orphan) for multiple myeloma and chronic lymphocytic leukemia (CLL)*

**Auralgan Otic** ear drops ℞ *local anes-thetic; analgesic* [benzocaine; antipy-rine] 1.4%•5.4% ☑ Allergan; allergen

**auranofin** USAN, INN, BAN, JAN *anti-rheumatic (29% gold)*

**aureoquin** [now: quinetolate]

**Auriculin** *investigational (orphan) for acute renal failure and renal trans-plants* [anaritide acetate]

**Auro Ear Drops** OTC *agent to emulsify and disperse ear wax* [carbamide per-oxide] 6.5%

**Auro-Dri** ear drops OTC *antibacterial; antifungal* [boric acid] 2.75%

**Auroguard Otic** ear drops ℞ *local anesthetic; analgesic* [benzocaine; antipyrine] 1.4%•5.4%

**Aurolate** IM injection ℞ *antirheumatic* [gold sodium thiomalate] 50 mg/mL

**aurolin** [see: gold sodium thiosulfate]

**auropin** [see: gold sodium thiosulfate]

**aurosan** [see: gold sodium thiosulfate]

**aurothioglucose** USP *antirheumatic (50% gold)*

**aurothioglycanide** INN, DCF

**aurothiomalate disodium** [see: gold sodium thiomalate]

**aurothiomalate sodium** [see: gold sodium thiomalate]

**Auroto Otic** ear drops ℞ *topical local anesthetic; analgesic* [antipyrine; ben-zocaine] 1.4%•5.4%

**Australian tea tree** *medicinal herb* [see: tea tree oil]

**Autohaler** (delivery form) *breath-acti-vated metered-dose inhaler*

**auto-injector** (delivery device) *auto-matic IM injection device*

**autologous cell (AC) vaccine** *inves-tigational (Phase III, orphan) therapeu-tic vaccine for adjuvant treatment of ovarian cancer*

**autolymphocyte therapy (ALT)** *investigational (orphan) for metastatic renal cell carcinoma*

**Autoplex T** IV injection or drip ℞ *antihemophilic to correct factor VIII deficiency and coagulation deficiency* [anti-inhibitor coagulant complex, heat treated] (each bottle is labeled with dosage)

**autoprothrombin I** [see: factor VII]

**autoprothrombin II** [see: factor IX]

**autumn crocus** (*Colchicum autum-nale; C. speciosum; C. vernum*) plant and corm *medicinal herb for edema, gonorrhea, gout, prostate enlargement, and rheumatism; not gen-erally regarded as safe and effective as it is highly toxic because of its colchicine content*

**AV (Adriamycin, vincristine)** *che-motherapy protocol*

**AVA (anthrax vaccine, adsorbed)** [q.v.]

**Avage** cream ℞ *retinoid pro-drug; adju-vant treatment for facial wrinkles, hyper- and hypopigmentation, and benign lentigines* [tazarotene] 0.1%

**Avail** tablets OTC *vitamin/mineral/iron supplement* [multiple vitamins & minerals; iron; folic acid] ≛•18•0.4 mg ☑ Advil

**Avalide** tablets ℞ *antihypertensive; angiotensin II receptor antagonist;*

*diuretic* [irbesartan; hydrochlorothiazide] 150•12.5, 300•12.5 mg

**Avandamet** film-coated tablets ℞ *antidiabetic combination for type 2 diabetes* [rosiglitazone maleate; metformin HCl] 1•500, 2•500, 2•1000, 4•500, 4•1000 mg

**Avandia** film-coated tablets ℞ *thiazolidinedione antidiabetic; increases cellular response to insulin without increasing insulin secretion* [rosiglitazone maleate] 2, 4, 8 mg

**Avapro** tablets ℞ *angiotensin II receptor antagonist for hypertension; treatment to delay the progression of diabetic nephropathy* [irbesartan] 75, 150, 300 mg

**Avar** cleanser, gel ℞ *acne treatment* [sulfacetamide sodium; sulfur] 10%•5%

**Avar Green** gel ℞ *acne treatment; tinted for "color correction"* [sulfacetamide sodium; sulfur] 10%•5%

**avasimbe** USAN *acylCoA transferase (ACAT) inhibitor for hyperlipidemia and atherosclerosis*

**Avastin** IV infusion ℞ *antineoplastic; angiogenesis inhibitor for metastatic colorectal cancer; investigational (Phase III) for metastatic breast cancer, cervical cancer, non–small cell lung cancer (NSCLC), and renal cell carcinoma* [bevacizumab] 100, 400 mg/vial

**Avaxim** ⒸⒶⓃ prefilled syringe for IM injection ℞ *immunization against hepatitis A virus (HAV)* [hepatitis A vaccine, inactivated] 0.5 mL

**AVC** vaginal cream, vaginal inserts (discontinued 2001) ℞ *broad-spectrum antibiotic* [sulfanilamide] 15%; 1.05 g

**Aveeno** lotion OTC *moisturizer; emollient* [colloidal oatmeal] 1%

**Aveeno Anti-Itch** cream, lotion (discontinued 2003) OTC *poison ivy treatment* [calamine; pramoxine HCl; camphor] 3%•1%•0.3%

**Aveeno Cleansing** bar OTC *soap-free therapeutic skin cleanser* [colloidal oatmeal] 51%

**Aveeno Cleansing for Acne-Prone Skin** bar OTC *medicated cleanser for acne* [salicylic acid; colloidal oatmeal]

**Aveeno Moisturizing** cream OTC *moisturizer; emollient* [colloidal oatmeal] 1%

**Aveeno Oilated Bath** packets OTC *bath emollient* [colloidal oatmeal; mineral oil] 43%• Ⓑ

**Aveeno Regular Bath** packets OTC *bath emollient* [colloidal oatmeal] 100%

**Aveeno Shave** gel OTC *moisturizer; emollient* [oatmeal flour]

**Aveeno Shower & Bath** oil OTC *bath emollient* [colloidal oatmeal] 5%

**Avelox** film-coated tablets, IV infusion ℞ *broad-spectrum fluoroquinolone antibiotic* [moxifloxacin HCl] 400 mg; 400 mg/bag

*Avena sativa* medicinal herb [see: oats]

**Aventyl HCl** Pulvules (capsules), oral solution ℞ *tricyclic antidepressant* [nortriptyline HCl] 10, 25 mg; 10 mg/5 mL Ⓑ Ambenyl; Bentyl

**avertin** [see: tribromoethanol]

**Aviane** tablets (in packs of 28) ℞ *monophasic oral contraceptive* [levonorgestrel; ethinyl estradiol] 0.1 mg•20 μg

**avicatonin** INN

**Avicine** ℞ *investigational (Phase III) theraccine for cervical and pancreatic cancer; investigational (Phase II) for prostate and advanced colorectal cancers* [CTP-37 (code name—generic name not yet assigned)]

**avilamycin** USAN, INN, BAN *antibacterial*

**avinar** [see: uredepa]

**Avinza** dual-release (immediate- plus extended-release) capsules ℞ *once-daily narcotic analgesic for treatment of chronic pain* [morphine sulfate] 30, 60, 90, 120 mg

**Avita** cream, gel ℞ *keratolytic for acne* [tretinoin] 0.025% Ⓑ Evista

**Avitene Hemostat** nonwoven web ℞ *topical hemostatic aid for surgery* [microfibrillar collagen hemostat] Ⓑ Ativan

**avitriptan fumarate** USAN *serotonin 5-HT₁ agonist for migraine*

**avizafone** INN, BAN

**avobenzone** USAN, INN *sunscreen*

**avocado** *(Persea americana; P. gratissima) fruit and seed medicinal herb for diarrhea, dysentery, inducing menstruation, lowering total cholesterol and improving overall lipid profile, promoting hair growth, and stimulating wound healing; also used as an aphrodisiac*

**avocado sugar extract** *natural weight-loss agent used to diminish carbohydrate cravings* [see also: D-mannoheptulose]

**Avodart** *capsules* ℞ *5α-reductase blocker for benign prostatic hyperplasia (BPH); investigational (Phase III) for prostate cancer* [dutasteride] 0.5 mg

**Avolean** *capsules* OTC *natural weight-loss agent used to diminish carbohydrate cravings* [avocado sugar extract] 50 mg

**Avonex** *powder for IM injection (multidose vials replaced by single-use prefilled syringes in 2003)*

**Avonex** *prefilled syringes for IM injection* ℞ *immunomodulator for relapsing remitting multiple sclerosis (orphan); investigational (orphan) for non-A, non-B hepatitis, Kaposi sarcoma, brain tumors, and various other cancers* [interferon beta-1a] 30 μg (6 MIU)/ 0.5 mL syringe

**avoparcin** USAN, INN, BAN *glycopeptide antibiotic*

**AVP (actinomycin D, vincristine, Platinol)** *chemotherapy protocol*

**avridine** USAN, INN *antiviral*

**Award** *hydrophilic contact lens material* [hilafilcon A]

**axamozide** INN

**axerophthol** [see: vitamin A]

**Axert** *tablets* ℞ *vascular serotonin HT₁ᵦ/₁ᴅ/₁ꜰ receptor agonist for the acute treatment of migraine* [almotriptan malate] 6.25, 12.5 mg

**axetil** USAN, INN *combining name for radicals or groups*

**Axid** *Pulvules (capsules)* ℞ *histamine H₂ antagonist for treatment of gastric and duodenal ulcers* [nizatidine] 150, 300 mg ▣ Biaxin

**Axid AR** ("acid reducer") *tablets* OTC *histamine H₂ antagonist for heartburn* [nizatidine] 75 mg

**axitirome** USAN *antihyperlipidemic*

**Axocet** *caplets (discontinued 2004)* ℞ *analgesic; barbiturate sedative* [acetaminophen; butalbital] 650•50 mg

**Axocet** *capsules (discontinued 2003)* ℞ *analgesic; barbiturate sedative* [acetaminophen; butalbital] 650•50 mg

**Axokine** ℞ *investigational (Phase III) second-generation ciliary neurotrophic factor for obesity associated with type 2 diabetes*

**Aygestin** *tablets* ℞ *progestin for amenorrhea, abnormal uterine bleeding, or endometriosis* [norethindrone acetate] 5 mg

**Ayr Saline** *nasal mist, nose drops, nasal gel* OTC *nasal moisturizer* [sodium chloride (saline solution)] 0.65%

**5-AZA (5-azacitidine)** [see: azacitidine]

**5-aza-2'-deoxycytidine** *investigational (orphan) for acute leukemia*

**azabon** USAN, INN *CNS stimulant*

**azabuperone** INN

**azacitidine (5-AZA; 5-AZC)** USAN, INN *demethylating antineoplastic for myelodysplastic syndrome (orphan)*

**azaclorzine** INN *coronary vasodilator* [also: azaclorzine HCl]

**azaclorzine HCl** USAN *coronary vasodilator* [also: azaclorzine]

**azaconazole** USAN, INN *antifungal*

**azacosterol** INN *avian chemosterilant* [also: azacosterol HCl]

**azacosterol HCl** USAN *avian chemosterilant* [also: azacosterol]

**AZA-CR** [see: azacitidine]

**Azactam** *powder for IV or IM injection* ℞ *monobactam bactericidal antibiotic* [aztreonam] 0.5, 1, 2 g

**azacyclonol** INN, BAN [also: azacyclonol HCl]

**azacyclonol HCl** NF [also: azacyclonol]

**5-azacytosine arabinoside (ara-AC)** [see: fazarabine]

**5-aza-2'-deoxycytidine** *investigational (orphan) for acute leukemia*

*Azadirachta indica* medicinal herb [see: neem tree]

**azaftozine** INN

**azalanstat dihydrochloride** USAN *hypolipidemic*

**azalomycin** INN, BAN

**azaloxan** INN *antidepressant* [also: azaloxan fumarate]

**azaloxan fumarate** USAN *antidepressant* [also: azaloxan]

**azamethiphos** BAN

**azamethonium bromide** INN, BAN

**azamulin** INN

**azanator** INN *bronchodilator* [also: azanator maleate]

**azanator maleate** USAN *bronchodilator* [also: azanator]

**azanidazole** USAN, INN, BAN *antiprotozoal*

**azaperone** USAN, INN, BAN *antipsychotic*

**azapetine** BAN

**azapetine phosphate** [see: azapetine]

**azaprocin** INN

**azapropazone** INN, BAN, DCF *antiinflammatory* [also: apazone]

**azaquinzole** INN

**azaribine** USAN, INN, BAN *antipsoriatic*

**azarole** USAN *immunoregulator*

**Azasan** tablets ℞ *immunosuppressant for organ transplantation (orphan) and rheumatoid arthritis* [azathioprine] 25, 50, 75, 100 mg

**azaserine** USAN, INN *antifungal*

**azasetron** INN

**azaspirium chloride** INN

**azaspirones** *a class of anxiolytics*

**azastene**

**azatadine** INN, BAN *piperidine antihistamine for allergic rhinitis and chronic urticaria* [also: azatadine maleate]

**azatadine maleate** USAN, USP *piperidine antihistamine for allergic rhinitis and chronic urticaria* [also: azatadine]

**azatepa** INN *antineoplastic* [also: azetepa]

**azathioprine** USAN, USP, INN, BAN, JAN *immunosuppressant for organ transplantation (orphan) and rheumatoid arthritis* 50 mg oral

**azathioprine sodium** USP *immunosuppressant for organ transplantation*

*(orphan) and rheumatoid arthritis* 100 mg injection

**5-AZC (5-azacitidine)** [see: azacitidine]

**Azdone** tablets ℞ *narcotic analgesic* [hydrocodone bitartrate; aspirin] 5• 500 mg

**azdU (3′-azido-2′,3′-dideoxyuridine)** [see: azidouridine]

**azelaic acid** USAN, INN *topical antimicrobial and keratolytic for acne and rosacea*

**azelastine** INN, BAN *peripherally selective phthalazinone antihistamine for allergic and vasomotor rhinitis; mast cell stabilizer; antiasthmatic* [also: azelastine HCl]

**azelastine HCl** USAN, JAN *peripherally selective phthalazinone antihistamine for allergic and vasomotor rhinitis; mast cell stabilizer; antiasthmatic* [also: azelastine]

**Azelex** cream ℞ *antimicrobial and keratolytic for inflammatory acne vulgaris* [azelaic acid] 20%

**azelnidipine** INN

**azepexole** INN, BAN

**azephine** [see: azapetine phosphate]

**azepinamide** [see: glypinamide]

**azepindole** USAN, INN *antidepressant*

**azetepa** USAN, BAN *antineoplastic* [also: azatepa]

**azetirelin** INN

**azidamfenicol** INN, BAN, DCF

**3′-azido-2′,3′-dideoxyuridine (azdU)** [see: azidouridine]

**azidoamphenicol** [see: azidamfenicol]

**azidocillin** INN, BAN

**azidothymidine (AZT)** [now: zidovudine]

**azidouridine (azdU)** *investigational (orphan) antiviral for HIV and AIDS*

**azimexon** INN

**azimilide dihydrochloride** USAN *investigational (NDA filed) antiarrhythmic and antifibrillatory*

**azintamide** INN

**azinthiamide** [see: azintamide]

**azipramine** INN *antidepressant* [also: azipramine HCl]

**azipramine HCl** USAN *antidepressant* [also: azipramine]

**aziridinyl benzoquinone** [see: diaziquone]

**azithromycin** USAN, USP, INN, BAN *macrolide antibiotic*

**azlocillin** USAN, INN, BAN *penicillin antibiotic*

**azlocillin sodium** USP *penicillin antibiotic*

**Azmacort** oral inhalation aerosol ℞ *corticosteroidal anti-inflammatory for chronic asthma* [triamcinolone acetonide] 100 μg/dose

**Azo Test Strips** reagent strips for home use *in vitro diagnostic aid for urinary tract infections*

**azoconazole** [now: azaconazole]

**azodisal sodium (ADS)** [now: olsalazine sodium]

**"azoles"** *a class of fungicides that include all with generic names ending in "azole," such clotrimazole, fluconazole, etc.*

**azolimine** USAN, INN *diuretic* 🔲 Azulfidine

**Azoline** ℞ *investigational (Phase III) oral triazole antifungal for fungal infections of the skin, hair, nails, and oral and genital mucosa*

**Azopt** eye drop suspension ℞ *carbonic anhydrase inhibitor for glaucoma* [brinzolamide] 1%

**azosemide** USAN, INN, JAN *diuretic*

**Azo-Standard** tablets OTC *urinary analgesic* [phenazopyridine HCl] 95 mg

**Azostix** reagent strips for professional use *in vitro diagnostic aid to estimate the amount of BUN in whole blood*

**Azo-Sulfisoxazole** tablets ℞ *urinary anti-infective; urinary analgesic* [sulfisoxazole; phenazopyridine HCl] 500•50 mg

**azotomycin** USAN, INN *antibiotic antineoplastic*

**azovan blue** BAN *blood volume test* [also: Evans blue]

**azovan sodium** [see: Evans blue]

**AZT (azidothymidine)** [now: zidovudine]

**Aztec** controlled release ℞ *investigational (Phase III) antiviral for early HIV and AIDS* [zidovudine]

**AZT-P-ddI** [see: zidovudine & didanosine]

**aztreonam** USAN, USP, INN, BAN, JAN *monobactam bactericidal antibiotic; investigational (orphan) inhalation therapy for cystic fibrosis*

**azulene sulfonate sodium** JAN [also: sodium gualenate]

**Azulfidine** tablets ℞ *broad-spectrum bacteriostatic; anti-inflammatory for ulcerative colitis* [sulfasalazine] 500 mg 🔲 Silvadene

**Azulfidine EN-tabs** enteric-coated delayed-release tablets ℞ *broad-spectrum bacteriostatic; anti-inflammatory for ulcerative colitis, rheumatoid arthritis (RA), and juvenile rheumatoid arthritis (JRA)* [sulfasalazine] 500 mg

**azumolene** INN *skeletal muscle relaxant* [also: azumolene sodium]

**azumolene sodium** USAN *skeletal muscle relaxant* [also: azumolene]

**azure A carbacrylic resin** [see: azuresin]

**azuresin** NF, BAN

**1,4-B (1,4-butanediol)** *a precursor to gamma hydroxybutyrate (GHB); a formerly legal alternative to GHB, now also illegal (Schedule I)* [see: gamma hydroxybutyrate (GHB)]

**B Complex + C** timed-release tablets OTC *vitamin supplement* [multiple B vitamins; vitamin C] ≜•500 mg

**B Complex with C and B-12** injection ℞ *parenteral vitamin supplement* [multiple vitamins]

**B Complex-50** sustained-release tablets OTC *vitamin supplement* [multiple B vitamins; folic acid; biotin] ≜• 400•50 μg

**B Complex-150** sustained-release tablets OTC *vitamin supplement* [multiple B vitamins; folic acid; biotin] ± •
400 • 150 μg

**B & O Supprettes No. 15A; B & O Supprettes No. 16A** suppositories ℞ *narcotic analgesic* [belladonna extract; opium] 16.2 • 30 mg; 16.2 • 60 mg

**B vitamins** [see: vitamin B]

**B₁ (vitamin B₁)** [see: thiamine HCl]

**B₂ (vitamin B₂)** [see: riboflavin]

**B₃ (vitamin B₃)** [see: niacin; niacinamide]

**B₅ (vitamin B₅)** [see: calcium pantothenate]

**B₆ (vitamin B₆)** [see: pyridoxine HCl]

**B₈ (vitamin B₈)** [see: adenosine phosphate]

**B₁₂ (vitamin B₁₂)** [see: cyanocobalamin]

**B₁₂ₐ (vitamin B₁₂ₐ)** [see: hydroxocobalamin]

**B₁₂ᵦ (vitamin B₁₂ᵦ)** [see: hydroxocobalamin]

**B-50** tablets OTC *vitamin supplement* [multiple B vitamins; folic acid; biotin] ± • 100 • 50 μg

**B-100** tablets, timed-release tablets OTC *vitamin supplement* [multiple B vitamins; folic acid; biotin] ± • 100 • 100 μg; ± • 400 • 50 μg

**Bᴄ (vitamin Bᴄ)** [see: folic acid]

**Bₜ (vitamin Bₜ)** [see: carnitine]

**Babee Teething** lotion OTC *topical oral anesthetic; antiseptic* [benzocaine; cetalkonium chloride] 2.5% • 0.02%

**baby brain I** *chemotherapy protocol for pediatric brain tumors* [see: COPE]

**Baby Vitamin** drops OTC *vitamin supplement* [multiple vitamins]

**Baby Vitamin with Iron** drops OTC *vitamin/iron supplement* [multiple vitamins; iron] ± • 10 mg/mL

**BabyBIG** powder for IV infusion ℞ *treatment for infant botulism type A or B (orphan)* [botulism immune globulin (BIG)] 100 mg/vial

**Babylax** [see: Fleet Babylax]

**BAC (BCNU, ara-C, cyclophosphamide)** *chemotherapy protocol*

**BAC (benzalkonium chloride)** [q.v.]

**bacampicillin** INN, BAN *aminopenicillin antibiotic* [also: bacampicillin HCl]

**bacampicillin HCl** USAN, USP, JAN *aminopenicillin antibiotic* [also: bacampicillin]

**bachelor's buttons** *medicinal herb* [see: cornflower; feverfew; tansy; buttercup]

**Bacid** capsules OTC *dietary supplement; fever blister treatment; not generally regarded as safe and effective as an antidiarrheal* [Lactobacillus acidophilus] 500 million cultures ⊘ Banacid

**Baciguent** ointment (discontinued 2003) OTC *antibiotic* [bacitracin] 500 U/g

**Baci-IM** powder for IM injection ℞ *bactericidal antibiotic* [bacitracin] 50 000 U

**bacillus Calmette-Guérin (BCG) vaccine** [see: BCG vaccine]

**bacitracin** USP, INN, BAN, JAN *bactericidal antibiotic; investigational (orphan) for pseudomembranous enterocolitis* 500 U/g topical; 50 000 U/vial injection ⊘ Bacitrin; Bactrim

**bacitracin zinc** USP, BAN *bactericidal antibiotic*

**bacitracin zinc & neomycin sulfate & polymyxin B sulfate** *topical antibiotic* 400 U • 5 mg • 10 000 U per g ophthalmic

**bacitracin zinc & polymyxin B sulfate** *topical antibiotic* 500 • 10 000 U/g ophthalmic

**bacitracins zinc complex** [see: bacitracin zinc]

**Backache Maximum Strength Relief** film-coated caplets OTC *analgesic; antirheumatic* [magnesium salicylate] 467 mg

**Back-Pack** (trademarked packaging form) *unit-of-use package*

**baclofen (L-baclofen)** USAN, USP, INN, BAN, JAN *skeletal muscle relaxant for intractable spasticity due to spinal cord injury or disease (orphan); investigational (orphan) for dystonia* 10, 20 mg oral

**bacmecillinam** INN

**Bacmin** tablets ℞ *vitamin/mineral/iron supplement* [multiple vitamins & minerals; iron; folic acid; biotin] ± • 27•0.8•0.15 mg

**BACOD (bleomycin, Adriamycin, CCNU, Oncovin, dexamethasone)** *chemotherapy protocol*

**BACON (bleomycin, Adriamycin, CCNU, Oncovin, nitrogen mustard)** *chemotherapy protocol*

**BACOP (bleomycin, Adriamycin, cyclophosphamide, Oncovin, prednisone)** *chemotherapy protocol*

**BACT (BCNU, ara-C, cyclophosphamide, thioguanine)** *chemotherapy protocol*

**bactericidal and permeability-increasing (BPI) protein, recombinant** *investigational (Phase III, orphan) treatment for gram-negative sepsis, hemorrhagic shock, and meningococcemia*

**bacteriostatic sodium chloride** [see: sodium chloride]

**Bacteriostatic Sodium Chloride Injection** ℞ *IV diluent* [sodium chloride (normal saline solution)] 0.9% (normal)

**Bacti-Cleanse** topical liquid OTC *soap-free therapeutic skin cleanser* [benzalkonium chloride]

**Bactigen B Streptococcus-CS** slide test for professional use *in vitro diagnostic aid for Group B streptococcal antigens in vaginal and cervical swabs*

**Bactigen Meningitis Panel** slide test for professional use *in vitro diagnostic aid for* H. influenzae, N. meningitidis, *and* S. pneumoniae *in various fluids* [latex agglutination test]

**Bactigen N. meningitidis** slide test for professional use (discontinued 2004) *in vitro diagnostic aid for* Neisseria meningitidis [latex agglutination test]

**Bactigen Salmonella-Shigella** slide test for professional use *in vitro diagnostic aid for salmonella and shigella* [latex agglutination test]

**Bactine Antiseptic Anesthetic** topical liquid, spray OTC *local anesthetic; antiseptic* [lidocaine HCl; benzalkonium chloride] 2.5%•0.13%

**Bactine First Aid Antibiotic Plus Anesthetic** ointment (discontinued 2001) OTC *antibiotic; local anesthetic* [polymyxin B sulfate; neomycin sulfate; bacitracin; diperodon HCl] 5000 U•3.5 mg•400 U•10 mg per g

**Bactine Hydrocortisone; Maximum Strength Bactine** cream OTC *corticosteroidal anti-inflammatory* [hydrocortisone] 0.5%; 1%

**Bactine Pain Relieving Cleansing Spray** OTC *local anesthetic; antiseptic* [lidocaine HCl; benzalkonium chloride] 2.5%•0.13%

**Bactine Pain Relieving Cleansing Wipes** OTC *local anesthetic; antiseptic* [pramoxine HCl; benzalkonium chloride] 1%•0.13%

**Bactocill** powder for IV or IM injection (discontinued 2002) ℞ *penicillinase-resistant penicillin antibiotic* [oxacillin sodium] 0.5, 1, 2, 4, 10 g ⊡ Pathocil

**BactoShield** aerosol foam, solution OTC *broad-spectrum antimicrobial; germicidal* [chlorhexidine gluconate; alcohol 4%] 4%

**BactoShield 2** solution OTC *broad-spectrum antimicrobial; germicidal* [chlorhexidine gluconate; alcohol 4%] 2%

**Bactrim; Bactrim DS** tablets ℞ *anti-infective; antibacterial* [trimethoprim; sulfamethoxazole] 80•400 mg; 160•800 mg ⊡ bacitracin

**Bactrim IV** infusion ℞ *anti-infective; antibacterial* [trimethoprim; sulfamethoxazole] 80•400 mg/5 mL

**Bactrim Pediatric** oral suspension ℞ *anti-infective; antibacterial* [trimethoprim; sulfamethoxazole] 40•200 mg/5 mL

**Bactroban** cream ℞ in the U.S.; OTC in Canada *antibiotic* [mupirocin calcium] 2.15% (=2% base)

**Bactroban** ointment ℞ *antibiotic for impetigo* [mupirocin] 2%

**Bactroban Nasal** ointment in single-use tubes ℞ *antibiotic for iatrogenic*

*methicillin-resistant* Staphylococcus aureus (MRSA) infections [mupirocin calcium] 2.15% (=2% base)

**Bagshawe protocol, modified** *chemotherapy protocol* [see: CHAMOCA]

**bakeprofen** INN

**baker's yeast** *natural source of protein and B-complex vitamins*

**BAL (British antilewisite)** [now: dimercaprol]

**BAL in Oil** deep IM injection ℞ *chelating agent for arsenic, gold, and mercury poisoning; adjunct to lead poisoning* [dimercaprol in peanut oil] 10% ② Balneol

**balafilcon A** USAN *hydrophilic contact lens material*

**Balamine DM** syrup, pediatric oral drops ℞ *antitussive; decongestant; antihistamine* [dextromethorphan hydrobromide; pseudoephedrine HCl; carbinoxamine maleate] 12.5•60•4 mg/5 mL; 3.5•25•2 mg/mL

**balipramine** BAN [also: depramine]

**balm** *medicinal herb* [see: lemon balm]

**balm, eye; eye root** *medicinal herb* [see: goldenseal]

**balm, mountain** *medicinal herb* [see: yerba santa]

**balm, squaw; squaw mint** *medicinal herb* [see: pennyroyal]

**balm of Gilead (*Populus balsamifera*; *P. candicans*)** buds *medicinal herb used as an antiscorbutic, balsamic, diuretic, stimulant, and vulnerary*

**Balmex** ointment OTC *astringent; moisturizer; emollient* [zinc oxide] 11.3%

**Balmex Baby** powder OTC *topical diaper rash treatment* [zinc oxide; peruvian balsam; corn starch]

**Balmex Emollient** lotion OTC *moisturizer; emollient*

**balmony** *medicinal herb* [see: turtlebloom]

**Balneol Perianal Cleansing** lotion OTC *emollient/protectant* [mineral oil; lanolin] ② BAL in Oil

**Balnetar** bath oil OTC *antipsoriatic; antipruritic; emollient* [coal tar] 2.5%

**balsalazide** INN, BAN *gastrointestinal anti-inflammatory for ulcerative colitis* [also: balsalazide disodium]

**balsalazide disodium** USAN *gastrointestinal anti-inflammatory for ulcerative colitis* [also: balsalazide]

**balsalazide sodium** [see: balsalazide disodium]

**balsalazine** [see: balsalazide disodium; balsalazide]

**balsam apple; balsam pear** *medicinal herb* [see: bitter melon]

**balsam Peru** [see: peruvian balsam; balsam tree]

**balsam poplar** *medicinal herb* [see: balm of Gilead]

**balsam tree** *medicinal herb* [see: Peruvian balsam]

**balsamics; balsams** *a class of agents that soothe or heal; balms; also, certain resinous substances of vegetable origin*

***Balsamodendron myrrha*** *medicinal herb* [see: myrrh]

**balsan** [see: peruvian balsam]

**Balziva** tablets (in packs of 21 or 28) ℞ *monophasic oral contraceptive* [norethindrone; ethinyl estradiol] 0.4 mg•35 μg

**bamaluzole** INN

**bambermycin** INN, BAN *antibacterial antibiotic* [also: bambermycins]

**bambermycins** USAN *antibacterial antibiotic* [also: bambermycin]

**bambuterol** INN, BAN

**bamethan** INN, BAN *vasodilator* [also: bamethan sulfate]

**bamethan sulfate** USAN, JAN *vasodilator* [also: bamethan]

**bamifylline** INN, BAN *bronchodilator* [also: bamifylline HCl]

**bamifylline HCl** USAN *bronchodilator* [also: bamifylline]

**bamipine** INN, BAN, DCF

**bamnidazole** USAN, INN *antiprotozoal (Trichomonas)*

**BAMON (bleomycin, Adriamycin, methotrexate, Oncovin, nitrogen mustard)** *chemotherapy protocol*

**Banadyne-3** solution OTC *topical oral anesthetic; analgesic; counterirritant;*

*antiseptic* [lidocaine; menthol; alcohol 45%] 4%•1%

**Banalg** lotion OTC *analgesic; counterirritant* [methyl salicylate; camphor; menthol] 4.9%•2%•1%

**Banalg Hospital Strength** lotion OTC *analgesic; counterirritant* [methyl salicylate; menthol] 14%•3%

**Bancap HC** capsules R̥ *narcotic analgesic* [hydrocodone bitartrate; acetaminophen] 5•500 mg

**bandage, adhesive** USP *surgical aid*

**bandage, gauze** USP *surgical aid*

**Band-Aid Plus** ointment (discontinued 2003) OTC *antibiotic; anesthetic* [polymyxin B sulfate; neomycin sulfate; bacitracin zinc; pramoxine HCl] 10 000 U•3.5 mg•500 U•10 mg per g

**Banflex** IV or IM injection R̥ *skeletal muscle relaxant* [orphenadrine citrate] 30 mg/mL

**banocide** [see: diethylcarbamazine citrate]

**Banophen** caplets, capsules OTC *antihistamine* [diphenhydramine HCl] 25 mg

**Banophen** elixir OTC *antihistamine* [diphenhydramine HCl] 12.5 mg/5 mL

**Banophen Allergy** elixir OTC *antihistamine* [diphenhydramine HCl] 12.5 mg/5 mL

**Banophen Decongestant** capsules (discontinued 2002) OTC *decongestant; antihistamine* [pseudoephedrine HCl; diphenhydramine HCl] 60•25 mg ② Barophen

**Banthīne** tablets (discontinued 2001) R̥ *anticholinergic; peptic ulcer treatment adjunct* [methantheline bromide] 50 mg ② Brethine; Vantin

*Baptisia tinctoria* medicinal herb [see: wild indigo]

**baquiloprim** INN, BAN

**Barbados aloe** *medicinal herb* [see: aloe]

**barbenyl** [see: phenobarbital]

**barberry (Berberis vulgaris)** bark *medicinal herb for bacteria-associated diarrhea, blood cleansing, cough, fever, indigestion, jaundice, liver disorders, sciatica, and sore throat*

**barberry, California** *medicinal herb* [see: Oregon grape]

**barbexaclone** INN

**Barbidonna; Barbidonna No. 2** tablets R̥ *GI antispasmodic; anticholinergic; sedative* [atropine sulfate; scopolamine hydrobromide; hyoscyamine hydrobromide; phenobarbital] 0.025•0.0074•0.1286•16 mg; 0.025•0.0074•0.1286•32 mg

**barbiphenyl** [see: phenobarbital]

**barbital** NF, INN, JAN [also: barbitone]

**barbital, soluble** [now: barbital sodium]

**barbital sodium** NF, INN [also: barbitone sodium]

**barbitone** BAN [also: barbital]

**barbitone sodium** BAN [also: barbital sodium]

**barbiturates** *a class of sedative/hypnotics that produce a wide range of mood alteration; also widely abused as addictive street drugs*

**Barc** topical liquid (discontinued 2003) OTC *pediculicide for lice* [pyrethrins; piperonyl butoxide; petroleum distillate] 0.18%•2.2%•5.52%

**bardana** *medicinal herb* [see: burdock]

**Baricon** powder for oral suspension R̥ *radiopaque contrast medium for gastrointestinal imaging* [barium sulfate] 98%

**Baridium** tablets R̥ *urinary analgesic* [phenazopyridine HCl] 100 mg

**barium** *element (Ba)*

**barium hydroxide lime** USP *carbon dioxide absorbent*

**barium sulfate** USP, JAN *oral/rectal radiopaque contrast medium for gastrointestinal imaging* 100% for oral/rectal suspension

**barley (Hordeum vulgare)** juice powder *medicinal herb for anemia, arthritis, blood cleansing, boils, bronchitis, cancer, metal poisoning, poor circulation, and reducing total and LDL cholesterol and increasing HDL cholesterol*

**barley malt soup extract** *bulk laxative*

**barmastine** USAN, INN *antihistamine*

**BarnesHind Saline for Sensitive Eyes** solution OTC *rinsing/storage* solution for soft contact lenses [sodium chloride (preserved saline solution)]

**barnidipine** INN

**Barobag** rectal suspension ℞ *radiopaque contrast medium for gastrointestinal imaging* [barium sulfate] 97%

**Baro-cat** oral suspension ℞ *radiopaque contrast medium for gastrointestinal imaging* [barium sulfate] 1.5%

**Baros** effervescent granules (discontinued 2004) ℞ *adjunct to gastrointestinal imaging* [sodium bicarbonate; tartaric acid; simethicone] 460• 420• ≟ mg/g

*Barosma betulina; B. cenulata; B. serratifolia* medicinal herb [see: buchu]

**barosmin** [see: diosmin]

**Barosperse** powder for oral suspension ℞ *radiopaque contrast medium for gastrointestinal imaging* [barium sulfate] 95%

**Barosperse, Liquid** oral/rectal suspension ℞ *radiopaque contrast medium for gastrointestinal imaging* [barium sulfate] 60%

**barucainide** INN

**BAS (benzyl analogue of serotonin)** [see: benanserin HCl]

**Basaljel** tablets, capsules, suspension (discontinued 2002) OTC *antacid* [aluminum carbonate gel, basic] 500 mg; 500 mg; 400 mg/5 mL

**base** [def.] *The active part of a compound. In* naproxen sodium, *for example, the base is* naproxen. [compare to: salt]

**Basen** ℞ *investigational α-glucosidase inhibitor for diabetes* [voglibose]

**basic aluminum acetate** [see: aluminum subacetate]

**basic aluminum aminoacetate** [see: dihydroxyaluminum aminoacetate]

**basic aluminum carbonate** [see: aluminum carbonate, basic]

**basic aluminum chloride** [see: aluminum sesquichlorohydrate]

**basic aluminum glycinate** [see: dihydroxyaluminum aminoacetate]

**basic bismuth carbonate** [see: bismuth subcarbonate]

**basic bismuth gallate** [see: bismuth subgallate]

**basic bismuth nitrate** [see: bismuth subnitrate]

**basic bismuth potassium bismuthotartrate** [see: bismuth potassium tartrate]

**basic bismuth salicylate** [see: bismuth subsalicylate]

**basic fibroblast growth factor (bFGF)** [see: ersofermin]

**basic fuchsin** [see: fuchsin, basic]

**basic zinc acetate** [see: zinc acetate, basic]

**basifungin** USAN, INN *antifungal*

**basil (Ocimum basilicum)** leaves *medicinal herb for colds, headache, indigestion, insect and snake bites, and whooping cough*

**basiliximab** USAN *immunosuppressant; IL-2 receptor antagonist for the prevention of acute rejection of renal transplants (orphan)*

**basswood; bast tree** *medicinal herb* [see: linden tree]

**bastard hemp** *medicinal herb* [see: hemp nettle]

**bastard saffron** *medicinal herb* [see: safflower]

**batanopride** INN *antiemetic* [also: batanopride HCl]

**batanopride HCl** USAN *antiemetic* [also: batanopride]

**batebulast** INN

**batelapine** INN *antipsychotic* [also: batelapine HCl]

**batelapine maleate** USAN *antipsychotic* [also: batelapine]

**batilol** INN

**batimastat** USAN, INN *investigational (Phase III) antineoplastic; matrix metalloproteinase (MMP) inhibitor*

**batoprazine** INN

**batroxobin** INN, JAN

**batyl alcohol** [see: batilol]

**batylol** [see: batilol]

**BAVIP (bleomycin, Adriamycin, vinblastine, imidazole carboxamide, prednisone)** *chemotherapy protocol*

**baxitozine** INN

**bay; bay laurel; bay tree; Indian bay; sweet bay** *medicinal herb* [see: laurel]

**bay, holly; red bay; white bay** *medicinal herb* [see: magnolia]

**bayberry (Myrica cerifera)** bark, berries, root bark *medicinal herb for cholera, diarrhea, dysentery, glands, goiter, indigestion, jaundice, excessive menstruation, scrofuloderma, and uterine hemorrhage; not generally regarded as safe and effective because of its high tannin content*

**Baycol** tablets (discontinued 2001 due to safety concerns) ℞ *HMG-CoA reductase inhibitor for hyperlipidemia and hypertriglyceridemia* [cerivastatin sodium] 0.2, 0.3, 0.4, 0.8 mg

**Bayer Arthritis Regimen** delayed-release enteric-coated tablets OTC *analgesic; antipyretic; anti-inflammatory; antirheumatic* [aspirin] 500 mg

**Bayer Aspirin, Genuine; Maximum Bayer Aspirin** film-coated tablets, film-coated caplets OTC *analgesic; antipyretic; anti-inflammatory; antirheumatic* [aspirin] 325 mg; 500 mg

**Bayer Aspirin Regimen** delayed-release enteric-coated tablets and caplets OTC *analgesic; antipyretic; anti-inflammatory; antirheumatic* [aspirin] 81, 325 mg

**Bayer Back & Body Pain** caplets OTC *analgesic; antipyretic; anti-inflammatory; antirheumatic* [aspirin; caffeine] 500•32.5 mg

**Bayer Buffered Aspirin** tablets OTC *analgesic; antipyretic; anti-inflammatory; antirheumatic* [aspirin, buffered] 325 mg

**Bayer Children's Aspirin** chewable tablets OTC *analgesic; antipyretic; anti-inflammatory; antirheumatic* [aspirin] 81 mg

**Bayer Muscle & Joint Cream** OTC *analgesic; counterirritant* [methyl salicylate; menthol; camphor] 30%•10%•4%

**Bayer Plus** caplets OTC *analgesic; antipyretic; anti-inflammatory; antirheu-*

*matic; antacid* [aspirin; calcium carbonate] 500•250 mg

**Bayer PM Aspirin Plus Sleep Aid** caplet OTC *analgesic; antipyretic; anti-inflammatory; antirheumatic; antihistaminic sleep aid* [aspirin; diphenhydramine HCl] 500•25 mg

**Bayer Select Allergy Sinus, Aspirin-Free** caplets (discontinued 2002) OTC *decongestant; antihistamine; analgesic; antipyretic* [pseudoephedrine HCl; chlorpheniramine maleate; acetaminophen] 30•2•500 mg

**Bayer Select Backache** caplets OTC *analgesic; antipyretic; anti-inflammatory; antirheumatic* [magnesium salicylate] 580 mg

**Bayer Select Chest Cold** caplets (discontinued 2002) OTC *antitussive; analgesic; antipyretic* [dextromethorphan hydrobromide; acetaminophen] 15•500 mg

**Bayer Select Flu Relief** caplets (discontinued 2002) OTC *antitussive; decongestant; antihistamine; analgesic; antipyretic* [dextromethorphan hydrobromide; pseudoephedrine HCl; chlorpheniramine maleate; acetaminophen] 15•30•2•500 mg

**Bayer Select Head & Chest Cold, Aspirin-Free** caplets (discontinued 2002) OTC *antitussive; decongestant; expectorant; analgesic; antipyretic* [dextromethorphan hydrobromide; pseudoephedrine HCl; guaifenesin; acetaminophen] 10•30•100•325 mg

**Bayer Select Head Cold; Bayer Select Sinus Pain Relief** caplets (discontinued 2002) OTC *decongestant; analgesic; antipyretic* [pseudoephedrine HCl; acetaminophen] 30•500 mg

**Bayer Select Headache** caplets (discontinued 2000) OTC *analgesic; antipyretic* [acetaminophen; caffeine] 500•65 mg

**Bayer Select Menstrual** caplets (discontinued 2000) OTC *analgesic; antipyretic; diuretic* [acetaminophen; pamabrom] 500•25 mg

**Bayer Select Night Time Cold** caplets (discontinued 2002) OTC *antitussive; decongestant; antihistamine; analgesic; antipyretic* [dextromethorphan hydrobromide; pseudoephedrine HCl; triprolidine HCl; acetaminophen] 15•30•1.25•500 mg

**Bayer Select Night Time Pain Relief** caplets (name changed to Bayer PM Aspirin Plus Sleep Aid in 2000)

**Bayer Select Pain Relief Formula** caplets (discontinued 2000) OTC *analgesic; antiarthritic; antipyretic; nonsteroidal anti-inflammatory drug (NSAID)* [ibuprofen] 200 mg

**Bayer Timed Release, 8-Hour** caplets OTC *analgesic; antipyretic; anti-inflammatory; antirheumatic* [aspirin] 650 mg

**Bayer Women's Aspirin Plus Calcium** caplets OTC *analgesic; antipyretic; anti-inflammatory; antirheumatic; calcium supplement* [aspirin; calcium] 81•300 mg

**BayGam** IM injection ℞ *immunizing agent for hepatitis A, measles, varicella, and rubella; treatment for immunoglobulin G deficiency and acquired agammaglobulinemia* [immune globulin, solvent/detergent treated] 2, 10 mL

**BayHep B** IM injection ℞ *hepatitis B immunizing agent* [hepatitis B immune globulin, solvent/detergent treated] 0.5, 1, 5 mL

**Baypress** ℞ *investigational (NDA filed) antihypertensive; calcium channel blocker* [nitrendipine]

**BayRab** IM injection ℞ *passive immunizing agent for rabies prophylaxis and treatment* [rabies immune globulin, solvent/detergent treated] 150 IU/mL

**BayRho-D Full Dose; BayRho-D Mini Dose** IM injection ℞ *obstetric Rh factor immunity suppressant* [Rh$_O$(D) immune globulin, solvent/detergent treated] 300 μg; 50 μg

**BayTet** IM injection ℞ *passive immunizing agent for post-exposure tetanus prophylaxis in patients with incomplete or uncertain pre-exposure immunization with tetanus toxoids* [tetanus immune globulin, solvent/detergent treated] 250 U

**bazedoxifene** *investigational (Phase III) selective estrogen receptor modulator (SERM) for the prevention and treatment of postmenopausal osteoporosis*

**bazinaprine** INN

**BBVP-M (BCNU, bleomycin, VePesid, prednisone, methotrexate)** *chemotherapy protocol*

**BC** powder OTC *analgesic; antipyretic; anti-inflammatory* [aspirin; salicylamide; caffeine] 650•195•33.3 mg/pkt.

**BC** tablets (discontinued 2000) OTC *analgesic; antipyretic; anti-inflammatory* [aspirin; salicylamide; caffeine] 325•95•16 mg

**B$_c$ (vitamin B$_c$)** [see: folic acid]

**BC Arthritis Strength** powder OTC *analgesic; antipyretic; anti-inflammatory* [aspirin; salicylamide; caffeine] 742•222•38 mg

**BC Cold-Sinus Powder** packets (discontinued 2001) OTC *decongestant; analgesic; antipyretic* [phenylpropanolamine HCl; aspirin] 25•650 mg

**BC Cold-Sinus-Allergy Powder** packets (discontinued 2001) OTC *decongestant; antihistamine; analgesic; antipyretic* [phenylpropanolamine HCl; chlorpheniramine maleate; aspirin] 25•4•650 mg

**B-C with Folic Acid** tablets ℞ *vitamin supplement* [multiple B vitamins; vitamin C; folic acid] ±•500•0.5 mg

**B-C with Folic Acid Plus** tablets ℞ *vitamin/mineral/iron supplement* [multiple vitamins & minerals; ferrous fumarate; folic acid; biotin] ±•27•0.8•0.15 mg

**BCAA (branched-chain amino acids)** [see: isoleucine; leucine; valine]

**BCAD 2** powder OTC *enteral nutritional therapy for maple syrup urine disease (MSUD)*

**BCAP (BCNU, cyclophosphamide, Adriamycin, prednisone)** *chemotherapy protocol*

**BCAVe; B-CAVe (bleomycin, CCNU, Adriamycin, Velban)** *chemotherapy protocol for Hodgkin lymphoma*

**B-C-Bid** caplets OTC *vitamin supplement* [multiple B vitamins; vitamin C] ≐ •300 mg

**BCD (bleomycin, cyclophosphamide, dactinomycin)** *chemotherapy protocol*

**BCG vaccine (bacillus Calmette-Guérin)** USP *active bacterin for tuberculosis prevention; antineoplastic for urinary bladder cancer*

**BCH 10652** *investigational (Phase II) reverse transcriptase inhibitor for HIV infection*

**B-CHOP (bleomycin, Cytoxin, hydroxydaunomycin, Oncovin, prednisone)** *chemotherapy protocol*

**BCMF (bleomycin, cyclophosphamide, methotrexate, fluorouracil)** *chemotherapy protocol*

**BCNU (bis-chloroethyl-nitrosourea)** [see: carmustine]

**B-Complex** elixir OTC *vitamin supplement* [multiple B vitamins]

**B-Complex and B-12** tablets OTC *vitamin supplement* [multiple B vitamins; protease] ≐ •10 mg

**B-Complex with B-12** tablets OTC *vitamin supplement* [multiple B vitamins]

**B-Complex/Vitamin C** caplets OTC *vitamin supplement* [multiple B vitamins; vitamin C] ≐ •300 mg

**BCOP (BCNU, cyclophosphamide, Oncovin, prednisone)** *chemotherapy protocol*

**BCP (BCNU, cyclophosphamide, prednisone)** *chemotherapy protocol*

**BCVP (BCNU, cyclophosphamide, vincristine, prednisone)** *chemotherapy protocol*

**BCVPP (BCNU, cyclophosphamide, vinblastine, procarbazine, prednisone)** *chemotherapy protocol for Hodgkin lymphoma*

**B-D glucose** chewable tablets OTC *glucose elevating agent* [glucose] 5 g

**BDO (1,4-butanediol)** *a precursor to gamma hydroxybutyrate (GHB); a formerly legal alternative to GHB, now also illegal (Schedule I)* [see: gamma hydroxybutyrate (GHB)]

**B-DOPA (bleomycin, DTIC, Oncovin, prednisone, Adriamycin)** *chemotherapy protocol*

**BDP (beclomethasone dipropionate)** [q.v.]

**BEAC (BCNU, etoposide, ara-C, cyclophosphamide)** *chemotherapy protocol*

**BEACOPP (bleomycin, etoposide, Adriamycin, cyclophosphamide, Oncovin, procarbazine, prednisone, [filgrastim])** *chemotherapy protocol for Hodgkin lymphoma*

**BEAM (BCNU, etoposide, ara-C, melphalan)** *chemotherapy protocol*

**bean herb** *medicinal herb* [see: summer savory]

**bean trefoil** *medicinal herb* [see: buckbean]

**Beano** oral liquid, tablets OTC *digestive aid* [alpha-D-galactosidase enzyme]

**bearberry** *medicinal herb* [see: uva ursi]

**beard, old man's** *medicinal herb* [see: fringe tree; woodbine]

**Bear-E-Bag Pediatric** rectal suspension (discontinued 2004) ℞ *radiopaque contrast medium for gastrointestinal imaging* [barium sulfate] 95%

**Bear-E-Yum CT** oral suspension ℞ *radiopaque contrast medium for gastrointestinal imaging* [barium sulfate] 1.5%

**Bear-E-Yum GI** oral/rectal suspension ℞ *radiopaque contrast medium for gastrointestinal imaging* [barium sulfate] 60%

**bear's grape** *medicinal herb* [see: uva ursi]

**bear's weed** *medicinal herb* [see: yerba santa]

**bearsfoot** *medicinal herb* [see: hellebore]

**Beaumont root** *medicinal herb* [see: Culver root]

**beaver tree** *medicinal herb* [see: magnolia]

**Bebulin VH** powder for injection ℞ *antihemophilic for hemophilia B (orphan)*

[coagulation factors II, IX, and X, heat treated]

**becanthone HCl** USAN *antischistosomal* [also: becantone]

**becantone** INN *antischistosomal* [also: becanthone HCl]

**becantone HCl** [see: becanthone HCl]

**becaplermin** USAN *recombinant platelet-derived growth factor B for chronic diabetic foot ulcers*

**Because** vaginal foam (discontinued 2002) OTC *spermicidal contraceptive* [nonoxynol 9] 8%

**beciparcil** INN

**beclamide** INN, BAN, DCF

**becliconazole** INN

**beclobrate** INN, BAN

**Becloforte Inhaler** Ⓒᴬᴺ oral inhalation aerosol (discontinued 2001) ℞ *corticosteroidal anti-inflammatory for chronic asthma* [beclomethasone dipropionate] 250 μg/dose

**beclometasone** INN *corticosteroidal inhalant for asthma; intranasal steroid* [also: beclomethasone dipropionate; beclomethasone; beclometasone dipropionate]

**beclometasone dipropionate** JAN *corticosteroidal inhalant for asthma; intranasal steroid* [also: beclomethasone dipropionate; beclomethasone; beclometasone]

**beclomethasone** BAN *corticosteroidal anti-inflammatory for chronic asthma* [also: beclomethasone dipropionate; beclometasone; beclometasone dipropionate]

**beclomethasone dipropionate (BDP)** USAN, USP *corticosteroidal anti-inflammatory for chronic asthma and rhinitis; investigational (orphan) oral treatment for intestinal graft vs. host disease* [also: beclometasone; beclomethasone; beclometasone dipropionate]

**beclotiamine** INN

**Beclovent** oral inhalation aerosol (discontinued 2001) ℞ *corticosteroidal anti-inflammatory for chronic asthma* [beclomethasone dipropionate] 42 μg/dose

**Beclovent Inhaler** Ⓒᴬᴺ oral inhalation aerosol (discontinued 2001) ℞ *corticosteroidal anti-inflammatory for chronic asthma* [beclomethasone dipropionate] 50 μg/dose

**Beconase** nasal inhalation aerosol (discontinued 2004) ℞ *corticosteroidal anti-inflammatory for seasonal or perennial rhinitis* [beclomethasone dipropionate] 42 μg/dose

**Beconase AQ** nasal spray ℞ *corticosteroidal anti-inflammatory for seasonal or perennial rhinitis* [beclomethasone dipropionate] 0.042% (42 μg/dose)

**bectumomab** USAN *monoclonal antibody; investigational (Phase III, orphan) diagnostic aid for non-Hodgkin lymphoma and AIDS-related lymphoma* [also: technetium Tc 99m bectumomab]

**Bedoz** Ⓒᴬᴺ injection ℞ *hematopoietic; vitamin $B_{12}$* [cyanocobalamin] 100 μg/mL

**bedstraw (Galium aparine; G. verum)** plant *medicinal herb used as an antispasmodic, aperient, diaphoretic, diuretic, and vulnerary*

**bee balm** *medicinal herb* [see: lemon balm]

**bee pollen** *natural remedy for anemia, bodily weakness, cerebral hemorrhage, colitis, constipation, enteritis, and weight loss; also used as an anti-aging agent and prenatal nutritional supplement; not generally regarded as safe and effective because of widespread allergic reactions*

**bee venom (derived from Apis mellifera)** *natural remedy for arthritis and multiple sclerosis, and for hyposensitization of persons highly sensitive to bee stings*

**beechwood creosote** [see: creosote carbonate]

**beef tallow** JAN

**Beelith** tablets OTC *dietary supplement* [vitamin $B_6$; magnesium oxide] 20•362 mg

**Beepen-VK** tablets, powder for oral solution (discontinued 2002) ℞ *nat-*

ural penicillin antibiotic [penicillin V potassium] 250, 500 mg; 125, 250 mg/5 mL

**bee's nest plant** medicinal herb [see: carrot]

**beeswax, white** JAN [also: wax, white]

**beeswax, yellow** JAN [also: wax, yellow]

**Bee-Zee** tablets OTC vitamin/zinc supplement [multiple vitamins; zinc] ± • 22.5 mg

**befiperide** INN

**befloxatone** INN

**befunolol** INN [also: befunolol HCl]

**befunolol HCl** JAN [also: befunolol]

**befuraline** INN

**behenyl alcohol** [see: docosanol]

**behepan** [see: cyanocobalamin]

**bekanamycin** INN antibiotic [also: bekanamycin sulfate]

**bekanamycin sulfate** JAN antibiotic [also: bekanamycin]

**belarizine** INN

**belfosdil** USAN, INN antihypertensive; calcium channel blocker

**Belganyl** (available only from the Centers for Disease Control) ℞ antiparasitic for African trypanosomiasis and onchocerciasis [suramin sodium]

**Bellacane** elixir ℞ GI antispasmodic; anticholinergic; sedative [atropine sulfate; scopolamine hydrobromide; hyoscyamine sulfate; phenobarbital] 0.0194•0.0065•0.1037•16.2 mg/5 mL

**Bellacane** tablets ℞ GI antispasmodic; anticholinergic; sedative [hyoscyamine sulfate; phenobarbital] 0.125•15 mg

**Bellacane SR** sustained-release tablets ℞ GI anticholinergic; sedative; analgesic [belladonna alkaloids; phenobarbital; ergotamine tartrate] 0.2•40•0.6 mg

**belladonna** (Atropa belladonna) leaves, tops, and berries medicinal herb used as an antispasmodic, calmative, diaphoretic, diuretic, and narcotic

**belladonna extract** USP GI/GU anticholinergic/antispasmodic; antiparkinsonian 27–33 mg/100 mL oral

**Bellahist-D LA** sustained-release caplets ℞ decongestant; antihistamine; anticholinergic to dry mucosal secretions [phenylephrine HCl; chlorpheniramine maleate; hyoscyamine sulfate; atropine sulfate; scopolamine hydrobromide] 20•8•0.19•0.04•0.01 mg

**Bellamine** tablets ℞ GI anticholinergic; sedative; analgesic [belladonna alkaloids; phenobarbital; ergotamine tartrate] 0.2•40•0.6 mg

**Bell/ans** tablets OTC antacid [sodium bicarbonate] 520 mg

**Bellatal** tablets ℞ long-acting barbiturate sedative, hypnotic, and anticonvulsant [phenobarbital] 16.2 mg

**Bellergal-S** tablets ℞ GI anticholinergic; sedative; analgesic [belladonna extract; phenobarbital; ergotamine tartrate] 0.2•40•0.6 mg

*Bellis perennis* medicinal herb [see: wild daisy]

**bells, May** medicinal herb [see: lily of the valley]

**beloxamide** USAN, INN antihyperlipoproteinemic

**beloxepin** USAN norepinephrine uptake inhibitor for depression

**Bel-Phen-Ergot SR** sustained-release tablets ℞ GI anticholinergic; sedative; analgesic [belladonna alkaloids; phenobarbital; ergotamine tartrate] 0.2•40•0.6 mg

**bemarinone** INN cardiotonic; positive inotropic; vasodilator [also: bemarinone HCl]

**bemarinone HCl** USAN cardiotonic; positive inotropic; vasodilator [also: bemarinone]

**bemegride** USP, INN, BAN, JAN

**bemesetron** USAN, INN antiemetic

**bemetizide** INN, BAN

**Beminal 500** tablets OTC vitamin supplement [multiple B vitamins; vitamin C] ± •500 mg ⓡ Benemid

**bemitradine** USAN, INN antihypertensive; diuretic

**bemoradan** USAN, INN cardiotonic

**BEMP (bleomycin, Eldisine, mitomycin, Platinol)** chemotherapy protocol

**benactyzine** INN, BAN

**benactyzine HCl** *mild antidepressant; anticholinergic*

**Benadryl** IV or IM injection ℞ *antihistamine; motion sickness preventative; sleep aid; antiparkinsonian* [diphenhydramine HCl] 50 mg/mL ⊠ Bentyl; Benylin; Caladryl

**Benadryl; Benadryl 2%** cream, spray OTC *topical antihistamine* [diphenhydramine HCl] 1%; 2% ⊠ Bentyl; Benylin; Caladryl

**Benadryl Allergy** Liqui-Gels (liquid-filled gelcaps), Kapseals (sealed capsules), Ultratabs (tablets), chewable tablets OTC *antihistamine* [diphenhydramine HCl] 25 mg; 25 mg; 25 mg; 12.5 mg ⊠ Bentyl; Benylin; Caladryl

**Benadryl Allergy & Cold** caplets OTC *decongestant; antihistamine; analgesic* [pseudoephedrine HCl; diphenhydramine HCl; acetaminophen] 30•12.5•500 mg

**Benadryl Allergy Decongestant** oral liquid (name changed to Benadryl Allergy & Sinus in 2002)

**Benadryl Allergy & Sinus** tablets, oral liquid OTC *decongestant; antihistamine* [pseudoephedrine HCl; diphenhydramine HCl] 60•25 mg; 60•25 mg/10 mL ⊠ Bentyl; Benylin; Caladryl

**Benadryl Allergy & Sinus Fastmelt** (orally dissolving tablets) OTC *decongestant; antihistamine* [pseudoephedrine HCl; diphenhydramine citrate] 30•19 mg ⊠ Bentyl; Benylin; Caladryl

**Benadryl Allergy & Sinus Headache** caplets, gelcaps OTC *decongestant; antihistamine; analgesic* [pseudoephedrine HCl; diphenhydramine HCl; acetaminophen] 30•12.5•500 mg ⊠ Bentyl; Benylin; Caladryl

**Benadryl Children's Allergy** oral liquid OTC *antihistamine* [diphenhydramine HCl] 12.5 mg/5 mL ⊠ Bentyl; Benylin; Caladryl

**Benadryl Children's Allergy Fastmelt** (orally disintegrating tablets) OTC *antihistamine* [diphenhydramine HCl] 19 mg

**Benadryl Children's Allergy & Sinus** oral liquid OTC *decongestant; antihistamine* [pseudoephedrine HCl; diphenhydramine HCl] 30•12.5 mg/5 mL

**Benadryl Children's Allergy/Cold Fastmelt** (orally dissolving tablets) OTC *decongestant; antihistamine* [pseudoephedrine HCl; diphenhydramine citrate] 30•19 mg

**Benadryl Decongestant Allergy** film-coated tablets OTC *decongestant; antihistamine* [pseudoephedrine HCl; diphenhydramine HCl] 60•25 mg ⊠ Bentyl; Benylin; Caladryl

**Benadryl Dye-Free Allergy** Liqui-Gels [see: Benadryl Allergy Liqui-Gels] ⊠ Bentyl; Benylin; Caladryl

**Benadryl Dye-Free Allergy** oral liquid (discontinued 2002) OTC *antihistamine* [diphenhydramine HCl] 6.25 mg/5 mL ⊠ Bentyl; Benylin; Caladryl

**Benadryl Itch Relief** spray, cream, stick OTC *antihistamine; astringent* [diphenhydramine HCl; zinc acetate] 2%•0.1% ⊠ Bentyl; Benylin; Caladryl

**Benadryl Itch Relief, Children's** spray, cream OTC *antihistamine; astringent* [diphenhydramine HCl; zinc acetate] 1%•0.1% ⊠ Bentyl; Benylin; Caladryl

**Benadryl Itch Stopping Gel; Benadryl Itch Stopping Gel Children's Formula** OTC *antihistamine; astringent* [diphenhydramine HCl; zinc acetate] 2%•1%; 1%•1% ⊠ Bentyl; Benylin; Caladryl

**Benadryl Itch Stopping Spray** OTC *antihistamine; astringent* [diphenhydramine HCl; zinc acetate; alcohol] 1%•0.1%•73.6%, 2%•0.1%•73.5%

**Benadryl Junior** ⓒ chewable tablets OTC *antihistamine* [diphenhydramine HCl] 12.5 mg

**Benadryl Severe Allergy & Sinus Headache** caplets OTC *decongestant; antihistamine; analgesic* [pseudoephedrine HCl; diphenhydramine HCl; acetaminophen] 30•25•500 mg

**benafentrine** INN

**benanserin HCl**

**benapen** [see: benethamine penicillin]

**benaprizine** INN *anticholinergic* [also: benapryzine HCl; benapryzine]

**benapryzine** BAN *anticholinergic* [also: benapryzine HCl; benaprizine]

**benapryzine HCl** USAN *anticholinergic* [also: benaprizine; benapryzine]

**benaxibine** INN

**benazepril** INN, BAN *antihypertensive; angiotensin-converting enzyme (ACE) inhibitor* [also: benazepril HCl]

**benazepril HCl** USAN *antihypertensive; angiotensin-converting enzyme (ACE) inhibitor* [also: benazepril] 5, 10, 20, 40 mg oral

**benazepril HCl & hydrochlorothiazide** *antihypertensive; angiotensin-converting enzyme (ACE) inhibitor; diuretic* 5•6.25, 10•12.5, 20•12.5, 20•25 mg oral

**benazeprilat** USAN, INN *angiotensin-converting enzyme inhibitor*

**bencianol** INN

**bencisteine** INN, DCF

**benclonidine** INN

**bencyclane** INN [also: bencyclane fumarate]

**bencyclane fumarate** JAN [also: bencyclane]

**bendacalol mesylate** USAN *antihypertensive*

**bendamustine** INN

**bendazac** USAN, INN, BAN, JAN *anti-inflammatory*

**bendazol** INN, DCF

**benderizine** INN

**bendrofluazide** BAN *diuretic; antihypertensive* [also: bendroflumethiazide]

**bendroflumethiazide** USP, INN *diuretic; antihypertensive* [also: bendrofluazide]

**Benefiber** powder for oral solution OTC *dietary fiber supplement* [guar gum] 3 g fiber per pkt. or tbsp.

**Benefix** powder for IV injection R *antihemophilic for factor IX deficiency (hemophilia B; Christmas disease) (orphan)* [nonacog alfa (synthetic coagulation factor IX)] 250, 500, 1000 IU

**Benemid** ⒸⒶⓃ tablets R *uricosuric for gout* [probenecid] 500 mg ② Beminal

**benethamine penicillin** INN, BAN

**benexate** INN

**benexate HCl** JAN

**benfluorex** INN, DCF

**benfosformin** INN, DCF

**benfotiamine** INN, JAN, DCF

**benfurodil hemisuccinate** INN, DCF

**bengal gelatin** [see: agar]

**Ben-Gay, Arthritis Formula** cream OTC *analgesic; counterirritant* [methyl salicylate; menthol] 30%•8%

**Ben-Gay Original** ointment OTC *analgesic; counterirritant* [methyl salicylate; menthol] 18.3%•16%

**Ben-Gay Patch** OTC *analgesic; counterirritant* [menthol] 1.4%

**Ben-Gay Regular Strength** cream OTC *analgesic; counterirritant* [methyl salicylate; menthol] 15%•10%

**Ben-Gay SPA** cream OTC *analgesic; counterirritant* [menthol] 10%

**Ben-Gay Ultra Strength** cream OTC *analgesic; counterirritant* [methyl salicylate; menthol; camphor] 30%•10%•4%

**Ben-Gay Vanishing Scent** gel OTC *analgesic; counterirritant* [menthol; camphor] 3%• ²

**benhepazone** INN

**Benicar** film-coated tablets R *antihypertensive; angiotensin II receptor antagonist* [olmesartan medoxomil] 5, 20, 40 mg

**Benicar HCT** film-coated tablets R *antihypertensive; angiotensin II receptor antagonist; diuretic* [olmesartan medoxomil; hydrochlorothiazide] 20•12.5, 40•12.5, 40•25 mg

**benidipine** INN

**benmoxin** INN, DCF

**benolizime** INN

**Benoquin** cream R *depigmenting agent for vitiligo* [monobenzone] 20%

**benorilate** INN, DCF [also: benorylate]

**benorterone** USAN, INN *antiandrogen*

**benorylate** BAN [also: benorilate]

**benoxafos** INN

**benoxaprofen** USAN, INN, BAN *anti-inflammatory; analgesic*

**benoxinate HCl** USP *topical ophthalmic anesthetic* [also: oxybuprocaine; oxybuprocaine HCl]

**Benoxyl 5** lotion, mask (discontinued 2003) OTC *keratolytic for acne* [benzoyl peroxide] 5% ☒ PanOxyl

**Benoxyl 10** lotion (discontinued 2003) OTC *topical keratolytic for acne* [benzoyl peroxide] 10%

**benpenolisin** INN

**benperidol** USAN, INN, BAN *antipsychotic*

**benproperine** INN [also: benproperine phosphate]

**benproperine phosphate** JAN [also: benproperine]

**benrixate** INN, DCF

**Bensal HP** ointment ℞ *antifungal; keratolytic* [benzoic acid; salicylic acid] 6%•3%

**bensalan** USAN, INN *disinfectant*

**benserazide** USAN, INN, BAN *decarboxylase inhibitor; antiparkinsonian adjunct* [also: benserazide HCl]

**benserazide HCl** JAN *decarboxylase inhibitor; antiparkinsonian adjunct* [also: benserazide]

**bensuldazic acid** INN, BAN

**Bensulfoid** cream OTC *topical acne treatment* [colloidal sulfur; resorcinol; alcohol] 8%•2%•12%

**bensylyte HCl** [see: phenoxybenzamine HCl]

**bentazepam** USAN, INN *sedative*

**bentemazole** INN

**bentiamine** INN

**bentipimine** INN

**bentiromide** USAN, INN, BAN, JAN *diagnostic aid for pancreas function*

**bentonite** NF, JAN *suspending agent*

**bentoquatam** USAN *topical skin protectant for allergic contact dermatitis and poison ivy exposure*

**Bentyl** capsules, tablets, IM injection, syrup ℞ *GI antispasmodic* [dicyclomine HCl] 10 mg; 20 mg; 10 mg/mL; 10 mg/5 mL ☒ Aventyl; Benadryl; Bontril

**benurestat** USAN, INN *urease enzyme inhibitor*

**Benuryl** ⓒⒶⓃ tablets ℞ *uricosuric for gout* [probenecid] 500 mg

**Benylin Adult** oral liquid OTC *antitussive* [dextromethorphan hydrobromide] 15 mg/5 mL ☒ Benadryl

**Benylin DM** syrup (discontinued 2002) OTC *antitussive* [dextromethorphan hydrobromide] 10 mg/5 mL ☒ Benadryl

**Benylin DM 12-Hour; Benylin DM for Children 12-Hour** ⓒⒶⓃ controlled-release syrup OTC *antitussive* [dextromethorphan polistirex] 30 mg/5 mL; 15 mg/5 mL ☒ Benadryl

**Benylin DM-D; Children's Benylin DM-D** ⓒⒶⓃ syrup OTC *antitussive; decongestant* [dextromethorphan hydrobromide; pseudoephedrine HCl] 15•30 mg/5 mL; 7.5•15 mg/5 mL ☒ Benadryl

**Benylin DM-D-E** ⓒⒶⓃ syrup OTC *antitussive; decongestant; expectorant* [dextromethorphan hydrobromide; pseudoephedrine HCl; guaifenesin; alcohol 5%] 15•30•100, 15•30•200 mg/5 mL ☒ Benadryl

**Benylin DM-E** ⓒⒶⓃ syrup OTC *antitussive; expectorant* [dextromethorphan hydrobromide; guaifenesin; alcohol 5%] 15•100 mg/5 mL ☒ Benadryl

**Benylin Expectorant** oral liquid OTC *antitussive; expectorant* [dextromethorphan hydrobromide; guaifenesin] 20•400 mg/20 mL ☒ Benadryl

**Benylin First Defense** ⓒⒶⓃ lozenges, syrup OTC *herbal remedy for coughs, nasal congestion, and sore throat due to cough or cold* [echinacea; menthol] 65•8 mg; 100•12.5 mg/10 mL

**Benylin Multi-Symptom** oral liquid (discontinued 2002) OTC *antitussive; decongestant; expectorant* [dextromethorphan hydrobromide; pseudoephedrine HCl; guaifenesin] 5•15•100 mg/5 mL ☒ Benadryl

**Benylin Pediatric** oral liquid OTC *antitussive* [dextromethorphan hydrobromide] 7.5 mg/5 mL ☒ Benadryl

**Benz 42** *hydrophilic contact lens material* [hefilcon A]

**Benza** solution OTC *topical antiseptic* [benzalkonium chloride] 1:750

**Benzac 5; Benzac 10** gel ℞ *keratolytic and antiseptic for acne* [benzoyl peroxide; alcohol] 5%•12%; 10%•12%

**Benzac AC 2½; Benzac W 2½; Benzac AC 5; Benzac W 5; Benzac AC 10; Benzac W 10** gel ℞ *keratolytic for acne* [benzoyl peroxide] 2.5%; 2.5%; 5%; 5%; 10%; 10%

**Benzac AC Wash 2½; Benzac AC Wash 5; Benzac W Wash 5; Benzac AC Wash 10; Benzac W Wash 10** topical liquid ℞ *keratolytic for acne* [benzoyl peroxide] 2.5%; 5%; 5%; 10%; 10%

**BenzaClin** gel ℞ *antibiotic and keratolytic for acne* [clindamycin phosphate; benzoyl peroxide] 1%•5%

**5 Benzagel; 10 Benzagel** gel (discontinued 2003) ℞ *keratolytic for acne* [benzoyl peroxide] 5%; 10%

**Benzagel Wash** gel ℞ *keratolytic and antiseptic for acne* [benzoyl peroxide; alcohol] 10%•14%

**benzaldehyde** NF *flavoring agent*

**benzalkonium chloride (BAC)** NF, INN, BAN, JAN *preservative; bacteriostatic antiseptic; surfactant/wetting agent* 17% topical

**Benzamycin** gel ℞ *antibiotic and keratolytic for acne* [erythromycin; benzoyl peroxide; alcohol 20%] 3%•5%

**benzaprinoxide** INN

**benzarone** INN, DCF

**Benzashave** shaving cream (discontinued 2003) ℞ *keratolytic for acne* [benzoyl peroxide] 5%, 10%

**benzathine benzylpenicillin** INN *natural penicillin antibiotic* [also: penicillin G benzathine; benzathine penicillin; benzylpenicillin benzathine]

**benzathine penicillin** BAN *natural penicillin antibiotic* [also: penicillin G benzathine; benzathine benzylpenicillin; benzylpenicillin benzathine]

**benzathine penicillin G** [see: penicillin G benzathine]

**benzatropine** INN *antiparkinsonian; anticholinergic* [also: benztropine mesylate; benztropine]

**benzazoline HCl** [see: tolazoline HCl]

**benzbromaron** JAN *uricosuric* [also: benzbromarone]

**benzbromarone** USAN, INN, BAN *uricosuric* [also: benzbromaron]

**benzchinamide** [see: benzquinamide]

**benzchlorpropamide** [see: beclamide]

**Benzedrex** inhaler ℞ *nasal decongestant* [propylhexedrine] 250 mg

**benzene ethanol** [see: phenylethyl alcohol]

**benzene hexachloride, gamma** [now: lindane]

**benzeneacetic acid, sodium salt** [see: sodium phenylacetate]

**benzenebutanoic acid, sodium salt** [see: sodium phenylbutyrate]

**1,3-benzenediol** [see: resorcinol]

**benzenemethanol** [see: benzyl alcohol]

**benzestrofol** [see: estradiol benzoate]

**benzestrol** USP, INN, BAN

**benzethacil** [see: penicillin G benzathine]

**benzethidine** INN, BAN, DCF

**benzethonium chloride** USP, INN, BAN, JAN *topical anti-infective; preservative*

**benzetimide** INN *anticholinergic* [also: benzetimide HCl]

**benzetimide HCl** USAN *anticholinergic* [also: benzetimide]

**benzfetamine** INN *anorexiant; CNS stimulant* [also: benzphetamine HCl; benzphetamine]

**benzhexol** BAN *anticholinergic; antiparkinsonian* [also: trihexyphenidyl HCl; trihexyphenidyl]

**N-benzhydryl-N-methylpiperazine** [see: cyclizine HCl]

**benzilone bromide** [see: benzilonium bromide]

**benzilonium bromide** USAN, INN, BAN *anticholinergic*

**benzimidavir** *investigational (Phase II) DNA inhibitor for AIDS-related cytomegalovirus infection*

**2-benzimidazolepropionic acid** [see: procodazole]

**benzimidazoles, substituted** *a class of gastric antisecretory agents that inhibit the ATPase "proton pump" within the cell* [also called: proton pump inhibitors; ATPase inhibitors]
**benzin, petroleum** JAN
**benzindamine HCl** [see: benzydamine HCl]
**benzindopyrine** INN *antipsychotic* [also: benzindopyrine HCl]
**benzindopyrine HCl** USAN *antipsychotic* [also: benzindopyrine]
**benzinoform** [see: carbon tetrachloride]
**benziodarone** INN, BAN, DCF
**benzisoxazoles** *a class of novel (atypical) antipsychotic agents*
**benzmalecene** INN
**benzmethoxazone** [see: chlorthenoxazine]
**benznidazole** INN
**benzoaric acid** [see: ellagic acid]
**benzoate & phenylacetate** [see: sodium benzoate & sodium phenylacetate]
**benzobarbital** INN
**benzocaine** USP, INN, BAN *topical anesthetic; nonprescription diet aid* [also: ethyl aminobenzoate] 5% topical
**benzoclidine** INN
**benzoctamine** INN, BAN *sedative; muscle relaxant* [also: benzoctamine HCl]
**benzoctamine HCl** USAN, INN *sedative; muscle relaxant* [also: benzoctamine]
**Benzodent** ointment OTC *topical oral anesthetic* [benzocaine] 20%
**benzodepa** USAN, INN *antineoplastic*
**benzodiazepine HCl** [see: medazepam HCl]
**benzodiazepines** *a class of nonbarbiturate sedative/hypnotics and anticonvulsants*
**benzododecinium chloride** INN
**benzogynestryl** [see: estradiol benzoate]
**benzoic acid** USP, JAN *antifungal; urinary acidifier*
**benzoic acid, phenylmethyl ester** [see: benzyl benzoate]
**benzoic acid, potassium salt** [see: potassium benzoate]

**benzoic acid, sodium salt** [see: sodium benzoate]
**benzoin** USP, JAN *topical protectant*
**Benzoin Compound** tincture OTC *skin protectant* [benzoin; aloe; alcohol 74–80%]
**benzol** [see: benzene ...]
**benzonatate** USP, INN, BAN *antitussive* 100 mg oral
**benzophenone**
**benzopyrrolate** [see: benzopyrronium]
**benzopyrronium bromide** INN
**benzoquinone amidoinohydrazone thiosemicarbazone hydrate** [see: ambazone]
**benzoquinonium chloride**
**benzorphanol** [see: levophenacylmorphan]
**benzosulfinide** [see: saccharin]
**benzosulphinide sodium** [see: saccharin sodium]
**benzothiazepines** *a class of calcium channel blockers*
**benzothiozon** [see: thioacetazone; thiacetazone]
**benzotript** INN
**Benzox-10** gel (discontinued 2003) ℞ *keratolytic for acne* [benzoyl peroxide] 10%
**benzoxiquine** USAN, INN *antiseptic/disinfectant*
**benzoxonium chloride** INN
**benzoyl p-aminosalicylate (B-PAS)** [see: benzoylpas calcium]
**benzoyl peroxide** USAN, USP *keratolytic* 2.5%, 5%, 10% topical
**benzoyl peroxide & erythromycin** *keratolytic and antibiotic for acne* 5%• 3% topical
**m-benzoylhydratropic acid** [see: ketoprofen]
**benzoylmethylecgonine** [see: cocaine]
**benzoylpas calcium** USAN, USP *antibacterial; tuberculostatic* [also: calcium benzamidosalicylate]
**benzoylsulfanilamide** [see: sulfabenzamide]
**benzoylthiamindisulfide** [see: bisbentiamine]

**benzoylthiaminmonophosphate**
[see: benfotiamine]

**benzphetamine** BAN *anorexiant; CNS stimulant* [also: benzphetamine HCl; benzfetamine]

**benzphetamine chloride** [see: benzphetamine HCl]

**benzphetamine HCl** NF *anorexiant; CNS stimulant* [also: benzfetamine; benzphetamine]

**benzpiperylon** [see: benzpiperylone]

**benzpiperylone** INN

**benzpyrinium bromide** NF, INN

**benzquercin** INN

**benzquinamide** USAN, INN, BAN *postanesthesia antinauseant and antiemetic*

**benzthiazide** USP, INN, BAN *diuretic; antihypertensive*

**benztropine** BAN *anticholinergic; antiparkinsonian* [also: benztropine mesylate; benzatropine]

**benztropine mesylate** USP *anticholinergic; antiparkinsonian* [also: benzatropine; benztropine] 0.5, 1, 2 mg oral

**benztropine methanesulfonate** [see: benztropine mesylate]

**benzydamine** INN, BAN *analgesic; antipyretic; anti-inflammatory* [also: benzydamine HCl]

**benzydamine HCl** USAN, JAN *analgesic; antipyretic; anti-inflammatory; investigational (orphan) radioprotectant for oral mucosa following radiation therapy for head and neck cancer* [also: benzydamine]

**benzydroflumethiazide** [see: bendroflumethiazide]

**benzyl alcohol** NF, INN, JAN *antimicrobial agent; antiseptic; local anesthetic*

**benzyl analogue of serotonin (BAS)** [see: benanserin HCl]

**benzyl antiserotonin** [see: benanserin HCl]

**benzyl benzoate** USP, JAN

**benzyl carbinol** [see: phenylethyl alcohol]

**S-benzyl thiobenzoate** [see: tibenzate]

**benzylamide** [see: beclamide]

**benzylamines** *a class of antifungals structurally related to the allylamines*

**N-benzylanilinoacetamidoxime** [see: cetoxime]

**2-benzylbenzimidazole** [see: bendazol]

**benzyldimethyltetradecylammonium chloride** [see: miristalkonium chloride]

**benzyldodecyldimethylammonium chloride** [see: benzododecinium chloride]

**0-6-benzylguanine** [see: alkylade]

**benzylhexadecyldimethylammonium** [see: cetalkonium]

**benzylhexadecyldimethylammonium chloride** [see: cetalkonium chloride]

**benzylhydrochlorothiazide** JAN

**p-benzyloxyphenol** [see: monobenzone]

**benzylpenicillin** INN, BAN *natural penicillin antibiotic; investigational (orphan) for penicillin hypersensitivity assessment*

**benzylpenicillin benzathine** JAN *natural penicillin antibiotic* [also: penicillin G benzathine; benzathine benzylpenicillin; benzathine penicillin]

**benzylpenicillin potassium** BAN, JAN *natural penicillin antibiotic* [also: penicillin G potassium]

**benzylpenicillin procaine** *natural penicillin antibiotic* [see: penicillin G procaine]

**benzylpenicillin sodium** BAN *natural penicillin antibiotic* [also: penicillin G sodium]

**benzylpenicilloic acid** [see: benzylpenicillin]

**benzylpenicilloyl polylysine** USP *diagnostic aid for penicillin sensitivity*

**benzylpenilloic acid** [see: benzylpenicillin]

**benzylsulfamide** INN, DCF

**benzylsulfanilamide** [see: benzylsulfamide]

**BEP (bleomycin, etoposide, Platinol)** *chemotherapy protocol for testicular cancer and germ cell tumors*

**bepafant** INN

**bepanthen** [see: panthenol]

**beperidium iodide** INN

**bephene oxinaphthoate** [see: bephenium hydroxynaphthoate]

**bephenium embonate** [see: bephenium hydroxynaphthoate]

**bephenium hydroxynaphthoate** USP, INN, BAN

**bepiastine** INN, DCF

**bepridil** INN, BAN *vasodilator; antianginal; calcium channel blocker* [also: bepridil HCl]

**bepridil HCl** USAN *vasodilator; antianginal; calcium channel blocker* [also: bepridil]

**beractant** USAN *pulmonary surfactant for neonatal respiratory distress syndrome or respiratory failure (orphan)*

**Beraprost** ℞ *investigational (Phase III) agent for peripheral vascular disease (PVD)*

**beraprost** USAN, INN *platelet aggregation inhibitor; peripheral vasodilator; investigational (Phase III) prostacyclin analogue for peripheral vascular disease (PVD); investigational (orphan) for pulmonary arterial hypertension (PAH)*

**beraprost sodium** USAN *platelet aggregation inhibitor*

**berberine chloride** JAN

**berberine sulfate** JAN

**berberine tannate** JAN

*Berberis vulgaris* medicinal herb [see: barberry]

**berculon A** [see: thioacetazone; thiacetazone]

**berefrine** USAN, INN *mydriatic*

**bergamot, scarlet** *medicinal herb* [see: Oswego tea]

**bergamot, wild** *medicinal herb* [see: wild bergamot]

**bergamot oil (Citrus aurantium; C. bergamia)** *fruit peel medicinal herb used in conjunction with long-wave UV light therapy for psoriasis and vitiligo; not generally regarded as safe and effective because of its photosensitizing properties*

**bergenin** JAN

**Berinert-P** ℞ *investigational (orphan) agent to prevent or treat acute attacks*

*of angioedema* [C1-esterase-inhibitor, human]

**berkelium** *element (Bk)*

**berlafenone** INN

**bermastine** [see: barmastine]

**bermoprofen** INN

**Berocca** tablets ℞ *vitamin supplement* [multiple B vitamins; vitamin C; folic acid] ± • 500 • 0.5 mg

**Berocca Plus** tablets ℞ *vitamin/mineral/iron supplement* [multiple vitamins & minerals; ferrous fumarate; folic acid; biotin] ± • 27 • 0.8 • 0.15 mg

**Berotec** (widely available outside the U.S.) ℞ *investigational (NDA filed) bronchodilator; antiasthmatic; β-blocker* [fenoterol hydrobromide]

**Berplex Plus** tablets (discontinued 2000) ℞ *vitamin/mineral/iron supplement* [multiple vitamins & minerals; ferrous fumarate; folic acid; biotin] ± • 27 • 0.8 • 0.15 mg

**bertosamil** INN

**beryllium** *element (Be)*

**berythromycin** USAN, INN *antiamebic; antibacterial*

**besigomsin** INN

**besilate** INN *combining name for radicals or groups* [also: besylate]

**besipirdine** INN *cognition enhancer for Alzheimer disease* [also: besipiridine HCl]

**besipirdine HCl** USAN *cognition enhancer for Alzheimer disease* [also: besipiridine]

**besulpamide** INN

**besunide** INN

**besylate** USAN *combining name for radicals or groups* [also: besilate]

**beta alethine** *investigational (Phase I/II, orphan) antineoplastic and immunostimulant for B-cell lymphoma, multiple myeloma, and metastatic melanoma*

**beta blockers** (β-blockers) *a class of cardiac agents characterized by their antihypertensive, antiarrhythmic, and antianginal actions; a class of topical antiglaucoma agents* [also called: beta-adrenergic antagonists]

**beta carotene** USAN, USP *vitamin A precursor* [also: betacarotene] 15 mg (25 000 IU) oral

**beta cyclodextrin (β-cyclodextrin)** *(previously used NF name)* [now: betadex]

**Beta LT** ℞ *investigational (Phase I/II, orphan) antineoplastic and immunostimulant for B cell lymphoma, multiple myeloma, and metastatic melanoma* [beta alethine]

**betacarotene** INN *vitamin A precursor* [also: beta carotene]

**betacetylmethadol** INN, BAN

**Betachron E-R** extended-release capsules (discontinued 2001) ℞ *antiarrhythmic; antihypertensive; antianginal; antiadrenergic (β-blocker); migraine prophylaxis* [propranolol HCl] 60, 80, 120, 160 mg

**betadex** USAN, INN *sequestering agent* [previous NF name: beta cyclodextrin]

**beta-D-galactosidase** *digestive enzyme* [see: tilactase]

**Betadine** aerosol, gauze pads, lubricating gel, cream, ointment, skin cleanser, foam, solution, swab, swabsticks OTC *broad-spectrum antimicrobial* [povidone-iodine] 5%; 10%; 5%; 5%; 10%; 7.5%; 7.5%; 10%; 10%; 10%

**Betadine** mouthwash, perineal wash, surgical scrub (discontinued 2003) OTC *broad-spectrum antimicrobial* [povidone-iodine] 0.5%; 10%; 7.5%

**Betadine** shampoo OTC *broad-spectrum antimicrobial for dandruff* [povidone-iodine] 7.5%

**Betadine 5% Sterile Ophthalmic Prep** solution ℞ *broad-spectrum antimicrobial for eye surgery* [povidone-iodine] 5%

**Betadine First Aid Antibiotics Plus Moisturizer** ointment OTC *antibiotic* [polymyxin B sulfate; bacitracin zinc] 10 000•500 IU/g

**Betadine Medicated** vaginal suppositories, vaginal gel OTC *antiseptic/germicidal; vaginal cleanser and deodorant* [povidone-iodine] 10%

**Betadine Medicated Douche; Betadine Medicated Disposable Douche; Betadine Premixed Medicated Disposable Douche** solution OTC *antiseptic/germicidal; vaginal cleanser and deodorant* [povidone-iodine] 10%

**Betadine Plus First Aid Antibiotics and Pain Reliever** ointment OTC *topical antibiotic and anesthetic* [polymyxin B sulfate; bacitracin zinc; pramoxine HCl] 10 000 IU•500 IU•10 mg per g

**Betadine PrepStick** swab OTC *broad-spectrum antimicrobial* [povidone-iodine] 10%

**Betadine PrepStick Plus** swab OTC *broad-spectrum antimicrobial* [povidone-iodine; alcohol] 10%• ²

**beta-estradiol** [see: estradiol]

**beta-estradiol benzoate** [see: estradiol benzoate]

**betaeucaine HCl** [now: eucaine HCl]

**Betagan Liquifilm** eye drops ℞ *topical antiglaucoma agent (β-blocker)* [levobunolol HCl] 0.25%, 0.5% ☒ Betagen

**Betagen** ointment, solution, surgical scrub OTC *broad-spectrum antimicrobial* [povidone-iodine] 1%; 10%; 7.5% ☒ Betagan

**beta-glucocerebrosidase** [see: alglucerase]

**betahistine** INN, BAN *vasodilator* [also: betahistine HCl; betahistine mesilate]

**betahistine HCl** USAN *vasodilator* [also: betahistine; betahistine mesilate]

**betahistine mesilate** JAN *vasodilator* [also: betahistine HCl; betahistine]

**beta-hypophamine** [see: vasopressin]

**betaine HCl** USP *electrolyte replenisher for homocystinuria (orphan)*

**Betaject** Ⓒᴬᴺ injection ℞ *corticosteroidal anti-inflammatory* [betamethasone sodium phosphate; betamethasone acetate] 3•3 mg/mL

**beta-lactams** *a class of antibiotics*

**beta-lactone** [see: propiolactone]

**betameprodine** INN, BAN, DCF

**betamethadol** INN, BAN, DCF

**betamethasone** USAN, USP, INN, BAN, JAN *corticosteroid; anti-inflammatory*

**betamethasone acetate** USP, JAN *corticosteroid; anti-inflammatory*

**betamethasone acibutate** INN, BAN *corticosteroid; anti-inflammatory*

**betamethasone benzoate** USAN, USP, BAN *topical corticosteroidal anti-inflammatory*

**betamethasone dipropionate** USAN, USP, BAN, JAN *topical corticosteroidal anti-inflammatory* 0.05% topical

**betamethasone dipropionate, augmented** *topical corticosteroidal anti-inflammatory* 0.05% topical

**betamethasone dipropionate & clotrimazole** *corticosteroidal anti-inflammatory; broad-spectrum antifungal* 0.05%•1% topical

**betamethasone sodium phosphate** USP, BAN, JAN *corticosteroid; anti-inflammatory*

**betamethasone valerate** USAN, USP, BAN, JAN *topical corticosteroidal anti-inflammatory; investigational (NDA filed) mousse for scalp psoriasis* 0.1% topical

**betamicin** INN *antibacterial* [also: betamicin sulfate]

**betamicin sulfate** USAN *antibacterial* [also: betamicin]

**betamipron** INN

**betanaphthol** NF

**betanidine** INN *antihypertensive* [also: bethanidine sulfate; bethanidine; betanidine sulfate]

**betanidine sulfate** JAN *antihypertensive* [also: bethanidine sulfate; betanidine; bethanidine]

**Betapace** tablets ℞ *antiarrhythmic (β-blocker) for life-threatening ventricular arrhythmias (orphan)* [sotalol HCl] 80, 120, 160, 240 mg

**Betapace AF** tablets ℞ *antiarrhythmic (β-blocker) for atrial fibrillation or atrial flutter* [sotalol HCl] 80, 120, 160 mg

**betaprodine** INN, BAN, DCF

**beta-propiolactone** [see: propiolactone]

**beta-pyridylcarbinol** [see: nicotinyl alcohol]

**BetaRx** *investigational (orphan) antidiabetic for type 1 patients on immunosuppression* [porcine islet preparation, encapsulated]

**Betasept** topical liquid OTC *broad-spectrum antimicrobial; germicidal* [chlorhexidine gluconate; alcohol 4%] 4%

**Betaseron** powder for subcu injection ℞ *immunomodulator for relapsing-remitting multiple sclerosis (orphan)* [interferon beta-1b] 0.25 mg (8 MIU)/dose

**BetaSite** ℞ *investigational (Phase III) agent for glaucoma* [levobunolol]

**Betathine** *investigational (orphan) antineoplastic and immunostimulant for multiple myeloma and metastatic melanoma* [beta alethine]

**Betatrex** cream, ointment, lotion (discontinued 2003) ℞ *corticosteroidal anti-inflammatory* [betamethasone valerate] 0.1%

**Beta-Val** cream, lotion ℞ *topical corticosteroidal anti-inflammatory* [betamethasone valerate] 0.1%

**betaxolol** INN, BAN *antianginal; antihypertensive; topical antiglaucoma agent (β-blocker)* [also: betaxolol HCl]

**betaxolol HCl** USAN, USP *antianginal; antihypertensive; topical antiglaucoma agent (β-blocker)* [also: betaxolol] 0.5% eye drops

**Betaxon** eye drops ℞ *topical antiglaucoma agent (β-blocker)* [levobetaxolol HCl] 0.5%

**betazole** INN [also: betazole HCl; ametazole]

**betazole HCl** USP [also: betazole; ametazole]

**betazolium chloride** [see: betazole HCl]

**betel nut** *(Areca catechu)* leaves and quids (a mixture of tobacco, powdered or sliced areca nut, and slaked lime wrapped in a *Piper betel* leaf) *medicinal herb used as a digestive aid and mild stimulant; not generally regarded as safe and effective as it causes leukoplakia and oral cancer*

**beth root** *medicinal herb* [see: birthroot]

**bethanechol chloride** USP, BAN, JAN *cholinergic urinary stimulant for post-surgical and postpartum urinary retention* 5, 10, 25, 50 mg oral

**bethanidine** BAN *antihypertensive* [also: bethanidine sulfate; betanidine; betanidine sulfate]

**bethanidine sulfate** USAN *antihypertensive; investigational (orphan) agent for the prevention and treatment of primary ventricular fibrillation* [also: betanidine; bethanidine; betanidine sulfate]

**betiatide** USAN, INN, BAN *pharmaceutic aid*

**Betimol** eye drops ℞ *antiglaucoma agent (β-blocker)* [timolol hemihydrate] 0.25%, 0.5%

*Betonica officinalis* medicinal herb [now: *Stachys officinalis*] [see: betony]

**betony (Stachys officinalis)** plant *medicinal herb for anxiety, delirium, diarrhea, fever, jaundice, liver and spleen sclerosis, migraine headache, mouth or throat irritation, nervousness, palpitations, and toothache; also used as a purgative and emetic agent*

**Betoptic; Betoptic S** Drop-Tainers (eye drops) ℞ *topical antiglaucoma agent (β-blocker)* [betaxolol HCl] 0.5%; 0.25%

**betoxycaine** INN

**betoxycaine HCl** [see: betoxycaine]

**betula oil** [see: methyl salicylate]

*Betula spp.* medicinal herb [see: birch]

**Betuline** lotion OTC *analgesic; counterirritant* [methyl salicylate; camphor; menthol; peppermint oil]

**bevacizumab** *antineoplastic; recombinant humanized monoclonal antibody (rhuMAb) to vascular endothelial growth factor (VEGF); angiogenesis inhibitor for metastatic colorectal cancer; investigational (Phase III) for breast, cervical, lung, and renal cancers*

**bevantolol** INN, BAN *antianginal; antihypertensive; antiarrhythmic* [also: bevantolol HCl]

**bevantolol HCl** USAN *antianginal; antihypertensive; antiarrhythmic* [also: bevantolol]

**bevonium methylsulphate** BAN [also: bevonium metilsulfate]

**bevonium metilsulfate** INN [also: bevonium methylsulphate]

**bexarotene** USAN *synthetic retinoid analogue antineoplastic for cutaneous T-cell lymphoma (orphan); investigational (Phase III) for lung cancer*

**bexlosteride** USAN *antineoplastic 5α-reductase inhibitor for prostate cancer*

**Bextra** film-coated caplets ℞ *COX-2 inhibitor; nonsteroidal anti-inflammatory drug (NSAID) for osteoarthritis (OA), rheumatoid arthritis (RA), and primary dysmenorrhea* [valdecoxib] 10, 20 mg

**Bexxar Dosimetric Package** IV infusion ℞ *first of two steps in the radiotherapeutic treatment of non-Hodgkin lymphoma (NHL)* [tositumomab; iodine I 131 tositumomab] 450•35 mg (5 mCi of radiation)

**Bexxar Therapeutic Package** IV infusion ℞ *second of two steps in the radiotherapeutic treatment of non-Hodgkin lymphoma (NHL)* [tositumomab; iodine I 131 tositumomab] 450•35 mg (delivers 65–75 cGy of radiation)

**bezafibrate** USAN, INN, BAN, JAN *antihyperlipidemic*

**bezitramide** INN, BAN, DCF

**bezomil** INN *combining name for radicals or groups*

**bFGF (basic fibroblast growth factor)** [see: ersofermin]

**B.F.I. Antiseptic** powder OTC *topical antiseptic* [bismuth-formic-iodide] 16%

**BGM-24** *investigational for prostatitis*

**BHA (butylated hydroxyanisole)** [q.v.]

**BHAPs (bisheteroarylpiperazines)** *a class of antiviral drugs*

**BHD (BCNU, hydroxyurea, dacarbazine)** *chemotherapy protocol*

**BHDV; BHD-V (BCNU, hydroxy-urea, dacarbazine, vincristine)** *chemotherapy protocol*

**BHT (butylated hydroxytoluene)** [q.v.]

**bialamicol** INN, BAN *antiamebic* [also: bialamicol HCl]

**bialamicol HCl** USAN *antiamebic* [also: bialamicol]

**biallylamicol** [see: bialamicol]

**biantrazole** [now: losoxantrone HCl]

**biapenem** USAN, INN *antibacterial*

**Biavax II** powder for subcu injection ℞ *mumps and rubella vaccine* [mumps and rubella virus vaccine, live] 1000•20 000 U/0.5 mL

**Biaxin** Filmtabs (film-coated tablets), granules for oral suspension ℞ *macrolide antibiotic* [clarithromycin] 250, 500 mg; 125, 187.5, 250 mg/5 mL ⊘ Axid

**Biaxin XL** film-coated extended-release tablets ℞ *once-daily macrolide antibiotic* [clarithromycin] 500 mg

**bibapcitide** USAN *glycoprotein (GP) IIb/IIIa receptor antagonist; investigational (Phase III) diagnostic imaging aid for deep vein thrombosis*

**bibenzonium bromide** INN, BAN

**bibrocathin** [see: bibrocathol]

**bibrocathol** INN, DCF

**bicalutamide** USAN, INN, BAN *antiandrogen antineoplastic for prostatic cancer*

**bicalutamide + LHRH-A (bicalutamide, goserelin acetate [Zoladex subcu implant])** *chemotherapy protocol for prostate cancer*

**bicalutamide + LHRH-A (bicalutamide, leuprolide acetate [Lupron Depot injection])** *chemotherapy protocol for prostate cancer*

**Bichloracetic Acid** topical liquid ℞ *cauterant; keratolytic* [dichloroacetic acid] 10 mL ⊘ dichloroacetic acid

**bicifadine** INN *analgesic* [also: bicifadine HCl]

**bicifadine HCl** USAN *analgesic* [also: bicifadine]

**Bicillin C-R; Bicillin C-R 900/300** Tubex (cartridge-needle unit) for deep IM injection ℞ *natural penicillin antibiotic* [penicillin G benzathine; penicillin G procaine] 300 000•300 000, 600 000•600 000, 1 200 000•1 200 000 U; 900 000•300 000 U ⊘ V-Cillin; Wycillin

**Bicillin L-A** Tubex (cartridge-needle unit) for deep IM injection ℞ *natural penicillin antibiotic* [penicillin G benzathine] 600 000, 1 200 000, 2 400 000 U

**biciromab** USAN, INN, BAN *antifibrin monoclonal antibody*

**Bicitra** oral solution ℞ *urinary alkalinizing agent* [sodium citrate; citric acid] 500•334 mg/5 mL

**biclodil** INN *antihypertensive; vasodilator* [also: biclodil HCl]

**biclodil HCl** USAN *antihypertensive; vasodilator* [also: biclodil]

**biclofibrate** INN, DCF

**biclotymol** INN, DCF

**BiCNU** powder for IV injection ℞ *nitrosourea-type alkylating antineoplastic for brain tumors, multiple myeloma, Hodgkin disease and non-Hodgkin lymphomas* [carmustine] 100 mg/dose

**bicozamycin** INN

**Bicozene** cream OTC *topical local anesthetic; antifungal* [benzocaine; resorcinol] 6%•1.67%

**bicyclomycin** [see: bicozamycin]

**bidCAP** (trademarked dosage form) *twice-daily capsule*

**Bidil** ℞ *investigational (NDA filed) nitric oxide donor; investigational vasodilator for congestive heart failure* [hydralazine; isosorbide dinitrate]

**bidimazium iodide** INN, BAN

**bidisomide** USAN, INN *antiarrhythmic*

**Biebrich scarlet red** [see: scarlet red]

**Biebrich scarlet-picroaniline blue**

**bietamiverine** INN

**bietamiverine HCl** [see: bietamiverine]

**bietaserpine** INN, DCF

**bifemelane** INN [also: bifemelane HCl]

**bifemelane HCl** JAN [also: bifemelane]

**bifepramide** INN

**bifeprofen** INN

**bifeprunox** *investigational (Phase III) dopamine agonist for schizophrenia*

*Bifidobacterium longum infantis* **35624** *investigational (orphan) agent for pediatric Crohn disease*

**bifluranol** INN, BAN

**bifonazole** USAN, INN, BAN, JAN *antifungal*

**Big Shot B-12** tablets OTC *vitamin B$_{12}$ supplement* [cyanocobalamin] 5000 μg

*Bignonia sempervirens medicinal herb* [see: gelsemium]

**bilberry (Myrtilli fructus; Vaccinium myrtillus)** *fruit medicinal herb for cold hands and feet, diarrhea, edema, increasing microvascular blood flow, gastroenteritis, mucous membrane inflammation, night blindness, and varicose veins*

**bile acid sequestrants** *a class of antihyperlipidemic agents*

**bile acids, conjugated** *investigational (orphan) agent for steatorrhea in short bowel syndrome*

**bile acids, oxidized** [see: dehydrocholic acid]

**bile salts** BAN *digestive enzymes; laxative*

**BiliCheck** breath analyzer device *in vitro diagnostic aid for infant jaundice*

**Bili-Labstix** reagent strips *in vitro diagnostic aid for multiple urine products*

**Bilopaque** capsules (discontinued 2001) R̸ *radiopaque contrast medium for cholecystography* [tyropanoate sodium (57.4% iodine)] 750 mg (430.5 mg)

**Biltricide** film-coated tablets R̸ *anthelmintic for schistosomiasis (flukes)* [praziquantel] 600 mg

**bimakalim** INN

**bimatoprost** *topical prostamide analogue for glaucoma and ocular hypertension*

**bimazol** [see: carbimazole]

**bimethadol** [see: dimepheptanol]

**bimethoxycaine lactate**

**bimosiamose disodium** USAN *anti-inflammatory for asthma, psoriasis, and reperfusion injury following transplants or coronary revascularization*

**bindarit** USAN, INN *antirheumatic; investigational (orphan) for lupus nephritis*

**bindazac** [see: bendazac]

**binedaline** INN

**binetrakin** USAN *immunomodulator for gastrointestinal carcinoma and rheumatoid arthritis*

**binfloxacin** USAN, INN *veterinary antibacterial*

**binifibrate** INN

**biniramycin** USAN, INN *antibacterial antibiotic*

**binizolast** INN

**binodaline** [see: binedaline]

**binospirone** INN *anxiolytic* [also: binospirone mesylate]

**binospirone mesylate** USAN *anxiolytic* [also: binospirone]

**bioallethrin** BAN *pediculicide*

**Biobrane** wound dressing *nylon fabric matrix bound to a silicon film*

**Biobrane-L** light adherence wound dressing *nylon fabric matrix bound to a silicon film*

**Biocef** capsules, powder for oral suspension R̸ *cephalosporin antibiotic* [cephalexin] 500 mg; 250 mg/5 mL

**Bioclate** powder for IV injection R̸ *antihemophilic to correct coagulation deficiency* [antihemophilic factor concentrate, recombinant] 250, 500, 1000 IU

**BioCox** intradermal injection (discontinued 2003) R̸ *diagnostic aid for coccidioidomycosis* [coccidioidin] 1:100, 1:10

**Biocult-GC** culture paddles for professional use *in vitro diagnostic aid for Neisseria gonorrhoeae*

**Biodine Topical** solution OTC *broad-spectrum antimicrobial* [povidone-iodine] 1%

**bioflavonoids (vitamin P)** *a group of more than 4000 natural substances with widespread biological activity, including anthelmintic, antimicrobial, antimalarial, antineoplastic, antioxidant, anti-inflammatory, and antiviral activity; historically named "vitamin P"*

**biogastrone** [see: carbenoxolone]

**BioGlue** R̸ *investigational (NDA filed) surgical adhesive for cardiovascular and pulmonary repair*

**Biohist-LA** sustained-release tablets R̸ *decongestant; antihistamine* [pseudoephedrine HCl; chlorpheniramine maleate] 120•12 mg

**Biojector 2000** (trademarked delivery system) ℞ *investigational (Phase I) jet injector for malaria DNA vaccine*

**biological indicator for dry-heat sterilization** USP *sterilization indicator*

**biological indicator for ethylene oxide sterilization** USP *sterilization indicator*

**biological indicator for steam sterilization** USP *sterilization indicator*

**Bion Tears** eye drops OTC *ophthalmic moisturizer/lubricant* [hydroxypropyl methylcellulose] 0.3%

**bioral** [see: carbenoxolone]

**Bio-Rescue** ℞ *investigational (orphan) chelating agent for acute iron poisoning* [dextran; deferoxamine]

**bioresmethrin** INN

**bios I** [see: inositol]

**bios II** [see: biotin]

**Biosafe HbA1c** (hemoglobin A1c) test kit for home use *in vitro diagnostic aid for glycemic control*

**Biosafe PSA** (prostate-specific antigen) test kit for home use *in vitro diagnostic aid for prostate function*

**Biosafe Total Cholesterol** (only) test kit for home use *in vitro diagnostic aid for hypercholesterolemia*

**Biosafe Total Cholesterol Panel** (includes HDL, LDL, and triglycerides) test kit for home use *in vitro diagnostic aid for hypercholesterolemia and hypertriglyceridemia*

**Biosafe TSH** (thyroid-stimulating hormone) test kit for home use *in vitro diagnostic aid for thyroid function*

**Biosynject** ℞ *investigational (orphan) for newborn hemolytic disease and ABO blood incompatibility of organ or bone marrow transplants* [trisaccharides A and B]

**biosynthetic human parathyroid hormone (1-34)** [see: teriparatide]

**Bio-Tab** film-coated tablets (discontinued 2003) ℞ *tetracycline antibiotic* [doxycycline hyclate] 100 mg

**Biotab** tablets (discontinued 2002) OTC *decongestant; antihistamine; analgesic* [phenylpropanolamine HCl; phenyltoloxamine citrate; acetaminophen]

**Biotel kidney** reagent strips *in vitro diagnostic aid for urine hemoglobin, RBCs, and albumin (predictor of kidney diseases)*

**biotexin** [see: novobiocin]

**Bio-Throid** capsules ℞ *thyroid replacement therapy for hypothyroidism or thyroid cancer* [thyroid, desiccated (porcine)] 7.5, 15, 30, 60, 90, 120, 150, 180, 240 mg

**biotin** USP, INN, JAN *B complex vitamin; vitamin H*

**Biotin Forte** tablets OTC *vitamin supplement* [multiple B vitamins; vitamin C; folic acid; biotin] ±•200• 0.8•3 mg, ±•100•0.8•5 mg

**BIP (bleomycin, ifosfamide [with mesna rescue], Platinol)** *chemotherapy protocol for cervical cancer*

**bipenamol** INN *antidepressant* [also: bipenamol HCl]

**bipenamol HCl** USAN *antidepressant* [also: bipenamol]

**biperiden** USP, INN, BAN, JAN *anticholinergic; antiparkinsonian*

**biperiden HCl** USP, BAN, JAN *anticholinergic; antiparkinsonian*

**biperiden lactate** USP, BAN, JAN *anticholinergic; antiparkinsonian*

**biphasic insulin** [see: insulin, biphasic]

**biphenamine HCl** USAN *topical anesthetic; antibacterial; antifungal* [also: xenysalate]

**biprofenide** [see: bifepramide]

**birch (*Betula* spp.)** bark and leaves *medicinal herb for bladder problems, blood cleansing, and eczema*

**birch oil, sweet** [see: methyl salicylate]

**bird lime** *medicinal herb* [see: mistletoe]

**bird pepper** *medicinal herb* [see: cayenne]

**bird's nest root** *medicinal herb* [see: carrot]

**biricodar dicitrate** USAN *investigational (Phase II) multi-drug–resistance inhibitor for prostate and ovarian cancers*

**biriperone** INN

**birthroot** *(Trillium erectum; T. grandiflorum; T. pendulum)* plant *medicinal herb for insect and snake bites, stimulating menses and diaphoresis, and stopping bleeding after childbirth; also used as an antiseptic and astringent*

**birthwort** *(Aristolochia clematitis)* root and flowering plant *medicinal herb used as a diaphoretic, emmenagogue, febrifuge, oxytocic, and stimulant*

**Bisac-Evac** enteric-coated tablets, suppositories OTC *stimulant laxative* [bisacodyl] 5 mg; 10 mg

**bisacodyl** USP, INN, BAN, JAN *stimulant laxative* 5 mg oral; 10 mg suppositories

**bisacodyl tannex** USAN *stimulant laxative*

**Bisa-Lax** enteric-coated tablets, suppositories OTC *stimulant laxative* [bisacodyl] 5 mg; 10 mg

**bisantrene** INN *antineoplastic* [also: bisantrene HCl]

**bisantrene HCl** USAN *antineoplastic* [also: bisantrene]

**bisaramil** INN

**bisatin** [see: oxyphenisatin acetate]

**bisbendazole** INN

**bisbentiamine** INN, JAN

**bisbutiamine** [see: bisbutitiamine]

**bisbutitiamine** JAN

**bis-chloroethyl-nitrosourea (BCNU)** [see: carmustine]

**bisdequalinium diacetate** JAN

**bisfenazone** INN, DCF

**bisfentidine** INN

**bisheteroarylpiperazines (BHAPs)** *a class of antiviral drugs*

**bishop's wort** *medicinal herb* [see: nutmeg; betony]

**bishydroxycoumarin** [now: dicumarol]

**bisibutiamine** JAN [also: sulbutiamine]

**Bismatrol** chewable tablets, oral liquid OTC *antidiarrheal; antinauseant* [bismuth subsalicylate] 262 mg; 524 mg/5 mL

**bismucatebrol** [see: bibrocathol]

**bismuth** *element (Bi)*

**bismuth, milk of** USP *antacid; astringent*

**bismuth aluminate** USAN

**bismuth betanaphthol** USP

**bismuth carbonate** USAN

**bismuth carbonate, basic** [see: bismuth subcarbonate]

**bismuth citrate** USP

**bismuth cream** [see: bismuth, milk of]

**bismuth gallate, basic** [see: bismuth subgallate]

**bismuth glycollylarsanilate** BAN [also: glycobiarsol]

**bismuth hydroxide** [see: bismuth, milk of]

**bismuth hydroxide nitrate oxide** [see: bismuth subnitrate]

**bismuth magma** [now: bismuth, milk of]

**bismuth magnesium aluminosilicate** JAN

**bismuth oxycarbonate** [see: bismuth subcarbonate]

**bismuth potassium tartrate** NF

**bismuth sodium triglycollamate** USP

**bismuth subcarbonate** USAN, JAN *antacid; GI adsorbent*

**bismuth subgallate** USAN, USP *antacid; GI adsorbent*

**bismuth subnitrate** USP, JAN *skin protectant*

**bismuth subsalicylate (BSS)** USAN, JAN *antiperistaltic; antacid; GI adsorbent*

**bisnafide dimesylate** USAN *antineoplastic; DNA and RNA synthesis inhibitor*

**bisobrin** INN *fibrinolytic* [also: bisobrin lactate]

**bisobrin lactate** USAN *fibrinolytic* [also: bisobrin]

**Bisolvon** ℞ *investigational (orphan) agent for keratoconjunctivitis sicca of Sjögren syndrome* [bromhexine HCl]

**bisoprolol** USAN, INN, BAN *antihypertensive (β-blocker)*

**bisoprolol fumarate** USAN, JAN *antihypertensive (β-blocker)* 5, 10 mg oral

**bisoprolol fumarate & hydrochlorothiazide** *antihypertensive; β-blocker; diuretic* 2.5•6.5, 5•6.5, 10•6.5 mg oral

**bisorcic** INN

**bisoxatin** INN, BAN *laxative* [also: bisoxatin acetate]

**bisoxatin acetate** USAN *laxative* [also: bisoxatin]

**Bispan** ℞ *investigational agent for rheumatoid arthritis* [IPL-423 (code name —generic name not yet assigned)]

**bispecific antibody 520C9x22** *investigational (orphan) for ovarian cancer*

**bisphosphonates** *a class of calcium-regulating agents that inhibit normal and abnormal bone resorption*

**bispyrithione magsulfex** USAN *antibacterial; antidandruff; antifungal*

**bistort (Polygonum bistorta)** root *medicinal herb for bleeding, cholera, cuts, diarrhea, dysentery, gum disease (mouthwash), and hemorrhoids*

**bis-tropamide** [now: tropicamide]

**Bite Rx** solution OTC *astringent wet dressing (Burow solution) for insect bites* [aluminum acetate] 0.5%

**bithionol** NF, INN, BAN, JAN *investigational anti-infective for paragonimiasis and fascioliasis*

**bithionolate sodium** USAN *topical anti-infective* [also: sodium bitionolate]

**bithionoloxide** INN

**Bitin** (available only from the Centers for Disease Control) ℞ *investigational anti-infective for paragonimiasis and fascioliasis* [bithionol]

**bitipazone** INN

**bitolterol** INN, BAN *sympathomimetic bronchodilator* [also: bitolterol mesylate; bitolterol mesilate]

**bitolterol mesilate** JAN *sympathomimetic bronchodilator* [also: bitolterol mesylate; bitolterol]

**bitolterol mesylate** USAN *sympathomimetic bronchodilator* [also: bitolterol; bitolterol mesilate]

**bitoscanate** INN

**bitter ash** *medicinal herb* [see: quassia; wahoo]

**bitter ash; bitter quassia; bitter wood** *medicinal herb* [see: quassia]

**bitter buttons** *medicinal herb* [see: tansy]

**bitter cardamom (Alpinia fructus; A. oxyphylla)** *medicinal herb for* dementia, excessive water loss, and gastric lesions

**bitter cucumber** *medicinal herb* [see: bitter melon]

**bitter dogbane** *medicinal herb* [see: dogbane]

**bitter grass** *medicinal herb* [see: star grass]

**bitter herb** *medicinal herb* [see: centaury]

**bitter melon (Momordica charantia)** fruit, leaves, seeds, oil *medicinal herb used as an antimicrobial and hypoglycemic; also used to reduce fertility in both males and females, and can act as an abortifacient*

**bitter quassia; bitter ash; bitter wood** *medicinal herb* [see: quassia tree]

**bitter tonics; bitters** *a class of agents that have a bitter taste, used as tonics, alteratives, or appetizers*

**bitter wintergreen** *medicinal herb* [see: pipsissewa]

**bitter wood; bitter ash; bitter quassia** *medicinal herb* [see: quassia tree]

**bitterroot; bitterwort** *medicinal herb* [see: dogbane; gentian]

**bitters; bitter tonics** *a class of agents that have a bitter taste, used as tonics, alteratives, or appetizers*

**bittersweet herb; bittersweet twigs** *medicinal herb* [see: bittersweet nightshade]

**bittersweet nightshade (Solanum dulcamara)** *medicinal herb for topical application on abrasions and felons; not generally regarded as safe and effective for internal use as it is highly toxic*

**bitterweed** *medicinal herb* [see: fleabane; horseweed]

**bitterwort; bitterroot** *medicinal herb* [see: gentian]

**bivalirudin** USAN *anticoagulant; thrombin inhibitor for DVT and unstable angina, and to prevent reocclusion in MI and angioplasty*

**bizelesin** USAN, INN *antineoplastic*

**B-Ject-100** injection ℞ *parenteral vitamin therapy* [multiple B vitamins]

**black alder (Alnus glutinosa)** bark and leaves *medicinal herb used as an*

*astringent, demulcent, emetic, hemo-
static, and tonic*

**black alder dogwood** *medicinal herb*
[see: buckthorn; cascara sagrada]

**black birch** *medicinal herb* [see: birch]

**black cherry; poison black cherry**
*medicinal herb* [see: belladonna]

**black choke** *medicinal herb* [see: wild
black cherry]

**black cohosh (Cimicifuga racemosa)**
root and rhizome *medicinal herb for
asthma, bronchitis, dysmenorrhea, dyspepsia, epilepsy, hypertension, hormone
imbalance, lung disorders, menopause,
rheumatism, snake bite, sore throat,
St. Vitus dance, and tuberculosis*

**black currant (Ribes nigrum)** *medicinal herb* [see: currant]

**black dogwood** *medicinal herb* [see:
buckthorn; cascara sagrada]

**black elder** *medicinal herb* [see: elder-
berry]

**black false hellebore (Veratrum
niger)** [see: hellebore]

**black ginger** *medicinal herb* [see: ginger]

**black hellebore (Helleborus niger)**
[see: hellebore]

**black mulberry (Morus nigra)** *medicinal herb* [see: mulberry]

**black oak (Quercus tinctoria)** *medicinal herb* [see: white oak]

**black poplar (Populus nigra; P. trem-
ula)** buds *medicinal herb used as a diaphoretic, diuretic, expectorant, and
vulnerary*

**black root** *medicinal herb* [see: Culver
root]

**black sanicle** *medicinal herb* [see: sani-
cle]

**black snakeroot** *medicinal herb* [see:
black cohosh; sanicle]

**black walnut (Juglans nigra)** hulls
and leaves *medicinal herb for parasites, ringworm, skin rashes, and stopping lactation; also used as an external
antiseptic*

**black widow spider antivenin** [see:
antivenin (Latrodectus mactans)]

**black willow (Salix nigra)** *medicinal
herb* [see: willow]

**blackberry (Rubus fructicosus; R.
villosus)** berries, leaves, and root bark
*medicinal herb for bleeding, cholera,
diarrhea in children, dysentery, sinus
drainage, and vomiting*

**Black-Draught** syrup (discontinued
2003) OTC *stimulant laxative* [casan-
thranol; senna extract; alcohol 5%]
90• ≗ mg/15 mL

**Black-Draught** tablets, granules OTC
*stimulant laxative* [sennosides] 6 mg;
20 mg/5 mL

**blackwort** *medicinal herb* [see: comfrey]

**bladder fucus; bladderwrack** *medicinal herb* [see: kelp (Fucus)]

**bladderpod** *medicinal herb* [see: lobelia]

**Blairex Lens Lubricant** solution OTC
*rewetting solution for soft contact lenses*

**Blairex Sterile Saline** aerosol solution OTC *rinsing/storage solution for
soft contact lenses* [sodium chloride
(saline solution)]

**blastomycin** NF

**blazing star** *medicinal herb* [see: star
grass]

**blazing star (Liatris scariosa; L. spi-
cata; L. squarrosa)** root *medicinal
herb used as a diuretic*

**BlemErase** lotion (discontinued 2003)
OTC *keratolytic for acne* [benzoyl per-
oxide] 10%

**Blenoxane** powder for IM, IV, subcu,
or intrapleural injection ℞ *antibiotic
antineoplastic for lymphomas, testicular
and squamous cell carcinomas and
malignant pleural effusion (orphan)*
[bleomycin sulfate] 15, 30 U

**BLEO-COMF (bleomycin, cyclo-
phosphamide, Oncovin, methotrexate, fluorouracil)** *chemotherapy
protocol*

**bleomycin (BLM)** INN, BAN *glycopeptide antibiotic antineoplastic* [also: bleomycin sulfate; bleomycin HCl] ⊘
Cleocin

**bleomycin HCl** JAN *glycopeptide antibiotic antineoplastic* [also: bleomycin
sulfate; bleomycin]

**bleomycin sulfate** USAN, USP, JAN
*glycopeptide antibiotic antineoplastic for*

*multiple carcinomas and malignant pleural effusion (orphan)* [also: bleomycin; bleomycin HCl] 15, 30 U injection

**Bleph-10** eye drops, ophthalmic ointment ℞ *antibiotic* [sulfacetamide sodium] 10%

**Blephamide** eye drop suspension, ophthalmic ointment ℞ *corticosteroidal anti-inflammatory; antibiotic* [prednisolone acetate; sulfacetamide sodium] 0.2%•10%

**blessed cardus; holy thistle** *medicinal herb* [see: blessed thistle]

**blessed thistle (*Cnicus benedictus*)** plant *medicinal herb for blood cleansing, digestive disorders, headache, hormonal imbalance, lactation disorders, liver and gallbladder ailments, menstrual disorders, poor circulation, and strengthening heart and lungs*

*Blighia sapida medicinal herb* [see: ackee]

**blind nettle (*Lamium album*)** plant and flowers *medicinal herb used as an antispasmodic, astringent, expectorant, and styptic*

**Blinx** ophthalmic solution OTC *extraocular irrigating solution* [sterile isotonic solution]

**BlisterGard** topical liquid OTC *skin protectant*

**Blistex** ointment OTC *topical antipruritic/counterirritant; mild local anesthetic; vulnerary* [camphor; phenol; allantoin] 0.5%•0.5%•1%

**Blistik** lip balm OTC *antipruritic/counterirritant; mild local anesthetic; skin protectant; sunscreen (SPF 10)* [camphor; phenol; allantoin; dimethicone; padimate O; oxybenzone] 0.5%•0.5%•1%•2%•6.6%•2.5%

**Blis-To-Sol** powder OTC *topical antifungal* [zinc undecylenate] 12%

**Blis-To-Sol** topical liquid OTC *antifungal; keratolytic* [tolnaftate] 1%

**BLM (bleomycin)** [q.v.]

**Blocadren** tablets ℞ *antihypertensive; antianginal; migraine preventative; β-blocker* [timolol maleate] 5, 10, 20 mg

**blocked ricin conjugated murine monoclonal antibodies (MAb)** [see: ricin (blocked) conjugated murine MAb]

**blood, whole** USP *blood replenisher*

**blood, whole human** [now: blood, whole]

**blood cells, human red** [now: blood cells, red]

**blood cells, red** USP *blood replenisher*

**blood group specific substances A, B & AB** USP *blood neutralizer*

**blood grouping serum, anti-A** [see: anti-A blood grouping serum]

**blood grouping serum, anti-B** [see: anti-B blood grouping serum]

**blood grouping serum, anti-C** USP *for in vitro blood testing*

**blood grouping serum, anti-c** USP *for in vitro blood testing*

**blood grouping serum, anti-D** USP *for in vitro blood testing*

**blood grouping serum, anti-E** USP *for in vitro blood testing*

**blood grouping serum, anti-e** USP *for in vitro blood testing*

**blood mononuclear cells, allogenic peripheral** *investigational (orphan) agent for pancreatic cancer*

**blood staunch** *medicinal herb* [see: fleabane; horseweed]

**blood volume expanders** *a class of therapeutic blood modifiers used to increase the volume of circulating blood* [also called: plasma expanders]

**bloodroot (*Sanguinaria canadensis*)** root and rhizome *medicinal herb for diuresis, fever, inducing emesis, nasal polyps, rheumatism, sedation, skin cancer, stimulating menstrual flow, and warts; also used in toothpaste and mouthwash; not generally regarded as safe and effective for internal use*

**Bluboro** powder packets OTC *astringent wet dressing (modified Burow solution)* [aluminum sulfate; calcium acetate]

**blue cohosh (*Caulophyllum thalictroides*)** root *medicinal herb for cramps, epilepsy, induction of labor,* menstrual flow stimulant, nerves, and chronic uterine problems

**blue curls** medicinal herb [see: woundwort]

**blue flag (Iris versicolor)** root medicinal herb used as a cathartic, diuretic, laxative, sialagogue, and vermifuge

**Blue Gel** (discontinued 2003) OTC pediculicide for lice [pyrethrins; piperonyl butoxide; petroleum distillate] 0.3% • 3% • 1.2%

**Blue Gel Muscular Pain Reliever** gel OTC topical analgesic; counterirritant [menthol]

**blue ginseng** medicinal herb [see: blue cohosh]

**blue gum tree** medicinal herb [see: eucalyptus]

**blue mountain tea** medicinal herb [see: goldenrod]

**blue pimpernel; blue skullcap** medicinal herb [see: skullcap]

**blue vervain (Verbena hastata)** plant medicinal herb for asthma, bladder and bowel disorders, bronchitis, colds, convulsions, cough, fever, insomnia, pulmonary tuberculosis, stomach upset, and worms

**blueberry** medicinal herb [see: bilberry; blue cohosh]

**bluebonnet; bluebottle** medicinal herb [see: cornflower]

**blue-green algae (Chloroplast membrane sulfolipids)** nutritional supplement for boosting the immune system

**bluensomycin** INN antibiotic

**BLyS (B lymphocyte stimulating) protein** investigational (orphan) natural immunostimulant for common variable immunodeficiency (CVI, CVID), autoimmune diseases, and B-cell tumors

**B-MOPP (bleomycin, nitrogen mustard, Oncovin, procarbazine, prednisone)** chemotherapy protocol

**BMP (BCNU, methotrexate, procarbazine)** chemotherapy protocol

**BMS 234475** investigational (Phase II) second-generation protease inhibitor for HIV infection

**BMY-45622** investigational (orphan) antineoplastic for ovarian cancer

**BOAP (bleomycin, Oncovin, Adriamycin, prednisone)** chemotherapy protocol

**Bo-Cal** tablets OTC dietary supplement [calcium; vitamin D; magnesium] 250 mg • 100 IU • 125 mg

**Body Fortress Natural Amino** tablets OTC protein supplement [protein; lactalbumin hydrolysate] 1.67 • 1.5 g

**boforsin** [see: colforsin]

**bofumustine** INN

**bogbean; bog myrtle** medicinal herb [see: buckbean]

**Boil-Ease** ointment OTC topical local anesthetic [benzocaine] 20%

**bolandiol** INN anabolic [also: bolandiol dipropionate]

**bolandiol dipropionate** USAN, JAN anabolic [also: bolandiol]

**bolasterone** USAN, INN anabolic steroid; also abused as a street drug

**bolazine** INN

**BOLD (bleomycin, Oncovin, lomustine, dacarbazine)** chemotherapy protocol

**Boldea fragrans** medicinal herb [see: boldo]

**boldenone** INN, BAN veterinary anabolic steroid; also abused as a street drug [also: boldenone undecylenate]

**boldenone undecylenate** USAN veterinary anabolic steroid; also abused as a street drug [also: boldenone]

**boldo (Peumus boldus)** plant and leaves medicinal herb for bile stimulation, colds, constipation, digestive disorders, earache, edema, gallstones, gonorrhea, gout, liver disease, rheumatism, syphilis, and worms

**Boldu boldus** medicinal herb [see: boldo]

**bolenol** USAN, INN anabolic

**bolmantalate** USAN, INN, BAN anabolic

**bolus alba** [see: kaolin]

**Bombay aloe** medicinal herb [see: aloe]

**bometolol** INN

**BOMP (bleomycin, Oncovin, Matulane, prednisone)** chemotherapy protocol

**BOMP; CLD-BOMP (bleomycin, Oncovin, mitomycin, Platinol)** *chemotherapy protocol for cervical cancer*

**Bonamil Infant Formula with Iron** powder, oral liquid OTC *total or supplementary infant feeding* 453 g; 384, 946 mL

**Bonamine** ⓒ chewable tablets OTC *anticholinergic; antihistamine; antivertigo agent; motion sickness preventative* [meclizine HCl] 25 mg ② Bonine

**bone ash** [see: calcium phosphate, tribasic]

**Bone Assure** capsules OTC *vitamin/mineral/calcium supplement to maintain bone mineral density* [calcium (from bis-glycinate); magnesium (from oxide); zinc (from citrate); manganese (from citrate); trimethylglycine; multiple vitamins and minerals] 1000•320•12•3•100• ± per 6 capsules

**Bone Meal** tablets OTC *dietary supplement* [calcium; phosphorus] 236•118 mg

**bone powder, purified** [see: calcium phosphate, tribasic]

**Bonefos** ⓒ capsules, IV infusion ℞ *bisphosphonate bone resorption inhibitor for hypercalcemia and osteolysis of malignancy (investigational (orphan) in the U.S.)* [clodronate disodium tetrahydrate] 400 mg; 60 mg/mL

**boneset (Eupatorium perfoliatum)** plant *medicinal herb for chills, colds, constipation, dengue fever, edema, fever, flu, pneumonia, and rheumatism*

**Bone-Up** capsules OTC *vitamin/mineral/calcium supplement to maintain bone mineral density* [calcium (hydroxyapatite); protein; magnesium (oxide); zinc (monomethionine); manganese; glucosamine HCl; multiple vitamins and minerals] 1000•1000•600•10•5•300• ± per 6 capsules

**Bonine** chewable tablets (discontinued 2004) OTC *anticholinergic; antihistamine; antivertigo agent; motion sickness preventative* [meclizine HCl] 25 mg

**Boniva** tablets ℞ *bone resorption inhibitor for postmenopausal osteoporosis, metastatic bone disease, hypercalcemia of malignancy, and Paget disease* [ibandronate sodium] 2.5 mg

**Boniva** extended-release (1, 3 month) tablets, IV depot ℞ *investigational (NDA filed) doseforms for postmenopausal osteoporosis* [ibandronate sodium]

**Bontril** slow-release capsules ℞ *anorexiant; CNS stimulant* [phendimetrazine tartrate] 105 mg ② Bentyl; Vontrol

**Bontril PDM** tablets ℞ *anorexiant; CNS stimulant* [phendimetrazine tartrate] 35 mg

**Bonviva** (European name for U.S. product Boniva)

**bookoo** *medicinal herb* [see: buchu]

**Boost** oral liquid, pudding OTC *enteral nutritional therapy* [milk-based formula] 237 mL

**BOP (BCNU, Oncovin, prednisone)** *chemotherapy protocol*

**BOPAM (bleomycin, Oncovin, prednisone, Adriamycin, mechlorethamine, methotrexate)** *chemotherapy protocol*

**bopindolol** INN

**BOPP (BCNU, Oncovin, procarbazine, prednisone)** *chemotherapy protocol*

**boracic acid** [see: boric acid]

**borage (Borago officinalis)** leaves *medicinal herb for bronchitis, colds, eye inflammation, hay fever, strengthening of heart, lactation stimulation, rashes, rheumatism, ringworm; not generally regarded as safe and effective*

**borax** [see: sodium borate]

**Borbonia pinifolia** *medicinal herb* [see: red bush tea]

**boric acid** NF, JAN *acidifying agent; ophthalmic emollient; antiseptic; astringent* 10% topical

**2-bornanone** [see: camphor]

**bornaprine** INN, BAN

**bornaprolol** INN

**bornelone** USAN, INN *ultraviolet screen*

**bornyl acetate** USAN

**borocaptate sodium B 10** USAN *antineoplastic; radioactive agent* [also: sodium borocaptate ($^{10}$B)]

**Borocell** ℞ *investigational (orphan) for boron neutron capture therapy (BNCT) for glioblastoma multiforme* [sodium monomercaptoundecahydro-closo-dodecaborate]

**Borofair Otic** ear drops ℞ *antibacterial; antifungal; astringent* [acetic acid; aluminum acetate] 2%•⍻

**Borofax Skin Protectant** ointment OTC *astringent* [zinc oxide] 15%

**boroglycerin** NF

**boron** *element (B); trace mineral for enhancing mental acuity and improving alertness; not generally regarded as safe and effective as it is highly toxic if taken internally or absorbed through broken skin*

**Boropak** powder packets OTC *astringent wet dressing (modified Burrow solution)* [aluminum sulfate; calcium acetate]

**bortezomib** *proteasome inhibitor; antineoplastic for multiple myeloma (orphan)*

**bosentan** USAN, INN *endothelin receptor antagonist (ERA) for pulmonary arterial hypertension (orphan)*

**Boston Advance Cleaner; Boston Cleaner** solution OTC *cleaning solution for rigid gas permeable contact lenses*

**Boston Advance Comfort Formula** solution OTC *disinfecting/wetting/soaking solution for rigid gas permeable contact lenses*

**Boston Conditioning Solution** OTC *disinfecting/wetting/soaking solution for rigid gas permeable contact lenses*

**Boston Rewetting Drops** OTC *rewetting solution for rigid gas permeable contact lenses*

**Boston Simplicity Multi-Action** solution OTC *disinfecting/wetting/soaking solution for rigid gas permeable contact lenses*

*Boswellia serrata* *medicinal herb* [see: frankincense]

**Botanol** ⓒᴬᴺ oral liquid OTC *dietary supplement* [potassium; magnesium; iron; iodine; herbal extracts] 779• 25.2•2.7•0.045•335 mg per 30 mL

**botiacrine** INN

**Botox; Botox Cosmetic** powder for injection ℞ *neurotoxin complex for blepharospasm and strabismus of dystonia (orphan), cervical dystonia (orphan), and cosmetic wrinkle treatments; investigational (orphan) for pediatric cerebral palsy* [botulinum toxin, type A] 100 U/vial

**BottomBetter** ointment OTC *topical diaper rash treatment*

**botulinum toxin, type A** *neurotoxin complex derived from* Clostridium botulinum, *type A; treatment for blepharospasm and strabismus of dystonia (orphan), cervical dystonia (orphan), and cosmetic wrinkle treatments; investigational (orphan) for pediatric cerebral palsy*

**botulinum toxin, type B** *neurotoxin complex derived from* Clostridium botulinum, *type B; symptomatic treatment of cervical dystonia (orphan)*

**botulinum toxin, type F** *investigational (orphan) neurotoxin for cervical dystonia and essential blepharospasm*

**botulinum toxoid, pentavalent (ABCDE)** (available only from the Centers for Disease Control and Prevention) *investigational vaccine*

**botulism antitoxin** USP *passive immunizing agent*

**botulism equine antitoxin, trivalent** *passive immunizing agent*

**botulism immune globulin intravenous (BIG-IV)** *treatment for infant botulism type A or B (orphan)*

**Bounty Bears** chewable tablets OTC *vitamin supplement* [multiple vitamins; folic acid] ⍻•0.3 mg

**Bounty Bears Plus Iron** chewable tablets OTC *vitamin/iron supplement* [multiple vitamins; iron; folic acid] ⍻•15•0.3 mg

**bourbonal** [see: ethyl vanillin]

**bovactant** BAN

**bovine colostrum** [see: *Cryptosporidium parvum* bovine colostrum IgG concentrate]

**bovine fibrin** BAN

**bovine immunoglobulin concentrate** [see: *Cryptosporidium parvum* bovine colostrum IgG concentrate]

**bovine superoxide dismutase (bSOD)** [see: orgotein]

**bovine whey protein concentrate** [see: *Cryptosporidium parvum* bovine colostrum IgG concentrate]

**bower, virgin's** *medicinal herb* [see: woodbine]

**Bowman's root** *medicinal herb* [see: Culver root]

**box, mountain** *medicinal herb* [see: uva ursi]

**boxberry** *medicinal herb* [see: wintergreen]

**boxidine** USAN, INN *antihyperlipoproteinemic*

**Boyol** salve OTC *topical anti-infective; anesthetic* [ichthammol; benzocaine] 10%•⚯ ⌸ boil

**B-PAS (benzoyl para-aminosalicylate)** [see: benzoylpas calcium]

**BPD-MA (benzoporphyrin derivative)** [see: verteporfin]

**B-Plex** tablets ℞ *vitamin supplement* [multiple B vitamins; vitamin C; folic acid] ⚯•500•0.5 mg

**BrachySeed I-125** implants ℞ *radioactive brachytherapy* [iodine I 125 ceramic beads] 0.19–0.65 mCi (7–24.1 MBq)

**BrachySeed Pd-103** implants ℞ *radioactive brachytherapy* [palladium Pd 103 ceramic beads] 1.0–1.8 mCi (37–66.6 MBq)

**brallobarbital** INN

**bramble** *medicinal herb* [see: blackberry]

**BranchAmin 4%** IV infusion ℞ *nutritional therapy for high metabolic stress* [multiple branched-chain essential amino acids]

**branched-chain amino acids (BCAA)** *investigational (orphan) for amyotrophic lateral sclerosis* [see: isoleucine; leucine; valine]

**brandy mint** *medicinal herb* [see: peppermint]

**Brasivol** cream OTC *abrasive cleanser for acne* [aluminum oxide]

**brasofensine maleate** USAN *investigational dopamine reuptake inhibitor for Parkinson disease*

**Brassica alba** *medicinal herb* [see: mustard]

**Bravelle** powder for subcu or IM injection ℞ *follicle-stimulating hormone (FSH); ovulation stimulant for polycystic ovary disease and assisted reproductive technologies (ART)* [urofollitropin] 75 IU

**brazergoline** INN

**Breathe Free** nasal spray OTC *nasal moisturizer* [sodium chloride (saline solution)] 0.65%

**Breezee Mist Aerosol** powder OTC *antifungal; analgesic; anhidrotic* [undecylenic acid; menthol; aluminum chlorohydrate]

**Breezee Mist Antifungal** powder OTC *antifungal* [miconazole nitrate] [note: one of two different products with the same name] 2%

**Breezee Mist Antifungal** powder OTC *antifungal* [tolnaftate] [note: one of two different products with the same name] 1%

**Breezee Mist Foot Powder** OTC *anhidrotic* [talc; aluminum chlorohydrate]

**brefonalol** INN

**bremazocine** INN

**Breonesin** capsules (discontinued 2002) OTC *expectorant* [guaifenesin] 200 mg

**brequinar** INN *antineoplastic* [also: brequinar sodium]

**brequinar sodium** USAN *antineoplastic* [also: brequinar]

**bretazenil** USAN, INN *anxiolytic*

**Brethaire** oral inhalation aerosol (discontinued 2001) ℞ *sympathomimetic bronchodilator* [terbutaline sulfate] 0.2 mg/dose

**Brethine** tablets, IV or subcu injection ℞ *sympathomimetic bronchodilator* [terbutaline sulfate] 2.5, 5 mg; 1 mg/mL ⌸ Banthine

**bretylium tosilate** INN *antiadrenergic; antiarrhythmic* [also: bretylium tosylate]

**bretylium tosylate** USAN, BAN *antiadrenergic; antiarrhythmic* [also: bretylium tosilate] 500, 1000 mg/vial injection

**Brevibloc; Brevibloc Double Strength** IV infusion ℞ *antiarrhythmic; β-blocker for supraventricular tachycardia* [esmolol HCl] 10, 250 mg/mL; 20 mg/mL

**Brevicon** tablets (in Wallettes of 28) ℞ *monophasic oral contraceptive* [norethindrone; ethinyl estradiol] 0.5 mg•35 μg

**Brevital Sodium** powder for IV injection ℞ *barbiturate general anesthetic* [methohexital sodium] 2.5 g ⬚ Bretylol

**Brevoxyl Cleansing Lotion** ℞ *keratolytic for acne* [benzoyl peroxide] 4%, 8%

**Brevoxyl-4; Brevoxyl-8** gel ℞ *keratolytic for acne* [benzoyl peroxide] 4%; 8%

**Brevoxyl-4 Creamy Wash; Brevoxyl-8 Creamy Wash** topical liquid ℞ *keratolytic for acne* [benzoyl peroxide] 4%; 8%

**brewer's yeast** *natural source of protein and B-complex vitamins*

**Brexidol 20** ⓒᵃⁿ tablets ℞ *analgesic; antirheumatic; nonsteroidal anti-inflammatory drug (NSAID)* [piroxicam betadex] 191.2 mg (=20 mg base)

**Brexin-L.A.** sustained-release capsules (discontinued 2003) ℞ *decongestant; antihistamine* [pseudoephedrine HCl; chlorpheniramine maleate] 120•8 mg

**Bricanyl** tablets, IV or subcu injection (discontinued 2001) ℞ *sympathomimetic bronchodilator* [terbutaline sulfate] 2.5, 5 mg; 1 mg/mL

**Brietal Sodium** ⓒᵃⁿ powder for IV injection (discontinued 2001) ℞ *barbiturate general anesthetic* [methohexital sodium] 10 mg/mL

**brifentanil** INN *narcotic analgesic* [also: brifentanil HCl]

**brifentanil HCl** USAN *narcotic analgesic* [also: brifentanil]

**Brigham tea; Brigham Young weed** *medicinal herb* [see: ephedra]

**Brik-Paks** (trademarked delivery form) *ready-to-use liquid containers*

**brimonidine** INN *ophthalmic $\alpha_2$-adrenergic agonist for open-angle glaucoma and ocular hypertension* [also: brimonidine tartrate]

**brimonidine tartrate** USAN *selective $\alpha_2$ agonist for open-angle glaucoma and ocular hypertension; investigational (orphan) for anterior ischemic optic neuropathy* [also: brimonidine] 0.2% eye drops

**brinaldix** [see: clopamide]

**brinase** INN [also: brinolase]

**brinazarone** INN

**brindoxime** INN

**brineurin** [now: abrineurin] [USAN changed 2000]

**brinolase** USAN *fibrinolytic enzyme* [also: brinase]

**brinzolamide** USAN, INN *topical carbonic anhydrase inhibitor for glaucoma*

**Bristoject** (trademarked delivery form) *prefilled disposable syringe*

**Brite Eyes II** eye drops OTC *moisturizer; lubricant; antioxidant and anti-glycation agent to prevent free radical damage in the lens* [N-acetyl-L-carnitine; glycerin; carboxymethylcellulose sodium] 1%•1%•0.3%

**British antilewisite (BAL)** [now: dimercaprol]

**British tobacco** *medicinal herb* [see: coltsfoot]

**brivudine** INN

**brobactam** INN

**brobenzoxaldine** [see: broxaldine]

**broclepride** INN

**brocresine** USAN, INN, BAN *histidine decarboxylase inhibitor*

**brocrinat** USAN, INN *diuretic*

**brodimoprim** INN

**brofaromine** INN *investigational reversible/selective MAO inhibitor*

**Brofed** oral liquid ℞ *decongestant; antihistamine* [pseudoephedrine HCl;

brompheniramine maleate] 60•8 mg/10 mL

**brofezil** INN, BAN

**brofoxine** USAN, INN *antipsychotic*

**brolaconazole** INN

**brolamfetamine** INN

**Brolene** eye drops *investigational (orphan) for* Acanthamoeba keratitis [propamidine isethionate] 0.1%

**bromacrylide** INN

**bromadel** [see: carbromal]

**Bromadine-DM** syrup (discontinued 2002) R *antitussive; decongestant; antihistamine* [dextromethorphan hydrobromide; pseudoephedrine HCl; brompheniramine maleate] 10•30•2 mg/5 mL

**Bromadine-DX** syrup R *antitussive; decongestant; antihistamine* [dextromethorphan hydrobromide; pseudoephedrine HCl; brompheniramine maleate] 10•30•2 mg/5 mL

**bromadoline** INN *analgesic* [also: bromadoline maleate]

**bromadoline maleate** USAN *analgesic* [also: bromadoline]

**Bromaline** elixir (discontinued 2001) OTC *decongestant; antihistamine* [phenylpropanolamine HCl; brompheniramine maleate] 12.5•2 mg/5 mL

**bromamid** INN

**Bromanate** pediatric elixir OTC *decongestant; antihistamine* [pseudoephedrine HCl; brompheniramine maleate] 30•2 mg/10 mL

**Bromanate DC Cough** syrup (discontinued 2002) R *narcotic antitussive; decongestant; antihistamine* [codeine phosphate; phenylpropanolamine HCl; brompheniramine maleate; alcohol] 10•12.5•2 mg/5 mL

**Bromanate DM Cold & Cough** pediatric elixir OTC *antitussive; decongestant; antihistamine* [dextromethorphan hydrobromide; pseudoephedrine HCl; brompheniramine maleate] 5•15•1 mg/5 mL

**Bromanyl** syrup (discontinued 2002) R *narcotic antitussive; antihistamine* [codeine phosphate; bromodiphenhydramine HCl] 10•12.5 mg/5 mL

**bromanylpromide** [see: bromamid]

**Bromarest DX Cough** syrup (discontinued 2002) R *antitussive; decongestant; antihistamine* [dextromethorphan hydrobromide; pseudoephedrine HCl; brompheniramine maleate; alcohol 0.95%] 10•30•2 mg/5 mL

**Bromatane DX Cough** syrup R *antitussive; decongestant; antihistamine* [dextromethorphan hydrobromide; pseudoephedrine HCl; brompheniramine maleate; alcohol 1%] 20•60•4 mg/10 mL

**Bromatapp** extended-release tablets (discontinued 2001) OTC *decongestant; antihistamine* [phenylpropanolamine HCl; brompheniramine maleate] 75•12 mg

**bromauric acid** NF

**bromazepam** USAN, INN, BAN, JAN *benzodiazepine anxiolytic; minor tranquilizer*

**bromazine** INN, DCF *antihistamine* [also: bromodiphenhydramine HCl; bromodiphenhydramine]

**bromazine HCl** [see: bromodiphenhydramine HCl]

**brombenzonium** [see: bromhexine HCl]

**bromchlorenone** USAN, INN *topical anti-infective*

**bromebric acid** INN, BAN

**bromelain** JAN *anti-inflammatory; proteolytic enzymes* [also: bromelains]

**bromelains** USAN, INN, BAN *anti-inflammatory; proteolytic enzymes* [also: bromelain]

**bromelin** [see: bromelains]

**bromerguride** INN

**brometenamine** INN, DCF

**bromethol** [see: tribromoethanol]

**Bromfed** extended-release capsules R *decongestant; antihistamine* [phenylephrine HCl; brompheniramine maleate] 15•12 mg

**Bromfed** syrup (discontinued 2003) OTC *decongestant; antihistamine* [pseudoephedrine HCl; brompheniramine

maleate] 60•4 mg/10 mL ⑨
Bromphen

**Bromfed** tablets ℞ *decongestant; antihistamine* [pseudoephedrine HCl; brompheniramine maleate] 60•4 mg

**Bromfed-DM Cough** syrup ℞ *antitussive; decongestant; antihistamine* [dextromethorphan hydrobromide; pseudoephedrine HCl; brompheniramine maleate] 20•60•4 mg/10 mL

**Bromfed-PD** extended-release pediatric capsules ℞ *decongestant; antihistamine* [phenylephrine HCl; brompheniramine maleate] 7.5•6 mg

**bromfenac** INN *long-acting nonsteroidal anti-inflammatory drug (NSAID); analgesic; antipyretic* [also: bromfenac sodium]

**bromfenac sodium** USAN *long-acting nonsteroidal anti-inflammatory drug (NSAID); analgesic; antipyretic; investigational (Phase III) topical treatment of ocular inflammation following cataract surgery* [also: bromfenac]

**Bromfenex** extended-release capsules ℞ *decongestant; antihistamine* [pseudoephedrine HCl; brompheniramine maleate] 120•12 mg

**Bromfenex PD** extended-release capsules ℞ *pediatric decongestant and antihistamine* [pseudoephedrine HCl; brompheniramine maleate] 60•6 mg

**bromhexine** INN, BAN *expectorant; mucolytic* [also: bromhexine HCl]

**bromhexine HCl** USAN, JAN *expectorant; mucolytic; investigational (orphan) for keratoconjunctivitis sicca of Sjögren syndrome* [also: bromhexine]

**bromindione** USAN, INN, BAN *anticoagulant*

**bromine** *element (Br)*

**bromisoval** INN [also: bromisovalum; bromvalerylurea; bromovaluree]

**bromisovalum** NF [also: bromisoval; bromvalerylurea; bromovaluree]

**2-bromo-α-ergocryptine** [see: bromocriptine]

**bromocamphor** [see: camphor, monobromated]

**bromociclen** INN [also: bromocyclen]

**bromocriptine** USAN, INN, BAN *dopamine agonist; prolactin enzyme inhibitor; antiparkinsonian*

**bromocriptine mesilate** JAN *dopamine agonist; prolactin enzyme inhibitor; antiparkinsonian* [also: bromocriptine mesylate]

**bromocriptine mesylate** USAN, USP *dopamine agonist; prolactin enzyme inhibitor; antiparkinsonian; investigational (NDA filed) agent for diabetic control of hypoglycemia; investigational (Phase II/III) treatment for obesity* [also: bromocriptine mesilate]

**bromocyclen** BAN [also: bromociclen]

**bromodeoxyuridine** [now: broxuridine]

**bromodiethylacetylurea** [see: carbromal]

**bromodiphenhydramine** BAN *antihistamine* [also: bromodiphenhydramine HCl; bromazine]

**bromodiphenhydramine HCl** USP *antihistamine* [also: bromazine; bromodiphenhydramine]

**bromofenofos** INN

**bromoform** USP

**bromofos** INN

**1-bromoheptadecafluorooctane** [see: perflubron]

**bromoisovaleryl urea (BVU)** [see: bromisovalum]

**Bromophen T.D.** sustained-release tablets (discontinued 2001) ℞ *decongestant; antihistamine* [phenylpropanolamine HCl; phenylephrine HCl; brompheniramine maleate] 15•15•12 mg ⑨ Bromphen

**bromophenol blue**

**bromophine** [see: apomorphine HCl]

**bromophos** [see: bromofos]

**bromopride** INN, DCF

**Bromo-Seltzer** effervescent granules OTC *antacid; analgesic; antipyretic* [sodium bicarbonate; citric acid; acetaminophen] 2781•2224•325 mg/dose

**bromotheophyllinate aminoisobutanol** [see: pamabrom]

**bromotheophyllinate pyranisamine** [see: pyrabrom]

**bromotheophyllinate pyrilamine**
[see: pyrabrom]

**8-bromotheophylline** [see: pamabrom]

**Bromotuss with Codeine** syrup (discontinued 2002) ℞ *narcotic antitussive; antihistamine* [codeine phosphate; bromodiphenhydramine HCl] 10•12.5 mg/5 mL

**bromovaluree** DCF [also: bromisovalum; bromisoval; bromvalerylurea]

**11-bromovincamine** [see: brovincamine]

**bromovinyl arabinosyluracil (BV-araU)** [see: sorivudine]

**bromoxanide** USAN, INN *anthelmintic*

**bromperidol** USAN, INN, BAN, JAN *antipsychotic*

**bromperidol decanoate** USAN, BAN *antipsychotic*

**Bromphen DC with Codeine Cough** syrup (discontinued 2002) ℞ *narcotic antitussive; decongestant; antihistamine* [codeine phosphate; phenylpropanolamine HCl; brompheniramine maleate] 10•12.5•2 mg/5 mL

**Bromphen DX Cough** syrup (discontinued 2002) ℞ *antitussive; decongestant; antihistamine* [dextromethorphan hydrobromide; pseudoephedrine HCl; brompheniramine maleate; alcohol 0.95%] 10•30•2 mg/5 mL

**brompheniramine** INN, BAN *alkylamine antihistamine* [also: brompheniramine maleate]

**Brompheniramine Cough** syrup (discontinued 2002) OTC *antitussive; decongestant; antihistamine* [dextromethorphan hydrobromide; pseudoephedrine HCl; brompheniramine maleate; alcohol 0.95%] 10•30•2 mg/5 mL

**Brompheniramine DC Cough** syrup (discontinued 2002) ℞ *narcotic antitussive; decongestant; antihistamine* [codeine phosphate; phenylpropanolamine HCl; brompheniramine maleate; alcohol 1.15%] 10•12.5•2 mg/5 mL

**brompheniramine maleate** USP *alkylamine antihistamine* [also: brompheniramine] 10 mg/mL injection

**brompheniramine maleate & pseudoephedrine HCl** *antihistamine; decongestant* 4•60 mg/5 mL oral

**brompheniramine tannate** *alkylamine antihistamine*

**Brompton's Cocktail; Brompton's Mixture** (refers to any oral narcotic/alcoholic solution containing morphine and either cocaine or a phenothiazine derivative) *prophylaxis for chronic, severe pain*

**bromvalerylurea** JAN [also: bromisovalum; bromisoval; bromovaluree]

**Bronalide** ⊛ oral inhalation aerosol (discontinued 2000) ℞ *corticosteroid for bronchial asthma* [flunisolide] 250 µg/dose

**Bronchial** capsules ℞ *antiasthmatic; bronchodilator; expectorant* [theophylline; guaifenesin] 150•90 mg

**Broncho Saline** solution (discontinued 2002) OTC *diluent for inhalation bronchodilators; solution for tracheal lavage* [sodium chloride (saline solution)] 0.9%

**Broncholate** softgels (discontinued 2002) ℞ *bronchodilator; decongestant; expectorant* [ephedrine HCl; guaifenesin] 12.5•200 mg ⃟ Brondelate

**Broncholate** syrup ℞ *bronchodilator; decongestant; expectorant* [ephedrine HCl; guaifenesin] 12.5•200 mg/10 mL ⃟ Brondelate

**Brondelate** elixir ℞ *antiasthmatic; bronchodilator; expectorant* [theophylline; guaifenesin] 192•150 mg/15 mL ⃟ Broncholate

**Bronkaid Dual Action** caplets OTC *bronchodilator; decongestant; expectorant* [ephedrine sulfate; guaifenesin] 25•400 mg

**Bronkodyl** capsules ℞ *antiasthmatic; bronchodilator* [theophylline] 100, 200 mg

**Bronkotuss Expectorant** oral liquid (discontinued 2002) ℞ *decongestant; antihistamine; expectorant* [ephedrine sulfate; chlorpheniramine maleate; guaifenesin; hydriodic acid; alcohol 5%] 8.2•4•100•1.67 mg/5 mL

**bronopol** INN, BAN, JAN

**Brontex** tablets, oral liquid (discontinued 2002) ℞ *narcotic antitussive; expectorant* [codeine phosphate; guaifenesin] 10•300 mg; 2.5•75 mg/5 mL

**brook bean** *medicinal herb* [see: buckbean]

**brooklime (Veronica beccabunga)** plant *medicinal herb used as a diuretic, emmenagogue, and febrifuge*

**broom (Cytisus scoparius)** plant and bloom *medicinal herb for inducing bowel evacuation, diuresis, and emesis; also used as a homeopathic remedy for arrhythmias, diphtheria, and head and throat congestion*

**broom, butcher's** *medicinal herb* [see: butcher's broom]

**broom, dyer's; green broom** *medicinal herb* [see: dyer's broom]

**broparestrol** INN, DCF

**broperamole** USAN, INN *anti-inflammatory*

**bropirimine** USAN, INN *antineoplastic; antiviral*

**broquinaldol** INN

**brosotamide** INN, DCF

**brosuximide** INN

**brotianide** INN, BAN

**brotizolam** USAN, INN, BAN, JAN *hypnotic*

**brovanexine** INN

**brovavir** [see: sorivudine]

**BrōveX** oral suspension ℞ *antihistamine* [brompheniramine tannate] 12 mg/5 mL

**BrōveX CT** chewable tablets ℞ *antihistamine* [brompheniramine tannate] 12 mg

**brovincamine** INN [also: brovincamine fumarate]

**brovincamine fumarate** JAN [also: brovincamine]

**brown algae** *medicinal herb* [see: kelp (Laminaria)]

**brownwort** *medicinal herb* [see: woundwort]

**broxaldine** INN, DCF

**broxaterol** INN

**Broxine** ℞ *investigational (NDA filed, orphan) radiosensitizer for primary brain tumors* [broxuridine]

**broxitalamic acid** INN

**broxuridine** INN *investigational (NDA filed, orphan) radiosensitizer for primary brain tumors*

**broxyquinoline** INN, DCF

**brucine sulfate** NF

**bruisewort** *medicinal herb* [see: comfrey; soapwort]

**bryony (Bryonia alba; B. dioica)** root *medicinal herb used as a pectoral and purgative; not generally regarded as safe and effective as root is poisonous in high doses (ingestion of as few as 40 berries can be fatal in adults, 15 in children)*

**bryostatin-1** *investigational (orphan) agent for esophageal cancer*

**B-Salt Forte** ophthalmic solution (discontinued 2004) ℞ *intraocular irrigating solution* [sodium chloride (balanced saline solution)]

**bSOD (bovine superoxide dismutase)** [see: orgotein]

**BSS (bismuth subsalicylate)** [q.v.]

**BSS; BSS Plus** ophthalmic solution ℞ *intraocular irrigating solution* [sodium chloride (balanced saline solution)]

**BTA Rapid Urine Test** test kit for professional use *in vitro diagnostic aid for bladder tumor analytes in the urine*

**BTA Stat Test** test kit for home use *in vitro diagnostic aid for bladder tumor analytes in the urine* [rapid immunoassay (RIA)]

**bucainide** INN *antiarrhythmic* [also: bucainide maleate]

**bucainide maleate** USAN *antiarrhythmic* [also: bucainide]

**bucco** *medicinal herb* [see: buchu]

**Bucet** capsules ℞ *sedative; barbiturate analgesic* [butalbital; acetaminophen] 50•650 mg

**bucetin** INN, BAN, JAN

**buchu** *(Agathosma betulina; Barosma betulina; B. cenulata; B. serratifolia)* leaves *medicinal herb for edema, gas, gout, inflammation, kidney and urinary tract infections, and prostatitis; also used as a douche for leukorrhea and vaginal yeast infections*

**buciclovir** INN

**bucillamine** INN, JAN

**bucindolol** INN, BAN *antihypertensive* [also: bucindolol HCl]

**bucindolol HCl** USAN *antihypertensive* [also: bucindolol]

**buckbean** *(Menyanthes trifoliata)* leaves *medicinal herb used as a tonic, cathartic, diuretic, anthelmintic, and emetic*

**buckeye; California buckeye; Ohio buckeye** *medicinal herb* [see: horse chestnut]

**buckhorn brake** *(Osmunda cinnamomea; O. regalis)* root *medicinal herb used as a demulcent and tonic*

**buckthorn** *(Rhamnus cathartica; R. frangula)* bark and berries *medicinal herb for bleeding, bowel disorders, chronic constipation, fever, gallstones, lead poisoning, and liver disorders* [also see: cascara sagrada]

**bucku** *medicinal herb* [see: buchu]

**bucladesine** INN [also: bucladesine sodium]

**bucladesine sodium** JAN [also: bucladesine]

**buclizine** INN, BAN *antinauseant; antiemetic; anticholinergic; motion sickness relief* [also: buclizine HCl]

**buclizine HCl** USAN *antinauseant; antiemetic; anticholinergic; motion sickness relief* [also: buclizine]

**buclosamide** INN, BAN, DCF

**bucloxic acid** INN, DCF

**bucolome** INN, JAN

**bucricaine** INN

**bucrilate** INN *tissue adhesive* [also: bucrylate]

**bucromarone** USAN, INN *antiarrhythmic*

**bucrylate** USAN *tissue adhesive* [also: bucrilate]

**bucumolol** INN [also: bucumolol HCl]

**bucumolol HCl** JAN [also: bucumolol]

**Budeprion SR** extended-release tablets ℞ *aminoketone antidepressant* [bupropion HCl] 100 mg

**budesonide** USAN, INN, BAN, JAN *corticosteroidal anti-inflammatory for chronic asthma, rhinitis, and inflammatory bowel disease*

**budipine** INN

**budotitane** INN

**budralazine** INN, JAN

**bufenadine** [see: bufenadrine]

**bufenadrine** INN

**bufeniode** INN, DCF

**bufetolol** INN [also: bufetolol HCl]

**bufetolol HCl** JAN [also: bufetolol]

**bufexamac** INN, BAN, JAN, DCF

**bufezolac** INN

**buffered aspirin** [see: aspirin, buffered]

**Bufferin** coated tablets, coated caplets OTC *analgesic; antipyretic; anti-inflammatory; antirheumatic* [aspirin (buffered with calcium carbonate, magnesium oxide, and magnesium carbonate)] 325, 500 mg

**Bufferin AF Nite Time** tablets OTC *antihistaminic sleep aid; analgesic* [diphenhydramine HCl; acetaminophen] 30•500 mg

**Buffets II** tablets (discontinued 2000) OTC *analgesic; antipyretic; anti-inflammatory; antacid* [acetaminophen; aspirin; caffeine; aluminum hydroxide] 162•227•32.4•50 mg

**Buffex** tablets OTC *analgesic; antipyretic; anti-inflammatory; antirheumatic* [aspirin (buffered with aluminum glycinate and magnesium carbonate)] 325 mg

**bufilcon A** USAN *hydrophilic contact lens material*

**buflomedil** INN, BAN, DCF

**bufogenin** INN

**buformin** USAN, INN *antidiabetic*

**bufrolin** INN, BAN

**bufuralol** INN, BAN

**bufylline** BAN *diuretic; smooth muscle relaxant* [also: ambuphylline]

**bugbane** *medicinal herb* [see: hellebore; black cohosh]

**bugleweed** *(Lycopus virginicus)* plant *medicinal herb for cough, excessive menses, nervous indigestion, and other nervous disorders*

**bugloss** *medicinal herb* [see: borage]

**Bugs Bunny Complete** chewable tablets OTC *vitamin/mineral/calcium/iron supplement* [multiple vitamins & minerals; calcium; iron; folic acid; biotin] ≛•100•18•0.4•0.04 mg

**Bugs Bunny Plus Iron** chewable tablets OTC *vitamin/iron supplement* [multiple vitamins; iron; folic acid] ≛•15•0.3 mg

**Bugs Bunny with Extra C Children's** chewable tablets OTC *vitamin supplement* [multiple vitamins; folic acid] ≛•0.3 mg

**bugwort** *medicinal herb* [see: black cohosh]

**buku** *medicinal herb* [see: buchu]

**Bulk Forming Fiber Laxative** film-coated tablets OTC *bulk laxative; antidiarrheal* [calcium polycarbophil] 625 mg

**bulk-producing laxatives** *a subclass of laxatives that work by increasing the hydration and volume of stool to stimulate peristalsis; also form an emollient gel to ease the movement of stool through the intestines* [see also: laxatives]

**bull's foot** *medicinal herb* [see: coltsfoot]

**bumadizone** INN, DCF

**bumecaine** INN

**bumepidil** INN

**bumetanide** USAN, USP, INN, BAN, JAN *loop diuretic* 0.25 mg/mL injection

**bumetrizole** USAN, INN *ultraviolet screen*

**Bumex** IV or IM injection (discontinued 2004) ℞ *loop diuretic* [bumetanide] 0.25 mg/mL

**Bumex** tablets ℞ *loop diuretic* [bumetanide] 0.5, 1, 2 mg

**Buminate 5%; Buminate 25%** IV infusion ℞ *blood volume expander for shock, burns, and hypoproteinemia* [human albumin] 5%; 25%

**bunaftine** INN

**bunamidine** INN, BAN *anthelmintic* [also: bunamidine HCl]

**bunamidine HCl** USAN *anthelmintic* [also: bunamidine]

**bunamiodyl** INN [also: buniodyl]

**bunamiodyl sodium** [see: bunamiodyl; buniodyl]

**bunaprolast** USAN, INN *antiasthmatic; 5-lipoxygenase inhibitor*

**bunapsilate** INN *combining name for radicals or groups*

**bunazosin** INN [also: bunazosin HCl]

**bunazosin HCl** JAN [also: bunazosin]

**bundlin** [now: sedecamycin]

**buniodyl** BAN [also: bunamiodyl]

**bunitrolol** INN [also: bunitrolol HCl]

**bunitrolol HCl** JAN [also: bunitrolol]

**bunolol** INN *antiadrenergic (β-receptor)* [also: bunolol HCl]

**bunolol HCl** USAN *antiadrenergic (β-receptor)* [also: bunolol]

**Bupap** caplets ℞ *analgesic; antipyretic; barbiturate sedative* [acetaminophen; butalbital] 650•50 mg

**buparvaquone** INN, BAN

**buphenine** INN, BAN *peripheral vasodilator* [also: nylidrin HCl]

**Buphenyl** tablets, powder for oral solution ℞ *antihyperammonemic for urea cycle disorders (orphan); investigational (orphan) for various sickling disorders* [sodium phenylbutyrate] 500 mg; 3 g/tsp., 8.6 g/tbsp.

**bupicomide** USAN, INN *antihypertensive*

**bupivacaine** INN, BAN *injectable local anesthetic* [also: bupivacaine HCl]

**bupivacaine HCl** USAN, USP, JAN *injectable local anesthetic* [also: bupivacaine] 0.25%, 0.5%, 0.75%

**bupivacaine HCl & epinephrine** *injectable local anesthetic; vasoconstrictor* 0.25%•1:200 000, 0.5%•1:200 000, 0.75%•1:200 000

**Bupivicaine Spinal** injection ℞ *injectable local anesthetic for obstetrical use* [bupivacaine HCl; dextrose] 0.75%•8.25%

**bupranol** [see: bupranolol]

**bupranolol** INN, DCF [also: bupranolol HCl]

**bupranolol HCl** JAN [also: bupranolol]

**Buprenex** IV or IM injection ℞ *narcotic agonist-antagonist analgesic* [buprenorphine HCl] 0.3 mg/mL

**buprenorphine** INN, BAN *narcotic agonist-antagonist analgesic* [also: buprenorphine HCl]

**buprenorphine HCl** USAN, JAN *narcotic agonist-antagonist analgesic for inpatient treatment of opiate dependence (orphan)* [also: buprenorphine] 0.3 mg/mL injection

**buprenorphine HCl & naloxone HCl** *investigational (orphan) for opiate addictions*

**bupropion** BAN *aminoketone antidepressant; non-nicotine aid to smoking cessation* [also: bupropion HCl; amfebutamone]

**bupropion HCl** USAN *aminoketone antidepressant; non-nicotine aid to smoking cessation* [also: amfebutamone; bupropion] 75, 100, 150 mg oral

**buquineran** INN, BAN

**buquinolate** USAN, INN *coccidiostat for poultry*

**buquiterine** INN

**buramate** USAN, INN *anticonvulsant; antipsychotic*

**burdock (*Arctium lappa; A. majus; A. minus*)** root *medicinal herb for arthritis, blood cleansing, dandruff, eczema, edema, fever, gout, kidney and lung disorders, rheumatism, skin diseases, and tumors; also used as an antimicrobial and diaphoretic*

**burefrine** [now: berefrine]

**burnet (*Pimpinella magna; P. saxifrage*)** root *medicinal herb used as an antispasmodic, astringent, carminative, diaphoretic, diuretic, stimulant, and stomachic*

**burning bush** *medicinal herb* [see: fraxinella; wahoo]

**burodiline** INN

**Buro-Sol** solution (discontinued 2004) OTC *astringent wet dressing (Burow solution)* [aluminum sulfate] 0.23%

**Burow solution** [see: aluminum acetate]

**burr seed; turkey burr seed; clotbur; hareburr; hurr-burr; thorny burr** *medicinal herb* [see: burdock]

**burrage** *medicinal herb* [see: borage]

**buserelin** INN, BAN *hormonal antineoplastic; gonad-stimulating principle; luteinizing hormone-releasing hormone analogue* [also: buserelin acetate]

**buserelin acetate** USAN, JAN *hormonal antineoplastic; gonad-stimulating principle; luteinizing hormone-releasing hormone analogue* [also: buserelin]

**BuSpar** tablets ℞ *nonsedating azaspirone anxiolytic* [buspirone HCl] 5, 10, 15, 30 mg

**buspirone** INN, BAN *nonsedating azaspirone anxiolytic* [also: buspirone HCl]

**buspirone HCl** USAN *nonsedating azaspirone anxiolytic* [also: buspirone] 5, 7.5, 10, 15, 30 mg oral

**busulfan** USP, INN, JAN *alkylating antineoplastic for chronic myelogenous leukemia (CML); pretreatment for bone marrow transplants (orphan); investigational (orphan) for neoplastic meningitis and primary brain malignancies* [also: busulphan]

**Busulfex** IV infusion ℞ *alkylating antineoplastic for chronic myelogenous leukemia (CML); pretreatment for bone marrow and stem cell transplants (orphan)* [busulfan] 6 mg/mL

**busulphan** BAN *alkylating antineoplastic* [also: busulfan]

**butabarbital** USP *sedative; hypnotic* [also: secbutobarbitone] 🔄 butalbital

**butabarbital sodium** USP *sedative; hypnotic* [also: secbutabarbital sodium] 15, 30 mg oral; 30 mg/5 mL oral

**butacaine** INN, BAN [also: butacaine sulfate]

**butacaine sulfate** USP [also: butacaine]

**butacetin** USAN *analgesic; antidepressant*

**butacetoluide** [see: butanilicaine]

**butaclamol** INN *antipsychotic* [also: butaclamol HCl]

**butaclamol HCl** USAN *antipsychotic* [also: butaclamol]

**butadiazamide** INN

**butafosfan** INN, BAN

**butalamine** INN, BAN

**butalbital** USAN, USP, INN *barbiturate sedative* ② butabarbital; Butibel

**butalbital & acetaminophen & caffeine** *analgesic; barbiturate sedative* 50•325•40, 50•500•40 mg oral

**butalbital & aspirin & caffeine** *analgesic; barbiturate sedative* 50•325•40 mg oral

**Butalbital Compound** tablets, capsules ℞ *analgesic; barbiturate sedative* [aspirin; caffeine; butalbital] 325• 40•50 mg

**butalgin** [see: methadone HCl]

**butallylonal** NF

**butamben** USAN, USP *topical anesthetic*

**butamben picrate** USAN *topical local anesthetic* 1% topical

**butamirate** INN *antitussive* [also: butamirate citrate; butamyrate]

**butamirate citrate** USAN *antitussive* [also: butamirate; butamyrate]

**butamisole** INN *veterinary anthelmintic* [also: butamisole HCl]

**butamisole HCl** USAN *veterinary anthelmintic* [also: butamisole]

**butamiverine** [see: butaverine]

**butamoxane** INN

**butamyrate** BAN *antitussive* [also: butamirate citrate; butamirate]

**butane (*n*-butane)** NF *aerosol propellant*

**1,4-butanediol (1,4-B; BDO); butane-1,4-diol** *precursor to gamma hydroxybutyrate (GHB); a formerly legal alternative to GHB, now also illegal (Schedule I)* [see: gamma hydroxybutyrate (GHB)]

**butanilicaine** INN, BAN

**butanixin** INN

**butanserin** INN

**butantrone** INN

**butaperazine** USAN, INN *antipsychotic*

**butaperazine maleate** USAN *antipsychotic*

**butaprost** USAN, INN, BAN *bronchodilator*

**butaverine** INN, DCF

**butaxamine** INN *antidiabetic; antihyperlipoproteinemic* [also: butoxamine HCl; butoxamine]

**butcher's broom (*Ruscus aculeatus*)** rhizomes *medicinal herb for atherosclerosis, circulatory disorders, hemorrhoids, thrombosis, varicose veins, and venous insufficiency; not generally regarded as safe and effective*

**butedronate tetrasodium** USAN *bone imaging aid*

**butedronic acid** INN

**butelline** [see: butacaine sulfate]

**butenafine** INN *antifungal*

**butenafine HCl** USAN *topical benzylamine antifungal*

**butenemal** [see: vinbarbital]

**buteprate** INN *former combining name for radicals or groups (name rescinded by the USAN)* [now: probutate]

**buterizine** USAN, INN *peripheral vasodilator*

**Butesin Picrate** ointment (discontinued 2004) OTC *local anesthetic* [butamben picrate] 1%

**butetamate** INN [also: butethamate]

**butethal** NF [also: butobarbitone]

**butethamate** BAN [also: butetamate]

**butethamine HCl** NF

**butethanol** [see: tetracaine]

**Butex Forte** capsules ℞ *analgesic; barbiturate sedative* [acetaminophen; butalbital] 650•50 mg

**buthalital sodium** INN [also: buthalitone sodium]

**buthalitone sodium** BAN [also: buthalital sodium]

**buthiazide** USAN *diuretic; antihypertensive* [also: butizide]

**Butibel** tablets, elixir ℞ *GI anticholinergic; sedative* [belladonna extract; butabarbital sodium] 15•15 mg; 15• 15 mg/5 mL ② butalbital

**butibufen** INN

**butidrine** INN, DCF

**butikacin** USAN, INN, BAN *antibacterial*

**butilfenin** USAN, INN *hepatic function test*

**butinazocine** INN

**butinoline** INN

**butirosin** INN *antibacterial antibiotic* [also: butirosin sulfate; butirosin sulphate]

**butirosin sulfate** USAN *antibacterial antibiotic* [also: butirosin; butirosin sulphate]

**butirosin sulphate** BAN *antibacterial antibiotic* [also: butirosin sulfate; butirosin]

**Butisol Sodium** tablets, elixir ℞ *sedative; hypnotic* [butabarbital sodium] 15, 30, 50, 100 mg; 30 mg/5 mL ⑨ Butazolidin

**butixirate** USAN, INN *analgesic; antirheumatic*

**butixocort** INN

**butizide** INN *diuretic; antihypertensive* [also: buthiazide]

**butobarbitone** BAN [also: butethal]

**butobendine** INN

**butoconazole** INN, BAN *topical antifungal* [also: butoconazole nitrate]

**butoconazole nitrate** USAN, USP *topical antifungal for vulvovaginal candidiasis* [also: butoconazole]

**butocrolol** INN

**butoctamide** INN [also: butoctamide semisuccinate]

**butoctamide semisuccinate** JAN [also: butoctamide]

**butofilolol** INN

**butonate** USAN, INN *anthelmintic*

**butopamine** USAN, INN *cardiotonic*

**butopiprine** INN, DCF

**butoprozine** INN *antiarrhythmic; antianginal* [also: butoprozine HCl]

**butoprozine HCl** USAN *antiarrhythmic; antianginal* [also: butoprozine]

**butopyrammonium iodide** INN

**butopyronoxyl** USP

**butorphanol** USAN, INN, BAN *analgesic; antitussive*

**butorphanol tartrate** USAN, USP, BAN, JAN *narcotic agonist-antagonist analgesic; antitussive* 10 mg nasal spray; 1, 2 mg/mL injection

**butoxamine** BAN *antidiabetic; antihyperlipoproteinemic* [also: butoxamine HCl; butaxamine]

**butoxamine HCl** USAN *antidiabetic; antihyperlipoproteinemic* [also: butaxamine; butoxamine]

**2-butoxyethyl nicotinate** [see: nicoboxil]

**butoxylate** INN

**butoxyphenylacethydroxamic acid** [see: bufexamac]

**butriptyline** INN, BAN *antidepressant* [also: butriptyline HCl]

**butriptyline HCl** USAN *antidepressant* [also: butriptyline]

**butropium bromide** INN, JAN

**butterbur (Petasites hybridus)** leaves and root *medicinal herb used as an analgesic for migraines and as an antispasmodic for asthma, cough, and gastrointestinal and urinary tract disorders; not generally regarded as safe and effective due to organ damage and carcinogenic properties*

**buttercup (Ranunculus acris; R. bulbosus; R. scleratus)** plant *medicinal herb used as an acrid, anodyne, antispasmodic, diaphoretic, and rubefacient*

**butterfly weed** *medicinal herb* [see: pleurisy root]

**butternut (Juglans cinerea)** bark, leaves, flowers *medicinal herb used as an anthelmintic, antiseptic, cathartic, cholagogue, and nervine*

**butterweed** *medicinal herb* [see: fleabane; horseweed]

**butydrine** [see: butidrine]

**butyl alcohol** NF *solvent*

**butyl aminobenzoate (butyl p-aminobenzoate)** [now: butamben]

**butyl p-aminobenzoate picrate** [see: butamben picrate]

**butyl chloride** NF

**butyl 2-cyanoacrylate** [see: enbucrilate]

**butyl DNJ (deoxynojirimycin)** [see: deoxynojirimycin]

**butyl p-hydroxybenzoate** [see: butylparaben]

**butyl methoxydibenzoylmethane** [see: avobenzone]

**butyl nitrite; isobutyl nitrite** *amyl nitrite substitutes, sold as euphoric street drugs, which produce a quick but short-lived "rush"* [see also: amyl nitrite; volatile nitrites]

**butyl parahydroxybenzoate** JAN *antifungal agent* [also: butylparaben]

***p*-butylaminobenzoyldiethylamino-ethyl HCl** JAN

**butylated hydroxyanisole (BHA)** NF, BAN *antioxidant*

**butylated hydroxytoluene (BHT)** NF, BAN *antioxidant*

**α-butylbenzyl alcohol** [see: fenipentol]

**1-butylbiguanide** [see: buformin]

**N-butyl-deoxynojirimycin** [see: deoxynojirimycin]

**1,4-butylene glycol (1,4-BG)** *precursor to gamma hydroxybutyrate (GHB); a formerly legal alternative to GHB, now also illegal (Schedule I)* [see: gamma hydroxybutyrate (GHB)]

**1,5-(butylimino)-1,5-dideoxy-D-glucitol** *investigational (orphan) for Fabry disease and Gaucher disease*

**butylmesityl oxide** [see: butopyronoxyl]

**butylparaben** NF *antifungal agent* [also: butyl parahydroxybenzoate]

**butylphenamide**

**butylphenylsalicylamide** [see: butylphenamide]

**butylscopolamine bromide** JAN

**butynamine** INN

**butyrate propionate** [see: probutate; buteprate]

**butyrophenones** *a class of dopamine receptor antagonists with conventional (typical) antipsychotic activity* [also called: phenylbutylpiperadines]

**butyrylcholesterinase** *investigational (orphan) agent for reduction and clearance of serum cocaine levels and postsurgical apnea*

**butyrylperazine** [see: butaperazine]

**O-butyrylthiamine disulfide** [see: bisbutitiamine]

**butyvinyl** [see: vinylbital]

**buzepide metiodide** INN, DCF

**BVAP (BCNU, vincristine, Adriamycin, prednisone)** *chemotherapy protocol*

**BV-araU (bromovinyl arabinosyluracil)** [see: sorivudine]

**BVCPP (BCNU, vinblastine, cyclophosphamide, procarbazine, prednisone)** *chemotherapy protocol*

**BVDS (bleomycin, Velban, doxorubicin, streptozocin)** *chemotherapy protocol*

**BVPP (BCNU, vincristine, procarbazine, prednisone)** *chemotherapy protocol*

**BVU (bromoisovaleryl urea)** [see: bromisovalum]

**BW 12C** *investigational (orphan) agent for sickle cell disease*

**Byclomine** capsules, tablets ℞ *GI antispasmodic* [dicyclomine HCl] 10 mg; 20 mg ⍰ Hycomine

# C

**C (vitamin C)** [see: ascorbic acid]

**C & E** softgels OTC *vitamin supplement* [vitamins C and E] 500•400 mg

**C Factors "1000" Plus** tablets OTC *vitamin C supplement with multiple bioflavonoids* [vitamin C; rose hips; citrus bioflavonoids; rutin; hesperidin] 1000•25•250•50•25 mg

**C vitamin** [see: ascorbic acid]

**14C urea** *diagnostic aid for H. pylori in the stomach* [also: carbon C 14 urea]

**C1-esterase-inhibitor, human** *investigational (orphan) agent to prevent or treat acute attacks of angioedema*

**CA (cyclophosphamide, Adriamycin)** *chemotherapy protocol*

**CA (cytarabine, asparaginase)** *chemotherapy protocol for acute myelocytic leukemia (AML)*

**cA2 monoclonal antibodies (chimeric A2 MAb)** [see: infliximab]

**45Ca** [see: calcium chloride Ca 45]

**<sup>47</sup>Ca** [see: calcium chloride Ca 47]

**cabastine** INN

**cabbage, cow** *medicinal herb* [see: masterwort; white pond lily]

**cabbage, meadow; swamp cabbage** *medicinal herb* [see: skunk cabbage]

**cabbage, water** *medicinal herb* [see: white pond lily]

**cabergoline** USAN, INN *dopamine agonist for hyperprolactinemia; investigational treatment for Parkinson disease and gynecologic disorders*

**cabis bromatum** [see: bibrocathol]

**CABO (cisplatin, Abitrexate, bleomycin, Oncovin)** *chemotherapy protocol for head and neck cancer*

**CABOP; CA-BOP (Cytoxin, Adriamycin, bleomycin, Oncovin, prednisone)** *chemotherapy protocol*

**CABS (CCNU, Adriamycin bleomycin, streptozocin)** *chemotherapy protocol*

**cabufocon A** USAN *hydrophobic contact lens material*

**cabufocon B** USAN *hydrophobic contact lens material*

**CAC (cisplatin, ara-C, caffeine)** *chemotherapy protocol*

**cacao butter** JAN

**Cachexon** Ŗ *investigational (orphan) for AIDS-related cachexia* [L-glutathione, reduced]

**cactinomycin** USAN, INN *antibiotic antineoplastic* [also: actinomycin C]

**CAD (cyclophosphamide, Adriamycin, dacarbazine)** *chemotherapy protocol*

**CAD (cytarabine [and] daunorubicin)** *chemotherapy protocol*

**cade oil** [see: juniper tar]

**cadexomer** INN

**cadexomer iodine** USAN, INN, BAN *antiseptic; antiulcerative wound dressing*

**cadmium** *element* (Cd)

**cadralazine** INN, BAN, JAN

**Ca-DTPA (calcium pentetate)** [see: pentetate calcium trisodium]

**Caduet** film-coated tablets Ŗ *calcium channel blocker and HMG-CoA reductase inhibitor for coronary artery disease (CAD)* [amlodipine besylate; atorvastatin] 5•10, 5•20, 5•40, 5•80, 10•10, 10•20, 10•40, 10•80 mg

**CAE (cyclophosphamide, Adriamycin, etoposide)** *chemotherapy protocol for small cell lung cancer (SCLC)* [also: ACE]

**Caelyx** ⒸⒶⓃ injection Ŗ *antineoplastic for ovarian carcinoma and AIDS-related Kaposi sarcoma* [doxorubicin HCl, liposome-encapsulated] 2 mg/mL

**CAF (cyclophosphamide, Adriamycin, fluorouracil)** *chemotherapy protocol for breast cancer*

**cafaminol** INN

**Cafatine** suppositories Ŗ *migraine-specific vasoconstrictor* [ergotamine tartrate; caffeine] 2•200 mg

**Cafatine-PB** tablets Ŗ *migraine treatment; vasoconstrictor; anticholinergic; sedative* [ergotamine tartrate; caffeine; pentobarbital sodium; belladonna extract] 1•100•30•0.125 mg

**Cafcit** oral solution, injectable Ŗ *analeptic; CNS stimulant for apnea of prematurity (orphan)* [caffeine citrate] 20 mg/mL

**cafedrine** INN, BAN

**Cafergot** tablets, suppositories Ŗ *migraine treatment; vasoconstrictor* [ergotamine tartrate; caffeine] 1•100 mg; 2•100 mg

**Cafetrate** suppositories (discontinued 2000) Ŗ *migraine-specific vasoconstrictor* [ergotamine tartrate; caffeine] 2•100 mg

**Caffedrine** tablets OTC *CNS stimulant; analeptic* [caffeine] 200 mg

**caffeic acid phenethyl ester (CAPE)** *antimicrobial substance found in bee propolis*

**caffeine** USP, BAN, JAN *methylxanthine analeptic; CNS stimulant; diuretic; treatment for apnea of prematurity (orphan); potentiator of various NSAIDs*

**caffeine citrate** *methylxanthine analeptic; CNS stimulant for apnea of prematurity (orphan)*

**caffeine monohydrate** [see: caffeine, citrated]

**caffeine nut** *medicinal herb* [see: kola nut]

**caffeine & sodium benzoate** *analeptic for respiratory depression due to an overdose of CNS depressants* 250 mg/mL injection

**CAFP (cyclophosphamide, Adriamycin, fluorouracil, prednisone)** *chemotherapy protocol*

**CAFTH (cyclophosphamide, Adriamycin, fluorouracil, tamoxifen, Halotestin)** *chemotherapy protocol*

**CAFVP (cyclophosphamide, Adriamycin, fluorouracil, vincristine, prednisone)** *chemotherapy protocol*

**Cal Carb-HD** powder for oral solution OTC *calcium supplement* [calcium carbonate] 2.5 g Ca/pkt.

**Caladryl** cream OTC *topical antihistamine; astringent; antipruritic/anesthetic* [diphenhydramine HCl; calamine] 1%•8% ☑ Benadryl

**Caladryl** lotion OTC *poison ivy treatment* [calamine; pramoxine HCl; alcohol 2.2%] 8%•1%

**Caladryl Clear** lotion OTC *poison ivy treatment* [pramoxine HCl; zinc acetate; alcohol 2%] 1%•0.1%

**Caladryl for Kids** cream (discontinued 2003) OTC *poison ivy treatment* [calamine; pramoxine HCl] 8%•1%

**Calafol** tablets ℞ *vitamin/calcium supplement* [vitamins $B_6$ and $B_{12}$; folic acid; vitamin $D_3$; calcium] 25 mg• 425 µg•1.6 mg•400 IU•400 mg

**Cala-gen** lotion (discontinued 2004) OTC *antipruritic; anesthetic; antihistamine* [diphenhydramine HCl; alcohol 2%] 1%

**Calamatum** spray (discontinued 2003) OTC *poison ivy treatment* [calamine; zinc oxide; menthol; camphor; benzocaine]

**calamine** USP, JAN *topical protectant; astringent; poison ivy treatment*

**Calamine, Phenolated** lotion OTC *poison ivy treatment* [calamine; zinc oxide; phenol] 8%•8%•1%

**Calamine Lotion** OTC *poison ivy treatment* [calamine; zinc oxide] 6.97%• 6.97%

**calamint (*Calamintha officinalis*)** *medicinal herb* [see: summer savory]

***Calamintha hortensis*** *medicinal herb* [see: summer savory]

***Calamintha montana*** *medicinal herb* [see: winter savory]

**Calamox** ointment (discontinued 2003) OTC *poison ivy treatment* [calamine] 17 g/100 g ☑ Camalox

**calamus (*Acorus calamus*)** rhizome *medicinal herb for anxiety, bad breath from smoking, colic, digestive disorders, fever, gas, irritated throat, and promoting wound healing; not generally regarded as safe and effective and is prohibited in the U.S. as a food additive or supplement*

**Calamycin** lotion OTC *antihistamine; astringent; anesthetic* [pyrilamine maleate; zinc oxide; calamine; benzocaine; chloroxylenol; alcohol 2%]

**Calan** film-coated tablets ℞ *antianginal; antiarrhythmic; antihypertensive; calcium channel blocker* [verapamil HCl] 40, 80, 120 mg ☑ kaolin; Kaon

**Calan SR** film-coated sustained-release tablets ℞ *antihypertensive; antianginal; antiarrhythmic; calcium channel blocker* [verapamil HCl] 120, 180, 240 mg ☑ kaolin; Kaon

**calanolide A** *investigational (Phase I/II) non-nucleoside reverse transcriptase inhibitor (NNRTI) for HIV infection*

**Calcarb 600 with Vitamin D** tablets OTC *calcium supplement* [calcium carbonate; vitamin D] 1.5 g (600 mg Ca)•125 IU

**Cal-Carb Forte** chewable tablets, caplets OTC *antacid; calcium supplement* [calcium carbonate] 1250 mg (500 mg Ca)

**Calcet** tablets OTC *dietary supplement* [calcium; vitamin D] 152.8 mg• 100 IU

**Calcet Plus** tablets OTC *vitamin/calcium/iron supplement* [multiple vita-

mins; calcium; iron; folic acid] ≜ •
152.8•18•0.8 mg

**Calcibind** powder for oral solution ℞ *antiurolithic to prevent stone formation in absorptive calciuria type I* [cellulose sodium phosphate] 300 g bulk pack

**CalciCaps** tablets OTC *dietary supplement* [dibasic calcium phosphate; calcium gluconate; calcium carbonate; vitamin D] 125 mg (Ca)•60 mg (P)•67 IU

**CalciCaps with Iron** tablets OTC *dietary supplement* [dibasic calcium phosphate; calcium gluconate; calcium carbonate; vitamin D; ferrous gluconate] 125 mg (Ca)•60 mg (P)•67 IU•7 mg

**Calci-Chew** chewable tablets OTC *calcium supplement* [calcium carbonate] 1250 mg (500 mg Ca)

**Calciday-667** tablets (discontinued 2002) OTC *calcium supplement* [calcium carbonate] 667 mg (250 mg Ca)

**calcidiol** [see: calcifediol]

**Calcidrine** syrup (discontinued 2002) ℞ *narcotic antitussive; expectorant* [codeine phosphate; calcium iodide; alcohol 6%] 8.4•152 mg/5 mL

**calcifediol (25-hydroxycholecalciferol; 25-hydroxyvitamin D₃)** USAN, USP, INN *vitamin D precursor (converted to calcitriol in the body); calcium regulator for treatment of metastatic bone disease or hypocalcemia of chronic renal dialysis*

**Calciferol** IM injection ℞ *vitamin deficiency therapy for refractory rickets, familial hypophosphatemia, and hypoparathyroidism* [ergocalciferol (vitamin D₂)] 500 000 IU/mL

**calciferol** [now: ergocalciferol]

**Calciferol Drops** OTC *vitamin supplement* [ergocalciferol (vitamin D₂)] 8000 IU/mL

**Calcijex** injection ℞ *vitamin D therapy for hypoparathyroidism and hypocalcemia of chronic renal dialysis* [calcitriol] 1, 2 μg/mL

**Calcimar** subcu or IM injection ℞ *calcium regulator for hypercalcemia, Paget disease, and postmenopausal osteoporosis* [calcitonin (salmon)] 200 IU/mL

**Calci-Mix** capsules OTC *calcium supplement* [calcium carbonate] 1250 mg (500 mg Ca)

**Calcionate** syrup OTC *calcium supplement* [calcium glubionate] 1.8 g/5 mL

**calcipotriene** USAN *topical antipsoriatic* [also: calcipotriol]

**calcipotriol** INN, BAN *topical antipsoriatic* [also: calcipotriene]

**Calciquid** syrup OTC *calcium supplement* [calcium glubionate] 1.8 g/5 mL

**calcitonin (human)** USAN, INN, BAN, JAN *calcium regulator for symptomatic Paget disease (osteitis deformans) (orphan)* ⚇ calcitriol

**calcitonin (salmon)** USAN, INN, BAN *calcium regulator for Paget disease (orphan), hypercalcemia, and postmenopausal osteoporosis*

**calcitonin salmon (synthesis)** JAN *synthetic analogue of calcitonin (salmon); calcium regulator* [also: salcatonin]

**calcitonin salmon, recombinant** *investigational (NDA filed) calcium regulator for hypercalcemia, postmenopausal osteoporosis, and Paget disease*

**Cal-Citrate** tablets, capsules OTC *calcium supplement* [calcium citrate] 250 mg Ca; 225 mg Ca

**calcitriol (1,25-hydroxycholecalciferol; 1,25-hydroxyvitamin D₃)** USAN, INN, BAN, JAN *physiologically active form of vitamin D; calcium regulator for hypoparathyroidism and hypocalcemia due to chronic renal dialysis; decreases the severity of psoriatic lesions* 0.25, 0.5 μg oral; 1 μg/mL oral; 1, 2 μg injection ⚇ calcitonin

**calcium** *element* (Ca)

**calcium, oyster shell** [see: calcium carbonate]

**Calcium 600** tablets OTC *calcium supplement* [calcium carbonate] 1500 mg (600 mg Ca)

**Calcium 600 + D** tablets OTC *dietary supplement* [calcium; vitamin D] 600 mg•125 IU

**Calcium 600 with Vitamin D** tablets OTC *dietary supplement* [calcium; vitamin D] 600 mg•100 IU

**calcium acetate** USP, JAN *dietary calcium supplement (25% elemental calcium); buffering agent for hyperphosphatemia of end-stage renal disease (orphan)*

**calcium alginate fiber** *topical local hemostatic*

**calcium aminacyl B-PAS (benzoyl para-aminosalicylate)** [see: benzoylpas calcium]

**calcium 4-aminosalicylate trihydrate** [see: aminosalicylate calcium]

**calcium amphomycin** [see: amphomycin]

**calcium antagonists** *a class of coronary vasodilators that inhibit cardiac muscle contraction and slow cardiac electrical conduction velocity* [also called: calcium channel blockers; slow channel blockers]

**calcium ascorbate (vitamin C)** USP *water-soluble vitamin; antiscorbutic* 500 mg oral; 3256 mg/tsp. oral

**calcium benzamidosalicylate** INN, BAN *antibacterial; tuberculostatic* [also: benzoylpas calcium]

**calcium benzoyl *p*-aminosalicylate (B-PAS)** [see: benzoylpas calcium]

**calcium benzoylpas** [see: benzoylpas calcium]

**calcium bis-dioctyl sulfosuccinate** [see: docusate calcium]

**calcium bis-glycinate** *dietary calcium supplement*

**calcium bromide** JAN

**calcium carbimide** INN [also: cyanamide]

**calcium carbonate** USP *antacid; dietary calcium supplement (40% elemental calcium); investigational (orphan) for hyperphosphatemia of end-stage renal disease* [also: precipitated calcium carbonate] 500, 600, 650, 1250 mg oral; 1250 mg/5 mL oral

**calcium carbonate, precipitated** [now: calcium carbonate]

**calcium carbophil** *bulk laxative*

**calcium caseinate** *dietary calcium supplement; infant formula modifier*

**calcium channel blockers** *a class of coronary vasodilators that inhibit cardiac muscle contraction and slow cardiac electrical conduction velocity* [also called: calcium antagonists; slow channel blockers]

**calcium chloride** USP, JAN *calcium replenisher*

**calcium chloride Ca 45** USAN *radioactive agent*

**calcium chloride Ca 47** USAN *radioactive agent*

**calcium chloride dihydrate** [see: calcium chloride]

**calcium citrate** USP *dietary calcium supplement (21% elemental calcium)* 1.2, 4.5 g oral; 3.6 g/5 mL oral

**calcium citrate tetrahydrate** [see: calcium citrate]

**calcium clofibrate** INN

**calcium cyanamide** [see: calcium carbimide]

**calcium D-glucarate tetrahydrate** [see: calcium saccharate]

**calcium D-gluconate lactobionate monohydrate** [see: calcium glubionate]

**calcium dioctyl sulfosuccinate** [see: docusate calcium]

**calcium disodium edathamil** [see: edetate calcium disodium]

**calcium disodium edetate** JAN *heavy metal chelating agent* [also: edetate calcium disodium; sodium calcium edetate; sodium calciumedetate]

**Calcium Disodium Versenate** IM, IV, or subcu injection ℞ *chelating agent for acute or chronic lead poisoning and lead encephalopathy* [edetate calcium disodium] 200 mg/mL

**calcium dobesilate** INN

**calcium doxybensylate** [see: calcium dobesilate]

**calcium edetate sodium** [see: edetate calcium disodium]

**calcium EDTA (ethylene diamine tetraacetic acid)** [see: edetate calcium disodium]

**calcium folinate** INN, BAN, JAN *anti-anemic; folate replenisher; antidote to folic acid antagonist* [also: leucovorin calcium]

**calcium glubionate** USAN, INN *dietary calcium supplement*

**calcium gluceptate** USP *parenteral calcium replenisher* [also: calcium glucoheptonate] 1100 mg/5 mL injection

**calcium glucoheptonate** INN, DCF *parenteral calcium replenisher* [also: calcium gluceptate]

**calcium gluconate (calcium D-gluconate)** USP *dietary calcium supplement (9% elemental calcium); investigational (orphan) wash for hydrofluoric acid burns* 500, 650, 975, 1000 mg oral; 3.85 g/15 mL oral; 10% injection

**calcium glycerinophosphate** [see: calcium glycerophosphate]

**calcium glycerophosphate** NF, JAN

**calcium hopantenate** JAN

**calcium hydroxide** USP *astringent*

**calcium hydroxide phosphate** [see: calcium phosphate, tribasic]

**calcium hypophosphite** NF

**calcium iodide** *expectorant*

**calcium iododocosanoate** [see: iodobehenate calcium]

**calcium lactate** USP, JAN *dietary calcium supplement (13% elemental calcium)* 325, 650, 770 mg oral

**calcium lactate hydrate** [see: calcium lactate]

**calcium lactate pentahydrate** [see: calcium lactate]

**calcium lactobionate** USP *dietary calcium supplement*

**calcium lactobionate dihydrate** [see: calcium lactobionate]

**calcium lactophosphate** NF

**calcium L-aspartate** JAN

**calcium levofolinate** [see: levoleucovorin calcium]

**calcium levulate** [see: calcium levulinate]

**calcium levulinate** USP *dietary calcium supplement*

**calcium levulinate dihydrate** [see: calcium levulinate]

**calcium mandelate** USP

**calcium oxide** [see: lime]

**calcium pantothenate (calcium D-pantothenate; vitamin B$_5$)** USP, INN, JAN *water-soluble vitamin; enzyme cofactor* [also: pantothenic acid] 100, 218, 545 mg oral

**calcium pantothenate, racemic (calcium DL-pantothenate)** USP *water-soluble vitamin; enzyme cofactor*

**calcium para-aminosalicylate** JAN [also: aminosalicylate calcium]

**calcium phosphate, dibasic** USP, JAN *dietary calcium supplement; tablet base*

**calcium phosphate, monocalcium** [see: calcium phosphate, dibasic]

**calcium phosphate, tribasic** NF *dietary calcium supplement (39% elemental calcium)* [also: durapatite; hydroxyapatite]

**Calcium +** Ⓒᴬᴺ oral liquid OTC *dietary supplement* [calcium; magnesium; vitamin D] 500 mg•200 mg•200 IU per 2 tsp. dose

**calcium polycarbophil** USAN, USP *bulk laxative; antidiarrheal*

**calcium polystyrene sulfonate** JAN *ion exchange resin for hyperkalemia*

**calcium polysulfide & calcium thiosulfate** [see: lime, sulfurated]

**calcium saccharate** USP, INN *stabilizer*

**calcium silicate** NF *tablet excipient*

**calcium sodium ferriclate** INN *hematinic* [also: ferriclate calcium sodium]

**calcium stearate** NF, JAN *tablet and capsule lubricant*

**calcium sulfate** NF *tablet and capsule diluent*

**calcium tetracemine disodium** [see: edetate calcium disodium]

**calcium trisodium pentetate** INN, BAN *plutonium chelating agent* [also: pentetate calcium trisodium]

**calcium 10-undecenoate** [see: calcium undecylenate]

**calcium undecylenate** USAN *antifungal*

**calciumedetate sodium** [see: edetate calcium disodium]

**Calderol** capsules ℞ *vitamin D therapy for metastatic bone disease or hypocal-*

*cemia of chronic renal dialysis* [calcife-diol] 20, 50 µg

**Caldesene** ointment OTC *moisturizer; emollient; astringent; antiseptic* [cod liver oil (vitamins A and D); zinc oxide; lanolin]

**Caldesene** powder OTC *topical antifungal* [calcium undecylenate] 10%

**caldiamide** INN *pharmaceutic aid* [also: caldiamide sodium]

**caldiamide sodium** USAN, BAN *pharmaceutic aid* [also: caldiamide]

**Calel D** tablets OTC *dietary supplement* [calcium carbonate; cholecalciferol] 500 mg•200 IU

*Calendula officinalis* *medicinal herb* [see: marigold]

**CALF (cyclophosphamide, Adriamycin, leucovorin [rescue], fluorouracil)** *chemotherapy protocol*

**calfactant** USAN *surface-active extract of saline lavage of calf lungs, used for prevention of respiratory distress syndrome (RDS) in premature infants (orphan)*

**CALF-E (cyclophosphamide, Adriamycin, leucovorin [rescue], fluorouracil, ethinyl estradiol)** *chemotherapy protocol*

**CAL-G (cyclophosphamide, asparaginase, leurocristine, daunorubicin, prednisone)** *chemotherapy protocol for acute lymphocytic leukemia (ALL)*

**Cal-Gest** chewable tablets OTC *calcium supplement* [calcium carbonate] 500 mg (200 mg Ca)

**Calgonate** wash ℞ *investigational (orphan) emergency treatment for hydrofluoric acid burns* [calcium gluconate]

**Cal-Guard** softgels (discontinued 2002) OTC *calcium supplement* [calcium carbonate] 125 mg (50 mg Ca)

**California barberry** *medicinal herb* [see: Oregon grape]

**California buckthorn** *medicinal herb* [see: buckthorn; cascara sagrada]

**California false hellebore (***Veratrum californicum***)** [see: hellebore]

**californium** *element (Cf)*

**calioben** [see: calcium iodobehenate]

**Cal-Lac** capsules OTC *calcium supplement* [calcium lactate] 500 mg

*Calluna vulgaris* *medicinal herb* [see: heather]

**calmatives** *a class of soothing agents that reduce excitement, nervousness, distress, or irritation* [also called: sedatives]

**Calmol 4** rectal suppositories OTC *emollient; astringent* [cocoa butter; zinc oxide] 80%•10%

**Calm-X** tablets OTC *anticholinergic; antiemetic; antivertigo agent; motion sickness preventative* [dimenhydrinate] 50 mg

**Calmylin** ⒸⒶⓃ oral solution (discontinued 2001) OTC *antitussive; decongestant; expectorant* [dextromethorphan hydrobromide; pseudoephedrine HCl; guaifenesin] 3•6•20 mg/mL

**Calmylin #1** ⒸⒶⓃ syrup (discontinued 2001) OTC *antihistamine* [dextromethorphan hydrobromide] 3 mg/mL

**Calmylin #2** ⒸⒶⓃ oral solution (discontinued 2001) OTC *antitussive; decongestant* [dextromethorphan hydrobromide; pseudoephedrine HCl] 3•6 mg/mL

**Calmylin #4** ⒸⒶⓃ oral solution (discontinued 2001) OTC *antitussive; antihistamine; expectorant* [dextromethorphan hydrobromide; diphenhydramine HCl; ammonium chloride] 2.5•3•25 mg/mL

**Calmylin Cough & Cold** ⒸⒶⓃ oral solution (discontinued 2001) OTC *antitussive; decongestant; expectorant; analgesic* [dextromethorphan hydrobromide; pseudoephedrine HCl; guaifenesin; acetaminophen] 1•2•6.67•21.67 mg/mL

**Calmylin Expectorant** ⒸⒶⓃ syrup (discontinued 2001) OTC *expectorant* [guaifenesin] 20 mg/mL

**Calmylin Pediatric** ⒸⒶⓃ syrup (discontinued 2001) OTC *pediatric antitussive and decongestant* [dextromethorphan hydrobromide; pseudoephedrine HCl] 1.5•3 mg/mL

**Calmylin with Codeine** (CAN) oral solution R narcotic antitussive; decongestant; expectorant [codeine phosphate; pseudoephedrine HCl; guaifenesin] 0.66•6•20 mg/mL

**Cal-Nate** tablets R vitamin/mineral/calcium/iron supplement; stool softener [multiple vitamins & minerals; calcium; iron; folic acid; docusate sodium] ≛•125•27•1•50 mg

**calomel** NF

**Calphosan** IV injection R calcium replacement [calcium glycerophosphate; calcium lactate] 50•50 mg/10 mL (0.08 mEq Ca/mL)

**Calphron** tablets (discontinued 2002) R calcium supplement; buffering agent for hyperphosphatemia in end-stage renal failure (orphan) [calcium acetate] 667 mg

**Cal-Plus** tablets (discontinued 2002) OTC calcium supplement [calcium carbonate] 1500 mg (600 mg Ca)

**calteridol** INN pharmaceutic aid [also: calteridol calcium]

**calteridol calcium** USAN, BAN pharmaceutic aid [also: calteridol]

*Caltha palustris* medicinal herb [see: cowslip]

**Caltrate 600** film-coated tablets OTC calcium supplement [calcium carbonate] 1500 mg (600 mg Ca)

**Caltrate 600 + D** tablets OTC dietary supplement [calcium carbonate; vitamin D] 600 mg•200 IU

**Caltrate 600 + Iron/Vitamin D** film-coated tablets OTC dietary supplement [calcium carbonate; ferrous fumarate; vitamin D] 600 mg•18 mg•125 IU

**Caltrate Jr.** chewable tablets (discontinued 2002) OTC calcium supplement [calcium carbonate] 750 mg (300 mg Ca)

**Caltrate Plus** tablets OTC dietary supplement [calcium carbonate; vitamin D; multiple minerals] 600 mg•200 IU• ≛

**Caltro** tablets OTC dietary supplement [calcium; vitamin D] 250 mg•125 IU

**calumba; calumba root; calumbo** medicinal herb [see: colombo]

**calusterone** USAN, INN antineoplastic

**Calypte** test kit for professional use urine test for HIV-1 antibodies

**CAM (cyclophosphamide, Adriamycin, methotrexate)** chemotherapy protocol

**Cama Arthritis Pain Reliever** tablets OTC analgesic; antipyretic; antiinflammatory; antirheumatic [aspirin (buffered with magnesium oxide and aluminum hydroxide)] 500 mg

**camazepam** INN

**CAMB (Cytoxin, Adriamycin, methotrexate, bleomycin)** chemotherapy protocol

**cambendazole** USAN, INN, BAN anthelmintic

**CAMELEON (cytosine arabinoside, methotrexate, Leukovorin, Oncovin)** chemotherapy protocol

**camellia oil** JAN

*Camellia sinensis* medicinal herb [see: green tea]

**CAMEO (cyclophosphamide, Adriamycin, methotrexate, etoposide, Oncovin)** chemotherapy protocol

**Cameo Oil** OTC bath emollient

**CAMF (cyclophosphamide, Adriamycin, methotrexate, folinic acid)** chemotherapy protocol

**camiglibose** USAN, INN antidiabetic

**Camila** tablets (in packs of 28) R oral contraceptive (progestin only) [norethindrone] 0.35 mg

**camiverine** INN

**camomile** medicinal herb [see: chamomile]

**camonagrel** INN

**camostat** INN [also: camostat mesilate]

**camostat mesilate** JAN [also: camostat]

**cAMP (cyclic adenosine monophosphate)** [see: adenosine phosphate]

**CAMP (cyclophosphamide, Adriamycin, methotrexate, procarbazine HCl)** chemotherapy protocol for non–small cell lung cancer (NSCLC)

**Campath** IV infusion R immunosuppressant for B-cell chronic lymphocytic leukemia (orphan); investigational (Phase II) for non-Hodgkin lymphoma, organ transplants, and multiple sclerosis [alemtuzumab] 30 mg/3 mL dose

**camphetamide** [see: camphotamide]

**Campho-Phenique** topical liquid, gel OTC *mild anesthetic; anti-infective; counterirritant* [camphor; phenol; eucalyptus oil] 10.8%•4.7%• ?

**Campho-Phenique Antibiotic Plus Pain Reliever** ointment (discontinued 2001) OTC *topical antibiotic; local anesthetic* [polymyxin B sulfate; neomycin sulfate; bacitracin zinc; lidocaine] 5000 U•3.5 mg•500 U•40 mg per g

**Campho-Phenique Cold Sore Treatment and Scab Relief** cream OTC *anesthetic for cold sores and fever blisters* [pramoxine HCl; petrolatum] 1%•30

**camphor (*d*-camphor; *dl*-camphor)** USP, JAN *topical antipruritic; mild local anesthetic; counterirritant* [also: trans-π-oxocamphor]

**camphor, monobromated** USP

**camphorated opium tincture** [now: paregoric]

**camphorated parachlorophenol** [see: parachlorophenol, camphorated]

**camphoric acid** USP

**camphotamide** INN, DCF

**Campral** delayed-release tablets ℞ *agent for the treatment of alcoholism* [acamprosate calcium]

**Camptosar** IV infusion ℞ *topoisomerase I inhibitor; antineoplastic for metastatic colorectal cancer* [irinotecan HCl] 20 mg/mL

**camptothecin-11 (CPT-11)** [see: irinotecan]

**Campyvax** ℞ *investigational (Phase II/III) Campylobacter vaccine*

**camsilate** INN *combining name for radicals or groups* [also: camsylate]

**camsylate** USAN, BAN *combining name for radicals or groups* [also: camsilate]

**Camvirex** ℞ *investigational (orphan) for pancreatic cancer and pediatric HIV/AIDS infections* [rubitecan]

**camylofin** INN, DCF

**Canada fleabane** *medicinal herb* [see: fleabane; horseweed]

**Canada pitch tree** *medicinal herb* [see: hemlock]

**Canada root** *medicinal herb* [see: pleurisy root]

**Canada tea** *medicinal herb* [see: wintergreen]

**canaigre (*Rumex hymenosepalus*)** *medicinal herb for a variety of disease states and used as a purported substitute for ginseng; not generally regarded as safe and effective because of high tannin content and possible mutagenic effect when used internally*

**Canasa** suppositories ℞ *anti-inflammatory for active ulcerative colitis, proctosigmoiditis, and proctitis* [mesalamine (5-aminosalicylic acid)] 500 mg

**canbisol** INN

**CancerVax** ℞ *investigational therapeutic vaccine for melanoma*

**Cancidas** powder for IV infusion ℞ *systemic antifungal for invasive aspergillosis and other resistant fungal infections* [caspofungin acetate] 50, 70 mg/vial

**candesartan** USAN, INN *antihypertensive; angiotensin II receptor antagonist*

**candesartan cilexetil** USAN *antihypertensive; angiotensin II receptor antagonist; investigational (Phase II) for the prevention of diabetic retinopathy*

**candicidin** USAN, USP, INN, BAN *polyene antifungal*

***Candida albicans* skin test antigen** *diagnostic aid for diminished cellular immunity; test for HIV patients to assess TB antigen response*

**CandidaSure** reagent slides for professional use *in vitro diagnostic aid for Candida albicans in the vagina*

**Candin** intradermal injection ℞ *diagnostic aid for diminished cellular immunity; test for HIV patients to assess TB antigen response* [Candida albicans skin test antigen] 0.1 mL

**candleberry; candleberry myrtle** *medicinal herb* [see: bayberry; tung seed]

**candocuronium iodide** INN

**candoxatril** USAN, INN, BAN *antihypertensive*

**candoxatrilat** USAN, INN, BAN *antihypertensive*

**Canesten Topical** ⒸⒶⓃ cream OTC *topical antifungal* [clotrimazole] 1%

**Cankaid** oral solution OTC *topical antiinflammatory and anti-infective* [carbamide peroxide] 10%

**cankerroot** *medicinal herb* [see: gold thread]

**canna; channa** *medicinal herb* [see: kanna]

**cannabinol** INN, BAN *antiemetic; antinauseant; a nonpsychoactive derivative of the Cannabis sativa plant*

*Cannabis sativa* **(marijuana; marihuana; hashish)** *euphoric/hallucinogenic street drug made from the resin or dried leaves and flowering tops of the cannabis plant; medicinal herb for asthma, analgesia, leprosy, and loss of appetite; investigational (Phase II) for pain relief and sleep enhancement*

**canrenoate potassium** USAN *aldosterone antagonist* [also: canrenoic acid; potassium canrenoate]

**canrenoic acid** INN, BAN *aldosterone antagonist* [also: canrenoate potassium; potassium canrenoate]

**canrenone** USAN, INN *aldosterone antagonist*

**cantharides** JAN

**cantharidin** *topical keratolytic*

**Cantil** tablets ℞ *GI antispasmodic; anticholinergic; peptic ulcer adjunct* [mepenzolate bromide] 25 mg

**Canvaxin** ℞ *investigational (Phase III) theraccine for malignant melanoma*

**CAO (cyclophosphamide, Adriamycin, Oncovin)** *chemotherapy protocol*

**CAP (cellulose acetate phthalate)** [q.v.]

**CAP (cyclophosphamide, Adriamycin, Platinol)** *chemotherapy protocol for non–small cell lung cancer (NSCLC)*

**CAP (cyclophosphamide, Adriamycin, prednisone)** *chemotherapy protocol*

**CAP; CAP-I (cyclophosphamide, Adriamycin, Platinol)** *chemotherapy protocol*

**CAP-II (cyclophosphamide, Adriamycin, high-dose Platinol)** *chemotherapy protocol*

**Capastat Sulfate** powder for IM injection ℞ *tuberculostatic* [capreomycin sulfate] 1 g/vial ② Cepastat

**CAP-BOP (cyclophosphamide, Adriamycin, procarbazine, bleomycin, Oncovin, prednisone)** *chemotherapy protocol*

**CAPE (caffeic acid phenethyl ester)** *antimicrobial substance found in bee propolis*

**Cape aloe** *medicinal herb* [see: aloe]

**cape gum** *medicinal herb* [see: acacia]

**capecitabine** USAN, INN *oral fluoropyrimidine (a 5-FU prodrug) antineoplastic for metastatic breast and colorectal cancer; investigational (Phase III) for pancreatic cancer*

**capers (*Capparis spinosa*)** flower buds and leaves *medicinal herb for skin disorders and reducing the effects of enlarged capillaries*

**Capex** shampoo ℞ *corticosteroidal antiinflammatory; antiseborrheic* [fluocinolone acetonide] 0.01% ② 12/00n

**capimorelin tartrate** [see: capromorelin tartrate]

**Capital with Codeine** oral suspension ℞ *narcotic antitussive; analgesic* [codeine phosphate; acetaminophen] 12•120 mg/5 mL

**Capitrol** shampoo ℞ *antiseborrheic; antibacterial; antifungal* [chloroxine] 2% ② captopril

**caplet** (dosage form) *capsule-shaped tablet*

**capmul 8210** [see: monoctanoin]

**capobenate sodium** USAN *antiarrhythmic*

**capobenic acid** USAN, INN *antiarrhythmic*

**Capoten** tablets ℞ *antihypertensive; angiotensin-converting enzyme (ACE) inhibitor; treatment for CHF and diabetic nephropathy* [captopril] 12.5, 25, 50, 100 mg

**Capozide 25/15; Capozide 25/25; Capozide 50/15; Capozide 50/25** tablets ℞ *antihypertensive; angiotensin-converting enzyme (ACE) inhibitor; diuretic* [captopril; hydrochlorothiazide] 25•15 mg; 25•25 mg; 50•15 mg; 50•25 mg

*Capparis spinosa medicinal herb* [see: capers]

**CAPPr (cyclophosphamide, Adriamycin, Platinol, prednisone)** *chemotherapy protocol*

**capreomycin** INN, BAN *bactericidal antibiotic; tuberculostatic* [also: capreomycin sulfate]

**capreomycin sulfate** USAN, USP, JAN *bactericidal antibiotic; tuberculostatic* [also: capreomycin]

**Caprogel** ℞ *investigational (orphan) topical treatment for traumatic hyphema of the eye* [aminocaproic acid]

**capromab** INN *monoclonal antibody for diagnosis of prostate cancer* [also: capromab pendetide]

**capromab pendetide** USAN *monoclonal antibody for diagnosis of prostate cancer* [also: capromab]

**capromorelin tartrate** USAN *growth hormone secretagogue for anti-aging, congestive heart failure, and catabolic illness* [previous USAN: capimorelin tartrate]

**caproxamine** INN, BAN

**capsaicin** *topical analgesic; counterirritant; investigational (orphan) for erythromelalgia and painful HIV-related neuropathy* 0.025%, 0.075% topical

*Capsella bursa-pastoris medicinal herb* [see: shepherd's purse]

*Capsicum frutescens; C. annuum medicinal herb* [see: cayenne]

**capsicum oleoresin** *topical analgesic; counterirritant*

**Capsin** lotion OTC *topical analgesic* [capsaicin] 0.025%, 0.075%

**Capsulets** (trademarked form) *sustained-release caplet*

**captab** (dosage form) *capsule-shaped tablet*

**captamine** INN *depigmentor* [also: captamine HCl]

**captamine HCl** USAN *depigmentor* [also: captamine]

**captodiame** INN, BAN

**captodiame HCl** [see: captodiame]

**captodiamine HCl** [see: captodiame]

**captopril** USAN, USP, INN, BAN, JAN *antihypertensive; angiotensin-converting enzyme (ACE) inhibitor; treatment for CHF and diabetic nephropathy* 12.5, 25, 50, 100 mg oral ② Capitrol

**captopril & hydrochlorothiazide** *antihypertensive; angiotensin-converting enzyme (ACE) inhibitor; diuretic* 25•15, 25•25, 50•15, 50•25 mg oral

**capuride** USAN, INN *hypnotic*

**Capzasin-P** cream OTC *topical analgesic* [capsaicin] 0.025%

**Carac** cream ℞ *antineoplastic for actinic keratoses and basal cell carcinomas* [fluorouracil] 0.5%

**caracemide** USAN, INN *antineoplastic*

**Carafate** tablets, oral suspension ℞ *treatment for duodenal ulcer* [sucralfate] 1 g; 1 g/10 mL

**caramel** NF *coloring agent*

**caramiphen** INN, BAN *antitussive*

**caramiphen edisylate** *antitussive*

**caramiphen HCl** [see: caramiphen]

**caraway (Carum carvi)** NF *seeds medicinal herb for acid indigestion, appetite stimulation, colic, gas, gastrointestinal spasms, and uterine cramps*

**caraway oil** NF

**carazolol** INN, BAN

**carbacephems** *a class of bactericidal antibiotics similar to second-generation cephalosporins (q.v.)*

**carbachol** USP, INN, BAN, JAN *ophthalmic cholinergic; miotic for surgery; antiglaucoma agent* [also: carbacholine chloride]

**carbacholine chloride** DCF *ophthalmic cholinergic; miotic for surgery; antiglaucoma agent* [also: carbachol]

**carbacrylamine resins**

**carbadipimidine HCl** [see: carpipramine dihydrochloride]

**carbadox** USAN, INN, BAN *antibacterial*

**carbaldrate** INN

**carbamate choline chloride** [see: carbachol]

**carbamazepine** USAN, USP, INN, BAN, JAN *anticonvulsant; analgesic for trigeminal neuralgia; antimanic* 100, 200 mg oral; 100 mg/5 mL oral

**carbamide** [see: urea]

**carbamide peroxide** USP *topical dental anti-infective; cerumenolytic to emulsify and disperse ear wax*

**N-carbamoylarsanilic acid** [see: carbarsone]

**carbamoylcholine chloride** [see: carbachol]

**O-carbamoylsalicylic acid lactam** [see: carsalam]

**carbamylcholine chloride** [see: carbachol]

**carbamylglutamic acid** *investigational (orphan) treatment for N-acetylglutamate synthetase deficiency*

**carbamylmethylcholine chloride** [see: bethanechol chloride]

**carbantel** INN *anthelmintic* [also: carbantel lauryl sulfate]

**carbantel lauryl sulfate** USAN *anthelmintic* [also: carbantel]

**carbaril** INN [also: carbaryl]

**carbarsone** USP, INN

**carbaryl** BAN [also: carbaril]

**carbasalate calcium** INN *analgesic* [also: carbaspirin calcium]

**carbaspirin calcium** USAN *analgesic* [also: carbasalate calcium]

**Carbastat** solution ℞ *direct-acting miotic for ophthalmic surgery* [carbachol] 0.01%

**Carbatrol** extended-release capsules ℞ *anticonvulsant; analgesic for trigeminal neuralgia; antipsychotic* [carbamazepine] 100, 200, 300 mg

**carbazeran** USAN, INN *cardiotonic*

**carbazochrome** INN, JAN

**carbazochrome salicylate** INN

**carbazochrome sodium sulfonate** INN

**carbazocine** INN

**carbenicillin** INN, BAN *extended-spectrum penicillin antibiotic* [also: carbenicillin disodium; carbenicillin sodium]

**carbenicillin disodium** USAN, USP *extended-spectrum penicillin antibiotic* [also: carbenicillin; carbenicillin sodium]

**carbenicillin indanyl sodium** USAN, USP *extended-spectrum penicillin antibiotic* [also: carindacillin]

**carbenicillin phenyl sodium** USAN *antibacterial* [also: carfecillin]

**carbenicillin potassium** USAN *antibacterial*

**carbenicillin sodium** JAN *antibacterial* [also: carbenicillin disodium; carbenicillin]

**carbenoxolone** INN, BAN *corticosteroid; anti-inflammatory* [also: carbenoxolone sodium]

**carbenoxolone sodium** USAN *corticosteroid; anti-inflammatory* [also: carbenoxolone]

**carbenzide** INN

**carbesilate** INN *combining name for radicals or groups*

**carbetapentane citrate** NF *antitussive* [also: pentoxyverine]

**carbetapentane tannate** *antitussive*

**carbetimer** USAN, INN *antineoplastic*

**carbetocin** INN, BAN *uterotonic agent to prevent postpartum hemorrhage following cesarean section*

**Carbex** tablets ℞ *dopaminergic antiparkinsonian* (orphan) [selegiline HCl] 5 mg

**carbidopa** USAN, USP, INN, BAN, JAN *decarboxylase inhibitor; antiparkinsonian adjunct*

**carbidopa & levodopa** *antiparkinsonian; dopamine precursor plus synergist* 10•100, 25•100, 25•250, 50•200 mg oral

**carbifene** INN *analgesic* [also: carbiphene HCl; carbiphene]

**carbimazole** INN, BAN

**carbinoxamine** INN, BAN *antihistamine for allergic rhinitis* [also: carbinoxamine maleate]

**Carbinoxamine** pediatric syrup, pediatric oral drops ℞ *decongestant; antihistamine* [pseudoephedrine HCl; carbinoxamine maleate] 60•4 mg/5 mL; 25•2 mg/mL

**Carbinoxamine Compound** syrup, pediatric oral drops (discontinued 2004) ℞ *antitussive; decongestant; antihistamine* [dextromethorphan hydrobromide; pseudoephedrine HCl; carbinoxamine maleate] 15•60•4 mg/5 mL; 4•25•2 mg/mL

**carbinoxamine maleate** USP *antihistamine for allergic rhinitis* [also: carbinoxamine]

**carbinoxamine maleate & hydrocodone bitartrate & pseudoephedrine HCl** *antihistamine; antitussive; decongestant* 2•5•30 mg/5 mL oral

**carbinoxamine maleate & pseudoephedrine HCl** *antihistamine; decongestant* 4•60 mg/5 mL oral; 2•25 mg/mL oral

**carbiphene** BAN *analgesic* [also: carbiphene HCl; carbifene]

**carbiphene HCl** USAN *analgesic* [also: carbifene; carbiphene]

**Carbiset** tablets (discontinued 2002) ℞ *decongestant; antihistamine* [pseudoephedrine HCl; carbinoxamine maleate] 60•4 mg

**Carbiset-TR** timed-release tablets (discontinued 2002) ℞ *decongestant; antihistamine* [pseudoephedrine HCl; carbinoxamine maleate] 120•8 mg

**Carbocaine** injection ℞ *injectable local anesthetic* [mepivacaine HCl] 1%, 1.5%, 2%, 3%

**Carbocaine with Neo-Cobefrin** injection ℞ *injectable local anesthetic; vasoconstrictor* [mepivacaine HCl; levonordefrin] 2%•1:20 000

**carbocisteine** INN, BAN *mucolytic* [also: carbocysteine]

**carbocloral** USAN, INN, BAN *hypnotic*

**carbocromen** INN *coronary vasodilator* [also: chromonar HCl]

**carbocysteine** USAN *mucolytic* [also: carbocisteine]

**Carbodec** tablets, syrup (discontinued 2002) ℞ *decongestant; antihistamine* [pseudoephedrine HCl; carbinoxamine maleate] 60•4 mg; 60•4 mg/5 mL

**Carbodec DM** syrup, pediatric drops (discontinued 2002) ℞ *antitussive; decongestant; antihistamine* [dextromethorphan hydrobromide; pseudoephedrine HCl; carbinoxamine maleate] 15•60•4 mg/5 mL; 4•25•2 mg/mL

**Carbodec TR** timed-release tablets (discontinued 2002) ℞ *decongestant; antihistamine* [pseudoephedrine HCl; carbinoxamine maleate] 120•8 mg

**Carbodex DM** pediatric oral drops ℞ *antitussive; decongestant; antihistamine* [dextromethorphan hydrobromide; pseudoephedrine HCl; carbinoxamine maleate] 4•15•2 mg/mL

**Carbodex DM** syrup ℞ *antitussive; decongestant; antihistamine* [dextromethorphan hydrobromide; pseudoephedrine HCl; brompheniramine maleate] 15•45•4 mg/5 mL

**carbodimid calcium** [see: calcium carbimide]

**Carbofed DM** pediatric oral drops ℞ *antitussive; decongestant; antihistamine* [dextromethorphan hydrobromide; pseudoephedrine HCl; carbinoxamine maleate] 4•15•1 mg/mL

**Carbofed DM** syrup ℞ *antitussive; decongestant; antihistamine* [dextromethorphan hydrobromide; pseudoephedrine HCl; brompheniramine maleate] 15•45•4 mg/5 mL

**carbofenotion** INN [also: carbophenothion]

**carbol-fuchsin solution (or paint)** USP *antifungal*

**carbolic acid** [see: phenol]

**carbolin** [see: carbachol]

**Carbolith** ⒸⒶ⒩ capsules ℞ *antipsychotic for manic episodes* [lithium carbonate] 150, 300, 600 mg

**carbolonium bromide** BAN [also: hexcarbacholine bromide]

**carbomer** INN, BAN *emulsifying and suspending agent* [also: carbomer 910]

**carbomer 1342** NF *emulsifying and suspending agent*

**carbomer 910** USAN, NF *emulsifying and suspending agent* [also: carbomer]

**carbomer 934** USAN, NF *emulsifying and suspending agent*

**carbomer 934P** USAN, NF *emulsifying and suspending agent*

**carbomer 940** USAN, NF *emulsifying and suspending agent*

**carbomer 941** USAN, NF *emulsifying and suspending agent*

**carbomycin** INN

**carbon** *element* (C)

**carbon, activated**

**carbon C 13 urea** *diagnostic aid for detection of H. pylori in the stomach*

**carbon C 14 urea** *diagnostic aid for H. pylori in the stomach* [also: $^{14}C$ urea]

**carbon dioxide ($CO_2$)** USP *respiratory stimulant*

**carbon tetrachloride** NF *solvent*

**carbonic acid, calcium salt** [see: calcium carbonate]

**carbonic acid, dilithium salt** [see: lithium carbonate]

**carbonic acid, dipotassium salt** [see: potassium carbonate]

**carbonic acid, disodium salt** [see: sodium carbonate]

**carbonic acid, magnesium salt** [see: magnesium carbonate]

**carbonic acid, monoammonium salt** [see: ammonium carbonate]

**carbonic acid, monopotassium salt** [see: potassium bicarbonate]

**carbonic acid, monosodium salt** [see: sodium bicarbonate]

**carbonic anhydrase inhibitors** *a class of diuretic agents that reduce the rate of aqueous humor formation, resulting in decreased intraocular pressure; available in both systemic (tablets) and topical (eye drops) forms*

**carbonis detergens, liquor (LCD)** [see: coal tar]

**carbonyl iron** *hematinic; dietary iron supplement (100% elemental iron as microparticles)*

**carbophenothion** BAN [also: carbofenotion]

**carboplatin** USAN, INN, BAN *alkylating antineoplastic for ovarian and other cancers* 10 mg/mL injection

**carboplatin & etoposide & paclitaxel** *chemotherapy protocol for primary adenocarcinoma and small cell lung cancer (SCLC)*

**carboplatin & gemcitabine** *chemotherapy protocol for non–small cell lung cancer (NSCLC)*

**carboprost** USAN, INN, BAN *oxytocic*

**carboprost methyl** USAN *oxytocic*

**carboprost trometanol** BAN *oxytocic; prostaglandin-type abortifacient* [also: carboprost tromethamine]

**carboprost tromethamine** USAN, USP *oxytocic; prostaglandin-type abortifacient* [also: carboprost trometanol]

**Carboptic** Drop-Tainers (eye drops) ℞ *topical antiglaucoma agent; direct-acting miotic* [carbachol] 3%

**carboquone** INN

**carbose D** [see: carboxymethylcellulose sodium]

**Carbo-Tax (carboplatin, Taxol)** *chemotherapy protocol for ovarian cancer* [also: CaT]

**carbovir** *investigational (orphan) agent for AIDS and symptomatic HIV infections*

**carboxyimamidate** [see: carbetimer]

**carboxymethylcellulose calcium** NF *tablet disintegrant*

**carboxymethylcellulose sodium** USP *bulk laxative; suspending and viscosity-increasing agent; ophthalmic moisturizer; tablet excipient* [also: carmellose; carmellose sodium]

**carboxymethylcellulose sodium 12** NF *suspending and viscosity-increasing agent*

**carboxypeptidase G2** *investigational (orphan) agent for methotrexate toxicity*

**carbromal** NF, INN

**carbubarb** INN

**carbubarbital** [see: carbubarb]

**carburazepam** INN
**carbutamide** INN, BAN
**carbuterol** INN, BAN *bronchodilator*
[also: carbuterol HCl]
**carbuterol HCl** USAN *bronchodilator*
[also: carbuterol]
**carcainium chloride** INN
**carcinoembryonic antigen (CEA)**
**cardamom seed** NF
**cardamom** [see: bitter cardamom]
**Cardec-DM** pediatric syrup, pediatric
drops (discontinued 2002) ℞ *antitussive; decongestant; antihistamine* [dex-
tromethorphan hydrobromide; pseudoephedrine HCl; carbinoxamine
maleate] 15•60•4 mg/5 mL; 4•25•
2 mg/mL
**Cardec-DM** syrup (discontinued 2004)
℞ *antitussive; decongestant; antihistamine* [dextromethorphan hydrobromide; pseudoephedrine HCl; carbinoxamine maleate] 15•60•4 mg/5 mL
**Cardec-S** oral liquid (discontinued
2004) ℞ *decongestant; antihistamine*
[pseudoephedrine HCl; carbinoxamine maleate] 60•4 mg/5 mL
**Cardene** capsules ℞ *antianginal; antihypertensive; calcium channel blocker*
[nicardipine HCl] 20, 30 mg ⊡ Cardizem
**Cardene I.V.** injection ℞ *antihypertensive; calcium channel blocker* [nicardi-
pine HCl] 2.5 mg/mL
**Cardene SR** sustained-release capsules
℞ *antihypertensive; calcium channel
blocker* [nicardipine HCl] 30, 45, 60
mg
**cardiac glycosides** a class of cardiovascular drugs that increase the force of
cardiac contractions [also called: digitalis glycosides]
**Cardiac T** test *in vitro diagnostic aid for
troponin T (indicator of cardiac damage) in whole blood*
**cardiacs** a class of agents that stimulate
or otherwise affect the heart (a term
used in folk medicine)
**cardiamid** [see: nikethamide]
**cardin** medicinal herb [see: blessed this-
tle]

**Cardio-Green (CG)** powder for IV
injection (discontinued 2004) ℞ *in
vivo diagnostic aid for cardiac output,
hepatic function, and ophthalmic angiography* [indocyanine green] 25, 50 mg
**Cardiolite** injection ℞ *myocardial perfusion agent for cardiac SPECT imaging*
[technetium Tc 99m sestamibi] 5 mL
**Cardi-Omega 3** capsules OTC *dietary
supplement* [omega-3 fatty acids;
multiple vitamins & minerals]
1000• ± mg
**cardioplegic solution (calcium
chloride, magnesium chloride,
potassium chloride, sodium chloride)** [q.v.]
**cardioprotective agents** a class of
potent intracellular chelating agents
which protect the heart from the effects
of doxorubicin
**Cardioquin** tablets (discontinued
2003) ℞ *antiarrhythmic* [quinidine
polygalacturonate] 275 mg
**Cardiotek Rx** coated tablets ℞ *dietary
supplement* [vitamins $B_6$ and $B_{12}$;
folic acid; L-arginine HCl] 50•0.5•
2• ± mg
**Cardizem** IV injection, Lyo-Ject (prefilled syringe) ℞ *calcium channel
blocker for atrial fibrillation or paroxysmal supraventricular tachycardia
(PSVT)* [diltiazem HCl] 5 mg/mL;
25 mg ⊡ Cardene
**Cardizem** Monovial (single-use vial)
(discontinued 2003) ℞ *calcium channel blocker for atrial fibrillation or
paroxysmal supraventricular tachycardia (PSVT)* [diltiazem HCl] 100 mg
⊡ Cardene
**Cardizem** tablets ℞ *antianginal; antihypertensive; antiarrhythmic; calcium
channel blocker* [diltiazem HCl] 30,
60, 90, 120 mg
**Cardizem LA** extended-release caplets
℞ *antihypertensive; antianginal; calcium channel blocker* [diltiazem HCl]
120, 180, 240, 300, 360, 420 mg
**Cardizem SR; Cardizem CD** sustained-release capsules ℞ *antihypertensive; antianginal; antiarrhythmic;*

calcium channel blocker [diltiazem HCl] 60, 90, 120 mg; 120, 180, 240, 300, 360 mg

**Cardizem XL** ℞ *investigational (NDA filed) h.s. dosing of Cardizem* [diltiazem HCl]

**cardophyllin** [see: aminophylline]

**Cardura** tablets ℞ *α₁-adrenergic blocker for hypertension and benign prostatic hyperplasia (BPH)* [doxazosin mesylate] 1, 2, 4, 8 mg

**Cardura XL** ℞ *investigational (NDA filed) sustained-release formulation* [doxazosin mesylate]

**carebastine** INN

**carena** [see: aminophylline]

**carfecillin** INN, BAN *antibacterial* [also: carbenicillin phenyl sodium]

**carfenazine** INN *antipsychotic* [also: carphenazine maleate; carphenazine]

**carfentanil** INN *narcotic analgesic* [also: carfentanil citrate]

**carfentanil citrate** USAN *narcotic analgesic* [also: carfentanil]

**carfimate** INN

**cargentos** [see: silver protein]

**cargutocin** INN

*Carica papaya* medicinal herb [see: papaya]

**Carimune NF** powder for IV infusion ℞ *passive immunizing agent for HIV and idiopathic thrombocytopenic purpura (ITP)* [immune globulin] 1, 3, 6, 12 g

**carindacillin** INN, BAN *extended-spectrum penicillin antibiotic* [also: carbenicillin indanyl sodium]

**Cariporide** ℞ *investigational (Phase III) for coronary artery bypass grafting*

**Carisolv** ⓒ gel ℞ *topical dissolution of dental caries* [sodium hypochlorite] 0.5%

**carisoprodol** USP, INN, BAN *skeletal muscle relaxant* 350 mg oral

**carline thistle (*Carlina acaulis*)** root *medicinal herb used as a carminative, diaphoretic, digestive, diuretic, febrifuge, and, in large doses, an emetic and purgative*

**carmantadine** USAN, INN *antiparkinsonian*

**carmellose** INN *suspending agent; tablet excipient* [also: carboxymethylcellulose sodium; carmellose sodium]

**carmellose sodium** BAN *suspending agent; tablet excipient* [also: carboxymethylcellulose sodium; carmellose]

**carmetizide** INN

**carminatives** *a class of agents that relieve flatulence*

**carminomycin HCl** [now: carubicin HCl]

**carmofur** INN

**Carmol 10** lotion OTC *moisturizer; emollient; keratolytic* [urea] 10%

**Carmol 20** cream OTC *moisturizer; emollient; keratolytic* [urea] 20%

**Carmol 40** cream, gel ℞ *moisturizer; emollient; keratolytic* [urea] 40%

**Carmol HC** cream ℞ *corticosteroidal anti-inflammatory; moisturizer; emollient* [hydrocortisone acetate; urea] 1%•10%

**carmoxirole** INN

**carmustine** USAN, INN, BAN *nitrosourea-type alkylating antineoplastic for brain tumors, multiple myeloma, Hodgkin disease, and non-Hodgkin lymphomas; polymer implant for recurrent malignant glioma (orphan)*

**Carnation Follow-Up; Carnation Good Start** oral liquid, powder for oral liquid OTC *total or supplementary infant feeding*

**carnauba wax** [see: wax, carnauba]

**carnidazole** USAN, INN, BAN *antiprotozoal*

**carnitine** INN *vitamin B_t*

**L-carnitine** [see: levocarnitine]

**Carnitor** tablets, oral solution, IV injection or infusion ℞ *dietary amino acid for primary and secondary genetic carnitine deficiency (orphan) and end-stage renal disease (orphan); investigational (orphan) for pediatric cardiomyopathy* [levocarnitine] 330 mg; 100 mg/mL; 500 mg/2.5 mL, 1 g/5 mL

**carnosine** *natural anti-carbonylation agent that prevents cross-linking of protein and collagen; antioxidant; dipeptide of β-alanine and L-histidine*

**carocainide** INN

**Caroid** enteric-coated tablets OTC *stimulant laxative* [bisacodyl] 5 mg

**β-carotene** [see: beta carotene]

**caroverine** INN

**caroxazone** USAN, INN *antidepressant*

**carpenter's herb** *medicinal herb* [see: woundwort]

**carpenter's square** *medicinal herb* [see: figwort]

**carperidine** INN, BAN

**carperone** INN

**carphenazine** BAN *antipsychotic* [also: carphenazine maleate; carfenazine]

**carphenazine maleate** USAN, USP *antipsychotic* [also: carfenazine; carphenazine]

**carpindolol** INN

**carpipramine** INN

**carpipramine dihydrochloride** [see: carpipramine]

**carpolene** [now: carbomer 934P]

**carprazidil** INN

**carprofen** USAN, INN, BAN *nonsteroidal anti-inflammatory drug (NSAID); analgesic; antipyretic*

**carpronium chloride** INN

**Carpuject** (trademarked delivery system) *prefilled cartridge-needle unit*

**Carpuject Smartpak** (trademarked delivery system) *prefilled cartridge-needle unit package*

**CarraFoam; CarraWash** topical liquid OTC *skin cleanser for incontinence care* [aloe vera; acemannan]

**carrageenan** NF *suspending and viscosity-increasing agent*

**CarraKlenz** topical liquid OTC *wound cleanser for intact skin* [aloe vera; acemannan]

**CarraSmart** gel OTC *hydrogel wound dressing* [acemannan]

**Carrasyn; Carrasyn V** gel OTC *hydrogel wound dressing* [acemannan]

**carrot** *(Daucus carota)* oil from the dried seed and root *medicinal herb for edema, gas, and worms; also used as a nutritional and vitamin supplement and stimulant; may possibly protect the heart and liver*

**carsalam** INN, BAN

**carsatrin** INN *cardiotonic* [also: carsatrin succinate]

**carsatrin succinate** USAN *cardiotonic* [also: carsatrin]

**cartazolate** USAN, INN *antidepressant*

**carteolol** INN, BAN *topical antiglaucoma agent (β-blocker)* [also: carteolol HCl]

**carteolol HCl** USAN *topical antiglaucoma agent (β-blocker)* [also: carteolol] 1%

*Carthamus tinctorius* *medicinal herb* [see: safflower]

**Cartia XT** extended-release capsules R *antihypertensive; antianginal; antiarrhythmic; calcium channel blocker* [diltiazem HCl] 120, 180, 240, 300 mg

**carticaine** BAN *amide local anesthetic for dentistry* [also: articaine]

**Carticel** R *investigational (NDA filed) process to grow autologous cartilage cells to correct cartilage damage due to acute or chronic trauma* [chondrocytes, cultured autologous]

**Cartrix** (delivery system) *prefilled syringes*

**Cartrol** Filmtabs (film-coated tablets) OTC *antihypertensive; β-blocker* [carteolol HCl] 2.5, 5 mg

**carubicin** INN *antineoplastic* [also: carubicin HCl]

**carubicin HCl** USAN *antineoplastic* [also: carubicin]

*Carum carvi* NF *medicinal herb* [see: caraway]

**carumonam** INN, BAN *antibacterial* [also: carumonam sodium]

**carumonam sodium** USAN *antibacterial* [also: carumonam]

**carvedilol** USAN, INN, BAN, JAN *antianginal; antihypertensive; α- and β-blocker for congestive heart failure*

**carvotroline HCl** USAN *antipsychotic*

*Caryophyllus aromaticus* *medicinal herb* [see: cloves]

**carzelesin** USAN *antineoplastic*

**carzenide** INN

**casanthranol** USAN, USP *stimulant laxative*

**Cascara Aromatic** oral liquid OTC *stimulant laxative* [cascara sagrada; alcohol 18%]

**cascara fluidextract, aromatic** USP *stimulant laxative; investigational (orphan) agent to speed the evacuation of an oral drug overdose* 2–6 mL oral

**cascara sagrada** USP *stimulant laxative* 325 mg oral

**cascara sagrada (Frangula purshiana; Rhamnus purshiana)** bark *medicinal herb for constipation, cough, and gallbladder, intestinal, and liver disorders; chronic use can cause hypokalemia and melanosis coli* [also see: buckthorn]

**cascarin** [see: casanthranol]

**Casec** powder OTC *protein supplement* [calcium caseinate]

**Casodex** film-coated tablets ℞ *antiandrogen antineoplastic for prostatic cancer* [bicalutamide] 50 mg

**caspofungin acetate** USAN *systemic echinocandin antifungal for invasive aspergillosis and other resistant fungal infections*

**Cassia acutifolia; C. angustifolia; C. senna** *medicinal herb* [see: senna]

**CAST (Color Allergy Screening Test)** reagent sticks for professional use *in vitro diagnostic aid for immunoglobulin E in serum*

**Castaderm** topical liquid OTC *antifungal; astringent; antiseptic* [resorcinol; boric acid; acetone; basic fuchsin; phenol; alcohol 9%]

**Castel Minus; Castel Plus** topical liquid OTC *antifungal* [resorcinol; acetone; basic fuchsin; alcohol 11.5%]

**Castellani Paint Modified** solution ℞ *topical antifungal; antibacterial; keratolytic* [basic fuchsin; phenol; resorcinol]

**Castellani's paint** [see: carbol-fuchsin solution]

**Castile soap**

**castor oil** USP *stimulant laxative*

**CaT (carboplatin, Taxol)** *chemotherapy protocol for adenocarcinoma, non–small cell lung cancer (NSCLC), and ovarian cancer* [also: Carbo-Tax]

**CAT (cytarabine, Adriamycin, thioguanine)** *chemotherapy protocol*

**Cataflam** tablets ℞ *analgesic; antiarthritic; nonsteroidal anti-inflammatory drug (NSAID) for ankylosing spondylitis* [diclofenac potassium] 50 mg

**Catapres** tablets ℞ *antihypertensive* [clonidine HCl] 0.1, 0.2, 0.3 mg ⊡ Catarase; Combipres; Ser-Ap-Es

**Catapres-TTS-1; Catapres-TTS-2; Catapres-TTS-3** 7-day transdermal patch ℞ *antihypertensive* [clonidine HCl] 0.1 mg/day (2.5 mg); 0.2 mg/day (5 mg); 0.3 mg/day (7.5 mg)

**Catatrol** ℞ *investigational (NDA filed) bicyclic antidepressant; investigational (orphan) for cataplexy and narcolepsy* [viloxazine]

**catchfly** *medicinal herb* [see: dogbane]

**catchweed** *medicinal herb* [see: bedstraw]

**catechol-O-methyltransferase (COMT)** [see: COMT inhibitors]

**catgut suture** [see: absorbable surgical suture]

**Catha edulis** *the plant from which cathinone, a naturally occurring stimulant, is derived* [see also: cathinone; methcathinone]

**Catharanthus roseus** *medicinal herb* [see: periwinkle]

**cathartics** *a class of agents that cause vigorous evacuation of the bowels by increasing bulk, stimulating peristaltic action, etc.* [also called: purgatives]

**Cathflo Activase** powder for intra-catheter instillation ℞ *tissue plasminogen activator (tPA) thrombolytic to keep open (TKO) central venous access devices (CVADs) (not therapeutic)* [alteplase] 2.2 mg/vial

**cathine** INN

**cathinone** INN *an extract of the* Catha edulis *plant, a naturally occurring stimulant* [see also: Catha edulis; methcathinone]

**cathomycin sodium** [see: novobiocin sodium]

**catkins willow** *medicinal herb* [see: willow]

**catmint** *medicinal herb* [see: catnip]

**catnip (Nepeta cataria)** plant *medicinal herb for colds, colic, convulsions, diarrhea, digestion, fever, flu, gas, hives, nervous conditions, and stimulating delayed menses*

**Catrix Correction** cream OTC *moisturizer; emollient*

**catrup** *medicinal herb* [see: catnip]

**cat's claw (Uncaria guianensis; U. tomentosa)** inner bark *medicinal herb for cancer, Candida infections, chronic fatigue, contraception, Crohn disease, diverticulitis, hypertension, irritable bowel, lupus, parasites, PMS, ulcers, and viral infections; also used as immune booster*

**catswort** *medicinal herb* [see: catnip]

**Caucasian walnut** *medicinal herb* [see: English walnut]

*Caulophyllum thalictroides* medicinal herb [see: blue cohosh]

**caustics** *a class of escharotic or corrosive agents that destroy living tissue* [also called: cauterants]

**cauterants** *a class of escharotic or corrosive agents that destroy living tissue* [also called: caustics]

**CAV (cyclophosphamide, Adriamycin, vinblastine)** *chemotherapy protocol*

**CAV (cyclophosphamide, Adriamycin, vincristine)** *chemotherapy protocol for small cell lung cancer (SCLC)* [also: VAC]

**CAVe; CA-Ve (CCNU, Adriamycin, vinblastine)** *chemotherapy protocol*

**CAVE (cyclophosphamide, Adriamycin, vincristine, etoposide)** *chemotherapy protocol for small cell lung cancer (SCLC)*

**CAV/EP (cyclophosphamide, Adriamycin, vincristine, etoposide, Platinol)** *chemotherapy protocol for small cell lung cancer (SCLC)*

**Caverject** intracavernosal injection, Luer-lock single-use autoinjector ℞ *vasodilator for erectile dysfunction* [alprostadil] 5, 10, 20, 40 μg/mL

**Caverject Impulse** powder for intracavernosal injection in prefilled syringe ℞ *vasodilator for erectile dysfunction* [alprostadil] 10, 20 μg/0.5 mL dose

**CA-VP16; CAVP16 (cyclophosphamide, Adriamycin, VP-16)** *chemotherapy protocol for small cell lung cancer (SCLC)*

**cayenne (Capsicum annuum; C. frutescens)** fruit *medicinal herb for arthritis, bleeding, cold feet, diabetes, high blood pressure, kidney disorders, rheumatism, poor circulation, strokes, topical neuritis syndromes, tumors, and ulcers*

**CBP-1011** *investigational (Phase III) orally administered steroid for idiopathic thrombocytopenic purpura*

**CBV (cyclophosphamide, BCNU, VePesid)** *chemotherapy protocol*

**CBV (cyclophosphamide, BCNU, VP-16-213)** *chemotherapy protocol*

**CC (carboplatin, cyclophosphamide)** *chemotherapy protocol for ovarian cancer*

**CC-Galactosidase** ℞ *investigational (orphan) enzyme replacement therapy for Fabry disease* [agalsidase alfa]

**CCM (cyclophosphamide, CCNU, methotrexate)** *chemotherapy protocol*

**CCNU (chloroethyl-cyclohexyl-nitrosourea)** [see: lomustine]

**CCV-AV (CCNU, cyclophosphamide, vincristine [alternates with] Adriamycin, vincristine)** *chemotherapy protocol*

**CCVPP (CCNU, cyclophosphamide, Velban, procarbazine, prednisone)** *chemotherapy protocol*

**CD (cytarabine, daunorubicin)** *chemotherapy protocol*

**CD4 human truncated 369 AA polypeptide** *investigational (orphan) treatment for AIDS*

**CD4 immunoglobulin G, recombinant human** *investigational (Phase I) antiviral for maternal/fetal transfer of HIV; investigational (orphan) for AIDS*

**CD4 recombinant soluble human (rCD4)** *investigational (Phase II, orphan) antiviral for AIDS*

**CD5-T lymphocyte immunotoxin** *investigational (orphan) agent for graft* *vs. host disease following bone marrow transplants*

**CD20** *investigational for low-grade non-Hodgkin lymphoma*

**CD-33** [see: ricin (blocked) conjugated murine MCA myeloid cells]

**CD-40 ligand (CD40L)** *investigational (Phase II) cytokine for renal cell carcinoma; investigational (Phase I) for rheumatoid arthritis, AIDS, and hyperimmunoglobulin M (HIM) syndrome*

**CdA (2-chloro-2′-deoxyadenosine)** [see: cladribine]

**CDB (cisplatin, dacarbazine, BCNU)** *chemotherapy protocol for malignant melanoma*

**CDC (carboplatin, doxorubicin, cyclophosphamide)** *chemotherapy protocol*

**CDDP; C-DDP (cis-diamminedichloroplatinum)** [see: cisplatin]

**CDDP/VP; CDDP/VP-16 (CDDP, VP-16)** *chemotherapy protocol for pediatric brain tumors*

**CDE (cyclophosphamide, doxorubicin, etoposide [filgrastim])** *chemotherapy protocol for HIV-related non-Hodgkin lymphoma*

**CDP-571** *investigational (Phase III, orphan) anti-TNFα (tumor necrosis factor alpha) antibody CB-0010 for steroid-dependent Crohn disease; investigational for rheumatoid arthritis*

**CDP-cholin** [see: citicoline]

**CEA (carcinoembryonic antigen)**

**CEA-Cide I-131** ℞ *investigational (orphan) antineoplastic for metastatic colorectal cancer* [iodine I 131–labeled labetuzumab]

**CEA-Cide Y-90** ℞ *investigational (orphan) antineoplastic for colorectal, pancreatic, ovarian, and small cell lung cancer* [yttrium Y 90–labeled labetuzumab]

*Ceanothus americanus* medicinal herb [see: New Jersey tea]

**CEA-Scan** powder for injection ℞ *investigational (orphan) imaging agent for detection of recurrent or metastatic thy-roid cancers; investigational (Phase III) for lung cancer* [arcitumomab] 1.25 mg

**CEA-Vac** ℞ *investigational (Phase III) vaccine for breast cancer*

**CEB (carboplatin, etoposide, bleomycin)** *chemotherapy protocol*

**CECA (cisplatin, etoposide, cyclophosphamide, Adriamycin)** *chemotherapy protocol*

**Ceclor** Pulvules (capsules), powder for oral suspension ℞ *cephalosporin antibiotic* [cefaclor] 250, 500 mg; 125, 187, 250, 375 mg/5 mL

**Ceclor CD** extended-release tablets (discontinued 2003) ℞ *cephalosporin antibiotic* [cefaclor] 375, 500 mg

**Ceclor CDpak** extended-release tablets (in compliance packs of 14) ℞ *cephalosporin antibiotic* [cefaclor] 500 mg

**Cecon** drops OTC *vitamin C supplement* [ascorbic acid] 100 mg/mL

**Cedax** capsules, oral suspension ℞ *cephalosporin antibiotic* [ceftibuten] 400 mg; 90, 180 mg/mL

**cedefingol** USAN *antipsoriatic; antineoplastic adjunct*

**cedelizumab** USAN *monoclonal antibody; prophylaxis of rejection of solid organ allograft; immunomodulator for autoimmune diseases*

**CEE (conjugated equine estrogen)** [see: estrogens, conjugated]

**CeeNu** capsules, dose pack ℞ *nitrosourea-type alkylating antineoplastic for brain tumors and Hodgkin disease* [lomustine] 10, 40, 100 mg; 2 × 100 mg + 2 × 40 mg + 2 × 10 mg

**CEF (cyclophosphamide, epirubicin, fluorouracil, [co-trimoxazole])** *chemotherapy protocol for breast cancer*

**cefacetrile** INN *antibacterial* [also: cephacetrile sodium]

**cefacetrile sodium** [see: cephacetrile sodium]

**cefaclor** USAN, USP, INN, BAN, JAN *second-generation cephalosporin antibiotic* 250, 500 mg oral; 125, 187, 250, 375 mg/5 mL oral

**cefadroxil** USAN, USP, INN, BAN *first-generation cephalosporin antibiotic* 500, 1000 mg oral

**Cefadyl** powder for IV or IM injection (discontinued 2004) ℞ *cephalosporin antibiotic* [cephapirin sodium] 1 g ⍰ Cefzil

**cefalexin** INN, JAN *first-generation cephalosporin antibiotic* [also: cephalexin]

**cefaloglycin** INN *antibacterial* [also: cephaloglycin]

**cefalonium** INN [also: cephalonium]

**cefaloram** INN [also: cephaloram]

**cefaloridine** INN *antibacterial* [also: cephaloridine]

**cefalotin** INN *first-generation cephalosporin antibiotic* [also: cephalothin sodium; cephalothin]

**cefalotin sodium** [see: cephalothin sodium]

**cefamandole** USAN, INN *second-generation cephalosporin antibiotic* [also: cephamandole]

**cefamandole nafate** USAN, USP *second-generation cephalosporin antibiotic* [also: cephamandole nafate]

**cefamandole sodium** USP *second-generation cephalosporin antibiotic*

**cefaparole** USAN, INN *antibacterial*

**cefapirin** INN, BAN *first-generation cephalosporin antibiotic* [also: cephapirin sodium]

**cefapirin sodium** [see: cephapirin sodium]

**cefatrizine** USAN, INN, BAN *antibacterial*

**cefazaflur** INN *antibacterial* [also: cefazaflur sodium]

**cefazaflur sodium** USAN *antibacterial* [also: cefazaflur]

**cefazedone** INN, BAN

**cefazolin** USP, INN *first-generation cephalosporin antibiotic* [also: cephazolin] ⍰ cephalothin; Zefazone

**cefazolin sodium** USAN, USP *first-generation cephalosporin antibiotic* [also: cephazolin sodium] 0.25, 0.5, 1, 5, 10, 20 g injection ⍰ cephalothin; Zefazone

**cefbuperazone** USAN, INN *antibacterial*

**cefcanel** INN

**cefcanel daloxate** INN

**cefdinir** USAN, INN *third-generation cephalosporin antibiotic*

**cefditoren pivoxil** *broad-spectrum cephalosporin antibiotic*

**cefedrolor** INN

**cefempidone** INN, BAN

**cefepime** USAN, INN *third-generation cephalosporin antibiotic*

**cefepime HCl** USAN *third-generation cephalosporin antibiotic*

**cefetamet** USAN, INN *veterinary antibacterial*

**cefetecol** USAN, INN, BAN *antibacterial*

**cefetrizole** INN

**cefivitril** INN

**cefixime** USAN, USP, INN, BAN *third-generation cephalosporin antibiotic*

**Cefizox** powder or frozen premix for IV or IM injection ℞ *cephalosporin antibiotic* [ceftizoxime sodium] 0.5, 1, 2, 10 g

**cefmenoxime** INN *antibacterial* [also: cefmenoxime HCl]

**cefmenoxime HCl** USAN, USP *antibacterial* [also: cefmenoxime]

**cefmepidium chloride** INN

**cefmetazole** USAN, INN *second-generation cephalosporin antibiotic*

**cefmetazole sodium** USAN, USP, JAN *second-generation cephalosporin antibiotic*

**cefminox** INN

**Cefobid** powder or frozen premix for IV or IM injection ℞ *cephalosporin antibiotic* [cefoperazone sodium] 1, 2, 10 g

**cefodizime** INN *investigational cephalosporin antibiotic*

**Cefol** Filmtabs (film-coated tablets) ℞ *vitamin supplement* [multiple vitamins; folic acid] ± •0.5 mg

**cefonicid** INN, BAN *second-generation cephalosporin antibiotic* [also: cefonicid monosodium]

**cefonicid monosodium** USAN *second-generation cephalosporin antibiotic* [also: cefonicid]

**cefonicid sodium** USAN, USP *second-generation cephalosporin antibiotic*

**cefoperazone** INN, BAN *third-generation cephalosporin antibiotic* [also: cefoperazone sodium]

**cefoperazone sodium** USAN, USP *third-generation cephalosporin antibiotic* [also: cefoperazone]

**ceforanide** USAN, USP, INN, BAN *bactericidal antibiotic*

**Cefotan** powder or frozen premix for IV or IM injection ℞ *cephamycin antibiotic* [cefotetan disodium] 1, 2, 10 g

**cefotaxime** INN, BAN *third-generation cephalosporin antibiotic* [also: cefotaxime sodium] ⧄ cefoxitin

**cefotaxime sodium** USAN, USP *third-generation cephalosporin antibiotic* [also: cefotaxime] 0.5, 1, 2, 10, 20 g injection

**cefotetan** USAN, INN, BAN *cephamycin antibiotic*

**cefotetan disodium** USAN, USP *cephamycin antibiotic*

**cefotiam** INN, BAN *antibacterial* [also: cefotiam HCl]

**cefotiam HCl** USAN *antibacterial* [also: cefotiam]

**cefoxazole** INN [also: cephoxazole]

**cefoxitin** USAN, INN, BAN *cephamycin antibiotic* ⧄ cefotaxime

**cefoxitin sodium** USAN, USP, BAN *cephamycin antibiotic* 1, 2, 10 g/vial injection

**cefpimizole** USAN, INN *antibacterial*

**cefpimizole sodium** USAN, JAN *antibacterial*

**cefpiramide** USAN, USP, INN *antibacterial*

**cefpiramide sodium** USAN, JAN *antibacterial*

**cefpirome** INN, BAN *antibacterial* [also: cefpirome sulfate]

**cefpirome sulfate** USAN, JAN *antibacterial* [also: cefpirome]

**cefpodoxime** INN, BAN *broad-spectrum third-generation cephalosporin antibiotic* [also: cefpodoxime proxetil]

**cefpodoxime proxetil** USAN, JAN *broad-spectrum third-generation cephalosporin antibiotic* [also: cefpodoxime]

**cefprozil** USAN, INN *second-generation cephalosporin antibiotic*

**cefprozil monohydrate**

**cefquinome** INN, BAN *veterinary antibacterial*

**cefquinome sulfate** USAN *veterinary antibacterial*

**cefradine** INN *first-generation cephalosporin antibiotic* [also: cephradine]

**cefrotil** INN

**cefroxadine** USAN, INN *antibacterial*

**cefsulodin** INN, BAN *antibacterial* [also: cefsulodin sodium]

**cefsulodin sodium** USAN *antibacterial* [also: cefsulodin]

**cefsumide** INN

**ceftazidime** USAN, USP, INN, BAN, JAN *third-generation cephalosporin antibiotic*

**cefteram** INN

**ceftezole** INN

**ceftibuten** USAN, INN, BAN *third-generation cephalosporin antibiotic*

**Ceftin** film-coated tablets, oral suspension ℞ *cephalosporin antibiotic* [cefuroxime axetil] 125, 250, 500 mg; 125, 250 mg/5 mL

**ceftiofur** INN, BAN *veterinary antibacterial* [also: ceftiofur HCl]

**ceftiofur HCl** USAN *veterinary antibacterial* [also: ceftiofur]

**ceftiofur sodium** USAN *veterinary antibacterial*

**ceftiolene** INN

**ceftioxide** INN

**ceftizoxime** INN, BAN *third-generation cephalosporin antibiotic* [also: ceftizoxime sodium] ⧄ cefuroxime

**ceftizoxime sodium** USAN, USP *third-generation cephalosporin antibiotic* [also: ceftizoxime]

**ceftriaxone** INN, BAN *third-generation cephalosporin antibiotic* [also: ceftriaxone sodium]

**ceftriaxone sodium** USAN, USP *third-generation cephalosporin antibiotic* [also: ceftriaxone]

**cefuracetime** INN, BAN

**cefuroxime** USAN, INN, BAN *second-generation cephalosporin antibiotic* ⧄ ceftizoxime

**cefuroxime axetil** USAN, USP, BAN *second-generation cephalosporin antibiotic* 125, 250, 500 mg oral

**cefuroxime pivoxetil** USAN *second-generation cephalosporin antibiotic*

**cefuroxime sodium** USP, BAN *second-generation cephalosporin antibiotic* 0.75, 1.5, 7.5 g injection

**cefuzonam** INN

**Cefzil** film-coated tablets, powder for oral suspension ℞ *cephalosporin antibiotic* [cefprozil] 250, 500 mg; 125, 250 mg/5 mL ② Cefadyl; Kefzol

**Cefzon** (foreign name for U.S. product Omnicef)

**celandine (Chelidonium majus)** root and plant *medicinal herb used as an analgesic, antispasmodic, caustic, diaphoretic, diuretic, narcotic, and purgative*

**Celebrex** capsules ℞ *antiarthritic; antipyretic; COX-2 inhibitor; nonsteroidal anti-inflammatory drug (NSAID); reduces polyp proliferation in familial adenomatous polyposis (FAP); investigational (Phase III) for bladder cancer* [celecoxib] 100, 200, 400 mg ② Celexa; Cerebyx

**celecoxib** USAN *antiarthritic; antipyretic; COX-2 inhibitor; nonsteroidal anti-inflammatory drug (NSAID); reduces polyp proliferation in familial adenomatous polyposis (FAP)*

**celery (Apium graveolens)** root, stem, and seeds *medicinal herb for aiding digestion, arthritis, cancer, diuresis, gas, headache, hysteria, inducing menstruation, lumbago, nervousness, rheumatism, and terminating lactation*

**Celestoderm-V; Celestoderm-V/2** ⒸⒶⓃ cream, ointment ℞ *corticosteroidal anti-inflammatory* [betamethasone valerate] 0.1%; 0.05%

**Celestone** tablets, syrup *corticosteroid; anti-inflammatory* [betamethasone] 0.6 mg; 0.6 mg/5 mL

**Celestone Phosphate** IV, IM injection ℞ *corticosteroid; anti-inflammatory* [betamethasone sodium phosphate] 4 mg/mL

**Celestone Soluspan** intrabursal, intra-articular, intralesional injection ℞ *corticosteroid; anti-inflammatory* [betamethasone sodium phosphate; betamethasone acetate] 3•3 mg/mL

**Celexa** film-coated tablets, oral solution ℞ *selective serotonin reuptake inhibitor (SSRI) for major depression* [citalopram hydrobromide] 10, 20, 40 mg; 10 mg/5 mL ② Celebrex

**celgosivir HCl** USAN *antiviral; α-glucosidase I inhibitor for HIV*

**celiprolol** INN, BAN *antihypertensive; antianginal; β-blocker* [also: celiprolol HCl]

**celiprolol HCl** USAN *investigational (NDA filed) antihypertensive; antianginal; β-blocker* [also: celiprolol]

**cellacefate** INN *tablet-coating agent* [also: cellulose acetate phthalate; cellacephate]

**cellacephate** BAN *tablet-coating agent* [also: cellulose acetate phthalate; cellacefate]

**CellCept** capsules, tablets, powder for oral suspension ℞ *immunosuppressant for allogenic renal, hepatic, or cardiac transplants* [mycophenolate mofetil] 250 mg; 500 mg; 200 mg/mL

**CellCept** powder for IV infusion ℞ *immunosuppressant for allogenic renal, hepatic, or cardiac transplants* [mycophenolate mofetil HCl] 500 mg

**cellulase** USAN *digestive enzyme*

**cellulolytic enzyme** [see: cellulase]

**cellulose** *bulk laxative*

**cellulose, absorbable** [see: cellulose, oxidized]

**cellulose, ethyl ester** [see: ethylcellulose]

**cellulose, hydroxypropyl methyl ether** [see: hydroxypropyl methylcellulose]

**cellulose, microcrystalline** NF *tablet and capsule diluent* [also: dispersible cellulose]

**cellulose, oxidized** USP *topical local hemostatic*

**cellulose, oxidized regenerated** USP *local hemostatic*

**cellulose, sodium carboxymethyl** [see: carboxymethylcellulose sodium]

**cellulose acetate** NF *tablet-coating agent; insoluble polymer membrane*

**cellulose acetate butyrate** [see: cabufocon A; cabufocon B]

**cellulose acetate dibutyrate** [see: porofocon A; porofocon B]

**cellulose acetate phthalate (CAP)** NF *tablet-coating agent* [also: cellacefate; cellacephate]

**cellulose carboxymethyl ether, sodium salt** [see: carboxymethylcellulose sodium]

**cellulose diacetate** [see: cellulose acetate]

**cellulose dihydrogen phosphate, disodium salt** [see: cellulose sodium phosphate]

**cellulose disodium phosphate** [see: cellulose sodium phosphate]

**cellulose ethyl ether** [see: ethylcellulose]

**cellulose gum, modified** [now: croscarmellose sodium]

**cellulose methyl ether** [see: methylcellulose]

**cellulose nitrate** [see: pyroxylin]

**cellulose sodium phosphate (CSP)** USAN, USP *antiurolithic to prevent stone formation in absorptive hypercalciuria Type I*

**cellulosic acid** [see: cellulose, oxidized]

**Celluvisc** solution OTC *ophthalmic moisturizer/lubricant* [carboxymethylcellulose] 1%

**celmoleukin** INN *immunostimulant*

**Celontin** Kapseals (capsules) ℞ *succinimide anticonvulsant for absence (petit mal) seizures* [methsuximide] 150, 300 mg

**celucloral** INN, BAN

**Cel·U·Jec** IV, IM injection (discontinued 2002) ℞ *corticosteroid; antiinflammatory* [betamethasone sodium phosphate] 4 mg/mL

**CEM (cytosine arabinoside, etoposide, methotrexate)** *chemotherapy protocol*

**Cenafed** tablets, syrup OTC *nasal decongestant* [pseudoephedrine HCl] 60 mg; 30 mg/5 mL

**Cenafed Plus** tablets OTC *decongestant; antihistamine* [pseudoephedrine HCl; triprolidine HCl] 60•2.5 mg

**Cena-K** oral liquid ℞ *potassium supplement* [potassium chloride] 20, 40 mEq K/15 mL

**Cenestin** film-coated tablets ℞ *a mixture of synthetic estrogens; hormone replacement therapy for the treatment of postmenopausal symptoms* [synthetic conjugated estrogens, A] 0.3, 0.45, 0.625, 0.9, 1.25 mg

**Cenogen Ultra** capsules ℞ *vitamin/ mineral/iron supplement* [multiple vitamins & minerals; iron; folic acid] ±•106•1 mg

**Cenogen-OB** capsules (discontinued 2004) ℞ *vitamin/mineral/iron supplement* [multiple vitamins & minerals; iron; folic acid] ±•106•1 mg

**Cenolate** IV, IM, or subcu injection ℞ *vitamin C therapy; antiscorbutic* [sodium ascorbate] 562.5 mg/mL

**Centany** ointment ℞ *antibiotic for impetigo due to* S. aureus *or* S. pyogenes [mupirocin] 2%

*Centaurea cyanus* *medicinal herb* [see: cornflower]

**centaury (Erythraea centaurium)** plant *medicinal herb for aiding digestion, blood cleansing, fever, and promoting menstruation*

*Centella asiatica* *medicinal herb* [see: gotu kola]

**Center-Al** subcu or IM injection ℞ *allergenic sensitivity testing (subcu); allergenic desensitization therapy (IM)* [allergenic extracts, alum-precipitated]

**Centoxin** ℞ *investigational (orphan) for gram-negative bacteremia in endotoxin shock* [nebacumab]

**centrazene** [see: simtrazene]

**centrophenoxine** [see: meclofenoxate]

**Centrum, Advanced Formula** oral liquid OTC *vitamin/mineral/iron supplement* [multiple vitamins & minerals; ferrous fumarate; biotin; alcohol 6.7%] ±•9•0.3 mg/15 mL

**Centrum, Advanced Formula** tablets OTC *vitamin/mineral/iron supple-*

ment [multiple vitamins & minerals; ferrous fumarate; folic acid; biotin] ± • 18 mg•0.4 mg•30 μg

**Centrum Jr. + Extra C; Centrum Jr. + Extra Calcium** chewable tablets OTC *vitamin/mineral/calcium/iron supplement* [multiple vitamins & minerals; calcium; iron; folic acid; biotin] ± • 108•18•0.4•0.045 mg; ± • 160• 18•0.4•0.045 mg

**Centrum Jr. with Iron** tablets OTC *vitamin/mineral/iron supplement* [multiple vitamins & minerals; iron; folic acid; biotin] ± • 18 mg•0.4 mg•45 μg

**Centrum Performance** tablets OTC *vitamin/mineral/calcium/iron supplement* [multiple vitamins & minerals; calcium; iron; folic acid; biotin] ± • 100•18 mg•0.4 mg•40 μg

**Centrum Silver** tablets OTC *geriatric vitamin/mineral supplement* [multiple vitamins & minerals; folic acid; biotin] ± •400•30 μg

**centruroides immune Fab 2** *investigational (orphan) antitoxin for scorpion stings*

**Ceo-Two** suppository OTC *CO₂-releasing laxative* [sodium bicarbonate; potassium bitartrate]

**CEP (CCNU, etoposide, prednimustine)** *chemotherapy protocol*

**Cēpacol** mouthwash/gargle OTC *oral antiseptic* [cetylpyridinium chloride] 0.05%

**Cēpacol, Children's** oral liquid (discontinued 2002) OTC *decongestant; analgesic* [pseudoephedrine HCl; acetaminophen] 15•160 mg/5 mL

**Cēpacol Anesthetic** troches OTC *topical oral anesthetic; antiseptic* [benzocaine; cetylpyridinium chloride] 10 mg•0.07%

**Cēpacol Maximum Strength** lozenges OTC *topical oral anesthetic* [benzocaine] 10 mg

**Cēpacol Sore Throat** oral liquid OTC *decongestant; analgesic* [pseudoephedrine HCl; acetaminophen] 60•640 mg/30 mL

**Cēpacol Throat** lozenges OTC *oral antiseptic* [cetylpyridinium chloride] 0.07%

**Cēpacol Viractin** cream, gel OTC *anesthetic for cold sores and fever blisters* [tetracaine HCl] 2%

**Cēpastat Sore Throat** lozenges OTC *topical antipruritic/counterirritant; mild local anesthetic* [phenol] 14.5, 29 mg ⃞ Capastat

**cephacetrile sodium** USAN, USP *antibacterial* [also: cefacetrile]

**cephalexin** USAN, USP, BAN *first-generation cephalosporin antibiotic* [also: cefalexin] 250, 500, 1000 mg oral; 125, 250 mg/5 mL oral ⃞ cefazolin; cephalothin

**cephalexin HCl** USAN, USP *first-generation cephalosporin antibiotic*

**cephaloglycin** USAN, USP, BAN *antibacterial* [also: cefaloglycin]

**cephalonium** BAN [also: cefalonium]

**cephaloram** BAN [also: cefaloram]

**cephaloridine** USAN, USP, BAN *antibacterial* [also: cefaloridine]

**cephalosporin N** [see: adicillin]

**cephalosporins** *a class of bactericidal antibiotics, divided into first-, second-, and third-generation cephalosporins; higher generations have increasing efficacy against gram-negative and decreasing efficacy against gram-positive bacteria*

**cephalothin** BAN *first-generation cephalosporin antibiotic* [also: cephalothin sodium; cefalotin] ⃞ cefazolin

**cephalothin sodium** USAN, USP *first-generation cephalosporin antibiotic* [also: cefalotin; cephalothin]

**cephamandole** BAN *second-generation cephalosporin antibiotic* [also: cefamandole]

**cephamandole nafate** BAN *second-generation cephalosporin antibiotic* [also: cefamandole nafate]

**cephamycins** *a class of bactericidal antibiotics similar to second-generation cephalosporins (q.v.)*

**cephapirin sodium** USAN, USP *first-generation cephalosporin antibiotic* [also: cefapirin] ⃞ cephradine

**cephazolin** BAN *first-generation cephalosporin antibiotic* [also: cefazolin]

**cephazolin sodium** BAN *first-generation cephalosporin antibiotic* [also: cefazolin sodium]

**cephoxazole** BAN [also: cefoxazole]

**cephradine** USAN, USP, BAN *first-generation cephalosporin antibiotic* [also: cefradine] 250, 500 mg oral; 125, 250 mg/5 mL oral ☒ cephapirin

**Cephulac** oral/rectal solution ℞ *synthetic disaccharide used to prevent and treat portal-systemic encephalopathy* [lactulose] 10 g/15 mL

**Ceplene** ℞ *investigational (Phase III) histamine $H_2$ receptor agonist for malignant melanoma and acute myeloid leukemia (AML); investigational (Phase II) for hepatitis C and renal cell carcinoma* [histamine dihydrochloride]

**Ceplene** ℞ *investigational (Phase III) treatment for advanced metastatic melanoma* [histamine dihydrochloride]

**CEPP (cyclophosphamide, etoposide, prednisone)** *chemotherapy protocol for non-Hodgkin lymphoma*

**CEPPB (cyclophosphamide, etoposide, prednisone, bleomycin)** *chemotherapy protocol for non-Hodgkin lymphoma*

**Ceptaz** powder for IV or IM injection ℞ *cephalosporin antibiotic* [ceftazidime pentahydrate] 1, 2 g

**CeraLyte** powder for oral liquid, ready-to-use oral liquid OTC *supplementary feeding to maintain hydration and electrolyte balance in infants with diarrhea or vomiting* [rice-based formula]

**ceramide trihexosidase (CTH) & agalsidase beta** *investigational (orphan) enzyme replacement therapy for Fabry disease*

**CerAxon** ℞ *investigational (Phase III) brain tissue protector for ischemic stroke* [citicoline sodium]

**Cerebyx** IV or IM injection ℞ *hydantoin anticonvulsant for grand mal status epilepticus (orphan)* [fosphenytoin sodium (phenytoin sodium equivalent)] 75 (50) mg/mL ☒ Celebrex

**Ceredase** IV infusion ℞ *glucocerebrosidase enzyme replacement in Gaucher disease type I (orphan); investigational (orphan) for types II and III* [alglucerase] 10, 80 U/mL

**Cerefolin** tablets ℞ *vitamin B supplement* [vitamins $B_2$, $B_6$, and $B_{12}$; L-methylfolate] 5•50•1•5.635 mg

**cerelose** [see: glucose]

**Cereport** ℞ *investigational (Phase III) blood-brain barrier permeability-enhancing agent for carrying carboplatin to brain tumors* [lobradimil]

**Ceresine** ℞ *investigational (orphan) pyruvate dehydrogenase activator for acute head trauma and neurologic injury* [sodium dichloroacetate]

**Cerezyme** powder for IV infusion ℞ *enzyme replacement therapy for types I, II, and III Gaucher disease (orphan)* [imiglucerase] 40 U/mL

**cerium** *element* (Ce)

**cerium oxalate** USP

**cerivastatin sodium** USAN *HMG-CoA reductase inhibitor for hyperlipidemia and hypertriglyceridemia (discontinued 2001 due to safety concerns)*

**Cernevit-12** powder for IV injection ℞ *parenteral vitamin therapy* [multiple vitamins; folic acid; biotin] ±•414•60 μg

**ceronapril** USAN, INN *antihypertensive*

**Cerose-DM** oral liquid (discontinued 2002) OTC *antitussive; decongestant; antihistamine* [dextromethorphan hydrobromide; phenylephrine HCl; chlorpheniramine maleate; alcohol 2.4%] 15•10•4 mg/5 mL

**Cerovite; Cerovite Advanced Formula** tablets OTC *vitamin/mineral/iron supplement* [multiple vitamins & minerals; ferrous fumarate; folic acid; biotin] ±•18 mg•0.4 mg•30 μg

**Cerovite Jr.** tablets OTC *vitamin/mineral/iron supplement* [multiple vitamins & minerals; ferrous fumarate; folic acid; biotin] ±•18 mg•0.4 mg•45 μg

**Cerovite Senior** tablets OTC *geriatric vitamin/mineral supplement* [multiple vitamins & minerals; folic acid; biotin] ±•200•30 μg

**Certagen** film-coated tablets OTC *vitamin/mineral/iron supplement* [multiple vitamins & minerals; ferrous fumarate; folic acid; biotin] ±•18 mg• 0.4 mg•30 μg

**Certagen** oral liquid OTC *vitamin/mineral/iron supplement* [multiple vitamins & minerals; iron; biotin; alcohol 6.6%] ±•9•0.3 mg

**Certagen Senior** tablets OTC *geriatric vitamin/mineral supplement* [multiple vitamins & minerals; folic acid; biotin] ±•200•30 μg

**CertaVite** tablets OTC *vitamin/mineral/ iron supplement* [multiple vitamins & minerals; ferrous fumarate; folic acid; biotin] ±•18 mg•0.4 mg•30 μg

**Certa-Vite Golden** tablets OTC *geriatric vitamin/mineral supplement* [multiple vitamins & minerals; biotin] ±•30 μg

**Certican** (approved in Europe) ℞ *investigational (NDA filed) agent for transplant rejection* [everolimus]

**Certiva** IM injection (discontinued 2002) ℞ *active immunizing agent for diphtheria, tetanus, and pertussis* [diphtheria & tetanus toxoids & acellular pertussis (DTaP) vaccine] 15 Lf•6 Lf•40 μg per 0.5 mL

**Cerubidine** powder for IV injection ℞ *antibiotic antineoplastic for multiple nonlymphocytic leukemias* [daunorubicin HCl] 20 mg

**ceruletide** USAN, INN, BAN *gastric secretory stimulant*

**ceruletide diethylamine** USAN *gastric secretory stimulant*

**Cerumenex** ear drops ℞ *cerumenolytic to emulsify and disperse ear wax* [trolamine polypeptide oleate-condensate] 10%

**Cervidil** vaginal insert ℞ *prostaglandin for cervical ripening at term* [dinoprostone] 10 mg

**C.E.S.** CAN sugar-coated tablets ℞ *estrogen replacement therapy for postmenopausal symptoms* [conjugated estrogens (from plants)] 0.4, 0.625, 0.9, 1.25 mg

**cesium** *element (Cs)*

**cesium (¹³¹Cs) chloride** INN *radioactive agent* [also: cesium chloride Cs 131]

**cesium chloride Cs 131** USAN *radioactive agent* [also: cesium (¹³¹Cs) chloride]

**Ceta** topical liquid OTC *soap-free therapeutic skin cleanser*

**Ceta Plus** capsules ℞ *narcotic analgesic* [hydrocodone bitartrate; acetaminophen] 5•500 mg

**cetaben** INN *antihyperlipoproteinemic* [also: cetaben sodium]

**cetaben sodium** USAN *antihyperlipoproteinemic* [also: cetaben]

**Cetacaine** topical liquid, gel, ointment, aerosol ℞ *local anesthetic; antiseptic* [benzocaine; tetracaine HCl; butamben] 14%•2%•2%

**Cetacort** lotion ℞ *topical corticosteroidal anti-inflammatory* [hydrocortisone] 0.25%, 0.5%

**cetalkonium** *antiseptic*

**cetalkonium chloride** USAN, INN, BAN *topical anti-infective*

**Cetamide** ophthalmic ointment ℞ *antibiotic* [sulfacetamide sodium] 10%

**cetamolol** INN *antiadrenergic (β-receptor)* [also: cetamolol HCl]

**cetamolol HCl** USAN *antiadrenergic (β-receptor)* [also: cetamolol]

**Cetaphil** cream, lotion, cleansing bar, cleansing solution OTC *soap-free therapeutic skin cleanser*

**Cetapred** ophthalmic ointment (discontinued 2003) ℞ *corticosteroidal anti-inflammatory; antibiotic* [prednisolone acetate; sulfacetamide sodium] 0.25%•10%

**cethexonium chloride** INN

**cetiedil** INN *peripheral vasodilator* [also: cetiedil citrate]

**cetiedil citrate** USAN *peripheral vasodilator; investigational (orphan) for sickle cell disease crisis* [also: cetiedil]

**cetirizine** INN, BAN *second-generation peripherally selective piperazine antihistamine for allergic rhinitis and chronic idiopathic urticaria* [also: cetirizine HCl]

**cetirizine HCl** USAN *second-generation peripherally selective piperazine antihistamine for allergic rhinitis and chronic idiopathic urticaria* [also: cetirizine]

**cetobemidone** [see: ketobemidone]

**cetocycline** INN *antibacterial* [also: cetocycline HCl]

**cetocycline HCl** USAN *antibacterial* [also: cetocycline]

**cetofenicol** INN *antibacterial* [also: cetophenicol]

**cetohexazine** INN

**cetomacrogol 1000** INN, BAN

**cetophenicol** USAN *antibacterial* [also: cetofenicol]

**cetophenylbutazone** [see: kebuzone]

**cetostearyl alcohol** NF *emulsifying agent*

**cetotetrine HCl** [now: cetocycline HCl]

**cetotiamine** INN

**cetoxime** INN, BAN

**cetoxime HCl** [see: cetoxime]

*Cetraria islandica* medicinal herb [see: Iceland moss]

**cetraxate** INN *GI antiulcerative* [also: cetraxate HCl]

**cetraxate HCl** USAN *GI antiulcerative* [also: cetraxate]

**cetrimide** INN, BAN *topical antiseptic*

**cetrimonium bromide** INN *topical antiseptic* [also: cetrimonium chloride]

**cetrimonium chloride** BAN *topical antiseptic* [also: cetrimonium bromide]

**cetrorelix acetate** USAN *gonadotropin-releasing hormone (GnRH) antagonist for infertility*

**Cetrotide** subcu injection R *gonadotropin-releasing hormone (GnRH) antagonist for infertility* [cetrorelix acetate] 0.25, 3 mg

**cetuximab** USAN *antineoplastic; epidermal growth factor receptor (EGFR) blocker; treatment for metastatic colorectal cancer; investigational (orphan) for squamous cell carcinoma of the head and neck; investigational (Phase III) for pancreatic cancer*

**cetyl alcohol** NF *emulsifying and stiffening agent*

**cetyl esters wax** NF *stiffening agent*

**cetyldimethylbenzyl ammonium chloride** [see: cetalkonium chloride]

**cetylpyridinium chloride** USP, INN, BAN *topical antiseptic; preservative*

**cetyltrimethyl ammonium bromide**

**CEV (cyclophosphamide, etoposide, vincristine)** *chemotherapy protocol for small cell lung cancer (SCLC)*

**Cevi-Bid** tablets OTC *vitamin C supplement* [ascorbic acid] 500 mg

**Cevi-Fer** timed-release capsules R *hematinic; iron/vitamin C supplement* [iron (from ferrous fumarate); ascorbic acid; folic acid] 20•300•1 mg

**cevimeline HCl** USAN *cholinergic and muscarinic receptor agonist for dry mouth due to Sjögren syndrome*

**cevitamic acid** [see: ascorbic acid]

**cevitan** [see: ascorbic acid]

**ceylon gelatin** [see: agar]

**Cezin-S** capsules R *geriatric vitamin/mineral supplement* [multiple vitamins & minerals; folic acid] ±•0.5 mg

**CF (carboplatin, fluorouracil)** *chemotherapy protocol for head and neck cancer*

**CF (cisplatin, fluorouracil)** *chemotherapy protocol for adenocarcinoma and head and neck cancer*

**CFL (cisplatin, fluorouracil, leucovorin [rescue])** *chemotherapy protocol*

**CFM (cyclophosphamide, fluorouracil, mitoxantrone)** *chemotherapy protocol for breast cancer* [also: CNF; FNC]

**CFP (cyclophosphamide, fluorouracil, prednisone)** *chemotherapy protocol*

**CFPT (cyclophosphamide, fluorouracil, prednisone, tamoxifen)** *chemotherapy protocol*

**CFTR (cystic fibrosis transmembrane conductance regulator)** [q.v.]

**CG (Cardio-Green)** [q.v.]

**CG (chorionic gonadotropin)** [see: gonadotropin, chorionic]

**CGF (*Chlorella* growth factor)** [q.v.]

**CGF (Control Gel Formula) dressing** [see: DuoDERM CGF]

**CGP-61755** *investigational (Phase I) protease inhibitor for HIV infection*

**CH1VPP; Ch1VPP (chlorambucil, vinblastine, procarbazine, prednisone)** *chemotherapy protocol*

**CHAD (cyclophosphamide, hexamethylmelamine, Adriamycin, DDP)** *chemotherapy protocol*

**chalk, precipitated** [see: calcium carbonate, precipitated]

*Chamaelirium luteum* *medicinal herb* [see: false unicorn]

**CHAMOCA (cyclophosphamide, hydroxyurea, actinomycin D, methotrexate, Oncovin, calcium folinate, Adriamycin)** *chemotherapy protocol for gestational trophoblastic neoplasm* [also known as: modified Bagshawe protocol]

**chamomile *(Anthemis nobilis; Matricaria chamomilla)*** *flowers medicinal herb for appetite stimulation, bronchitis, excessive menstruation with cramps, fever, gastrointestinal cramps, hysteria, inflammation, insomnia, nervousness, rheumatic disorders, and parasites*

**channa; canna** *medicinal herb* [see: kanna]

**CHAP (cyclophosphamide, Hexalen, Adriamycin, Platinol)** *chemotherapy protocol for ovarian cancer*

**CHAP (cyclophosphamide, hexamethylmelamine, Adriamycin, Platinol)** *chemotherapy protocol*

**Chap Stick Medicated Lip Balm** stick, jar, squeezable tube OTC *topical analgesic; counterirritant; moisturizer; protectant; emollient* [camphor; menthol; phenol] 1%•0.6%•0.5%

**chaparral *(Larrea divaricata; L. glutinosa; L. tridentata)*** *leaves and stems medicinal herb for arthritis, blood cleansing, bronchitis, cancer, chickenpox, colds, leukemia, rheumatic pain, stomach pain, and tumors; not generally regarded as safe and effective because of liver toxicity and stimulation of some tumors*

**CharcoAid** oral suspension OTC *adsorbent antidote for poisoning* [activated charcoal] 15 g/120 mL, 30 g/150 mL

**CharcoAid 2000** oral liquid, granules OTC *adsorbent antidote for poisoning* [activated charcoal] 15 g/120 mL, 50 g/240 mL; 15 g

**charcoal** *gastric adsorbent/detoxicant; antiflatulent* 260 mg oral

**charcoal, activated** USP *general purpose antidote/adsorbent* 15, 30, 40, 120, 240 g, 208 mg/mL oral

**Charcoal Plus** enteric-coated tablets OTC *adsorbent; detoxicant* [activated charcoal] 250 mg

**CharcoCaps** capsules OTC *adsorbent; detoxicant; antiflatulent* [charcoal] 260 mg

**Chardonna-2** tablets ℞ *GI anticholinergic; sedative* [belladonna extract; phenobarbital] 15•15 mg

**chaste tree *(Vitex agnus-castus)*** dried ripe fruit *medicinal herb for acne, balancing progesterone and estrogen production, increasing lactation, ovarian insufficiency, premenstrual breast pain, regulating menstrual cycle, and uterine bleeding*

**chaulmosulfone** INN

**checkerberry** *medicinal herb* [see: squaw vine; wintergreen]

**cheese plant; cheeseflower** *medicinal herb* [see: mallow]

**cheese rennet** *medicinal herb* [see: bedstraw]

**Cheetah** oral suspension ℞ *radiopaque contrast medium for gastrointestinal imaging* [barium sulfate] 2.2%

**chelafrin** [see: epinephrine]

**Chelated Magnesium** tablets (discontinued 2002) OTC *magnesium supplement* [magnesium amino acid chelate] 500 mg

**Chelated Manganese** tablets OTC *manganese supplement* [manganese] 20, 50 mg

**chelating agents** *a class of agents that prevent bodily absorption of and cause the excretion of substances such as heavy metals*

**chelen** [see: ethyl chloride]

*Chelidonium majus* *medicinal herb* [see: celandine]

**Chelone glabra** *medicinal herb* [see: turtlebloom]

**Chemet** *capsules* ℞ *heavy metal chelating agent for lead poisoning (orphan); investigational (orphan) for cystine kidney stones and mercury poisoning* [succimer] 100 mg

**Chemo-Pin** (trademarked form) *chemical-dispensing pin*

**Chemstrip 2 GP; Chemstrip 2 LN; Chemstrip 4 the OB; Chemstrip 6; Chemstrip 7; Chemstrip 8; Chemstrip 9; Chemstrip 10 with SG; Chemstrip uGK** *reagent strips in vitro diagnostic aid for multiple urine products*

**Chemstrip bG** *reagent strips for home use in vitro diagnostic aid for blood glucose*

**Chemstrip K** *reagent strips for professional use in vitro diagnostic aid for acetone (ketones) in the urine*

**Chemstrip Micral** *reagent strips for professional use in vitro diagnostic aid for albumin (protein) in the urine*

**Chemstrip uG** *reagent strips for home use in vitro diagnostic aid for urine glucose*

**chenic acid** [now: chenodiol]

**Chenix** *tablets* ℞ *anticholelithogenic for radiolucent gallstones (orphan)* [chenodiol] 250 mg

**chenodeoxycholic acid** INN, BAN *anticholelithogenic* [also: chenodiol]

**chenodiol** USAN *anticholelithogenic for radiolucent gallstones (orphan); investigational (orphan) for cerebrotendinous xanthomatosis* [also: chenodeoxycholic acid]

**Chenofalk** ℞ *investigational (orphan) agent for cerebrotendinous xanthomatosis* [chenodiol]

**Cheracol Cough** *syrup* ℞ *narcotic antitussive; expectorant* [codeine phosphate; guaifenesin; alcohol 4.75%] 20•200 mg/10 mL

**Cheracol D Cough Formula; Cheracol Plus** *syrup* OTC *antitussive; expectorant* [dextromethorphan hydrobromide; guaifenesin; alcohol 4.75%] 20•200 mg/10 mL

**Cheracol Nasal** *spray* (discontinued 2001) OTC *nasal decongestant* [oxymetazoline HCl] 0.05%

**Cheracol Sore Throat** *spray* OTC *topical antipruritic/counterirritant; mild local anesthetic* [phenol] 1.4%

**cherry, black; choke cherry; rum cherry** *medicinal herb* [see: wild black cherry]

**cherry, black; poison black cherry** *medicinal herb* [see: belladonna]

**cherry birch** *medicinal herb* [see: birch]

**cherry juice** NF

**chervil (Anthriscus cerefolium)** *flowering plant medicinal herb used as a digestive, diuretic, expectorant, and stimulant*

**chervil, sweet** *medicinal herb* [see: sweet cicely]

**chestnut** *medicinal herb* [see: horse chestnut]

**Chewable Multivitamins with Fluoride** *tablets* ℞ *pediatric vitamin supplement and dental caries preventative* [multiple vitamins; fluoride; folic acid] ±•1•0.3 mg

**Chewable Triple Vitamins with Fluoride** *tablets* ℞ *pediatric vitamin supplement and dental caries preventative* [vitamins A, C, and D; fluoride] 2500 IU•60 mg•400 IU•1 mg

**Chewable Vitamin C** *chewable tablets* OTC *vitamin C supplement* [ascorbic acid and sodium ascorbate] 250, 500 mg

**Chew-C** *chewable tablets* OTC *vitamin supplement* [vitamin C (as ascorbic acid and sodium ascorbate)] 500 mg

**ChexUP; Chex-Up; CHEX-UP (cyclophosphamide, hexamethylmelamine, fluorouracil, Platinol)** *chemotherapy protocol*

**CHF (cyclophosphamide, hexamethylmelamine, fluorouracil)** *chemotherapy protocol*

**Chibroxin** *Ocumeter (eye drops)* (discontinued 2002) ℞ *topical fluoro-*

quinolone antibiotic for bacterial conjunctivitis [norfloxacin] 0.3%

**chicken's toes** *medicinal herb* [see:
coral root]

**chickweed (Stellaria media)** *plant
medicinal herb for appetite suppression,
bleeding, blood cleansing, convulsions,
obesity, skin rashes, and ulcers; also
used as a homeopathic remedy for psoriasis and rheumatic pain*

**chicory (Chicorium intybus)** *plant
and root medicinal herb for blood
cleansing, cardiac disease, jaundice,
liver disorders, promoting expectoration, and removal of calcium deposits*

**Chiggerex** ointment OTC *topical local
anesthetic; analgesic; counterirritant*
[benzocaine; camphor; menthol]

**Chigger-Tox** topical liquid OTC *local
anesthetic* [benzocaine]

**Chikusetsu ginseng (Panax pseudo-
ginseng)** *medicinal herb* [see: ginseng]

**Children's Elixir DM Cough &
Cold** OTC *antitussive; decongestant;
antihistamine* [dextromethorphan
hydrobromide; pseudoephedrine
HCl; brompheniramine maleate]
10•30•2 mg/10 mL

**Children's Formula Cough** syrup (discontinued 2002) OTC *antitussive;
expectorant* [dextromethorphan hydrobromide; guaifenesin] 5•50 mg/5 mL

**Children's Ibuprofen Cold** oral suspension OTC *analgesic; antipyretic;
nonsteroidal anti-inflammatory drug;
nasal decongestant* [ibuprofen; pseu-
doephedrine] 100•15 mg/5 mL

**chili pepper; chilies** *medicinal herb*
[see: cayenne]

**chillifolinum** [see: quillifoline]

*Chimaphila umbellata* *medicinal herb*
[see: pipsissewa]

**chimeric (human-murine) G250
IgG monoclonal antibodies
(MAb)** *investigational (orphan) agent
for renal cell carcinoma*

**chimeric A2 (human-murine) IgG
monoclonal anti-TNF antibody
(cA2)** [see: infliximab]

**chimeric humanized monoclonal
antibodies (MAb) to** *Staphylococcus investigational (orphan) prophylaxis of S. epidermidis sepsis in low
birth weight infants*

**chimeric M-T412 (human-murine)
IgG monoclonal anti-CD4** [now:
priliximab]

**chinchona** *medicinal herb* [see: quinine]

**Chinese cucumber (Trichosanthes
kirilowii)** *gourd and root medicinal
herb for abscesses, amenorrhea, cough,
diabetes, edema, fever, inducing abortion, invasive moles, jaundice, poly-
uria, and tumors*

**Chinese gelatin** [see: agar]

**Chinese isinglass** [see: chiniofon]

**Chinese rhubarb** *medicinal herb* [see:
rhubarb]

**chinethazone** [see: quinethazone]

**chiniofon** NF, INN

*Chionanthus virginica* *medicinal herb*
[see: fringe tree]

**Chirocaine** local or epidural injection
R *long-acting local anesthetic* [levobu-
pivacaine HCl] 2.5, 5, 7.5 mg/mL

**chitosamine** [see: glucosamine]

**chitosan** *natural cellulose-like biopoly-
mer extracted from marine animal
exoskeletons and used as a treatment
for hypercholesterolemia, hyperlipidemia, and obesity; also used topically
as an antimicrobial and vulnerary*

**chittem bark** *medicinal herb* [see:
buckthorn; cascara sagrada]

**CHL + PRED (chlorambucil, pred-
nisone)** *chemotherapy protocol*

**Chlamydiazyme** reagent kit for professional use *in vitro diagnostic aid for
Chlamydia trachomatis* [solid phase
enzyme immunoassay]

**Chlo-Amine** chewable tablets OTC
*antihistamine* [chlorpheniramine mal-
eate] 2 mg

**chlophedianol** BAN *antitussive* [also:
chlophedianol HCl; clofedanol]

**chlophedianol HCl** USAN *antitussive*
[also: clofedanol; chlophedianol]

**chlophenadione** [see: clorindione]

**chloquinate** [see: cloquinate]

**chloracyzine** INN

**Chlorafed** oral liquid (discontinued 2002) OTC *decongestant; antihistamine* [pseudoephedrine HCl; chlorpheniramine maleate] 30•2 mg/5 mL

**Chlorafed; Chlorafed HS** Timecelles (sustained-release capsules) (discontinued 2002) ℞ *decongestant; antihistamine* [pseudoephedrine HCl; chlorpheniramine maleate] 120•8 mg; 60•4 mg

**chloral betaine** USAN, NF, BAN *sedative* [also: cloral betaine]

**chloral hydrate** USP, BAN *hypnotic; sedative; also abused as a street drug* 500 mg oral; 250, 500 mg/5 mL oral

**chloral hydrate betaine** [see: chloral betaine]

**chloralformamide** USP

**chloralodol** INN [also: chlorhexadol]

**chloralose (α-chloralose)** INN

**chloralurethane** [see: carbocloral]

**chlorambucil** USP, INN, BAN *nitrogen mustard-type alkylating antineoplastic for multiple leukemias and lymphomas*

**chloramidobenzol** [see: clofenamide]

**chloramine** [now: chloramine-T]

**chloramine-T** NF [also: tosylchloramide sodium]

**chloramiphene** [see: clomiphene citrate]

**chloramphenicol** USP, INN, BAN, JAN *bacteriostatic antibiotic; antirickettsial* 5 mg/mL eye drops; 10 mg/g topical

**chloramphenicol palmitate** USP, JAN *antibacterial; antirickettsial* 150 mg/5 mL oral

**chloramphenicol pantothenate complex** USAN *antibacterial; antirickettsial* [also: cloramfenicol pantotenate complex]

**chloramphenicol sodium succinate** USP, JAN *antibacterial; antirickettsial* 100 mg/mL injection

**chloranautine** [see: dimenhydrinate]

**ChloraPrep One-Step** swabs *topical antiseptic* [chlorhexidine gluconate; isopropyl alcohol] 2%•70%

**chlorarsen** [see: dichlorophenarsine HCl]

**Chloraseptic** mouthwash/gargle OTC *topical antipruritic/counterirritant; mild local anesthetic* [phenol] 1.4%

**Chloraseptic, Children's** lozenges OTC *topical oral anesthetic* [benzocaine] 5 mg

**Chloraseptic, Children's** throat spray OTC *topical antipruritic/counterirritant; mild local anesthetic* [phenol] 0.5%

**Chloraseptic Sore Throat** lozenges OTC *topical oral anesthetic; analgesic; counterirritant* [benzocaine; menthol] 6•10 mg

**chlorazanil** INN

**chlorazanil HCl** [see: chlorazanil]

**chlorazodin** INN [also: chloroazodin]

**chlorazone** [see: chloramine-T]

**chlorbenzoxamine** INN

**chlorbenzoxamine HCl** [see: chlorbenzoxamine]

**chlorbetamide** INN, BAN

**chlorbutanol** [see: chlorobutanol]

**chlorbutin** [see: chlorambucil]

**chlorbutol** BAN *antimicrobial agent* [also: chlorobutanol]

**chlorcinnazine** [see: clocinizine]

**chlorcyclizine** INN, BAN *topical antihistamine* [also: chlorcyclizine HCl]

**chlorcyclizine HCl** USP *topical antihistamine* [also: chlorcyclizine]

**chlordantoin** USAN, BAN *antifungal* [also: clodantoin]

**chlordiazepoxide** USP, INN, BAN, JAN *benzodiazepine anxiolytic; sedative; alcohol withdrawal aid*

**chlordiazepoxide HCl** USAN, USP, BAN, JAN *benzodiazepine anxiolytic; sedative; alcohol withdrawal aid; sometimes abused as a street drug* 5, 10, 25 mg oral

**chlordiazepoxide HCl & clidinium bromide** *anxiolytic; GI anticholinergic* 5•2.5 mg

**chlordimorine** INN

**Chlordrine S.R.** sustained-release capsules (discontinued 2002) ℞ *decongestant; antihistamine* [pseudoephedrine HCl; chlorpheniramine maleate] 120•8 mg

*Chlorella* a genus of single-cell algae used as a source of multiple vitamins and minerals, protein, chlorellin, chloro-phyll and Chlorella *growth factor (q.v.); immune enhancer and chelator of heavy metals*

**Chlorella growth factor (CGF)** *natural extract of the nucleus of* Chlorella *algae (q.v.) that is widely used in wound healing and skin disorders*

**Chloresium** ointment, solution OTC *vulnerary and deodorant for wounds, burns, and ulcers* [chlorophyllin copper complex] 0.5%; 0.2%

**Chloresium** tablets OTC *systemic deodorant for ostomy, breath, and body odors* [chlorophyllin copper complex] 14 mg

**chlorethate** [see: clorethate]

**chlorethyl** [see: ethyl chloride]

**chlorfenisate** [see: clofibrate]

**chlorfenvinphos** BAN [also: clofenvinfos]

**chlorguanide HCl** [see: chloroguanide HCl]

**chlorhexadol** BAN [also: chloralodol]

**chlorhexidine** INN, BAN *antimicrobial* [also: chlorhexidine gluconate]

**chlorhexidine gluconate** USAN *antimicrobial; investigational (orphan) for oral mucositis in bone marrow transplant patients* [also: chlorhexidine]

**chlorhexidine HCl** USAN, BAN *topical anti-infective*

**chlorhexidine phosphanilate** USAN *antibacterial*

**chlorimiphenin** [see: imiclopazine]

**chlorimpiphenine** [see: imiclopazine]

**chlorinated & iodized peanut oil** [see: chloriodized oil]

**chlorindanol** USAN *spermaticide* [also: clorindanol]

**chlorine** *element (Cl)*

**chloriodized oil** USP

**chlorisondamine chloride** INN, BAN

**chlorisondamone chloride** [see: chlorisondamine chloride]

**chlormadinone** INN, BAN *progestin* [also: chlormadinone acetate]

**chlormadinone acetate** USAN, NF *progestin* [also: chlormadinone]

**chlormerodrin** NF, INN, BAN

**chlormerodrin ($^{197}$Hg)** INN *renal function test; radioactive agent* [also: chlormerodrin Hg 197]

**chlormerodrin Hg 197** USAN, USP *renal function test; radioactive agent* [also: chlormerodrin ($^{197}$Hg)]

**chlormerodrin Hg 203** USAN, USP *renal function test; radioactive agent*

**chlormeroprin** [see: chlormerodrin]

**chlormethazanone** [see: chlormezanone]

**chlormethiazole** BAN [also: clomethiazole]

**chlormethine** INN *nitrogen mustard-type alkylating antineoplastic* [also: mechlorethamine HCl; mustine; nitrogen mustard N-oxide HCl]

**chlormethylencycline** [see: clomocycline]

**chlormezanone** INN, BAN *mild anxiolytic*

**chlormidazole** INN, BAN

**chlornaphazine** INN

**chloroacetic acid** [see: monochloroacetic, dichloroacetic, or trichloroacetic acid]

**8-chloroadenosine monophosphate, cyclic (8-Cl cAMP)** [see: tocladesine]

**chloroazodin** USP [also: chlorazodin]

**5-chlorobenzoxazolinone** [see: chlorzoxazone]

**chlorobutanol** NF, INN *antimicrobial agent; preservative* [also: chlorbutol]

**chlorochine** [see: chloroquine]

**chlorocresol** USAN, NF, INN *antiseptic; disinfectant*

**2-chloro-2'-deoxyadenosine (CdA)** [now: cladribine]

**chlorodeoxylincomycin** [see: clindamycin]

**chloroethane** [see: ethyl chloride]

**2-chloroethyl-3-sarcosinamide-1-nitrosourea** *investigational (orphan) for malignant glioma*

**chloroform** NF *solvent*

**chloroguanide HCl** USP *antimalarial; dihydrofolate reductase inhibitor* [also: proguanil]

**chloroguanide triazine pamoate** [see: cycloguanil pamoate]

**chloro-iodohydroxyquinoline** [see: clioquinol]

**chlorolincomycin** [see: clindamycin]

**chloromethapyrilene citrate** [see: chlorothen citrate]

**Chloromycetin** powder for eye drops, ophthalmic ointment ℞ *topical ophthalmic antibiotic* [chloramphenicol] 25 mg/15 mL; 10 mg/g

**Chloromycetin Hydrocortisone** powder for eye drops (discontinued 2000) ℞ *topical ophthalmic corticosteroidal anti-inflammatory; broad-spectrum antibiotic* [hydrocortisone acetate; chloramphenicol] 0.5%•0.25%

**Chloromycetin Otic** ear drops (discontinued 2003) ℞ *broad-spectrum antibiotic* [chloramphenicol] 0.5%

**Chloromycetin Sodium Succinate** powder for IV injection ℞ *broad-spectrum bacteriostatic antibiotic* [chloramphenicol sodium succinate] 100 mg/mL

*p*-**chlorophenol** [see: parachlorophenol]

**chlorophenothane** NF [also: clofenotane; dicophane]

**chlorophenoxamide** [see: clefamide]

**chlorophenylmercury** [see: phenylmercuric chloride]

**chlorophyll, water soluble** [see: chlorophyllin]

**chlorophyllin** *vulnerary; oral deodorant for ostomy, breath, and body odors; topical deodorant for wounds and ulcers* 20 mg oral

**chlorophyllin copper complex** USAN *oral deodorant for ostomy, breath, and body odors; topical deodorant for wounds and ulcers*

**chloroprednisone** INN

**chloroprednisone acetate** [see: chloroprednisone]

**chloroprocaine** INN *local anesthetic* [also: chloroprocaine HCl]

**chloroprocaine HCl** USP *injectable local anesthetic* [also: chloroprocaine]

**Chloroptic** eye drops ℞ *topical ophthalmic antibiotic* [chloramphenicol] 5 mg/mL

**Chloroptic S.O.P.** ophthalmic ointment ℞ *topical ophthalmic antibiotic* [chloramphenicol] 10 mg/g

**chloropyramine** INN [also: halopyramine]

**chloropyrilene** INN, BAN [also: chlorothen citrate]

**chloroquine** USP, INN, BAN *amebicide; antimalarial*

**chloroquine diphosphate** [see: chloroquine phosphate]

**chloroquine HCl** USP *amebicide; antimalarial* [also: chloroquine]

**chloroquine phosphate** USP, BAN *amebicide; antimalarial; lupus erythematosus suppressant* 250 mg oral

**chloroserpidine** INN

**N-chlorosuccinimide** [see: succinchlorimide]

**chlorothen citrate** NF [also: chloropyrilene]

**chlorothenium citrate** [see: chlorothen citrate]

**chlorothenylpyramine** [see: chlorothen]

**chlorothiazide** USP, INN, BAN *diuretic; antihypertensive* 250, 500 mg oral

**chlorothiazide sodium** USAN, USP *diuretic; antihypertensive*

**chlorothymol** NF

**chlorotrianisene** USP, INN, BAN *estrogen for hormone replacement therapy or inoperable prostatic cancer*

**chloroxine** USAN *antiseborrheic*

**chloroxylenol** USP, INN, BAN *bacteriostatic*

**chlorozone** [see: chloramine-T]

**chlorpenthixol** [see: clopenthixol]

**Chlorphed-LA** nasal spray (discontinued 2002) OTC *nasal decongestant* [oxymetazoline HCl] 0.05%

**Chlorphedrine SR** sustained-release capsules (discontinued 2002) ℞ *decongestant; antihistamine* [pseudoephedrine HCl; chlorpheniramine maleate] 120•8 mg

**chlorphenamine** INN *antihistamine* [also: chlorpheniramine maleate; chlorpheniramine]

**chlorphenamine maleate** [see: chlorpheniramine maleate]

**chlorphenecyclane** [see: clofenciclan]

**chlorphenesin** INN, BAN *skeletal muscle relaxant* [also: chlorphenesin carbamate]

**chlorphenesin carbamate** USAN, JAN *skeletal muscle relaxant* [also: chlorphenesin]

**chlorphenindione** [see: clorindione]

**chlorpheniramine** BAN *alkylamine antihistamine* [also: chlorpheniramine maleate; chlorphenamine] 🔟 chlorphentermine

**chlorpheniramine maleate** USP *alkylamine antihistamine* [also: chlorphenamine; chlorpheniramine] 4, 8, 12 mg oral

**chlorpheniramine maleate & phenylpropanolamine HCl** *antihistamine; decongestant* PPA banned in all OTC products in 2001

**chlorpheniramine maleate & pseudoephedrine HCl** *antihistamine; decongestant* 8•120 mg oral

**chlorpheniramine polistirex** USAN *alkylamine antihistamine*

**chlorpheniramine tannate & pseudoephedrine tannate** *antihistamine; decongestant* 75•4.5 mg/5 mL oral

**chlorpheniramine tannate & pyrilamine tannate & phenylephrine tannate** *antihistamine; decongestant* 2•12.5•5 mg/5 mL oral

**chlorphenoctium amsonate** INN, BAN

**chlorphenotane** [see: chlorophenothane]

**chlorphenoxamine** INN, BAN [also: chlorphenoxamine HCl]

**chlorphenoxamine HCl** USP [also: chlorphenoxamine]

**chlorphentermine** INN, BAN *anorectic* [also: chlorphentermine HCl] 🔟 chlorpheniramine

**chlorphentermine HCl** USAN *anorectic* [also: chlorphentermine]

**chlorphenylindandione** [see: clorindione]

**chlorphthalidone** [see: chlorthalidone]

**chlorprocaine chloride** [see: chloroprocaine HCl]

**chlorproethazine** INN [also: chlorproethazine HCl]

**chlorproethazine HCl** [also: chlorproethazine]

**chlorproguanil** INN, BAN

**chlorproguanil HCl** [see: chlorproguanil]

**chlorpromazine** USP, INN, BAN *phenothiazine antipsychotic; antiemetic; intractable hiccough relief*

**chlorpromazine HCl** USP, BAN, JAN *phenothiazine antipsychotic; antiemetic; intractable hiccough relief* 10, 25, 50, 100, 200 mg oral; 100 mg/mL oral; 25 mg/mL injection

**chlorpromazine hibenzate** JAN *phenothiazine antipsychotic; antiemetic*

**chlorpromazine phenolphthalinate** JAN *phenothiazine antipsychotic; antiemetic*

**chlorpromazine tannate** USP, INN, BAN *phenothiazine antipsychotic; antiemetic*

**chlorpropamide** USP, INN, BAN, JAN *sulfonylurea antidiabetic* 100, 250 mg oral

**chlorprophenpyridamine maleate** [see: chlorpheniramine maleate]

**chlorprothixene** USAN, USP, INN, BAN *thioxanthene antipsychotic*

**chlorpyrifos** BAN

**chlorquinaldol** INN, BAN

**Chlor-Rest** tablets (discontinued 2001) OTC *decongestant; antihistamine* [phenylpropanolamine HCl; chlorpheniramine maleate] 18.7•2 mg

**chlortalidone** INN *antihypertensive; diuretic* [also: chlorthalidone]

**chlortetracycline** INN, BAN *antibiotic; antiprotozoal* [also: chlortetracycline bisulfate]

**chlortetracycline bisulfate** USP *antibiotic; antiprotozoal* [also: chlortetracycline]

**chlortetracycline calcium** *antibiotic; antiprotozoal*

**chlortetracycline HCl** USP, BAN *antibiotic; antiprotozoal*

**chlorthalidone** USAN, USP, BAN *antihypertensive; diuretic* [also: chlortalidone] 25, 50, 100 mg oral

**chlorthenoxazin** BAN [also: chlorthenoxazine]

**chlorthenoxazine** INN [also: chlorthenoxazin]

**chlorthiazide** [see: chlorothiazide]

**chlortrianisestrol** [see: chlorotrianisene]

**Chlor-Trimeton Allergy 4 Hour** syrup (discontinued 2001) OTC *antihistamine* [chlorpheniramine maleate] 2 mg/5 mL

**Chlor-Trimeton Allergy 4 Hour** tablets OTC *antihistamine* [chlorpheniramine maleate] 4 mg

**Chlor-Trimeton Allergy 8 Hour; Chlor-Trimeton Allergy 12 Hour** timed-release tablets OTC *antihistamine* [chlorpheniramine maleate] 8 mg; 12 mg

**Chlor-Trimeton Allergy-D 4 Hour** tablets OTC *decongestant; antihistamine* [pseudoephedrine sulfate; chlorpheniramine maleate] 60•4 mg

**Chlor-Trimeton Allergy-D 12 Hour** sustained-release tablets OTC *decongestant; antihistamine* [pseudoephedrine sulfate; chlorpheniramine maleate] 120•8 mg

**Chlor-Trimeton Allergy-Sinus** caplets (discontinued 2001) OTC *decongestant; antihistamine; analgesic* [phenylpropanolamine HCl; chlorpheniramine maleate; acetaminophen] 12.5•2•500 mg

**chlorzoxazone** USP, INN, BAN, JAN *skeletal muscle relaxant* 250, 500 mg oral

**chlosudimeprimylum** [see: clopamide]

**ChlVPP (chlorambucil, vinblastine, procarbazine, prednisone/prednisolone)** *chemotherapy protocol for Hodgkin lymphoma* [note: prednisone is preferred in the U.S.; prednisolone is preferred in England]

**ChlVPP/EVA (chlorambucil, vinblastine, procarbazine, prednisone/prednisolone, etoposide, vincristine, Adriamycin)** *chemotherapy protocol for Hodgkin lymphoma* [note: prednisone is preferred in the U.S.; prednisolone is preferred in England]

**CHO (cyclophosphamide, hydroxydaunomycin, Oncovin)** *chemotherapy protocol*

**CHO cells, recombinant** [see: CD4, human truncated]

**CHOB (cyclophosphamide, hydroxydaunomycin, Oncovin, bleomycin)** *chemotherapy protocol*

**CHOD (cyclophosphamide, hydroxydaunomycin, Oncovin, dexamethasone)** *chemotherapy protocol*

**choice dielytra** *medicinal herb* [see: turkey corn]

**Choice dm** oral liquid OTC *enteral nutritional therapy for abnormal glucose tolerance* [lactose-free formula] 240 mL

**choke cherry; black choke** *medicinal herb* [see: wild black cherry]

**Cholac** oral/rectal solution ℞ *synthetic disaccharide used to prevent and treat portal-systemic encephalopathy* [lactulose] 10 g/15 mL

**cholagogues** *a class of agents that stimulate the flow of bile into the duodenum*

**cholalic acid** [see: dehydrocholic acid]

**cholecalciferol (vitamin D₃)** USP, BAN, JAN *fat-soluble vitamin* [also: colecalciferol] 1000 IU oral

**Choledyl SA** sustained-action tablets (discontinued 2004) ℞ *antiasthmatic; bronchodilator* [oxtriphylline] 400, 600 mg

**cholera vaccine** USP *active bacterin for cholera (Vibrio cholerae)*

**CholestaGel** (name changed to WelChol upon marketing release in 2000)

**cholesterin** [see: cholesterol]

**cholesterol** NF *emulsifying agent*

**cholestrin** [see: cholesterol]

**cholestyramine** BAN *bile salts ion-exchange resin; antihyperlipoproteinemic* [also: cholestyramine resin; colestyramine]

**Cholestyramine Light** powder for oral suspension ℞ *cholesterol-lowering antihyperlipidemic; also used for biliary* *obstruction* [cholestyramine resin] 4 g/dose

**cholestyramine resin** USP *bile salts ion-exchange resin; cholesterol-lowering antihyperlipidemic; also used for biliary obstruction* [also: colestyramine; cholestyramine] 4 g powder for oral solution

**cholic acid** [see: dehydrocholic acid]

**Cholidase** tablets OTC *dietary lipotropic with vitamin supplementation* [choline; inositol; vitamins $B_6$, $B_{12}$, and E] 185•150•2.5•0.005•7.5 mg

**choline** *dietary lipotropic supplement* 250, 300, 500, 650 mg oral

**choline alfoscerate** INN

**choline bitartrate** NF 250 mg oral

**choline bromide hexamethylenedi-carbamate** [see: hexacarbacholine bromide]

**choline chloride** INN *investigational (orphan) for choline deficiency of long-term parenteral nutrition*

**choline chloride acetate** [see: acetyl-choline chloride]

**choline chloride carbamate** [see: carbachol]

**choline chloride succinate** [see: succinylcholine chloride]

**choline dihydrogen citrate** NF 650 mg oral

**choline gluconate** INN

**choline glycerophosphate** [see: choline alfoscerate]

**choline perchlorate, nitrate ester** [see: nitricholine perchlorate]

**choline salicylate** USAN, INN, BAN *analgesic; antipyretic; anti-inflammatory; antirheumatic*

**choline theophyllinate** INN, BAN *bronchodilator* [also: oxtriphylline]

**cholinergic agonists** *a class of agents that produce effects similar to those of the parasympathetic nervous system* [also called: parasympathomimetics]

**cholinesterase inhibitors** *a class of drugs which increase acetylcholine neurotransmitters, used as a cognition adjuvant in Alzheimer dementia* [also

called: acetylcholinesterase (AChE) inhibitors]

**Cholinoid** capsules OTC *dietary lipotropic with vitamin supplementation* [choline; inositol; multiple B vitamins; vitamin C; lemon bioflavonoids] 111•111•±•100•100 mg

**Cholografin Meglumine** injection ℞ *radiopaque contrast medium for cholecystography and cholangiography* [iodipamide meglumine (49.2% iodine)] 520 mg/mL (257 mg/mL)

**chondodendron tomentosum** [see: tubocurarine chloride]

**chondrocyte-alginate** *investigational (orphan) gel suspension for vesicoureteral reflux in children*

**chondroitin 4-sulfate** [see: danaparoid sodium]

**chondroitin 6-sulfate** [see: danaparoid sodium]

**chondroitin sulfate** *natural remedy for arthritis, blood clots, and extravasation from needle sticks after certain chemotherapy treatments*

**chondroitin sulfate sodium** JAN

**chondroitin sulfuric acid** *natural remedy* [see: chondroitin sulfate]

**chondroitinase** *investigational (orphan) agent for vitrectomy*

**Chondrox** capsules OTC *dietary supplement for osteoarthritis; protects and rebuilds cartilage in joints* [N-acetyl-D-glucosamine; glucosamine sulfate; chondroitin sulfate; manganese (from manganese aspartate)] 500•500•800•0.17 mg

*Chondrus crispus* *medicinal herb* [see: Irish moss]

**chonsurid** *natural remedy* [see: chondroitin sulfate]

**Chooz** chewable tablets OTC *antacid* [calcium carbonate] 500 mg

**CHOP (cyclophosphamide, hydroxydaunomycin, Oncovin, prednisone)** *chemotherapy protocol for non-Hodgkin lymphoma*

**CHOP-BLEO (cyclophosphamide, hydroxydaunomycin, Oncovin,**

**prednisone, bleomycin)** *chemotherapy protocol for non-Hodgkin lymphoma*

**CHOPE (cyclophosphamide, hydroxydaunomycin, Oncovin, prednisone, etoposide)** *chemotherapy protocol*

**CHOR (cyclophosphamide, hydroxydaunomycin, Oncovin, radiation therapy)** *chemotherapy protocol*

**Chorex-5; Chorex-10** powder for IM injection ℞ *hormone for prepubertal cryptorchidism and hypogonadism; ovulation stimulant* [chorionic gonadotropin] 500 U/mL; 1000 U/mL

**choriogonadotropin alfa** USAN *recombinant human chorionic gonadotropin (rhCG); fertility stimulant for anovulatory women; adjuvant therapy for cryptorchidism*

**chorionic gonadotrophin** [see: gonadotropin, chorionic]

**chorionic gonadotropin (CG)** [see: gonadotropin, chorionic]

**Choron-10** powder for IM injection ℞ *hormone for prepubertal cryptorchidism and hypogonadism; ovulation stimulant* [chorionic gonadotropin] 1000 U/mL

**CHP (chlorhexidine phosphanilate)** [q.v.]

**Christmas factor** [see: factor IX complex]

**Chromagen** capsules ℞ *hematinic* [ferrous fumarate; cyanocobalamin; ascorbic acid; intrinsic factor concentrate] 70•0.01•150•100 mg

**Chromagen FA; Chromagen Forte** capsules ℞ *vitamin/iron supplement* [vitamins $B_{12}$ & C; iron; folic acid] 0.01•150•70•1 mg; 0.01•60•151•1 mg

**Chromagen OB** capsules OTC *prenatal vitamin/mineral/iron supplement* [multiple vitamins & minerals; iron; folic acid] ≐•28•1 mg

**Chroma-Pak** IV injection ℞ *chromium supplement* [chromic chloride hexahydrate (20% elemental chromium)] 20.5, 102.5 μg/mL (4, 20 μg Cr/mL)

**chromargyre** [see: merbromin]

**chromated albumin** [see: albumin, chromated Cr 51 serum]

**Chromelin Complexion Blender** topical suspension OTC *skin darkening agent for vitiligo and hypopigmented areas* [dihydroxyacetone] 5%

**chromic acid, disodium salt** [see: sodium chromate Cr 51]

**chromic chloride** USP *dietary chromium supplement (20% elemental chromium)* 20.5, 102.5 μg/mL (4, 20 μg Cr/mL) injection

**chromic chloride Cr 51** USAN *radioactive agent*

**chromic chloride hexahydrate** [see: chromic chloride]

**chromic phosphate Cr 51** USAN *radioactive agent*

**chromic phosphate P 32** USAN, USP *antineoplastic; radioactive agent*

**chromium** *element (Cr); trace mineral important in glucose metabolism*

**Chromium Chloride** IV injection ℞ *intravenous nutritional therapy* [chromic chloride hexahydrate] 4 μg/mL

**chromium chloride** [see: chromic chloride Cr 51]

**chromium chloride hexahydrate** [see: chromic chloride]

**chromium picolinate** *dietary chromium supplement*

**chromium polynicotinate** *dietary chromium supplement*

**chromocarb** INN

**chromonar HCl** USAN *coronary vasodilator* [also: carbocromen]

**Chronoforte** capsules OTC *anti-aging supplement* [acetyl-L-carnitine; alpha lipoic acid; carnosine; nettle leaf; quercetin; biotin] 333.3•50•166.7•166.7•12.5•0.5 mg

**Chronogesic** ℞ *investigational (Phase III) narcotic analgesic for cancer-related pain* [sufentanil]

**Chronosule** (trademarked dosage form) *sustained-action capsule*

**Chronotab** (trademarked dosage form) *sustained-action tablet*

**Chronovera** ⒸⒶⓃ delayed-onset, extended-release tablets ℞ *antihypertensive; calcium channel blocker* [verapamil HCl] 180, 240 mg

**Chronulac** oral/rectal solution ℞ *hyperosmotic laxative* [lactulose] 10 g/15 mL

***Chrysanthemum parthenium*** *medicinal herb* [see: feverfew]

***Chrysanthemum vulgare*** *medicinal herb* [see: tansy]

**chrysazin** *(withdrawn from market by FDA)* [see: danthron]

**chrysin** *natural aromatase inhibitor used to block the conversion of testosterone to estrogen*

**CHVP (cyclophosphamide, hydroxydaunomycin, VM-26, prednisone)** *chemotherapy protocol*

**Chymodiactin** powder for intradiscal injection (discontinued 2003) ℞ *proteolytic enzyme for herniated nucleus pulposus* [chymopapain] 4 nKat

**chymopapain** USAN, INN, BAN *proteolytic enzyme for herniated lumbar discs*

**chymotrypsin** USP, INN, BAN *proteolytic enzyme; zonulolytic for intracapsular lens extraction*

**C.I. acid orange 24 monosodium salt (color index)** [see: resorcin brown]

**C.I. basic violet 3 (color index)** [see: gentian violet]

**C.I. basic violet 14 monohydrochloride (color index)** [see: fuchsin, basic]

**C.I. direct blue 53 tetrasodium salt (color index)** [see: Evans blue]

**C.I. mordant yellow 5, disodium salt (color index)** [see: olsalazine sodium]

**ciadox** INN

**Cialis** film-coated tablets ℞ *phosphodiesterase type 5 (PDE5) inhibitor; selective vasodilator for erectile dysfunction (ED); investigational for female sexual dysfunction* [tadalafil] 5, 10, 20 mg

**ciamexon** INN, BAN

**cianergoline** INN

**cianidanol** INN

**cianidol** [see: cianidanol]

**cianopramine** INN

**ciapilome** INN

**Ciba Vision Cleaner for Sensitive Eyes** solution OTC *surfactant cleaning solution for soft contact lenses*

**Ciba Vision Saline** aerosol solution OTC *rinsing/storage solution for soft contact lenses* [sodium chloride (saline solution)]

**Cibacalcin** subcu or IM injection ℞ *calcium regulator for Paget disease (osteitis deformans) (orphan)* [calcitonin (human)] 0.5 mg/vial

**cibenzoline** INN, BAN *antiarrhythmic* [also: cifenline]

**cibenzoline succinate** JAN *antiarrhythmic* [also: cifenline succinate]

**cicaprost** INN *prostacyclin analogue*

**cicarperone** INN

**cicely, sweet** *medicinal herb* [see: sweet cicely]

***Cichorium intybus*** *medicinal herb* [see: chicory]

**ciclacillin** INN, BAN *antibacterial* [also: cyclacillin]

**ciclactate** INN

**ciclafrine** INN *antihypotensive* [also: ciclafrine HCl]

**ciclafrine HCl** USAN *antihypotensive* [also: ciclafrine]

**ciclazindol** USAN, INN, BAN *antidepressant*

**Ciclesonide** ℞ *investigational (Phase III) for asthma*

**ciclesonide** *investigational (NDA filed) inhaled corticosteroid for asthma*

**cicletanine** USAN, INN, BAN *antihypertensive*

**ciclindole** INN *antidepressant* [also: cyclindole]

**cicliomenol** INN

**ciclobendazole** INN, BAN *anthelmintic* [also: cyclobendazole]

**ciclofenazine** INN *antipsychotic* [also: cyclophenazine HCl]

**ciclofenazine HCl** [see: cyclophenazine HCl]

**cicloheximide** INN *antipsoriatic* [also: cycloheximide]

**ciclonicate** INN

**ciclonium bromide** INN

**ciclopirox** USAN, INN, BAN *topical antifungal for tinea pedis, tinea cruris, tinea corporis, tinea versicolor, candidiasis, seborrheic dermatitis, and onychomycosis*

**ciclopirox olamine** USAN, USP, JAN *topical antifungal*

**ciclopramine** INN

**cicloprofen** USAN, INN, BAN *antiinflammatory*

**cicloprolol** INN *antiadrenergic (β-receptor)* [also: cicloprolol HCl; cycloprolol]

**cicloprolol HCl** USAN *antiadrenergic (β-receptor)* [also: cicloprolol; cycloprolol]

**ciclosidomine** INN, BAN

**ciclosporin** INN *immunosuppressive* [also: cyclosporine; cyclosporin]

**ciclotate** INN *combining name for radicals or groups*

**ciclotizolam** INN, BAN

**ciclotropium bromide** INN

**cicloxilic acid** INN

**cicloxolone** INN, BAN

**cicortonide** INN

**cicrotoic acid** INN

**Cidecin** injection (name changed to Cubicin upon marketing release in 2003)

**cideferron** INN

**Cidex; Cidex-7; Cidex Plus 28** solution OTC *broad-spectrum antimicrobial* [glutaral] 2%; 2%; 3.2%

**cidofovir** USAN, INN *nucleoside antiviral for AIDS-related cytomegalovirus retinitis; investigational (Phase I/II) gel for AIDS-related genital herpes and Kaposi sarcoma*

**cidoxepin** INN *antidepressant* [also: cidoxepin HCl]

**cidoxepin HCl** USAN *antidepressant* [also: cidoxepin]

**cifenline** USAN *antiarrhythmic* [also: cibenzoline]

**cifenline succinate** USAN *antiarrhythmic* [also: cibenzoline succinate]

**cifostodine** INN

**ciglitazone** USAN, INN *antidiabetic*

**cignolin** [see: anthralin]

**ciheptolane** INN

**ciladopa** INN, BAN *antiparkinsonian; dopaminergic agent* [also: ciladopa HCl]

**ciladopa HCl** USAN *antiparkinsonian; dopaminergic agent* [also: ciladopa]

**cilansetron** INN *investigational treatment for irritable bowel syndrome*

**cilastatin** INN, BAN *enzyme inhibitor* [also: cilastatin sodium]

**cilastatin sodium** USAN, JAN *enzyme inhibitor* [also: cilastatin]

**cilazapril** USAN, INN, BAN, JAN *antihypertensive; ACE inhibitor*

**cilazaprilat** INN, BAN

**cilexetil** USAN *combining name for radicals or groups*

**ciliary neurotrophic factor** *investigational (orphan) agent for amyotrophic lateral sclerosis and other spinal muscular atrophies; investigational (Phase III) treatment for obesity in type 2 diabetics*

**"cillins"** *brief term for a class of antibiotics derived from various strains of the fungus Penicillium, or their semi-synthetic analogues, whose generic names end in "cillin," such as ampicillin* [properly called: penicillins]

**cilmostim** USAN *hematopoietic; macrophage colony-stimulating factor*

**cilobamine** INN *antidepressant* [also: cilobamine mesylate]

**cilobamine mesylate** USAN *antidepressant* [also: cilobamine]

**cilofungin** USAN, INN *antifungal*

**cilomilast** *phosphodiesterase type IV (PDE-IV) inhibitor; investigational (NDA filed) pulmonary anti-inflammatory for COPD*

**ciloprost** [see: iloprost]

**cilostamide** INN

**cilostazol** USAN, INN *vasodilator; antithrombotic; phosphodiesterase (PDE) III platelet aggregation inhibitor for intermittent claudication*

**Ciloxan** Drop-Tainers (eye drops), ointment ℞ *ophthalmic antibiotic* [ciprofloxacin HCl] 3.5 mg/mL; 0.3%

**ciltoprazine** INN

**cilutazoline** INN

**cimaterol** USAN, INN *repartitioning agent*

**cimemoxin** INN

**cimepanol** INN

**cimetidine** USAN, USP, INN, BAN, JAN *histamine H₂ antagonist for gastric ulcers* 200, 300, 400, 800 mg oral ▣ dimethicone

**cimetidine HCl** USAN *histamine H₂ antagonist for gastric ulcers* 300 mg/5 mL oral; 300 mg/2 mL injection

**cimetropium bromide** INN

*Cimicifuga racemosa* medicinal herb [see: black cohosh]

**cimoxatone** INN

**cinacalcet HCl** *oral calcimimetic agent for hypercalcemia due to parathyroid carcinoma (orphan) and secondary hyperparathyroidism (SHPT) due to chronic kidney disease* (base=91%)

**cinalukast** USAN, INN *antiasthmatic*

**cinametic acid** INN

**cinamolol** INN

**cinanserin** INN *serotonin inhibitor* [also: cinanserin HCl]

**cinanserin HCl** USAN *serotonin inhibitor* [also: cinanserin]

**cinaproxen** INN

**cincaine chloride** [see: dibucaine HCl]

**cinchocaine** INN, BAN *local anesthetic* [also: dibucaine]

**cinchocaine HCl** BAN *local anesthetic* [also: dibucaine HCl]

*Cinchona succirubra; C. ledgeriana; C. calisaya* medicinal herb [see: quinine]

**cinchonidine sulfate** NF

**cinchonine sulfate** NF

**cinchophen** NF, INN, BAN

**cinecromen** INN

**cinepaxadil** INN

**cinepazet** INN, BAN *antianginal* [also: cinepazet maleate]

**cinepazet maleate** USAN *antianginal* [also: cinepazet]

**cinepazic acid** INN

**cinepazide** INN, BAN

**cinfenine** INN

**cinfenoac** INN, BAN

**cinflumide** USAN, INN *muscle relaxant*

**cingestol** USAN, INN *progestin*

**cinitapride** INN

**cinmetacin** INN

**cinnamaldehyde** NF

**cinnamaverine** INN

**cinnamedrine** USAN, INN *smooth muscle relaxant*

**cinnamedrine HCl** *smooth muscle relaxant*

**cinnamic aldehyde** [now: cinnamaldehyde]

**cinnamon** NF

**cinnamon oil** NF

**cinnamon (Cinnamonum zeylanicum)** bark and oil *medicinal herb for diarrhea, dysmenorrhea, gastrointestinal upset, microbial and fungal infections, and gas pain; also used as an aromatic, astringent, and stimulant*

**cinnamon wood** *medicinal herb* [see: sassafras]

**cinnarizine** USAN, INN, BAN *antihistamine*

**cinnarizine clofibrate** INN

**cinnofuradione** INN

**cinnofuron** [see: cinnofuradione]

**cinnopentazone** INN *anti-inflammatory* [also: cintazone]

**cinnopropazone** [see: apazone]

**Cinobac** capsules ℞ *urinary antibacterial* [cinoxacin] 250 mg

**cinoctramide** INN

**cinodine HCl** USAN *veterinary antibacterial*

**cinolazepam** INN

**cinoquidox** INN

**cinoxacin** USAN, USP, INN, BAN *urinary antibacterial*

**cinoxate** USAN, USP, INN *ultraviolet screen*

**cinoxolone** INN, BAN

**cinoxopazide** INN

**cinperene** USAN, INN *antipsychotic*

**cinprazole** INN

**cinpropazide** INN

**cinquefoil (Potentilla anserina; P. canadensis; P. reptans)** plant *medicinal herb used as an antispasmodic and astringent*

**cinromide** USAN, INN *anticonvulsant*

**cintazone** USAN *anti-inflammatory* [also: cinnopentazone]

**cintramide** INN *antipsychotic* [also: cintriamide]

**cintriamide** USAN *antipsychotic* [also: cintramide]

**cinuperone** INN

**cioteronel** USAN, INN *antiandrogen*

**cipamfylline** USAN *antiviral agent; tumor necrosis factor alpha inhibitor*

**cipemastat** USAN *matrix metalloproteinase inhibitor; investigational cartilage protective agent for rheumatoid arthritis*

**cipionate** INN *combining name for radicals or groups* [also: cypionate]

**ciprafamide** INN

**Cipralan** ℞ *investigational antiarrhythmic* [cifenline succinate]

**Cipralex** (name changed to Lexapro upon marketing release in 2002)

**ciprazafone** INN

**ciprefadol** INN *analgesic* [also: ciprefadol succinate]

**ciprefadol succinate** USAN *analgesic* [also: ciprefadol]

**Cipro Cystitis Pack** (6 film-coated tablets) ℞ *broad-spectrum fluoroquinolone antibiotic* [ciprofloxacin] 100 mg ⚕ Septa; Septra

**Cipro** film-coated tablets, powder for oral suspension ℞ *broad-spectrum fluoroquinolone antibiotic* [ciprofloxacin] 250, 500, 750 mg; 250, 500 mg/5 mL ⚕ Septa; Septra

**Cipro HC Otic** ear drop suspension ℞ *topical broad-spectrum fluoroquinolone antibiotic; corticosteroidal anti-inflammatory* [ciprofloxacin; hydrocortisone] 0.2%•1% (2•10 mg/mL)

**Cipro I.V.** ℞ *broad-spectrum fluoroquinolone antibiotic* [ciprofloxacin] 200, 400 mg/vial ⚕ Septa; Septra

**Cipro XR** film-coated extended-release tablets ℞ *broad-spectrum fluoroquinolone antibiotic* [ciprofloxacin] 500, 1000 mg

**ciprocinonide** USAN, INN *adrenocortical steroid*

**Ciprodex** ear drop suspension ℞ *broad-spectrum fluoroquinolone antibiotic; corticosteroidal anti-inflammatory* [ciprofloxacin HCl; dexamethasone] 0.3%•0.1%

**ciprofibrate** USAN, INN, BAN *antihyperlipoproteinemic*

**ciprofloxacin** USAN, INN, BAN *broad-spectrum fluoroquinolone antibiotic* 100, 250, 500, 750 mg oral; 250, 500 mg/5 mL oral; 0.3% eye drops

**ciprofloxacin HCl** USAN, USP, JAN *broad-spectrum bactericidal antibiotic*

**cipropride** INN

**ciproquazone** INN

**ciproquinate** INN *coccidiostat for poultry* [also: cyproquinate]

**ciprostene** INN *platelet antiaggregatory agent* [also: ciprostene calcium]

**ciprostene calcium** USAN *platelet antiaggregatory agent* [also: ciprostene]

**ciproximide** INN *antipsychotic; antidepressant* [also: cyproximide]

**ciramadol** USAN, INN *analgesic*

**ciramadol HCl** USAN *analgesic*

**cirazoline** INN

**Circavite-T** tablets OTC *vitamin/mineral/iron supplement* [multiple vitamins & minerals; iron] ≛•12 mg

**cirolemycin** USAN, INN *antineoplastic; antibacterial*

**cisapride** USAN, INN, BAN, JAN *peristaltic stimulant; treatment for nocturnal heartburn due to gastroesophageal reflux disease; (withdrawn from U.S. markets in 2000 due to increased cardiac arrhythmias)*

**cisatracurium besylate** USAN *nondepolarizing neuromuscular blocker*

**CISCA; CisCA (cisplatin, cyclophosphamide, Adriamycin)** *chemotherapy protocol for bladder cancer*

**CISCA$_{II}$/VB$_{IV}$ (cisplatin, cyclophosphamide, Adriamycin, vinblastine, bleomycin)** *chemotherapy protocol for germ cell tumors*

**cisclomiphene** [now: enclomiphene]

**cisconazole** USAN, INN *antifungal*

*cis*-**DDP (diamminedichloroplatinum)** [see: cisplatin]

*cis*-**diamminedichloroplatinum (DDP)** [see: cisplatin]

**cismadinone** INN

**cisplatin** USAN, USP, INN, BAN *alkylating antineoplastic for testicular, ovar-*

ian, and bladder cancer 1 mg/mL injection

**cisplatin & docetaxel** chemotherapy protocol for bladder cancer and non–small cell lung cancer (NSCLC)

**cisplatin & fluorouracil** chemotherapy protocol for cervical cancer, used in conjunction with radiation therapy

**cisplatin & gemcitabine** chemotherapy protocol for metastatic bladder cancer

**cisplatin & vinorelbine** chemotherapy protocol for cervical cancer and non–small cell lung cancer (NSCLC)

**cis-platinum** [now: cisplatin]

**cis-platinum II** [now: cisplatin]

**9-cis-retinoic acid** [see: alitretinoin]

**13-cis-retinoic acid** [see: isotretinoin]

**cistinexine** INN

**citalopram** INN, BAN selective serotonin reuptake inhibitor (SSRI) for major depression

**citalopram hydrobromide** USAN selective serotonin reuptake inhibitor (SSRI) for major depression

**Citanest Forte** injection ℞ injectable local anesthetic for dental procedures [prilocaine HCl; epinephrine] 4%• 1:200 000

**Citanest Plain** injection ℞ injectable local anesthetic for dental procedures [prilocaine HCl] 4%

**citatepine** INN

**citenamide** USAN, INN anticonvulsant

**citenazone** INN

**citicoline** INN, JAN investigational (Phase III) oral treatment for ischemic stroke and head trauma [also: citicoline sodium]

**citicoline & dizocilpine maleate** investigational (Phase III) neuroprotective treatment for stroke

**citicoline sodium** USAN investigational (Phase III) oral treatment for ischemic stroke and head trauma [also: citicoline]

**citiolone** INN, DCF

**Citra pH** oral solution OTC antacid [sodium citrate] 450 mg/5 mL

**Citracal** tablets OTC calcium supplement [calcium citrate] 200 mg Ca ⊡ Citrucel

**Citracal Caplets + D** OTC dietary supplement [calcium citrate; vitamin D] 315 mg•200 IU ⊡ Citrucel

**Citracal Liquitab** effervescent tablets OTC calcium supplement [calcium citrate] 500 mg Ca ⊡ Citrucel

**Citracal Plus with Magnesium** tablets OTC dietary supplement [calcium citrate; vitamin D; multiple minerals] 250 mg Ca•125 IU• ±

**Citracal Prenatal** tablets ℞ calcium/iron supplement [calcium citrate; iron; folic acid; docusate sodium] 125•1•27•50 mg

**Citralax** effervescent granules OTC saline laxative [magnesium citrate; magnesium sulfate]

**citrate dextrose** [see: ACD solution]

**citrate of magnesia** [see: magnesium citrate]

**citrate phosphate dextrose** [see: anticoagulant citrate phosphate dextrose solution]

**citrate phosphate dextrose adenine** [see: anticoagulant citrate phosphate dextrose adenine solution]

**citrated caffeine** NF [see: caffeine citrate]

**citric acid** USP pH adjusting agent; urinary acidifier

**citric acid, magnesium oxide & sodium carbonate** [see: Suby solution G]

**citrin** [see: bioflavonoids]

**Citrocarbonate** effervescent granules OTC antacid [sodium bicarbonate; sodium citrate] 780•1820 mg/dose

**Citrolith** tablets ℞ urinary alkalinizing agent [potassium citrate; sodium citrate] 50•950 mg

**citronella (Cymbopogon nardus; C. winterianus)** oil medicinal herb for gastrointestinal spasms, promoting diuresis, and worms; also used as an antibacterial; not generally regarded as safe and effective for internal use as it is highly toxic

**Citrotein** oral liquid, powder for oral liquid OTC enteral nutritional therapy [lactose-free formula]

**citrovorum factor** [see: leucovorin calcium]

**Citrucel** powder, tablets OTC *bulk laxative* [methylcellulose] 2 g/tbsp. or scoop; 500 mg ⊠ Citracal

**Citrucel Sugar Free** powder OTC *bulk laxative* [methylcellulose; phenylalanine] 2 g•52 mg per tbsp. ⊠ Citracal

*Citrus bergamia; C. aurantium* medicinal herb [see: bergamot oil]

**citrus bioflavonoids** [see: bioflavonoids]

**Citrus Calcium** coated tablets OTC *calcium supplement* [calcium citrate] 200 mg Ca

*Citrus limon* medicinal herb [see: lemon]

*Citrus paradisi* medicinal herb [see: grapefruit]

**civamide** *investigational (orphan) agent for postherpetic neuralgia of the trigeminal nerve*

**CIVPP (chlorambucil, vinblastine, procarbazine, prednisone)** *chemotherapy protocol*

**8-Cl cAMP (8-chloroadenosine monophosphate, cyclic)** [see: tocladesine]

**CLA (conjugated linoleic acid)** [q.v.]

**cladribine** *antimetabolite antineoplastic for hairy-cell leukemia (orphan); investigational (orphan) for chronic lymphocytic leukemia, myeloid leukemia, multiple sclerosis, and non-Hodgkin lymphoma* 1 mg/mL injection

**Claforan** powder or frozen premix for IV or IM injection ℞ *cephalosporin antibiotic* [cefotaxime sodium] 0.5, 1, 2, 10 g

**clamidoxic acid** INN, BAN

**clamoxyquin** BAN *antiamebic* [also: clamoxyquin HCl; clamoxyquine]

**clamoxyquin HCl** USAN *antiamebic* [also: clamoxyquine; clamoxyquin]

**clamoxyquine** INN *antiamebic* [also: clamoxyquin HCl; clamoxyquin]

**clanfenur** INN

**clanobutin** INN

**clantifen** INN

**clara cell 10kDa protein** *investigational (orphan) for prevention of bronchopulmonary dysplasia in neonates*

*with respiratory distress syndrome* ⊠ Clearasil

**Claravis** capsules ℞ *keratolytic for severe recalcitrant cystic acne* [isotretinoin] 10, 20, 40 mg

**claretin-12** [see: cyanocobalamin] ⊠ Claritin; Clarityne

**Clarinex** film-coated tablets, syrup ℞ *nonsedating antihistamine for allergic rhinitis and chronic idiopathic urticaria* [desloratadine] 5 mg; 5 mg/5 mL

**Clarinex RediTabs** (rapidly disintegrating tablets) ℞ *nonsedating antihistamine for allergic rhinitis and chronic idiopathic urticaria* [desloratadine] 5 mg

**Claripel** cream ℞ *hyperpigmentation bleaching agent* [hydroquinone] 4%

**clarithromycin** USAN, INN, BAN, JAN *macrolide antibiotic* ⊠ dirithromycin; erythromycin

**Claritin** tablets, syrup OTC *nonsedating antihistamine for allergic rhinitis and chronic idiopathic urticaria* [loratadine] 10 mg; 1 mg/mL ⊠ claretin; Clarityne

**Claritin Hives Relief** tablets OTC *nonsedating antihistamine for hives* [loratadine] 10 mg

**Claritin Non-Drowsy Allergy** tablets OTC *nonsedating antihistamine for allergic rhinitis and chronic idiopathic urticaria* [loratadine] 10 mg

**Claritin RediTabs** (rapidly disintegrating tablets) OTC *nonsedating antihistamine for allergic rhinitis and chronic idiopathic urticaria* [loratadine] 10 mg ⊠ claretin; Clarityne

**Claritin-D 12 Hour; Claritin-D 24 Hour** extended-release tablets OTC *decongestant; nonsedating antihistamine* [pseudoephedrine sulfate; loratadine] 120•5 mg; 240•10 mg

**Clarityne** (Mexican name for U.S. product Claritin) ⊠ claretin; Claritin

*Claviceps purpurea* medicinal herb [see: ergot]

**clavulanate potassium** USAN, USP *β-lactamase inhibitor; penicillin synergist*

**clavulanic acid** INN, BAN *β-lactamase inhibitor; penicillin synergist*

**claw, scaly dragon's; turkey claw** *medicinal herb* [see: coral root]

**clay, kaolin** *natural material* [see: kaolin]

**clazolam** USAN, INN *minor tranquilizer*

**clazolimine** USAN, INN *diuretic*

**clazuril** USAN, INN, BAN *coccidiostat for pigeons*

**CLD-BOMP** *chemotherapy protocol for cervical cancer* [see: BOMP]

**Clean-N-Soak** solution OTC *cleaning/ soaking solution for hard contact lenses*

**Clear By Design** gel (discontinued 2003) OTC *keratolytic for acne* [benzoyl peroxide] 2.5%

**Clear Eyes** eye drops OTC *topical ophthalmic decongestant and vasoconstrictor* [naphazoline HCl] 0.012%

**Clear Eyes ACR** eye drops OTC *topical ophthalmic decongestant and astringent* [naphazoline HCl; zinc sulfate] 0.012%•0.25%

**Clear Total Lice Elimination System** kit (shampoo + egg remover enzymes + nit comb) (discontinued 2003) OTC *pediculicide for lice* [pyrethrins; piperonyl butoxide] 0.3%•3%

**Clear Tussin 30** oral liquid (discontinued 2002) OTC *antitussive; expectorant* [dextromethorphan hydrobromide; guaifenesin] 15•100 mg/5 mL

**Clearasil** lotion (discontinued 2003) OTC *keratolytic for acne* [benzoyl peroxide] 10% ℞ clara cell

**Clearasil Acne Treatment** cream OTC *keratolytic for acne* [benzoyl peroxide] 10% ℞ clara cell

**Clearasil Acne-Fighting Pads** OTC *keratolytic for acne* [salicylic acid; alcohol 2%] 2%

**Clearasil Adult Care** cream OTC *acne treatment* [sulfur; resorcinol; alcohol 10%]

**Clearasil Antibacterial Soap** bar OTC *medicated cleanser for acne* [triclosan]

**Clearasil Clearstick** topical liquid OTC *keratolytic for acne* [salicylic acid; alcohol 39%] 1.25%, 2%

**Clearasil Daily Face Wash** topical liquid OTC *medicated cleanser for acne* [triclosan] 0.3%

**Clearasil Double Clear; Clearasil Double Textured** medicated pads OTC *keratolytic for acne* [salicylic acid; alcohol 40%] 1.25%, 2%; 2%

**Clearasil Medicated Deep Cleanser** topical liquid OTC *keratolytic cleanser for acne* [salicylic acid; alcohol 42%] 0.5%

**Clearblue Easy Digital Pregnancy Test** test stick plus digital readout for home use *in vitro diagnostic aid; urine pregnancy test*

**Clearblue Easy Pregnancy Test** test stick for home use *in vitro diagnostic aid; urine pregnancy test*

**Clearly Cala-gel** OTC *topical antihistamine* [diphenhydramine HCl]

**Clearplan Easy** test kit for home use *in vitro diagnostic aid to predict ovulation time*

**Clearview Chlamydia** test for professional use *in vitro diagnostic aid for Chlamydia trachomatis* [color-label immunoassay]

**cleavers; cleaverwort** *medicinal herb* [see: bedstraw]

**clebopride** USAN, INN *antiemetic*

**clefamide** INN, BAN

**clemastine** USAN, BAN *ethanolamine antihistamine*

**clemastine fumarate** USAN, USP, BAN *ethanolamine antihistamine* 1.34, 2.68 mg oral; 0.67 mg/5 mL

*Clematis cirrhosa; C. virginiana* *medicinal herb* [see: woodbine]

**clemeprol** INN, BAN

**clemizole** INN, BAN

**clemizole penicillin** INN, BAN

**clenbuterol** INN, BAN

**Clenia** cream, foaming wash ℞ *treatment for acne, rosacea, and seborrheic dermatitis* [sulfacetamide sodium; sulfur] 10%•5%

**clenoliximab** *investigational (Phase I/ II) anti-CD4 antibody for the treatment of rheumatoid arthritis*

**clenpirin** INN [also: clenpyrin]

**clenpyrin** BAN [also: clenpirin]

**clentiazem** INN *calcium channel antagonist* [also: clentiazem maleate]

**clentiazem maleate** USAN *calcium channel antagonist* [also: clentiazem]

**Cleocin** capsules ℞ *lincosamide antibiotic; investigational (orphan) for AIDS-related* Pneumocystis carinii *pneumonia* [clindamycin HCl] 75, 150, 300 mg ⧫ bleomycin; Lincocin

**Cleocin** vaginal cream, vaginal ovules (suppositories) ℞ *lincosamide antibiotic for bacterial vaginosis* [clindamycin phosphate] 2%; 100 mg

**Cleocin Pediatric** granules for oral solution ℞ *lincosamide antibiotic* [clindamycin palmitate HCl] 75 mg/5 mL

**Cleocin Phosphate** IV infusion, IM injection ℞ *lincosamide antibiotic; investigational (orphan) for AIDS-related* Pneumocystis carinii *pneumonia* [clindamycin phosphate] 150 mg/mL

**Cleocin T** gel, lotion, topical suspension, pledgets ℞ *antibiotic for acne* [clindamycin phosphate] 1%

**Clerz 2; Clerz Plus** solution OTC *rewetting solution for hard or soft contact lenses*

**cletoquine** INN, BAN

**Clexane** (European name for U.S. product Lovenox)

**clibucaine** INN

**clidafidine** INN

**clidanac** INN

**clidinium bromide** USAN, USP, INN, BAN *GI anticholinergic; peptic ulcer adjunct*

**clidinium bromide & chlordiazepoxide HCl** *GI anticholinergic; anxiolytic* 2.5•5 mg

**Climara** transdermal patch ℞ *estrogen replacement therapy for the treatment of postmenopausal symptoms and prevention of postmenopausal osteoporosis* [estradiol] 25, 37.5, 50, 60, 75, 100 μg/day

**ClimaraPro** transdermal patch ℞ *hormone replacement therapy for the treatment of postmenopausal symptoms and prevention of postmenopausal osteoporosis* [levonorgestrel; estradiol] 15•45 μg/day

**climazolam** INN

**climbazole** INN, BAN

**climiqualine** INN

**Clinac BPO** gel ℞ *keratolytic for acne* [benzoyl peroxide] 7%

**clinafloxacin HCl** USAN *quinolone antibacterial*

**Clinda-Derm** topical solution (discontinued 2003) ℞ *antibiotic for acne* [clindamycin phosphate] 1%

**Clindagel** gel ℞ *antibiotic for acne* [clindamycin phosphate] 1%

**ClindaMax** gel, lotion, topical suspension ℞ *antibiotic for acne* [clindamycin phosphate] 1%

**clindamycin** USAN, INN, BAN *lincosamide antibiotic; investigational (orphan) for AIDS-related* Pneumocystis carinii *pneumonia*

**clindamycin HCl** USP, BAN *lincosamide antibiotic; investigational (orphan) for AIDS-related* Pneumocystis carinii *pneumonia* 75, 150, 300 mg oral

**clindamycin HCl & primaquine phosphate** *investigational (orphan) for AIDS-associated* Pneumocystis carinii *pneumonia*

**clindamycin palmitate HCl** USAN, USP *lincosamide antibiotic*

**clindamycin phosphate** USAN, USP *lincosamide antibiotic* 1% topical; 150 mg/mL injection

**Clindets** topical suspension, pledgets ℞ *antibiotic for acne* [clindamycin; alcohol 52%] 1%

**Clinipak** (trademarked packaging form) *unit dose package*

**Clinistix** reagent strips for home use *in vitro diagnostic aid for urine glucose*

**Clinitest** reagent tablets for home use *in vitro diagnostic aid for urine glucose*

**clinocaine HCl** [see: procaine HCl]

**clinofibrate** INN

**clinolamide** INN

**Clinoril** tablets ℞ *antiarthritic; nonsteroidal anti-inflammatory drug (NSAID) for ankylosing spondylitis and acute bursitis/tendinitis* [sulindac] 150, 200 mg

**clioquinol** USP, INN, BAN *topical antibacterial and antifungal* 3% topical

**clioxanide** USAN, INN, BAN *anthelmintic* ⏃ Clinoxide
**clipoxamine** [see: cliropamine]
**cliprofen** USAN, INN *anti-inflammatory*
**cliropamine** INN
**clobamine mesylate** [now: cilobamine mesylate]
**clobazam** USAN, INN, BAN *minor benzodiazepine tranquilizer; anxiolytic*
**clobedolum** [see: clonitazene]
**clobenoside** INN
**clobenzepam** INN
**clobenzorex** INN
**clobenztropine** INN
**clobetasol** INN, BAN *topical corticosteroidal anti-inflammatory* [also: clobetasol propionate]
**clobetasol propionate** USAN *topical corticosteroidal anti-inflammatory for scalp dermatoses and plaque psoriasis* [also: clobetasol] 0.05% topical
**clobetasone** INN, BAN *topical corticosteroidal anti-inflammatory* [also: clobetasone butyrate]
**clobetasone butyrate** USAN *topical corticosteroidal anti-inflammatory* [also: clobetasone]
**Clobex** lotion, shampoo ℞ *corticosteroidal anti-inflammatory* [clobetasol propionate] 0.05%
**clobutinol** INN
**clobuzarit** INN, BAN
**clocanfamide** INN
**clocapramine** INN
**clociguanil** INN, BAN
**clocinizine** INN
**clocortolone** INN *topical corticosteroid* [also: clocortolone acetate]
**clocortolone acetate** USAN *topical corticosteroid* [also: clocortolone]
**clocortolone pivalate** USAN, USP *topical corticosteroid*
**clocoumarol** INN
**Clocream** cream OTC *moisturizer; emollient* [cod liver oil (vitamins A and E); cholecalciferol; vitamin A palmitate]
**clodacaine** INN
**clodanolene** USAN, INN *skeletal muscle relaxant*

**clodantoin** INN *antifungal* [also: chlordantoin]
**clodazon** INN *antidepressant* [also: clodazon HCl]
**clodazon HCl** USAN *antidepressant* [also: clodazon]
**Cloderm** cream ℞ *corticosteroidal anti-inflammatory* [clocortolone pivalate] 0.1%
**clodoxopone** INN
**clodronate disodium** *bisphosphonate bone resorption inhibitor for hypercalcemia of malignancy* [also: disodium clodronate]
**clodronic acid** USAN, INN, BAN *calcium regulator*
**clofarabine** *investigational (Phase II, orphan) purine nucleoside antimetabolite antineoplastic for acute myelogenous leukemia (AML) and acute lymphoblastic leukemia (ALL)*
**Clofarex** ℞ *investigational (Phase II, orphan) purine nucleoside antimetabolite antineoplastic for acute myelogenous leukemia (AML) and acute lymphoblastic leukemia (ALL)* [clofarabine]
**clofazimine** USAN, INN, BAN *bactericidal; tuberculostatic; leprostatic (orphan)*
**clofedanol** INN *antitussive* [also: chlophedianol HCl; chlophedianol]
**clofedanol HCl** [see: chlophedianol HCl]
**clofenamic acid** INN
**clofenamide** INN
**clofenciclan** INN
**clofenetamine** INN
**clofenetamine HCl** [see: clofenetamine]
**clofenotane** INN [also: chlorophenothane; dicophane]
**clofenoxyde** INN
**clofenpyride** [see: nicofibrate]
**clofenvinfos** INN [also: chlorfenvinphos]
**cloveverine** INN
**clofexamide** INN
**clofezone** INN
**clofibrate** USAN, USP, INN, BAN *triglyceride-lowering antihyperlipidemic for*

*primary dysbetalipoproteinemia (type III hyperlipidemia) and hypertriglyceridemia (types IV and V hyperlipidemia)*

**clofibric acid** INN

**clofibride** INN

**clofilium phosphate** USAN, INN *antiarrhythmic*

**clofinol** [see: nicofibrate]

**cloflucarban** USAN *disinfectant* [also: halocarban]

**clofluperol** INN, BAN *antipsychotic* [also: seperidol HCl]

**clofluperol HCl** [see: seperidol HCl]

**clofoctol** INN

**cloforex** INN

**clofurac** INN

**clogestone** INN, BAN *progestin* [also: clogestone acetate]

**clogestone acetate** USAN *progestin* [also: clogestone]

**cloguanamil** INN, BAN [also: cloguanamile]

**cloguanamile** BAN [also: cloguanamil]

**clomacran** INN, BAN *antipsychotic* [also: clomacran phosphate]

**clomacran phosphate** USAN *antipsychotic* [also: clomacran]

**clomegestone** INN *progestin* [also: clomegestone acetate]

**clomegestone acetate** USAN *progestin* [also: clomegestone]

**clometacin** INN

**clometerone** INN *antiestrogen* [also: clometherone]

**clometherone** USAN *antiestrogen* [also: clometerone]

**clomethiazole** INN [also: chlormethiazole]

**clomethiazole edisylate** USAN *GABA (A) receptor modulator for acute ischemic stroke*

**clometocillin** INN

**Clomid** tablets ℞ *ovulation stimulant* [clomiphene citrate] 50 mg

**clomide** [see: aklomide]

**clomifene** INN *gonad-stimulating principle; ovulation stimulant* [also: clomiphene citrate; clomiphene]

**clomifenoxide** INN

**clominorex** USAN, INN *anorectic*

**clomiphene** BAN *gonad-stimulating principle; ovulation stimulant* [also: clomiphene citrate; clomifene] ⑨

**clonidine**

**clomiphene citrate** USAN, USP *gonad-stimulating principle; ovulation stimulant* [also: clomifene; clomiphene] 50 mg oral

**clomipramine** INN, BAN *tricyclic antidepressant for obsessive-compulsive disorders* [also: clomipramine HCl]

**clomipramine HCl** USAN *tricyclic antidepressant for obsessive-compulsive disorders* [also: clomipramine] 25, 50, 75 mg oral

**clomocycline** INN, BAN

**clomoxir** INN

**Clomycin** ointment (discontinued 2001) OTC *topical antibiotic; anesthetic* [polymyxin B sulfate; bacitracin; neomycin sulfate; lidocaine] 5000 U•500 U•3.5 mg•40 mg per g

**clonazepam** USAN, USP, INN, BAN *anticonvulsant; anxiolytic for panic disorder; investigational (orphan) for hyperexplexia (startle disease)* 0.5, 1, 2 mg oral

**clonazoline** INN

**clonidine** USAN, INN, BAN *centrally acting antiadrenergic antihypertensive; adjunct to epidural opioid analgesics for severe cancer pain (orphan)* ⑨ clomiphene; Klonopin; quinidine

**clonidine HCl** USAN, USP, BAN *centrally acting antiadrenergic antihypertensive; adjunct to epidural opioid analgesics for severe cancer pain (orphan)* 0.1, 0.2, 0.3 mg oral

**clonitazene** INN, BAN

**clonitrate** USAN, INN *coronary vasodilator*

**clonixeril** USAN, INN *analgesic*

**clonixin** USAN, INN *analgesic*

**clopamide** USAN, INN, BAN *antihypertensive; diuretic*

**clopenthixol** USAN, INN, BAN *antipsychotic*

**cloperastine** INN

**cloperidone** INN *sedative* [also: cloperidone HCl]

**cloperidone HCl** USAN *sedative* [also: cloperidone]

clophenoxate [see: meclofenoxate]

clopidogrel INN, BAN *platelet aggregation inhibitor for stroke, myocardial infarction, peripheral artery disease, and acute coronary syndrome*

clopidogrel bisulfate USAN *platelet aggregation inhibitor for stroke, myocardial infarction, peripheral artery disease, and acute coronary syndrome*

clopidol USAN, INN, BAN *coccidiostat for poultry*

clopimozide USAN, INN *antipsychotic*

clopipazan INN *antipsychotic* [also: clopipazan mesylate]

clopipazan mesylate USAN *antipsychotic* [also: clopipazan]

clopirac USAN, INN, BAN *anti-inflammatory*

cloponone INN, BAN

clopoxide [see: chlordiazepoxide]

clopoxide chloride [see: chlordiazepoxide HCl]

Clopra tablets ℞ *antidopaminergic; antiemetic for chemotherapy; peristaltic* [metoclopramide HCl] 10 mg

cloprednol USAN, INN, BAN *corticosteroid; anti-inflammatory*

cloprostenol INN, BAN *prostaglandin* [also: cloprostenol sodium]

cloprostenol sodium USAN *prostaglandin* [also: cloprostenol]

cloprothiazole INN

cloquinate INN, BAN

cloquinozine INN

cloracetadol INN

cloral betaine INN *sedative* [also: chloral betaine]

cloramfenicol pantotenate complex INN *antibacterial; antirickettsial* [also: chloramphenicol pantothenate complex]

cloranolol INN

clorarsen [see: dichlorophenarsine HCl]

clorazepate dipotassium USAN, USP *benzodiazepine anxiolytic; minor tranquilizer; alcohol withdrawal aid; anticonvulsant adjunct* [also: dipotassium clorazepate] 3.75, 7.5, 15 mg oral

clorazepate monopotassium USAN *minor tranquilizer*

clorazepic acid BAN

cloretate INN *sedative; hypnotic* [also: clorethate]

clorethate USAN *sedative; hypnotic* [also: cloretate]

clorexolone USAN, INN, BAN *diuretic*

Clorfed extended-release tablets ℞ *decongestant; antihistamine* [pseudoephedrine HCl; chlorpheniramine maleate] 60•4 mg

clorgiline INN [also: clorgyline]

clorgyline BAN [also: clorgiline]

cloricromen INN

cloridarol INN

clorindanic acid INN

clorindanol INN *spermaticide* [also: chlorindanol]

clorindione INN, BAN

clormecaine INN

clorofene INN *disinfectant* [also: clorophene]

cloroperone INN *antipsychotic* [also: cloroperone HCl]

cloroperone HCl USAN *antipsychotic* [also: cloroperone]

clorophene USAN *disinfectant* [also: clorofene]

cloroqualone INN

clorotepine INN

Clorpactin WCS-90 powder for solution OTC *topical antimicrobial* [oxychlorosene sodium] 2 g

clorprenaline INN, BAN *adrenergic; bronchodilator* [also: clorprenaline HCl]

clorprenaline HCl USAN *adrenergic; bronchodilator* [also: clorprenaline]

Clorpres tablets ℞ *antihypertensive; diuretic* [clonidine HCl; chlorthalidone] 0.1•15 mg; 0.2•15 mg; 0.3•15 mg

clorquinaldol [see: chlorquinaldol]

clorsulon USAN, INN *antiparasitic; fasciolicide*

clortermine INN *anorectic* [also: clortermine HCl]

clortermine HCl USAN *anorectic* [also: clortermine]

closantel USAN, INN, BAN *anthelmintic*

closilate INN *combining name for radicals or groups* [also: closylate]

**closiramine** INN *antihistamine* [also: closiramine aceturate]

**closiramine aceturate** USAN *antihistamine* [also: closiramine]

**clostebol** INN [also: clostebol acetate]

**clostebol acetate** BAN [also: clostebol]

**clostridial collagenase** *investigational (Phase II, orphan) agent for advanced Dupuytren disease*

**Clostridium botulinum toxin** [see: botulinum toxin]

**closylate** USAN, BAN *combining name for radicals or groups* [also: closilate]

**clotbur** *medicinal herb* [see: burdock]

**clothiapine** USAN, BAN *antipsychotic* [also: clotiapine]

**clothixamide maleate** USAN *antipsychotic* [also: clotixamide]

**clotiapine** INN *antipsychotic* [also: clothiapine]

**clotiazepam** INN

**cloticasone** INN, BAN *anti-inflammatory* [also: cloticasone propionate]

**cloticasone propionate** USAN *anti-inflammatory* [also: cloticasone]

**clotioxone** INN

**clotixamide** INN *antipsychotic* [also: clothixamide maleate]

**clotixamide maleate** [see: clothixamide maleate]

**Clotrimaderm** ⒸⒶⓃ cream, topical solution, vaginal cream OTC *topical antifungal* [clotrimazole] 1%

**clotrimazole (CLT)** USAN, USP, INN, BAN, JAN *broad-spectrum antifungal; investigational (orphan) for sickle cell disease* 1% topical; 100 mg vaginal 🔊 co-trimoxazole

**clotrimazole & betamethasone dipropionate** *broad-spectrum antifungal; corticosteroidal anti-inflammatory* 1%•0.05% topical

**clotrimidazole** *investigational (orphan) for sickle cell disease*

**cloudberry** *medicinal herb* [see: blackberry]

**clove oil** NF

**clover, king's; sweet clover** *medicinal herb* [see: melilot]

**clover, marsh** *medicinal herb* [see: buckbean]

**clover, purple; wild clover** *medicinal herb* [see: red clover]

**clover, winter** *medicinal herb* [see: squaw vine]

**cloves** (*Caryophyllus aromaticus; Eugenia caryophyllata; Syzygium aromaticum*) seed and oil *medicinal herb for bad breath, bronchial secretions, dizziness, earache, fever, nausea, platelet aggregation inhibition, poor circulation, and thrombosis; also used topically as an analgesic and antiseptic*

**clovoxamine** INN

**cloxacepride** INN

**cloxacillin** INN, BAN *penicillinase-resistant penicillin antibiotic* [also: cloxacillin benzathine]

**cloxacillin benzathine** USP *penicillinase-resistant penicillin antibiotic* [also: cloxacillin]

**cloxacillin sodium** USAN, USP *penicillinase-resistant penicillin antibiotic*

**Cloxapen** capsules (discontinued 2002) ℞ *penicillinase-resistant penicillin antibiotic* [cloxacillin sodium] 250, 500 mg

**cloxazolam** INN

**cloxestradiol** INN

**cloxifenol** [see: triclosan]

**cloximate** INN

**cloxiquine** INN *antibacterial* [also: cloxyquin]

**cloxotestosterone** INN

**cloxphendyl** [see: cloxypendyl]

**cloxypendyl** INN

**cloxyquin** USAN *antibacterial* [also: cloxiquine]

**clozapine** USAN, INN, BAN *dibenzapine antipsychotic for severe schizophrenia; sedative* 12.5, 25, 100 mg oral

**Clozaril** tablets ℞ *novel (atypical) antipsychotic for severe schizophrenia* [clozapine] 25, 100 mg

**CLT (clotrimazole)** [q.v.]

**club, shepherd's** *medicinal herb* [see: mullein]

**club moss** *(Lycopodium clavatum)* spores *medicinal herb used as a hemostatic and vulnerary*

**cluster, wax** *medicinal herb* [see: wintergreen]

**C-Max** gradual-release tablets OTC *vitamin/mineral supplement* [vitamin C; multiple minerals] 1 • ± g

**CMC (carboxymethylcellulose) gum** [see: carboxymethylcellulose sodium]

**CMC (cyclophosphamide, methotrexate, CCNU)** *chemotherapy protocol*

**CMC-VAP (cyclophosphamide, methotrexate, CCNU, vincristine, Adriamycin, procarbazine)** *chemotherapy protocol*

**CMF; CMF-IV (cyclophosphamide, methotrexate, fluorouracil)** *chemotherapy protocol for breast cancer*

**CMF/AV (cyclophosphamide, methotrexate, fluorouracil, Adriamycin, Oncovin)** *chemotherapy protocol*

**CMFAVP (cyclophosphamide, methotrexate, fluorouracil, Adriamycin, vincristine, prednisone)** *chemotherapy protocol*

**CMFP; CMF-P (cyclophosphamide, methotrexate, fluorouracil, prednisone)** *chemotherapy protocol for breast cancer*

**CMFPT (cyclophosphamide, methotrexate, fluorouracil, prednisone, tamoxifen)** *chemotherapy protocol*

**CMFPTH (cyclophosphamide, methotrexate, fluorouracil, prednisone, tamoxifen, Halotestin)** *chemotherapy protocol*

**CMFT (cyclophosphamide, methotrexate, fluorouracil, tamoxifen)** *chemotherapy protocol*

**CMFVAT (cyclophosphamide, methotrexate, fluorouracil, vincristine, Adriamycin, testosterone)** *chemotherapy protocol*

**CMFVP (cyclophosphamide, methotrexate, fluorouracil, vincristine, prednisone)** *chemotherapy protocol for breast cancer* [two dosing protocols: Cooper protocol and SWOG protocol]

**CMH (cyclophosphamide, *m*-AMSA, hydroxyurea)** *chemotherapy protocol*

**C-MOPP (cyclophosphamide, mechlorethamine, Oncovin, procarbazine, prednisone)** *chemotherapy protocol for Hodgkin or non-Hodgkin lymphoma*

**CMV (cisplatin, methotrexate, vinblastine)** *chemotherapy protocol for bladder cancer*

**CMV-IGIV (cytomegalovirus immune globulin intravenous)** [see: globulin, immune]

**CN2 HCl** [see: mechlorethamine HCl]

**CNF (cyclophosphamide, Novantrone, fluorouracil)** *chemotherapy protocol for breast cancer* [also: CFM; FNC]

*Cnicus benedictus* *medicinal herb* [see: blessed thistle]

**CNOP (cyclophosphamide, Novantrone, Oncovin, prednisone)** *chemotherapy protocol for non-Hodgkin lymphoma*

**CO Fluoxetine** ⓒ capsules ℞ *selective serotonin reuptake inhibitor (SSRI) for depression, obsessive-compulsive disorder (OCD), and bulimia nervosa* [fluoxetine HCl] 10, 20 mg

**Co I (coenzyme I)** [see: nadide]

**CO₂ (carbon dioxide)** [q.v.]

**⁵⁷Co** [see: cobaltous chloride Co 57]

**⁵⁷Co** [see: cyanocobalamin Co 57]

**⁵⁸Co** [see: cyanocobalamin (⁵⁸Co)]

**⁶⁰Co** [see: cobaltous chloride Co 60]

**⁶⁰Co** [see: cyanocobalamin Co 60]

**coachweed** *medicinal herb* [see: bedstraw]

**Coactinon** ℞ *investigational (NDA filed) non-nucleoside reverse transcriptase inhibitor for naive HIV infection* [emivirine]

**coagulants** *a class of agents that promote or accelerate clotting of the blood*

**coagulation factor VIIa** [see: factor VIIa, recombinant]

**coagulation factor IX (human)** [see: factor IX complex; nonacog alfa]

**Coagulin-B** ℞ *investigational (orphan) agent for moderate to severe hemophilia* [adeno-associated viral vector containing the gene for human coagulation Factor IX]

**coakum** *medicinal herb* [see: pokeweed]

**coal tar** USP *topical antieczematic; antiseborrheic*

**co-amoxiclav (amoxicillin & potassium clavulanate)** [q.v.]

**COAP (cyclophosphamide, Oncovin, ara-C, prednisone)** *chemotherapy protocol*

**Co-Apap** tablets (discontinued 2002) OTC *antitussive; decongestant; antihistamine; analgesic* [dextromethorphan hydrobromide; pseudoephedrine HCl; chlorpheniramine maleate; acetaminophen] 15•30•2•325 mg

**COAP-BLEO (cyclophosphamide, Oncovin, ara-C, prednisone, bleomycin)** *chemotherapy protocol*

**Coated Aspirin; Coated Aspirin Extra Strength; Coated Aspirin Arthritis Pain Relief; Coated Aspirin Daily Low Dose** ⒸⒶⓃ OTC *analgesic; antipyretic; anti-inflammatory; antirheumatic* [aspirin] 235 mg; 500 mg; 650 mg; 81 mg

**COB (cisplatin, Oncovin, bleomycin)** *chemotherapy protocol for head and neck cancer*

**cobalamin concentrate** USP *vitamin $B_{12}$; hematopoietic*

**cobalt** *element (Co)*

**cobalt-labeled vitamin $B_{12}$** [see: cyanocobalamin Co 57 & Co 60]

**cobaltous chloride Co 57** USAN *radioactive agent*

**cobaltous chloride Co 60** USAN *radioactive agent*

**cobamamide** INN

**COBARTin** ℞ *investigational (orphan) agent for steatorrhea in short bowel syndrome* [bile acids, conjugated]

**cocaine** USP, BAN *topical anesthetic for mucous membranes; widely abused as*

*a street drug, derived from coca leaves* 4%, 10% *topical*

**cocaine, crack** *street drug made by converting cocaine HCl into a form that can be smoked, which causes a faster, more intense effect*

**cocaine HCl** USP *topical anesthetic for mucous membranes; widely abused as a street drug, derived from coca leaves* 135 mg *oral;* 4%, 10% *topical*

**Cocaine Viscous** *topical solution* ℞ *topical mucosal anesthesia* [cocaine] 4%, 10%

**cocarboxylase** INN [also: co-carboxylase]

**co-carboxylase** BAN [also: cocarboxylase]

**cocashweed** *medicinal herb* [see: life root]

**coccidioidin** USP *dermal coccidioidomycosis test*

**cocculin** [see: picrotoxin]

***Cocculus lacunosus; C. suberosus*** *medicinal herb* [see: levant berry]

***Cocculus palmatus*** *medicinal herb* [see: colombo]

***Cochlearia armoracia*** *medicinal herb* [see: horseradish]

**cocklebur** *medicinal herb* [see: agrimony; burdock]

**cockspur pepper** *medicinal herb* [see: cayenne]

**cockspur rye** *medicinal herb* [see: ergot]

**cocoa** NF

**cocoa (*Theobromo cacao*)** *bean medicinal herb used as a cardiac stimulant, diuretic, and vasodilator*

**cocoa butter** NF *suppository base; emollient/protectant*

**cocowort** *medicinal herb* [see: shepherd's purse]

**cod liver oil** USP, BAN *vitamins A and D source; emollient/protectant*

**cod liver oil, nondestearinated** NF

**codactide** INN, BAN

**Codal-DH** syrup ℞ *narcotic antitussive; decongestant; antihistamine* [hydrocodone bitartrate; phenylephrine HCl; pyrilamine maleate] 1.66•5•8.33 mg/5 mL

**Codal-DM** syrup OTC *antitussive; decongestant; antihistamine* [dextromethorphan hydrobromide; phenylephrine HCl; pyrilamine maleate] 20•10•16.67 mg/10 mL

**Codamine** syrup, pediatric syrup (discontinued 2002) R *narcotic antitussive; decongestant* [hydrocodone bitartrate; phenylpropanolamine HCl] 5•25 mg/5 mL; 2.5•12.5 mg/5 mL

**CODE (cisplatin, Oncovin, doxorubicin, etoposide)** *chemotherapy protocol for small cell lung cancer (SCLC)*

**Codegest Expectorant** oral liquid (discontinued 2002) R *narcotic antitussive; decongestant; expectorant* [codeine phosphate; phenylpropanolamine HCl; guaifenesin] 10•12.5•100 mg/5 mL ⧉ Codehist

**Codehist DH** elixir (discontinued 2002) R *narcotic antitussive; decongestant; antihistamine* [codeine phosphate; pseudoephedrine HCl; chlorpheniramine maleate; alcohol 5.7%] 10•30•2 mg/5 mL ⧉ Codegest

**codehydrogenase I** [see: nadide]

**codeine** USP, BAN *narcotic analgesic used as an antitussive; sometimes abused as a street drug* ⧉ Kaodene

**codeine & acetaminophen** *narcotic analgesic* 15•300, 30•300, 60•300 mg oral; 12•30 mg/5 mL oral

**codeine phosphate** USP, BAN *narcotic analgesic used as an antitussive* 15 mg/5 mL oral; 30, 60 mg injection

**codeine phosphate & aspirin** *narcotic antitussive; analgesic; antipyretic* 325•15 mg oral

**codeine phosphate & guaifenesin** *antitussive; narcotic analgesic; expectorant* 10•300 mg oral; 10•100 mg/5 mL oral

**codeine phosphate & promethazine HCl** *narcotic antitussive; antihistamine* 10•6.25 mg/5 mL oral

**codeine polistirex** USAN *narcotic analgesic used as an antitussive*

**codeine sulfate** USP *narcotic analgesic used as an antitussive* 15, 30, 60 mg oral

**codelcortone** [see: prednisolone]

**co-dergocrine mesylate** BAN *cognition adjuvant* [also: ergoloid mesylates]

**Codiclear DH** syrup R *narcotic antitussive; expectorant* [hydrocodone bitartrate; guaifenesin] 5•100 mg/5 mL

**Codimal** capsules, film-coated tablets (discontinued 2002) OTC *decongestant; antihistamine; analgesic* [pseudoephedrine HCl; chlorpheniramine maleate; acetaminophen] 30•2•325 mg

**Codimal DH** syrup R *narcotic antitussive; decongestant; antihistamine* [hydrocodone bitartrate; phenylephrine HCl; pyrilamine maleate] 1.66•5•8.33 mg/5 mL

**Codimal DM** syrup OTC *antitussive; decongestant; antihistamine* [dextromethorphan hydrobromide; phenylephrine HCl; pyrilamine maleate] 20•10•16.67 mg/10 mL

**Codimal PH** syrup R *narcotic antitussive; decongestant; antihistamine* [codeine phosphate; phenylephrine HCl; pyrilamine maleate] 20•10•16.66 mg/10 mL

**Codimal-L.A.; Codimal-L.A. Half** extended-release capsules (discontinued 2002) R *decongestant; antihistamine* [pseudoephedrine HCl; chlorpheniramine maleate] 120•8 mg; 60•4 mg

**codorphone** [now: conorphone HCl]

**codoxime** USAN, INN *antitussive*

**Coease** intraocular injection R *viscoelastic agent for ophthalmic surgery* [hyaluronate sodium] 12 mg/mL

**coenzyme Q10** *natural enzyme cofactor used as a cardiac protectant, free radical scavenger, membrane stabilizer; investigational (orphan) for Huntington disease*

**COF/COM (cyclophosphamide, Oncovin, fluorouracil + cyclophosphamide, Oncovin, methotrexate)** *chemotherapy protocol*

**coffeine** [see: caffeine]

**cofisatin** INN

**cofisatine** [see: cofisatin]

**cogazocine** INN

**Cogentin** tablets, IV or IM injection ℞ *anticholinergic; antiparkinsonian* [benztropine mesylate] 0.5, 1, 2 mg; 1 mg/mL

**Co-Gesic** tablets ℞ *narcotic analgesic* [hydrocodone bitartrate; acetaminophen] 5•500 mg

**Cognex** capsules ℞ *reversible cholinesterase inhibitor; cognition adjuvant for Alzheimer dementia* [tacrine HCl] 10, 20, 30, 40 mg

**Cognitex; Cognitex with Pregnenolone** softgels OTC *anti-aging supplement for improving mental function* [glyceryl phosphorylcholine; choline dihydrogen citrate; choline bitartrate; phosphatidylserine; vinpocetine; pantothenic acid; RNA/DNA; (pregnenolone)] 100•250•200• 16.7•2.5•83.3•70.8•(8.3) mg

**Co-Hist** tablets (discontinued 2002) OTC *decongestant; antihistamine; analgesic* [pseudoephedrine HCl; chlorpheniramine maleate; acetaminophen] 30•2•325 mg

**cohosh** *medicinal herb* [see: black cohosh; blue cohosh; white cohosh]

*Cola acuminata medicinal herb* [see: kola nut]

**Colace** capsules, syrup, oral liquid OTC *laxative; stool softener* [docusate sodium] 50, 100 mg; 60 mg/15 mL; 150 mg/15 mL

**Colace; Colace Infant/Child** suppositories OTC *hyperosmolar laxative* [glycerin]

**colaspase** BAN *antineoplastic for acute lymphocytic leukemia (ALL)* [also: asparaginase]

**Colazal** capsules ℞ *gastrointestinal anti-inflammatory for ulcerative colitis* [balsalazide disodium] 750 mg

**Colazide** (European name for U.S. product Colazal)

**colchamine** [see: demecolcine]

**colchicine** USP, JAN *gout suppressant; investigational (orphan) to stop the progression of multiple sclerosis* 0.6 mg oral; 1 mg injection

*Colchicum autumnale; C. speciosum; C. vernum medicinal herb* [see: autumn crocus]

**Cold & Allergy** elixir (discontinued 2001) OTC *decongestant; antihistamine* [phenylpropanolamine HCl; brompheniramine maleate] 12.5•2 mg/ 5 mL

**cold cream** USP

**Cold Relief** tablets (discontinued 2002) OTC *antitussive; decongestant; antihistamine; analgesic* [dextromethorphan hydrobromide; phenylpropanolamine HCl; chlorpheniramine maleate; acetaminophen] 10•12.5• 2•325 mg

**Cold Symptoms Relief** tablets OTC *antitussive; decongestant; antihistamine; analgesic* [dextromethorphan hydrobromide; pseudoephedrine HCl; chlorpheniramine maleate; acetaminophen] 10•30•2•325 mg

**Coldec D** extended-release caplets ℞ *decongestant; antihistamine* [pseudoephedrine HCl; carbinoxamine maleate] 80•8 mg

**Coldec DM** oral liquid ℞ *antitussive; decongestant; antihistamine* [dextromethorphan hydrobromide; pseudoephedrine HCl; brompheniramine maleate] 15•60•4 mg/5 mL

**Cold-Gest** sustained-release capsules (discontinued 2001) OTC *decongestant; antihistamine* [phenylpropanolamine HCl; chlorpheniramine maleate] 75•8 mg

**Coldloc** oral liquid (discontinued 2002) ℞ *decongestant; expectorant* [phenylpropanolamine HCl; phenylephrine HCl; guaifenesin] 20•5• 100 mg/5 mL

**Coldloc-LA** sustained-release caplets (discontinued 2002) ℞ *decongestant; expectorant* [phenylpropanolamine HCl; guaifenesin] 75•600 mg

**Coldmist JR** sustained-release tablets ℞ *decongestant; expectorant* [pseudoephedrine HCl; guaifenesin] 45•600 mg

**Coldmist LA** extended-release caplets ℞ *decongestant; expectorant* [pseudoephedrine HCl; guaifenesin] 80•800 mg

**Coldrine** tablets (discontinued 2002) OTC *decongestant; analgesic* [pseudoephedrine HCl; acetaminophen] 30•325 mg

**colecalciferol (vitamin D₃)** INN *fat-soluble vitamin* [also: cholecalciferol]

**colesevelam HCl** USAN *bile acid sequestrant; nonabsorbable cholesterol-lowering polymer for hyperlipidemia*

**Colestid** tablets, granules ℞ *cholesterol-lowering antihyperlipidemic* [colestipol HCl] 1 g; 5 g/dose ☑ colistin

**colestipol** INN, BAN *bile acid sequestrant; cholesterol-lowering antihyperlipidemic* [also: colestipol HCl] ☑ colistin

**colestipol HCl** USAN, USP *bile acid sequestrant; cholesterol-lowering antihyperlipidemic* [also: colestipol] ☑ colistin

**colestolone** USAN, INN *hypolipidemic*

**colestyramine** INN *bile salt ion-exchange resin; antihyperlipoproteinemic* [also: cholestyramine resin; cholestyramine]

**colestyramine resin** [see: cholestyramine]

**colextran** INN

**Colfed-A** sustained-release capsules ℞ *decongestant; antihistamine* [pseudoephedrine HCl; chlorpheniramine maleate] 120•8 mg

**colfenamate** INN

**colforsin** USAN, INN *antiglaucoma agent*

**colfosceril palmitate** USAN, INN, BAN *pulmonary surfactant for hyaline membrane disease and neonatal respiratory distress syndrome (orphan); investigational (orphan) for adult respiratory distress syndrome (ARDS)*

**colic root** *medicinal herb* [see: blazing star; star grass; wild yam]

**colimecycline** INN

**colistimethate sodium** USAN, USP, INN *bactericidal antibiotic* [also: colistin sulphomethate]

**colistin** INN, BAN *bactericidal antibiotic* [also: colistin sulfate] ☑ Colestid; colestipol

**colistin methanesulfonate** [see: colistimethate sodium]

**colistin sulfate** USP *bactericidal antibiotic* [also: colistin]

**colistin sulphomethate** BAN *bactericidal antibiotic* [also: colistimethate sodium]

**collagen** *ophthalmic implant to block puncta and retain moisture; urethral injection for stress urinary incontinence*

**collagen, purified bovine** *injectable dermal filler for scars, wrinkles, and facial folds*

**collagen, purified human** *injectable dermal filler for scars, wrinkles, and facial folds*

**collagen, purified type II** *investigational (Phase III, orphan) oral treatment for juvenile rheumatoid arthritis*

**collagen sponge, absorbable** *topical local hemostat for surgery*

**collagenase** *topical proteolytic enzymes for necrotic tissue debridement; investigational (orphan) for Peyronie disease*

**collagenase, clostridial** [see: clostridial collagenase]

**Collagenase Santyl** ointment ℞ *proteolytic enzymes for debriding dermal ulcers* [collagenase] 250 U/g

**collard** *medicinal herb* [see: skunk cabbage]

**Collinsonia canadensis** *medicinal herb* [see: stone root]

**collodion** USP *topical protectant*

**colloidal aluminum hydroxide** [see: aluminum hydroxide gel]

**colloidal oatmeal** *demulcent*

**colloidal silicon dioxide** [see: silicon dioxide, colloidal]

**Colloral** *investigational (Phase III, orphan) collagen derivative for treatment of juvenile rheumatoid arthritis* [trinecol (pullus)]

**Collyrium for Fresh Eyes** *ophthalmic solution* OTC *extraocular irrigating solution* [sterile isotonic solution]

**Collyrium Fresh** eye drops OTC *topical ophthalmic decongestant and vasoconstrictor* [tetrahydrozoline HCl] 0.05%

**ColoCare** test kit for home use *in vitro diagnostic aid for fecal occult blood*

**colombo (*Cocculus palmatus*)** root *medicinal herb used as an antiemetic and febrifuge*

**Colomed** enema ℞ *investigational (orphan) for left-sided ulcerative colitis and chronic radiation proctitis* [short chain fatty acids]

**colony-stimulating factors** *a class of glycoproteins that stimulate the production of granulocytes and macrophages*

**Color Allergy Screening Test (CAST)** reagent assay tubes *in vitro diagnostic aid for immunoglobulin E in serum*

**Color Ovulation Test** kit for home use *in vitro diagnostic aid to predict ovulation time*

**ColoScreen** slide test for professional use *in vitro diagnostic aid for fecal occult blood*

**colterol** INN *bronchodilator* [also: colterol mesylate]

**colterol mesylate** USAN *bronchodilator* [also: colterol]

**colt's tail** *medicinal herb* [see: fleabane; horseweed]

**coltsfoot (*Tussilago farfara*)** buds, flowers, and leaves *medicinal herb for asthma, bronchitis, dry cough, hay fever, lung disorders, excess mucus, and throat irritation*

**Columbia Antiseptic** powder OTC *astringent; antiseptic* [zinc oxide; talc; carbolic acid; boric acid]

**columbine (*Aquilegia vulgaris*)** plant *medicinal herb used as an astringent, diaphoretic, and diuretic*

**Coly-Mycin M** powder for IV or IM injection ℞ *bactericidal antibiotic* [colistimethate sodium] 150 mg

**Coly-Mycin S Otic** suspension ℞ *corticosteroidal anti-inflammatory; antibiotic* [hydrocortisone acetate; neomycin sulfate; colistin sulfate] 1%•4.71 mg•3 mg per mL

**CoLyte** powder for oral solution ℞ *pre-procedure bowel evacuant* [polyethylene glycol–electrolyte solution (PEG 3350)] 60 g/L

**COM (cyclophosphamide, Oncovin, MeCCNU)** *chemotherapy protocol*

**COM (cyclophosphamide, Oncovin, methotrexate)** *chemotherapy protocol*

**COMA-A (cyclophosphamide, Oncovin, methotrexate/citrovorum factor, Adriamycin, ara-C)** *chemotherapy protocol*

**COMB (cyclophosphamide, Oncovin, MeCCNU, bleomycin)** *chemotherapy protocol*

**COMB (Cytoxin, Oncovin, methotrexate, bleomycin)** *chemotherapy protocol*

**ComBgen** tablets ℞ *vitamin B supplement* [vitamins $B_6$ and $B_{12}$; folic acid] 25•0.5•2.2 mg

**Combidex** ℞ *investigational (NDA filed) MRI diagnostic aid for lymph node metastases* [ferumoxtran-10]

**CombiPatch** transdermal patch ℞ *estrogen/progesterone for hormone replacement therapy* [estradiol; norethindrone acetate] 0.05•0.14, 0.05•0.25 mg/day

**Combipres 0.1; Combipres 0.2; Combipres 0.3** tablets ℞ *antihypertensive; diuretic* [clonidine HCl; chlorthalidone] 0.1•15 mg; 0.2•15 mg; 0.3•15 mg ℞ Catapres

**Combistix** reagent strips *in vitro diagnostic aid for multiple urine products*

**Combivent** oral inhalation aerosol ℞ *anticholinergic bronchodilator for chronic bronchospasm with COPD* [ipratropium bromide; albuterol sulfate] 18•103 μg/dose

**Combivir** film-coated caplets ℞ *nucleoside reverse transcriptase inhibitor combination for HIV* [lamivudine; zidovudine] 150•300 mg

**combretastatin A4 phosphate** *investigational (orphan) agent for anaplastic, medullary, papillary, or follicular thyroid cancer*

**COMe (Cytoxin, Oncovin, methotrexate)** *chemotherapy protocol*

**COMF (cyclophosphamide, Oncovin, methotrexate, fluorouracil)** *chemotherapy protocol*

**Comfort** eye drops OTC *topical ophthalmic decongestant and vasoconstrictor* [naphazoline HCl] 0.03%

**Comfort Tears** eye drops OTC *ocular moisturizer/lubricant* [hydroxyethylcellulose]

**ComfortCare GP Wetting & Soaking** solution OTC *disinfecting/wetting/soaking solution for rigid gas permeable contact lenses*

**Comfortine** ointment (discontinued 2004) OTC *moisturizer; emollient; astringent; antiseptic* [vitamins A and D; lanolin; zinc oxide]

**comfrey (Symphytum officinale; S. tuberosum)** leaves and roots *medicinal herb for anemia, arthritis, blood cleansing, boils and sores, bruises, burns, edema, emphysema, fractures, gastric ulcers, hemorrhoids, and sprains; not generally regarded as safe and effective as it may be carcinogenic and hepatotoxic*

**comfrey, spotted** *medicinal herb* [see: lungwort]

**Comhist** tablets (discontinued 2002) ℞ *decongestant; antihistamine* [phenylephrine HCl; chlorpheniramine maleate; phenyltoloxamine citrate] 10•2•25 mg

**Comhist LA** long-acting capsules (discontinued 2002) ℞ *decongestant; antihistamine* [phenylephrine HCl; chlorpheniramine maleate; phenyltoloxamine citrate] 20•4•50 mg

**COMLA (cyclophosphamide, Oncovin, methotrexate, leucovorin [rescue], ara-C)** *chemotherapy protocol for non-Hodgkin lymphoma*

*Commiphora abssynica; C. molmol; C. myrrha* medicinal herb [see: myrrh]

*Commiphora mukul* medicinal herb [see: guggul]

**Commit** lozenges OTC *smoking deterrent; nicotine withdrawal aid* [nicotine polacrilex] 2, 4 mg

**common bugloss** *medicinal herb* [see: borage]

**common elder** *medicinal herb* [see: elderberry]

**common flax** *medicinal herb* [see: flaxseed]

**comosain** *investigational (orphan) proteolytic enzymes for debridement of severe burns*

**COMP (CCNU, Oncovin, methotrexate, procarbazine)** *chemotherapy protocol*

**COMP (cyclophosphamide, Oncovin, methotrexate, prednisone)** *chemotherapy protocol for pediatric Hodgkin lymphoma*

**Compack** (trademarked packaging form) *patient compliance package for oral contraceptives*

**Compazine** suppositories ℞ *conventional (typical) antipsychotic; antiemetic* [prochlorperazine] 2.5, 5, 25 mg

**Compazine** syrup, IV or IM injection ℞ *conventional (typical) antipsychotic; antiemetic* [prochlorperazine edisylate] 5 mg/5 mL; 5 mg/mL

**Compazine** tablets, Spansules (sustained-release capsules) ℞ *conventional (typical) antipsychotic; antiemetic* [prochlorperazine maleate] 5, 10 mg; 10, 15 mg

**Compete** tablets OTC *vitamin/iron supplement* [multiple vitamins; ferrous gluconate; folic acid] ±•27•0.4 mg

**Compleat Modified Formula** closed system containers OTC *enteral nutritional therapy* [lactose-free formula]

**Compleat Modified Formula** ready-to-use oral liquid OTC *enteral nutritional therapy* [lactose-free formula]

**Compleat Regular Formula** ready-to-use oral liquid OTC *enteral nutritional therapy* [milk-based formula]

**complement receptor type I, soluble recombinant human** *investigational (orphan) for adult respiratory distress syndrome*

172    Complete

**Complete** solution OTC *rewetting solution for soft contact lenses*

**Complete All-in-One** solution OTC *cleaning/disinfecting/rinsing/storage solution for soft contact lenses*

**Complete Weekly Enzymatic Cleaner** effervescent tablets OTC *enzymatic cleaner for soft contact lenses* [subtilisin A]

**Complex 15 Face** cream OTC *moisturizer; emollient*

**Complex 15 Hand & Body** cream, lotion OTC *moisturizer; emollient*

**Comply** oral liquid OTC *enteral nutritional therapy* [lactose-free formula]

**component pertussis vaccine** (alternate name for acellular pertussis vaccine) [see: diphtheria & tetanus toxoids & acellular pertussis (DTaP) vaccine, adsorbed]

**Compound 347** liquid for vaporization ℞ *inhalation general anesthetic* [enflurane]

**compound 42** [see: warfarin]

**compound CB3025** [see: melphalan]

**compound E** [see: cortisone acetate]

**compound F** [see: hydrocortisone]

**compound orange spirit** [see: orange spirit, compound]

**compound Q** [see: trichosanthin]

**compound S** [see: zidovudine]

**compound solution of sodium chloride** INN *fluid and electrolyte replenisher* [also: Ringer injection]

**compound solution of sodium lactate** INN *electrolyte and fluid replenisher; systemic alkalizer* [also: Ringer injection, lactated]

**Compound W** topical liquid, gel OTC *keratolytic* [salicylic acid in collodion] 17%

**Compound W One Step Wart Remover for Kids** pad OTC *keratolytic* [salicylic acid] 40%

**Compoz** gelcaps OTC *antihistaminic sleep aid* [diphenhydramine HCl] 25 mg

**Compoz Nighttime Sleep Aid** tablets OTC *antihistaminic sleep aid* [diphenhydramine HCl] 50 mg

**compressible sugar** [see: sugar, compressible]

**Compro** suppositories ℞ *conventional (typical) antipsychotic; antiemetic* [prochlorperazine] 25 mg

**Computer Eye Drops** OTC *ophthalmic moisturizer and emollient* [glycerin] 1%

**COMT (catechol-O-methyltransferase) inhibitors** *a class of antiparkinson agents that stabilize serum levodopa levels by inhibiting an enzyme that breaks down the levodopa before it reaches the brain*

**Comtan** film-coated tablets ℞ *COMT inhibitor for Parkinson disease* [entacapone] 200 mg

**Comtrex** oral liquid (discontinued 2002) OTC *antitussive; decongestant; antihistamine; analgesic* [dextromethorphan hydrobromide; pseudoephedrine HCl; chlorpheniramine maleate; acetaminophen] 3.3•10•0.67•108.3 mg/5 mL

**Comtrex, Cough Formula** oral liquid (discontinued 2002) OTC *antitussive; decongestant; expectorant; analgesic* [dextromethorphan hydrobromide; pseudoephedrine HCl; guaifenesin; acetaminophen; alcohol 20%] 7.5•15•50•125 mg/5 mL

**Comtrex Acute Head Cold & Sinus Pressure Relief, Multi-Symptom** tablets OTC *decongestant; antihistamine; analgesic* [pseudoephedrine HCl; brompheniramine maleate; acetaminophen] 30•2•500 mg

**Comtrex Allergy-Sinus Treatment** caplets, tablets OTC *decongestant; antihistamine; analgesic* [pseudoephedrine HCl; chlorpheniramine maleate; acetaminophen] 30•2•500 mg

**Comtrex Cold & Cough Relief, Multi-Symptom; Multi-Symptom Comtrex Day & Night Cold & Cough Relief** caplets OTC *antitussive; decongestant; antihistamine; analgesic* [dextromethorphan hydrobromide; pseudoephedrine HCl; chlorpheniramine maleate; acetaminophen] 15•30•2•500 mg

**Comtrex Flu Therapy & Fever Relief Day & Night, Multi-Symptom** caplets OTC *decongestant; analgesic; antihistamine added* PM [pseudoephedrine HCl; acetaminophen; chlorpheniramine maleate added PM] 30•500 mg AM; 30•500•2 mg PM

**Comtrex Liqui-Gels** (liquid-filled capsules) (discontinued 2002) OTC *antitussive; decongestant; antihistamine; analgesic* [dextromethorphan hydrobromide; phenylpropanolamine HCl; chlorpheniramine maleate; acetaminophen] 10•12.5•2•325, 15•12.5•2•500 mg

**Comtrex Multi-Symptom Cold & Flu Relief** tablets, caplets (name changed to Comtrex Cough & Cold Relief, Multi-Symptom and/or Comtrex Day & Night Cold & Cough Relief, Multi-Symptom in 2002)

**Comtrex Multi-Symptom Cold & Flu Relief Liqui-Gels** (capsules) (discontinued 2002) OTC *antitussive; decongestant; antihistamine; analgesic* [dextromethorphan hydrobromide; phenylpropanolamine HCl; chlorpheniramine maleate; acetaminophen] 15•12.5•2•500 mg

**Comtrex Multi-Symptom Deep Chest Cold & Congestion Relief** softgels OTC *antitussive; decongestant; expectorant; analgesic* [dextromethorphan hydrobromide; pseudoephedrine HCl; guaifenesin; acetaminophen] 10•30•100•250 mg

**Comtrex Multi-Symptom Non-Drowsy Cold & Cough Relief** caplets OTC *antitussive; decongestant; analgesic* [dextromethorphan hydrobromide; pseudoephedrine HCl; acetaminophen] 15•30•500 mg

**Comtrex Non-Drowsy** caplets (name changed to Comtrex Multi-Symptom Non-Drowsy Cold & Cough Relief in 2002)

**Comtussin HC** syrup ℞ *narcotic antitussive; decongestant; antihistamine* [hydrocodone bitartrate; phenylephrine HCl; chlorpheniramine maleate] 5•10•4 mg/10 mL

**Comvax** IM injection ℞ *infant (1½–15 months) vaccine for* H. influenzae *and hepatitis B* [Hemophilus b purified capsular polysaccharide; *Neisseria meningitidis* OMPC; hepatitis B virus vaccine] 7.5•125•5 μg/0.5 mL

**Conceive Ovulation Predictor** 5-day test kit for professional use *in vitro diagnostic aid to predict ovulation time*

**Conceive Pregnancy** test kit for home use *in vitro diagnostic aid; urine pregnancy test*

**Concentrated Cleaner** solution OTC *cleaning solution for rigid gas permeable contact lenses*

**Conceptrol Contraceptive Inserts** vaginal suppositories (discontinued 2002) OTC *spermicidal contraceptive* [nonoxynol 9] 150 mg

**Conceptrol Disposable Contraceptive** vaginal gel OTC *spermicidal contraceptive* [nonoxynol 9] 4%

**Concerta** dual-release tablets ℞ *CNS stimulant; once-daily treatment for attention-deficit hyperactivity disorder (ADHD)* [methylphenidate HCl] 18, 27, 36, 54 mg (22% immediate release, 78% extended release)

**Condylox** solution, gel ℞ *topical antimitotic for external genital and perianal warts* [podofilox] 0.5%

**cone flower, purple** *medicinal herb* [see: echinacea]

**conessine** INN

**conessine hydrobromide** [see: conessine]

**Conex** syrup (discontinued 2002) OTC *decongestant; expectorant* [phenylpropanolamine HCl; guaifenesin] 12.5•100 mg/5 mL

**Conex with Codeine** syrup (discontinued 2002) ℞ *narcotic antitussive; decongestant; expectorant* [codeine phosphate; phenylpropanolamine HCl; guaifenesin] 10•12.5•100 mg/5 mL

**confectioner's sugar** [see: sugar, confectioner's]

**Confide** test kit for home use *in vitro diagnostic aid for HIV in the blood*

**congazone sodium** [see: Congo red]

**Congess JR** capsules (discontinued 2002) ℞ *decongestant; expectorant* [pseudoephedrine HCl; guaifenesin] 60•125 mg

**Congess SR** sustained-release capsules (discontinued 2002) ℞ *decongestant; expectorant* [pseudoephedrine HCl; guaifenesin] 120•250 mg

**Congestac** caplets OTC *decongestant; expectorant* [pseudoephedrine HCl; guaifenesin] 60•400 mg

**Congestaid** tablets OTC *nasal decongestant* [pseudoephedrine HCl] 30 mg

**Congestant D** tablets (discontinued 2001) OTC *decongestant; antihistamine; analgesic* [phenylpropanolamine HCl; chlorpheniramine maleate; acetaminophen] 12.5•2•325 mg

**Congestion Relief** tablets (discontinued 2000) OTC *nasal decongestant* [pseudoephedrine HCl] 30, 60 mg

**Congestion Relief, Children's** oral liquid (discontinued 2002) OTC *nasal decongestant* [pseudoephedrine HCl] 30 mg/5 mL

**Congo red** USP

**conivaptan** *investigational (NDA filed) vasopressin antagonist for hyponatremia*

**conjugated equine estrogen CEE)** [see: estrogens, conjugated]

**conjugated estrogens** [see: estrogens, conjugated]

**conjugated linoleic acid (CLA)** *natural omega-6 essential fatty acid shown to be effective in weight management and cancer prevention*

**conorfone** INN *analgesic* [also: conorphone HCl]

**conorfone HCl** [see: conorphone HCl]

**conorphone HCl** USAN *analgesic* [also: conorfone]

**CONPADRI; CONPADRI-I (cyclophosphamide, Oncovin, L-phenylalanine mustard, Adriamycin)** *chemotherapy protocol*

**Conray; Conray 30; Conray 43** injection ℞ *radiopaque contrast*

medium [iothalamate meglumine (47% iodine)] 600 mg/mL (282 mg/mL); 300 mg/mL (141 mg/mL); 430 mg/mL (202 mg/mL)

**Conray 400** injection (discontinued 2001) ℞ *radiopaque contrast medium* [iothalamate sodium (59.9% iodine)] 668 mg/mL (400 mg/mL)

**Consonar** ℞ *investigational reversible/ selective MAO inhibitor, type A* [brofaromine]

**Constilac** oral/rectal solution ℞ *hyperosmotic laxative* [lactulose] 10 g/15 mL

**Constulose** oral/rectal solution ℞ *hyperosmotic laxative* [lactulose] 10 g/15 mL

**consumptive's weed** *medicinal herb* [see: yerba santa]

**Contac 12 Hour** sustained-release capsules, sustained-release caplets (discontinued 2001) OTC *decongestant; antihistamine* [phenylpropanolamine HCl; chlorpheniramine maleate] 75•8 mg; 75•12 mg

**Contac Cough & Chest Cold** oral liquid (discontinued 2002) OTC *antitussive; decongestant; expectorant; analgesic* [dextromethorphan hydrobromide; pseudoephedrine HCl; guaifenesin; acetaminophen; alcohol 10%] 5•15•50•125 mg/5 mL

**Contac Cough & Sore Throat** oral liquid (discontinued 2002) OTC *antitussive; analgesic* [dextromethorphan hydrobromide; acetaminophen; alcohol 10%] 5•125 mg/5 mL

**Contac Day & Night Allergy/Sinus Relief** daytime caplets + nighttime caplets OTC *decongestant; analgesic; antihistamine/sleep aid added PM* [pseudoephedrine HCl; acetaminophen; diphenhydramine HCl added PM] 03/02 60•650 mg AM; 60•650•50 mg PM

**Contac Day & Night Cold & Flu** daytime caplets + nighttime caplets OTC *decongestant; analgesic; (antitussive added daytime; antihistamine/sleep aid added nighttime)* [pseudoephedrine HCl; acetaminophen; (dextromethorphan hydrobromide added daytime; diphenhydramine HCl added nighttime)] 60•650•30 mg daytime; 60•650•50 mg nighttime

**Contac Severe Cold & Flu** caplets OTC *antitussive; decongestant; antihistamine; analgesic* [dextromethorphan hydrobromide; pseudoephedrine HCl; chlorpheniramine maleate; acetaminophen] 15•30•2•500 mg

**Contac Severe Cold & Flu Nighttime** oral liquid (discontinued 2002) OTC *antitussive; decongestant; antihistamine; analgesic* [dextromethorphan hydrobromide; pseudoephedrine HCl; chlorpheniramine maleate; acetaminophen; alcohol 18.5%] 5• 10•0.67•167 mg/5 mL

**conteben** [see: thioacetazone; thiacetazone]

**ConTE-Pak-4** IV injection (discontinued 2003) ℞ *intravenous nutritional therapy* [multiple trace elements (metals)]

**ContolRx** toothpaste ℞ *dental caries preventative* [sodium fluoride] 1.1%

**Contrin** capsules ℞ *hematinic* [ferrous fumarate; cyanocobalamin; ascorbic acid; intrinsic factor concentrate; folic acid] 110 mg•15 µg•75 mg• 240 mg•0.5 mg

**Control** timed-release capsules (discontinued 2001) OTC *diet aid* [phenylpropanolamine HCl] 75 mg

**ControlPak** (trademarked packaging form) *tamper-resistant unit-dose package*

**Contuss** oral liquid (discontinued 2002) ℞ *decongestant; expectorant* [phenylpropanolamine HCl; phenylephrine HCl; guaifenesin; alcohol 5%] 20•5•100 mg/5 mL

**conval lily** *medicinal herb* [see: lily of the valley]

***Convallaria majalis*** *medicinal herb* [see: lily of the valley]

**conventional (typical) antipsychotics** *a class of dopamine receptor antagonists with a higher affinity to the $D_2$ than $D_1$ receptors and little affinity to the nondopaminergic receptors; high incidence of extrapyramidal side effects*

*(EPS)* [compare to: novel (atypical) antipsychotics]

***Convolvulus sepium*** *medicinal herb* [see: hedge bindweed]

**convulsion root; convulsion weed** *medicinal herb* [see: fit root]

**ConXn** *investigational (Phase II/III) for scleroderma* [relaxin H2, recombinant human]

***Conyza canadensis*** *medicinal herb* [see: horseweed]

**cool.click** (trademarked device) *needle-free subcutaneous injector*

**Cooper regimen** *chemotherapy protocol for breast cancer* [see: CMFVP]

**COP** [see: creatinolfosfate]

**COP (cyclophosphamide, Oncovin, prednisone)** *chemotherapy protocol for non-Hodgkin lymphoma*

**COP 1 (copolymer 1)** [see: glatiramer acetate]

**COPA (Cytoxin, Oncovin, prednisone, Adriamycin)** *chemotherapy protocol*

**COPA-BLEO (cyclophosphamide, Oncovin, prednisone, Adriamycin, bleomycin)** *chemotherapy protocol*

**COPAC (CCNU, Oncovin, prednisone, Adriamycin, cyclophosphamide)** *chemotherapy protocol*

**Copaxone** subcu injection in Autoject2 (prefilled glass syringe) ℞ *immunomodulator for relapsing-remitting multiple sclerosis (orphan)* [glatiramer acetate] 20 mg

**COPB (cyclophosphamide, Oncovin, prednisone, bleomycin)** *chemotherapy protocol*

**COP-BLAM (cyclophosphamide, Oncovin, prednisone, bleomycin, Adriamycin, Matulane)** *chemotherapy protocol*

**COP-BLEO (cyclophosphamide, Oncovin, prednisone, bleomycin)** *chemotherapy protocol*

**Cope** tablets OTC *analgesic; antipyretic; anti-inflammatory; antacid* [aspirin; caffeine; magnesium hydroxide; aluminum hydroxide] 421•32•50•25 mg

**COPE (cyclophosphamide, Oncovin, Platinol, etoposide)** *chemotherapy protocol for small cell lung cancer (SCLC) and pediatric brain tumors*

**Copegus** film-coated tablets ℞ *nucleoside antiviral; combination therapy for chronic hepatitis C infection* [ribavirin] 200 mg

**Cophene No. 2** sustained-release capsules (discontinued 2002) ℞ *decongestant; antihistamine* [pseudoephedrine HCl; chlorpheniramine maleate] 120•12 mg

**Cophene XP** oral liquid (discontinued 2002) ℞ *narcotic antitussive; decongestant; expectorant* [hydrocodone bitartrate; pseudoephedrine HCl; guaifenesin; alcohol 12.5%] 5•60•200 mg/5 mL

**Cophene-X** capsules (discontinued 2002) ℞ *antitussive; decongestant; expectorant* [carbetapentane citrate; phenylephrine HCl; phenylpropanolamine HCl; potassium guaiacolsulfonate] 20•10•10•45 mg

**copolymer 1 (COP 1)** [see: glatiramer acetate]

**copovithane** BAN

**COPP (CCNU, Oncovin, procarbazine, prednisone)** *chemotherapy protocol*

**COPP (cyclophosphamide, Oncovin, procarbazine, prednisone)** *chemotherapy protocol for Hodgkin or non-Hodgkin lymphoma*

**copper** *element (Cu)*

**copper chloride dihydrate** [see: cupric chloride]

**copper gluconate (copper D-gluconate)** USP *dietary copper supplement*

**copper sulfate pentahydrate** [see: cupric sulfate]

**copper 10-undecenoate** [see: copper undecylenate]

**copper undecylenate** USAN

**copperhead snake antivenin** [see: antivenin (Crotalidae) polyvalent]

*Coptis trifolia* medicinal herb [see: gold thread]

**Co-Pyronil 2** Pulvules (capsules) (discontinued 2002) OTC *decongestant; antihistamine* [pseudoephedrine HCl; chlorpheniramine maleate] 60•4 mg

**CoQ10** [see: coenzyme Q10]

**coral (*Goniopora* spp.; *Porite* spp.)** *natural material used as a substrate for bone grafts and fractures and in reconstructive surgery*

**coral root (*Corallorhiza odontorhiza*)** *medicinal herb for diaphoresis, fever, insomnia, and sedation*

**coral snake antivenin** [see: antivenin (Micrurus fulvius)]

**corbadrine** INN *adrenergic; vasoconstrictor* [also: levonordefrin]

**Cordarone** tablets, IV infusion ℞ *antiarrhythmic for acute ventricular tachycardia and fibrillation (orphan)* [amiodarone HCl] 200 mg; 50 mg/mL

**Cordox** ℞ *investigational (Phase III) adjunct to coronary artery bypass graft (CABG) surgery; investigational (Phase III, orphan) cytoprotective agent for vaso-occlusive episodes of sickle cell disease* [fructose-1,6-diphosphate]

**Cordran** ointment, lotion, tape ℞ *corticosteroidal anti-inflammatory* [flurandrenolide] 0.05%; 0.05%; 4 μg/cm$^2$

**Cordran SP** cream ℞ *corticosteroidal anti-inflammatory* [flurandrenolide] 0.05%

**Coreg** Tiltab (film-coated tablets) ℞ *antihypertensive; α- and β-blocker for congestive heart failure* [carvedilol] 3.125, 6.25, 12.5, 25 mg

**Corgard** tablets ℞ *antihypertensive; antianginal; β-blocker* [nadolol] 20, 40, 80, 120, 160 mg

**Corgenic** ℞ *investigational AC-6 gene therapy for congestive heart failure*

**coriander (*Coriandrum sativum*)** *seed medicinal herb used as antispasmodic, appetizer, carminative, and stomachic*

**coriander oil** NF

**Coricidin D Cold, Flu, & Sinus** tablets OTC *decongestant; antihistamine; analgesic* [pseudoephedrine HCl; chlorpheniramine maleate; acetaminophen] 30•2•325 mg

**Coricidin HBP Chest Congestion & Cough** softgels OTC *antitussive; expectorant* [dextromethorphan hydrobromide; guaifenesin] 10•200 mg

**Coricidin HBP Cold & Flu** tablets OTC *antihistamine; analgesic* [chlorpheniramine maleate; acetaminophen] 2•325 mg

**Coricidin HBP Cough & Cold** tablets OTC *antitussive; antihistamine* [dextromethorphan hydrobromide; chlorpheniramine maleate] 30•4 mg

**Coricidin HBP Flu** tablets OTC *antitussive; antihistamine; analgesic* [dextromethorphan hydrobromide; chlorpheniramine maleate; acetaminophen] 15•2•500 mg

**Coricidin Sinus Headache** tablets (discontinued 2001) OTC *decongestant; antihistamine; analgesic* [phenylpropanolamine HCl; chlorpheniramine maleate; acetaminophen] 12.5•2•500 mg

**corkwood tree** *(Duboisia myoporoides)* leaves *medicinal herb used as a central nervous system stimulant and in homeopathic therapy for eye disorders; not generally regarded as safe and effective as it contains scopolamine and related alkaloids, which may be fatal in high doses*

**Corlopam** IV infusion ℞ *rapid-acting vasodilator for in-hospital management of severe hypertension* [fenoldopam mesylate] 10 mg/mL

**Cormax** ointment ℞ *corticosteroidal anti-inflammatory* [clobetasol propionate] 0.05%

**cormed** [see: nikethamide]

**cormetasone** INN *topical anti-inflammatory* [also: cormethasone acetate]

**cormetasone acetate** [see: cormethasone acetate]

**cormethasone acetate** USAN *topical anti-inflammatory* [also: cormetasone]

**corn, turkey** *medicinal herb* [see: turkey corn]

**corn cockle** *(Agrostemma githago)* seeds and root *medicinal herb for cancer, edema, exanthema, hemorrhoids,*

*jaundice, and worms; also used as an emmenagogue and expectorant, and in homeopathic remedies for gastritis and paralysis; not generally regarded as safe and effective as it is extremely poisonous*

**Corn Huskers** lotion OTC *moisturizer; emollient*

**corn oil** NF *solvent; caloric replacement*

**corn silk (stigmata maidis)** *medicinal herb* [see: Indian corn]

**cornflower** *(Centaurea cyanus)* plant *medicinal herb for conjunctivitis, corneal ulcers and other eye disorders and for nervous disorders and poisonous bites and stings*

**corpse plant** *medicinal herb* [see: fit root]

**corpus luteum extract** [see: progesterone]

**Corque** cream ℞ *topical corticosteroidal anti-inflammatory; antifungal; antibacterial* [hydrocortisone; clioquinol] 1%•3%

**Correctol** enteric-coated tablets OTC *stimulant laxative* [bisacodyl] 5 mg

**CortaGel** OTC *corticosteroidal anti-inflammatory* [hydrocortisone] 1%

**Cortaid** cream, ointment OTC *corticosteroidal anti-inflammatory* [hydrocortisone acetate] 1%

**Cortaid** pump spray OTC *corticosteroidal anti-inflammatory* [hydrocortisone] 1%

**Cortaid Faststick** roll-on stick OTC *corticosteroidal anti-inflammatory* [hydrocortisone; alcohol 55%] 1%

**Cortaid Intensive Therapy** cream (discontinued 2004) OTC *corticosteroidal anti-inflammatory* [hydrocortisone] 1%

**Cortaid with Aloe** cream, ointment OTC *corticosteroidal anti-inflammatory* [hydrocortisone acetate] 0.5%

**Cortane-B** lotion ℞ *corticosteroidal anti-inflammatory; local anesthetic; antiseptic* [hydrocortisone acetate; pramoxine HCl; chloroxylenol] 1%•1%•0.1%

**Cortane-B Aqueous; Cortane-B Otic** ear drops ℞ *corticosteroidal anti-inflammatory; local anesthetic; bacte-*

riostatic [hydrocortisone; pramoxine HCl; chloroxylenol] 1%•1%•0.1%

**Cortate** Ⓒ cream, ointment ℞ *corticosteroidal anti-inflammatory* [hydrocortisone acetate] 1%

**Cortatrigen Modified** ear drops, otic suspension ℞ *corticosteroidal anti-inflammatory; antibiotic* [hydrocortisone; neomycin sulfate; polymyxin B sulfate] 1%•5 mg•10 000 U per mL

**Cort-Dome** cream ℞ *corticosteroidal anti-inflammatory* [hydrocortisone] 0.5%, 1% ② Cortone

**Cort-Dome High Potency** rectal suppositories ℞ *corticosteroidal anti-inflammatory* [hydrocortisone acetate] 25 mg

**Cortef** tablets, oral suspension ℞ *corticosteroid; anti-inflammatory* [hydrocortisone] 5, 10, 20 mg; 10 mg/5 mL

**Cortef Feminine Itch** cream OTC *corticosteroidal anti-inflammatory* [hydrocortisone acetate] 0.5%

**Cortenema** retention enema ℞ *corticosteroidal anti-inflammatory for ulcerative colitis* [hydrocortisone] 100 mg/60 mL ② quart enema

**cortenil** [see: desoxycorticosterone acetate]

**cortexolone** [see: cortodoxone]

**Cortic-ND** ear drops ℞ *corticosteroidal anti-inflammatory; local anesthetic; bacteriostatic* [hydrocortisone; pramoxine HCl; chloroxylenol] 1%•1%•0.1%

**Corticaine** cream OTC *corticosteroidal anti-inflammatory* [hydrocortisone acetate] 0.5%

**corticorelin ovine triflutate** USAN, INN *corticotropin-releasing hormone; diagnostic aid for Cushing syndrome and adrenocortical insufficiency* (orphan)

**corticosteroids** *a class of anti-inflammatory drugs*

**corticotrophin** INN, BAN *adrenocorticotropic hormone; corticosteroid; anti-inflammatory; diagnostic aid* [also: corticotropin]

**corticotrophin-zinc hydroxide** INN *adrenocorticotropic hormone; corticosteroid; anti-inflammatory; diagnostic aid* [also: corticotropin zinc hydroxide]

**corticotropin** USP *adrenocorticotropic hormone; corticosteroid; anti-inflammatory; diagnostic aid* [also: corticotrophin]

**corticotropin, repository** USP *adrenocorticotropic hormone; corticosteroid; anti-inflammatory; diagnostic aid*

**corticotropin tetracosapeptide** [see: cosyntropin]

**corticotropin zinc hydroxide** USP *adrenocorticotropic hormone; corticosteroid; anti-inflammatory; diagnostic aid* [also: corticotrophin-zinc hydroxide]

**corticotropin-releasing factor** *investigational (Phase I/II, orphan) agent for peritumoral brain edema*

**Cortifoam** intrarectal foam aerosol ℞ *corticosteroidal anti-inflammatory for ulcerative proctitis* [hydrocortisone acetate] 90 mg/dose

**cortisol** [see: hydrocortisone]

**cortisol 21-acetate** [see: hydrocortisone acetate]

**cortisol 21-butyrate** [see: hydrocortisone butyrate]

**cortisol 21-cyclopentanepropionate** [see: hydrocortisone cypionate]

**cortisol cyclopentylpropionate** [see: hydrocortisone cypionate]

**cortisol 21-valerate** [see: hydrocortisone valerate]

**cortisone** INN, BAN *corticosteroid; anti-inflammatory* [also: cortisone acetate] ② Cortizone

**cortisone acetate** USP *corticosteroid; anti-inflammatory* [also: cortisone] 5, 10, 25 mg oral

**Cortisporin** cream ℞ *corticosteroidal anti-inflammatory; antibiotic* [hydrocortisone acetate; neomycin sulfate; polymyxin B sulfate] 0.5%•0.5%•10 000 U per g

**Cortisporin** eye drop suspension ℞ *ophthalmic corticosteroidal anti-inflammatory; antibiotic* [hydrocortisone;

neomycin sulfate; polymyxin B sulfate] 1%•0.35%•10 000 U per mL

**Cortisporin** ointment ℞ *corticosteroidal anti-inflammatory; antibiotic* [hydrocortisone; neomycin sulfate; bacitracin zinc; polymyxin B sulfate] 1%•0.5%•400 U•5000 U per g

**Cortisporin** ophthalmic ointment ℞ *ophthalmic corticosteroidal anti-inflammatory; antibiotic* [hydrocortisone; neomycin sulfate; bacitracin zinc; polymyxin B sulfate] 1%•0.35%•400 U/g•10 000 U/g

**Cortisporin Otic** ear drops, otic suspension ℞ *corticosteroidal anti-inflammatory; antibiotic* [hydrocortisone; neomycin sulfate; polymyxin B sulfate] 1%•5 mg•10 000 U per mL

**Cortisporin-TC** ear drop suspension ℞ *corticosteroidal anti-inflammatory; antibiotic; surface-active synergist* [hydrocortisone acetate; neomycin sulfate; colistin sulfate; thonzonium bromide] 10•3.3•3•0.5 mg/mL

**cortisuzol** INN

**cortivazol** USAN, INN *corticosteroid; anti-inflammatory*

**Cortizone for Kids** cream OTC *corticosteroidal anti-inflammatory* [hydrocortisone] 0.5%

**Cortizone-5** ointment, cream OTC *corticosteroidal anti-inflammatory* [hydrocortisone] 0.5%; 1% ⑨ cortisone

**Cortizone-10** ointment OTC *corticosteroidal anti-inflammatory* [hydrocortisone] 1%

**Cortizone-10 Plus** cream OTC *corticosteroidal anti-inflammatory* [hydrocortisone] 1%

**Cortizone-10 Quickshot** spray OTC *corticosteroidal anti-inflammatory* [hydrocortisone] 1%

**cortodoxone** USAN, INN, BAN *anti-inflammatory*

**Cortone Acetate** intra-articular or intralesional injection ℞ *corticosteroidal anti-inflammatory* [cortisone acetate] 50 mg/mL ⑨ Cort-Dome

**Cortrosyn** powder for IM or IV injection ℞ *multiple sclerosis; diagnostic aid for adrenal function; treatment for infantile spasms* [cosyntropin] 0.25 mg

**Corvert** IV infusion ℞ *antiarrhythmic for atrial fibrillation/flutter* [ibutilide fumarate] 0.1 mg/mL

**corydalis (*Corydalis cava*)** root *medicinal herb used as an antispasmodic, hypnotic, and antiparkinsonian*

***Corydalis formosa*** *medicinal herb* [see: turkey corn]

***Corynanthe johimbe*** *medicinal herb* [see: yohimbe]

**Corzide 40/5; Corzide 80/5** tablets ℞ *antihypertensive; β-blocker; diuretic* [nadolol; bendroflumethiazide] 40•5 mg; 80•5 mg

**Cosmederm-7** Ⓒᴬᴺ (trademarked ingredient) *topical anti-irritant* [strontium chloride]

**Cosmegen** powder for IV injection ℞ *antibiotic antineoplastic for melanomas, sarcomas, testicular and trophoblastic tumors* [dactinomycin] 0.5 mg

**CosmoDerm** gel for subcu injection ℞ *dermal filler for shallow scars and fine wrinkles* [collagen, purified human] 35 mg/mL

**cosmoline** [see: petrolatum]

**CosmoPlast** gel for subcu injection ℞ *dermal filler for scars, deep wrinkles, and facial folds* [collagen, purified human, cross-linked] 35 mg/mL

**Cosopt** eye drops ℞ *topical carbonic anhydrase inhibitor and beta-blocker for glaucoma* [dorzolamide HCl; timolol maleate] 2%•0.5%

**cosyntropin** USAN *adrenocorticotropic hormone; diagnostic aid for adrenal function* [also: tetracosactide; tetracosactrin]

**Cotara** ℞ *investigational (Phase III) agent for glioblastoma multiforme; investigational (Phase I/II) tumor necrosis therapy (TNT) for solid tumors; investigational (Phase I/II) for pancreatic, prostate, and liver cancers* [chimeric monoclonal antibody labeled with iodine-131]

**cotarnine chloride** NF

**cotarnine HCl** [see: cotarnine chloride]

**Cotazym** capsules (discontinued 2002) R̥ *digestive enzymes; antacid* [lipase; protease; amylase; calcium carbonate] 8000 U•30 000 U•30 000 U•25 mg

**Cotazym-S** capsules containing enteric-coated spheres (discontinued 2002) R̥ *digestive enzymes* [lipase; protease; amylase] 5000•20 000•20 000 USP units

**cotinine** INN *antidepressant* [also: cotinine fumarate]

**cotinine fumarate** USAN *antidepressant* [also: cotinine]

**Cotridin** Ⓒᴬᴺ syrup R̥ *narcotic antitussive; decongestant; antihistamine* [codeine phosphate; pseudoephedrine HCl; triprolidine HCl] 2•6•0.4 mg/mL

**Cotridin Expectorant** Ⓒᴬᴺ oral solution R̥ *narcotic antitussive; decongestant; antihistamine* [codeine phosphate; pseudoephedrine HCl; triprolidine HCl; guaifenesin] 2•6•0.4•20 mg/mL

**Cotrim; Cotrim D.S.** tablets R̥ *anti-infective; antibacterial* [trimethoprim; sulfamethoxazole] 80•400 mg; 160•800 mg ⑦ Cortin

**Cotrim Pediatric** oral suspension R̥ *anti-infective; antibacterial* [trimethoprim; sulfamethoxazole] 40•200 mg/5 mL

**co-trimoxazole** BAN [also: trimethoprim + sulfamethoxazole] ⑦ clotrimazole

**cotriptyline** INN

**cotton, purified** USP *surgical aid*

**cottonseed oil** NF *solvent*

**cottonweed** *medicinal herb* [see: milkweed]

**Co-Tuss V** oral liquid (discontinued 2002) R̥ *narcotic antitussive; expectorant* [hydrocodone bitartrate; guaifenesin] 5•100 mg

**couch grass (Agropyron repens)** rhizomes, roots, and stems *medicinal herb for blood cleansing, cystitis, diabetes, jaundice, kidney problems, upper respiratory tract inflammation with mucous discharge, rheumatism, and urinary infections*

**Cough** syrup (discontinued 2002) OTC *antitussive; decongestant; expectorant* [dextromethorphan hydrobromide; phenylephrine HCl; guaifenesin] 10•5•100 mg/5 mL

**Cough Formula** oral liquid (discontinued 2002) OTC *antitussive; antihistamine* [dextromethorphan hydrobromide; chlorpheniramine maleate; alcohol 10%] 15•2 mg/5 mL

**Cough Formula with Decongestant** oral liquid (discontinued 2002) OTC *antitussive; decongestant* [dextromethorphan hydrobromide; pseudoephedrine HCl; alcohol 10%] 10•20 mg/5 mL

**coughroot** *medicinal herb* [see: birthroot]

**coughweed** *medicinal herb* [see: life root]

**coughwort** *medicinal herb* [see: coltsfoot]

**Cough-X** lozenges OTC *antitussive; topical oral anesthetic* [dextromethorphan hydrobromide; benzocaine] 5•2 mg

**Coumadin** tablets, powder for IV injection R̥ *coumarin-derivative anticoagulant* [warfarin sodium] 1, 2, 2.5, 3, 4, 5, 6, 7.5, 10 mg; 2 mg/mL ⑦ Kemadrin

**coumafos** INN [also: coumaphos]

**coumamycin** INN *antibacterial* [also: coumermycin]

**coumaphos** BAN [also: coumafos]

**coumarin** NF *anticoagulant; investigational (orphan) for renal cell carcinoma*

**coumarins** *a class of anticoagulants that interfere with vitamin K-dependent clotting factors*

**coumazoline** INN

**coumermycin** USAN *antibacterial* [also: coumamycin]

**coumermycin sodium** USAN *antibacterial*

**coumetarol** INN [also: cumetharol]

**counterirritants** *a class of agents that produce superficial irritation in one part of the body to relieve irritation in another part*

**Covangesic** tablets (discontinued 2001) OTC *decongestant; antihistamine; analgesic* [phenylpropanolamine HCl; phenylephrine HCl; chlorpheniramine maleate; pyrilamine maleate; acetaminophen] 12.5•7.5•2•12.5•275 mg

**covatin HCl** [see: captodiame HCl]

**Covera-HS** extended-release film-coated tablets ℞ *antihypertensive; antianginal; antiarrhythmic; calcium channel blocker* [verapamil HCl] 180, 240 mg ⊡ Provera

**Coversyl** ⓒ tablets ℞ *angiotensin-converting enzyme (ACE) inhibitor for essential hypertension; treatment for congestive heart failure (CHF)* [perindopril erbumine] 2, 4 mg

**Coviracil** (name changed to Emtriva upon marketing release in 2003) ℞

**cow cabbage** *medicinal herb* [see: masterwort; white pond lily]

**cow parsnip** *medicinal herb* [see: masterwort]

**cowslip (*Caltha palustris*)** plant *medicinal herb used as an analgesic, antispasmodic, diaphoretic, diuretic, expectorant, and rubefacient*

**cowslip, Jerusalem** *medicinal herb* [see: lungwort]

**COX-2 (cyclooxygenase-2) inhibitors** *a class of nonsteroidal anti-inflammatory drugs (NSAIDs) for osteoarthritis, rheumatoid arthritis, acute pain, and primary dysmenorrhea; these agents also have antipyretic activity*

**Cozaar** film-coated tablets ℞ *angiotensin II receptor antagonist for hypertension; treatment to delay the progression of diabetic nephropathy* [losartan potassium] 25, 50, 100 mg

**CP (chlorambucil, prednisone)** *chemotherapy protocol for chronic lymphocytic leukemia (CLL)*

**CP (cyclophosphamide, Platinol)** *chemotherapy protocol for ovarian cancer*

**CP (cyclophosphamide, prednisone)** *chemotherapy protocol*

**CPB (cyclophosphamide, Platinol, BCNU)** *chemotherapy protocol*

**CPC (cyclophosphamide, Platinol, carboplatin)** *chemotherapy protocol*

**C.P.-DM** pediatric oral drops ℞ *antitussive; decongestant; antihistamine* [dextromethorphan hydrobromide;

pseudoephedrine HCl; carbinoxamine maleate] 4•15•1 mg/mL

**C-Phed Tannate** oral suspension ℞ *decongestant; antihistamine* [pseudoephedrine tannate; chlorpheniramine tannate] 150•9 mg/10 mL

**CPI-1189** *investigational (Phase II) agent for cognitive impairment in Parkinson disease*

**CPM (CCNU, procarbazine, methotrexate)** *chemotherapy protocol*

**CPM 8/PSE 90/MSC 2.5** sustained-release tablets ℞ *antihistamine; decongestant; anticholinergic to dry mucosal secretions* [chlorpheniramine maleate; pseudoephedrine HCl; methscopolamine nitrate] 8•90•2.5 mg

**CPOB (cyclophosphamide, prednisone, Oncovin, bleomycin)** *chemotherapy protocol*

**CPT-11 (camptothecin-11)** [see: irinotecan]

**CP-Tannic** oral suspension ℞ *decongestant; antihistamine* [pseudoephedrine tannate; chlorpheniramine tannate] 150•9 mg/10 mL

**⁵¹Cr** [see: albumin, chromated Cr 51 serum]

**⁵¹Cr** [see: chromic chloride Cr 51]

**⁵¹Cr** [see: chromic phosphate Cr 51]

**⁵¹Cr** [see: sodium chromate Cr 51]

**cramp bark (*Viburnum opulus*)** bark and berries *medicinal herb for asthma, convulsions, cramps, heart palpitations, hypertension, hysteria, leg cramps, nervousness, spasm, and urinary disorders*

**crampweed** *medicinal herb* [see: cinquefoil]

**cranberry (*Vaccinium edule; V. erythrocarpum; V. macrocarpon; V. oxycoccos; V. vitis*)** fruit *medicinal herb for bladder, kidney, and urinary tract infections; also used to decrease the rate of urine degradation and odor formation in incontinent patients*

**cranesbill; spotted cranesbill** *medicinal herb* [see: alum root]

***Crataegus laevigata; C. monogyna; C. oxyacantha*** *medicinal herb* [see: hawthorn]

**crawley; crawley root** *medicinal herb*
[see: coral root]

**Creamy Tar** shampoo OTC *antiseborrheic; antipsoriatic; antipruritic; antibacterial* [coal tar] 8.65%

**Creapure** ℞ *investigational (orphan)
agent for amyotrophic lateral sclerosis
(ALS)* [creatine]

**creatine** *investigational (orphan) agent
for amyotrophic lateral sclerosis (ALS)*

**creatinolfosfate** INN

**Creon** delayed-release capsules containing enteric-coated microspheres
(discontinued 2002) ℞ *porcine-
derived digestive enzymes* [pancreatin
(lipase; protease; amylase)] 300 mg
(8000•13 000•30 000 USP units)

**Creon 5; Creon 10: Creon 20**
delayed-release capsules containing
enteric-coated microspheres ℞ in
the U.S; OTC in Canada *porcine-
derived digestive enzymes* [lipase;
protease; amylase] 5000•18 750•
16 600 USP units; 10 000•37 500•
33 200 USP units; 20 000•75 000•
66 400 USP units

**Creon 25** ⒸⒶⓃ delayed-release capsules
containing enteric-coated microspheres OTC *porcine-derived digestive
enzymes* [pancreatin (lipase; protease; amylase)] 300 mg (25 000•
62 500•74 700 USP units)

**creosote carbonate** USP

**Creo-Terpin** oral liquid OTC *antitussive*
[dextromethorphan hydrobromide;
alcohol 25%] 10 mg/15 mL

**cresol** NF *disinfectant*

**cresotamide** INN

**cresoxydiol** [see: mephenesin]

**crestomycin sulfate** [see: paromomycin sulfate]

**Crestor** tablets ℞ *HMG-CoA reductase inhibitor for hypercholesterolemia,
mixed dyslipidemia, and hypertriglyceridemia* [rosuvastatin calcium] 5, 10,
20, 40 mg

**Cresylate** ear drops ℞ *antibacterial;
antifungal* [m-cresyl acetate; chlorobutanol; alcohol] 25%•25%•1%

**cresylic acid** [see: cresol]

**crilanomer** INN

**crilvastatin** USAN, INN *antihyperlipidemic*

**Crinone** vaginal gel ℞ *natural progestin; hormone replacement or supplementation for assisted reproductive
technology (ART) treatments* [proges-
terone] 4%, 8%

**crisnatol** INN *antineoplastic* [also: crisnatol mesylate]

**crisnatol mesylate** USAN *antineoplastic*
[also: crisnatol]

**Criticare HN** ready-to-use oral liquid
OTC *enteral nutritional therapy* [lac-
tose-free formula]

**Crixivan** capsules ℞ *antiviral; HIV
protease inhibitor* [indinavir sulfate]
100, 200, 333, 400 mg

**crobefate** INN *combining name for radicals or groups*

**croconazole** INN

**crocus, autumn** *medicinal herb* [see:
autumn crocus]

**Crocus sativus** *medicinal herb* [see: saf-
fron]

**CroFab** injection ℞ *treatment of pit
viper (rattlesnake, copperhead, and cottonmouth moccasin) snake bites (orphan)*
[antivenin (Crotalidae) polyvalent
(ovine) Fab]

**crofelemer** USAN *investigational (Phase
III) treatment for AIDS-related diarrhea; investigational (Phase II) antiviral for AIDS-related genital herpes*

**crofilcon A** USAN *hydrophilic contact
lens material*

**Crolom** eye drops ℞ *mast cell stabilizer;
ocular antiallergic and antiviral for vernal keratoconjunctivitis (orphan)* [cro-
molyn sodium] 4%

**cromacate** INN *combining name for
radicals or groups*

**cromakalim** INN, BAN

**Cro-Man-Zin** tablets OTC *mineral supplement* [chromium; manganese;
zinc] 0.2•5•25 mg

**cromesilate** INN *combining name for
radicals or groups*

**cromitrile** INN *antiasthmatic* [also: cromitrile sodium]

**cromitrile sodium** USAN *antiasthmatic* [also: cromitrile]

**cromoglicic acid** INN *prophylactic antiasthmatic* [also: cromolyn sodium; cromoglycic acid]

**cromoglycic acid** BAN *prophylactic antiasthmatic* [also: cromolyn sodium; cromoglicic acid]

**cromolyn sodium** USAN, USP *antiinflammatory; mast cell stabilizer for prophylactic treatment of allergy, asthma, and bronchospasm; treatment for mastocytosis and vernal keratoconjunctivitis (orphan)* [also: cromoglicic acid; cromoglycic acid] 20 mg/2 mL inhalation

**Cronassial** *investigational (orphan) agent for retinitis pigmentosa* [gangliosides, sodium salts]

**cronetal** [see: disulfiram]

**cronidipine** INN

**cropropamide** INN, BAN

**croscarmellose** INN *tablet disintegrant* [also: croscarmellose sodium]

**croscarmellose sodium** USAN, NF *tablet disintegrant* [also: croscarmellose]

**crosfumaril** [see: hemoglobin crosfumaril]

**crospovidone** NF *tablet excipient*

**cross-linked carboxymethylcellulose sodium** [now: croscarmellose sodium]

**cross-linked carmellose sodium** [see: croscarmellose sodium]

**crotaline antivenin** [see: antivenin (Crotalidae) polyvalent]

**crotamiton** USP, INN, BAN *scabicide; antipruritic*

**crotetamide** INN [also: crotethamide]

**crotethamide** BAN [also: crotetamide]

**crotoniazide** INN

**crotonylidenisoniazid** [see: crotoniazide]

**crotoxyfos** BAN

**crowfoot** *medicinal herb* [see: alum root; buttercup]

**crowfoot buttercup; acrid crowfoot; cursed crowfoot; marsh crowfoot; meadow crowfoot; tall crowfoot; water crowfoot** *medicinal herb* [see: buttercup]

**crown, priest's** *medicinal herb* [see: dandelion]

**crude tuberculin** [see: tuberculin, old]

**Cruex** cream OTC *antifungal* [clotrimazole] 1%

**Cruex** cream, aerosol powder OTC *topical antifungal* [undecylenic acid; zinc undecylenate] 20% total; 19% total

**Cruex** powder OTC *antifungal* [calcium undecylenate] 10%

**crufomate** USAN, INN, BAN *veterinary anthelmintic*

**cryofluorane** INN *aerosol propellant* [also: dichlorotetrafluoroethane]

**cryptenamine acetates**

**Crypto-LA** slide test for professional use *in vitro diagnostic aid for Cryptococcus neoformans antigens*

*Cryptosporidium parvum* **bovine colostrum IgG concentrate** *investigational (orphan) treatment of cryptosporidiosis-induced diarrhea in immunocompromised patients*

**Cryselle** tablets (in packs of 21 and 28) ℞ *monophasic oral contraceptive; emergency postcoital contraceptive* [norgestrel; ethinyl estradiol] 0.3 mg•30 μg

**crystal violet** [see: gentian violet]

**crystallized trypsin** [see: trypsin, crystallized]

**Crystamine** IM or subcu injection ℞ *hematinic; vitamin B$_{12}$ supplement* [cyanocobalamin] 1000 μg/mL

**Crysti 1000** IM or subcu injection ℞ *hematinic; vitamin B$_{12}$ supplement* [cyanocobalamin] 1000 μg/mL

**Crystodigin** tablets (discontinued 2000) ℞ *cardiac glycoside to increase cardiac output; antiarrhythmic* [digitoxin] 0.05, 0.1 mg

**crystografin** [see: meglumine diatriazole]

$^{131}$**Cs** [see: cesium chloride Cs 131]

**CS-92** *investigational (Phase I/II) nucleoside reverse transcriptase inhibitor (NRTI) for HIV infection*

**C-Solve** OTC *lotion base*

**CSP (cellulose sodium phosphate)** [q.v.]

**CT (cisplatin, Taxol)** *chemotherapy protocol for ovarian cancer*

**CT (cytarabine, thioguanine)** *chemotherapy protocol*

**CT-2584 mesylate** *investigational (Phase II, orphan) antineoplastic for soft tissue sarcomas and malignant mesothelioma*

**CT-3** *investigational anti-inflammatory*

**CTAB (cetyltrimethyl ammonium bromide)**

**C-Tanna 12D** tablets, oral suspension ℞ *pediatric antitussive, decongestant, and antihistamine* [carbetapentane tannate; phenylephrine tannate; pyrilamine tannate] 60•10•40 mg; 30•5•30 mg/5 mL

**CTCb (cyclophosphamide, thiotepa, carboplatin)** *chemotherapy protocol*

**CTH (ceramide trihexosidase)** [q.v.]

**CTP-37** *investigational (Phase III) theraccine for cervical and pancreatic cancer; investigational (Phase II) for prostate and advanced colorectal cancers*

**C/T/S** topical solution (discontinued 2003) ℞ *antibiotic for acne* [clindamycin phosphate] 1%

**CTX (cyclophosphamide)** [q.v.]

**Ctx-Plat (cyclophosphamide, Platinol)** *chemotherapy protocol*

**⁶⁴Cu** [see: cupric acetate Cu 64]

**cubeb (Piper cubeba)** unripe berries *medicinal herb used as an antiseptic, antisyphilitic, carminative, diuretic, expectorant, stimulant, and stomachic*

**Cubicin** powder for IV infusion ℞ *cyclic lipopeptide antibiotic for skin and skin structure infections* [daptomycin] 250, 500 mg/vial

**cucurbita (Cucurbita maxima; C. moschata; C. pepa)** seeds *medicinal herb for prophylaxis, immobilizing, and aiding in the expulsion of intestinal worms and parasites; also used in prostate gland disorders*

**Culturette 10 Minute Group A Strep ID** slide test for professional use *in vitro diagnostic test for Group A streptococcal antigens in throat swabs* [latex agglutination test]

**Culver physic** *medicinal herb* [see: Culver root]

**Culver root (Varonicastrum virginicum)** *medicinal herb for blood cleansing, diarrhea, and liver and stomach disorders*

**cumetharol** BAN [also: coumetarol]

**cumin (Cuminum cyminum; C. odorum)** seeds and oil *medicinal herb for gastric cancer; also used as an antioxidant*

**cupric acetate Cu 64** USAN *radioactive agent*

**cupric chloride** USP *dietary copper supplement*

**cupric sulfate** USP *antidote to phosphorus; dietary copper supplement (40% elemental copper)* 0.4, 2 mg/mL injection

**Cuprimine** capsules ℞ *metal chelating agent for rheumatoid arthritis, Wilson disease, and cystinuria* [penicillamine] 125, 250 mg

**cuprimyxin** USAN, INN *veterinary antibacterial; antifungal*

**cuproxoline** INN, BAN

**Curaçao aloe** *medicinal herb* [see: aloe]

**curare** [see: tubocurarine chloride]

**Curcuma domestica; C. longa** *medicinal herb* [see: turmeric]

**cure-all** *medicinal herb* [see: lemon balm]

**curium** *element (Cm)*

**curled dock; curly dock** *medicinal herb* [see: yellow dock]

**curled mint** *medicinal herb* [see: peppermint]

**curls, blue** *medicinal herb* [see: woundwort]

**Curosurf** intratracheal suspension ℞ *porcine lung extract for respiratory distress syndrome (RDS) in premature infants (orphan)* [poractant alfa] 1.5, 3 mL (120, 240 mg phospholipids)

**curral** [see: diallylbarbituric acid]

**currant (Ribes nigrum; R. rubrum)** leaves and fruit *medicinal herb used as a diaphoretic and diuretic*

**Curretab** tablets (discontinued 2004) ℞ *synthetic progestin for secondary* amenorrhea, abnormal uterine bleeding, and endometrial hyperplasia [medroxyprogesterone acetate] 10 mg

**custard apple** medicinal herb [see: pawpaw]

**Cūtar Bath Oil Emulsion** OTC antipsoriatic; antiseborrheic; antipruritic; emollient [coal tar] 7.5%

**Cūtemol** cream OTC moisturizer; emollient [allantoin]

**Cuticura Medicated Soap** bar OTC therapeutic skin cleanser [triclocarban] 1%

**Cutivate** cream, ointment ℞ corticosteroidal anti-inflammatory [fluticasone propionate] 0.05%; 0.005%

**CV (cisplatin, VePesid)** chemotherapy protocol

**CVA (cyclophosphamide, vincristine, Adriamycin)** chemotherapy protocol

**CVA-BMP; CVA + BMP (cyclophosphamide, vincristine, Adriamycin, BCNU, methotrexate, procarbazine)** chemotherapy protocol

**CVAD; C-VAD (cyclophosphamide, vincristine, Adriamycin, dexamethasone)** chemotherapy protocol

**CVB (CCNU, vinblastine, bleomycin)** chemotherapy protocol

**CVBD (CCNU, bleomycin, vinblastine, dexamethasone)** chemotherapy protocol

**CVD (cisplatin, vinblastine, dacarbazine)** chemotherapy protocol for malignant melanoma

**CVD+IL-2I (cisplatin, vinblastine, dacarbazine, interleukin-2, interferon alfa)** chemotherapy protocol for malignant melanoma

**CVEB (cisplatin, vinblastine, etoposide, bleomycin)** chemotherapy protocol

**CVI (carboplatin, VePesid, ifosfamide [with mesna rescue])** chemotherapy protocol for non–small cell lung cancer (NSCLC) [also: VIC]

**CVM (cyclophosphamide, vincristine, methotrexate)** chemotherapy protocol

**CVP (cyclophosphamide, vincristine, prednisone)** chemotherapy protocol for non-Hodgkin lymphoma and chronic lymphocytic leukemia (CLL)

**CVPP (CCNU, vinblastine, procarbazine, prednisone)** chemotherapy protocol for Hodgkin lymphoma

**CVPP (cyclophosphamide, Velban, procarbazine, prednisone)** chemotherapy protocol

**CVPP-CCNU (cyclophosphamide, vinblastine, procarbazine, prednisone, CCNU)** chemotherapy protocol

**CVT-510** investigational (Phase I) selective adenosine $A_1$ receptor agonist for atrial arrhythmias; investigational (Phase III) for paroxysmal supraventricular tachycardia

**CY-1503** investigational (Phase III, orphan) adjunct to surgery for congenital heart defects in newborns; investigational (orphan) for postischemic pulmonary reperfusion edema

**CY-1899** investigational (orphan) agent for chronic active hepatitis B

**cyacetacide** INN [also: cyacetazide]

**cyacetazide** BAN [also: cyacetacide]

**CyADIC (cyclophosphamide, Adriamycin, DIC)** chemotherapy protocol

**cyamemazine** INN

**cyamepromazine** [see: cyamemazine]

**cyanamide** JAN [also: calcium carbimide]

**cyani** medicinal herb [see: cornflower]

**Cyanide Antidote Package** ℞ emergency treatment of cyanide poisoning [sodium nitrite; sodium thiosulfate; amyl nitrite inhalant] 300 mg•12.5 g•0.3 mL

**cyanoacetohydrazide** [see: cyacetazide]

**cyanoacrylate** topical skin adhesive for closing surgical incisions and traumatic lacerations; topical mucous membrane sealant and protectant for canker and mouth sores

**cyanocobalamin (vitamin B$_{12}$)** USP, INN, BAN, JAN water-soluble vitamin; hematopoietic 50, 100, 250, 500, 1000 μg oral; 100, 1000 μg/mL injection cyanocobalamin ($^{57}$Co) INN *pernicious anemia test; radioactive agent* [also: cyanocobalamin Co 57]

cyanocobalamin ($^{58}$Co) INN

cyanocobalamin ($^{60}$Co) INN *pernicious anemia test; radioactive agent* [also: cyanocobalamin Co 60]

cyanocobalamin Co 57 USAN, USP *pernicious anemia test; radioactive agent* [also: cyanocobalamin ($^{57}$Co)]

cyanocobalamin Co 60 USAN, USP *pernicious anemia test; radioactive agent* [also: cyanocobalamin ($^{60}$Co)]

Cyanoject IM or subcu injection ℞ *hematinic; vitamin B$_{12}$ supplement* [cyanocobalamin] 1000 μg/mL

cyclacillin USAN, USP *antibacterial* [also: ciclacillin]

cyclamate calcium NF

cyclamic acid USAN, BAN *non-nutritive sweetener (banned in the U.S.)*

cyclamide [see: glycyclamide]

cyclandelate INN, BAN, JAN *peripheral vasodilator; vascular smooth muscle relaxant*

cyclarbamate INN, BAN

cyclazocine USAN, INN *analgesic*

cyclazodone INN

Cyclessa tablets (in packs of 28) ℞ *triphasic oral contraceptive; emergency postcoital contraceptive* [desogestrel; ethinyl estradiol]
Phase 1 (7 days): 100•25 μg;
Phase 2 (7 days): 125•25 μg;
Phase 3 (7 days): 150•25 μg

cyclexanone INN

cyclic adenosine monophosphate (cAMP) [see: adenosine phosphate]

cyclic lipopeptides *a class of antibiotics that binds to bacterial membranes and causes a rapid depolarization of membrane potential, which inhibits RNA/DNA synthesis, leading to bacterial cell death*

cyclic propylene carbonate [see: propylene carbonate]

cyclindole USAN *antidepressant* [also: ciclindole]

Cyclinex-1 powder OTC *formula for infants with urea cycle disorders or gyrate atrophy*

Cyclinex-2 powder OTC *enteral nutritional therapy for urea cycle disorders or gyrate atrophy* [multiple essential amino acids]

cycliramine INN *antihistamine* [also: cycliramine maleate]

cycliramine maleate USAN *antihistamine* [also: cycliramine]

cyclizine USP, INN, BAN *antihistamine; antiemetic; anticholinergic; motion sickness relief*

cyclizine HCl USP, BAN *antiemetic*

cyclizine lactate USP, BAN *antinauseant*

cyclobarbital NF, INN [also: cyclobarbitone]

cyclobarbital calcium NF

cyclobarbitone BAN [also: cyclobarbital]

cyclobendazole USAN *anthelmintic* [also: ciclobendazole]

cyclobenzaprine INN *skeletal muscle relaxant* [also: cyclobenzaprine HCl]

cyclobenzaprine HCl USAN, USP *skeletal muscle relaxant* [also: cyclobenzaprine] 10 mg oral

cyclobutoic acid INN

cyclobutyrol INN

cyclocarbothiamine [see: cycotiamine]

Cyclocort ointment, cream, lotion ℞ *topical corticosteroidal anti-inflammatory* [amcinonide] 0.1%

cyclocoumarol BAN

cyclocumarol [see: cyclocoumarol]

α-cyclodextrin [see: alfadex]

Cyclofed Pediatric syrup ℞ *pediatric narcotic antitussive, decongestant, and expectorant* [codeine phosphate; pseudoephedrine HCl; guaifenesin; alcohol 6%] 10•30•100 mg/5 mL

cyclofenil INN, BAN

cyclofilcon A USAN *hydrophilic contact lens material*

cycloguanil embonate INN, BAN *antimalarial* [also: cycloguanil pamoate]

cycloguanil pamoate USAN *antimalarial* [also: cycloguanil embonate]

**Cyclogyl** Drop-Tainers (eye drops) ℞ *cycloplegic; mydriatic* [cyclopentolate HCl] 0.5%, 1%, 2%

**cyclohexanehexol** [see: inositol]

**cyclohexanesulfamate dihydrate** [see: sodium cyclamate]

**cyclohexanesulfamic acid** *(banned in the U.S.)* [see: cyclamic acid]

**cycloheximide** USAN *antipsoriatic* [also: cicloheximide]

***p*-cyclohexylhydratropic acid** [see: hexaprofen]

**N-cyclohexyllinoleamide** [see: clinolamide]

**4-cyclohexyloxybenzoate** [see: cyclomethycaine]

**1-cyclohexylpropyl carbamate** [see: procymate]

**N-cyclohexylsulfamic acid** *(banned in the U.S.)* [see: cyclamic acid]

**cyclomenol** INN

**cyclomethicone** NF *wetting agent*

**cyclomethycaine** INN, BAN *local anesthetic* [also: cyclomethycaine sulfate]

**cyclomethycaine sulfate** USP *local anesthetic* [also: cyclomethycaine]

**Cyclomydril** Drop-Tainers (eye drops) ℞ *cycloplegic; mydriatic* [cyclopentolate HCl; phenylephrine HCl] 0.2%•1%

**cyclonium iodide** [see: oxapium iodide]

**cyclooxygenase-2 (COX-2) inhibitors** *a class of investigational anti-inflammatory drugs*

**cyclopentamine** INN, BAN [also: cyclopentamine HCl]

**cyclopentamine HCl** USP [also: cyclopentamine]

**cyclopentaphene** [see: cyclarbamate]

**cyclopenthiazide** USAN, INN, BAN *antihypertensive*

**cyclopentolate** INN, BAN *ophthalmic anticholinergic* [also: cyclopentolate HCl]

**cyclopentolate HCl** USP *ophthalmic anticholinergic; mydriatic; cycloplegic* [also: cyclopentolate] 1% eye drops

**8-cyclopentyl 1,3-dipropylxanthine** *investigational (orphan) for cystic fibrosis*

**cyclophenazine HCl** USAN *antipsychotic* [also: ciclofenazine]

**cyclophosphamide** USP, INN, BAN, JAN *nitrogen mustard–type alkylating antineoplastic; immunosuppressive* 25, 50 mg oral

**cycloplegics** *a class of drugs that paralyze the ciliary muscles of the eye*

**cyclopolydimethylsiloxane** [see: cyclomethicone]

**cyclopregnol** INN

**cycloprolol** BAN *antiadrenergic (β-receptor)* [also: cicloprolol HCl; cicloprolol]

**cyclopropane** USP, INN *inhalation general anesthetic*

**Cycloprostin** ℞ *investigational (orphan) heparin replacement for hemodialysis* [epoprostenol]

**cyclopyrronium bromide** INN

**cycloserine (L-cycloserine)** USP, INN, BAN, JAN *bacteriostatic; tuberculosis retreatment; investigational (orphan) for Gaucher disease*

**cyclosporin** BAN *immunosuppressant* [also: cyclosporine; ciclosporin]

**cyclosporin A** [now: cyclosporine]

**cyclosporine** USAN, USP *immunosuppressant for transplants (orphan), rheumatoid arthritis, and psoriasis; tear stimulant for Sjögren keratoconjunctivitis sicca (orphan); investigational (orphan) for corneal melting syndrome* [also: ciclosporin; cyclosporin] 25, 100 mg oral; 100 mg/mL oral; 50 mg/mL injection

**CycloTech** (trademarked delivery device) *provides premeasured doses of oral liquids and records dosing times*

**cyclothiazide** USAN, USP, INN, BAN *diuretic; antihypertensive*

**cyclovalone** INN

**cycobemin** [see: cyanocobalamin]

**Cycofed** syrup ℞ *narcotic antitussive; decongestant* [codeine phosphate; pseudoephedrine HCl] 20•60 mg/5 mL

**Cycofed Pediatric** syrup (discontinued 2002) ℞ *narcotic antitussive; decongestant; expectorant* [codeine phosphate; pseudoephedrine HCl; guaifenesin; alcohol 6%] 10•30•100 mg

**cycotiamine** INN

**cycrimine** INN, BAN [also: cycrimine HCl]

**cycrimine HCl** USP [also: cycrimine]

**Cycrin** tablets (discontinued 2004) ℞ *synthetic progestin for secondary amenorrhea, abnormal uterine bleeding, and endometrial hyperplasia* [medroxyprogesterone acetate] 2.5, 5, 10 mg

**Cydec** pediatric oral drops ℞ *decongestant; antihistamine* [pseudoephedrine HCl; carbinoxamine maleate] 25•2 mg/mL

**Cydec-DM** syrup, pediatric oral drops ℞ *antitussive; decongestant; antihistamine* [dextromethorphan hydrobromide; pseudoephedrine HCl; carbinoxamine maleate] 15•60•4 mg/5 mL; 4•25•2 mg/mL

**cyfluthrin** BAN

**cyhalothrin** BAN

**cyheptamide** USAN, INN *anticonvulsant*

**cyheptropine** INN

**CyHOP (cyclophosphamide, Halotestin, Oncovin, prednisone)** *chemotherapy protocol*

**Cyklokapron** tablets, IV injection ℞ *systemic hemostatic* [tranexamic acid] 500 mg; 100 mg/mL

**Cylert** tablets, chewable tablets ℞ *CNS stimulant for attention-deficit hyperactivity disorder (ADHD)* [pemoline] 18.75, 37.5, 75 mg; 37.5 mg

**Cylex; Cylex Sugar-Free** throat lozenges OTC *topical oral anesthetic; antiseptic* [benzocaine; cetylpyridinium chloride] 15•5 mg

**Cylexin** ℞ *investigational (Phase III, orphan) adjunct to surgery for congenital heart defects in newborns; investigational (orphan) for postischemic pulmonary reperfusion edema* [CY-1503 (code name—generic name not yet assigned)]

**Cymbalta** capsules ℞ *selective serotonin and norepinephrine reuptake inhibitor (SSNRI) for major depression; analgesic for diabetic neuropathy; investigational (Phase II) for urinary incontinence* [duloxetine HCl] 20, 30, 60 mg

**Cymbopogon citratus** *medicinal herb* [see: lemongrass]

**Cymbopogon nardus; C. winterianus** *medicinal herb* [see: citronella]

**cymemoxine** [see: cimemoxin]

**Cymeval** (name changed to Valcyte upon marketing release in 2001)

**Cymevene** (foreign name for U.S. product Cytovene)

**Cynara scolymus** *medicinal herb* [see: artichoke]

**cynarine** INN

**Cyomin** IM or subcu injection ℞ *hematinic; vitamin B$_{12}$ supplement* [cyanocobalamin] 1000 μg/mL

**CyPat** ℞ *investigational (Phase III) antineoplastic for prostate cancer*

**cypenamine** INN, BAN *antidepressant* [also: cypenamine HCl]

**cypenamine HCl** USAN *antidepressant* [also: cypenamine]

**cypionate** USAN, BAN *combining name for radicals or groups* [also: cipionate]

**cypothrin** USAN *veterinary insecticide*

**cyprazepam** USAN, INN *sedative*

**cyprenorphine** INN, BAN

**cyprenorphine HCl** [see: cyprenorphine]

**Cypripedium pubescens** *medicinal herb* [see: lady's slipper]

**cyprodemanol** [see: cyprodenate]

**cyprodenate** INN

**cyproheptadine** INN, BAN *piperidine antihistamine for hypersensitivity reactions; antipruritic* [also: cyproheptadine HCl]

**cyproheptadine HCl** USP, JAN *nonselective piperidine antihistamine for allergic rhinitis and type I hypersensitivity reactions; antipruritic; adjunctive anaphylactic therapy* [also: cyproheptadine] 4 mg oral; 2 mg/5 mL oral

**cyprolidol** INN *antidepressant* [also: cyprolidol HCl]

**cyprolidol HCl** USAN *antidepressant* [also: cyprolidol]

**cyproquinate** USAN *coccidiostat for poultry* [also: ciproquinate]

**cyproterone** INN, BAN *antiandrogen* [also: cyproterone acetate]

**cyproterone acetate** USAN *antiandrogen; investigational (orphan) for severe hirsutism* [also: cyproterone]

**cyproximide** USAN *antipsychotic; antidepressant* [also: ciproximide]

**cyren A** [see: diethylstilbestrol]

**cyren B** [see: diethylstilbestrol dipropionate]

**cyromazine** INN, BAN

**Cystadane** powder for oral solution ℞ *electrolyte replenisher for homocystinuria (orphan)* [betaine HCl] 1 g

**Cystagon** capsules ℞ *antiurolithic for nephropathic cystinosis (orphan)* [cysteamine bitartrate] 50, 150 mg

**cystamin** [see: methenamine]

**cysteamine** USAN, BAN *antiurolithic for nephropathic cystinosis (orphan)* [also: mercaptamine]

**cysteamine bitartrate** *antiurolithic for nephropathic cystinosis (orphan)*

**cysteamine HCl** USAN *antiurolithic; investigational (orphan) for corneal cystine crystal accumulation in cystinosis patients*

**cysteine (L-cysteine)** INN *nonessential amino acid; symbols: Cys, C; investigational (orphan) for erythropoietic protoporphyria photosensitivity* [also: cysteine HCl]

**cysteine HCl (L-cysteine HCl)** USP *nonessential amino acid* [also: cysteine] 50 mg/mL injection

**L-cysteine HCl monohydrate** [see: cysteine HCl]

**Cystex** tablets ℞ *urinary antibiotic; analgesic; acidifier* [methenamine; sodium salicylate; benzoic acid] 162•162.5•32 mg

**cystic fibrosis gene therapy** *investigational (orphan) agent for cystic fibrosis*

**cystic fibrosis transmembrane conductance regulator (CFTR)** *investigational (orphan) agent for cystic fibrosis*

**cystic fibrosis transmembrane conductance regulator, recombinant adenovirus (AdGV-CFTR)** *investigational (orphan) agent for cystic fibrosis*

**cystine (L-cystine)** USAN *amino acid*

**Cysto-Conray; Cysto-Conray II** intracavitary instillation ℞ *radiopaque contrast medium for urological imaging* [iothalamate meglumine (47% iodine)] 430 mg/mL (202 mg/mL); 172 mg/mL (81 mg/mL)

**cystogen** [see: methenamine]

**Cystografin; Cystografin Dilute** intracavitary instillation ℞ *radiopaque contrast medium for urological imaging* [diatrizoate meglumine (46.67% iodine)] 300 mg/mL (141 mg/mL); 180 mg/mL (85 mg/mL)

**Cystospaz** tablets ℞ *GI/GU antispasmodic; antiparkinsonian; anticholinergic "drying agent" for allergic rhinitis and hyperhidrosis* [hyoscyamine sulfate] 0.15 mg

**Cystospaz-M** timed-release capsules (discontinued 2004) ℞ *GI/GU antispasmodic; antiparkinsonian; anticholinergic "drying agent" for allergic rhinitis and hyperhidrosis* [hyoscyamine sulfate] 0.375 mg

**CYTABOM (cytarabine, bleomycin, Oncovin, mechlorethamine)** *chemotherapy protocol*

**Cytadren** tablets ℞ *adrenal steroid inhibitor; antisteroidal antineoplastic for corticotropin-producing tumors* [aminoglutethimide] 250 mg

**cytarabine** USAN, USP, INN, BAN *antimetabolite antineoplastic for various leukemias* 100, 500, 1000, 2000 mg injection ⃞ vidarabine

**cytarabine, liposomal** *antimetabolite antineoplastic for lymphomatous neoplastic meningitis (orphan)*

**cytarabine HCl** USAN *antiviral*

**Cytisus scoparius** *medicinal herb* [see: broom]

**CytoGam** IV infusion ℞ *prevention of primary cytomegalovirus in bone marrow and organ transplants from a CMV seropositive donor to an immunocompromised CMV seronegative recipient (orphan)* [cytomegalovirus immune globulin, solvent/detergent treated] 50 mg/mL

**CytoImplant** ℞ *investigational (orphan) agent for pancreatic cancer* [blood mononuclear cells, allogenic peripheral]

**cytolin** *investigational (Phase I/II) monoclonal antibody for AIDS*

**cytomegalovirus immune globulin, human** *prevention of primary cytomegalovirus in bone marrow and organ transplants from a CMV seropositive donor to an immunocompromised CMV seronegative recipient (orphan)*

**cytomegalovirus immune globulin intravenous (CMV-IGIV) & ganciclovir sodium** *investigational (orphan) for cytomegalovirus pneumonia in bone marrow transplant patients*

**Cytomel** tablets ℞ *synthetic thyroid hormone (T₃ fraction only)* [liothyronine sodium] 5, 25, 50 μg

**cytoprotective agents** *a class of drugs that provide prophylaxis against the side effects of antineoplastic agents*

**Cytosar-U** powder for subcu, intrathecal or IV injection ℞ *antimetabolite antineoplastic for various leukemias* [cytarabine] 100, 500, 1000, 2000 mg/vial

**cytosine arabinoside (ara-C)** [see: cytarabine]

**cytosine arabinoside HCl** [now: cytarabine HCl]

**Cytosol** topical liquid ℞ *sterile irrigant* [physiological irrigating solution]

**Cytotec** tablets ℞ *prevents NSAID-induced gastric ulcers; has been used for cervical ripening and induction of labor; use by pregnant women can cause abortion, premature birth, or birth defects* [misoprostol] 100, 200 μg

**cytotoxic lymphocyte maturation factor** [see: edodekin alfa]

**Cytovene** capsules ℞ *antiviral for AIDS-related cytomegalovirus (CMV) infections (orphan) and CMV retinitis (orphan)* [ganciclovir] 250, 500 mg

**Cytovene** powder for IV infusion ℞ *antiviral for AIDS-related cytomegalovirus (CMV) infections (orphan)* [ganciclovir sodium] 500 mg/vial

**Cytoxan** tablets, powder for IV injection ℞ *nitrogen mustard-type alkylating antineoplastic for multiple leukemias, lymphomas, blastomas, sarcomas and organ cancers* [cyclophosphamide] 25, 50 mg; 100 mg

**Cytra-2** solution ℞ *urinary alkalizing agent* [sodium citrate; citric acid] 500•334 mg/5 mL

**Cytra-3** syrup ℞ *urinary alkalinizing agent* [potassium citrate; sodium citrate; citric acid] 550•500•334 mg/5 mL

**Cytra-K** oral solution ℞ *urinary alkalizing agent* [potassium citrate; citric acid] 1100•334 mg/5 mL

**Cytra-LC** solution ℞ *urinary alkalizing agent* [potassium citrate; sodium citrate; citric acid] 550•500•334 mg/5 mL

**Cytuss HC** oral liquid ℞ *narcotic antitussive; decongestant; antihistamine* [hydrocodone bitartrate; phenylephrine HCl; chlorpheniramine maleate] 5•10•4 mg/10 mL

**CY-VA-DACT (Cytoxin, vincristine, Adriamycin, dactinomycin)** *chemotherapy protocol*

**CYVADIC; CY-VA-DIC; CyVADIC (cyclophosphamide, vincristine, Adriamycin, DIC)** *chemotherapy protocol for bone and soft tissue sarcomas*

**CYVMAD (cyclophosphamide, vincristine, methotrexate, Adriamycin, DTIC)** *chemotherapy protocol*

**D (vitamin D)** [q.v.]

**D-2.5-W; D-5-W; D-10-W; D-20-W; D-25-W; D-30-W; D-40-W; D-50-W; D-60-W; D-70-W** ℞ *intravenous nutritional therapy* [dextrose]

**D₂ (vitamin D₂)** [see: ergocalciferol]

**D₃ (vitamin D₃)** [see: cholecalciferol]

**d4T** [see: stavudine]

**D.A.** chewable tablets ℞ *decongestant; antihistamine; anticholinergic to dry mucosal secretions* [phenylephrine HCl; chlorpheniramine maleate; methscopolamine nitrate] 10•2•1.25 mg

**DA (daunorubicin, ara-C)** *chemotherapy protocol for acute myelocytic leukemia (AML)*

**D.A. II** tablets ℞ *decongestant; antihistamine; anticholinergic to dry mucosal secretions* [phenylephrine HCl; chlorpheniramine maleate; methscopolamine nitrate] 10•4•1.25 mg

**DAA (dihydroxyaluminum aminoacetate)** [q.v.]

**dacarbazine** USAN, USP, INN, BAN *alkylating antineoplastic for metastatic malignant melanoma and Hodgkin disease* 100, 200 mg injection ⚠ Dicarbosil; procarbazine

**dacemazine** INN

**dacisteine** INN

**dacliximab** [see: daclizumab] [USAN changed 2000]

**daclizumab** USAN, INN, BAN *immunosuppressant; monoclonal antibodies (MAb) to prevent acute rejection of organ and bone marrow transplants (orphan)*

**Dacriose** ophthalmic solution OTC *extraocular irrigating solution* [sterile isotonic solution]

**dactinomycin** USAN, USP, BAN *antibiotic antineoplastic* [also: actinomycin D]

**dacuronium bromide** INN, BAN

**DADDS (diacetyl diaminodiphenylsulfone)** [see: acedapsone]

**dagapamil** INN

**Daily Vitamins** oral liquid OTC *vitamin supplement* [multiple vitamins]

0.4• ± mg

**Dairy Ease** chewable tablets OTC *digestive aid for lactose intolerance* [lactase enzyme] 3000 U

**daisy, wild** *medicinal herb* [see: wild daisy]

**Dakin solution** [see: sodium hypochlorite]

**DAL (daunorubicin, ara-C, L-asparaginase)** *chemotherapy protocol*

**Dalacin** ⓒᴬᴺ vaginal cream ℞ *lincosamide antibiotic for bacterial vaginosis* [clindamycin phosphate] 2% (100 mg/5 g dose)

**Dalacin C** ⓒᴬᴺ capsules ℞ *lincosamide antibiotic* [clindamycin HCl] 150, 300 mg

**Dalacin C** ⓒᴬᴺ granules for oral solution ℞ *lincosamide antibiotic* [clindamycin palmitate HCl] 75 mg/5 mL

**Dalacin C Phosphate** ⓒᴬᴺ IV infusion, IM injection ℞ *lincosamide antibiotic; treatment for AIDS-related Pneumocystis carinii pneumonia* [clindamycin phosphate] 150 mg/mL

**Dalacin T** ⓒᴬᴺ topical solution ℞ *topical antibiotic for acne* [clindamycin phosphate]

**Dalalone** intra-articular, intralesional, soft tissue, or IM injection ℞ *corticosteroid; anti-inflammatory* [dexamethasone sodium phosphate] 4 mg/mL

**Dalalone D.P.** intra-articular, soft tissue, or IM injection ℞ *corticosteroid; anti-inflammatory* [dexamethasone acetate] 16 mg/mL

**Dalalone L.A.** intralesional, intra-articular, soft tissue, or IM injection ℞ *corticosteroid; anti-inflammatory* [dexamethasone acetate] 8 mg/mL

**dalanated insulin** [see: insulin, dalanated]

**dalbraminol** INN

**daledalin** INN *antidepressant* [also: daledalin tosylate]

**daledalin tosylate** USAN *antidepressant* [also: daledalin]

**dalfopristin** USAN, INN *streptogramin antibacterial antibiotic for life-threatening infections*

**dalfopristin & quinupristin** *two streptogramin antibiotics that are synergistically bactericidal to gram-positive infections; investigational (NDA filed) for pneumonia*

**Dalgan** IV, subcu, or IM injection (discontinued 2000) ℞ *narcotic agonist-antagonist analgesic* [dezocine] 5, 10, 15 mg/mL

**Dallergy** tablets, sustained-release caplets, syrup ℞ *decongestant; antihistamine; anticholinergic to dry mucosal secretions* [phenylephrine HCl; chlorpheniramine maleate; methscopolamine nitrate] 10•4•1.25 mg; 20•12•2.5 mg; 20•4•1.25 mg/10 mL

**Dallergy-D** syrup (discontinued 2002) OTC *decongestant; antihistamine* [phenylephrine HCl; chlorpheniramine maleate] 5•2 mg/5 mL

**Dallergy-JR** extended-release pediatric capsules ℞ *decongestant; antihistamine* [phenylephrine HCl; chlorpheniramine maleate] 20•4 mg

**Dalmane** capsules ℞ *benzodiazepine sedative; hypnotic; sometimes abused as a street drug* [flurazepam HCl] 15, 30 mg ⓢ Dialume

**d'Alpha E 400; d'Alpha E 1000** softgels (discontinued 2004) OTC *vitamin supplement* [vitamin E (as d-alpha tocopherol)] 400 IU; 1000 IU

**dalteparin sodium** USAN, INN, BAN *a low molecular weight heparin–type anticoagulant and antithrombotic for prevention of deep vein thrombosis (DVT), unstable angina, and myocardial infarction*

**daltroban** USAN, INN *immunosuppressive*

**Damason-P** tablets ℞ *narcotic analgesic* [hydrocodone bitartrate; aspirin] 5•500 mg

**dambose** [see: inositol]

**dametralast** INN

**damiana** *(Turnera aphrodisiaca; T. diffusa; T. microphylla)* leaves *medicinal herb for bed-wetting, bronchitis, emphysema, headache, hormonal imbalance, hot flashes, menopause, and Parkinson disease; also used as an aphrodisiac*

**damotepine** INN

**danaparoid sodium** USAN, BAN *glycosaminoglycan anticoagulant and antithrombotic for prevention of deep vein thrombosis (DVT)*

**danazol** USAN, USP, INN, BAN *anterior pituitary suppressant; gonadotropin inhibitor for endometriosis, fibrocystic breast disease, and hereditary angioedema* 50, 100, 200 mg oral

**dandelion** *(Leontodon taraxacum; Taraxacum officinale)* leaves and root *medicinal herb for anemia, analgesia, blisters, blood cleansing, blood glucose regulation, constipation, diaphoresis, dyspepsia, edema, endurance, gallbladder disease, hypertension, and liver disorders*

**daniplestim** USAN *treatment for chemotherapy-induced bone marrow suppression*

**daniquidone** BAN

**danitamon** [see: menadione]

**danitracen** INN

**Danocrine** capsules ℞ *gonadotropin inhibitor for endometriosis, fibrocystic breast disease, and hereditary angioedema* [danazol] 50, 100, 200 mg

**danofloxacin** INN *veterinary antibacterial* [also: danofloxacin mesylate]

**danofloxacin mesylate** USAN *veterinary antibacterial* [also: danofloxacin]

**danosteine** INN

**danshen** *(Salvia miltiorrhiza)* medicinal herb for abdominal pain, bruises, circulatory problems, insomnia, menstrual irregularity, and stroke; also used as an aid in granulation of wounds

**danthron** USP, BAN *(withdrawn from market by FDA)* [also: dantron] ⓢ Dantrium

**Dantrium** capsules, powder for IV injection ℞ *skeletal muscle relaxant; investigational (orphan) for neuroleptic malignant syndrome* [dantrolene sodium] 25, 50, 100 mg; 20 mg/vial (0.32 mg/mL) ⓡ danthron

**dantrolene** USAN, INN, BAN *skeletal muscle relaxant*

**dantrolene sodium** USAN, BAN *skeletal muscle relaxant; investigational (orphan) for neuroleptic malignant syndrome*

**dantron** INN *(withdrawn from market by FDA)* [also: danthron]

**Dapacin Cold** capsules (discontinued 2001) OTC *decongestant; antihistamine; analgesic* [phenylpropanolamine HCl; chlorpheniramine maleate; acetaminophen] 12.5•2•325 mg

*Daphne mezereum* medicinal herb [see: mezereon]

**dapiprazole** INN *α-adrenergic blocker; miotic; neuroleptic* [also: dapiprazole HCl]

**dapoxetine** *investigational (Phase III) agent for various urogenital indications, including premature ejaculation (PE)*

**dapsone** USAN, USP, BAN *bactericidal; leprostatic; herpetiform dermatitis suppressant; investigational (Phase III, orphan) for* Pneumocystis carinii *and* toxoplasmosis 25, 100 mg oral

**dapsone & trimethoprim** *investigational (Phase III) for* Pneumocystis carinii pneumonia

**Daptacel** IM injection ℞ *active immunizing agent for diphtheria, tetanus, and pertussis* [diphtheria & tetanus toxoids & acellular pertussis (DTaP) vaccine, adsorbed] 15 Lf•5 Lf•10 μg per 0.5 mL dose

**daptazole** [see: amiphenazole]

**daptomycin** USAN, INN, BAN *cyclic lipopeptide antibiotic for skin and skin structure infections*

**Daranide** tablets (discontinued 2004) ℞ *carbonic anhydrase inhibitor; diuretic* [dichlorphenamide] 50 mg ⓡ Daraprim

**Daraprim** tablets ℞ *antimalarial; toxoplasmosis treatment adjunct* [pyrimethamine] 25 mg ⓡ Daranide

**darbepoetin alfa** USAN *hematopoietic; recombinant erythropoietin analogue for anemia associated with chronic renal failure*

**darbufelone mesylate** USAN *antiinflammatory; antiarthritic; cyclooxygenase inhibitor; 5-lipoxygenase inhibitor*

**darenzepine** INN

**darglitazone sodium** USAN *oral hypoglycemic*

**darifenacin hydrobromide** *investigational (NDA filed) selective muscarinic $M_3$ receptor antagonist for urinary frequency, urgency, and incontinence*

**darodipine** USAN, INN *antihypertensive; bronchodilator; vasodilator*

**Darvocet A500** film-coated tablets ℞ *narcotic analgesic* [propoxyphene napsylate; acetaminophen] 100•500 mg

**Darvocet-N 50; Darvocet-N 100** tablets ℞ *narcotic analgesic* [propoxyphene napsylate; acetaminophen] 50•325 mg; 100•650 mg ⓡ Darvon-N

**Darvon** Pulvules (capsules) ℞ *narcotic analgesic* [propoxyphene HCl] 65 mg ⓡ Diovan

**Darvon Compound 32; Darvon Compound 65** Pulvules (capsules) ℞ *narcotic analgesic* [propoxyphene HCl; aspirin; caffeine] 32•389•32.4 mg; 65•389•32.4 mg ⓡ Diovan

**Darvon-N** film-coated tablets ℞ *narcotic analgesic* [propoxyphene napsylate] 100 mg ⓡ Diovan

**DAT (daunorubicin, ara-C, thioguanine)** *chemotherapy protocol for acute myelocytic leukemia (AML)* [also: DCT; TAD]

**datelliptium chloride** INN

*Datura stramonium* medicinal herb [see: jimsonweed]

**daturine hydrobromide** [see: hyoscyamine hydrobromide]

**DATVP (daunorubicin, ara-C, thioguanine, vincristine, prednisone)** *chemotherapy protocol*

*Daucus carota* medicinal herb [see: carrot]

**daunomycin** [see: daunorubicin HCl]

**daunorubicin (DNR)** INN, BAN
*anthracycline antibiotic antineoplastic for various leukemias* [also: daunorubicin HCl] ② doxorubicin

**daunorubicin citrate, liposomal**
*anthracycline antibiotic antineoplastic for advanced HIV-related Kaposi sarcoma (orphan)*

**daunorubicin HCl** USAN, USP, JAN
*anthracycline antibiotic antineoplastic for various leukemias* [also: daunorubicin] 20, 50 mg injection ② doxorubicin

**DaunoXome** IV infusion ℞ *antibiotic antineoplastic for advanced AIDS-related Kaposi sarcoma (orphan)* [daunorubicin citrate, liposomal] 2 mg/mL (50 mg/dose)

**DAV (daunorubicin, ara-C, VePesid)** *chemotherapy protocol for acute myelocytic leukemia (AML)*

**DAVA (desacetyl vinblastine amide)** [see: vindesine]

**DAVH (dibromodulcitol, Adriamycin, vincristine, Halotestin)** *chemotherapy protocol*

**davitamon** [see: menadione]

**Dayalets** Filmtabs (film-coated tablets) OTC *vitamin supplement* [multiple vitamins; folic acid] ± •0.4 mg

**Dayalets + Iron** Filmtabs (film-coated tablets) OTC *vitamin/iron supplement* [multiple vitamins; ferrous sulfate; folic acid] ± •18•0.4 mg

**Dayhist-1** tablets OTC *antihistamine* [clemastine fumarate] 1.34 mg

**Daypro** film-coated caplets ℞ *antiarthritic; nonsteroidal anti-inflammatory drug (NSAID)* [oxaprozin] 600 mg

**Daypro Alta** film-coated caplets ℞ *antiarthritic; nonsteroidal anti-inflammatory drug (NSAID)* [oxaprozin potassium] 678 mg (=600 mg base)

**DayQuil** LiquiCaps (liquid-filled gelcaps), oral liquid (discontinued 2002) OTC *antitussive; decongestant; expectorant; analgesic* [dextromethorphan hydrobromide; pseudoephedrine HCl; guaifenesin; acetamino-

phen] 10•30•100•250 mg; 3.3•10•33.3•108.3 mg/5 mL

**DayQuil Allergy Relief 4 Hour** tablets (discontinued 2001) OTC *decongestant; antihistamine* [phenylpropanolamine HCl; brompheniramine maleate] 25•4 mg

**DayQuil Allergy Relief 12 Hour** extended-release tablets (discontinued 2001) OTC *decongestant; antihistamine* [phenylpropanolamine HCl; brompheniramine maleate] 75•12 mg

**DayQuil Multi-Symptom Cold/Flu Relief** LiquiCaps (liquid-filled gelcaps), oral liquid OTC *antitussive; decongestant; analgesic* [dextromethorphan hydrobromide; pseudoephedrine HCl; acetaminophen] 10•30•250 mg; 20•60•650 mg/30 mL

**DayQuil Sinus Pressure & Pain Relief** caplets (discontinued 2002) OTC *decongestant; analgesic; antipyretic* [pseudoephedrine HCl; acetaminophen] 30•500 mg

**Dayto Himbin** tablets (discontinued 2003) ℞ *alpha$_2$-adrenergic blocker for impotence; sympatholytic; mydriatic; may have aphrodisiac activity; no FDA-approved indications* [yohimbine HCl] 5.4 mg

**Dayto Sulf** vaginal cream (discontinued 2001) ℞ *broad-spectrum bacteriostatic* [sulfathiazole; sulfacetamide; sulfabenzamide] 3.42%•2.86%•3.7%

**dazadrol** INN *antidepressant* [also: dazadrol maleate]

**dazadrol maleate** USAN *antidepressant* [also: dazadrol]

**Dazamide** tablets ℞ *carbonic anhydrase inhibitor diuretic; treatment for acute mountain sickness* [acetazolamide] 250 mg

**dazepinil** INN *antidepressant* [also: dazepinil HCl]

**dazepinil HCl** USAN *antidepressant* [also: dazepinil]

**dazidamine** INN

**dazmegrel** USAN, INN, BAN *thromboxane synthetase inhibitor*

**dazolicine** INN

**dazopride** INN *peristaltic stimulant* [also: dazopride fumarate]

**dazopride fumarate** USAN *peristaltic stimulant* [also: dazopride]

**dazoquinast** INN

**dazoxiben** INN, BAN *antithrombotic* [also: dazoxiben HCl]

**dazoxiben HCl** USAN *antithrombotic* [also: dazoxiben]

**DBED (dibenzylethylenediamine dipenicillin G)** [see: penicillin G benzathine]

**DBM (dibromomannitol)** [see: mitobronitol]

**DC** softgels OTC *laxative; stool softener* [docusate calcium] 240 mg

**DC (daunorubicin, cytarabine)** *chemotherapy protocol*

**D&C Brown No. 1 (drugs & cosmetics)** [see: resorcin brown]

**DCA (desoxycorticosterone acetate)** [q.v.]

**DCA (dichloroacetate)** [see: sodium dichloroacetate]

**DCF (2′-deoxycoformycin)** [see: pentostatin]

**DCL (descarboethoxyloratadine)** [q.v.]

**DCMP (daunorubicin, cytarabine, mercaptopurine, prednisone)** *chemotherapy protocol*

**DCPM (daunorubicin, cytarabine, prednisone, mercaptopurine)** *chemotherapy protocol*

**DCT (daunorubicin, cytarabine, thioguanine)** *chemotherapy protocol for acute myelocytic leukemia (AML)* [also: DAT; TAD]

**DCV (DTIC, CCNU, vincristine)** *chemotherapy protocol*

**DCVax-Brain** ℞ *investigational (Phase II, orphan) vaccine for glioblastoma multiforme* [dendritic cells pulsed with glioblastoma multiforme acid-eluted tumor antigens]

**DCVax-Prostate** ℞ *investigational (Phase II, orphan) vaccine for prostate cancer*

**DDAVP** tablets, nasal spray, rhinal tube, subcu or IV injection ℞ *posterior pituitary hormone for hemophilia A (orphan), von Willebrand disease (orphan), central diabetes insipidus, and nocturnal enuresis* [desmopressin acetate] 0.1, 0.2 mg; 10 μg/dose; 0.1 mg/mL; 15 μg/mL

**DDAVP (1-deamino-8-D-arginine-vasopressin)** [see: desmopressin acetate]

**DDC; ddC (dideoxycytidine)** [see: zalcitabine]

*o,p′*-**DDD** [now: mitotane]

**DDI; ddI (dideoxyinosine)** [see: didanosine]

**DDP; *cis*-DDP (diamminedichloroplatinum)** [see: cisplatin]

**DDS (diaminodiphenylsulfone)** [now: dapsone]

**DDT (dichlorodiphenyltrichloroethane)** [see: chlorophenothane]

**DDVP (dichlorovinyl dimethyl phosphate)** [see: dichlorvos]

**DEA (diethanolamine)** [q.v.]

**deacetyllanatoside C** [see: deslanoside]

**17-deacylnorgestimate** [see: norelgestromin]

**deadly nightshade** *medicinal herb* [see: belladonna]

**deadly nightshade leaf** [see: belladonna extract]

**deal pine** *medicinal herb* [see: white pine]

**1-deamino-8-D-arginine-vasopressin (DDAVP)** [see: desmopressin acetate]

**deanil** INN *combining name for radicals or groups*

**deanol** BAN [also: deanol aceglumate]

**deanol aceglumate** INN [also: deanol]

**deanol acetamidobenzoate**

**deba** [see: barbital]

**Debacterol** oral solution with swab applicator ℞ *antiseptic and analgesic for ulcerating mouth and gum lesions such as aphthous ulcers (canker sores) and necrotizing ulcerative gingivitis (pyorrhea)* [sulfuric acid; sulfonated phenol; mixed sulfonated phenolics] 50%•4%•24%

**deboxamet** INN

**debrase** *investigational (orphan) agent for debridement of acute, deep dermal burns*

**Debridase** ℞ *investigational (orphan) agent for debridement of acute, deep dermal burns* [debrase]

**Debrisan** beads, paste ℞ *debrider and cleanser for wet wounds* [dextranomer]

**debrisoquin sulfate** USAN *antihypertensive* [also: debrisoquine]

**debrisoquine** INN, BAN *antihypertensive* [also: debrisoquin sulfate]

**Debrox** ear drops OTC *agent to emulsify and disperse ear wax* [carbamide peroxide] 6.5%

**Decadron** tablets, elixir ℞ *corticosteroid; anti-inflammatory* [dexamethasone] 0.5, 0.75, 1.5, 4 mg; 0.5 mg/5 mL ⊡ Decaderm; Percodan

**Decadron Phosphate** intra-articular, intralesional, soft tissue or IM injection ℞ *corticosteroid; anti-inflammatory* [dexamethasone sodium phosphate] 4 mg/mL

**Decadron Phosphate** IV injection ℞ *corticosteroid; anti-inflammatory* [dexamethasone sodium phosphate] 24 mg/mL

**Decadron Phosphate** Ocumeter (eye drops) ℞ *topical ophthalmic corticosteroidal anti-inflammatory* [dexamethasone sodium phosphate] 0.1%

**Decadron Phosphate** ophthalmic ointment (discontinued 2000) ℞ *topical ophthalmic corticosteroidal anti-inflammatory* [dexamethasone sodium phosphate] 0.05%

**Decadron with Xylocaine** soft tissue injection ℞ *corticosteroid; anti-inflammatory* [dexamethasone sodium phosphate; lidocaine HCl] 4•10 mg/mL

**Decadron-LA** intralesional, intra-articular, soft tissue, or IM injection (discontinued 2004) ℞ *corticosteroid; anti-inflammatory* [dexamethasone acetate] 8 mg/mL

**Deca-Durabolin** IM injection ℞ *anabolic steroid for anemia of renal insufficiency; sometimes abused as a street drug* [nandrolone decanoate (in oil)] 100, 200 mg/mL

**Decagen** tablets OTC *vitamin/mineral/iron supplement* [multiple vitamins & minerals; iron; folic acid; biotin] ≛• 18 mg•0.4 mg•30 μg

**Decaject** intra-articular, intralesional, soft tissue, or IM injection ℞ *corticosteroid; anti-inflammatory* [dexamethasone sodium phosphate] 4 mg/mL

**Decaject-L.A.** intralesional, intra-articular, soft tissue, or IM injection ℞ *corticosteroid; anti-inflammatory* [dexamethasone acetate] 8 mg/mL

**DECAL (dexamethasone, etoposide, cisplatin, ara-C, L-asparaginase)** *chemotherapy protocol*

**decamethonium bromide** USP, INN [also: decamethonium iodide]

**decamethonium iodide** BAN [also: decamethonium bromide]

**decapinol** [see: delmopinol]

**decavitamin** USP

**Decholin** tablets OTC *laxative; hydrocholeretic* [dehydrocholic acid] 250 mg

**decicain** [see: tetracaine HCl]

**decil** INN *combining name for radicals or groups*

**decimemide** INN

**decitabine** USAN, INN, BAN *antineoplastic; investigational (orphan) for myelodysplastic syndromes, chronic myelogenous leukemia, and sickle cell anemia; investigational (Phase III) for multiple myeloma*

**decitropine** INN

**declaben** [now: lodelaben]

**declenperone** USAN, INN *veterinary sedative*

**Declomycin** capsules (discontinued 2003) ℞ *broad-spectrum antibiotic* [demeclocycline HCl] 150 mg

**Declomycin** film-coated tablets ℞ *broad-spectrum antibiotic* [demeclocycline HCl] 150, 300 mg

**decloxizine** INN

**Decodult** tablets OTC *decongestant; antihistamine; analgesic* [phenylephrine HCl; chlorpheniramine maleate; acetaminophen] 5•2•300 mg

**Decofed** syrup OTC *nasal decongestant* [pseudoephedrine HCl] 30 mg/5 mL

**Decohistine DH** oral liquid ℞ *narcotic antitussive; decongestant; antihis-*

*tamine* [codeine phosphate; pseudo-ephedrine HCl; chlorpheniramine maleate; alcohol 5.8%] 10•30•2 mg/5 mL

**Decolate** tablets ℞ *decongestant; antihistamine; expectorant* [phenylephrine HCl; chlorpheniramine maleate; guaifenesin] 5•4•100 mg

**decominol** INN

**Deconamine** tablets, syrup ℞ *decongestant; antihistamine* [pseudoephedrine HCl; chlorpheniramine maleate] 60•4 mg; 30•2 mg/5 mL

**Deconamine CX** tablets, oral liquid (discontinued 2002) ℞ *narcotic antitussive; decongestant; expectorant* [hydrocodone bitartrate; pseudoephedrine HCl; guaifenesin] 5•30•300 mg; 5•60•200 mg/5 mL

**Deconamine SR** sustained-release capsules ℞ *decongestant; antihistamine* [pseudoephedrine HCl; chlorpheniramine maleate] 120•8 mg

**Decongestabs** sustained-release tablets (discontinued 2001) ℞ *decongestant; antihistamine* [phenylpropanolamine HCl; phenylephrine HCl; chlorpheniramine maleate; phenyltoloxamine citrate] 40•10•5•15 mg

**Decongestant** sustained-release tablets (discontinued 2001) ℞ *decongestant; antihistamine* [phenylpropanolamine HCl; phenylephrine HCl; chlorpheniramine maleate; phenyltoloxamine citrate] 40•10•5•15 mg

**Decongestant** tablets (discontinued 2002) OTC *decongestant; antihistamine; analgesic* [phenylephrine HCl; chlorpheniramine maleate; acetaminophen] 5•2•325 mg

**Decongestant Expectorant** oral liquid (discontinued 2000) ℞ *narcotic antitussive; decongestant; expectorant* [codeine phosphate; pseudoephedrine HCl; guaifenesin; alcohol 7.5%] 10•30•100 mg/5 mL

**Deconhist L.A.** sustained-release tablets (discontinued 2001) ℞ *decongestant; antihistamine; anticholinergic* [phenylpropanolamine HCl; phenyl-

ephrine HCl; chlorpheniramine maleate; hyoscyamine sulfate; atropine sulfate; scopolamine hydrobromide] 50•25•8•0.19•0.04•0.01 mg

**Deconomed SR** sustained-release capsules ℞ *decongestant; antihistamine* [pseudoephedrine HCl; chlorpheniramine maleate] 120•8 mg

**Deconsal II** extended-release capsules ℞ *decongestant; expectorant* [phenylephrine HCl; guaifenesin] 20•375 mg

**Deconsal II** sustained-release tablets (discontinued 2004) ℞ *decongestant; expectorant* [pseudoephedrine HCl; guaifenesin] 60•600 mg ⊡ Deconal

**Deconsal Sprinkle** sustained-release capsules (discontinued 2002) ℞ *decongestant; expectorant* [phenylephrine HCl; guaifenesin] 10•300 mg ⊡ Deconal

**decoquinate** USAN, INN, BAN *coccidiostat for poultry*

**dectaflur** USAN, INN *dental caries prophylactic*

**Decylenes** ointment OTC *topical antifungal* [undecylenic acid; zinc undecylenate]

**deditonium bromide** INN

**Deep-Down Rub** OTC *analgesic; counterirritant* [methyl salicylate; menthol; camphor] 15%•5%•0.5%

**deer musk *(Moschus moschiferus)*** *natural remedy in ancient Chinese medicine; reported to have antianginal, antibacterial, antihistaminic, anti-inflammatory, CNS-depressant, and stimulant activity in clinical studies*

**deerberry** *medicinal herb* [see: holly; squaw vine; wintergreen]

**DEET (diethyltoluamide)** [q.v.]

**DeFed-60** tablets (discontinued 2002) OTC *nasal decongestant* [pseudoephedrine HCl] 60 mg

**Defen-LA** sustained-release tablets (discontinued 2004) ℞ *decongestant; expectorant* [pseudoephedrine HCl; guaifenesin] 60•600 mg

**deferasirox** *investigational (orphan) agent for chronic iron overload due to transfusion-dependent anemias*

**deferiprone** *investigational (orphan) agent for chronic iron overload due to transfusion-dependent anemias*

**deferoxamine** USAN, INN *chelating agent for acute or chronic iron poisoning* [also: desferrioxamine]

**deferoxamine HCl** USAN *chelating agent for acute or chronic iron poisoning*

**deferoxamine mesylate** USAN, USP *chelating agent for acute or chronic iron poisoning* [also: desferrioxamine mesylate]

**defibrotide** INN, BAN *investigational (orphan) agent for thrombotic thrombocytopenic purpura and hepatic veno-occlusive disease*

**Definity** injection ℞ *ultrasound contrast medium for cardiac imaging; investigational (NDA filed) for gynecologic imaging* [perflutren] 6.52 mg/mL

**deflazacort** USAN, INN, BAN *anti-inflammatory*

**Deflux** injectable gel ℞ *investigational treatment for pediatric vesicoureteral reflux (VUR)* [dextranomer microspheres in a NASHA carrier] 50 mg/mL

**defosfamide** INN

**defungit sodium salt** [see: bensuldazic acid]

**Defy** eye drops ℞ *topical ophthalmic antibiotic* [tobramycin] 0.3%

**Degas** chewable tablets OTC *antiflatulent* [simethicone] 80 mg

**Degest 2** eye drops OTC *topical ophthalmic decongestant and vasoconstrictor* [naphazoline HCl] 0.012%

**Dehistine** syrup ℞ *decongestant; antihistamine; anticholinergic to dry mucosal secretions* [phenylephrine HCl; chlorpheniramine maleate; methscopolamine nitrate] 20•4•2.5 mg/10 mL

**DEHOP (diethylhomospermine)** [q.v.]

**dehydrated alcohol** [see: alcohol, dehydrated]

**dehydrex** *investigational (orphan) for recurrent corneal erosion*

**Dehydrex** drops ℞ *investigational (orphan) treatment for recurrent corneal erosion* [dextran 70]

**dehydroacetic acid** NF *preservative*

**dehydroandrosterone** [see: prasterone]

**dehydrocholate sodium** USP [also: sodium dehydrocholate]

**7-dehydrocholesterol, activated** [now: cholecalciferol]

**dehydrocholic acid** USP, INN, BAN, JAN *choleretic; laxative; investigational (orphan) agent for congenital errors of cholesterol and bile acid synthesis* 250 mg oral

**dehydrocholin** [see: dehydrocholic acid]

**dehydroemetine** INN, BAN, DCF *investigational anti-infective for amebiasis and amebic dysentery*

**dehydroepiandrosterone (DHEA)** *natural hormone precursor; investigational (NDA filed, orphan) for systemic lupus erythematosus (SLE); investigational (orphan) replacement therapy for adrenal insufficiency*

**dehydroepiandrosterone sulfate (DHEAS)** *investigational (Phase II) injectable antiasthmatic*

**dehydroepiandrosterone sulfate sodium** *investigational (orphan) agent for re-epithelialization of serious burns and skin graft donor sites*

**Del Aqua-5; Del Aqua-10** gel (discontinued 2003) ℞ *keratolytic for acne* [benzoyl peroxide] 5%; 10%

**delanterone** INN

**Delaprem** (approved in several foreign countries) ℞ *investigational (NDA filed) tocolytic and bronchodilator* [hexoprenaline sulfate]

**delapril** INN *antihypertensive; angiotensin-converting enzyme inhibitor* [also: delapril HCl]

**delapril HCl** USAN *antihypertensive; angiotensin-converting enzyme inhibitor* [also: delapril]

**Delatestryl** IM injection ℞ *androgen replacement for testosterone deficiency in men, delayed puberty in boys, and metastatic breast cancer in women; some-*

times abused as a street drug [testosterone enanthate (in oil)] 200 mg/mL

**delavirdine** INN *antiviral; non-nucleoside reverse transcriptase inhibitor (NNRTI) for HIV and AIDS* [also: delavirdine mesylate]

**delavirdine mesylate** USAN *antiviral; investigational (Phase III) non-nucleoside reverse transcriptase inhibitor (NNRTI) for HIV and AIDS* [also: delavirdine]

**delayed-release aspirin** [see: aspirin]

**Delcap** (trademarked dosage form) *unit dispensing cap*

**Delcort** cream OTC *topical corticosteroidal anti-inflammatory* [hydrocortisone] 0.5%, 1% ☑ Dilacor

**delequamine** INN $\alpha_2$ *adrenoreceptor antagonist for sexual dysfunction* [also: delequamine HCl]

**delequamine HCl** USAN $\alpha_2$ *adrenoreceptor antagonist for sexual dysfunction* [also: delequamine]

**delergotrile** INN

**Delestrogen** IM injection ℞ *estrogen replacement therapy for the treatment of postmenopausal symptoms and prevention of postmenopausal osteoporosis; hormonal antineoplastic for prostate and metastatic breast cancers* [estradiol valerate in oil] 10, 20, 40 mg/mL

**delfantrine** INN

**delfaprazine** INN

**Delfen Contraceptive** vaginal foam OTC *spermicidal contraceptive* [nonoxynol 9] 12.5%

**delmadinone** INN, BAN *progestin; antiandrogen; antiestrogen* [also: delmadinone acetate]

**delmadinone acetate** USAN *progestin; antiandrogen; antiestrogen* [also: delmadinone]

**delmetacin** INN

**delmopinol** INN

**Del·Mycin** topical solution (discontinued 2003) ℞ *antibiotic for acne* [erythromycin] 2%

**delnav** [see: dioxathion]

**delorazepam** INN

**deloxolone** INN

*m*-**delphene** [see: diethyltoluamide]

**delprostenate** INN, BAN

**Delsym** extended-release oral suspension OTC *antitussive* [dextromethorphan polistirex] 30 mg/5 mL

**Delta-Cortef** tablets ℞ *corticosteroid; anti-inflammatory* [prednisolone] 5 mg

**deltacortone** [see: prednisone]

**Delta-D** tablets OTC *vitamin supplement* [cholecalciferol (vitamin $D_3$)] 400 IU

**deltafilcon A** USAN *hydrophilic contact lens material*

**deltafilcon B** USAN *hydrophilic contact lens material*

**delta-1-hydrocortisone** [see: prednisolone]

**Deltasone** tablets ℞ *corticosteroid; anti-inflammatory* [prednisone] 2.5, 5, 10, 20 mg

**delta-9-tetrahydrocannabinol (THC)** [see: dronabinol]

**delta-9-THC (tetrahydrocannabinol)** [see: dronabinol]

**Delta-Tritex** cream, ointment ℞ *topical corticosteroidal anti-inflammatory* [triamcinolone acetonide] 0.1%

**Deltavac** vaginal cream ℞ *broad-spectrum antibiotic; antiseptic; vulnerary* [sulfanilamide; aminacrine HCl; allantoin] 15%•0.2%•2%

**deltibant** USAN *bradykinin antagonist for treatment of systemic inflammatory response syndrome*

**deltra-stab** [see: prednisolone]

**delucemine HCl** USAN *NMDA receptor antagonist; neuroprotectant*

**Demadex** tablets, IV injection ℞ *antihypertensive; loop diuretic* [torsemide] 5, 10, 20, 100 mg; 10 mg/mL

**Demazin** Repetabs (repeat-action tablets), syrup (discontinued 2001) OTC *decongestant; antihistamine* [phenylpropanolamine HCl; chlorpheniramine maleate] 25•4 mg; 12.5•2 mg/5 mL

**dembrexine** INN, BAN

**dembroxol** [see: dembrexine]

**demecarium bromide** USP, INN, BAN *antiglaucoma agent; reversible cholinesterase inhibitor miotic*

**demeclocycline** USP, BAN *tetracycline antibiotic*

**demeclocycline HCl** USP, BAN *tetracycline antibiotic; antirickettsial* 150, 300 mg oral

**demecolcine** INN, BAN

**demecycline** USAN, INN *antibacterial*

**demegestone** INN

**demekastigmine bromide** [see: demecarium bromide]

**demelverine** INN

**Demerol** tablets, syrup, IV or IM injection ℞ *narcotic analgesic; also abused as a street drug* [meperidine HCl] 50, 100 mg; 50 mg/5 mL; 25, 50, 75, 100 mg/mL

**demetacin** [see: delmetacin]

**11-demethoxyreserpine** [see: deserpidine]

**demethylchlortetracycline (DMCT)** [now: demeclocycline]

**demethylchlortetracycline HCl** [see: demeclocycline HCl]

**N-demethylcodeine** [see: norcodeine]

**demexiptiline** INN

**Demi-Regroton** tablets ℞ *antihypertensive; diuretic* [chlorthalidone; reserpine] 25•0.125 mg

**democonazole** INN

**demoxepam** USAN, INN *minor tranquilizer*

**demoxytocin** INN

**Demser** capsules ℞ *antihypertensive for pheochromocytoma* [metyrosine] 250 mg

**demulcents** *a class of agents that soothe irritated or abraded tissues, particularly mucous membranes*

**Demulen 1/35; Demulen 1/50** tablets (in Compacks of 21 or 28) ℞ *monophasic oral contraceptive* [ethynodiol diacetate; ethinyl estradiol] 1 mg•35 μg; 1 mg•50 μg ⊘ Demerol; Demolin

**denatonium benzoate** USAN, NF, INN, BAN *alcohol denaturant; flavoring agent*

**denaverine** INN

**Denavir** cream ℞ *antiviral for recurrent herpes labialis* [penciclovir] 1%

**denbufylline** INN, BAN

**dendritic cells pulsed with glioblastoma multiforme acid-eluted tumor antigens** *investigational (orphan) agent for glioblastoma multiforme*

**denileukin diftitox** USAN, INN *antineoplastic for cutaneous T-cell lymphoma (orphan)*

**denipride** INN

**denofungin** USAN *antifungal; antibacterial*

**denopamine** INN

**Denorex** shampoo (discontinued 2003) OTC *antiseborrheic; antipsoriatic; antipruritic; antibacterial* [coal tar; menthol; alcohol] 9%•1.5•7.5%; 12.5%•1.5%•10.4%

**Denorex Everyday Dandruff** shampoo OTC *antiseborrheic; antibacterial; antifungal* [pyrithione zinc] 2%

**denpidazone** INN

**Denquel** toothpaste OTC *tooth desensitizer* [potassium nitrate] 5%

**Denta 5000 Plus** dental cream ℞ *topical caries preventative* [sodium fluoride] 1.1%

**DentaGel** ℞ *topical dental caries preventative* [sodium fluoride] 1.1%

**dental antiformin** [see: antiformin, dental]

**dental-type silica** [see: silica, dental-type]

**Dentipatch** transmucosal patch ℞ *mucous membrane anesthetic* [lidocaine HCl] 23, 46.1 mg

**Dent's Lotion-Jel** lotion/gel OTC *mucous membrane anesthetic* [benzocaine]

**Dent's Toothache Gum; Dent's Toothache Drops** OTC *topical oral anesthetic* [benzocaine]

**denyl sodium** [see: phenytoin sodium]

**denzimol** INN

**deodorants** *a class of agents that mask undesirable or offensive odors* [also called: antibromics]

**2'-deoxycoformycin (DCF)** [see: pentostatin]

**deoxycorticosterone acetate** [see: desoxycorticosterone acetate]

**deoxycorticosterone pivalate** [see: desoxycorticosterone pivalate]

**deoxycortolone pivalate** BAN *salt-regulating adrenocortical steroid* [also: desoxycorticosterone pivalate]

**deoxycortone** BAN *salt-regulating adrenocortical steroid* [also: desoxycorticosterone acetate; desoxycortone]

**2′-deoxycytidine** *investigational (orphan) host-protective agent in acute myelogenous leukemia*

**deoxyephedrine HCl** [see: methamphetamine HCl]

**12-deoxyerythromycin** [see: berythromycin]

**deoxyribonuclease, recombinant human (rhDNase)** [see: dornase alfa]

**deoxyribonucleic acid (DNA)**

**15-deoxyspergualin trihydrochloride** [now: gusperimus trihydrochloride]

**Depacin** capsules OTC *analgesic; antipyretic* [acetaminophen] 325 mg

**Depacon** IV infusion R *anticonvulsant* [valproate sodium] 500 mg/vial

**Depade** tablets R *narcotic antagonist for opiate dependence or overdose (orphan) and alcoholism* [naltrexone HCl] 50 mg

**Depakene** capsules R *anticonvulsant* [valproic acid] 250 mg

**Depakene** syrup R *anticonvulsant* [valproate sodium] 250 mg/5 mL

**Depakote** delayed-release enteric-coated tablets R *anticonvulsant; antipsychotic for manic episodes of a bipolar disorder; migraine prophylaxis* [divalproex sodium] 125, 250, 500 mg

**Depakote** sprinkle capsules R *anticonvulsant* [divalproex sodium] 125 mg

**Depakote ER** extended-release tablets R *anticonvulsant; antipsychotic for manic episodes of a bipolar disorder; migraine prophylaxis* [divalproex sodium] 250, 500 mg

**depAndro 100; depAndro 200** IM injection (discontinued 2001) R *androgen replacement for delayed puberty or breast cancer* [testosterone cypionate] 100 mg/mL; 200 mg/mL

**Depen** titratable tablets R *metal chelating agent for rheumatoid arthritis, Wilson disease, and cystinuria* [penicillamine] 250 mg

**depepsen** [see: sodium amylosulfate]

**depGynogen** IM injection (discontinued 2003) R *estrogen replacement therapy for the treatment of postmenopausal symptoms* [estradiol cypionate in oil] 5 mg/mL

**depMedalone 40; depMedalone 80** intralesional, soft tissue, and IM injection R *corticosteroid; anti-inflammatory; immunosuppressant* [methylprednisolone acetate] 40 mg/mL; 80 mg/mL

**DepoCyt** sustained-release intrathecal injection R *antineoplastic for lymphomatous neoplastic meningitis (NM) arising from solid tumors or non-Hodgkin lymphoma (orphan)* [cytarabine, liposomal] 10 mg/mL

**DepoDur** extended-release injection R *narcotic analgesic* [morphine sulfate] 10 mg/mL

**Depo-Estradiol** IM injection R *synthetic estrogen; hormone replacement therapy for the treatment of postmenopausal symptoms* [estradiol cypionate in oil] 5 mg/mL

**DepoGen** IM injection (discontinued 2003) R *estrogen replacement therapy for the treatment of postmenopausal symptoms* [estradiol cypionate in oil] 5 mg/mL

**Depoject** intralesional, soft tissue, and IM injection R *corticosteroid; anti-inflammatory; immunosuppressant* [methylprednisolone acetate] 40, 80 mg/mL

**Depo-Medrol** intralesional, soft tissue, and IM injection R *corticosteroid; anti-inflammatory; immunosuppressant* [methylprednisolone acetate] 20, 40, 80 mg/mL

**DepoMorphine** R *investigational (Phase II) sustained-release, encapsulated formulation to treat severe postsurgical pain* [morphine sulfate]

**Deponit** transdermal patch ℞ *antianginal; vasodilator* [nitroglycerin] 16, 32 mg (0.2, 0.4 mg/hr.)

**Depopred-40; Depopred-80** intralesional, soft tissue, and IM injection ℞ *corticosteroid; anti-inflammatory; immunosuppressant* [methylprednisolone acetate] 40 mg/mL; 80 mg/mL

**Depo-Provera** IM injection ℞ *hormonal antineoplastic adjunct for metastatic endometrial and renal carcinoma; long-term injectable contraceptive* [medroxyprogesterone acetate] 150, 400 mg/mL

**Depotest 100; Depotest 200** IM injection (discontinued 2001) ℞ *androgen replacement for delayed puberty or breast cancer* [testosterone cypionate] 100 mg/mL; 200 mg/mL

**Depo-Testadiol** IM injection (discontinued 2004) ℞ *hormone replacement therapy for postmenopausal symptoms* [estradiol cypionate; testosterone cypionate] 2•50 mg/mL

**Depotestogen** IM injection (discontinued 2003) ℞ *hormone replacement therapy for postmenopausal symptoms* [estradiol cypionate; testosterone cypionate] 2•50 mg/mL

**Depo-Testosterone** IM injection ℞ *androgen replacement for testosterone deficiency in men; sometimes abused as a street drug* [testosterone cypionate (in oil)] 100, 200 mg/mL

**depramine** INN [also: balipramine]

**deprenyl (L-deprenyl)** [see: selegiline HCl]

**depreotide** USAN *radiopharmaceutical imaging agent for lung cancer; investigational (NDA filed) for malignant melanoma and neuroendocrine tumors*

**depressants** *a class of agents that reduce functional activity and vital energy in general by producing muscular relaxation and diaphoresis*

**deprodone** INN, BAN

**Deproic** ⓒᴬᴺ capsules, syrup (discontinued 2001) ℞ *anticonvulsant* [valproic acid] 250, 500 mg; 250 mg/5 mL

**Deproist Expectorant with Codeine** oral liquid (discontinued 2002) ℞ *narcotic antitussive; decongestant; expectorant* [codeine phosphate; pseudoephedrine HCl; guaifenesin; alcohol 8.2%] 10•30•100 mg/5 mL

**deprostil** USAN, INN *gastric antisecretory*

**deptropine** INN, BAN

**deptropine citrate** [see: deptropine]

**depurants; depuratives** *a class of agents that purify or cleanse the system, particularly the blood* [also called: pellants]

**dequalinium chloride** INN, BAN

**Dequasine** tablets OTC *dietary supplement* [multiple minerals & amino acids; vitamin C] ≜•200 mg

**deracoxib** USAN *COX-2 inhibitor anti-inflammatory and analgesic for osteoarthritis and rheumatoid arthritis*

**deramciclane** *serotonin 5-HT₂ receptor antagonist; investigational (Phase III) antidepressant and anxiolytic for general anxiety disorder (GAD)*

**Derifil** tablets OTC *systemic deodorant for ostomy, breath, and body odors* [chlorophyllin] 100 mg

**Derma Viva** lotion (discontinued 2004) OTC *moisturizer; emollient*

**Dermabase** OTC *cream base*

**Dermabond** topical liquid OTC *skin adhesive for closing surgical incisions and traumatic lacerations*

**Dermacoat** aerosol OTC *topical local anesthetic* [benzocaine] 4.5%

**Dermacort** cream, lotion ℞ *corticosteroidal anti-inflammatory* [hydrocortisone] 1% ⊡ DermiCort

**DermaFlex** gel OTC *local anesthetic* [lidocaine] 2.5%

**Dermal-Rub** balm OTC *analgesic; counterirritant* [methyl salicylate; camphor; racemic manthol; cajuput oil]

**Dermamycin** cream, spray OTC *antihistamine* [diphenhydramine HCl] 2%

**Derma-Pax** lotion OTC *antihistamine; antiseptic; antipruritic* [pyrilamine maleate; chlorpheniramine maleate; alcohol 35%] 0.44%•0.06%

**Dermarest** gel OTC *antihistamine; antifungal* [diphenhydramine HCl; resorcinol] 2%•2%

**Dermarest Dricort Creme** OTC *corticosteroidal anti-inflammatory* [hydrocortisone acetate] 1%

**Dermarest Plus** gel, spray OTC *antihistamine; analgesic; counterirritant* [diphenhydramine HCl; menthol] 2%•1%

**Dermasept Antifungal** spray liquid OTC *antifungal; antiseptic; anesthetic; astringent* [tolnaftate; tannic acid; zinc chloride; benzocaine; methylbenzethonium HCl; undecylenic acid; alcohol 58.54%] 1.017%•6.098%•5.081%•2.032%•3.049%•5.081%

**Dermasil** lotion OTC *bath emollient*

**Derma-Smoothe/FS** oil R *corticosteroidal anti-inflammatory; emollient* [fluocinolone acetonide] 0.01%

**dermatan sulfate** [see: danaparoid sodium]

**dermatol** [see: bismuth subgallate]

**Dermatop E** cream, ointment R *corticosteroidal anti-inflammatory* [prednicarbate] 0.1%

**DermaVite** tablets OTC *vitamin/mineral supplement* [multiple vitamins & minerals; folic acid; biotin] ≐•400•600 μg

**Dermazinc** shampoo OTC *antiseborrheic; antibacterial; antifungal* [pyrithione zinc] 0.25%

**Derm-Cleanse** topical liquid OTC *soap-free therapeutic skin cleanser*

**Dermol HC** anorectal cream, anorectal ointment R *corticosteroidal anti-inflammatory* [hydrocortisone] 1%, 2.5%; 1%

**Dermolate Anti-Itch** cream OTC *corticosteroidal anti-inflammatory* [hydrocortisone] 0.5%

**Dermolin** liniment OTC *analgesic; counterirritant; antiseptic* [methyl salicylate; camphor; racemic menthol; mustard oil; alcohol 8%]

**Dermoplast** aerosol spray, lotion OTC *local anesthetic; analgesic* [benzocaine; menthol] 20%•0.5%; 8%•0.5%

**Dermovan** OTC *cream base*

**Dermprotective Factor (DPF)** (trademarked ingredient) *aromatic syrup* [eriodictyon]

**Dermtex HC with Aloe** cream OTC *corticosteroidal anti-inflammatory* [hydrocortisone] 0.5%

**Dermuspray** aerosol spray R *enzyme for wound debridement* [trypsin; peruvian balsam] 0.1•72.5 mg/0.82 mL

**derpanicate** INN

**DES (diethylstilbestrol)** [q.v.]

**desacetyl vinblastine amide (DAVA)** [see: vindesine]

**desacetyl-lanatoside C** [see: deslanoside]

**desaglybuzole** [see: glybuzole]

**desamino-oxytocin** [see: demoxytocin]

**desaspidin** INN

**descarboethoxyloratadine (DCL)** *investigational antihistamine for allergy*

**desciclovir** USAN, INN *antiviral*

**descinolone** INN *corticosteroid; anti-inflammatory* [also: descinolone acetonide]

**descinolone acetonide** USAN *corticosteroid; anti-inflammatory* [also: descinolone]

**Desenex** cream OTC *antifungal* [clotrimazole] 1%

**Desenex** foam, soap OTC *antifungal* [undecylenic acid] 10%

**Desenex** powder, aerosol powder, ointment, cream OTC *antifungal* [undecylenic acid; zinc undecylenate] 25% total

**Desenex, Prescription Strength** spray liquid, spray powder OTC *antifungal* [miconazole nitrate] 2%

**Desenex Antifungal** cream OTC *antifungal* [miconazole nitrate] 2%

**DesenexMax** cream OTC *allylamine antifungal* [terbinafine HCl] 1%

**deserpidine** INN, BAN *antihypertensive; peripheral antiadrenergic; rauwolfia derivative* ☒ desipramine

**desert herb; desert tea** *medicinal herb* [see: ephedra]

**Desert Pure Calcium** film-coated tablets OTC *calcium supplement* [calcium carbonate; vitamin D] 500 mg•125 IU

**Desferal** powder for IM, IV, or subcu injection ℞ *chelating agent for acute or chronic iron poisoning* [deferoxamine mesylate] 500, 2000 mg ☒ Disophrol

**desferrioxamine** BAN *chelating agent for acute or chronic iron poisoning* [also: deferoxamine]

**desferrioxamine mesylate** BAN *chelating agent for acute or chronic iron poisoning* [also: deferoxamine mesylate]

**desflurane** USAN, INN *inhalation general anesthetic*

**desglugastrin** INN

**desipramine** INN, BAN *tricyclic antidepressant* [also: desipramine HCl] ☒ deserpidine

**desipramine HCl** USAN, USP *tricyclic antidepressant* [also: desipramine] 10, 25, 50, 75, 100, 150 mg oral

**desirudin** USAN *anticoagulant; thrombin inhibitor for the prevention of deep vein thrombosis (DVT) in elective hip replacement surgery*

**Desitin** ointment OTC *moisturizer; emollient; astringent; antiseptic* [cod liver oil; zinc oxide]

**Desitin Creamy** ointment OTC *topical diaper rash treatment* [zinc oxide] 10%

**Desitin with Zinc Oxide** powder OTC *topical diaper rash treatment* [zinc oxide; corn starch] 10%•88.2%

**deslanoside** USP, INN, BAN *cardiotonic; cardiac glycoside*

**desloratadine** USAN *second-generation peripherally selective piperidine antihistamine for allergic rhinitis and chronic idiopathic urticaria; active metabolite of loratadine*

**deslorelin** USAN, INN *LHRH agonist; investigational (orphan) for central precocious puberty*

**desmethylmoramide** INN

**desmophosphamide** [see: defosfamide]

**desmopressin** INN, BAN *posterior pituitary antidiuretic hormone (ADH)* [also: desmopressin acetate]

**desmopressin acetate** USAN *antidiuretic; posterior pituitary antidiuretic hormone for hemophilia A (orphan), von Willebrand disease (orphan), and nocturnal enuresis* [also: desmopressin] 4 μg/mL injection; 10 μg nasal spray

**desocriptine** INN

**Desogen** tablets (in packs of 28) ℞ *monophasic oral contraceptive* [desogestrel; ethinyl estradiol] 0.15 mg•30 μg

**desogestrel** USAN, INN, BAN *progestin*

**desolone** [see: deprodone]

**desomorphine** INN, BAN

**desonide** USAN, INN, BAN *topical corticosteroidal anti-inflammatory* 0.05% topical

**DesOwen** ointment, cream, lotion ℞ *corticosteroidal anti-inflammatory* [desonide] 0.05%

**Desoxi** ⓐ cream, gel ℞ *corticosteroidal anti-inflammatory* [desoximetasone] 0.05%, 0.25%; 0.05%

**desoximetasone** USAN, USP, INN *topical corticosteroidal anti-inflammatory* [also: desoxymethasone] 0.05%, 0.25% topical ☒ dexamethasone

**desoxycholic acid** *increases secretion of bile acids*

**desoxycorticosterone acetate (DCA; DOCA)** USP *salt-regulating adrenocortical steroid* [also: desoxycortone; deoxycortone]

**desoxycorticosterone pivalate** USP *salt-regulating adrenocortical steroid* [also: deoxycortolone pivalate]

**desoxycorticosterone trimethylacetate** USP

**desoxycortone** INN *salt-regulating adrenocortical steroid* [also: desoxycorticosterone acetate; deoxycortone]

**l-desoxyephedrine** [see: levmetamfetamine]

**desoxyephedrine HCl** [see: methamphetamine HCl]

**desoxymethasone** BAN *topical corticosteroidal anti-inflammatory* [also: desoximetasone]

**Desoxyn** Gradumets (sustained-release tablets) (discontinued 2002) ℞ *CNS* stimulant; sometimes abused as a street drug [methamphetamine HCl] 5, 10, 15 mg ⊘ digitoxin; digoxin

**Desoxyn** tablets ℞ *CNS stimulant; sometimes abused as a street drug* [methamphetamine HCl] 5 mg ⊘ digitoxin; digoxin

**desoxyribonuclease** [see: fibrinolysin & desoxyribonuclease]

**Despec** oral liquid (discontinued 2002) ℞ *decongestant; expectorant* [phenylephrine HCl; phenylpropanolamine HCl; guaifenesin] 20•5•100 mg/5 mL

**Desquam-E** gel (discontinued 2003) ℞ *keratolytic for acne* [benzoyl peroxide] 2.5%

**Desquam-E 5; Desquam-E 10** gel ℞ *keratolytic for acne* [benzoyl peroxide] 5%; 10%

**Desquam-X** cleansing bar ℞ *keratolytic for acne* [benzoyl peroxide] 10%

**Desquam-X 5; Desquam-X 10** gel ℞ *keratolytic for acne* [benzoyl peroxide] 5%; 10%

**Desquam-X 5 Wash; Desquam-X 10 Wash** topical liquid (discontinued 2003) ℞ *keratolytic for acne* [benzoyl peroxide] 5%; 10%

**de-Stat 3; de-Stat 4** solution OTC *cleaning/disinfecting/soaking solution for rigid gas permeable contact lenses*

**destradiol** [see: estradiol]

**63-desulfohirudin** [see: desirudin]

**Desyrel** film-coated tablets, Dividose (multiple-scored tablets) ℞ *antidepressant used for panic disorders, aggressive behavior, alcoholism, and cocaine withdrawal* [trazodone HCl] 50, 100 mg; 150, 300 mg

**DET (diethyltryptamine)** [q.v.]

**Detachol** topical liquid OTC *adhesive remover for the skin*

**detajmium bitartrate** INN

**Detane** gel OTC *topical local anesthetic* [benzocaine] 7.5%

**detanosal** INN

**Detect-A-Strep** slide tests for professional use *in vitro diagnostic aid for streptococcal antigens in throat swabs*

**Detecto-Seal** (trademarked packaging form) *tamper-resistant parenteral package*

**deterenol** INN *ophthalmic adrenergic* [also: deterenol HCl]

**deterenol HCl** USAN *ophthalmic adrenergic* [also: deterenol]

**detergents** *a class of agents that cleanse wounds and sores*

**detigon HCl** [see: chlophedianol HCl]

**detirelix** INN *luteinizing hormone-releasing hormone (LHRH) antagonist* [also: detirelix acetate]

**detirelix acetate** USAN *luteinizing hormone-releasing hormone (LHRH) antagonist* [also: detirelix]

**detomidine** INN, BAN *veterinary analgesic; sedative* [also: detomidine HCl]

**detomidine HCl** USAN *veterinary analgesic; sedative* [also: detomidine]

**detorubicin** INN

**Detox-B** ℞ *investigational (Phase III) adjuvant to Theratope-STn for breast cancer*

**detralfate** INN

**Detrol** film-coated tablets ℞ *muscarinic receptor antagonist for urinary frequency, urgency, and incontinence* [tolterodine tartrate] 1, 2 mg

**Detrol LA** extended-release capsules ℞ *muscarinic receptor antagonist for urinary frequency, urgency, and incontinence* [tolterodine tartrate] 2, 4 mg

**detrothyronine** INN

**Detrusitol** (European name for U.S. product Detrol)

**Detussin** oral liquid ℞ *narcotic antitussive; decongestant* [hydrocodone bitartrate; pseudoephedrine HCl; alcohol 5%] 5•60 mg/5 mL

**Detussin Expectorant** oral liquid (discontinued 2002) ℞ *narcotic antitussive; decongestant; expectorant* [hydrocodone bitartrate; pseudoephedrine HCl; guaifenesin; alcohol] 5•60•200 mg/5 mL

**deuterium oxide** USAN *radioactive agent*

**devapamil** INN

**devazepide** USAN *cholecystokinin antagonist*

**devil's bones** *medicinal herb* [see: wild yam]

**devil's claw (Harpagophytum procumbens)** root *medicinal herb for arrhythmias, arteriosclerosis, arthritis, blood cleansing, diabetes, hypertension, liver disease, lowering cholesterol, rheumatism, stomach disorders, and strengthening bladder and kidneys*

**devil's club (Echinopanax horridum; Fatsia horrida; Oplopanax horridus; Panax horridum)** cambium and stem *medicinal herb for arthritis, burns and cuts, colds, cough, fever, inducing vomiting and bowel evacuation, pneumonia, and tuberculosis*

**devil's dung** *medicinal herb* [see: asafetida]

**devil's eye** *medicinal herb* [see: henbane]

**devil's fuge** *medicinal herb* [see: mistletoe]

**devil's shrub** *medicinal herb* [see: Siberian ginseng]

**Devrom** chewable tablets OTC *systemic deodorizer for ostomy and incontinence odors* [bismuth subgallate] 200 mg

**dewberry** *medicinal herb* [see: blackberry]

**Dex GG TR** timed-release tablets ℞ *antitussive; expectorant* [dextromethorphan hydrobromide; guaifenesin] 60•1000 mg

**Dex4 Glucose** chewable tablets OTC *glucose elevating agent* [glucose]

**dexa** [see: dexamethasone]

**Dexacidin** eye drop suspension ℞ *ophthalmic corticosteroidal anti-inflammatory; antibiotic* [dexamethasone; neomycin sulfate; polymyxin B sulfate] 0.1%•0.35%•10 000 U/mL

**Dexacidin** ophthalmic ointment (name changed to Dexacine in 2002)

**Dexacine** ophthalmic ointment (discontinued 2004) ℞ *corticosteroidal anti-inflammatory; antibiotic* [dexamethasone; neomycin sulfate; polymyxin B sulfate] 0.1%•0.35%•10 000 U/g

**Dexacort Phosphate** Respihaler (oral inhalation aerosol) ℞ *corticosteroid for bronchial asthma* [dexamethasone sodium phosphate] 84 μg/dose

**Dexacort Phosphate** Turbinaire (nasal inhalation aerosol) ℞ *intranasal corticosteroidal anti-inflammatory* [dexamethasone sodium phosphate; alcohol 2%] 84 μg/dose

**Dexafed Cough** syrup (discontinued 2002) OTC *antitussive; decongestant; expectorant* [dextromethorphan hydrobromide; phenylephrine HCl; guaifenesin] 10•5•100 mg/5 mL

**DexAlone** liquid-filled gelcaps OTC *antitussive* [dextromethorphan hydrobromide] 30 mg

**Dexameth** tablets ℞ *corticosteroid; anti-inflammatory* [dexamethasone] 0.5, 0.75, 1.5, 4 mg

**dexamethasone** USP, INN, BAN *corticosteroidal anti-inflammatory; investigational (orphan) for idiopathic intermediate uveitis* 0.25, 0.5, 0.75, 1, 1.5, 2, 4, 6 mg oral; 0.5 mg/5 mL oral; 0.5 mg/0.5 mL oral ⊡ desoximetasone

**dexamethasone acefurate** USAN, INN *corticosteroidal anti-inflammatory*

**dexamethasone acetate** USAN, USP, BAN *corticosteroidal anti-inflammatory* 8 mg/mL injection

**dexamethasone dipropionate** USAN *corticosteroidal anti-inflammatory*

**dexamethasone & neomycin sulfate & polymyxin B sulfate** *topical ophthalmic corticosteroidal anti-inflammatory and antibiotic* 0.1%•0.35%•10 000 U/mL eye drops

**dexamethasone sodium phosphate** USP, BAN *corticosteroid; anti-inflammatory* 0.05%, 0.1% eye drops; 4, 10 mg/mL injection

**dexamfetamine** INN *CNS stimulant* [also: dextroamphetamine; dexamphetamine]

**dexamisole** USAN, INN *antidepressant*

**dexamphetamine** BAN *CNS stimulant* [also: dextroamphetamine; dexamfetamine]

**Dexaphen S.A.** sustained-release tablets (discontinued 2002) ℞ *decongestant; antihistamine* [pseudoephedrine sulfate; dexbrompheniramine maleate] 120•6 mg

**Dexasone** intra-articular, intralesional, soft tissue, or IM injection ℞ *corticosteroid; anti-inflammatory* [dexamethasone sodium phosphate] 4 mg/mL

**Dexasone L.A.** intralesional, intra-articular, soft tissue, or IM injection ℞ *corticosteroid; anti-inflammatory* [dexamethasone acetate] 8 mg/mL

**Dexasporin** ophthalmic ointment ℞ *topical ophthalmic corticosteroidal anti-inflammatory; antibiotic* [dexamethasone; neomycin sulfate; polymyxin B sulfate] 0.1%•0.35%•10 000 U/g

**Dexatrim** extended-release tablets, timed-release capsules (discontinued 2001) OTC *diet aid* [phenylpropanolamine HCl] 75 mg

**Dexatrim plus Vitamin C** timed-release capsules (discontinued 2001) OTC *diet aid* [phenylpropanolamine HCl; vitamin C] 75•180 mg

**Dexatrim Pre-Meal** timed-release capsules (discontinued 2001) OTC *diet aid* [phenylpropanolamine HCl] 25 mg

**dexbrompheniramine** INN, BAN *alkylamine antihistamine* [also: dexbrompheniramine maleate]

**dexbrompheniramine maleate** USP *alkylamine antihistamine* [also: dexbrompheniramine]

**dexchlorpheniramine** INN *alkylamine antihistamine* [also: dexchlorpheniramine maleate]

**dexchlorpheniramine maleate** USP *alkylamine antihistamine* [also: dexchlorpheniramine] 4, 6 mg oral

**dexchlorpheniramine tannate** *alkylamine antihistamine*

**dexclamol** INN *sedative* [also: dexclamol HCl]

**dexclamol HCl** USAN *sedative* [also: dexclamol]

**Dexedrine** Spansules (sustained-release capsules), tablets ℞ *amphetamine; CNS stimulant; widely abused as a street drug* [dextroamphetamine sulfate] 5, 10, 15 mg; 5 mg Ⓓ dextran

**dexetimide** USAN, INN, BAN *anticholinergic*

**dexetozoline** INN

**dexfenfluramine** INN, BAN *anorexiant; appetite suppressant; serotonin reuptake inhibitor* [also: dexfenfluramine HCl]

**dexfenfluramine HCl** USAN *anorexiant; appetite suppressant; serotonin reuptake inhibitor* [also: dexfenfluramine]

**DexFerrum** IV or IM injection ℞ *hematinic* [iron dextran] 50 mg/mL

**DexFol** tablets ℞ *vitamin B supplement* [vitamins B$_1$, B$_2$, B$_3$, B$_5$, B$_6$, B$_{12}$, and C; folic acid; biotin] 1.5•1.5•20•10•50•1•60•5•0.3 mg

**dexibuprofen** USAN, INN *analgesic; cyclooxygenase inhibitor; anti-inflammatory*

**dexibuprofen lysine** USAN *analgesic; cyclooxygenase inhibitor; anti-inflammatory* [also: dexibuprofen]

**deximafen** USAN, INN *antidepressant*

**dexindoprofen** INN

**Dexiron** Ⓒ IM injection ℞ *hematinic* [iron dextran] 50 mg/mL

**dexivacaine** USAN, INN *anesthetic*

**dexlofexidine** INN

**dexmedetomidine** USAN, INN, BAN *sedative*

**dexmedetomidine HCl** *sedative for intubated and ventilated patients in an intensive care setting; premedication to anesthesia*

**dexmethylphenidate HCl** CNS *stimulant for attention-deficit hyperactivity disorder (ADHD) and narcolepsy; active isomer of methylphenidate HCl*

**dexnorgestrel acetime** [now: norgestimate]

**Dexone** intra-articular, intralesional, soft tissue, or IM injection ℞ *corticosteroid; anti-inflammatory* [dexamethasone sodium phosphate] 4 mg/mL

**Dexone** tablets ℞ *corticosteroid; anti-inflammatory* [dexamethasone] 0.5, 0.75, 1.5, 4 mg

**Dexone LA** intralesional, intra-articular, soft tissue, or IM injection ℞

corticosteroid; anti-inflammatory [dex-amethasone acetate] 8 mg/mL

**dexormaplatin** USAN, INN antineoplastic

**dexoxadrol** INN CNS stimulant; analgesic [also: dexoxadrol HCl]

**dexoxadrol HCl** USAN CNS stimulant; analgesic [also: dexoxadrol]

**dexpanthenol** USAN, USP, INN, BAN cholinergic; antipruritic; postoperative prophylaxis for paralytic ileus 250 mg/mL injection

**dexpemedolac** USAN analgesic

**dexpropranolol HCl** USAN antiarrhythmic; antiadrenergic (β-receptor) [also: dexpropranolol]

**dexproxibutene** INN

**dexrazoxane** USAN, INN, BAN cardioprotectant for doxorubicin-induced cardiomyopathy (orphan); chelates intracellular iron

**dexsecoverine** INN

**dexsotalol HCl** USAN class III antiarrhythmic

**dextilidine** INN

**dextran** INN, BAN blood flow adjuvant; plasma volume extender [also: dextran 40] ⑨ Dexedrine; dextrin

**dextran, high molecular weight** [see: dextran 70]

**dextran, low molecular weight** [see: dextran 40]

**dextran 1** monovalent hapten for prevention of dextran-induced anaphylactic reactions; investigational (orphan) for cystic fibrosis

**dextran 40** USAN blood flow adjuvant; plasma volume extender [also: dextran] 10% injection

**dextran 70** USAN plasma volume extender; viscosity-increasing agent; investigational (orphan) for recurrent corneal erosion 6% injection

**dextran 75** USAN plasma volume extender; viscosity-increasing agent 6% injection

**dextran sulfate** investigational (orphan) inhalant for cystic fibrosis

**dextran sulfate, sodium salt, aluminum complex** [see: detralfate]

**dextran sulfate sodium** investigational (orphan) agent for AIDS

**dextranomer** INN, BAN wound cleanser and debrider

**dextrates** USAN, NF tablet binder and diluent

**dextriferron** NF, INN, BAN

**dextrin** NF, BAN suspending agent; tablet binder and diluent ⑨ dextran

**dextroamphetamine** USAN CNS stimulant; widely abused as a street drug, which causes strong psychic dependence [also: dexamfetamine; dexamphetamine]

**dextroamphetamine phosphate** USP CNS stimulant

**dextroamphetamine saccharate** CNS stimulant

**dextroamphetamine sulfate** USP CNS stimulant; widely abused as a street drug, which causes psychic dependence 5, 10, 15 mg oral

**dextrobrompheniramine maleate** [see: dexbrompheniramine maleate]

**dextrochlorpheniramine maleate** [see: dexchlorpheniramine maleate]

**dextrofemine** INN

**dextromethorphan** USP, INN, BAN antitussive

**dextromethorphan hydrobromide** USP, BAN antitussive

**dextromethorphan hydrobromide & guaifenesin** antitussive; expectorant 30•500, 60•1000 mg oral

**dextromethorphan polistirex** USAN antitussive

**dextromethorphan tannate** antitussive

**dextromoramide** INN, BAN

**dextromoramide tartrate** [see: dextromoramide]

**dextro-pantothenyl alcohol** [see: dexpanthenol]

**dextropropoxiphene chloride** [see: propoxyphene HCl]

**dextropropoxyphene** INN, BAN narcotic analgesic [also: propoxyphene HCl]

**dextropropoxyphene HCl** BAN [also: propoxyphene HCl]

**dextrorphan** INN, BAN adjunct to vasospastic therapy; investigational glutamate receptor antagonist for neurodegenerative disorders [also: dextrorphan HCl]

**dextrorphan HCl** USAN *adjunct to vasospastic therapy; investigational glutamate receptor antagonist for neurodegenerative disorders* [also: dextrorphan]

**dextrose** USP *fluid and nutrient replenisher; parenteral antihypoglycemic*

**5% Dextrose and Electrolyte #48; 5% Dextrose and Electrolyte #75; 10% Dextrose and Electrolyte #48** IV infusion ℞ *intravenous nutritional/electrolyte therapy* [combined electrolyte solution; dextrose]

**dextrose excipient** NF *tablet excipient*

**50% Dextrose with Electrolyte Pattern A (or N)** IV infusion (discontinued 2001) ℞ *intravenous nutritional/electrolyte therapy* [combined electrolyte solution; dextrose]

**Dextrostat** tablets ℞ *amphetamine; CNS stimulant* [dextroamphetamine sulfate] 5, 10 mg

**Dextrostix** reagent strips for home use (discontinued 2004) *in vitro diagnostic aid for blood glucose*

**dextrothyronine** [see: detrothyronine]

**dextrothyroxine** BAN *antihyperlipidemic* [also: dextrothyroxine sodium]

**dextrothyroxine sodium** USAN, USP, INN *antihyperlipidemic* [also: dextrothyroxine]

**dexverapamil** INN *investigational adjunct to chemotherapy*

**Dey-Dose** (delivery system) *nebulizer*

**Dey-Lute** (delivery system) *nebulizer*

**Dey-Pak Sodium Chloride 3% & 10%** solution ℞ *for inducing sputum production for specimen collection* [sodium chloride] 3%; 10%

**dezaguanine** USAN, INN *antineoplastic*

**dezaguanine mesylate** USAN *antineoplastic*

**dezinamide** USAN, INN *anticonvulsant*

**dezocine** USAN, INN *narcotic analgesic*

**DFMO (difluoromethylornithine)** [see: eflornithine]

**DFMO (difluoromethylornithine) HCl** [see: eflornithine HCl]

**DFMO-MGBG (eflornithine, mitoguazone)** *chemotherapy protocol* [also see: DFMO; MGBG]

**DFP (diisopropyl flurophosphate)** [see: isoflurophate]

**DFV (DDP, fluorouracil, VePesid)** *chemotherapy protocol*

**DHA (docosahexaenoic acid)** [q.v.; also: doconexent]

**DHAP (dexamethasone, high-dose ara-C, Platinol)** *chemotherapy protocol for non-Hodgkin lymphoma*

**DHC Plus** capsules ℞ *narcotic analgesic* [dihydrocodeine bitartrate; acetaminophen; caffeine] 16•356.4•30 mg

**DHE (dihydroergotamine)** [see: dihydroergotamine mesylate]

**D.H.E. 45** IV or IM injection ℞ *prophylaxis or treatment of migraine and cluster headaches* [dihydroergotamine mesylate] 1 mg/mL

**DHEA (dehydroepiandrosterone)** [q.v.]

**DHPG (dihydroxy propoxymethyl guanine)** [see: ganciclovir]

**DHS Tar** liquid shampoo, gel shampoo OTC *antiseborrheic; antipsoriatic; antipruritic; antibacterial* [coal tar] 0.5%

**DHS Zinc** shampoo OTC *antiseborrheic; antibacterial; antifungal* [pyrithione zinc] 2%

**DHT** tablets, Intensol (concentrated oral solution) ℞ *vitamin D therapy for tetany and hypoparathyroidism* [dihydrotachysterol] 0.125, 0.2, 0.4 mg; 0.2 mg/mL

**DHT (dihydrotachysterol)** [q.v.]

**DHT (dihydrotestosterone)** [see: androstanolone; stanolone]

**DI (doxorubicin, ifosfamide [with mesna rescue])** *chemotherapy protocol for soft tissue sarcoma*

**Diaβeta (or DiaBeta)** tablets ℞ *sulfonylurea antidiabetic* [glyburide] 1.25, 2.5, 5 mg

**Diabetic Tussin** oral liquid OTC *expectorant* [guaifenesin] 100 mg/5 mL

**Diabetic Tussin** oral liquid (discontinued 2002) OTC *antitussive; decongestant; expectorant* [dextromethorphan hydrobromide; phenylephrine HCl; guaifenesin] 10•5•100 mg/5 mL

**Diabetic Tussin DM** oral liquid OTC *antitussive; expectorant* [dextromethorphan hydrobromide; guaifenesin] 20•200, 20•400 mg/10 mL

**Diabetic Tussin EX** oral liquid (discontinued 2002) OTC *expectorant* [guaifenesin] 100 mg/5 mL

**Diabinese** tablets ℞ *sulfonylurea antidiabetic* [chlorpropamide] 100, 250 mg

**diacerein** INN

**diacetamate** INN, BAN

**diacetolol** INN, BAN *antiadrenergic (β-receptor)* [also: diacetolol HCl]

**diacetolol HCl** USAN *antiadrenergic (β-receptor)* [also: diacetolol]

**diacetoxyphenylisatin** [see: oxyphenisatin acetate]

**diacetoxyphenyloxindol** [see: oxyphenisatin acetate]

**diacetrizoate sodium** [see: diatrizoate sodium]

**diacetyl diaminodiphenylsulfone (DADDS)** [see: acedapsone]

**diacetylated monoglycerides** NF *plasticizer*

**diacetylcholine chloride** [see: succinylcholine chloride]

**diacetyl-dihydroxydiphenylisatin** [see: oxyphenisatin acetate]

**diacetyldioxphenylisatin** [see: oxyphenisatin acetate]

**diacetylmorphine HCl** USP *(heroin; banned in USA)* [also: diamorphine]

**diacetylmorphine salts** *(heroin; banned in USA)*

**diacetylsalicylic acid** [see: dipyrocetyl]

**diacetyltannic acid** [see: acetyltannic acid]

**diacetylthiamine** [see: acetiamine]

**diagniol** [see: sodium acetrizoate]

**diallybarbituric acid** [see: allobarbital]

**diallylbarbituric acid** [now: allobarbital]

**diallylnortoxiferene dichloride** [see: alcuronium chloride]

**diallymal** [see: allobarbital]

**Dialpak** (trademarked packaging form) *reusable patient compliance package for oral contraceptives*

**Dialume** capsules ℞ *antacid* [aluminum hydroxide gel] 500 mg ⟳ Dalmane

**Dialyte Pattern LM** solution ℞ *peritoneal dialysis solution* [multiple electrolytes; dextrose] 1.5%•≛, 2.5%•≛, 4.5%•≛

**Dialyvite 3000** tablets OTC *vitamin/mineral supplement* [multiple vitamins & minerals; folic acid; biotin] ≛•3•0.3 mg

**dia-mer-sulfonamides (sulfadiazine & sulfamerazine)** [q.v.]

**diamethine** [see: dimethyltubocurarinium chloride; dimethyltubocurarine]

**diamfenetide** INN [also: diamphenethide]

**diaminedipenicillin G** [see: penicillin G benzathine]

**diaminodiphenylsulfone (DDS)** [now: dapsone]

**3,4-diaminopyridine** *investigational (orphan) for Lambert-Eaton myasthenic syndrome*

**cis-diamminedichloroplatinum (DDP)** [see: cisplatin]

**diammonium phosphate** [see: ammonium phosphate]

**diamocaine** INN, BAN *local anesthetic* [also: diamocaine cyclamate]

**diamocaine cyclamate** USAN *local anesthetic* [also: diamocaine]

**diamorphine** BAN *(heroin; banned in the U.S.)* [also: diacetylmorphine HCl]

**Diamox** powder for IV injection ℞ *carbonic anhydrase inhibitor diuretic; antiglaucoma; anticonvulsant; treatment for acute mountain sickness* [acetazolamide sodium] 500 mg

**Diamox** tablets, Sequels (sustained-release capsules) ℞ *carbonic anhydrase inhibitor diuretic; antiglaucoma; anticonvulsant; treatment for acute mountain sickness* [acetazolamide] 125, 250 mg; 500 mg

**diamphenethide** BAN [also: diamfenetide]

**diampromide** INN, BAN

**diampron** [see: amicarbalide]

**diamthazole** BAN [also: dimazole]

**diamthazole dihydrochloride** [see: diamthazole]

**Dianabol** tablets (discontinued 1982) ℞ *steroid; discontinued for human use, but the veterinary product is still available and sometimes abused as a street drug* [methandrostenolone] 2.5, 5 mg

**Diane-35** ⓒᴬᴺ sugar-coated tablets ℞ *antiandrogen/estrogen for severe acne in women* [cyproterone acetate; ethinyl estradiol] 2•0.035 mg

**Dianeal Peritoneal Dialysis Solution with 1.1% Amino Acids** ℞ *investigational (orphan) nutritional supplement for continuous ambulatory peritoneal dialysis patients*

**diapamide** USAN *diuretic; antihypertensive* [also: tiamizide]

**Diaparene Baby** cream OTC *topical diaper rash treatment*

**Diaparene Cornstarch Baby** powder OTC *topical diaper rash treatment* [corn starch; aloe]

**Diaparene Diaper Rash** ointment OTC *diaper rash treatment* [zinc oxide]

**Diaper Guard** ointment OTC *diaper rash treatment* [dimethicone; vitamins A, D, and E; zinc oxide] 1%• ± • 2

**Diaper Rash** ointment OTC *diaper rash treatment* [zinc oxide]

**diaphene** [see: dibromsalan]

**diaphenylsulfone** [see: dapsone]

**diaphoretics** *a class of agents that promote profuse perspiration* [also called: sudorifics]

**Diapid** nasal spray (discontinued 2001) ℞ *pituitary antidiuretic hormone for diabetes insipidus* [lypressin] 50 U/mL

**Diar-Aid** tablets OTC *antidiarrheal; GI adsorbent* [loperamide HCl] 2 mg

**diarbarone** INN

**Diascan** reagent strips for home use *in vitro diagnostic aid for blood glucose*

**DiaScreen** reagent strips for professional use *in vitro diagnostic aid for multiple disease markers in the urine*

**Diasorb** tablets, oral liquid OTC *antidiarrheal; GI adsorbent* [activated attapulgite] 750 mg; 750 mg/5 mL

**Diastat** rectal gel in a disposable applicator ("pediatric" and "adult" refer to the length of the applicator tip) ℞ *benzodiazepine anticonvulsant for acute repetitive seizures (orphan)* [diazepam] 2.5, 5, 10 mg (pediatric); 10, 15, 20 mg (adult)

**Diastix** reagent strips for home use *in vitro diagnostic aid for urine glucose*

**diathymosulfone** INN

**diatrizoate meglumine** USP *oral/ parenteral radiopaque contrast medium (46.67% iodine)* [also: meglumine diatrizoate] 76% injection

**diatrizoate methylglucamine** [see: diatrizoate meglumine]

**diatrizoate sodium** USP *oral/rectal/ parenteral radiopaque contrast medium (59.87% iodine)* [also: sodium amidotrizoate; sodium diatrizoate]

**diatrizoate sodium I 125** USAN *radioactive agent*

**diatrizoate sodium I 131** USAN *radioactive agent*

**diatrizoic acid** USAN, USP, BAN *radiopaque contrast medium* [also: amidotrizoic acid]

**Diatx** tablets ℞ *hematinic* [multiple B vitamins; folic acid; biotin] ± •5• 0.3 mg

**Diatx Fe** tablets ℞ *vitamin/mineral supplement for anemia* [multiple B vitamins; folic acid; biotin; ferrous fumarate] ± •5•0.3•100 mg

**diaveridine** USAN, INN, BAN *antibacterial*

**diazacholesterol dihydrochloride** [see: azacosterol HCl]

**diazepam** USAN, USP, INN, BAN, JAN *benzodiazepine anxiolytic; sedative; skeletal muscle relaxant; anticonvulsant for acute repetitive seizures (orphan); alcohol withdrawal aid; also abused as a street drug* 2, 5, 10 mg oral; 5 mg/5 mL oral; 5 mg/mL injection

**Diazepam Intensol** oral drops ℞ *benzodiazepine sedative; anxiolytic; skeletal muscle relaxant; anticonvulsant;*

*also abused as a street drug* [diazepam; alcohol 19%] 5 mg/mL

**diazinon** BAN [also: dimpylate]

**diaziquone** USAN, INN *antineoplastic; investigational (orphan) for primary brain malignancies (astrocytomas)*

**diazoxide** USAN, USP, INN, BAN *emergency antihypertensive; vasodilator; glucose-elevating agent*

**dibasic calcium phosphate** [see: calcium phosphate, dibasic]

**dibasic potassium phosphate** [see: potassium phosphate, dibasic]

**dibasic sodium phosphate** [see: sodium phosphate, dibasic]

**dibasol** [see: bendazol]

**dibazol** [see: bendazol]

**dibekacin** INN, BAN

**dibemethine** INN

**dibencil** [see: penicillin G benzathine]

**dibencozide** [see: cobamamide]

**Dibent** IM injection ℞ *GI antispasmodic* [dicyclomine HCl] 10 mg/mL

**dibenthiamine** [see: bentiamine]

**dibenzathione** [see: sulbentine]

**dibenzepin** INN, BAN *antidepressant* [also: dibenzepin HCl]

**dibenzepin HCl** USAN *antidepressant* [also: dibenzepin]

**dibenzodiazepines** *a class of novel (atypical) antipsychotic agents*

**dibenzothiazepines** *a class of novel (atypical) antipsychotic agents*

**dibenzothiazine** [see: phenothiazine]

**dibenzothiophene** USAN *keratolytic*

**dibenzoxazepines** *a class of dopamine receptor antagonists with antipsychotic, hypotensive, antiemetic, antispasmodic, and antihistaminic activity*

**dibenzoyl peroxide** [see: benzoyl peroxide]

**dibenzoylthiamin** [see: bentiamine]

**dibenzthion** [see: sulbentine]

**dibenzylethylenediamine dipenicillin G (DBED)** [see: penicillin G benzathine]

**Dibenzyline** capsules ℞ *antihypertensive for pheochromocytoma* [phenoxybenzamine HCl] 10 mg

**N,N-dibenzylmethylamine** [see: dibemethine]

**dibromodulcitol** [see: mitolactol]

**dibromohydroxyquinoline** [see: broxyquinoline]

**dibromomannitol (DBM)** [see: mitobronitol]

**dibromopropamidine** BAN [also: dibrompropamidine]

**4,5-dibromorhodamine 123** *investigational (orphan) for chronic myelogenous leukemia*

**dibrompropamidine** INN [also: dibromopropamidine]

**dibromsalan** USAN, INN *disinfectant*

**dibrospidium chloride** INN

**dibucaine** USP *topical local anesthetic* [also: cinchocaine] 1% topical

**dibucaine HCl** USP *local anesthetic* [also: cinchocaine HCl]

**dibudinate** INN *combining name for radicals or groups*

**dibunate** INN *combining name for radicals or groups*

**dibuprol** INN

**dibupyrone** INN, BAN

**dibusadol** INN

**dibutoline sulfate**

**DIC (dimethyl imidazole carboxamide)** [see: dacarbazine]

**Dical** CapTabs (capsule-shaped tablets) OTC *dietary supplement* [dibasic calcium phosphate; vitamin D] 117 mg (Ca)•90 mg (P)•133 IU

**dicalcium phosphate** [see: calcium phosphate, dibasic]

**Dical-D** tablets, chewable wafers OTC *dietary supplement* [dibasic calcium phosphate; vitamin D] 117 mg (Ca) •90 mg (P)•133 IU; 232 mg (Ca)• 180 mg (P)•200 IU

**dicarbine** INN

**dicarfen** INN

**dichlofenthion** BAN

**dichloralantipyrine** [see: dichloralphenazone]

**dichloralphenazone (chloral hydrate & phenazone)** BAN *mild sedative*

**dichloralphenazone & acetaminophen & isometheptane mucate**

cerebral vasoconstrictor and analgesic
for vascular and tension headaches;
"possibly effective" for migraine headaches 100•325•65 mg oral

**dichloralpyrine** [see: dichloralphena-
zone]

**dichloramine-T** NF

**dichloranilino imidazolin** [see: clonidine HCl]

**dichloren** [see: mechlorethamine HCl]

**dichlorisone** INN

**dichlorisone acetate** [see: dichlorisone]

**dichlormethazanone** [see: dichlor-
mezanone]

**dichlormezanone** INN

**dichloroacetic acid** *strong keratolytic/
cauterant* ⚠ Bichloracetic acid

**dichlorodifluoromethane** NF *aerosol
propellant; topical refrigerant anesthetic*

**dichlorodiphenyl trichloroethane
(DDT)** [see: chlorophenothane]

**dichlorometaxylenol** [see: dichloro-
xylenol]

**dichloromethane** [see: methylene
chloride]

**dichlorophen** INN, BAN

**dichlorophenarsine** INN, BAN [also:
dichlorophenarsine HCl]

**dichlorophenarsine HCl** USP [also:
dichlorophenarsine]

**dichlorotetrafluoroethane** NF *aerosol
propellant; topical refrigerant anesthetic*
[also: cryofluorane]

**dichlorovinyl dimethyl phosphate
(DDVP)** [see: dichlorvos]

**dichloroxylenol** INN, BAN

**dichlorphenamide** USP, BAN *carbonic
anhydrase inhibitor; diuretic* [also:
diclofenamide]

**dichlorvos** USAN, INN, BAN *anthelmintic*

**dichysterol** [see: dihydrotachysterol]

**diciferron** INN

**dicirenone** USAN, INN *hypotensive;
aldosterone antagonist*

**Dick test (scarlet fever streptococ-
cus toxin)**

**diclazuril** USAN, INN, BAN *coccidiostat
for poultry; investigational for crypto-
sporidiosis in AIDS*

**diclofenac** INN, BAN *analgesic; antiarthritic; nonsteroidal anti-inflammatory
drug (NSAID) for ankylosing spondylitis* [also: diclofenac potassium]

**diclofenac potassium** USAN *analgesic;
antiarthritic; nonsteroidal anti-inflammatory drug (NSAID) for ankylosing
spondylitis; topical treatment for actinic
keratoses* [also: diclofenac] 50 mg oral

**diclofenac sodium** USAN, JAN *analgesic; antiarthritic; nonsteroidal anti-
inflammatory drug (NSAID) for ankylosing spondylitis; ocular treatment for
cataract extraction; topical treatment
for actinic keratoses (AK)* 25, 50, 75,
100 mg oral

**diclofenamide** INN *carbonic anhydrase
inhibitor* [also: dichlorphenamide]

**diclofensine** INN

**diclofibrate** [see: simfibrate]

**diclofurime** INN

**diclometide** INN

**diclonixin** INN

**dicloralurea** USAN, INN *veterinary food
additive*

**Diclotec** ⒸⒶⓃ suppositories ℞ *nonsteroidal
anti-inflammatory drug (NSAID); antiarthritic; analgesic* [diclofenac sodium]
50, 100 mg

**dicloxacillin** USAN, INN, BAN *penicillinase-resistant penicillin antibiotic*

**dicloxacillin sodium** USAN, USP, BAN
*penicillinase-resistant penicillin antibi-
otic* 250, 500 mg oral

**dicobalt edetate** INN, BAN

**dicolinium iodide** INN

**Dicomal-DH** syrup ℞ *narcotic antitussive; decongestant; antihistamine*
[hydrocodone bitartrate; phenylephrine HCl; pyrilamine maleate] 1.66•
5•8.33 mg/5 mL

**Dicomal-DM** syrup OTC *antitussive;
decongestant; antihistamine* [dextro-
methorphan hydrobromide; phenylephrine HCl; pyrilamine maleate]
20•10•16.67 mg/10 mL

**dicophane** BAN [also: chlorophenothane; clofenotane]

**dicoumarin** [see: dicumarol]

**dicoumarol** INN *coumarin-derivative anticoagulant* [also: dicumarol]

**dicresulene** INN

*Dictamnus albus medicinal herb* [see: fraxinella]

**dicumarol** USAN, USP *coumarin-derivative anticoagulant* [also: dicoumarol] ⑨ Demerol

**dicyclomine** BAN *anticholinergic* [also: dicyclomine HCl; dicycloverine]

**dicyclomine HCl** USP *GI antispasmodic; anticholinergic* [also: dicycloverine; dicyclomine] 10, 20 mg oral; 10 mg/5 mL oral; 10 mg/mL injection

**dicycloverine** INN *anticholinergic* [also: dicyclomine HCl; dicyclomine]

**dicycloverine HCl** [see: dicyclomine HCl]

**dicysteine** [see: cystine]

**didanosine** USAN, INN, BAN *antiviral nucleoside reverse transcriptase inhibitor for HIV-1 infections (orphan)*

**didanosine & nevirapine & zidovudine** *investigational (Phase III) antiviral combination for HIV infection*

**didanosine & zidovudine** *investigational (Phase II) heterodimer antiviral combination for AIDS*

**didehydrodideoxythymidine** [see: stavudine]

**Di-Delamine** gel, spray OTC *topical antihistamine; bacteriostatic* [diphenhydramine HCl; tripelennamine HCl] 1%•0.5%•

**2′,3′-dideoxyadenosine (ddA)** *investigational (orphan) treatment for AIDS*

**dideoxycytidine (DDC; ddC)** [see: zalcitabine]

**dideoxyinosine (DDI; ddI)** [see: didanosine]

**Didrex** tablets ℞ *anorexiant* [benzphetamine HCl] 50 mg

**Didrocal** ⓒ tablets (in a 90-day therapy pack) ℞ *bisphosphonate bone resorption inhibitor plus calcium supplement for established postmenopausal osteoporosis* [Phase 1 (14 days): etidronate disodium; Phase 2 (76 days): calcium carbonate] 400 mg; 1250 mg

**Didro-Kit** (Italian name for U.S. product Didronel)

**Didronel** IV infusion ℞ *bisphosphonate bone resorption inhibitor for hypercalcemia of malignancy (orphan); investigational (orphan) for metabolic bone disease* [etidronate disodium] 300 mg/ampule

**Didronel** tablets ℞ *bisphosphonate bone resorption inhibitor for Paget disease, heterotopic ossification, and hypercalcemia of malignancy (orphan)* [etidronate disodium] 200, 400 mg

**didrovaltrate** INN

**didroxane** [see: dichlorophen]

**dieldrin** INN, BAN

**dielytra; choice dielytra** *medicinal herb* [see: turkey corn]

**diemal** [see: barbital]

**dienestrol** USP, INN *estrogen* [also: dienoestrol]

**dienoestrol** BAN *estrogen* [also: dienestrol]

**dienogest** INN

**Diet Ayds** candy (discontinued 2001) OTC *decrease taste perception of sweetness* [benzocaine] 6 mg

**dietamiphylline** [see: etamiphyllin]

**dietamiverine HCl** [see: bietamiverine HCl]

**diethadione** INN, BAN

**diethanolamine** NF *alkalizing agent*

**diethazine** INN, BAN

**diethazine HCl** [see: diethazine]

**diethyl phthalate** NF *plasticizer*

**diethylamine *p*-aminobenzenestibonate** [see: stibosamine]

**3-diethylaminobutyranilide** [see: octacaine]

**diethylbarbiturate monosodium** [see: barbital sodium]

**diethylbarbituric acid** [see: barbital]

**diethylcarbamazine** INN, BAN *anthelmintic for Bancroft filariasis, onchocerciasis, tropical eosinophilia, and loiasis* [also: diethylcarbamazine citrate]

**diethylcarbamazine citrate** USP *anthelmintic for Bancroft filariasis, onchocerciasis, tropical eosinophilia, and loiasis* [also: diethylcarbamazine]

**diethylcarbamazine dihydrogen citrate** [see: diethylcarbamazine citrate]

**diethyldithiocarbamate** *investigational (Phase II/III, orphan) immunomodulator for HIV and AIDS*

**diethyldixanthogen** [see: dixanthogen]

**diethylenediamine citrate** [see: piperazine citrate]

**diethylenetriaminepentaacetic acid (DTPA)** [see: pentetic acid]

**diethylhomospermine (DEHOP; DEHSPM)** *investigational (Phase II) polyamine analogue for AIDS-related non-Hodgkin lymphoma and uncontrolled, refractory diarrhea*

**N,N-diethyllysergamide** [see: lysergide]

**diethylmalonylurea** [see: barbital]

**diethylmalonylurea sodium** [see: barbital sodium]

**N,N-diethylnicotinamide** [see: nikethamide]

**diethylnorspermine** *investigational (Phase I) anticancer agent*

**diethylpropion** BAN *anorexiant; CNS stimulant* [also: diethylpropion HCl; amfepramone] 75 mg oral

**diethylpropion HCl** USP *anorexiant; CNS stimulant* [also: amfepramone; diethylpropion] 25 mg oral

**diethylstilbestrol (DES)** USP, INN *hormonal antineoplastic for inoperable prostatic and breast cancer* [also: stilboestrol]

**diethylstilbestrol diphosphate** USP *hormonal antineoplastic* [also: fosfestrol]

**diethylstilbestrol dipropionate** NF

**p-diethylsulfamoylbenzoic acid** [see: etebenecid; ethebenecid]

**diethylthiambutene** INN, BAN

**diethyltoluamide (DEET)** USP, BAN *arthropod repellent*

**diethyltryptamine (DET)** *a hallucinogenic street drug closely related to dimethyltryptamine (DMT), but prepared synthetically*

**N,N-diethylvanillamide** [see: ethamivan]

**dietifen** INN

**dietroxine** [see: diethadione]

**Dieutrim T.D.** timed-release capsules (discontinued 2001) OTC *diet aid; decrease perception of sweetness* [phenylpropanolamine HCl; benzocaine] 75•9 mg

**diexanthogen** [see: dixanthogen]

**difebarbamate** INN

**difemerine** INN [also: difemerine HCl]

**difemerine HCl** [also: difemerine]

**difemetorex** INN

**difenamizole** INN

**difencloxazine** INN

**difencloxazine HCl** [see: difencloxazine]

**difenidol** INN *antiemetic; antivertigo* [also: diphenidol]

**difenoximide** INN *antiperistaltic* [also: difenoximide HCl]

**difenoximide HCl** USAN *antiperistaltic* [also: difenoximide]

**difenoxin** USAN, INN, BAN *antiperistaltic*

**difenoxin HCl** *antiperistaltic*

**diferuloylmethane** *investigational (orphan) agent for cystic fibrosis*

**difetarsone** INN, BAN

**difeterol** INN

**Differin** solution, gel, cream, single-use pledgets R *synthetic retinoid analogue for acne* [adapalene] 0.1%

**diflorasone** INN, BAN *topical corticosteroidal anti-inflammatory* [also: diflorasone diacetate]

**diflorasone diacetate** USAN, USP *topical corticosteroidal anti-inflammatory* [also: diflorasone] 0.05% topical

**difloxacin** INN *anti-infective; DNA gyrase inhibitor* [also: difloxacin HCl]

**difloxacin HCl** USAN *anti-infective; DNA gyrase inhibitor* [also: difloxacin]

**difluanazine** INN *CNS stimulant* [also: difluanine HCl]

**difluanazine HCl** [see: difluanine HCl]

**difluanine HCl** USAN *CNS stimulant* [also: difluanazine]

**Diflucan** tablets, powder for oral suspension, IV infusion R *systemic triazole antifungal* [fluconazole] 50, 100, 150, 200 mg; 10, 40 mg/mL; 2 mg/mL

**diflucortolone** USAN, INN, BAN *corticosteroid; anti-inflammatory*

**diflucortolone pivalate** USAN *corticosteroid; anti-inflammatory*
**diflumidone** INN, BAN *anti-inflammatory* [also: diflumidone sodium]
**diflumidone sodium** USAN *anti-inflammatory* [also: diflumidone]
**diflunisal** USAN, USP, INN, BAN *anti-inflammatory; analgesic; antipyretic; antiarthritic; antirheumatic* 250, 500 mg oral
**difluoromethylornithine (DFMO)** [see: eflornithine]
**difluoromethylornithine HCl** [see: eflornithine HCl]
**difluprednate** USAN, INN *anti-inflammatory*
**difolliculin** [see: estradiol benzoate]
**diftalone** USAN, INN *anti-inflammatory*
**digalloyl trioleate** USAN
**Di-Gel** oral liquid OTC *antacid; antiflatulent* [aluminum hydroxide; magnesium hydroxide; simethicone] 200•200•20 mg/5 mL
**Di-Gel, Advanced Formula** chewable tablets OTC *antacid; antiflatulent* [magnesium hydroxide; calcium carbonate; simethicone] 128•280•20 mg
**Digepepsin** dual-coated tablets (discontinued 2002) ℞ *digestive enzymes* [pancreatin; pepsin; bile salts] 300•250•150 mg
**digestants; digestives** *a class of agents that promote or aid in digestion*
**Digestozyme** tablets (discontinued 2002) ℞ *digestive enzymes; laxative; choleretic* [pancreatin; pepsin; dehydrocholic acid] 300•250•25 mg
**Digibind** powder for IV injection ℞ *antidote to digoxin/digitoxin overdose (orphan)* [digoxin immune Fab (ovine)] 38 mg/vial
**Digidote** ℞ *investigational (orphan) antidote to cardiac glycoside intoxication* [digoxin immune Fab (ovine)]
**DigiFab** powder for IV injection ℞ *antidote to digoxin/digitoxin overdose (orphan)* [digoxin immune Fab (ovine)] 40 mg/vial
**digitalis** USP *cardiotonic*

*Digitalis ambigua; D. ferriginea; D. grandiflora; D. lanata; D. lutea; D. purpurea* medicinal herb [see: foxglove]
**digitalis glycosides** *a class of cardiovascular drugs that increase the force of cardiac contractions* [also called: cardiac glycosides]
**Digitek** tablets ℞ *cardiac glycoside to increase cardiac output; antiarrhythmic* [digoxin] 0.125, 0.25 mg
**digitoxin** USP, INN, BAN *cardiotonic; cardiac glycoside; investigational (orphan) for soft tissue sarcomas and ovarian cancer* ⑨ Desoxyn; digoxin
**digitoxin, acetyl** [see: acetyldigitoxin]
**α-digitoxin monoacetate** [see: acetyldigitoxin]
**digitoxoside** [see: digitoxin]
**digolil** INN *combining name for radicals or groups*
**digoxin** USP, INN, BAN *cardiotonic; cardiac glycoside antiarrhythmic* 0.125, 0.25 mg oral, 0.05 mg/mL oral, 0.1, 0.25 mg/mL injection ⑨ Desoxyn; digitoxin
**digoxin antibody** [see: digoxin immune Fab]
**digoxin immune Fab (ovine)** *antidote to digoxin/digitoxin intoxication (orphan); investigational (orphan) for other cardiac glycoside intoxication*
**Digoxin Injection C.S.D.** ⓒⒶⓃ ℞ *cardiac glycoside to increase cardiac output; antiarrhythmic* [digoxin] 0.25 mg/mL
**Digoxin Pediatric Injection C.S.D.** ⓒⒶⓃ ℞ *cardiac glycoside to increase cardiac output; antiarrhythmic* [digoxin] 0.05 mg/mL
**dihexyverine** INN *anticholinergic* [also: dihexyverine HCl]
**dihexyverine HCl** USAN *anticholinergic* [also: dihexyverine]
**Dihistine DH** elixir ℞ *narcotic antitussive; decongestant; antihistamine* [codeine phosphate; pseudoephedrine HCl; chlorpheniramine maleate] 20•60•4 mg/10 mL
**Dihistine Expectorant** oral liquid (discontinued 2002) ℞ *narcotic antitussive; decongestant; expectorant*

[codeine phosphate; pseudoephedrine HCl; guaifenesin; alcohol] 10•30•100 mg/5 mL

**dihydan soluble** [see: phenytoin sodium]

**dihydralazine** INN, BAN

**dihydralazine sulfate** [see: dihydralazine]

**5,6-dihydro-5-azacytidine** *investigational (orphan) for malignant mesothelioma*

**dihydrobenzthiazide** [see: hydrobentizide]

**dihydrocodeine** INN, BAN *narcotic analgesic* [also: dihydrocodeine bitartrate]

**dihydrocodeine bitartrate** USP *narcotic analgesic* [also: dihydrocodeine]

**dihydrocodeinone bitartrate** [see: hydrocodone bitartrate]

**dihydroergocornine** [see: ergoloid mesylates]

**dihydroergocristine** [see: ergoloid mesylates]

**dihydroergocryptine** [see: ergoloid mesylates]

**dihydroergotamine (DHE)** INN, BAN *antiadrenergic; anticoagulant; ergot alkaloid for rapid control of migraines* [also: dihydroergotamine mesylate; dihydroergotamine mesilate]

**dihydroergotamine mesilate** JAN *antiadrenergic; anticoagulant; ergot alkaloid for rapid control of migraines* [also: dihydroergotamine mesylate; dihydroergotamine]

**dihydroergotamine mesylate** USAN, USP *antiadrenergic; anticoagulant; ergot alkaloid for rapid control of migraines* [also: dihydroergotamine; dihydroergotamine mesilate] 1 mg/mL injection

**dihydroergotamine methanesulfonate** [see: dihydroergotamine mesylate]

**dihydroergotoxine mesylate** [now: ergoloid mesylates]

**dihydroergotoxine methanesulfonate** [now: ergoloid mesylates]

**dihydroethaverine** [see: drotaverine]

**dihydrofollicular hormone** [see: estradiol]

**dihydrofolliculine** [see: estradiol]

**dihydrogenated ergot alkaloids** [now: ergoloid mesylates]

**dihydrohydroxycodeinone** [see: oxycodone]

**dihydrohydroxycodeinone HCl** [see: oxycodone HCl]

**6-dihydro-6-iminopurine** [see: adenine]

**dihydroindolones** *a class of dopamine receptor antagonists with conventional (typical) antipsychotic activity* [also called: indolones]

**dihydroisoperparine** [see: drotaverine]

**dihydromorphinone HCl** [now: hydromorphone HCl]

**dihydroneopine** [see: dihydrocodeine bitartrate]

**dihydropyridines** *a class of calcium channel blockers*

**dihydrostreptomycin (DST)** INN *antibacterial* [also: dihydrostreptomycin sulfate]

**dihydrostreptomycin sulfate** USP *antibacterial* [also: dihydrostreptomycin]

**dihydrostreptomycin-streptomycin** [see: streptoduocin]

**dihydrotachysterol (DHT)** USP, INN, BAN, JAN *fat-soluble vitamin; synthetic reduction product of a vitamin D isomer; calcium regulator for tetany and hypoparathyroidism* 0.125, 0.2, 0.4 mg oral; 0.2 mg/mL oral

**dihydrotestosterone (DHT)** *investigational (Phase II, orphan) steroid for AIDS-wasting syndrome* [see: androstanolone; stanolone]

**dihydrotheelin** [see: estradiol]

**dihydroxy(stearato)aluminum** [see: aluminum monostearate]

**dihydroxy propoxymethyl guanine (DHPG)** [see: gancyclovir]

**dihydroxyacetone** *skin darkener for vitiligo and hypopigmented areas*

**dihydroxyaluminum aminoacetate (DAA)** USP *antacid*

**dihydroxyaluminum sodium carbonate** USP *antacid*

**dihydroxyanthranol** [see: anthralin]

**dihydroxyanthraquinone** *(withdrawn from market)* [see: danthron]

**1,25-dihydroxycholecalciferol** [see: calcitriol]

**24,25-dihydroxycholecalciferol** *investigational (orphan) for uremic osteodystrophy*

**dihydroxyestrin** [see: estradiol]

**5,7-dihydroxyflavone** [see: chrysin]

**dihydroxyfluorane** [see: fluorescein]

**dihydroxyphenylalanine (DOPA)** [see: levodopa]

**dihydroxyphenylisatin** [see: oxyphenisatin acetate]

**dihydroxyphenyloxindol** [see: oxyphenisatin acetate]

**dihydroxyprogesterone acetophenide** [see: algestone acetophenide]

**dihydroxypropyl theophylline** [see: dyphylline]

**diiodobuphenine** [see: bufeniode]

**diiodohydroxyquin** [now: iodoquinol]

**diiodohydroxyquinoline** INN, BAN *antiamebic* [also: iodoquinol]

**diisopromine** INN

**diisopromine HCl** [see: diisopromine]

**diisopropanolamine** NF *alkalizing agent*

**diisopropyl flurophosphate (DFP)** [see: isoflurophate]

**diisopropyl flurophosphonate** [see: isoflurophate]

**diisopropyl phosphorofluoridate** [see: isoflurophate]

**2,6-diisopropylphenol** [see: propofol]

**Dilacor XR** sustained-release capsules ℞ *antihypertensive; antianginal; antiarrhythmic; calcium channel blocker* [diltiazem HCl] 120, 180, 240 mg ⊠ Delcort

**Dilantin** Infatabs (chewable tablets) ℞ *hydantoin anticonvulsant* [phenytoin] 50 mg ⊠ Milontin; Mylanta; Xalatan

**Dilantin** Kapseals (capsules) ℞ *hydantoin anticonvulsant* [phenytoin sodium] 30, 100 mg ⊠ Milontin; Mylanta; Xalatan

**Dilantin-125** oral suspension ℞ *hydantoin anticonvulsant* [phenytoin] 125

mg/5 mL ⊠ Milontin; Mylanta; Xalatan

**Dilatrate-SR** sustained-release capsules ℞ *antianginal; vasodilator* [isosorbide dinitrate] 40 mg

**Dilatrend** ℞ *antihypertensive; α- and β-blocker for congestive heart failure* [carvedilol]

**Dilaudid** tablets, oral liquid, subcu or IM injection, suppositories ℞ *narcotic analgesic; widely abused as a street drug* [hydromorphone HCl] 2, 4, 8 mg; 5 mg/5 mL; 2, 4 mg/mL; 3 mg

**Dilaudid Cough** syrup ℞ *narcotic antitussive; expectorant* [hydromorphone HCl; guaifenesin; alcohol 5%] 1• 100 mg/5 mL

**Dilaudid-HP** subcu or IM injection ℞ *narcotic analgesic* [hydromorphone HCl] 10 mg/mL (250 mg/vial)

**dilazep** INN

**dilevalol** INN, BAN *antihypertensive; antiadrenergic (β-receptor)* [also: dilevalol HCl]

**dilevalol HCl** USAN, JAN *antihypertensive; antiadrenergic (β-receptor)* [also: dilevalol]

**dilithium carbonate** [see: lithium carbonate]

**dill** *(Anethum graveolens)* fruit and seed *medicinal herb used as an aromatic, carminative, diaphoretic, stimulant, and stomachic*

**dilmefone** INN

**Dilocaine** injection (discontinued 2002) ℞ *injectable local anesthetic* [lidocaine HCl] 1%, 2%

**Dilor** tablets, elixir, IM injection ℞ *antiasthmatic; bronchodilator* [dyphylline] 200 mg; 160 mg/15 mL; 250 mg/mL

**Dilor 400** tablets ℞ *antiasthmatic; bronchodilator* [dyphylline] 400 mg

**Dilor-G** tablets, oral liquid (discontinued 2003) ℞ *antiasthmatic; bronchodilator; expectorant* [dyphylline; guaifenesin] 200•200 mg; 300•300 mg/15 mL

**Dilotab** tablets OTC *decongestant; analgesic; antipyretic* [pseudoephedrine HCl; acetaminophen] 30•500 mg

**diloxanide** INN, BAN, DCF

**Diltia XT** sustained-release capsules ℞ *antihypertensive; calcium channel blocker* [diltiazem HCl] 120, 180, 240 mg

**diltiazem** INN, BAN *coronary vasodilator; calcium channel blocker; antianginal; antihypertensive* [also: diltiazem HCl]

**diltiazem HCl** USAN, USP, JAN *coronary vasodilator; calcium channel blocker; antianginal; antihypertensive; antiarrhythmic* [also: diltiazem] 30, 60, 90, 120, 180, 240, 300, 360 mg oral; 5 mg/mL injection

**diltiazem malate** USAN *coronary vasodilator; calcium channel blocker; antianginal; antihypertensive; antiarrhythmic*

**Dilusol** Ⓒᴬᴺ OTC *topical solution base* [ethyl alcohol] 38.7%

**Dilusol AHA** Ⓒᴬᴺ OTC *topical solution base* [ethyl alcohol with 8% glycolic acid (alpha hydroxy acid)]

**diluted acetic acid** [see: acetic acid, diluted]

**diluted alcohol** [see: alcohol, diluted]

**diluted hydrochloric acid** [see: hydrochloric acid, diluted]

**diluted sodium hypochlorite** [see: sodium hypochlorite, diluted]

**dimabefylline** INN

**Dimacol** caplets (discontinued 2002) OTC *antitussive; decongestant; expectorant* [dextromethorphan hydrobromide; pseudoephedrine HCl; guaifenesin] 10•30•100 mg ⎙ dimercaprol

**dimantine** INN *anthelmintic* [also: dymanthine HCl]

**dimantine HCl** INN [also: dymanthine HCl]

**Dimaphen** pediatric elixir OTC *decongestant; antihistamine* [pseudoephedrine HCl; brompheniramine maleate] 30•2 mg/10 mL

**Dimaphen** tablets, Release-Tabs (timed-release tablets) (discontinued 2001) OTC *decongestant; antihistamine* [phenylpropanolamine HCl; brompheniramine maleate] 25•4 mg; 75•12 mg

**Dimaphen DM Cold & Cough** pediatric elixir OTC *antitussive; decongestant; antihistamine* [dextromethorphan hydrobromide; pseudoephedrine

HCl; brompheniramine maleate] 10•30•2 mg/10 mL

**dimazole** INN [also: diamthazole]

**dimazole dihydrochloride** [see: dimazole; diamthazole]

**dimecamine** INN

**dimecolonium iodide** INN

**dimecrotic acid** INN

**dimedrol** [see: diphenhydramine HCl]

**dimefadane** USAN, INN *analgesic*

**dimefilcon A** USAN *hydrophilic contact lens material*

**dimefline** INN, BAN *respiratory stimulant* [also: dimefline HCl]

**dimefline HCl** USAN *respiratory stimulant* [also: dimefline]

**dimefocon A** USAN *hydrophobic contact lens material*

**dimekolin** [see: dimecolonium iodide]

**dimelazine** INN

**dimelin** [see: dimecolonium iodide]

**dimemorfan** INN

**dimenhydrinate** USP, INN, BAN *antiemetic; anticholinergic; antivertigo; motion sickness prophylaxis* 50 mg oral; 12.5 mg/4 mL oral; 50 mg/mL injection ⎙ diphenhydramine

**dimenoxadol** INN [also: dimenoxadole]

**dimenoxadole** BAN [also: dimenoxadol]

**dimepheptanol** INN, BAN

**dimepranol** INN *immunomodulator* [also: dimepranol acedoben]

**dimepranol acedoben** USAN *immunomodulator* [also: dimepranol]

**dimepregnen** INN, BAN

**dimepropion** BAN [also: metamfepramone]

**dimeprozan** INN

**dimeprozinum** [see: dimeprozan]

**dimercaprol** USP, INN *chelating agent for arsenic, gold, and mercury poisoning; adjunct to lead poisoning* ⎙ Dimacol

**dimercaptopropanol** [see: dimercaprol]

**2,3-dimercaptosuccinic acid (DMSA)** [see: succimer]

**dimesna** INN

**dimesone** INN, BAN

**Dimetabs** tablets ℞ *anticholinergic; antiemetic; antivertigo agent; motion* *sickness preventative* [dimenhydrinate] 50 mg ☒ Dimetane; Dimetapp

**dimetacrine** INN

**dimetamfetamine** INN

**Dimetane Decongestant** caplets, elixir (discontinued 2002) OTC *decongestant; antihistamine* [phenylephrine HCl; brompheniramine maleate] 10•4 mg; 5•2 mg/5 mL

**Dimetane-DC Cough** syrup (discontinued 2002) ℞ *narcotic antitussive; decongestant; antihistamine* [codeine phosphate; phenylpropanolamine HCl; brompheniramine maleate; alcohol 0.95%] 10•12.5•2 mg/5 mL

**Dimetane-DX Cough** syrup (discontinued 2004) ℞ *antitussive; decongestant; antihistamine* [dextromethorphan hydrobromide; pseudoephedrine HCl; brompheniramine maleate; alcohol 1%] 20•60•4 mg/10 mL

**Dimetapp** tablets, Extentabs (long-acting tablets), elixir (discontinued 2001) OTC *decongestant; antihistamine* [phenylpropanolamine HCl; brompheniramine maleate] 25•4 mg; 75• 12 mg; 12.5•2 mg/5 mL ☒ Dimetabs

**Dimetapp 4-Hour Liqui-Gels** (liquid-filled capsules) (discontinued 2001) OTC *decongestant; antihistamine* [phenylpropanolamine HCl; brompheniramine maleate] 25•4 mg

**Dimetapp 12-Hour Non-Drowsy** Extentabs (extended-release tablets) OTC *decongestant* [pseudoephedrine HCl] 120 mg

**Dimetapp Allergy** liqui-gels (discontinued 2001) OTC *antihistamine* [brompheniramine maleate] 4 mg

**Dimetapp Children's Nighttime Flu** syrup OTC *antitussive; decongestant; antihistamine; analgesic* [dextromethorphan hydrobromide; pseudoephedrine HCl; brompheniramine maleate; acetaminophen] 10•30•2•320 mg/10 mL

**Dimetapp Children's Non-Drowsy Flu** syrup OTC *antitussive; decongestant; analgesic* [dextromethorphan hydrobromide; pseudoephedrine

HCl; acetaminophen] 5•15•160 mg/5 mL

**Dimetapp Cold & Allergy** pediatric chewable tablets, quick-dissolve tablets (discontinued 2001) OTC *decongestant; antihistamine* [phenylpropanolamine HCl; brompheniramine maleate] 6.25•1 mg

**Dimetapp Cold & Allergy** pediatric elixir OTC *decongestant; antihistamine* [pseudoephedrine HCl; brompheniramine maleate] 30•2 mg/10 mL

**Dimetapp Cold & Flu** caplets (discontinued 2001) OTC *decongestant; antihistamine; analgesic* [phenylpropanolamine HCl; brompheniramine maleate; acetaminophen] 12.5•2• 500 mg

**Dimetapp Decongestant Pediatric** oral drops OTC *nasal decongestant* [pseudoephedrine HCl] 7.5 mg/0.8 mL

**Dimetapp Decongestant Plus Cough** pediatric oral drops OTC *antitussive; decongestant* [dextromethorphan hydrobromide; pseudoephedrine HCl] 5•15 mg/1.6 mL

**Dimetapp DM** elixir (discontinued 2002) OTC *antitussive; decongestant; antihistamine* [dextromethorphan hydrobromide; phenylpropanolamine HCl; brompheniramine maleate] 10•12.5•2 mg/5 mL

**Dimetapp DM Children's Cold & Cough** elixir OTC *antitussive; decongestant; antihistamine* [dextromethorphan hydrobromide; pseudoephedrine HCl; brompheniramine maleate] 10•30•2 mg/10 mL

**Dimetapp Long Acting Cough Plus Cold** syrup OTC *antitussive; decongestant* [dextromethorphan hydrobromide; pseudoephedrine HCl] 7.5•15 mg/5 mL

**Dimetapp Non-Drowsy** Liqui-Gels (liquid-filled softgels) OTC *decongestant* [pseudoephedrine HCl] 30 mg

**Dimetapp Sinus** caplets OTC *decongestant; analgesic* [pseudoephedrine HCl; ibuprofen] 30•200 mg

**dimethadione** USAN, INN *anticonvulsant*

dimethazan

dimethazine [see: mebolazine]

dimethicone USAN, NF, BAN *lubricant and hydrophobing agent; soft tissue prosthetic aid* [also: dimeticone] ⑨ cimetidine

dimethicone 350 USAN *soft tissue prosthetic aid*

dimethindene BAN *antihistamine* [also: dimethindene maleate; dimetindene]

dimethindene maleate USP *antihistamine* [also: dimetindene; dimethindene]

dimethiodal sodium INN

dimethisoquin BAN [also: dimethisoquin HCl; quinisocaine]

dimethisoquin HCl USAN [also: quinisocaine; dimethisoquin]

dimethisterone USAN, NF, INN, BAN *progestin*

dimetholizine INN

dimethothiazine BAN *serotonin inhibitor* [also: fonazine mesylate; dimetotiazine]

dimethoxanate INN, BAN

dimethoxanate HCl [see: dimethoxanate]

2,5-dimethoxy-4-methylamphetamine (DOM) *a hallucinogenic street drug derived from amphetamine, popularly called STP*

dimethoxyphenyl penicillin sodium [see: methicillin sodium]

dimethpyridene maleate [see: dimethindene maleate]

dimethyl ketone [see: acetone]

dimethyl phthalate USP

dimethyl polysiloxane [see: dimethicone]

dimethyl sulfoxide (DMSO) USAN, USP, INN *solvent; anti-inflammatory for symptomatic relief of interstitial cystitis; investigational (orphan) for traumatic brain coma; investigational (orphan) topical treatment for scleroderma and extravasation of cytotoxic drugs* [also: dimethyl sulphoxide]

dimethyl sulphoxide BAN *topical anti-inflammatory; solvent* [also: dimethyl sulfoxide]

dimethyl triazeno imidazole carboxamide (DIC; DTIC) [see: dacarbazine]

3-(3,5-dimethyl-1H-methylene)-1,3-dihydro-indole-2-one *investigational (orphan) for Kaposi sarcoma and von Hippel-Lindau disease*

dimethylaminoethanol (DMAE) *natural precursor to the neurotransmitter acetylcholine; readily crosses the blood-brain barrier to enhance memory and cognitive function*

dimethylaminoethanol bitartrate *natural precursor to the neurotransmitter acetylcholine; readily crosses the blood-brain barrier to enhance memory and cognitive function* (base=37%)

dimethylaminophenazone [see: aminopyrine]

dimethylcysteine [see: penicillamine]

dimethylglycine HCl

dimethylhexestrol [see: methestrol]

1,5-dimethylhexylamine [see: octodrine]

5,5-dimethyl-2,4-oxazolidinedione (DMO) [see: dimethadione]

dimethyloxyquinazine [see: antipyrine]

o,α-dimethylphenethylamine [see: ortetamine]

dimethylsiloxane polymers [see: dimethicone]

dimethylthiambutene INN, BAN

dimethyltryptamine (DMT) *hallucinogenic street drug derived from a plant native to South America and the West Indies*

dimethyltubocurarine BAN [also: dimethyltubocurarinium chloride]

dimethyltubocurarine iodide [see: metocurine iodide]

dimethyltubocurarinium chloride INN [also: dimethyltubocurarine]

dimethylxanthine [see: theophylline]

dimeticone INN *lubricant and hydrophobing agent; soft tissue prosthetic aid* [also: dimethicone]

dimetindene INN *antihistamine* [also: dimethindene maleate; dimethindene]

**dimetindene maleate** [see: dimethindene maleate]

**dimetipirium bromide** INN

**dimetofrine** INN

**dimetotiazine** INN *serotonin inhibitor* [also: fonazine mesylate; dimethothiazine]

**dimetridazole** INN, BAN

**dimevamide** INN

**dimevamide sulfate** [see: dimevamide]

**diminazene** INN, BAN

**dimoxamine HCl** USAN *memory adjuvant*

**dimoxaprost** INN

**dimoxyline** INN

**dimpylate** INN [also: diazinon]

**dinaline** INN

**Dinate** IV or IM injection ℞ *anticholinergic; antiemetic; antivertigo agent; motion sickness preventative* [dimenhydrinate] 50 mg/mL

**dinazafone** INN

**diniprofylline** INN

**dinitolmide** INN, BAN

**dinitrotoluamide** [see: dinitolmide]

**dinoprost** USAN, INN, BAN *oxytocic; prostaglandin*

**dinoprost trometamol** BAN *oxytocic; prostaglandin* [also: dinoprost tromethamine]

**dinoprost tromethamine** USAN *oxytocic; prostaglandin-type abortifacient* [also: dinoprost trometamol]

**dinoprostone** USAN, INN, BAN *oxytocic for induction of labor; prostaglandin-type abortifacient; cervical ripening agent*

**dinsed** USAN, INN *coccidiostat for poultry*

**Diocto** oral liquid, syrup (discontinued 2004) OTC *laxative; stool softener* [docusate sodium] 150 mg/15 mL; 60 mg/15 mL

**Diocto-C** syrup (discontinued 2003) OTC *stimulant laxative; stool softener* [casanthranol; docusate sodium] 30•60 mg/15 mL

**dioctyl calcium sulfosuccinate** [now: docusate calcium]

**dioctyl potassium sulfosuccinate** [now: docusate potassium]

**dioctyl sodium sulfosuccinate (DSS)** [now: docusate sodium]

**Diodex** ⓒᴬᴺ eye drops ℞ *topical ophthalmic corticosteroidal anti-inflammatory* [dexamethasone sodium phosphate] 0.1%

**diodone** INN [also: iodopyracet]

**diohippuric acid I 125** USAN *radioactive agent*

**diohippuric acid I 131** USAN *radioactive agent*

**diolamine** USAN, INN *combining name for radicals or groups*

**diolostene** [see: methandriol]

**dionin** [see: ethylmorphine HCl]

**diophyllin** [see: aminophylline]

*Dioscorea villosa* medicinal herb [see: wild yam]

**diosmin** INN

**Diostate D** tablets OTC *dietary supplement* [calcium; phosphorus; vitamin D] 114 mg•88 mg•133 IU

**diotyrosine I 125** USAN *radioactive agent*

**diotyrosine I 131** USAN *radioactive agent*

**Diovan** capsules (discontinued 2002) ℞ *angiotensin II receptor antagonist; antihypertensive; treatment for congestive heart failure (CHF)* [valsartan] 80, 160 mg ② Darvon

**Diovan** tablets ℞ *angiotensin II receptor antagonist; antihypertensive; treatment for congestive heart failure (CHF)* [valsartan] 40, 80, 160, 320 mg ② Darvon

**Diovan HCT** tablets ℞ *antihypertensive; angiotensin II receptor antagonist; diuretic* [valsartan; hydrochlorothiazide] 80•12.5, 160•12.5, 160•25 mg ② Darvon

**dioxadilol** INN

**dioxadrol** INN *antidepressant* [also: dioxadrol HCl]

**dioxadrol HCl** USAN *antidepressant* [also: dioxadrol]

*d*-**dioxadrol HCl** [see: dexoxadrol HCl]

**dioxamate** INN, BAN

**dioxaphetyl butyrate** INN, BAN

**dioxathion** BAN [also: dioxation]

**dioxation** INN [also: dioxathion]

**dioxethedrin** INN

**dioxethedrin HCl** [see: dioxethedrin]

**dioxifedrine** INN

**dioxindol** [see: oxyphenisatin acetate]

**dioxyanthranol** [see: anthralin]

**dioxyanthraquinone** *(withdrawn from market)* [see: danthron]

**dioxybenzone** USAN, USP, INN *ultraviolet screen*

**dipalmitoylphosphatidylcholine (DPPC)** [see: colfosceril palmitate]

**diparcol HCl** [see: diethazine HCl]

**dipegyl** [see: niacinamide]

**dipenicillin G** [see: penicillin G benzathine]

**dipenine bromide** BAN [also: diponium bromide]

**Dipentum** capsules ℞ *anti-inflammatory for ulcerative colitis* [olsalazine sodium] 250 mg

**diperodon** USP, INN, BAN *topical anesthetic*

**diperodon HCl** *topical anesthetic*

**diphemanil methylsulfate** USP *anticholinergic* [also: diphemanil metilsulfate; diphemanil methylsulphate]

**diphemanil methylsulphate** BAN *anticholinergic* [also: diphemanil methylsulfate; diphemanil metilsulfate]

**diphemanil metilsulfate** INN *anticholinergic* [also: diphemanil methylsulfate; diphemanil methylsulphate]

**Diphen AF** oral liquid OTC *antihistamine* [diphenhydramine HCl] 12.5 mg/5 mL

**Diphen Cough** syrup (discontinued 2002) OTC *antihistamine; antitussive* [diphenhydramine HCl; alcohol 5%] 12.5 mg/5 mL

**diphenadione** USP, INN, BAN

**diphenan** INN

**diphenatil** [see: diphemanil methylsulfate]

**diphenchloxazine HCl** [see: difencloxazine HCl]

**diphenesenic acid** [see: xenyhexenic acid]

**Diphenhist** caplets, oral liquid OTC *antihistamine* [diphenhydramine HCl] 25 mg; 12.5 mg/5 mL

**Diphenhist** softgels (discontinued 2002) OTC *antihistamine* [diphenhydramine HCl] 25 mg

**diphenhydramine** INN, BAN *ethanolamine antihistamine; anticholinergic; antiparkinsonian; motion sickness relief* [also: diphenhydramine citrate] ☑ dimenhydrinate

**Diphenhydramine 50** capsules (discontinued 2001) OTC *antihistamine* [diphenhydramine HCl] 50 mg

**diphenhydramine citrate** USP *ethanolamine antihistamine; anticholinergic; antiparkinsonian; motion sickness relief* [also: diphenhydramine]

**diphenhydramine HCl** USP, BAN *ethanolamine antihistamine; antitussive; motion sickness preventative; sleep aid* 25, 50 mg oral; 50 mg/mL injection

**diphenhydramine tannate** *ethanolamine antihistamine; anticholinergic; antiparkinsonian; motion sickness relief*

**diphenhydramine theoclate** [see: dimenhydrinate]

**diphenidol** USAN, BAN *antiemetic; antivertigo* [also: difenidol]

**diphenidol HCl** USAN *antiemetic*

**diphenidol pamoate** USAN *antiemetic*

**diphenmethanil methylsulfate** [see: diphemanil methylsulfate]

**diphenoxylate** INN, BAN *antiperistaltic* [also: diphenoxylate HCl]

**diphenoxylate HCl** USP *antiperistaltic* [also: diphenoxylate]

**diphenylacetylindandione** [see: diphenadione]

**diphenylalkylamines** *a class of calcium channel blockers*

**Diphenylan Sodium** capsules ℞ *anticonvulsant* [phenytoin sodium] 30, 100 mg ☑ Diphenylin

**diphenylbutazone** [see: phenylbutazone]

**diphenylbutylpiperidines** [see: phenylbutylpiperidines]

**diphenylcyclopenone** *investigational (orphan) agent for severe alopecia areata, alopecia totalis, and alopecia universalis*

**diphenylhydantoin** [now: phenytoin]

**diphenylhydantoin sodium** [now: phenytoin sodium]

**diphenylisatin** [see: oxyphenisatin]

**diphenylpyraline** INN, BAN *antihistamine* [also: diphenylpyraline HCl]

**diphenylpyraline HCl** USP *antihistamine* [also: diphenylpyraline]

**diphetarsone** [see: difetarsone]

**diphexamide iodomethylate** [see: buzepide metiodide]

**diphosphonic acid** [see: etidronic acid]

**diphosphopyridine nucleotide (DPN)** [now: nadide]

**diphosphoric acid, tetrasodium salt** [see: sodium pyrophosphate]

**diphosphothiamin** [see: co-carboxylase]

**diphoxazide** INN

**diphtheria antitoxin** USP *passive immunizing agent for diphtheria* [also: diphtheria toxoid] 500 U/mL injection

**diphtheria CRM$_{197}$ conjugate** *carrier protein for hemophilus b and pneumococcal vaccines*

**diphtheria equine antitoxin** *investigational passive immunizing agent (available only from the Centers for Disease Control and Prevention)*

**diphtheria & tetanus toxoids, adsorbed (DT; Td)** USP *active immunizing agent for diphtheria and tetanus* 2•2, 2•5, 2•10, 6.6•5, 7.5•7.5, 10•5, 12.5•5, 15•10 LfU/0.5 mL injection

**diphtheria & tetanus toxoids & acellular pertussis (DTaP) vaccine** *active immunizing agent for diphtheria, tetanus, and pertussis*

**diphtheria & tetanus toxoids & pertussis vaccine (DTP)** USP *active immunizing agent for diphtheria, tetanus, and pertussis*

**diphtheria & tetanus toxoids & whole-cell pertussis vaccine (DTwP)** *active immunizing agent for diphtheria, tetanus, and pertussis* 6.5•5•4, 10•5.5•4 LfU/0.5 mL injection

**diphtheria toxin, diagnostic** [now: diphtheria toxin for Schick test]

**diphtheria toxin, inactivated diagnostic** [now: Schick test control] ·

**diphtheria toxin for Schick test** USP *dermal diphtheria immunity test*

**diphtheria toxoid** USP *active immunizing agent for diphtheria* [also: diphtheria antitoxin]

**diphtheria toxoid, adsorbed** USP *active immunizing agent for diphtheria* 15 LfU/0.5 mL injection

**dipipanone** INN, BAN

**dipipanone HCl** [see: dipipanone]

**dipiproverine** INN

**dipiproverine HCl** [see: dipiproverine]

**dipivalyl epinephrine (DPE)** [now: dipivefrin]

**dipivefrin** USAN *ophthalmic adrenergic* [also: dipivefrine]

**dipivefrin HCl** USP *topical antiglaucoma agent* 0.1% eye drops

**dipivefrine** INN, BAN *ophthalmic adrenergic* [also: dipivefrin]

**diponium bromide** INN [also: dipenine bromide]

**dipotassium carbonate** [see: potassium carbonate]

**dipotassium clorazepate** INN *benzodiazepine anxiolytic; minor tranquilizer; anticonvulsant adjunct; alcohol withdrawal aid* [also: clorazepate dipotassium]

**dipotassium hydrogen phosphate** [see: potassium phosphate, dibasic]

**dipotassium phosphate** [see: potassium phosphate, dibasic]

**dipotassium pyrosulfite** [see: potassium metabisulfite]

**diprafenone** INN

**diprenorphine** INN, BAN

**Diprivan** emulsion for IV ℞ *general anesthetic* [propofol] 10 mg/mL

**diprobutine** INN, BAN

**diprofene** INN

**diprogulic acid** INN

**diproleandomycin** INN

**Diprolene** ointment, gel, lotion ℞ *topical corticosteroidal anti-inflammatory* [betamethasone dipropionate, augmented] 0.05%

**Diprolene AF** cream ℞ *topical corticosteroidal anti-inflammatory* [betamethasone dipropionate, augmented] 0.05%

**diprophylline** INN, BAN *bronchodilator* [also: dyphylline]

**dipropylacetic acid** [see: valproic acid]

**2-dipropylaminoethyl diphenylth-ioacetate** [see: diprofene]

**1,1-dipropylbutylamine** [see: diprobutine]

**diproqualone** INN

**Diprosone** ointment, cream, lotion, aerosol ℞ *corticosteroidal anti-inflammatory* [betamethasone dipropionate] 0.05%; 0.05%; 0.05%; 0.1%

**diproteverine** INN, BAN

**diprothazine** [see: dimelazine]

**diprotrizoate sodium** USP [also: sodium diprotrizoate]

**diproxadol** INN

*Dipteryx odorata; D. oppositifolia* medicinal herb [see: tonka bean]

**dipyridamole** USAN, USP, INN, BAN *coronary vasodilator; platelet aggregation inhibitor; diagnostic aid for coronary artery function* 25, 50, 75 mg oral

**dipyrithione** USAN, INN *antibacterial; antifungal*

**dipyrocetyl** INN

**dipyrone** USAN, BAN *analgesic; antipyretic* [also: metamizole sodium]

**diquafosol tetrasodium** *investigational (NDA filed) treatment for dry eye*

**Dirame** ℞ *investigational (Phase III) narcotic agonist-antagonist analgesic for moderate to severe pain* [propiram fumarate]

**dirithromycin** USAN, INN, BAN *macrolide antibiotic* ⏃ clarithromycin; erythromycin

**disaccharide tripeptide glycerol dipalmitoyl** *investigational (orphan) immunostimulant for pulmonary and hepatic metastases of colorectal adenocarcinoma*

**Disalcid** film-coated tablets, capsules ℞ *analgesic; antipyretic; anti-inflammatory; antirheumatic* [salsalate] 500, 750 mg; 500 mg

**disalicylic acid** [see: salsalate]

**Dis-Co Pack** (trademarked packaging form) *unit-dose package*

**discutients** *a class of agents that cause a dispersal or disappearance of a pathological condition, such as a tumor*

**disease-modifying antirheumatic drugs (DMARDs)** *a class of agents that slow the progression of rheumatic arthritis (RA) by modifying immune system response; this is in contrast to NSAIDs, which treat only the symptoms of the disease*

**disinfectants** *a class of agents that inhibit the growth and development of microorganisms, usually on an inanimate surface, without necessarily killing them* [see also: antiseptics; germicides]

**Disinfecting Solution** OTC *chemical disinfecting solution for soft contact lenses*

**Disipal** Ⓒᴬᴺ film-coated tablets (discontinued 2001) ℞ *anticholinergic; antiparkinsonian* [orphenadrine HCl] 50 mg

**disiquonium chloride** USAN, INN *antiseptic*

**Disket** (trademarked dosage form) *dispersible tablet*

**Diskhaler** (trademarked device) *inhalation powder dispenser* [used with a Rotadisk]

**Diskus** (trademarked device) *breath-activated inhalation powder dispenser*

**Disobrom** sustained-release tablets (discontinued 2002) ℞ *decongestant; antihistamine* [pseudoephedrine sulfate; dexbrompheniramine maleate] 120•6 mg

**disobutamide** USAN, INN *antiarrhythmic*

**disodium carbenicillin** [see: carbenicillin disodium]

**disodium carbonate** [see: sodium carbonate]

**disodium cefotetan** [see: cefotetan disodium]

**disodium chromate** [see: sodium chromate]

**disodium clodronate tetrahydrate** *bisphosphonate bone resorption inhibitor for hypercalcemia and osteolysis of malignancy* [approved in Canada; investigational (orphan) in the U.S.]

**disodium cromoglycate (DSC; DSCG)** [see: cromolyn sodium]

**disodium dihydrogen methylenediphosphonate** [see: medronate disodium]

**disodium edathamil** [see: edathamil disodium]

**disodium edetate** BAN *metal-chelating agent* [also: edetate disodium]

**disodium ethylenediamine tetraacetate** [see: edetate disodium]

**disodium hydrogen phosphate** [see: sodium phosphate]

**disodium hydrogen phosphate heptahydrate** [see: sodium phosphate, dibasic]

**disodium hydrogen phosphate hydrate** [see: sodium phosphate, dibasic]

**(disodium) methylene diphosphonate (MDP)** [now: medronate disodium]

**disodium phosphate** [see: sodium phosphate, dibasic]

**disodium phosphate heptahydrate** [see: sodium phosphate]

**disodium phosphonoacetate monohydrate** [see: fosfonet sodium]

**disodium phosphorofluoridate** [see: sodium monofluorophosphate]

**disodium pyrosulfite** [see: sodium metabisulfite]

**disodium silibinin dihemisuccinate** *investigational (orphan) antitoxin for* Amanita phalloides *(mushroom) intoxication*

**disodium sulfate decahydrate** [see: sodium sulfate]

**disodium thiosulfate pentahydrate** [see: sodium thiosulfate]

**disofenin** USAN, INN, BAN *carrier agent in diagnostic tests*

**disogluside** INN

**Disophrol** tablets, Chronotabs (sustained-action tablets) (discontinued 2002) OTC *decongestant; antihistamine* [pseudoephedrine sulfate; dexbrompheniramine maleate] 60•2 mg; 120•6 mg ② Desferal; disoprofol; Stilphostrol

**disoprofol** [see: propofol] ② Disophrol

**disopromine HCl** [see: diisopromine HCl]

**disoproxil** *combining name for radicals or groups* [also: soproxil]

**disopyramide** USAN, INN, BAN *antiarrhythmic*

**disopyramide phosphate** USAN, USP, BAN *antiarrhythmic* 100, 150 mg oral

**Disotate** IV infusion (discontinued 2000) ℞ *chelating agent for hypercalcemia and ventricular arrhythmias due to digitalis toxicity* [edetate disodium] 150 mg/mL

**disoxaril** USAN, INN *antiviral*

**Di-Spaz** capsules, IM injection ℞ *GI antispasmodic* [dicyclomine HCl] 10 mg; 10 mg/mL

**Dispenserpak** (trademarked packaging form) *unit-of-use package*

**DisperMox** tablets for oral suspension ℞ *aminopenicillin antibiotic* [amoxicillin] 200, 400 mg

**dispersible cellulose** BAN *tablet and capsule diluent* [also: cellulose, microcrystalline]

**Dispertab** (trademarked dosage form) *delayed-release tablet*

**Dispette** (trademarked delivery system) *disposable pipette*

**Dispos-a-Med** (trademarked delivery form) *solution for inhalation*

**distaquaine** [see: penicillin V]

**distigmine bromide** INN, BAN

**disulergine** INN

**disulfamide** INN [also: disulphamide]

**disulfiram** USP, INN, BAN *deterrent to alcohol consumption*

**disulfurous acid, dipotassium salt** [see: potassium metabisulfite]

**disulfurous acid, disodium salt** [see: sodium metabisulfite]

**disulphamide** BAN [also: disulfamide]

**disuprazole** INN

**Ital** slow-release capsules (discontinued 2001) ℞ *anorexiant; CNS stimulant* [phendimetrazine tartrate] 105 mg

**ditazole** INN

**ditekiren** USAN *antihypertensive; renin inhibitor*

**ditercalinium chloride** INN

**dithiazanine** BAN [also: dithiazanine iodide]

**dithiazanine iodide** USP, INN [also: dithiazanine]

**dithranol** INN, BAN *topical antipsoriatic* [also: anthralin]

**D.I.T.I.-2** vaginal cream ℞ *broad-spectrum antibiotic; antiseptic; vulnerary* [sulfanilamide; aminacrine HCl; allantoin] 15%•0.2%•2%

**ditiocarb sodium** INN

**ditiomustine** INN

**ditolamide** INN

**ditophal** INN, BAN

**Ditropan** tablets, syrup ℞ *urinary antispasmodic for urge urinary incontinence and frequency* [oxybutynin chloride] 5 mg; 5 mg/5 mL ☒ Intropin

**Ditropan XL** extended-release tablets ℞ *urinary antispasmodic for urge urinary incontinence and frequency* [oxybutynin chloride] 5, 10, 15 mg

**Diucardin** tablets (discontinued 2003) ℞ *diuretic; antihypertensive* [hydroflumethiazide] 50 mg

**Diurese** tablets ℞ *diuretic; antihypertensive* [trichlormethiazide] 4 mg

**diuretics** *a class of agents that stimulate increased excretion of urine*

**Diurigen** tablets ℞ *diuretic* [chlorothiazide] 500 mg

**Diuril** tablets, oral suspension ℞ *diuretic* [chlorothiazide] 250, 500 mg; 250 mg/5 mL

**Diutensen-R** tablets ℞ *antihypertensive* [methyclothiazide; reserpine] 2.5•0.1 mg ☒ Salutensin

**divabuterol** INN

**divalproex sodium** USAN *anticonvulsant; antipsychotic for manic episodes; migraine prophylaxis* [also: valproate semisodium; semisodium valproate]

**divanilliden cyclohexanone** [see: cyclovalone]

**divaplon** INN

**Divide-Tab** (trademarked dosage form) *scored tablet*

**Dividose** (trademarked dosage form) *multiple-scored tablets*

**diviminol** [see: viminol]

**divinyl ether** [see: vinyl ether]

**divinyl oxide** [see: vinyl ether]

**dixamone bromide** [see: methantheline bromide]

**dixanthogen** INN

**dixarit** [see: clonidine]

**dizatrifone** INN

**Dizmiss** chewable tablets (discontinued 2000) OTC *anticholinergic; antivertigo agent; motion sickness preventative* [meclizine HCl] 25 mg

**dizocilpine** INN *neuroprotective; NMDA (N-methyl-D-aspartate) antagonist* [also: dizocilpine maleate]

**dizocilpine maleate** USAN *neuroprotective; NMDA (N-methyl-D-aspartate) antagonist* [also: dizocilpine]

**dizocilpine maleate & citicoline** *investigational (Phase III) neuroprotective treatment for stroke*

**D-Lay** (trademarked dosage form) *timed-release tablet*

**DMAE (dimethylaminoethanol)** [q.v.]

**DMARDs (disease-modifying antirheumatic drugs)** *a class of agents that slow the progression of rheumatic arthritis (RA) by modifying immune system response; this is in contrast to NSAIDs, which treat only the symptoms of the disease*

**DMax** syrup ℞ *antitussive; decongestant; antihistamine* [dextromethorphan hydrobromide; phenylephrine HCl; carbinoxamine maleate] 15•8•4 mg/5 mL

**DMax Pediatric** oral drops ℞ *antitussive; decongestant; antihistamine* [dextromethorphan hydrobromide; phenylephrine HCl; carbinoxamine maleate] 4•2•1 mg/mL

**DMC (dactinomycin, methotrexate, cyclophosphamide)** *chemotherapy protocol*

**DMCT (demethylchlortetracycline)** [see: demeclocycline]

**DML** lotion OTC *moisturizer; emollient*

**DML Forte** cream OTC *moisturizer; emollient*

**DMO (dimethyl oxazolidinedione)**
[see: dimethadione]

**DMP 450** *investigational (Phase I/II)*
*second-generation protease inhibitor for*
*HIV infection*

**DMP 777** *investigational (orphan) agent*
*for the management of cystic fibrosis*
*lung disease*

**d-MPH (d-methylphenidate HCl)**
[q.v.]

**DMSA (dimercaptosuccinic acid)**
[see: succimer]

**DMSO (dimethyl sulfoxide)** [q.v.]

**DMT (dimethyltryptamine)** *street*
*drug* [q.v.]

**DNA (deoxyribonucleic acid)**

**DNA polymerase** [see: reverse transcriptase inhibitors; non-nucleoside
reverse transcriptase inhibitors]

**DNase (recombinant human deoxy-
ribonuclease I)** [see: dornase alfa]

**DNP-conjugated tumor vaccine**
*investigational (Phase III, orphan)*
*theraccine for postsurgical stage III*
*malignant melanoma*

**DNR (daunorubicin)** [q.v.]

**Doak Tar** bath oil, lotion (discontinued 2003) OTC *antiseborrheic; antipso-*
*riatic; antipruritic; antibacterial* [coal
tar] 0.8%; 2%

**Doak Tar** shampoo OTC *antiseborrheic;*
*antipsoriatic; antipruritic; antibacterial*
[coal tar] 1.2%

**Doak Tar Distillate** topical liquid
(discontinued 2003) OTC *antiseibor-*
*rheic; antipsoriatic; antipruritic; anti-*
*bacterial* [coal tar] 40%

**Doak Tar Oil** topical liquid OTC *anti-*
*seborrheic; antipsoriatic; antipruritic;*
*antibacterial* [coal tar] 0.8%, 2%

**Doan's Pills** caplets OTC *analgesic;*
*antirheumatic* [magnesium salicylate]
325, 500 mg

**Doan's P.M.** caplets OTC *analgesic;*
*antirheumatic; antihistaminic sleep aid*
[magnesium salicylate; diphenhydramine HCl] 500•25 mg

**DOAP (daunorubicin, Oncovin,
ara-C, prednisone)** *chemotherapy*
*protocol*

**dobupride** INN

**dobutamine** USAN, INN, BAN *cardio-*
*tonic; vasopressor for shock* ② dopamine

**dobutamine HCl** USAN, USP, BAN *car-*
*diotonic; vasopressor for shock* 12.5
mg/mL injection

**dobutamine lactobionate** USAN *car-*
*diotonic*

**dobutamine tartrate** USAN *cardiotonic*

**Dobutrex** IV infusion ℞ *vasopressor*
*for cardiac shock* [dobutamine HCl]
12.5 mg/mL

**DOCA (desoxycorticosterone ace-
tate)** [q.v.]

**docarpamine** INN

**docebenone** USAN, INN *5-lipoxygenase*
*inhibitor*

**docetaxel** USAN, INN *antineoplastic for*
*advanced or metastatic breast, prostate,*
*and non–small cell lung cancer*
*(NSCLC); analogue to paclitaxel;*
*investigational (Phase III) for head and*
*neck cancers*

**docetaxel & cisplatin** *chemotherapy*
*protocol for bladder cancer and non–*
*small cell lung cancer (NSCLC)*

**dock, curled; curly dock; narrow
dock; sour dock** *medicinal herb*
[see: yellow dock]

**dock, patience; sweet dock** *medici-*
*nal herb* [see: bistort]

**doconazole** USAN, INN *antifungal*

**doconexent** INN *omega-3 marine tri-*
*glyceride* [also: docosahexaenoic acid
(DHA)]

**docosahexaenoic acid (DHA)** *natu-*
*ral omega-3 fatty acid used to prevent a*
*wide range of degenerative diseases;*
*high concentrations are found in the*
*brain, where supplementation may*
*increase brain function; effective in*
*treating depression and other brain dis-*
*orders* [also: doconexent]

**docosanol (n-docosanol)** USAN *antivi-*
*ral for herpes simplex labialis; topical*
*treatment of oral herpes simplex type 1;*
*investigational (Phase II) for HIV infec-*
*tion and AIDS-related Kaposi sarcoma*

**docosil** INN *combining name for radicals*
*or groups*

**Doctar** shampoo (discontinued 2003) OTC *antiseborrheic; antipsoriatic; antipruritic; antibacterial* [coal tar] 0.5%

**Docu** oral liquid; syrup OTC *laxative; stool softener* [docusate sodium] 150 mg/15 mL; 20 mg/5 mL

**docusate calcium** USAN, USP *laxative; stool softener* 240 mg oral

**docusate potassium** USAN, USP *laxative; stool softener*

**docusate sodium** USAN, USP, BAN *stool softener; surfactant/wetting agent* [also: sodium dioctyl sulfosuccinate] 50, 100, 250 mg oral; 50 mg/15 mL oral

**Docusate with Casanthranol** capsules OTC *stool softener; stimulant laxative* [docusate sodium; casanthranol] 100•30 mg

**dodecafluoropentane** [see: perflenapent]

**dodeclonium bromide** INN

**1-(11-dodecylamino-10-hydroxyundecyl)-3,7-dimethylxanthine hydrogen methanesulfonate** *investigational (orphan) for hormone refractory prostate cancer*

**2-dodecylisoquinolinium bromide** [see: lauryl isoquinolinium bromide]

**dofamium chloride** INN, BAN

**dofetilide** USAN, INN, BAN *antiarrhythmic; potassium channel blocker*

**dofosfate** INN *combining name for radicals or groups*

**dog grass** *medicinal herb* [see: couch grass]

**dog poison (Aethusa cynapium)** plant *medicinal herb used as an antispasmodic and emetic in homeopathic remedies; not generally regarded as safe and effective as ingestion may be fatal*

**dogbane (Apocynum androsaemifolium)** root *medicinal herb used as a cathartic, diuretic, emetic, expectorant, stimulant, and sudorific*

**dogwood, black; black alder dogwood** *medicinal herb* [see: buckthorn; cascara sagrada]

**DOK-Plus** syrup OTC *stimulant laxative; stool softener* [casanthranol; doc-usate sodium; alcohol 10%] 30•60 mg/15 mL

**Dolacet** capsules ℞ *narcotic analgesic* [hydrocodone bitartrate; acetaminophen] 5•500 mg

**dolantal** [see: meperidine HCl]

**dolantin** [see: meperidine HCl]

**dolasetron** INN *serotonin 5-HT₃ receptor antagonist; antiemetic for nausea following chemotherapy, radiation, or surgery* [also: dolasetron mesylate]

**dolasetron mesylate** USAN *serotonin 5-HT₃ receptor antagonist; antiemetic for nausea following chemotherapy, radiation, or surgery* [also: dolasetron]

**Dolgic** caplets ℞ *analgesic; antipyretic; barbiturate sedative* [acetaminophen; butalbital] 650•50 mg

**Dolgic LQ** oral solution ℞ *analgesic; antipyretic; barbiturate sedative* [acetaminophen; butalbital; caffeine; alcohol 7.4%] 325•50•40 mg/15 mL

**doliracetam** INN

**Dolobid** film-coated tablets ℞ *analgesic; antiarthritic; antirheumatic; antiinflammatory; antipyretic* [diflunisal] 250, 500 mg

**dolomite** *nutritional supplement; source of calcium and magnesium*

**Dolomite** tablets OTC *mineral supplement* [calcium; magnesium] 130•78 mg

**Dolono** elixir OTC *analgesic; antipyretic* [acetaminophen] 160 mg/5 mL

**Dolophine HCl** tablets, subcu or IM injection (discontinued 2004) ℞ *narcotic analgesic; narcotic addiction detoxicant; often abused as a street drug* [methadone HCl] 5, 10 mg; 10 mg/mL

**Dolorac** cream OTC *topical analgesic* [capsaicin] 0.025%

**dolosal** [see: meperidine HCl]

**Dolsed** sugar-coated tablets ℞ *urinary antibiotic; analgesic; antispasmodic; acidifier* [methenamine; phenyl salicylate; atropine sulfate; methylene blue; hyoscyamine sulfate; benzoic acid] 40.8•18.1•0.03•5.4•0.03•4.5 mg

**dolvanol** [see: meperidine HCl]

**DOM (2,5-dimethoxy-4-methylamphetamine)** *a hallucinogenic street* *drug derived from amphetamine, popularly called STP*

**domazoline** INN *anticholinergic* [also: domazoline fumarate]

**domazoline fumarate** USAN *anticholinergic* [also: domazoline]

**Domeboro** powder packets, effervescent tablets OTC *astringent wet dressing (modified Burow solution)* [aluminum sulfate; calcium acetate]

**Domeboro Otic** [see: Otic Domeboro]

**Dome-Paste** medicated gauze bandage OTC *protection and support of extremities* [zinc oxide; calamine; gelatin]

**domestrol** [see: diethylstilbestrol]

**domibrom** [see: domiphen bromide]

**domiodol** USAN, INN *mucolytic*

**domiphen bromide** USAN, BAN *topical anti-infective*

**domipizone** INN

**Domol Bath and Shower Oil** OTC *bath emollient*

**domoprednate** INN

**domoxin** INN

**domperidone** USAN, INN, BAN, JAN *antiemetic for diabetic gastroparesis and chronic gastritis*

**Donatussin** pediatric oral drops ℞ *decongestant; antihistamine; expectorant* [phenylephrine HCl; chlorpheniramine maleate; guaifenesin] 2•1•20 mg/mL

**Donatussin** syrup ℞ *antitussive; decongestant; antihistamine; expectorant* [dextromethorphan hydrobromide; phenylephrine HCl; chlorpheniramine maleate; guaifenesin] 15•10•2•100 mg/5 mL

**Donatussin DC** syrup ℞ *narcotic antitussive; decongestant; expectorant* [hydrocodone bitartrate; phenylephrine HCl; guaifenesin] 5•15•100 mg/10 mL

**donepezil HCl** USAN *reversible acetylcholinesterase (AChE) inhibitor; cognition adjuvant for Alzheimer dementia*

**donetidine** USAN, INN, BAN *antagonist to histamine $H_2$ receptors*

**dong quai (Angelica polymorpha; A. sinensis; A. dahurica)** root *medicinal herb for allergies, anemia, blood cleansing, constipation, female hormonal problems, hypertension, internal bleeding, menopausal symptoms, nourishing brain, and ulcers; not generally regarded as safe and effective as it contains coumarins and safrole*

**Donnagel** chewable tablets, oral liquid (discontinued 2004) OTC *antidiarrheal; GI adsorbent* [attapulgite] 600 mg; 600 mg/15 mL ⑨ Donnatal

**Donnamar** tablets (discontinued 2004) ℞ *GI/GU antispasmodic; antiparkinsonian; anticholinergic "drying agent" for allergic rhinitis and hyperhidrosis* [hyoscyamine sulfate] 0.125 mg

**Donna-Sed** elixir ℞ *GI antispasmodic; anticholinergic; sedative* [atropine sulfate; scopolamine hydrobromide; hyoscyamine hydrobromide; phenobarbital] 0.0194•0.0065•0.1037•16.2 mg/5 mL

**Donnatal** capsules & tablets, elixir, Extentabs (extended-release tablets) (discontinued 2004) ℞ *GI antispasmodic; anticholinergic; sedative* [atropine sulfate; scopolamine hydrobromide; hyoscyamine sulfate; phenobarbital] 0.0194•0.0065•0.1037•16.2 mg; 0.0194•0.0065•0.1037•16.2 mg/5 mL; 0.0582•0.0195•0.3111•48.6 mg ⑨ Donnagel

**Donnatal No. 2** tablets (discontinued 2004) ℞ *GI antispasmodic; anticholinergic; sedative* [atropine sulfate; scopolamine hydrobromide; hyoscyamine sulfate; phenobarbital] 0.0194•0.0065•0.1037•32.4 mg

**Donnazyme** tablets (discontinued 2002) ℞ *digestive enzymes* [pancreatin (lipase; protease; amylase)] 500 mg (1000•12 500•12 500 USP units) ⑨ Entozyme

**DOPA (dihydroxyphenylalanine)** [see: levodopa]

**L-dopa** [see: levodopa]

**dopamantine** USAN, INN *antiparkinsonian*

**dopamine** INN, BAN *adrenergic; vasopressor for shock* [also: dopamine HCl] ⍰ dobutamine; Dopram

**dopamine HCl** USAN, USP *adrenergic; vasopressor for shock* [also: dopamine] 40, 80, 160 mg/mL injection

**dopamine HCl in 5% dextrose** *adrenergic; vasopressor for shock* 80, 160, 320 mg/100 mL injection

**dopaminergics** *a class of antiparkinsonian agents that affect the dopamine neurotransmitters in the brain*

**Dopar** capsules ℞ *dopamine precursor; antiparkinsonian* [levodopa] 100, 250, 500 mg ⍰ Dopram

**Dopascan** injection *investigational (Phase III) diagnostic imaging aid for dopamine and serotonin transporter sites* [iometopane I 123]

**dopexamine** USAN, INN, BAN *cardiovascular agent*

**dopexamine HCl** USAN, BAN *cardiovascular agent*

**Dopram** IV injection or infusion ℞ *CNS stimulant; analeptic; adjunct to postanesthesia "stir-up"* [doxapram HCl] 20 mg/mL ⍰ dopamine; Dopar

**dopropidil** INN

**doqualast** INN

**Doral** tablets ℞ *sedative; hypnotic* [quazepam] 7.5, 15 mg

**dorastine** INN *antihistamine* [also: dorastine HCl]

**dorastine HCl** USAN *antihistamine* [also: dorastine]

**Dorcol Children's Cold Formula** oral liquid (discontinued 2002) OTC *pediatric decongestant and antihistamine* [pseudoephedrine HCl; chlorpheniramine maleate] 15•1 mg/5 mL

**Dorcol Children's Cough** syrup (discontinued 2002) OTC *pediatric antitussive, decongestant, and expectorant* [dextromethorphan hydrobromide; pseudoephedrine HCl; guaifenesin] 5•15•50 mg/5 mL

**Dorcol Children's Decongestant** oral liquid (discontinued 2002) OTC *nasal decongestant* [pseudoephedrine HCl] 15 mg/5 mL

**doreptide** INN

**doretinel** USAN, INN *antikeratinizing agent*

**Dormarex 2** tablets OTC *antihistaminic sleep aid; motion sickness preventative* [diphenhydramine HCl] 50 mg

**dormethan** [see: dextromethorphan hydrobromide]

**Dormin** caplets, capsules OTC *antihistaminic sleep aid* [diphenhydramine HCl] 25 mg

**dormiral** [see: phenobarbital]

**dormonal** [see: barbital]

**dornase alfa** USAN, INN *reduces respiratory viscoelasticity of sputum in cystic fibrosis (orphan)*

**Doryx** coated pellets in capsules ℞ *tetracycline antibiotic* [doxycycline hyclate] 75, 100 mg

**dorzolamide HCl** USAN *topical carbonic anhydrase inhibitor for glaucoma*

**D.O.S.** softgels OTC *laxative; stool softener* [docusate sodium] 100, 250 mg

**Dosa-Trol Pack** (trademarked dosage form) *unit-of-use package*

**Dosepak** (trademarked dosage form) *unit-of-use package*

**dosergoside** INN

**Dosette** (trademarked dosage form) *injectable unit-of-use system (vials, ampules, syringes, etc.)*

**Dospan** (trademarked form) *controlled-release tablets*

**Dostinex** tablets ℞ *dopamine agonist for hyperprolactinemia; investigational treatment for Parkinson disease and gynecologic disorders* [cabergoline] 0.5 mg

**dosulepin** INN *antidepressant* [also: dothiepin HCl; dothiepin; dosulepin HCl]

**dosulepin HCl** JAN *antidepressant* [also: dothiepin HCl; dosulepin; dothiepin]

**dotarizine** INN

**dotefonium bromide** INN

**dothiepin** BAN *antidepressant* [also: dothiepin HCl; dosulepin; dosulepin HCl]

**dothiepin HCl** USAN *antidepressant* [also: dosulepin; dothiepin; dosulepin HCl]

**Double Antibiotic** ointment OTC *antibiotic* [polymyxin B sulfate; bacitracin zinc] 10 000•500 U/g

**Double Antibiotic Plus** cream (discontinued 2003) OTC *antibiotic; local anesthetic* [polymyxin B sulfate; neomycin sulfate; pramoxine HCl] 5000 U•3.5 mg•10 mg per g

**Double Ice ArthriCare** [see: ArthriCare, Double Ice]

**Double-Action Toothache Kit** tablets + topical liquid OTC *analgesic; oral anesthetic* [(acetaminophen) + (benzocaine; alcohol 74%)] (325 mg) + ( ≟ )

**Dovobet** (approved in 23 countries) ℞ *investigational (NDA filed) topical antipsoriatic and steroidal anti-inflammatory for plaque psoriasis* [calcipotriene; betamethasone dipropionate] 50 μg•0.5 mg

**Dovonex** cream, ointment, scalp solution ℞ *antipsoriatic* [calcipotriene] 0.005%

**DOX→ CMF, sequential (doxorubicin; cyclophosphamide, methotrexate, fluorouracil)** *chemotherapy protocol for breast cancer*

**doxacurium chloride** USAN, INN, BAN *nondepolarizing neuromuscular blocker; muscle relaxant; adjunct to anesthesia*

**doxaminol** INN

**doxapram** INN, BAN *respiratory stimulant; analeptic* [also: doxapram HCl]

**doxapram HCl** USAN, USP *respiratory stimulant; analeptic* [also: doxapram] 20 mg/mL injection

**doxaprost** USAN, INN *bronchodilator*

**doxate** [see: docusate sodium]

**doxazosin** INN, BAN *alpha$_1$-adrenergic blocker for hypertension and benign prostatic hyperplasia (BPH)* [also: doxazosin mesylate]

**doxazosin mesylate** USAN *alpha$_1$-adrenergic blocker for hypertension and benign prostatic hyperplasia (BPH)* [also: doxazosin] 1, 2, 4, 8 mg oral

**doxefazepam** INN

**doxenitoin** INN

**doxepin** INN, BAN *tricyclic antidepressant; anxiolytic; topical antihistamine* [also: doxepin HCl] ☒ Doxidan; Loxitane

**doxepin HCl** USAN, USP *tricyclic antidepressant; anxiolytic; topical antihistamine* [also: doxepin] 10, 25, 50, 75, 100, 150 mg oral; 10 mg/mL oral

**doxercalciferol** USAN *synthetic vitamin D analogue; serum calcium regulator for hyperparathyroidism of chronic renal dialysis*

**doxibetasol** INN [also: doxybetasol]

**Doxidan** capsules (discontinued 2003) OTC *stimulant laxative; stool softener* [casanthranol; docusate sodium] 30•100 mg

**Doxidan** delayed-release tablets OTC *stimulant laxative* [bisacodyl] 5 mg

**doxifluridine** INN, JAN *investigational antineoplastic*

**Doxil** IV injection ℞ *anthracycline antibiotic antineoplastic for ovarian cancer (orphan) and Kaposi sarcoma; investigational (NDA filed) for prostate cancer; investigational (Phase III) for breast cancer and multiple myeloma* [doxorubicin HCl, liposome-encapsulated] 20 mg/vial

**doxofylline** USAN, INN *bronchodilator*

**doxorubicin** USAN, INN, BAN *anthracycline antibiotic antineoplastic* ☒ daunorubicin

**doxorubicin HCl** USP *anthracycline antibiotic antineoplastic* 10, 20, 50 mg, 2 mg/mL injection

**doxorubicin HCl, liposome-encapsulated (LED)** *anthracycline antibiotic antineoplastic for ovarian cancer (orphan) and Kaposi sarcoma; investigational (NDA filed) for prostate cancer; investigational (Phase III) for breast cancer*

**doxorubicin & vinorelbine** *chemotherapy protocol for breast cancer*

**Doxovir** ℞ *investigational (Phase II) prophylaxis for genital herpes* [CTC-96 (code name—generic name not yet assigned)]

**doxpicodin HCl** [now: doxpicomine HCl]

**doxpicomine** INN *analgesic* [also: doxpicomine HCl]

**doxpicomine HCl** USAN *analgesic* [also: doxpicomine]

**Doxy 100; Doxy 200** powder for IV infusion ℞ *tetracycline antibiotic* [doxycycline hyclate] 100 mg/vial; 200 mg/vial

**Doxy Caps** capsules (discontinued 2003) ℞ *tetracycline antibiotic* [doxycycline hyclate] 100 mg

**doxybetasol** BAN [also: doxibetasol]

**Doxychel Hyclate** capsules, tablets, powder for IV injection (discontinued 2003) ℞ *tetracycline antibiotic* [doxycycline hyclate] 50, 100 mg; 50, 100 mg; 100, 200 mg

**doxycycline** USAN, USP, INN, BAN *tetracycline antibiotic; antirickettsial; malaria prophylaxis*

**doxycycline calcium** USP *tetracycline antibiotic; antiprotozoal*

**doxycycline fosfatex** USAN, BAN *tetracycline antibiotic*

**doxycycline hyclate** USP *tetracycline antibiotic; periodontitis treatment* 50, 100 mg oral; 100 mg/vial injection

**doxycycline monohydrate** *tetracycline antibiotic*

**doxylamine** INN, BAN *antihistamine; sleep aid* [also: doxylamine succinate]

**doxylamine succinate** USP *antihistamine; sleep aid* [also: doxylamine]

**DPE (dipivalyl epinephrine)** [now: dipivefrin]

**DPF** [see: Dermprotective Factor]

**DPN (diphosphopyridine nucleotide)** [now: nadide]

**DPPC (dipalmitoylphosphatidylcholine)** [see: colfosceril palmitate]

**DPPE (diethyl-phenylmethyl-phenoxy ethenamine) HCl** [see: tesmilifene HCl]

**Dr. Brown's Home Drug Testing System** *in vitro diagnostic aid for detection of multiple illicit drugs in the urine*

**Dr. Dermi-Heal** ointment OTC *vulnerary; antipruritic; astringent* [allantoin;

zinc oxide; peruvian balsam] 1% • 2 • 2

**Dr. Scholl's Advanced Pain Relief Corn Removers; Dr. Scholl's Callus Removers; Dr Scholl's Clear Away; Dr. Scholl's Corn Removers** medicated discs OTC *keratolytic* [salicylic acid in a rubber-based vehicle] 40%

**Dr. Scholl's Athlete's Foot** powder, spray powder, spray liquid OTC *topical antifungal* [tolnaftate] 1%

**Dr. Scholl's Clear Away OneStep; Dr. Scholl's OneStep Corn Removers** medicated strips OTC *keratolytic* [salicylic acid in a rubber-based vehicle] 40%

**Dr. Scholl's Corn/Callus Remover** topical liquid OTC *keratolytic* [salicylic acid in flexible collodion] 17%

**Dr. Scholl's Cracked Heel Relief** cream OTC *topical local anesthetic; antiseptic* [lidocaine HCl; benzalkonium chloride] 2% • 0.13%

**Dr. Scholl's Moisturizing Corn Remover Kit** medicated discs + cushions + moisturizing cream OTC *keratolytic* [salicylic acid in a rubber-based vehicle] 40%

**Dr. Scholl's Tritin** powder, spray powder OTC *topical antifungal* [tolnaftate] 1%

**Dr. Scholl's Wart Remover Kit** topical liquid + adhesive pads OTC *keratolytic* [salicylic acid in flexible collodion] 17%

**Dr. Smith's Adult Care; Dr. Smith's Diaper** ointment OTC *astringent; moisturizer; emollient* [zinc oxide] 10%

**draflazine** USAN *cardioprotectant*

**dragée** (French for "sugar plum") *a sugar-coated pill or medicated confection* [pronounced "drah zhá"]

**dragon's claw, scaly** *medicinal herb* [see: coral root]

**dragonwort** *medicinal herb* [see: bistort]

**Dramamine** oral liquid ℞ *antinauseant; antiemetic; antivertigo agent; motion sickness preventative* [dimenhydrinate] 15.62 mg/5 mL

**Dramamine** tablets, chewable tablets, oral liquid OTC *antinauseant; antiemetic; antivertigo agent; motion sickness preventative* [dimenhydrinate] 50 mg; 50 mg; 12.5 mg/4 mL

**Dramamine, Children's** oral liquid OTC *antinauseant; antiemetic; antivertigo agent; motion sickness preventative* [dimenhydrinate; alcohol 5%] 12.5 mg/5 mL

**Dramamine II** tablets (name changed to Dramamine Less Drowsy Formula in 2000)

**Dramamine Less Drowsy Formula** tablets OTC *anticholinergic; antihistamine; antivertigo agent; motion sickness preventative* [meclizine HCl] 25 mg

**Dramanate** IV or IM injection ℞ *antinauseant; antiemetic; antivertigo agent; motion sickness preventative* [dimenhydrinate] 50 mg/mL ② Dommanate

**dramarin** [see: dimenhydrate]

**dramedilol** INN

**Dramilin** IV or IM injection ℞ *antinauseant; antiemetic; antivertigo agent; motion sickness preventative* [dimenhydrinate] 50 mg/mL

**dramyl** [see: dimenhydrate]

**draquinolol** INN

**drazidox** INN

**Drepanol** ℞ *investigational (orphan) for prophylactic treatment of sickle cell disease* [OM 401 (code name—generic name not yet assigned)]

**dribendazole** USAN, INN *anthelmintic*

**dricol** [see: amidephrine]

**Dri/Ear** ear drops OTC *antibacterial; antifungal* [boric acid] 2.75%

**dried aluminum hydroxide gel** [see: aluminum hydroxide gel, dried]

**dried basic aluminum carbonate** [see: aluminum carbonate, basic]

**dried ferrous sulfate** [see: ferrous sulfate, dried]

**dried yeast** [see: yeast, dried]

**DriHist SR** sustained-release caplets ℞ *decongestant; antihistamine; anticholinergic to dry mucosal secretions* [phenylephrine HCl; chlorphenir-amine maleate; methscopolamine nitrate] 20•8•2.5 mg

**drinidene** USAN, INN *analgesic*

**Drisdol** capsules ℞ *vitamin deficiency therapy for refractory rickets, familial hypophosphatemia, and hypoparathyroidism* [ergocalciferol (vitamin $D_2$)] 50 000 IU

**Drisdol Drops** OTC *vitamin supplement* [ergocalciferol (vitamin $D_2$)] 8000 IU/mL

**Dristan 12-Hr.** nasal spray OTC *nasal decongestant* [oxymetazoline HCl] 0.05%

**Dristan Cold, Maximum Strength** caplets OTC *decongestant; antihistamine; analgesic* [pseudoephedrine HCl; brompheniramine maleate; acetaminophen] 30•2•500 mg

**Dristan Cold Multi-Symptom Formula** tablets OTC *decongestant; antihistamine; analgesic* [phenylephrine HCl; chlorpheniramine maleate; acetaminophen] 5•2•325 mg

**Dristan Cold Non-Drowsy** caplets OTC *decongestant; analgesic; antipyretic* [pseudoephedrine HCl; acetaminophen] 30•500 mg

**Dristan Fast Acting Formula** nasal spray OTC *nasal decongestant; antihistamine* [phenylephrine HCl; pheniramine maleate] 0.5%•0.2%

**Dristan Saline Spray** (discontinued 2002) OTC *nasal moisturizer* [sodium chloride (saline solution)]

**Dristan Sinus** caplets OTC *decongestant; analgesic* [pseudoephedrine HCl; ibuprofen] 30•200 mg

**Drithocreme; Drithocreme HP 1%; Dritho-Scalp** cream ℞ *topical antipsoriatic* [anthralin] 0.1%, 0.25%, 0.5%; 1%; 0.5%

**Drixomed** sustained-release tablets ℞ *decongestant; antihistamine* [pseudoephedrine sulfate; dexbrompheniramine maleate] 120•6 mg

**Drixoral** syrup (discontinued 2002) OTC *decongestant; antihistamine* [pseudoephedrine sulfate; brompheniramine maleate] 30•2 mg/5 mL

**Drixoral 12 hour Non-Drowsy Formula** extended-release tablets OTC *nasal decongestant* [pseudoephedrine sulfate] 120 mg

**Drixoral Allergy Sinus** extended-release tablets OTC *decongestant; antihistamine; analgesic* [pseudoephedrine sulfate; dexbrompheniramine maleate; acetaminophen] 60•3•500 mg

**Drixoral Cold & Allergy** sustained-action tablets OTC *decongestant; antihistamine* [pseudoephedrine sulfate; dexbrompheniramine maleate] 120•6 mg

**Drixoral Cold & Flu; Drixoral Plus** extended-release tablets (name changed to Drixoral Allergy Sinus in 2002)

**Drixoral Cough & Congestion Liquid Caps** (capsules) (discontinued 2002) OTC *antitussive; decongestant* [dextromethorphan hydrobromide; pseudoephedrine HCl] 30•60 mg

**Drixoral Cough & Sore Throat Liquid Caps** (liquid-filled capsules) (discontinued 2002) OTC *antitussive; analgesic* [dextromethorphan hydrobromide; acetaminophen] 15•325 mg

**Drixoral Day; Drixoral N.D.** ⓒᴀɴ sustained-action tablets OTC *decongestant* [pseudoephedrine sulfate] 120 mg

**Drixoral Night** ⓒᴀɴ tablets OTC *decongestant; antihistamine* [pseudoephedrine sulfate; dexbrompheniramine maleate] 60•2 mg

**Drize** sustained-release capsules (discontinued 2001) ℞ *decongestant; antihistamine* [phenylpropanolamine HCl; chlorpheniramine maleate] 75•12 mg

**drobuline** USAN, INN *antiarrhythmic*

**drocarbil** NF

**drocinonide** USAN, INN *anti-inflammatory*

**droclidinium bromide** INN

**drocode** [see: dihydrocodeine]

**drofenine** INN

**droloxifene** INN *investigational (Phase III) antineoplastic for breast cancer; investigational (Phase III) antiestrogen for postmenopausal osteoporosis*

**droloxifene citrate** USAN *antineoplastic; antiestrogen*

**drometrizole** USAN, INN *ultraviolet screen*

**dromostanolone propionate** USAN, USP *antineoplastic* [also: drostanolone]

**dronabinol** USAN, USP, INN *antiemetic for chemotherapy; appetite stimulant for AIDS patients (orphan); investigational (Phase II) for pain relief and sleep enhancement*

**drop chalk** [see: calcium carbonate]

**dropberry** *medicinal herb* [see: Solomon's seal]

**Drop-Dose** (trademarked delivery system) *prefilled eye drop dispenser*

**dropempine** INN

**droperidol** USAN, USP, INN, BAN *general anesthetic; antiemetic; antipsychotic*

**Dropperettes** (delivery system) *prefilled droppers*

**droprenilamine** USAN, INN *coronary vasodilator*

**dropropizine** INN, BAN

**Drop-Tainers** (trademarked packaging form) *prefilled eye drop dispenser*

**drospirenone** USAN *progestin; spironolactone analogue; aldosterone antagonist*

**drostanolone** INN, BAN *antineoplastic* [also: dromostanolone propionate]

**drotaverine** INN

**drotebanol** INN, BAN

**Drotic** ear drops ℞ *topical corticosteroidal anti-inflammatory; antibiotic* [hydrocortisone; neomycin sulfate; polymyxin B sulfate] 1%•5 mg• 10 000 U per mL

**drotrecogin alfa** *recombinant human activated protein C (rhAPC) for severe sepsis*

**droxacin** INN *antibacterial* [also: droxacin sodium]

**droxacin sodium** USAN *antibacterial* [also: droxacin]

**Droxia** capsules ℞ *sickle cell anemia treatment (orphan)* [hydroxyurea] 200, 300, 400 mg

**droxicainide** INN

**droxicam** INN

**droxidopa** INN

**droxifilcon A** USAN *hydrophilic contact lens material*

**droxinavir HCl** USAN *antiviral; HIV-1 protease inhibitor*

**droxypropine** INN, BAN

**Dry E 400** tablets (discontinued 2004) OTC *vitamin supplement* [vitamin E (as *d*-alpha tocopheryl acid succinate)] 400 IU

**Dry Eyes** eye drops OTC *ophthalmic moisturizer/lubricant* [polyvinyl alcohol] 1.4%

**Dry Eyes** ophthalmic ointment OTC *ocular moisturizer/lubricant* [white petrolatum; mineral oil]

*Dryopteris filix-mas medicinal herb* [see: aspidium]

**Dryox 2.5; Dryox 5; Dryox 10; Dryox 20** gel (discontinued 2003) OTC *keratolytic for acne* [benzoyl peroxide] 2.5%; 5%; 10%; 20%

**Dryox 10S 5; Dryox 20S 10** gel (discontinued 2003) OTC *keratolytic for acne* [benzoyl peroxide; sulfur] 10%•5%; 20%•10%

**Dryox Wash 5; Dryox Wash 10** topical liquid (discontinued 2003) OTC *keratolytic for acne* [benzoyl peroxide] 5%; 10%

**Dryphen Multi-Symptom Formula** tablets OTC *decongestant; antihistamine; analgesic* [phenylephrine HCl; chlorpheniramine maleate; acetaminophen] 5•2•325 mg

**Drysol** solution ℞ *astringent for hyperhidrosis* [aluminum chloride] 20%

**Drytergent** topical liquid OTC *soapfree therapeutic skin cleanser*

**Drytex** lotion OTC *keratolytic cleanser for acne* [salicylic acid; acetone; isopropyl alcohol] ≟•10%•40%

**Dryvax** powder for reconstitution ℞ *active immunization against smallpox using the multiple-puncture technique (scarification); licensed for restricted use and available only from the CDC* [smallpox vaccine] 100 million infectious vaccinia viruses/mL

**DSC; DSCG (disodium cromoglycate)** [see: cromolyn sodium]

**D-S-S** capsules OTC *laxative; stool softener* [docusate sodium] 100 mg

**DSS (dioctyl sodium sulfosuccinate)** [now: docusate sodium]

**DSS 100 Plus** capsules (discontinued 2003) OTC *stimulant laxative; stool softener* [casanthranol; docusate sodium] 30•100 mg

**DST (dihydrostreptomycin)** [q.v.]

**DT; Td (diphtheria & tetanus [toxoids])** *the designation DT (or TD) denotes the pediatric vaccine; Td denotes the adult vaccine* [see: diphtheria & tetanus toxoids, adsorbed]

**DTaP (diphtheria & tetanus [toxoids] & acellular pertussis [vaccine])** [q.v.]

**DTI-015** *investigational (orphan) antineoplastic for glioblastoma multiforme*

**DTIC (dimethyl triazeno imidazole carboxamide)** [see: dacarbazine]

**DTIC & tamoxifen** *chemotherapy protocol for malignant melanoma*

**DTIC-ACTD; DTIC-ACT-D (DTIC, actinomycin D)** *chemotherapy protocol*

**DTIC-Dome** IV injection ℞ *antineoplastic for metastatic malignant melanoma and Hodgkin disease* [dacarbazine] 100, 200 mg

**DTP (diphtheria & tetanus [toxoids] & pertussis [vaccine])** [q.v.]

**DTPA (diethylenetriaminepentaacetic acid)** [see: pentetic acid]

**DTPA (diethylenetriaminepentaacetic acid) technetium ($^{99m}$Tc), human serum albumin** [see: technetium Tc 99m pentetate]

**DTwP (diphtheria & tetanus [toxoids] & whole-cell pertussis [vaccine])** [q.v.]

**Duac** gel ℞ *antibiotic and keratolytic for acne* [clindamycin; benzoyl peroxide] 1%•5%

**Duadacin** capsules (discontinued 2001) OTC *decongestant; antihistamine; analgesic* [phenylpropanolamine HCl; chlorpheniramine maleate; acetaminophen] 12.5•2•325 mg

**Duadacin Cold & Flu** caplets (discontinued 2004) OTC *decongestant; antihistamine; analgesic* [pseudoephedrine HCl; chlorpheniramine maleate; acetaminophen] 30•2•500 mg

**duazomycin** USAN, INN *antineoplastic*

**duazomycin A** [see: duazomycin]

**duazomycin B** [see: azotomycin]

**duazomycin C** [see: ambomycin]

*Duboisia myoporoides* medicinal herb [see: corkwood]

**duck's foot** medicinal herb [see: mandrake]

**ducodal** [see: oxycodone]

**Duet** tablets ℞ *vitamin/mineral/calcium/iron supplement* [multiple vitamins & minerals; calcium; iron] ≛•200•29 mg

**Dulcet** (trademarked dosage form) *chewable tablet*

**Dulcolax** enteric-coated tablets, suppositories OTC *stimulant laxative* [bisacodyl] 5 mg; 10 mg

**Dull-C** powder OTC *vitamin C supplement* [ascorbic acid] 4.24 g/tsp.

**dulofibrate** INN

**duloxetine** INN *serotonin and norepinephrine reuptake inhibitor for depression* [also: duloxetine HCl]

**duloxetine HCl** USAN *selective serotonin and norepinephrine reuptake inhibitor (SSNRI) for major depression; analgesic for diabetic neuropathy; investigational (Phase II) for urinary incontinence* [also: duloxetine]

**dulozafone** INN

**dumorelin** INN

**duneryl** [see: phenobarbital]

**Duocaine** injection ℞ *injectable local anesthetic* [bupivacaine HCl; lidocaine HCl]

**Duocet** tablets ℞ *narcotic analgesic* [hydrocodone bitartrate; acetaminophen] 5•500 mg

**Duo-Cyp** IM injection (discontinued 2003) ℞ *hormone replacement therapy for postmenopausal symptoms* [estradiol cypionate; testosterone cypionate] 2•50 mg/mL

**DuoDerm CGF; DuoDerm Extra Thin; DuoDerm Hydroactive** adhesive dressings OTC *occlusive wound dressing* [hydrocolloid gel]

**DuoDerm Hydroactive** paste, granules OTC *wound dressing* [hydrocolloid gel] 30 g; 5 g

**DuoFilm** patch OTC *keratolytic* [salicylic acid in a rubber-based vehicle] 40%

**DuoFilm** topical liquid OTC *keratolytic* [salicylic acid in flexible collodion] 17%

**DuoFilm Gel for Kids** ⒞ OTC *topical keratolytic* [salicylic acid in flexible collodion] 11%

**duometacin** INN

**duomycin** [see: chlortetracycline HCl]

**Duonate-12** pediatric oral suspension ℞ *decongestant; antihistamine* [phenylephrine tannate; pyrilamine tannate] 5•30 mg/5 mL

**DuoNeb** oral inhalation aerosol ℞ *anticholinergic bronchodilator for chronic obstructive pulmonary disease (COPD)* [ipratropium bromide; albuterol sulfate] 0.5•3 mg/dose

**duoperone** INN *neuroleptic* [also: duoperone fumarate]

**duoperone fumarate** USAN *neuroleptic* [also: duoperone]

**DuoPlant** gel ℞ *keratolytic* [salicylic acid in flexible collodion] 17%

**duotal** [see: guaiacol carbonate]

**Duo-Trach Kit** pre-filled syringe with cannula (discontinued 2002) ℞ *injectable local anesthetic* [lidocaine HCl] 4%

**DuoVisc** prefilled syringes ℞ *dispersive/cohesive viscoelastic agent for ophthalmic surgery* [Viscoat (q.v.); ProVisc (q.v.)] 0.35•0.4, 0.5•0.55 mL

**Duphalac** oral/rectal solution ℞ *hyperosmotic laxative* [lactulose] 10 g/15 mL

**Duplex** topical liquid OTC *soap-free therapeutic skin cleanser* [sodium lauryl sulfate] 15%

**Duplex T** shampoo (discontinued 2003) OTC *antiseborrheic; antipsoriatic; antipruritic; antibacterial* [coal tar] 10%

**duponol** [see: sodium lauryl sulfate]

**dupracetam** INN

**Durabolin** IM injection (discontinued 2000) ℞ *anabolic steroid for metastatic breast cancer in women; also abused as a street drug* [nandrolone phenpropionate (in oil)] 25, 50 mg/mL

**Duracaps** (dosage form) *sustained-release capsules*

**DURAcare II** solution OTC *surfactant cleaning solution for soft contact lenses*

**Duraclon** continuous epidural infusion ℞ *central analgesic; adjunct to opioid analgesics for severe cancer pain (orphan)* [clonidine HCl] 500 μg/mL

**Duradrin** capsules ℞ *cerebral vasoconstrictor and analgesic for vascular and tension headaches; "possibly effective" for migraine headaches* [isomethepene mucate; dichloralphenazone; acetaminophen] 65•100•325 mg

**Duradryl** syrup ℞ *decongestant; antihistamine; anticholinergic to dry mucosal secretions* [phenylephrine HCl; chlorpheniramine maleate; methscopolamine nitrate] 10•2•1.25 mg/5 mL

**Duradryl JR** pediatric capsules (discontinued 2004) ℞ *decongestant; antihistamine; anticholinergic to dry mucosal secretions* [phenylephrine HCl; chlorpheniramine maleate; methscopolamine nitrate] 10•4•1.25 mg

**Duraflu** tablets ℞ *antitussive; decongestant; expectorant; analgesic* [dextromethorphan hydrobromide; pseudoephedrine HCl; guaifenesin; acetaminophen] 20•60•200•500 mg

**DuraGen** ℞ *resorbable graft matrix to repair the dura mater following brain surgery or traumatic injury*

**Duragesic-25; Duragesic-50; Duragesic-75; Duragesic-100** transdermal patch ℞ *narcotic analgesic* [fentanyl] 25 μg/hr.; 50 μg/hr.; 75 μg/hr.; 100 μg/hr.

**Dura-Gest** capsules (discontinued 2002) ℞ *decongestant; expectorant* [phenylephrine HCl; phenylpropanolamine HCl; guaifenesin] 45•5•200 mg

**Durahist** sustained-release tablets ℞ *decongestant; antihistamine; anticholinergic* [pseudoephedrine HCl; chlorpheniramine maleate; methscopolamine bromide] 60•8•1.25 mg

**Duralex** sustained-release capsules (discontinued 2002) ℞ *decongestant; antihistamine* [pseudoephedrine HCl; chlorpheniramine maleate] 120•8 mg

**Duralith** ⒸⒶⓃ sustained-release tablets ℞ *antipsychotic for manic episodes* [lithium carbonate] 300 mg

**Duralone-40; Duralone-80** intralesional, soft tissue, and IM injection (discontinued 2004) ℞ *corticosteroid; anti-inflammatory; immunosuppressant* [methylprednisolone acetate] 40 mg/mL; 80 mg/mL

**Duramist Plus 12-Hour Decongestant** nasal spray OTC *nasal decongestant* [oxymetazoline HCl] 0.05%

**Duramorph** IV, subcu or IM injection ℞ *narcotic analgesic* [morphine sulfate] 0.5, 1 mg/mL

**duramycin** *investigational (orphan) agent for cystic fibrosis*

**Duranest; Duranest MPF** injection (discontinued 2002) ℞ *injectable local anesthetic* [etidocaine HCl] [note: one of two different products with the same name] 1% ② Duratest

**Duranest; Duranest MPF** injection (discontinued 2002) ℞ *injectable local anesthetic* [etidocaine; epinephrine] [note: one of two different products with the same name] 1%• 1:200 000, 1.5%•1:200 000 ② Duratest

**durapatite** USAN *prosthetic aid* [also: calcium phosphate, tribasic; hydroxyapatite]

**DuraPrep Surgical Solution** self-contained applicator OTC *broad-spectrum antimicrobial prep for surgical procedures* [iodine; isopropyl alcohol] 0.7%•74%

**Durasal II** sustained-release tablets ℞ *decongestant; expectorant* [pseudoephedrine HCl; guaifenesin] 60•600 mg

**DuraSite** (delivery system) *polymer-based eye drops*

**DuraSolv** (trademarked delivery system) *orally disintegrating tablets*

**Durasphere** injection ℞ *tissue-bulking agent for female stress urinary incontinence* [carbon-coated beads]

**Dura-Tab** (trademarked dosage form) *sustained-release tablet*

**Dura-Tap/PD** prolonged-action capsule (discontinued 2002) ℞ *pediatric decongestant and antihistamine* [pseudoephedrine HCl; chlorpheniramine maleate] 60•4 mg

**Duratears Naturale** ophthalmic ointment OTC *ocular moisturizer/lubricant* [white petrolatum; mineral oil; lanolin]

**Duratest 100; Duratest 200** IM injection (discontinued 2001) ℞• *androgen replacement for delayed puberty or breast cancer* [testosterone cypionate] 100 mg/mL; 200 mg/mL ⓓ Duranest; Duratuss

**Durathate-200** IM injection (discontinued 2001) ℞ *androgen replacement for delayed puberty or breast cancer* [testosterone enanthate] 200 mg/mL

**Duration** nasal spray OTC *nasal decongestant* [oxymetazoline HCl] 0.05%

**Duratocin** ⓒⒶⓃ IV injection ℞ *uterotonic agent to prevent postpartum hemorrhage following cesarean section* [carbetocin] 100 μg/mL

**Duratuss; Duratuss GP** sustained-release film-coated tablets (discontinued 2003) ℞ *decongestant; expectorant* [pseudoephedrine HCl; guaifenesin] 120•600 mg; 120•1200 mg ⓓ Duratest

**Duratuss DM** elixir (discontinued 2003) ℞ *antitussive; expectorant* [dextromethorphan hydrobromide; guaifenesin; alcohol 5%] 20•200 mg/5 mL

**Duratuss G** sustained-release film-coated caplets (discontinued 2003) ℞ *expectorant* [guaifenesin] 1200 mg

**Duratuss HD** elixir (discontinued 2003) ℞ *narcotic antitussive; decongestant; expectorant* [hydrocodone bitartrate; pseudoephedrine HCl; guaifenesin] 5•60•200 mg/10 mL

**Dura-Vent** long-acting tablets (discontinued 2002) ℞ *decongestant; expectorant* [phenylpropanolamine HCl; guaifenesin] 75•600 mg

**Dura-Vent/A** continuous-release capsule (discontinued 2001) ℞ *decongestant; antihistamine* [phenylpropanolamine HCl; chlorpheniramine maleate] 75•10 mg

**Dura-Vent/DA** sustained-release tablets ℞ *decongestant; antihistamine; anticholinergic to dry mucosal secretions* [phenylephrine HCl; chlorpheniramine maleate; methscopolamine nitrate] 20•8•2.5 mg

**Duraxin** capsules ℞ *antihistamine; analgesic* [phenyltoloxamine citrate; acetaminophen; salicylamide] 25•325•200 mg

**Duricef** capsules, tablets, powder for oral suspension ℞ *cephalosporin antibiotic* [cefadroxil] 500 mg; 1000 mg; 125, 250, 500 mg/5 mL

**dusting powder, absorbable** USP *surgical glove lubricant*

**dutasteride** USAN *5α-reductase blocker; inhibits the conversion of testosterone to dihydrotestosterone (DHT); treatment for benign prostatic hyperplasia (BPH); investigational (Phase III) for prostate cancer*

**Dutonin** (British name for U.S. product Serzone)

**Duvoid** tablets (discontinued 2001) ℞ *cholinergic urinary stimulant for postsurgical and postpartum urinary retention* [bethanechol chloride] 10, 25, 50 mg

**DVB (DDP, vindesine, bleomycin)** *chemotherapy protocol*

**DVP (daunorubicin, vincristine, prednisone)** *chemotherapy protocol for acute lymphocytic leukemia (ALL)*

**DVPL-ASP (daunorubicin, vincristine, prednisone, L-asparaginase)** *chemotherapy protocol*

**dwarf ginseng (*Panax trifolius*)** *medicinal herb* [see: ginseng]

**dwarf palm; dwarf palmetto** *medicinal herb* [see: saw palmetto]

**dwarf sumach** *medicinal herb* [see: sumach]

**Dyazide** capsules ℞ *antihypertensive; diuretic* [triamterene; hydrochlorothiazide] 37.5•25 mg ⊡ thiazides; Tiazac

**Dycill** capsules (discontinued 2002) ℞ *penicillinase-resistant penicillin antibiotic* [dicloxacillin sodium] 250, 500 mg

**dyclocaine** BAN *topical anesthetic* [also: dyclonine HCl; dyclonine]

**Dyclone** solution (discontinued 2004) ℞ *anesthetic prior to upper GI and respiratory endoscopies* [dyclonine HCl] 0.5%, 1%

**dyclonine** INN *topical anesthetic* [also: dyclonine HCl; dyclocaine]

**dyclonine HCl** USP *topical anesthetic* [also: dyclonine; dyclocaine]

**dydrogesterone** USAN, USP, INN, BAN *progestin*

**dyer's broom** *(Genista tinctoria)* flowering twigs *medicinal herb used as an aperient, diuretic, stimulant, and vasoconstrictor*

**dyer's bugloss** *medicinal herb* [see: henna *(Alkanna)*]

**dyer's saffron** *medicinal herb* [see: safflower]

**dyer's weed** *medicinal herb* [see: goldenrod]

**Dyflex-G** tablets ℞ *antiasthmatic; bronchodilator; expectorant* [dyphylline; guaifenesin] 200•200 mg

**dyflos** BAN *antiglaucoma agent; irreversible cholinesterase inhibitor miotic* [also: isoflurophate]

**Dy-G** oral liquid ℞ *antiasthmatic; bronchodilator; expectorant* [dyphylline; guaifenesin] 100•100 mg/5 mL

**dylate** [see: clonitrate]

**Dyline-GG** tablets, oral liquid ℞ *antiasthmatic; bronchodilator; expectorant* [dyphylline; guaifenesin] 200•200 mg; 300•300 mg/15 mL

**dymanthine HCl** USAN *anthelmintic* [also: dimantine HCl]

**Dymelor** tablets ℞ *sulfonylurea antidiabetic* [acetohexamide] 250, 500 mg ⊡ Demerol; Pamelor

**Dymenate** IV or IM injection ℞ *antinauseant; antiemetic; antivertigo; motion sickness preventative* [dimenhydrinate] 50 mg/mL

**Dynabac** enteric-coated tablets ℞ *once-daily macrolide antibiotic for respiratory and dermatological infections* [dirithromycin] 250 mg

**Dynacin** capsules, film-coated tablets ℞ *tetracycline antibiotic* [minocycline HCl] 50, 75, 100 mg

**DynaCirc** capsules ℞ *antihypertensive; dihydropyridine calcium channel blocker* [isradipine] 2.5, 5 mg

**DynaCirc CR** controlled-release tablets ℞ *once-daily antihypertensive; dihydropyridine calcium channel blocker* [isradipine] 5, 10 mg

**dynacoryl** [see: nikethamide]

**Dynafed; Dynafed Plus** tablets (discontinued 2002) OTC *decongestant; analgesic; antipyretic* [pseudoephedrine HCl; acetaminophen] 30•500 mg

**Dynafed Asthma Relief** tablets OTC *bronchodilator; decongestant; expectorant* [ephedrine HCl; guaifenesin] 25•200 mg

**Dynafed E.X.** tablets OTC *analgesic; antipyretic* [acetaminophen] 500 mg

**Dynafed IB** tablets (discontinued 2000) OTC *analgesic; antiarthritic; nonsteroidal anti-inflammatory drug (NSAID)* [ibuprofen] 200 mg

**Dynafed Jr., Children's** chewable tablets OTC *analgesic; antipyretic* [acetaminophen] 80 mg

**Dynafed Pseudo** tablets (discontinued 2000) OTC *nasal decongestant* [pseudoephedrine HCl] 60 mg

**Dyna-Hex Skin Cleanser; Dyna-Hex 2 Skin Cleanser** topical liquid OTC *broad-spectrum antimicrobial; germicidal* [chlorhexidine gluconate; alcohol 4%] 4%; 2%

**dynamine** *investigational (orphan) agent for Lambert-Eaton myasthenic syndrome and Charcot-Marie-Tooth disease*

**Dynapen** capsules, powder for oral suspension (discontinued 2002) ℞ *penicillinase-resistant penicillin antibi-*

*otic* [dicloxacillin sodium] 125, 250, 500 mg; 62.5 mg/5 mL

**dynarsan** [see: acetarsone]

**Dynepo** (approved in Europe) ℞ *investigational (NDA filed) gene therapy for anemia of renal failure* [erythropoietin, gene-activated]

**Dynex** sustained-release caplets ℞ *decongestant; expectorant* [pseudoephedrine HCl; guaifenesin] 90• 1200 mg

**dyphylline** USP *antiasthmatic; bronchodilator* [also: diprophylline] 200, 400 mg oral

**dyphylline & guaifenesin** *antiasthmatic; bronchodilator; expectorant* 200•200 mg oral

**Dyphylline-GG** elixir OTC *antiasthmatic; bronchodilator; expectorant* [dyphylline; guaifenesin] 100•100 mg/15 mL

**Dyprotex** pads OTC *topical diaper rash treatment* [zinc oxide; dimethicone] 40%•2.5%

**Dyrenium** capsules ℞ *antihypertensive; potassium-sparing diuretic* [triamterene] 50, 100 mg 🄯 Pyridium

**Dyrexan-OD** sustained-release capsules (discontinued 2001) ℞ *anorexiant; CNS stimulant* [phendimetrazine tartrate] 105 mg

**Dysport** ℞ *investigational (orphan) agent for blepharospasm and strabismus of dystonia, pediatric cerebral palsy, and cervical dystonia* [botulinum toxin, type A]

**dysprosium** *element (Dy)*

**Dytan-D** chewable tablets ℞ *decongestant; antihistamine* [phenylephrine tannate; diphenhydramine tannate] 10•25 mg

**DZAPO (daunorubicin, azacitidine, ara-C, prednisone, Oncovin)** *chemotherapy protocol*

**E2II** transdermal patch ℞ *investigational (NDA filed) hormone replacement therapy* [estradiol]

**E₂C (estradiol cypionate)** [q.v.]

**E5 monoclonal antibodies (MAb)** [now: edobacomab]

**EACA (epsilon-aminocaproic acid)** [see: aminocaproic acid]

**EAP (etoposide, Adriamycin, Platinol)** *chemotherapy protocol for gastric and small bowel cancer*

**ear, lion's** *medicinal herb* [see: motherwort]

**Ear-Dry** ear drops OTC *antibacterial; antifungal* [boric acid] 2.75%

**Ear-Eze** ear drops ℞ *topical corticosteroidal anti-inflammatory; antibiotic* [hydrocortisone; neomycin sulfate; polymyxin B sulfate] 1%•5 mg• 10 000 U per mL

**EarSol** ear drops (discontinued 2003) OTC *antiseptic* [alcohol] 44%

**EarSol-HC** ear drops OTC *topical corticosteroidal anti-inflammatory; antiseptic* [hydrocortisone; alcohol 44%] 1%

**earthnut oil** [see: peanut oil]

**Easprin** delayed-release enteric-coated tablets ℞ *analgesic; antipyretic; anti-inflammatory; antirheumatic* [aspirin] 975 mg

**Easter giant** *medicinal herb* [see: bistort]

**Easy A1C** fingerstick test kit for home use *in vitro diagnostic aid for glycosylated hemoglobin levels*

**EasyInjector** (trademarked device) *self-injector*

**E-Base** delayed-release enteric-coated caplets and tablets ℞ *macrolide antibiotic* [erythromycin] 333, 500 mg

**ebastine** USAN, INN *antihistamine*

**ebiratide** INN

**ebrotidine** INN

**ebselen** INN

**EC (etoposide, carboplatin)** *chemotherapy protocol for lung cancer*

**ecadotril** USAN, INN *antihypertensive*

**ecalcidene** USAN *antipsoriatic*

**ecamsule** USAN *UVA sunscreen*

**ecarazine** [see: todralazine]

**EC-ASA (enteric-coated aspirin)** [see: aspirin]

**ecastolol** INN

**Ecee Plus** tablets OTC *vitamin/mineral supplement* [vitamins C and E; zinc sulfate; magnesium sulfate] 100•165•80•70 mg

**echinacea** (*Echinacea angustifolia; E. purpurea; E. pallida*) root *medicinal herb for anemia, blood diseases, blood poisoning, boils, dizziness, immune system stimulation, lymph disorders, promoting wound healing, prostate disorders, skin infections, and snake bites*

**echinocandins** *a class of antifungals* [also: glucan synthesis inhibitors]

*Echinopanax horridum medicinal herb* [see: devil's club]

**ECHO (etoposide, cyclophosphamide, hydroxydaunomycin, Oncovin)** *chemotherapy protocol*

**EchoGen** emulsion ℞ *investigational (NDA filed) ultrasound contrast agent for stress cardiography and transrectal prostate imaging* [perflenapent; perflisopent] 85%•15%

**echothiophate iodide** USP *antiglaucoma agent; irreversible cholinesterase inhibitor miotic* [also: ecothiopate iodide]

**Echovist** ⓒ *intrauterine suspension* ℞ *ultrasound contrast medium for gynecological imaging* [galactose]

**ecipramidil** INN

**eclanamine** INN *antidepressant* [also: eclanamine maleate]

**eclanamine maleate** USAN *antidepressant* [also: eclanamine]

**eclazolast** USAN, INN *antiallergic; mediator release inhibitor*

**EC-Naprosyn** enteric-coated delayed-release tablets ℞ *antiarthritic; nonste-*

*roidal anti-inflammatory drug (NSAID)* [naproxen] 375, 500 mg

**ecogramostim** BAN

**ecomustine** INN

**econazole** USAN, INN, BAN *topical antifungal*

**econazole nitrate** USAN, USP, BAN *topical antifungal* 1% topical

**Econo B & C** caplets OTC *vitamin supplement* [multiple B vitamins; vitamin C] ±•300 mg

**Econopred; Econopred Plus** Drop-Tainers (eye drop suspension) ℞ *topical ophthalmic corticosteroidal anti-inflammatory* [prednisolone acetate] 0.125%; 1%

**ecopipam HCl** USAN *selective dopamine receptor antagonist for addiction*

**ecostigmine iodide** [see: echothiophate iodide]

**ecothiopate iodide** INN, BAN *antiglaucoma agent; irreversible cholinesterase inhibitor miotic* [also: echothiophate iodide]

**Ecotrin** enteric-coated tablets, enteric-coated caplets OTC *analgesic; antipyretic; anti-inflammatory; antiarthritic* [aspirin] 325, 500 mg ⓔ Edecrin

**Ecotrin Adult Low Strength** enteric-coated tablets OTC *analgesic; antipyretic; anti-inflammatory; antiarthritic* [aspirin] 81 mg

**ecraprost** USAN *treatment of peripheral occlusive disease*

**ecteinascidin** *investigational (Phase III) tetrahydroisoquinoline alkaloid for sarcoma*

**ectylurea** BAN

**eculizumab** *investigational (orphan) agent for idiopathic membranous glomerular nephropathy and paroxysmal nocturnal hemoglobinuria*

**Ed A-Hist** sustained-release tablets, oral liquid ℞ *decongestant; antihistamine* [phenylephrine HCl; chlorpheniramine maleate] 20•8 mg; 10•4 mg/5 mL

**ED Tuss HC** syrup ℞ *narcotic antitussive; decongestant; antihistamine* [hydrocodone bitartrate; phenylephrine HCl; chlorpheniramine maleate] 2.5•10•4 mg/5 mL

**edamine** [see: ethylenediamine]

**EDAP (etoposide, dexamethasone, ara-C, Platinol)** *chemotherapy protocol*

**edathamil** [now: edetate calcium disodium]

**edathamil calcium disodium** [now: edetate calcium disodium]

**edathamil disodium** [now: edetate disodium]

**edatrexate** USAN, INN *antineoplastic; methotrexate analogue*

**Edecrin** tablets ℞ *antihypertensive; loop diuretic* [ethacrynic acid] 25, 50 mg ⊞ Ecotrin; Ethaquin

**Edecrin Sodium** powder for IV injection ℞ *antihypertensive; loop diuretic* [ethacrynate sodium] 50 mg

**edelfosine** INN

**edetate calcium disodium** USAN, USP *heavy metal chelating agent for acute or chronic lead poisoning and lead encephalopathy* [also: sodium calcium edetate; sodium calciumedetate; calcium disodium edetate]

**edetate dipotassium** USAN *chelating agent*

**edetate disodium** USP *chelating agent; preservative; antioxidant* [also: disodium edetate] 150 mg/mL injection

**edetate magnesium disodium** *chelating agent for atherosclerosis*

**edetate sodium** USAN *chelating agent*

**edetate trisodium** USAN *chelating agent*

**edetic acid** NF, INN, BAN *chelating agent*

**edetol** USAN, INN *alkalizing agent*

**Edex** injection, pre-filled syringes ℞ *vasodilator for erectile dysfunction* [alprostadil] 10, 20, 40 μg/mL

**Ed-Flex** capsules ℞ *antihistamine; analgesic* [phenyltoloxamine citrate; acetaminophen; salicylamide] 20•300•200 mg

**edifolone** INN *antiarrhythmic* [also: edifolone acetate]

**edifolone acetate** USAN *antiarrhythmic* [also: edifolone]

**Ed-In-Sol** drops OTC *hematinic* [ferrous sulfate (source of iron)] 75 mg/0.6 mL (15 mg/0.6 mL)

**edisilate** INN *combining name for radicals or groups* [also: edisylate]

**edisylate** USAN, BAN *combining name for radicals or groups* [also: edisilate]

**edithamil** [see: edetate ...]

**edobacomab** USAN *antiendotoxin monoclonal antibody for gram-negative sepsis; clinical trials discontinued 1997*

**edodekin alfa** USAN *antiasthmatic; investigational (Phase I/II) immunomodulator for AIDS-related Kaposi sarcoma; investigational (orphan) for renal cell carcinoma* [previously: interleukin 12 (IL-12)]

**edogestrone** INN, BAN

**edonentan** USAN *endothelin A (ETA) inhibitor for heart failure*

**edoxudine** USAN, INN *antiviral*

**edrecolomab** USAN *monoclonal antibody; antineoplastic adjuvant*

**edrofuradene** [see: nifurdazil]

**Edronax** (approved in England) ℞ *investigational (NDA filed) fast-acting selective norepinephrine reuptake inhibitor for depression* [reboxetine mesylate]

**edrophone chloride** [see: edrophonium chloride]

**edrophonium chloride** USP, INN, BAN *cholinergic/anticholinesterase muscle stimulant; antidote to curare; myasthenia gravis diagnostic aid*

**Ed-Spaz** tablets ℞ *GI/GU antispasmodic; antiparkinsonian; anticholinergic "drying agent" for allergic rhinitis and hyperhidrosis* [hyoscyamine sulfate] 0.125 mg

**EDTA (ethylenediaminetetraacetic acid)** [see: edetate disodium]

**EDTA calcium** [see: edetate calcium disodium]

**ED-TLC** oral liquid ℞ *narcotic antitussive; decongestant; antihistamine* [hydrocodone bitartrate; phenylephrine HCl; chlorpheniramine maleate] 3.33•10•4 mg/10 mL

**E.E.S.** granules for oral suspension ℞ *macrolide antibiotic* [erythromycin ethylsuccinate] 200 mg/5 mL

**EES (erythromycin ethylsuccinate)** [q.v.]

**E.E.S. 200** oral suspension ℞ *macrolide antibiotic* [erythromycin ethylsuccinate] 200 mg/5 mL

**E.E.S. 400** film-coated tablets, oral suspension ℞ *macrolide antibiotic* [erythromycin ethylsuccinate] 400 mg; 400 mg/5 mL

**efalizumab** *recombinant humanized monoclonal antibody (rhuMAb) to leukocyte function–associated antigen-1 (LFA-1); immunosuppressant for moderate to severe plaque psoriasis*

**efaproxiral** *investigational (NDA filed) radiosensitizer for breast, lung, and brain tumors*

**Efaproxyn** ℞ *investigational (NDA filed) radiosensitizer for breast, lung, and brain tumors* [efaproxiral]

**efaroxan** INN, BAN

**efavirenz** *antiviral non-nucleoside reverse transcriptase inhibitor (NNRTI) for HIV infection*

**efavirenz & lamivudine & zidovudine** *investigational (Phase III) antiviral combination for HIV and AIDS*

**efegatran sulfate** USAN *antithrombotic*

**efetozole** INN

**Effer-K** effervescent tablets ℞ *potassium supplement* [potassium bicarbonate; potassium citrate] 25 mEq K

**Effervescent Potassium** effervescent tablets ℞ *potassium supplement* [potassium bicarbonate; potassium citrate] 25 mEq K

**Effexor** tablets ℞ *antidepressant for major depression* [venlafaxine HCl] 25, 37.5, 50, 75, 100 mg

**Effexor XR** extended-release capsules ℞ *antidepressant for major depression; anxiolytic for generalized anxiety disorder (GAD) and social anxiety disorder (SAD)* [venlafaxine HCl] 37.5, 75, 150 mg

**Efidac 24 Chlorpheniramine** dual-release tablets OTC *antihistamine* [chlorpheniramine maleate] 16 mg (4 mg immediate release, 12 mg extended release)

**Efidac 24 Pseudoephedrine** dual-release tablets OTC *nasal decongestant* [pseudoephedrine HCl] 240 mg (60 mg immediate release, 180 mg extended release)

**Eflone** eye drop suspension ℞ *topical ophthalmic corticosteroidal anti-inflammatory* [fluorometholone acetate] 0.1%

**eflornithine** INN, BAN *antineoplastic; antiprotozoal; topical hair growth inhibitor* [also: eflornithine HCl]

**eflornithine HCl** USAN *antiprotozoal for* Trypanosoma brucei *gambiense (sleeping sickness) infection (orphan); topical hair growth inhibitor; investigational (Phase III) for bladder cancer; investigational (orphan) for AIDS-related* Pneumocystis carinii *pneumonia (PCP)* [also: eflornithine]

**efloxate** INN

**eflumast** INN

**Efodine** ointment OTC *broad-spectrum antimicrobial* [povidone-iodine] 1%

**eformoterol fumarate** BAN *bronchodilator* [also: formoterol; formoterol fumarate]

**EFP (etoposide, fluorouracil, Platinol)** *chemotherapy protocol for gastric and small bowel cancer*

**efrotomycin** USAN, INN, BAN *veterinary growth stimulant*

**Efudex** cream, topical solution ℞ *antineoplastic for actinic keratoses and basal cell carcinomas* [fluorouracil] 5%; 2%, 5%

**egtazic acid** USAN, INN *pharmaceutic aid*

**Egyptian privet** *medicinal herb* [see: henna (Lawsonia)]

**Egyptian thorn** *medicinal herb* [see: acacia]

**EHDP (ethane hydroxydiphosphonate)** [see: etidronate disodium]

**Ehrlich 594** [see: acetarsone]

**Ehrlich 606** [see: arsphenamine]

**eicosapentaenoic acid (EPA)** *natural omega-3 fatty acid used to prevent a* wide range of degenerative diseases; precursor to the anti-inflammatory and anticoagulant series 3 prostaglandins; effective in treating depression and other mental disorders [also: icosapent]

**8 in 1 (methylprednisolone, vincristine, lomustine, procarbazine, hydroxyurea, cisplatin, cytarabine, cyclophosphamide)** chemotherapy protocol

**8 in 1 (methylprednisolone, vincristine, lomustine, procarbazine, hydroxyurea, cisplatin, cytarabine, dacarbazine)** chemotherapy protocol for pediatric brain tumors

**8-MOP** capsules ℞ systemic psoralens for psoriasis, repigmentation of idiopathic vitiligo, and cutaneous T-cell lymphoma (CTCL); used to increase tolerance to sunlight and enhance pigmentation [methoxsalen] 10 mg

**einsteinium** element (Es)

**eIPV (enhanced, inactivated polio vaccine)** [see: poliovirus vaccine, enhanced inactivated]

**elacridar HCl** USAN chemotherapy potentiator; multi–drug-resistance inhibitor

**ELA-Max** cream (name changed to L-M-X4 in 2003) OTC local anesthetic [lidocaine] 4%

**elantrine** USAN, INN anticholinergic

**elanzepine** INN

**elastofilcon A** USAN hydrophilic contact lens material

**Elavil** film-coated tablets (discontinued 2004) ℞ tricyclic antidepressant [amitriptyline HCl] 10, 25, 50, 75, 100, 150 mg ☑ Aldoril; Elidel; Eldepryl; Enovil; Equanil; Mellaril

**Elavil** IM injection (discontinued 2003) ℞ tricyclic antidepressant [amitriptyline HCl] 10 mg/mL ☑ Aldoril; Eldepryl; Enovil; Equanil; Mellaril

**elbanizine** INN

**elcatonin** INN, JAN investigational (orphan) intrathecal treatment of intractable pain

**eldacimibe** USAN antihyperlipidemic; antiatherosclerotic; AcylCoA transferase (ACAT) inhibitor

**Eldepryl** capsules ℞ dopaminergic antiparkinsonian (orphan) [selegiline HCl] 5 mg ☑ Aldoril; Elavil; Enovil; Equanil; Mellaril

**elder flower; elderberry (Sambucus canadensis; S. ebulus; S. nigra; S. racemosa)** berries and flowers medicinal herb for allergies, asthma, bronchitis, colds, constipation, edema, fever, hay fever, pneumonia, and sinus congestion; also used topically as an astringent

**Eldercaps** capsules ℞ vitamin/mineral supplement [multiple vitamins & minerals; folic acid] ≛•1 mg

**Eldertonic** oral liquid OTC vitamin/mineral supplement [multiple B vitamins & minerals; alcohol 13.5%]

**eldexomer** INN

**Eldisine** ℞ investigational (NDA filed) antineoplastic for leukemia, melanoma, breast and lung cancers [vindesine sulfate]

**Eldopaque; Eldopaque-Forte** cream OTC hyperpigmentation bleaching agent; sunscreen [hydroquinone in a sunblock base] 2%; 4%

**Eldoquin** cream (discontinued 2003) OTC hyperpigmentation bleaching agent [hydroquinone] 2%

**Eldoquin-Forte** cream OTC hyperpigmentation bleaching agent [hydroquinone] 4%

**elecampane (Inula helenium)** root medicinal herb for chronic bronchitis and cough

**electrocortin** [see: aldosterone]

**eledoisin** INN

**Elestat** eye drops ℞ selective $H_1$ antagonist; antihistamine; mast cell stabilizer [epinastine HCl]

**eletriptan hydrobromide** USAN vascular serotonin 5-HT$_{1B/1D/1F}$-receptor agonist for the acute treatment of migraine (base=82.5%)

**Eleutherococcus senticosus** medicinal herb [see: Siberian ginseng]

**ELF (etoposide, leucovorin [rescue], fluorouracil)** chemotherapy protocol for gastric cancer

**elfazepam** USAN, INN *veterinary appetite stimulant*

**elfdock; elfwort** *medicinal herb* [see: elecampane]

**elgodipine** INN

**Elidel** cream ℞ *nonsteroidal anti-inflammatory for atopic dermatitis* [pimecrolimus] 1% ☑ Elavil

**Eligard** sustained-release subcu injection ℞ *antihormonal antineoplastic for advanced prostate cancer* [leuprolide acetate] 7.5 mg (1-month depot), 22.5 mg (3-month depot), 30 mg (4-month depot)

**Elimite** cream ℞ *pediculicide for lice; scabicide* [permethrin] 5%

**eliprodil** INN *investigational treatment for ischemic stroke*

**Elitek** powder for IV infusion ℞ *antimetabolite antineoplastic for leukemia, lymphoma, and solid tumor malignancies* [rasburicase] 1.5 mg/vial

**Elixomin** elixir ℞ *antiasthmatic; bronchodilator* [theophylline] 80 mg/15 mL

**Elixophyllin** capsules, elixir ℞ *antiasthmatic; bronchodilator* [theophylline] 100, 200 mg; 80 mg/15 mL

**Elixophyllin GG** oral liquid ℞ *antiasthmatic; bronchodilator; expectorant* [theophylline; guaifenesin] 100•100 mg/15 mL

**Elixophyllin-KI** elixir ℞ *antiasthmatic; bronchodilator; expectorant* [theophylline; potassium iodide] 80•130 mg/15 mL

**ElixSure Congestion** syrup OTC *decongestant* [pseudoephedrine HCl] 15 mg/5 mL

**ElixSure Cough** syrup OTC *antitussive* [dextromethorphan hydrobromide] 7.5 mg/5 mL

**ElixSure Fever/Pain** syrup OTC *analgesic; antipyretic* [acetaminophen] 160 mg/5 mL

**ElixSure IB** oral suspension OTC *analgesic; antipyretic* [ibuprofen] 100 mg/5 mL

**ellagic acid** INN

**Ellence** IV infusion ℞ *anthracycline antibiotic antineoplastic for breast cancer (orphan)* [epirubicin HCl] 2 mg/mL

**Elliott's B solution** *investigational (orphan) intrathecal chemotherapy diluent*

**elliptinium acetate** INN, BAN

**elm, American; Indian elm; moose elm; red elm; rock elm; sweet elm; winged elm** *medicinal herb* [see: slippery elm]

**Elmiron** capsules ℞ *urinary tract anti-inflammatory and analgesic for interstitial cystitis (orphan)* [pentosan polysulfate sodium] 100 mg

**elmustine** INN

**elnadipine** INN

**Elocom** ⒸⒶⓃ ointment, cream, lotion ℞ *topical corticosteroidal anti-inflammatory* [mometasone furoate] 0.1%

**Elocon** ointment, cream, lotion ℞ *topical corticosteroidal anti-inflammatory* [mometasone furoate] 0.1%

**Eloxatin** powder for IV infusion ℞ *alkylating antineoplastic for metastatic ovarian and colorectal cancers (orphan); investigational (Phase III) for pancreatic cancer* [oxaliplatin] 50, 100 mg

**elsamitrucin** USAN, INN *antineoplastic*

**Elspar** powder for IV or IM injection ℞ *antineoplastic adjunct for acute lymphocytic leukemia* [asparaginase] 10 000 IU

**eltanolone** INN *investigational IV anesthetic*

**eltenac** INN

**eltoprazine** INN

**Eltroxin** tablets (discontinued 2003) ℞ *synthetic thyroid hormone ($T_4$ fraction only)* [levothyroxine sodium] 50, 75, 100, 125, 150, 200, 300 μg

**elucaine** USAN, INN *gastric anticholinergic*

**Elymus repens** *medicinal herb* [see: couch grass]

**elziverine** INN

**EMA (estramustine L-alanine)** [q.v.]

**EMA 86 (etoposide, mitoxantrone, ara-C)** *chemotherapy protocol for acute myelocytic leukemia (AML)*

**EMACO (etoposide, methotrexate, actinomycin D, cyclophospha-**

**mide, Oncovin)** *chemotherapy protocol*

**Emadine** eye drops ℞ *topical antihistamine for allergic conjunctivitis* [emedastine difumarate] 0.05%

**Embeline** ointment, gel, cream, scalp application ℞ *corticosteroidal antiinflammatory* [clobetasol propionate] 0.05%

**embinal** [see: barbital sodium]

**embonate** INN, BAN *combining name for radicals or groups* [also: pamoate]

**embramine** INN, BAN

**embramine HCl** [see: embramine]

**Embrex 600** chewable tablets ℞ *vitamin/mineral/calcium/iron supplement* [multiple vitamins & minerals; calcium; iron; folic acid] ≛•240•90•1 mg

**embutramide** USAN, INN, BAN *veterinary anesthetic; veterinary euthanasia*

**Emcyt** capsules ℞ *nitrogen mustard-type alkylating antineoplastic for metastatic or progressive prostatic carcinoma* [estramustine phosphate sodium] 140 mg

**Emdogain** ℞ *investigational (NDA filed) freeze-dried enamel matrix protein for wound healing*

**emedastine** INN *ophthalmic antihistamine* [also: emedastine difumarate]

**emedastine difumarate** USAN, JAN *ophthalmic antihistamine* [also: emedastine]

**Emend** capsules ℞ *antiemetic for chemotherapy* [aprepitant] 80, 125 mg

**emepronium bromide** INN, BAN

**emepronium carrageenate** BAN

**Emergent-Ez Kit** (discontinued 2002) *carry-kit for medical personnel* [multiple drugs and devices for emergencies]

**Emersal** topical emulsion (discontinued 2004) ℞ *antipsoriatic; antiseborrheic* [ammoniated mercury; salicylic acid] 5%•2.5%

**emetic herb; emetic weed** *medicinal herb* [see: lobelia]

**emetics** *a class of agents that induce vomiting*

**emetine** BAN *antiamebic* [also: emetine HCl] ⑨ Emetrol

**emetine bismuth iodide** [see: emetine HCl]

**emetine HCl** USP *amebicide* [also: emetine]

**Emetrol** oral solution OTC *antiemetic for nausea associated with influenza, morning sickness, motion sickness, inhalation anesthesia, or food and drink indiscretions* [phosphorated carbohydrate solution (fructose, dextrose, and phosphoric acid)] 1.87 g•1.87 g•21.5 mg ⑨ emetine

**EMF** oral liquid OTC *protein supplement* [multiple amino acids] 15 g protein

**Emgel** gel ℞ *antibiotic for acne* [erythromycin; alcohol 77%] 2%

**emiglitate** INN, BAN

**emilium tosilate** INN *antiarrhythmic* [also: emilium tosylate]

**emilium tosylate** USAN *antiarrhythmic* [also: emilium tosilate]

**Eminase** powder for IV injection (discontinued 2003) ℞ *thrombolytic enzyme for acute myocardial infarction* [anistreplase] 30 U/vial

**emitefur** USAN *antineoplastic for stomach, colorectal, breast, pancreatic, and non–small cell lung cancers (NSCLC)*

**emivirine** *investigational (NDA filed) non-nucleoside reverse transcriptase inhibitor for naive HIV infection*

**Emko; Emko Pre-Fil** vaginal foam (discontinued 2002) OTC *spermicidal contraceptive* [nonoxynol 9] 8%

**EMLA** cream, adhesive disc ℞ *local anesthetic* [lidocaine; prilocaine] 2.5%•2.5%

**emmenagogues** *a class of agents that induce or increase menstruation*

**Emollia** lotion OTC *moisturizer; emollient*

**emollient laxatives** *a subclass of laxatives that work by retarding colonic absorption of fecal water to soften the stool and ease its movement through the intestines* [see also: laxatives]

**emollients** *a class of dermatological agents that soften and soothe the skin*

**emonapride** INN

**emopamil** INN

**emorfazone** INN

**Empirin** tablets OTC *analgesic; antipyretic; anti-inflammatory; antirheumatic* [aspirin] 325 mg

**Empirin with Codeine No. 3 & No. 4** tablets ℞ *narcotic antitussive; analgesic; sometimes abused as a street drug* [codeine phosphate; aspirin] 30•325 mg; 60•325 mg

**emtricitabine** USAN *antiviral; nucleoside analogue reverse transcriptase inhibitor for HIV-1 infection; synthetic cytosine analogue*

**Emtriva** capsules, ℞ *antiviral for HIV-1 infection* [emtricitabine] 200 mg

**emtryl** [see: dimetridazole]

**emu oil** *natural remedy for arthritis pain, hair loss prevention, and chronic skin disorders*

**emulsifying wax** [see: wax, emulsifying]

**Emulsoil** oral emulsion OTC *stimulant laxative* [castor oil] 95%

**E-Mycin** enteric-coated tablets ℞ *macrolide antibiotic* [erythromycin] 250, 333 mg

**emylcamate** INN, BAN

**Enable** ℞ *investigational (NDA filed) anti-inflammatory for rheumatoid arthritis and osteoarthritis* [tenidap]

**Enablex** ℞ *investigational (NDA filed) selective muscarinic M₃ receptor antagonist for urinary frequency, urgency, and incontinence* [darifenacin hydrobromide] 7.5, 15 mg

**enadoline** INN *analgesic* [also: enadoline HCl]

**enadoline HCl** USAN *analgesic; investigational (orphan) for severe head injury* [also: enadoline]

**enalapril** INN, BAN *antihypertensive; angiotensin-converting enzyme (ACE) inhibitor* [also: enalapril maleate]

**enalapril maleate** USAN, USP *antihypertensive; angiotensin-converting enzyme (ACE) inhibitor; treatment for CHF* [also: enalapril] 2.5, 5, 10, 20 mg oral

**enalapril maleate & hydrochlorothiazide** *antihypertensive; angiotensin-converting enzyme (ACE) inhibitor; diuretic* 5•12.5, 10•25 mg oral

**enalaprilat** USAN, USP, INN, BAN *antihypertensive; angiotensin-converting enzyme (ACE) inhibitor* 1.25 mg/mL injection

**enalkiren** USAN, INN *antihypertensive; renin inhibitor*

**enallynymal sodium** [see: methohexital sodium]

**enantate** INN *combining name for radicals or groups* [also: enanthate]

**enanthate** USAN, USP, BAN *combining name for radicals or groups* [also: enantate]

**enantiomer** [def.] *One of a pair of chemical compounds having the same molecular formula, but with the atoms arranged in mirror image. Subdivided into (+) (formerly d- or dextro-) and (−) (formerly l- or levo-).* [see also: isomer; racemic]

**Enbrel** powder for subcu injection ℞ *soluble tumor necrosis factor receptor (sTNFR) inhibitor for rheumatoid arthritis, juvenile rheumatoid arthritis (orphan), psoriatic arthritis, and ankylosing spondylitis; investigational (NDA filed) for congestive heart failure; investigational (orphan) for Wegener granulomatosis* [etanercept] 25 mg/vial ⚕ Incel

**enbucrilate** INN, BAN

**encainide** INN, BAN *antiarrhythmic* [also: encainide HCl]

**encainide HCl** USAN *antiarrhythmic* [also: encainide]

**Encare** vaginal suppositories OTC *spermicidal contraceptive* [nonoxynol 9] 2.27%

**enciprazine** INN, BAN *minor tranquilizer* [also: enciprazine HCl]

**enciprazine HCl** USAN *minor tranquilizer* [also: enciprazine]

**enclomifene** INN [also: enclomiphene]

**enclomiphene** USAN [also: enclomifene]

**encyprate** USAN, INN *antidepressant*

**End Lice** topical liquid (discontinued 2003) OTC *pediculicide for lice* [pyrethrins; piperonyl butoxide] 0.3%•3%

**Endafed** sustained-release capsules (discontinued 2002) ℞ *decongestant; antihistamine* [pseudoephedrine HCl; brompheniramine maleate] 120•12 mg

**Endagen-HD** oral liquid ℞ *narcotic antitussive; decongestant; antihistamine* [hydrocodone bitartrate; phenylephrine HCl; chlorpheniramine maleate] 3.33•10•4 mg/10 mL

**Endal Expectorant** syrup ℞ *narcotic antitussive; decongestant; expectorant* [codeine phosphate; phenylephrine HCl; guaifenesin; alcohol 5%] 12.5•4•125 mg/5 mL

**Endal Nasal Decongestant** timed-release caplets ℞ *decongestant; expectorant* [phenylephrine HCl; guaifenesin] 20•300 mg ⃞ Intal

**Endal-HD** syrup ℞ *narcotic antitussive; decongestant; antihistamine* [hydrocodone bitartrate; phenylephrine HCl; diphenhydramine HCl] 2•7.5•12.5 mg/5 mL

**Endal-HD Plus** syrup ℞ *narcotic antitussive; decongestant; antihistamine* [hydrocodone bitartrate; phenylephrine HCl; chlorpheniramine maleate] 3.5•7.5•2.5 mg/5 mL

**endiemal** [see: metharbital]

**endive** *medicinal herb* [see: chicory]

**endive, white; wild endive** *medicinal herb* [see: dandelion]

**endixaprine** INN

**endobenzyline bromide**

**endocaine** [see: pyrrocaine]

**Endocet** tablets ℞ *narcotic analgesic* [oxycodone HCl; acetaminophen] 5•325, 7.5•325, 10•325 mg

**Endocodone** tablets ℞ *narcotic analgesic* [oxycodone HCl] 5 mg

**endolate** [see: meperidine HCl]

**Endolor** capsules (discontinued 2000) ℞ *analgesic; barbiturate sedative* [acetaminophen; caffeine; butalbital] 325•40•50 mg

**endomide** INN

**endomycin**

**Endospray** ⓒ metered-dose spray OTC *topical anesthetic for oropharyngeal and endotracheal areas* [benzocaine; tetracaine] 18•2 mg/spray

**endothelin-1 receptor antagonists** *a class of vasodilator antihypertensives that block the action of endothelin-1 (ET-1), a vascular vasoconstrictor more potent than angiotensin II*

**endralazine** INN, BAN *antihypertensive* [also: endralazine mesylate]

**endralazine mesylate** USAN *antihypertensive* [also: endralazine]

**Endrate** IV infusion ℞ *chelating agent for hypercalcemia and ventricular arrhythmias due to digitalis toxicity* [edetate disodium] 150 mg/mL

**endrisone** INN *topical ophthalmic anti-inflammatory* [also: endryson]

**endryson** USAN *topical ophthalmic anti-inflammatory* [also: endrisone]

**Enduret** (trademarked dosage form) *prolonged-action tablet*

**Enduron** tablets ℞ *diuretic; antihypertensive* [methyclothiazide] 5 mg ⃞ Imuran; Inderal

**Enduronyl; Enduronyl Forte** tablets (discontinued 2003) ℞ *antihypertensive* [methyclothiazide; deserpidine] 5•0.25 mg; 5•0.5 mg ⃞ Inderal

**Enecat CT** concentrated rectal suspension ℞ *radiopaque contrast medium for gastrointestinal imaging* [barium sulfate] 5%

**enefexine** INN

**Enerjets** lozenges OTC *CNS stimulant; analeptic* [caffeine] 75 mg

**enestebol** INN

**EnfaCare** [see: Enfamil EnfaCare]

**Enfalac AR** ⓒ powder OTC *total or supplementary infant feeding; thickened formula* [cow's milk–based formula]

**Enfalac Iron Fortified** ⓒ oral liquid, powder for oral liquid OTC *total or supplementary infant feeding* [milk-based formula]

**Enfalac ProSobee Soy** ⓒ oral liquid, powder for oral liquid OTC *hypoallergenic infant food* [soy protein formula]

**Enfalac Regular** ⓒ oral liquid, powder for oral liquid OTC *total or supple-*

mentary infant feeding [milk-based formula]

**Enfalyte** ready-to-use oral liquid OTC *supplementary feeding to maintain hydration and electrolyte balance in infants with diarrhea or vomiting* 33.8 oz bottles

**Enfamil** oral liquid, powder for oral liquid OTC *total or supplementary infant feeding*

**Enfamil EnfaCare** oral liquid, powder for oral liquid OTC *enriched formula for premature infants* [milk-based formula] 3 oz bottles; 14 oz cans

**Enfamil Human Milk Fortifier** powder OTC *supplement to breast milk*

**Enfamil LactoFree** oral liquid, concentrate for oral liquid, powder for oral liquid OTC *hypoallergenic infant formula* [milk-based formula, lactose free] 946 mL; 384 mL; 397 g

**Enfamil LIPIL with Iron** Nursette bottles, ready-to-use oral liquid, concentrate for oral liquid, powder for oral liquid OTC *infant formula fortified with omega-3 fatty acids* 3, 6 oz. bottles; 32 oz. cans; 13 oz. cans; 12.9, 25.9 oz. cans

**Enfamil Low Iron** oral liquid (discontinued 2003) OTC *total or supplementary infant feeding*

**Enfamil Next Step** oral liquid, powder for oral liquid OTC *total or supplementary infant feeding*

**Enfamil Premature Formula** oral liquid OTC *total or supplementary infant feeding*

**Enfamil with Iron** oral liquid, powder for oral liquid OTC *total or supplementary infant feeding*

**enfenamic acid** INN

**enflurane** USAN, USP, INN, BAN *inhalation general anesthetic* 125, 250 mL

**enfuvirtide** *fusion inhibitor that prevents HIV from binding to T-cells, thus preventing viral entry into healthy cells*

**Engerix-B** adult IM injection, pediatric IM injection R *active immunizing agent for hepatitis B and D* [hepa-

titis B virus vaccine, recombinant] 20 µg/mL, 10 µg/0.5 mL

**English elm** *(Ulmus campestris) medicinal herb* [see: slippery elm]

**English hawthorn** *medicinal herb* [see: hawthorn]

**English ivy** *(Hedera helix)* leaves *medicinal herb used as an antispasmodic and antiexanthematous agent*

**English oak** *(Quercus robur) medicinal herb* [see: white oak]

**English valerian** *medicinal herb* [see: valerian]

**English walnut** *(Juglans regia)* leaves *medicinal herb used as an astringent*

**englitazone** INN *antidiabetic* [also: englitazone sodium]

**englitazone sodium** USAN *antidiabetic* [also: englitazone]

**enhanced, inactivated polio vaccine (eIPV)** [see: poliovirus vaccine, enhanced inactivated]

**Enhancer** oral suspension R *radiopaque contrast medium for gastrointestinal imaging* [barium sulfate] 98%

**enhexymal** [see: hexobarbital]

**eniclobrate** INN

**enilconazole** USAN, INN, BAN *antifungal*

**enilospirone** INN

**eniluracil** USAN *antineoplastic potentiator for fluorouracil; uracil reductase inhibitor*

**enisoprost** USAN, INN *antiulcerative; investigational (orphan) to reduce cyclosporine nephrotoxicity following organ transplants*

**Enisyl** tablets OTC *dietary amino acid supplement* [L-lysine] 334, 500 mg

**Enjuvia** film-coated tablets R *a mixture of synthetic estrogens; hormone replacement therapy for severe postmenopausal vasomotor symptoms* [synthetic conjugated estrogens, B] 0.625, 1.25 mg

**Enlive!** ready-to-use oral liquid OTC *enteral nutritional therapy* 240 mL

**Enlon** IV or IM injection R *myasthenia gravis treatment; antidote to curare overdose* [edrophonium chloride] 10 mg/mL

**Enlon Plus** IV or IM injection ℞ *muscle stimulant; neuromuscular blocker antagonist* [edrophonium chloride; atropine sulfate] 10•0.14 mg

**enloplatin** USAN, INN *antineoplastic*

**enocitabine** INN

**enofelast** USAN, INN *antiasthmatic*

**enolicam** INN *anti-inflammatory; antirheumatic* [also: enolicam sodium]

**enolicam sodium** USAN *anti-inflammatory; antirheumatic* [also: enolicam]

**Enomine** capsules (discontinued 2002) ℞ *decongestant; expectorant* [phenylpropanolamine HCl; phenylephrine HCl; guaifenesin] 45•5•200 mg

**enoxacin** USAN, INN, BAN, JAN *broadspectrum fluoroquinolone antibiotic*

**enoxamast** INN

**enoxaparin** BAN *a low molecular weight heparin–type anticoagulant and antithrombotic for the prevention of deep vein thrombosis (DVT), unstable angina, and myocardial infarction* [also: enoxaparin sodium]

**enoxaparin sodium** USAN, INN *a low molecular weight heparin–type anticoagulant and antithrombotic for the prevention of deep vein thrombosis (DVT), unstable angina, and myocardial infarction* [also: enoxaparin]

**enoximone** USAN, INN, BAN *cardiotonic*

**enoxolone** INN, BAN

**enphenemal** [see: mephobarbital]

**enpiprazole** INN, BAN

**enpiroline** INN *antimalarial* [also: enpiroline phosphate]

**enpiroline phosphate** USAN *antimalarial* [also: enpiroline]

**enprazepine** INN

**Enpresse** tablets (in packs of 28) ℞ *triphasic oral contraceptive; emergency postcoital contraceptive* [levonorgestrel; ethinyl estradiol]
Phase 1 (6 days): 50•30 μg;
Phase 2 (5 days): 75•40 μg;
Phase 3 (10 days): 125•30 μg

**enprofen** [now: furaprofen]

**enprofylline** USAN, INN *bronchodilator*

**enpromate** USAN, INN *antineoplastic*

**enprostil** USAN, INN, BAN *investigational antisecretory and antiulcerative for acute peptic ulcers*

**enramycin** INN

**enrofloxacin** USAN, INN, BAN *veterinary antibacterial*

**Enseal** (trademarked dosage form) *enteric-coated tablet*

**Ensure** oral liquid, powder for oral liquid OTC *enteral nutritional therapy* [lactose-free formula]

**Ensure** pudding OTC *enteral nutritional therapy* [milk-based formula] 150 g

**Ensure Glucerna** beverage, bars OTC *diabetic nutritional supplements/snacks*

**Ensure High Calcium** ready-to-use oral liquid OTC *enteral nutritional therapy for postmenopausal women*

**Ensure High Protein** ready-to-use oral liquid OTC *enteral nutritional therapy* [lactose-free formula] 237 mL

**Ensure HN; Ensure with Fiber** ready-to-use oral liquid OTC *enteral nutritional therapy* [lactose-free formula]

**Ensure Plus; Ensure Plus HN** oral liquid OTC *enteral nutritional therapy* [lactose-free formula]

**EN-tab** (trademarked dosage form) *enteric-coated tablet*

**entacapone** USAN *catechol-O-methyltransferase (COMT) inhibitor for Parkinson disease*

**entecavir** USAN *antiviral for hepatitis B infection*

**enteramine** [see: serotonin]

**Entero-Test; Entero-Test Pediatric** string capsules for professional use *in vitro diagnostic aid for GI disorders*

**Entertainer's Secret** oral spray OTC *saliva substitute*

**Entex** capsules (discontinued 2001) ℞ *decongestant; expectorant* [phenylephrine HCl; phenylpropanolamine HCl; guaifenesin] 5•45•200 mg

**Entex** oral liquid ℞ *decongestant; expectorant* [phenylephrine HCl; guaifenesin] 7.5•100 mg/5 mL

**Entex ER** extended-release capsules ℞ *decongestant; expectorant* [phenylephrine HCl; guaifenesin] 10•300 mg

**Entex HC** oral liquid ℞ *narcotic antitussive; decongestant; expectorant* [hydrocodone bitartrate; phenylephrine HCl; guaifenesin] 5•7.5•100 mg/5 mL

**Entex LA** dual-release capsules ℞ *decongestant; expectorant* [phenylephrine HCl (extended release); guaifenesin (immediate release)] 30•400 mg

**Entex LA** long-acting tablets ℞ *decongestant; expectorant* [phenylephrine HCl; guaifenesin] 30•600 mg

**Entex PSE** dual-release capsules ℞ *decongestant; expectorant* [pseudoephedrine HCl (extended release); guaifenesin (immediate release)] 120•400 mg

**Entex PSE** sustained-release tablets ℞ *decongestant; expectorant* [pseudoephedrine HCl; guaifenesin] 120•600 mg

**Entocort** ⒸⒶⓃ oral capsules for ileal release, retention enema ℞ *steroidal anti-inflammatory for Crohn disease* [budesonide] 3 mg; 2 mg

**Entocort EC** oral capsules for ileal release ℞ *corticosteroidal anti-inflammatory for Crohn disease* [budesonide] 3 mg

**Entri-Pak** (dosage form) *liquid-filled pouch*

**Entrition 0.5** oral liquid OTC *enteral nutritional therapy* [lactose-free formula]

**Entrition HN** Entri-Pak (liquid-filled pouch) OTC *enteral nutritional therapy* [lactose-free formula]

**Entrobar** oral suspension ℞ *radiopaque contrast medium for gastrointestinal imaging* [barium sulfate] 50% (500 mL)

**EntroEase** oral suspension ℞ *radiopaque contrast medium for gastrointestinal imaging* [barium sulfate] 13%

**EntroEase Dry** powder for oral suspension ℞ *radiopaque contrast medium for gastrointestinal imaging* [barium sulfate] 92%

**Entrophen** ⒸⒶⓃ enteric-coated tablets, enteric-coated caplets OTC *analgesic; antipyretic; anti-inflammatory; anti-rheumatic* [aspirin] 325, 500, 650 mg; 325, 650 mg

**entsufon** INN *detergent* [also: entsufon sodium]

**entsufon sodium** USAN *detergent* [also: entsufon]

**Entuss Expectorant** oral liquid (discontinued 2002) ℞ *narcotic antitussive; expectorant* [hydrocodone bitartrate; potassium guaiacolsulfonate] 5•300 mg/5 mL

**Entuss Expectorant** tablets (discontinued 2002) ℞ *narcotic antitussive; expectorant* [hydrocodone bitartrate; guaifenesin] 5•300 mg

**Entuss-D** oral liquid (discontinued 2002) ℞ *narcotic antitussive; decongestant* [hydrocodone bitartrate; pseudoephedrine HCl] 5•30 mg/5 mL

**Entuss-D** tablets (discontinued 2002) ℞ *narcotic antitussive; decongestant; expectorant* [hydrocodone bitartrate; pseudoephedrine HCl; guaifenesin] 5•30•300 mg

**Entuss-D Jr.** pediatric oral liquid (discontinued 2002) ℞ *narcotic antitussive; decongestant; expectorant* [hydrocodone bitartrate; pseudoephedrine HCl; guaifenesin; alcohol 5%] 2.5•30•100 mg/5 mL

**Enuclene** eye drops OTC *cleaning, wetting and lubricating agent for artificial eyes* [tyloxapol] 0.25%

**Enulose** oral/rectal solution ℞ *synthetic disaccharide used to prevent and treat portal-systemic encephalopathy* [lactulose] 10 g/15 mL

**enviomycin** INN

**enviradene** USAN, INN *antiviral*

**Enviro-Stress** slow-release tablets OTC *vitamin/mineral supplement* [multiple vitamins & minerals; folic acid] ≛•0.4 mg

**enviroxime** USAN, INN *antiviral*

**enzacamene** USAN *ultraviolet sunscreen*

**Enzone** cream ℞ *topical corticosteroidal anti-inflammatory; local anesthetic* [hydrocortisone acetate; pramoxine HCl] 1%•1%

**Enzymatic Cleaner for Extended Wear** tablets OTC *enzymatic cleaner for soft contact lenses* [pork pancreatin]

**Enzyme** chewable tablets (discontinued 2002) OTC *digestive enzymes* [amylase; protease; lipase; cellulase] 30•6•2•25 mg

**EP (etoposide, Platinol)** *chemotherapy protocol for adenocarcinoma, lung cancer, and testicular cancer*

**EPA** capsules OTC *dietary supplement* [omega-3 fatty acids] 1000 mg

**EPA (eicosapentaenoic acid)** [q.v.; also: icosapent]

**epalrestat** INN *investigational treatment for diabetic neuropathy*

**epanolol** INN, BAN

**Epaxal Berna** ⓐ suspension for IM injection OTC *active immunizing agent for hepatitis A* [hepatitis A vaccine, inactivated] 0.5 mL

**eperezolid** USAN *antibacterial*

**eperisone** INN

**epervudine** INN

**ephedra (Ephedra spp.)** plant *medicinal herb for asthma, blood cleansing, bronchitis, bursitis, chills, colds, edema, fever, flu, headache, kidney disorders, nasal congestion, and venereal disease*

**ephedrine** USP, BAN *sympathomimetic bronchodilator; nasal decongestant; vasopressor for shock* ⚠ Appedrine; aprindine

**ephedrine HCl** USP, BAN *sympathomimetic bronchodilator; nasal decongestant; vasopressor for shock* ⚠ Appedrine; aprindine

**ephedrine sulfate** USP *sympathomimetic bronchodilator; nasal decongestant; vasopressor for acute hypotensive shock* [also: ephedrine sulphate] 25 mg oral; 50 mg/mL injection ⚠ Appedrine; aprindine

**ephedrine sulphate** BAN *sympathomimetic bronchodilator; nasal decongestant* [also: ephedrine sulfate] ⚠ Appedrine; aprindine

**ephedrine tannate** *sympathomimetic bronchodilator; nasal decongestant* ⚠ Appedrine; aprindine

**Epi-C** concentrated oral suspension ℞ *radiopaque contrast medium for gastrointestinal imaging* [barium sulfate] 150%

**epicainide** INN

**epicillin** USAN, INN, BAN *antibacterial*

**epicriptine** INN

**epidermal growth factor, human** *investigational (orphan) for acceleration of corneal regeneration and the healing of severe burns*

**epidermal growth factor receptor inhibitors** *a class of antineoplastics*

**epiestriol** INN [also: epioestriol]

**Epifoam** aerosol foam ℞ *topical corticosteroidal anti-inflammatory; local anesthetic* [hydrocortisone acetate; pramoxine] 1%•1%

**Epifrin** eye drops (discontinued 2004) ℞ *antiglaucoma agent* [epinephrine HCl] 0.5%, 1%, 2% ⚠ epinephrine; EpiPen

**Epiject** ⓐ IV infusion ℞ *anticonvulsant* [valproate sodium] 100 mg/mL

**epilin** [see: dietifen]

**E-Pilo-1; E-Pilo-2; E-Pilo-4; E-Pilo-6** eye drops (discontinued 2004) ℞ *antiglaucoma agent* [pilocarpine HCl; epinephrine bitartrate] 1%•1%; 2%•1%; 4%•1%; 6%•1%

**Epilyt** lotion concentrate OTC *moisturizer; emollient*

**epimestrol** USAN, INN, BAN *anterior pituitary activator*

**Epinal** eye drops ℞ *topical antiglaucoma agent* [epinephryl borate] 0.5%, 1% ⚠ Epitol

**epinastine** INN *ophthalmic antihistamine* [also: epinastine HCl]

**epinastine HCl** *ophthalmic antihistamine* [also: epinastine]

**epinephran** [see: epinephrine]

**epinephrine** USP, INN *vasoconstrictor; sympathomimetic bronchodilator; topical antiglaucoma agent; vasopressor for shock* [also: adrenaline] 1:1000, 1:10 000 (1, 0.1 mg/mL) injection ⚠ Epifrin

**epinephrine bitartrate** USP *sympathomimetic bronchodilator; ophthalmic adrenergic; topical antiglaucoma agent*

**epinephrine borate** *topical antiglaucoma agent*

**epinephrine HCl** *sympathomimetic bronchodilator; nasal decongestant; topical antiglaucoma agent; vasopressor for shock* 0.1% eye drops

**Epinephrine Mist** inhalation aerosol OTC *sympathomimetic bronchodilator* [epinephrine] 0.22 mg/spray

**Epinephrine Pediatric** subcu injection (discontinued 2000) ℞ *bronchodilator for bronchial asthma or bronchospasm; vasopressor for shock* [epinephrine HCl] 1:100 000 (0.01 mg/mL)

**epinephryl borate** USAN, USP *adrenergic; topical antiglaucoma agent*

**epioestriol** BAN [also: epiestriol]

**EpiPen; EpiPen Jr.** auto-injector (automatic IM injection device) (discontinued 2002) ℞ *emergency treatment of anaphylaxis; vasopressor for shock* [epinephrine] 1:1000 (1 mg/mL); 1:2000 (0.5 mg/mL) ⎙ Epifrin

**epipropidine** USAN, INN *antineoplastic*

**EpiQuin Micro** cream ℞ *hyperpigmentation bleaching agent* [hydroquinone (in a base containing vitamins A, C, and E)] 4%

**epirizole** USAN, INN *analgesic; anti-inflammatory*

**epiroprim** INN

**epirubicin** INN, BAN *anthracycline antibiotic antineoplastic* [also: epirubicin HCl]

**epirubicin HCl** USAN, JAN *anthracycline antibiotic antineoplastic for breast cancer (orphan)* [also: epirubicin]

**epirubicin & tamoxifen** *chemotherapy protocol for breast cancer*

**epitetracycline HCl** USP *antibacterial*

**epithiazide** USAN, BAN *antihypertensive; diuretic* [also: epitizide]

**epithioandrostanol** [see: epitiostanol]

**epitiostanol** INN

**epitizide** INN *antihypertensive; diuretic* [also: epithiazide]

**Epitol** tablets ℞ *anticonvulsant; analgesic for trigeminal neuralgia; antipsychotic* [carbamazepine] 200 mg ⎙ Epinal

**Epival** ⒸⒶⓃ enteric-coated tablets ℞ *anticonvulsant; antipsychotic for manic episodes of a bipolar disorder* [divalproex sodium] 125, 250, 500 mg

**Epival ER** ⒸⒶⓃ extended-release tablets ℞ *anticonvulsant* [divalproex sodium] 500 mg

**Epivir** film-coated tablets, oral solution ℞ *antiviral for HIV infection* [lamivudine] 150, 300 mg; 10 mg/mL

**Epivir-HBV** film-coated caplets, oral solution ℞ *antiviral for hepatitis B virus (HBV) infection* [lamivudine] 100 mg; 5 mg/mL

**eplerenone** USAN *aldosterone receptor antagonist for hypertension and congestive heart failure (CHF); improves survival after a cardiovascular event*

**EPO (epoetin alfa)** [q.v.]

**EPO (evening primrose oil)** [see: evening primrose]

**EPOCH (etoposide, prednisone, Oncovin, cyclophosphamide, Halotestin)** *chemotherapy protocol*

**epoetin alfa (EPO)** USAN, INN, BAN, JAN *hematopoietic for anemia of chronic renal failure, HIV, and chemotherapy (orphan); also given to reduce the need for blood transfusions in surgery; investigational (orphan) for myelodysplastic syndrome*

**epoetin beta** USAN, INN, BAN, JAN *investigational (orphan) hematinic for anemia of end-stage renal disease*

**Epogen** IV or subcu injection ℞ *hematopoietic to stimulate RBC production for anemia of chronic renal failure, HIV, or chemotherapy (orphan)* [epoetin alfa] 2000, 3000, 4000, 10 000, 20 000, 40 000 U/mL ⎙ "amp and gent" (ampicillin & gentamicin)

**epoprostenol** USAN, INN *platelet aggregation inhibitor and vasodilator for primary pulmonary hypertension (orphan); investigational (orphan) heparin replacement for hemodialysis*

**epoprostenol sodium** USAN, BAN *platelet aggregation inhibitor and vasodilator for hypertension*

**epostane** USAN, INN, BAN *interceptive*

**epoxytropine tropate methylbromide** [see: methscopolamine bromide]

**epratuzumab** *monoclonal antibody to CD22; investigational (Phase III, orphan) for AIDS-related non-Hodgkin lymphoma*

**eprazinone** INN

**eprinomectin** USAN *veterinary antiparasitic*

**epristeride** USAN, INN, BAN *alpha reductase inhibitor for benign prostatic hypertrophy*

**eprosartan** USAN *antihypertensive; angiotensin II receptor antagonist*

**eprosartan mesylate** USAN *antihypertensive; angiotensin II receptor antagonist*

**eprovafen** INN

**eproxindine** INN

**eprozinol** INN

**epsikapron** [see: aminocaproic acid]

**epsilon-aminocaproic acid (EACA)** [see: aminocaproic acid]

**epsiprantel** INN, BAN

**Epsom salt** *granules* OTC *saline laxative* [magnesium sulfate]

**Epsom salt** [see: magnesium sulfate]

**e.p.t. Quick Stick** *test stick for home use* in vitro *diagnostic aid; urine pregnancy test*

**eptacog alfa (activated)** *activated recombinant human blood coagulation Factor VII (rFVIIa) for hemophilia A and B*

**eptaloprost** INN

**eptamestrol** [see: etamestrol]

**eptaprost** [see: eptaloprost]

**eptastatin sodium** [see: pravastatin sodium]

**eptastigmine** INN *investigational treatment for Alzheimer disease*

**eptazocine** INN

**eptifibatide** *glycoprotein (GP) IIb/IIIa receptor antagonist; platelet aggregation inhibitor for acute coronary syndrome, unstable angina, myocardial infarction, and cardiac surgery*

**Epulor** *oral liquid* OTC *enteral nutritional therapy* [milk-based formula]

**Equagesic** *tablets (discontinued 2004)* R̶ *analgesic; antipyretic; anti-inflammatory; anxiolytic; sedative* [aspirin; meprobamate] 325•200 mg

**Equalactin** *chewable tablets* OTC *bulk laxative; antidiarrheal* [calcium polycarbophil] 625 mg

**Equanil** *tablets (discontinued 2004)* R̶ *anxiolytic* [meprobamate] 200, 400 mg ⚎ Aldoril; Elavil; Eldepryl; Enovil; Mellaril

**Equilet** *chewable tablets* OTC *antacid* [calcium carbonate] 500 mg

**equilin** USP *estrogen*

**Equipoise** *brand name for boldenone undecylenate, a veterinary anabolic steroid abused as a street drug*

**Equisetum arvens** *medicinal herb* [see: horsetail]

**Erbitux** *IV infusion* R̶ *antineoplastic for metastatic colorectal cancer;investigational (orphan) for squamous cell carcinoma of the head and neck; investigational (Phase III) for pancreatic cancer* [cetuximab] 100 mg/vial

**erbium** *element (Er)*

**erbulozole** USAN, INN *antineoplastic adjunct*

**erbumine** USAN, INN, BAN *combining name for radicals or groups*

**Ercaf** *tablets* R̶ *migraine-specific vasoconstrictor* [ergotamine tartrate; caffeine] 1•100 mg

**erdosteine** INN

**Erechtites hieracfolia** *medicinal herb* [see: pilewort]

**Ergamisol** *tablets* R̶ *biological response modifier; antineoplastic adjunct for colon cancer* [levamisole HCl] 50 mg

**ergocalciferol (vitamin D$_2$)** USP, INN, BAN, JAN *fat-soluble vitamin for refractory rickets, familial hypophosphatemia, and hypoparathyroidism*

**ergoloid mesylates** USAN, USP *cognition adjuvant for age-related mental capacity decline* [also: co-dergocrine mesylate] 0.5, 1 mg oral

**Ergomar** *sublingual tablets* R̶ *prophylaxis or treatment of migraine and other vascular headaches* [ergotamine tartrate] 2 mg

**ergometrine** INN, BAN *oxytocic for induction of labor* [also: ergonovine maleate]

**ergonovine maleate** USP *oxytocic for the induction of labor and prevention of postpartum and postabortal hemorrhage* [also: ergometrine]

**ergosterol, activated** [see: ergocalciferol]

**ergot (Claviceps purpurea)** *dried sclerotia medicinal herb used as an abortifacient, emmenagogue, hemostatic, oxytocic, and vasoconstrictor; source of ergotamine and LSD*

**ergot alkaloids** [see: ergoloid mesylates]

**ergotamine** INN, BAN *migraine-specific analgesic* [also: ergotamine tartrate]

**ergotamine tartrate** USP *prophylaxis or treatment of migraine and other vascular headaches* [also: ergotamine]

**Ergotrate Maleate** IM or IV injection (discontinued 2004) ℞ *oxytocic for the induction of labor and prevention of postpartum and postabortal hemorrhage* [ergonovine maleate] 0.2 mg/mL

**Ergotrate Maleate** tablets ℞ *oxytocic for the induction of labor and prevention of postpartum and postabortal hemorrhage* [ergonovine maleate] 0.2 mg

**ericolol** INN

*Erigeron canadensis medicinal herb* [see: fleabane; horseweed]

**eriodictyon** NF

*Eriodictyon californicum medicinal herb* [see: yerba santa]

**eritrityl tetranitrate** INN *coronary vasodilator* [also: erythrityl tetranitrate]

**erizepine** INN

**erlizumab** USAN *monoclonal antibody to treat reperfusion injury following acute myocardial infarction*

**erlotinib HCl** *investigational (Phase III) antineoplastic for lung, breast, and pancreatic cancers; investigational (orphan) for non-Hodgkin lymphoma*

**E-R-O Ear Drops** OTC *agent to emulsify and disperse ear wax* [carbamide peroxide] 6.5%

**erocainide** INN

**errhines** *a class of agents that promote nasal discharge or secretion*

**Errin** tablets (in packs of 28) ℞ *oral contraceptive (progestin only)* [norethindrone] 0.35 mg

**ersofermin** USAN, INN *wound healing agent; transglutaminase inhibitor for the treatment of scar tissue*

**Ertaczo** cream ℞ *antifungal* [sertaconazole nitrate] 2%

**ertapenem sodium** USAN *antibiotic*

**Erwinase** ℞ *investigational (orphan) antineoplastic for acute lymphocytic leukemia* [erwinia L-asparaginase]

**erwinia L-asparaginase** *investigational (orphan) antineoplastic for acute lymphocytic leukemia*

**Ery Pads** pledgets ℞ *antibiotic for acne* [erythromycin; alcohol 60.5%] 2%

**ERYC** delayed-release capsules containing enteric-coated pellets ℞ *macrolide antibiotic* [erythromycin] 250 mg ⊡ ara-C

**Erycette** topical solution (discontinued 2003) ℞ *antibiotic for acne* [erythromycin] 2% ⊡ Aricept

**EryDerm 2%** topical solution ℞ *antibiotic for acne* [erythromycin; alcohol 77%] 2%

**Erygel** gel (discontinued 2004) ℞ *antibiotic for acne* [erythromycin; alcohol 92%] 2%

**Erymax** topical solution (discontinued 2003) ℞ *antibiotic for acne* [erythromycin] 2%

*Eryngium aquaticum medicinal herb* [see: water eryngo]

**EryPed** chewable tablets (discontinued 2003) ℞ *macrolide antibiotic* [erythromycin ethylsuccinate] 200 mg

**EryPed** drops ℞ *macrolide antibiotic* [erythromycin ethylsuccinate] 100 mg/2.5 mL

**EryPed 200; EryPed 400** oral suspension ℞ *macrolide antibiotic* [erythromycin ethylsuccinate] 200 mg/5 mL; 400 mg/5 mL

**Ery-Tab** delayed-release enteric-coated tablets ℞ *macrolide antibiotic* [erythromycin] 250, 333, 500 mg

**erythorbic acid**

**Erythra-Derm** topical solution (discontinued 2003) ℞ *antibiotic for acne* [erythromycin] 2%

*Erythraea centaurium* *medicinal herb* [see: centaury]

**erythrityl tetranitrate** USAN, USP *coronary vasodilator; antianginal* [also: eritrityl tetranitrate]

**Erythrocin** powder for IV injection ℞ *macrolide antibiotic* [erythromycin lactobionate] 500, 1000 mg/vial

**Erythrocin Stearate** Filmtabs (film-coated tablets) ℞ *macrolide antibiotic* [erythromycin stearate] 250, 500 mg

**erythrol tetranitrate** [now: erythrityl tetranitrate]

**erythromycin** USP, INN, BAN *macrolide antibiotic* 250, 500 mg oral; 2% topical; 0.5% ophthalmic ⊡ clarithromycin; dirithromycin

**erythromycin 2′-acetate octadecanoate** [see: erythromycin acistrate]

**erythromycin 2′-acetate stearate** [see: erythromycin acistrate]

**erythromycin acistrate** USAN, INN *macrolide antibiotic*

**erythromycin B** [see: berythromycin]

**erythromycin & benzoyl peroxide** *antibiotic and keratolytic for acne* 3%•5% topical

**erythromycin estolate** USAN, USP, BAN *macrolide antibiotic* 250 mg oral; 125, 250 mg/5 mL oral

**erythromycin ethyl succinate** BAN *macrolide antibiotic* [also: erythromycin ethylsuccinate]

**erythromycin ethylcarbonate** USP *macrolide antibiotic*

**erythromycin ethylsuccinate (EES)** USP *macrolide antibiotic* [also: erythromycin ethyl succinate] 400 mg oral; 200, 400 mg/5 mL oral

**erythromycin gluceptate** USP *macrolide antibiotic*

**erythromycin glucoheptonate** [see: erythromycin gluceptate]

**erythromycin lactobionate** USP *macrolide antibiotic* 500, 1000 mg/vial injection

**erythromycin lauryl sulfate, propionyl** [now: erythromycin estolate]

**erythromycin monoglucoheptonate** [see: erythromycin gluceptate]

**erythromycin octadecanoate** [see: erythromycin stearate]

**erythromycin 2′-propanoate** [see: erythromycin propionate]

**erythromycin propionate** USAN *macrolide antibiotic*

**erythromycin 2′-propionate dodecyl sulfate** [see: erythromycin estolate]

**erythromycin propionate lauryl sulfate** [now: erythromycin estolate]

**erythromycin salnacedin** USAN *macrolide antibiotic for acne vulgaris*

**erythromycin stearate** USP, BAN *macrolide antibiotic* 250, 500 mg oral

**erythromycin stinoprate** INN *macrolide antibiotic*

*Erythronium americanum* *medicinal herb* [see: adder's tongue]

**erythropoietin, gene-activated (GA-EPO)** *investigational (NDA filed) gene therapy for anemia of renal failure*

**erythropoietin, recombinant human (rEPO)** [see: epoetin alfa; epoetin beta]

**erythrosine sodium** USP *dental disclosing agent*

**Eryzole** granules for oral suspension ℞ *antibiotic* [erythromycin ethylsuccinate; sulfisoxazole acetyl] 200•600 mg/5 mL

**esafloxacin** INN

**esaprazole** INN

**escitalopram oxalate** USAN *selective serotonin reuptake inhibitor (SSRI) for major depression and generalized anxiety disorder; isomer of citalopram*

**Esclim** transdermal patch ℞ *estrogen replacement therapy for the treatment of postmenopausal symptoms* [estradiol] 25, 37.5, 50, 75, 100 µg/day

**esculamine** INN

**eseridine** INN

**eserine** [see: physostigmine]

**esflurbiprofen** INN, BAN

**Esgic** caplets, capsules ℞ *analgesic; barbiturate sedative* [acetaminophen; caffeine; butalbital] 325•40•50 mg

**Esgic-Plus** caplets, capsules ℞ *analgesic; barbiturate sedative* [acetaminophen; caffeine; butalbital] 500•40•50 mg

**ESHAP (etoposide, Solu-Medrol, high-dose ara-C, Platinol)** *chemotherapy protocol for non-Hodgkin lymphoma*

**ESHAP-MINE (alternating cycles of ESHAP and MINE)** *chemotherapy protocol*

**Esidrix** tablets ℞ *antihypertensive; diuretic* [hydrochlorothiazide] 25, 50, 100 mg ② Lasix

**esilate** INN *combining name for radicals or groups* [also: esylate]

**Esimil** tablets ℞ *antihypertensive; diuretic* [hydrochlorothiazide; guanethidine monosulfate] 25•10 mg ② Estinyl; Isomil

**Eskalith** capsules, tablets ℞ *antipsychotic for manic episodes* [lithium carbonate] 300 mg

**Eskalith CR** controlled-release tablets ℞ *antipsychotic for manic episodes* [lithium carbonate] 450 mg

**esmolol** INN, BAN *antihypertensive; antiadrenergic (β-receptor)* [also: esmolol HCl]

**esmolol HCl** USAN *antihypertensive; antiarrhythmic; antiadrenergic (β-receptor)* [also: esmolol] 10 mg/mL injection

**E-Solve** OTC *lotion base*

**esomeprazole magnesium** USAN *proton pump inhibitor for gastric and duodenal ulcers, erosive esophagitis, GERD, and other gastroesophageal disorders; isomer of omeprazole*

**esopiclone** *non-benzodiazepine sedative and hypnotic*

**esorubicin** INN *antineoplastic* [also: esorubicin HCl]

**esorubicin HCl** USAN *antineoplastic* [also: esorubicin]

**Esotérica Dry Skin Treatment** lotion OTC *moisturizer; emollient*

**Esotérica Facial; Esotérica Regular** cream OTC *hyperpigmentation bleaching agent* [hydroquinone] 2%

**Esotérica Fortified** cream (discontinued 2003) OTC *hyperpigmentation bleaching agent; sunscreen* [hydroquinone; padimate O; oxybenzone] 2%•3.3%•2.5%

**Esotérica Sensitive Skin Formula** cream (discontinued 2003) OTC *hyperpigmentation bleaching agent* [hydroquinone] 1.5%

**Esotérica Soap** OTC *bath emollient*

**Esotérica Sunscreen** cream OTC *hyperpigmentation bleaching agent; sunscreen* [hydroquinone; padimate O; oxybenzone] 2%•3.3%•2.5%

**esprolol** *investigational (Phase II) beta-adrenoreceptor antagonist for angina pectoris*

**esproquin HCl** USAN *adrenergic* [also: esproquine]

**esproquine** INN *adrenergic* [also: esproquin HCl]

**Essential ProPlus** powder for oral solution OTC *oral protein supplement with vitamins and minerals* [soy protein; multiple vitamins and minerals]

**Essential Protein** powder OTC *oral protein supplement* [soy protein]

**Estalis 140/50; Estalis 250/50** ⓒᴬᴺ transdermal patch ℞ *hormone replacement therapy for postmenopausal symptoms* [norethindrone acetate; estradiol-17β] 140•50 μg/day; 250•50 μg/day

**Estar** gel OTC *antipsoriatic; antiseborrheic* [coal tar] 5%

**estazolam** USAN, INN *hypnotic* 1, 2 mg oral

**Ester-C Plus Multi-Mineral** capsules OTC *vitamin C/mineral supplement with multiple bioflavonoids* [vitamin C; acerola; rose hips; multiple minerals; citrus bioflavonoids; rutin] 425•12.5•12.5•≛•50•5 mg

**Ester-C Plus Vitamin C** capsules OTC *vitamin C/calcium supplement with multiple bioflavonoids* [vitamin C; acerola; rose hips; calcium; citrus

bioflavonoids; rutin] 500•10•10•
62•25•5 mg; 1000•25•25•125•
200•25 mg

**esterified estrogens** [see: estrogens, esterified]

**esterifilcon A** USAN *hydrophilic contact lens material*

**Esterom** solution ℞ *investigational (Phase III) topical treatment for acute impaired shoulder function*

**estilben** [see: diethylstilbestrol dipropionate]

**Estinyl** tablets (discontinued 2003) ℞ *estrogen replacement therapy for the treatment of postmenopausal symptoms; palliative therapy for breast and prostate cancers* [ethinyl estradiol] 0.02, 0.05, 0.5 mg ⊡ Esimil

**estolate** INN *combining name for radicals or groups*

**estomycin sulfate** [see: paromomycin sulfate]

**Estorra** tablets ℞ *non-benzodiazepine sedative and hypnotic* [esopiclone] 1, 2, 3 mg

**Estrace** tablets ℞ *estrogen replacement therapy for the treatment of postmenopausal symptoms and prevention of postmenopausal osteoporosis; palliative therapy for prostate and metastatic breast cancers* [estradiol, soy-derived] 0.5, 1, 2 mg

**Estrace Vaginal** cream ℞ *estrogen replacement for postmenopausal atrophic vaginitis* [estradiol] 0.1 mg/g

**Estraderm** transdermal patch ℞ *estrogen replacement therapy for the treatment of postmenopausal symptoms and prevention of postmenopausal osteoporosis* [estradiol] 50, 100 μg/day ⊡ Estradurin

**estradiol** USP, INN *estrogen replacement therapy for the treatment of postmenopausal disorders and the prevention of postmenopausal osteoporosis; palliative therapy for breast and prostate cancers; may be naturally derived or a synthetic analogue* [also: oestradiol] 0.5, 1, 2 mg oral

**estradiol acetate** *synthetic estrogen; hormone replacement therapy for the treatment of postmenopausal symptoms*

**estradiol-17β** *estrogen replacement therapy for postmenopausal disorders*

**estradiol benzoate** USP, INN, JAN [also: oestradiol benzoate]

**estradiol 17-cyclopentanepropionate** [see: estradiol cypionate]

**estradiol cypionate** USP *synthetic estrogen; hormone replacement therapy for the treatment of postmenopausal symptoms*

**estradiol dipropionate** NF, JAN

**estradiol enanthate** USAN *estrogen*

**estradiol hemihydrate** *synthetic estrogen; topical hormone therapy for atrophic vaginitis*

**estradiol 17-heptanoate** [see: estradiol enanthate]

**estradiol monobenzoate** [see: estradiol benzoate]

**estradiol 17-nicotinate 3-propionate** [see: estrapronicate]

**estradiol phosphate polymer** [see: polyestradiol phosphate]

**Estradiol Transdermal System** patch ℞ *estrogen replacement therapy for the treatment of postmenopausal symptoms and prevention of postmenopausal osteoporosis* [estradiol] 50, 100 μg/day

**estradiol 17-undecanoate** [see: estradiol undecylate]

**estradiol undecylate** USAN, INN *estrogen*

**estradiol valerate** USP, INN, JAN *synthetic estrogen; hormone replacement therapy for the treatment of postmenopausal symptoms and the prevention of postmenopausal osteoporosis; hormonal antineoplastic for breast and prostate cancers* [also: oestradiol valerate]

**Estra-L 40** IM injection ℞ *estrogen replacement therapy for postmenopausal symptoms; antineoplastic for prostatic cancer* [estradiol valerate in oil] 40 mg/mL

**estramustine** USAN, INN, BAN *nitrogen mustard-type alkylating antineoplastic*

**estramustine phosphate sodium**
USAN, BAN, JAN *nitrogen mustard-type alkylating antineoplastic for prostate cancer*

**estramustine & vinblastine sulfate**
*chemotherapy protocol for prostate cancer*

**estrapronicate** INN

**Estrasorb** topical emulsion ℞ *estrogen replacement therapy for postmenopausal symptoms* [estradiol hemihydrate] 2.5 mg/g (4.35 mg/pouch = 25 µg base/pouch)

**Estratab** tablets (discontinued 2003) ℞ *estrogen replacement therapy for the treatment of postmenopausal symptoms; palliative therapy for breast and prostate cancers* [esterified estrogens] 0.3, 0.625, 2.5 mg ⃞ Ethatab

**Estratest; Estratest H.S.** sugar-coated tablets ℞ *hormone replacement therapy for postmenopausal symptoms* [esterified estrogens; methyltestosterone] 1.25•2.5 mg; 0.625•1.25 mg

**estrazinol** INN *estrogen* [also: estrazinol hydrobromide]

**estrazinol hydrobromide** USAN *estrogen* [also: estrazinol]

**Estring** vaginal ring ℞ *three-month estrogen replacement for postmenopausal atrophic vaginitis* [estradiol] 2 mg (7.5 µg/day)

**estriol** USP *estrogen* [also: estriol succinate; oestriol succinate]

**estriol succinate** INN *estrogen* [also: estriol; oestriol succinate]

**estrobene** [see: diethylstilbestrol]

**estrobene DP** [see: diethylstilbestrol dipropionate]

**estrofurate** USAN, INN *estrogen*

**Estrogel** transdermal gel ℞ *estrogen replacement therapy for postmenopausal symptoms* [estradiol] 0.06%

**Estrogel** ⓒᴬᴺ transdermal gel ℞ *estrogen replacement therapy for postmenopausal symptoms* [estrogen-17β] 0.06% (1.25 g/metered actuation)

**estrogenic substances, conjugated** [see: estrogens, conjugated]

**estrogenine** [see: diethylstilbestrol]

**estrogens** *a class of sex hormones that includes estradiol, estrone, and estriol, also used as an antineoplastic*

**estrogens, conjugated** USP, JAN *a mixture of equine estrogens; hormone replacement therapy for the treatment of postmenopausal symptoms and prevention of postmenopausal osteoporosis; palliative therapy for breast and prostate cancers*

**estrogens, esterified** USP *a mixture of equine estrogens; hormone replacement therapy for the treatment of postmenopausal disorders; palliative therapy for breast and prostate cancers*

**estrogens, synthetic conjugated, A** *a mixture of 9 synthetic estrogenic substances; hormone replacement therapy for postmenopausal symptoms*

**estrogens, synthetic conjugated, B** *a mixture of 10 synthetic estrogenic substances; hormone replacement therapy for severe postmenopausal vasomotor symptoms*

**estromenin** [see: diethylstilbestrol]

**estrone** USP, INN *bioidentical human estrogen; natural hormone replacement therapy for postmenopausal disorders; palliative therapy for breast and prostate cancers* [also: oestrone]

**Estrone Aqueous** IM injection (discontinued 2003) ℞ *estrogen replacement therapy for postmenopausal symptoms; palliative therapy for breast and prostate cancers* [estrone] 5 mg/mL

**estrone hydrogen sulfate** [see: estrone sodium sulfate]

**estrone sodium sulfate** *synthetic estrogen*

**Estrophasic** (trademarked/patented dosing regimen) *gradual estrogen intake with steady progestin intake*

**estropipate** USP *natural estrogen replacement therapy for the treatment of postmenopausal symptoms and prevention of postmenopausal osteoporosis; a stabilized form of estrone, the bioidentical human estrogen* 0.75, 1.5, 3, 6 mg oral

**Estrostep 21** tablets (in packs of 21) ℞ *triphasic oral contraceptive; treatment*

*for acne vulgaris in females* [norethindrone acetate; ethinyl estradiol]
Phase 1 (5 days): 1000•20 μg;
Phase 2 (7 days): 1000•30 μg;
Phase 3 (9 days): 1000•35 μg

**Estrostep Fe** tablets (in packs of 28) ℞ *triphasic oral contraceptive; iron supplement* [norethindrone acetate; ethinyl estradiol; ferrous fumarate]
Phase 1 (5 days): 1•0.02•75 mg;
Phase 2 (7 days): 1•0.03•75 mg;
Phase 3 (9 days): 1•0.035•75 mg;
Counters (7 days): 0•0•75 mg

**esuprone** INN

**esylate** USAN, BAN *combining name for radicals or groups* [also: esilate]

**etabenzarone** INN

**etabonate** USAN, INN *combining name for radicals or groups*

**etacepride** INN

**etacrynic acid** INN, JAN *antihypertensive; loop diuretic* [also: ethacrynic acid]

**etafedrine** INN, BAN *adrenergic* [also: etafedrine HCl]

**etafedrine HCl** USAN *adrenergic* [also: etafedrine]

**etafenone** INN

**etafilcon A** USAN *hydrophilic contact lens material*

**etamestrol** INN

**etaminile** INN

**etamiphyllin** INN [also: etamiphylline]

**etamiphyllin methesculetol** [see: metescufylline]

**etamiphylline** BAN [also: etamiphyllin]

**etamivan** INN *central and respiratory stimulant* [also: ethamivan]

**etamocycline** INN

**etamsylate** INN *hemostatic* [also: ethamsylate]

**etanercept** USAN *soluble tumor necrosis factor receptor (sTNFR) inhibitor for rheumatoid arthritis, juvenile rheumatoid arthritis (orphan), psoriatic arthritis, and ankylosing spondylitis; investigational (NDA filed) for congestive heart failure; investigational (orphan) for Wegener granulomatosis*

**etanidazole** USAN, INN *antineoplastic; hypoxic cell radiosensitizer*

**etanterol** INN

**etaperazine** [see: perphenazine]

**etaqualone** INN

**etarotene** USAN, INN *keratolytic*

**etasuline** INN

**etazepine** INN

**etazolate** INN *antipsychotic* [also: etazolate HCl]

**etazolate HCl** USAN *antipsychotic* [also: etazolate]

**etebenecid** INN [also: ethebenecid]

**etenzamide** BAN [also: ethenzamide]

**eterobarb** USAN, INN, BAN *anticonvulsant*

**etersalate** INN

**ethacridine** INN [also: ethacridine lactate; acrinol] ② ethacrynic

**ethacridine lactate** [also: ethacridine; acrinol]

**ethacrynate sodium** USAN, USP *antihypertensive; loop diuretic*

**ethacrynic acid** USAN, USP, BAN *antihypertensive; loop diuretic* [also: etacrynic acid] ② ethacridine

**ethambutol** INN, BAN *bacteriostatic; primary tuberculostatic* [also: ethambutol HCl]

**ethambutol HCl** USAN, USP *bacteriostatic; primary tuberculostatic* [also: ethambutol] 400 mg oral

**ethamivan** USAN, USP, BAN *central and respiratory stimulant* [also: etamivan]

**Ethamolin** IV injection ℞ *sclerosing agent for bleeding esophageal varices (orphan)* [ethanolamine oleate] 5%

**ethamsylate** USAN, BAN *hemostatic* [also: etamsylate]

**ethanol** JAN *topical anti-infective/antiseptic; astringent; solvent; a widely abused "legal street drug" used to produce euphoria* [also: alcohol]

**ethanol, dehydrated** JAN *antidote* [also: alcohol, dehydrated]

**ethanolamine oleate** USAN *sclerosing agent for bleeding esophageal varices (orphan)* [also: monoethanolamine oleate]

**ethanolamines** *a class of antihistamines that includes diphenhydramine HCl and clemastine fumarate*

**ethaverine** INN *peripheral vasodilator*

**ethaverine HCl** *peripheral vasodilator* [see: ethaverine]

**ethchlorvynol** USP, INN, BAN *sedative; hypnotic*

**ethebenecid** BAN [also: etebenecid]

**EtheDent** chewable tablets ℞ *dental caries preventative* [sodium fluoride] 0.25, 0.5, 1 mg

**EtheDent** dental cream ℞ *topical caries preventative* [sodium fluoride] 1.1%

**ethenzamide** INN, JAN [also: etenzamide]

**ether** USP *inhalation anesthetic*

**Ethezyme 830** ointment ℞ *enzyme for wound debridement; vulnerary* [papain; urea] 830 000 IU/g•10%

**ethiazide** INN, BAN

**ethidium bromide** [see: homidium bromide]

**ethinamate** USP, INN, BAN *sedative; hypnotic* ⓩ ethionamide

**ethinyl estradiol** USP *estrogen replacement therapy for the treatment of post-menopausal disorders; palliative therapy for prostate and breast cancers; investigational (orphan) for Turner syndrome* [also: ethinylestradiol; ethinyloestradiol]

**ethinylestradiol** INN *estrogen replacement therapy for the treatment of post-menopausal disorders; palliative therapy for prostate and breast cancers* [also: ethinyl estradiol; ethinyloestradiol]

**ethinyloestradiol** BAN *estrogen replacement therapy for the treatment of post-menopausal disorders; palliative therapy for prostate and breast cancers* [also: ethinyl estradiol; ethinylestradiol]

**ethiodized oil** USP *parenteral radiopaque contrast medium (37% iodine)*

**ethiodized oil (¹³¹I)** INN *antineoplastic; radioactive agent* [also: ethiodized oil I 131]

**ethiodized oil I 131** USAN *antineoplastic; radioactive agent* [also: ethiodized oil (¹³¹I)]

**Ethiodol** intracavitary instillation ℞ *radiopaque contrast medium for lymphography and gynecological imaging*

[ethiodized oil (37% iodine)] 1284 mg/mL (475 mg/mL) ⓩ ethynodiol

**ethiofos** [now: amifostine]

**ethionamide** USAN, USP, INN, BAN *bacteriostatic; tuberculosis retreatment* ⓩ ethinamate

**ethisterone** NF, INN, BAN

**Ethmozine** film-coated tablets ℞ *antiarrhythmic* [moricizine HCl] 200, 250, 300 mg

**ethodryl** [see: diethylcarbamazine citrate]

**ethoglucid** BAN [also: etoglucid]

**ethoheptazine** BAN [also: ethoheptazine citrate]

**ethoheptazine citrate** NF, INN [also: ethoheptazine]

**ethohexadiol** USP

**ethomoxane** INN, BAN

**ethomoxane HCl** [see: ethomoxane]

**ethonam nitrate** USAN *antifungal* [also: etonam]

**ethopabate** BAN

**ethopropazine** BAN *anticholinergic; antiparkinsonian* [also: ethopropazine HCl; profenamine]

**ethopropazine HCl** USP *anticholinergic; antiparkinsonian* [also: profenamine; ethopropazine]

**ethosalamide** BAN [also: etosalamide]

**ethosuximide** USAN, USP, INN, BAN *anticonvulsant* 250 mg oral; 250 mg/ 5 mL oral

**ethotoin** USP, INN, BAN *hydantoin anticonvulsant*

**ethoxarutine** [see: ethoxazorutoside]

**ethoxazene HCl** USAN *analgesic* [also: etoxazene]

**ethoxazorutoside** INN

**ethoxyacetanilide** *(withdrawn from market)* [see: phenacetin]

**o-ethoxybenzamide** [see: ethenzamide; etenzamide]

**ethoxzolamide** USP

**Ethrane** liquid for vaporization ℞ *inhalation general anesthetic* [enflurane]

**ethybenztropine** USAN, BAN *anticholinergic* [also: etybenzatropine]

**ethyl acetate** NF *solvent*

ethyl alcohol (EtOH; ETOH) [now: alcohol; ethanol]

ethyl aminobenzoate (ethyl *p*-aminobenzoate) JAN *topical anesthetic; nonprescription diet aid* [also: benzocaine]

ethyl 2-benzimidazolecarbamate [see: lobendazole]

ethyl *N*-benzylcyclopropanecarbamate [see: encyprate]

ethyl biscoumacetate NF, INN, BAN

ethyl biscumacetate [see: ethyl biscoumacetate]

ethyl carbamate [now: urethane]

ethyl carfluzepate INN

ethyl cartrizoate INN

ethyl chloride USP *topical local anesthetic; topical vapo-coolant*

ethyl dibunate USAN, INN, BAN *antitussive*

ethyl dirazepate INN

ethyl eicosapentaenoate *investigational (orphan) agent for Huntington disease*

ethyl ether [see: ether]

ethyl *p*-fluorophenyl sulfone [see: fluoresone]

ethyl *p*-hydroxybenzoate [see: ethylparaben]

ethyl loflazepate INN

ethyl nitrite NF

ethyl oleate NF *vehicle*

ethyl oxide [see: ether]

ethyl vanillin NF *flavoring agent*

ethylcellulose NF *tablet binder*

ethylchlordiphene [see: etofamide]

ethyldicoumarol [see: ethyl biscoumacetate]

ethylene NF *inhalation general anesthesia*

ethylene disterate [see: glycol distearate]

ethylenediamine USP, JAN

ethylenediaminetetraacetate [see: edetate disodium]

ethylenediaminetetraacetic acid (EDTA) [see: edetate disodium]

N,N-ethylenediarsanilic acid [see: difetarsone]

ethylenedinitrilotetraacetate disodium [see: edetate disodium]

ethylestrenol USAN, INN *anabolic steroid; also abused as a street drug* [also: ethyloestrenol; ethylnandrol]

ethylhexanediol [see: ethohexadiol]

2-ethylhexyl diphenyl phosphate [see: octicizer]

2-ethylhexyl *p*-methoxycinnamate [see: octinoxate]

2-ethylhexyl salicylate [see: octisalate]

ethylhydrocupreine HCl NF

ethylmethylthiambutene INN, BAN

ethylmorphine BAN [also: ethylmorphine HCl]

ethylmorphine HCl NF [also: ethylmorphine]

ethylnandrol JAN *anabolic steroid; also abused as a street drug* [also: ethylestrenol; ethyloestrenol]

ethylnorepinephrine HCl USP *sympathomimetic bronchodilator*

ethyloestradiol BAN *estrogen* [also: ethinyl estradiol]

ethyloestrenol BAN *anabolic steroid; also abused as a street drug* [also: ethylestrenol; ethylnandrol]

ethylpapaverine HCl [see: ethaverine HCl]

ethylparaben NF *antifungal agent*

ethylphenacemide [see: pheneturide]

ethylstibamine [see: stibosamine]

2-ethylthioisonicotinamide [see: ethionamide]

ethynerone USAN, INN *progestin*

ethynodiol BAN *progestin* [also: ethynodiol diacetate; etynodiol] ⧉ Ethiodol

ethynodiol diacetate USAN, USP *progestin* [also: etynodiol; ethynodiol]

5-ethynyluracil [see: eniluracil]

Ethyol *powder for IV infusion* ℞ *chemoprotective agent for cisplatin and paclitaxel chemotherapy (orphan); investigational (orphan) for cyclophosphamide; treatment for moderate to severe xerostomia following postoperative radiation therapy (orphan)* [amifostine] 500 mg/vial

ethypicone INN

ethypropymal sodium [see: probarbital sodium]

**etibendazole** USAN, INN *anthelmintic*

**eticlopride** INN

**eticyclidine** INN

**etidocaine** USAN, INN, BAN *injectable local anesthetic*

**etidocaine HCl** *injectable local anesthetic*

**etidronate disodium** USAN, USP *bisphosphonate bone resorption inhibitor for Paget disease, heterotopic ossification, and hypercalcemia of malignancy (orphan); investigational (orphan) for metabolic bone disease*

**etidronate monosodium**

**etidronate sodium** *(this term is used only when the form of sodium cannot be more accurately identified)*

**etidronate tetrasodium**

**etidronate trisodium**

**etidronic acid** USAN, INN, BAN *calcium regulator*

**etifelmine** INN

**etifenin** USAN, INN, BAN *diagnostic aid*

**etifoxin** BAN [also: etifoxine]

**etifoxine** INN [also: etifoxin]

**etilamfetamine** INN

**etilefrine** INN

**etilefrine pivalate** INN

**etilevodopa** *investigational (Phase III) antiparkinsonian agent*

**etintidine** INN *antagonist to histamine $H_2$ receptors* [also: etintidine HCl]

**etintidine HCl** USAN *antagonist to histamine $H_2$ receptors* [also: etintidine]

**etiocholanedione** *investigational (orphan) for aplastic anemia and Prader-Willi syndrome*

**etipirium iodide** INN

**etiproston** INN

**etiracetam** INN

**etiroxate** INN

**etisazole** INN, BAN

**etisomicin** INN, BAN

**etisulergine** INN

**etizolam** INN

**etobedolum** [see: etonitazene]

**etocarlide** INN

**etocrilene** INN *ultraviolet screen* [also: etocrylene]

**etocrylene** USAN *ultraviolet screen* [also: etocrilene]

**etodolac** USAN, INN, BAN *analgesic; antiarthritic; nonsteroidal anti-inflammatory drug (NSAID)* [also: etodolic acid] 200, 300, 400, 500, 600 mg oral

**etodolic acid** INN *analgesic; antiarthritic; nonsteroidal anti-inflammatory drug (NSAID)* [also: etodolac]

**etodroxizine** INN

**etofamide** INN

**etofenamate** USAN, INN, BAN *analgesic; anti-inflammatory*

**etofenprox** INN

**etofibrate** INN

**etoformin** INN *antidiabetic* [also: etoformin HCl]

**etoformin HCl** USAN *antidiabetic* [also: etoformin]

**etofuradine** INN

**etofylline** INN

**etofylline clofibrate** INN *antihyperlipoproteinemic* [also: theofibrate]

**etoglucid** INN [also: ethoglucid]

**EtOH; ETOH (ethyl alcohol)** [now: alcohol]

**etolorex** INN

**etolotifen** INN

**etoloxamine** INN

**etomidate** USAN, INN, BAN *rapid-acting nonbarbiturate general anesthetic; hypnotic*

**etomidoline** INN

**etomoxir** INN

**etonam** INN *antifungal* [also: ethonam nitrate]

**etonam nitrate** [see: ethonam nitrate]

**etonitazene** INN, BAN

**etonogestrel** USAN, INN *progestin*

**etoperidone** INN *antidepressant* [also: etoperidone HCl]

**etoperidone HCl** USAN *antidepressant* [also: etoperidone]

**etophylate** [see: acepifylline]

**Etopophos** *powder for IV injection* ℞ *antineoplastic for testicular and small cell lung cancers* [etoposide phosphate diethanolate] 119.3 mg/vial

**etoposide** USAN, INN, BAN *antineoplastic* 20, 30 mg/mL injection

**etoposide & paclitaxel & carboplatin** *chemotherapy protocol for pri-*

mary adenocarcinoma and small cell lung cancer (SCLC)

**etoposide phosphate** USAN *antineoplastic*

**etoprindole** INN

**etoprine** USAN *antineoplastic*

**etoricoxib** USAN *antiarthritic; antipyretic; COX-2 inhibitor; nonsteroidal anti-inflammatory drug (NSAID); investigational (NDA filed) for osteoarthritis, rheumatoid arthritis, musculoskeletal pain, and gout*

**etorphine** INN, BAN

**etosalamide** INN [also: ethosalamide]

**etoxadrol** INN *anesthetic* [also: etoxadrol HCl]

**etoxadrol HCl** USAN *anesthetic* [also: etoxadrol]

**etoxazene** INN *analgesic* [also: ethoxazene HCl]

**etoxazene HCl** [see: ethoxazene HCl]

**etoxeridine** INN, BAN

**etozolin** USAN, INN *diuretic*

**etrabamine** INN

**Etrafon; Etrafon 2–10; Etrafon-A; Etrafon-Forte** tablets R̶ *conventional (typical) antipsychotic; antidepressant* [perphenazine; amitriptyline HCl] 2•25 mg; 2•10 mg; 4•10 mg; 4•25 mg

**etretin** [see: acitretin]

**etretinate** USAN, INN, BAN, JAN *systemic antipsoriatic; retinoic acid analogue*

**etryptamine** INN, BAN *CNS stimulant* [also: etryptamine acetate]

**etryptamine acetate** USAN *CNS stimulant* [also: etryptamine]

**etybenzatropine** INN *anticholinergic* [also: ethybenztropine]

**etymemazine** INN

**etymemazine HCl** [see: etymemazine]

**etynodiol** INN *progestin* [also: ethynodiol diacetate; ethynodiol]

**etyprenaline** [see: isoetharine]

**eucaine HCl** NF

**Eucalyptamint** ointment, gel OTC *topical analgesic; counterirritant; antiseptic* [menthol; eucalyptus oil] 16%•⸮; 8%•⸮

**eucalyptol** USAN *topical bacteriostatic antiseptic/germicidal*

**eucalyptus (Eucalyptus globulus)** oil *medicinal herb for bronchitis, lung disorders, neuralgia, and skin sores; source of bioflavonoids*

**eucalyptus oil** NF *topical antiseptic*

**eucatropine** INN, BAN *ophthalmic anticholinergic* [also: eucatropine HCl]

**eucatropine HCl** USP *ophthalmic anticholinergic* [also: eucatropine]

**Eucerin** cream, lotion OTC *moisturizer; emollient*

**Eucerin** OTC *cream base*

**Eucerin Itch-Relief Moisturizing** spray OTC *counterirritant* [menthol] 0.15%

**Eucerin Plus** lotion OTC *moisturizer; emollient* [sodium lactate; urea] 5%•5%

**eucodal** [see: oxycodone]

**Eudal-SR** sustained-release tablets (discontinued 2002) R̶ *decongestant; expectorant* [pseudoephedrine HCl; guaifenesin] 120•400 mg

**euflavine** [see: acriflavine]

**Euflex** ⊛ tablets R̶ *antiandrogen antineoplastic adjunct to metastatic prostate cancer* [flutamide] 250 mg

**Eugenia caryophyllata** *medicinal herb* [see: cloves]

**Eugenia pimenta** *medicinal herb* [see: allspice]

**eugenol** USP *dental analgesic*

**Euglucon** ⊛ tablets R̶ *sulfonylurea antidiabetic* [glyburide] 2.5, 5 mg

**eukadol** [see: oxycodone]

**Eulexin** capsules R̶ *antiandrogen antineoplastic adjunct to metastatic prostate cancer* [flutamide] 125 mg

**Euonymus atropurpureus** *medicinal herb* [see: wahoo]

**Eupatorium cannabinum** *medicinal herb* [see: hemp agrimony]

**Eupatorium perfoliatum** *medicinal herb* [see: boneset]

**Eupatorium purpureum** *medicinal herb* [see: queen of the meadow]

**Euphorbia poinsettia; E. pulcherrima** *medicinal herb* [see: poinsettia]

**euphoretics; euphoriants; euphora-
gens** *a class of agents that produce
euphoria*
*Euphrasia officinalis; E. rostkoviana;
E. strica* medicinal herb [see: eyebright]
**euprocin** INN *topical anesthetic* [also:
euprocin HCl]
**euprocin HCl** USAN *topical anesthetic*
[also: euprocin]
**euquinine** [see: quinine ethylcarbonate]
**Eurax** cream, lotion ℞ *scabicide; antipruritic* [crotamiton] 10% ⧄ Serax; Urex
**European alder; European black
alder; European buckthorn** *medicinal herb* [see: buckthorn]
**European aspen** *medicinal herb* [see:
black poplar]
**europium** *element (Eu)*
**EVA (etoposide, vinblastine, Adria-
mycin)** *chemotherapy protocol for
Hodgkin lymphoma*
**Evac-Q-Kwik** suppositories (discontinued 2003) OTC *stimulant laxative*
[bisacodyl] 10 mg ⧄ Evac-Q-Kit
**Evac-Q-Kwik Kit** oral solution + 2
tablets + 1 suppository (discontinued
2003) OTC *pre-procedure bowel evacuant* [Evac-Q-Mag (q.v.); Evac-Q-
Tabs (q.v.); Evac-Q-Kwik suppository (q.v.)]
**Evac-Q-Mag** carbonated oral solution
OTC *saline laxative* [magnesium citrate; citric acid; potassium citrate]
**Evac-Q-Tabs** tablets OTC *stimulant laxative* [bisacodyl] 5 mg
**evandamine** INN
**Evans blue** USP *diagnostic aid for blood
volume* [also: azovan blue] 5 mL
injection
**evening primrose (*Oenothera bien-
nis*)** bark, leaves, oil *medicinal herb
for cardiovascular health, hypertension,
mastalgia, multiple sclerosis, nerves,
obesity, premenstrual syndrome, prostate disorders, rheumatoid arthritis, and
skin disorders*
**everlasting (*Anaphalis margaritacea;
Gnaphalium polycephalum; G.
uliginosum*)** plant *medicinal herb used
as an astringent, diaphoretic, febrifuge,
pectoral, vermifuge, and vulnerary*
**evernimicin** USAN *investigational antibiotic*
**everolimus** *investigational agent for
transplant rejection*
**Everone 200** IM injection (discontinued 2001) ℞ *androgen replacement
for delayed puberty or breast cancer*
[testosterone enanthate] 200 mg/mL
**Evista** film-coated tablets ℞ *selective
estrogen receptor modulator (SERM)
for the prevention and treatment of
postmenopausal osteoporosis; investigational (Phase III) for breast cancer*
[raloxifene HCl] 60 mg ⧄ Avita
**E-Vitamin** ointment OTC *emollient*
[vitamin E] 30 mg/g
**E-VMAC (escalated methotrexate,
vinblastine, Adriamycin, cisplatin)** *chemotherapy protocol*
**E-VMAC (escalated methotrexate,
vinblastine, Adriamycin, cyclophosphamide)** *chemotherapy protocol*
**Evoxac** capsules ℞ *cholinergic and muscarinic receptor agonist for treatment of
dry mouth due to Sjögren syndrome*
[cevimeline HCl] 30 mg
**Evra** [see: Ortho Evra]
**Exact** topical liquid (discontinued
2003) OTC *keratolytic cleanser for acne*
[salicylic acid] 2%
**Exact** vanishing cream OTC *keratolytic
for acne* [benzoyl peroxide] 5%
**exalamide** INN
**exametazime** USAN, INN, BAN *regional
cerebral perfusion imaging aid*
**Exanta** tablets (approved in 14 European countries) ℞ *investigational
(NDA filed) oral anticoagulant and
direct thrombin inhibitor for the prevention of stroke due to atrial fibrillation
and the prevention and treatment of a
venous thromboembolic event (VTE)*
[ximelagatran]
**exaprolol** INN *antiadrenergic (β-receptor)* [also: exaprolol HCl]
**exaprolol HCl** USAN *antiadrenergic (β-
receptor)* [also: exaprolol]

**exatecan mesylate** USAN *antineoplastic; topoisomerase I inhibitor for skin cancer*

**Excedrin Aspirin Free** caplets, geltabs OTC *analgesic; antipyretic; anti-inflammatory* [acetaminophen; caffeine] 500•65 mg

**Excedrin Dual, Aspirin Free** film-coated caplets (discontinued 2000) OTC *analgesic; antipyretic; antacid* [acetaminophen; calcium carbonate; magnesium carbonate; magnesium oxide] 500•111•64•30 mg

**Excedrin Extra Strength** caplets, tablets, geltabs OTC *analgesic; antipyretic; anti-inflammatory* [acetaminophen; aspirin; caffeine] 250•250•65 mg

**Excedrin Migraine** tablets OTC *analgesic for relief of migraine headache syndrome, including prodrome, pain, and associated symptoms* [acetaminophen; aspirin; caffeine] 250•250•65 mg

**Excedrin P.M.** oral liquid, liquigels OTC *antihistaminic sleep aid; analgesic* [diphenhydramine HCl; acetaminophen] 50•1000 mg/30 mL; 25•500 mg

**Excedrin P.M.** tablets, caplets, geltabs OTC *antihistaminic sleep aid; analgesic* [diphenhydramine citrate; acetaminophen] 38•500 mg

**Excedrin QuickTabs** (orally dissolving tablets) OTC *analgesic; antipyretic; anti-inflammatory* [acetaminophen; caffeine] 500•65 mg

**Excedrin Sinus** tablets, caplets (discontinued 2002) OTC *decongestant; analgesic; antipyretic* [pseudoephedrine HCl; acetaminophen] 30•500 mg

**Excedrin Tension Headache** caplets, geltabs OTC *analgesic; antipyretic; anti-inflammatory* [acetaminophen; caffeine] 500•65 mg

**Excita Extra** premedicated condom OTC *spermicidal/barrier contraceptive* [nonoxynol 9] 8%

**Exelderm** solution ℞ *topical antifungal* [sulconazole nitrate] 1%

**Exelon** capsules, oral solution ℞ *acetylcholinesterase inhibitor to increase cognition in Alzheimer disease* [rivastigmine tartrate] 1.5, 3, 4.5, 6 mg; 2 mg/mL

**exemestane** INN *aromatase inhibitor; antihormonal antineoplastic for advanced breast cancer in postmenopausal women* (orphan)

**exenatide** *incretin memetic agent; investigational (NDA filed) synthetic exendin-4 analogue to reduce blood sugar levels and control obesity in type 2 diabetics*

**exepanol** INN

**Exgest LA** long-acting tablets (discontinued 2002) ℞ *decongestant; expectorant* [phenylpropanolamine HCl; guaifenesin] 75•400 mg

**Ex-Histine** syrup ℞ *decongestant; antihistamine; anticholinergic to dry mucosal secretions* [phenylephrine HCl; chlorpheniramine maleate; methscopolamine bromide] 20•4•2.5 mg/10 mL

**Exidine Skin Cleanser; Exidine-2 Scrub; Exidine-4 Scrub** topical liquid OTC *broad-spectrum antimicrobial; germicidal* [chlorhexidine gluconate; alcohol 4%] 4%; 2%; 4%

**exifone** INN

**exiproben** INN

**exisulind** *investigational (NDA filed, orphan) antineoplastic for familial adenomatous polyposis (FAP; also known as adenomatous polyposis coli, or APC); investigational (Phase III) for lung cancer*

**Ex-Lax** tablets, chocolated chewable tablets OTC *stimulant laxative* [sennosides] 15 mg

**Ex-Lax Gentle Strength** caplets OTC *stimulant laxative; stool softener* [sennosides; docusate sodium] 10•65 mg

**Ex-Lax Maximum Relief** tablets OTC *stimulant laxative* [sennosides] 25 mg

**Ex-Lax Stool Softener** caplets OTC *laxative; stool softener* [docusate sodium] 100 mg

**Exna** tablets (discontinued 2003) ℞ *diuretic; antihypertensive* [benzthiazide] 50 mg

**EXO-226** *investigational (Phase III) albumin glycation inhibitor for the prevention and treatment of diabetes-related kidney disease*

**Exocaine Medicated Rub; Exocaine Plus Rub** OTC *analgesic; counterirritant* [methyl salicylate] 25%; 30%

**Exosurf** Ɽ *investigational (orphan) pulmonary surfactant for adult respiratory distress syndrome (ARDS)* [colfosceril palmitate]

**Exosurf Neonatal** intratracheal suspension Ɽ *pulmonary surfactant for hyaline membrane disease and respiratory distress syndrome (orphan)* [colfosceril palmitate] 108 mg

**Exosurf Neonatal** powder for injection (discontinued 2003) Ɽ *pulmonary surfactant for hyaline membrane disease and respiratory distress syndrome (orphan)* [colfosceril palmitate] 108 mg

**expectorants** *a class of drugs that promote the ejection of mucus from the respiratory tract*

**Expidet** (trademarked dosage form) *fast-dissolving dose*

**Exsel** lotion/shampoo (discontinued 2004) Ɽ *antiseborrheic; dandruff treatment* [selenium sulfide] 2.5%

**exsiccated sodium arsenate** [see: sodium arsenate, exsiccated]

**Extencap** (trademarked dosage form) *extended-release capsule*

**extended insulin zinc** [see: insulin zinc, extended]

**Extendryl** chewable tablets, syrup Ɽ *decongestant; antihistamine; anticholinergic to dry mucosal secretions* [phenylephrine HCl; chlorpheniramine maleate; methscopolamine nitrate] 10•2•1.25 mg; 20•4•2.5 mg/10 mL

**Extendryl JR** sustained-release pediatric capsules Ɽ *decongestant; antihistamine; anticholinergic to dry mucosal secretions* [phenylephrine HCl; chlorpheniramine maleate; methscopolamine nitrate] 10•4•1.25 mg

**Extendryl SR** sustained-release capsules Ɽ *decongestant; antihistamine; anticholinergic to dry mucosal secretions* [phenylephrine HCl; chlorpheniramine maleate; methscopolamine nitrate] 20•8•2.5 mg

**Extentab** (trademarked dosage form) *extended-release tablet*

**Extina** foam Ɽ *investigational (Phase III) antifungal for seborrheic dermatitis* [ketoconazole]

**Extra Action Cough** syrup OTC *antitussive; expectorant* [dextromethorphan hydrobromide; guaifenesin] 20•200 mg/10 mL

**"Extra Strength"** products [see under product name]

**Extraneal** IV infusion (supplied in Ultrabag and Ambu-Flex) Ɽ *peritoneal dialysis solution for end-stage renal disease (orphan)* [icodextrin] 75 g

**Exubera** Ɽ *investigational (Phase III) inhaled aerosol dry powder insulin*

**eye balm; eye root** *medicinal herb* [see: goldenseal]

**Eye Drops** OTC *topical ophthalmic decongestant and vasoconstrictor* [tetrahydrozoline HCl] 0.05%

**Eye Irrigating Solution** OTC *extraocular irrigating solution* [sterile isotonic solution]

**Eye Irrigating Wash** OTC *extraocular irrigating solution* [sterile isotonic solution]

**Eye Scrub** solution OTC *eyelid cleanser for blepharitis or contact lenses*

**Eye Stream** ophthalmic solution OTC *extraocular irrigating solution* [sterile isotonic solution]

**Eye Wash** ophthalmic solution OTC *extraocular irrigating solution* [sterile isotonic solution]

**eyebright (Euphrasia officinalis; E. rostkoviana; E. strica)** *plant medicinal herb for blood cleansing, cataracts, colds, conjunctivitis, eye disorders and infections, and stimulating liver function; not generally regarded as safe and effective for topical ophthalmic use*

**Eye-Lube-A** eye drops OTC *ophthalmic moisturizer/lubricant* [glycerin] 0.25%

**Eye-Sed** eye drops (discontinued 2001) OTC *ophthalmic astringent* [zinc sulfate] 0.25%

**Eyesine** eye drops (discontinued 2003) OTC *ophthalmic decongestant;*

vasoconstrictor [tetrahydrozoline HCl] 0.05%

**EZ Detect** test kit for home use *in vitro diagnostic aid for fecal occult blood*

**ezetimibe** USAN *antihyperlipidemic; intestinal cholesterol absorption inhibitor*

**Ezide** tablets ℞ *antihypertensive; diuretic* [hydrochlorothiazide] 50 mg

**ezlopitant** USAN *substance P receptor antagonist for emesis, pain, and inflammation*

# F

**1+1-F Creme** ℞ *topical corticosteroidal anti-inflammatory; antifungal; antibacterial; local anesthetic* [hydrocortisone; clioquinol; pramoxine] 1%•3%•1%

**¹⁸F** [see: fludeoxyglucose F 18]

**¹⁸F** [see: sodium fluoride F 18]

**FABRase** ℞ *investigational (orphan) enzyme replacement therapy for Fabry disease* [agalsidase alfa]

**Fabrazyme** powder for IV infusion ℞ *enzyme replacement therapy for Fabry disease (orphan)* [agalsidase beta] 5.5, 37 mg/dose

**FAC (fluorouracil, Adriamycin, cyclophosphamide)** *chemotherapy protocol for breast cancer*

**FAC-LEV (fluorouracil, Adriamycin, Cytoxin, levamisole)** *chemotherapy protocol*

**FAC-M (fluorouracil, Adriamycin, cyclophosphamide, methotrexate)** *chemotherapy protocol*

**Fact Plus** test kit for home use *in vitro diagnostic aid; urine pregnancy test*

**Factive** film-coated tablets ℞ *broadspectrum fluoroquinolone antibiotic for respiratory tract infections* [gemifloxacin mesylate] 320 mg

**factor II (prothrombin)**

**factor III** [see: thromboplastin]

**factor VIIa, recombinant** *coagulant for hemophilia A and B (orphan)*

**factor VIII** [see: antihemophilic factor]

**factor VIII (rDNA)** BAN *blood coagulating factor*

**factor VIII fraction** BAN *blood coagulating factor*

**fact**[...] *[...] A [...]*

**fact**[...] *static; antihemophilic for hemophilia B (orphan)* [also: factor IX fraction; nonacog alfa]

**factor IX fraction** BAN *systemic hemostatic; antihemophilic* [also: factor IX complex; nonacog alfa]

**factor XIII, plasma-derived** *investigational (orphan) hemostatic for congenital factor XIII deficiency*

**factor XIII, recombinant** *investigational (orphan) hemostatic for congenital factor XIII deficiency*

**Factrel** powder for subcu or IV injection ℞ *gonadotropin releasing hormone* [gonadorelin HCl] 100, 500 μg

**fadrozole** INN *antineoplastic; aromatase inhibitor* [also: fadrozole HCl]

**fadrozole HCl** USAN *antineoplastic; aromatase inhibitor* [also: fadrozole]

**falintolol** INN

**falipamil** INN

**Falkochol** ℞ *investigational (orphan) agent for congenital errors of cholesterol and bile acid synthesis* [dehydrocholic acid]

**false foxglove** *medicinal herb* [see: feverweed]

**false unicorn (Chamaelirium luteum)** root *medicinal herb used for amenorrhea, morning sickness, and preventing miscarriages; also used for colic, cough, and digestive, kidney, and prostate problems; emetic in high doses*

**false valerian** *medicinal herb* [see: life root]

**false vervain** *medicinal herb* [see: blue vervain]

**FAM (fluorouracil, Adriamycin, mitomycin)** *chemotherapy protocol for adenocarcinoma and gastric cancer*

**FAM-CF (fluorouracil, Adriamycin, mitomycin, citrovorum factor)** *chemotherapy protocol*

**famciclovir** USAN, INN, BAN *oral antiviral for herpes simplex type 2 (HSV-2, genital herpes) and herpes zoster (shingles) infections; suppressive therapy for recurrent outbreaks*

**FAME; FAMe (fluorouracil, Adriamycin, MeCCNU)** *chemotherapy protocol*

**famiraprinium chloride** INN

**FAMMe (fluorouracil, Adriamycin, mitomycin, MeCCNU)** *chemotherapy protocol*

**famotidine** USAN, USP, INN, BAN *histamine $H_2$ antagonist for gastric ulcers* 10, 20, 40 mg oral; 10 mg/mL injection

**famotine** INN *antiviral* [also: famotine HCl]

**famotine HCl** USAN *antiviral* [also: famotine]

**fampridine** USAN, INN *investigational (orphan) agent for multiple sclerosis and spinal cord injury*

**famprofazone** INN, BAN

**FAM-S (fluorouracil, Adriamycin, mitomycin, streptozocin)** *chemotherapy protocol*

**FAMTX (fluorouracil, Adriamycin, methotrexate [with leucovorin rescue])** *chemotherapy protocol for gastric cancer*

**Famvir** film-coated tablets ℞ *antiviral for herpes simplex virus type 2 (HSV-2, genital herpes) and herpes zoster (shingles) infections; suppressive therapy for recurrent outbreaks* [famciclovir] 125, 250, 500 mg

**fananserin** USAN *antipsychotic; antischizophrenic; dopamine $D_2$ and serotonin $5-HT_2$ receptor antagonist*

**fanetizole** INN, BAN *immunoregulator* [also: fanetizole mesylate]

**fanetizole mesylate** USAN *immunoregulator* [also: fanetizole]

**Fansidar** tablets ℞ *antimalarial* [sulfadoxine; pyrimethamine] 500•25 mg

**fanthridone** BAN *antidepressant* [also: fantridone HCl; fantridone]

**fantridone** INN *antidepressant* [also: fantridone HCl; fanthridone]

**fantridone HCl** USAN *antidepressant* [also: fantridone; fanthridone]

**FAP (fluorouracil, Adriamycin, Platinol)** *chemotherapy protocol for gastric cancer*

**Farbee with Vitamin C** caplets OTC *vitamin supplement* [multiple B vitamins; vitamin C] ±•300 mg

**Fareston** tablets ℞ *antiestrogen antineoplastic for metastatic breast cancer in postmenopausal women (orphan); investigational (orphan) for desmoid tumors* [toremifene citrate] 60 mg

**farglitazar** USAN *thiazolidinedione antidiabetic; increases cellular response to insulin without increasing insulin secretion*

**farnesil** INN *combining name for radicals or groups*

**fasiplon** INN

**Faslodex** prefilled syringe for IM injection (once monthly) ℞ *antiestrogen antineoplastic for metastatic breast cancer in postmenopausal women* [fulvestrant] 50 mg/mL

**Faspak** (trademarked form) *flexible plastic bag*

**Fastic** (Japanese name for U.S. product Starlix)

**Fastin** capsules (discontinued 2001) ℞ *anorexiant; CNS stimulant* [phentermine HCl] 30 mg

**Fast-Trak** (trademarked delivery system) *quick-loading syringe*

**fat, hard** NF *suppository base*

**fat emulsion, intravenous** *parenteral essential fatty acid replacement*

**Father John's Medicine Plus** oral liquid OTC *antitussive; decongestant; antihistamine* [dextromethorphan hydrobromide; phenylephrine HCl;

chlorpheniramine maleate] 10•10•4 mg/30 mL

*Fatsia horrida medicinal herb* [see: devil's club]

**Fazaclo** orally disintegrating tablets ℞ *novel (atypical) antipsychotic for severe schizophrenia* [clozapine] 25, 100 mg

**fazadinium bromide** INN, BAN

**fazarabine** USAN, INN *antineoplastic*

**5-FC (5-fluorocytosine)** [see: flucytosine]

**FCAP (fluorouracil, cyclophosphamide, Adriamycin, Platinol)** *chemotherapy protocol*

**FCE (fluorouracil, cisplatin, etoposide)** *chemotherapy protocol*

**F-CL (fluorouracil, leucovorin calcium [rescue])** *chemotherapy protocol for colorectal cancer* [also: FU/LV]

**FCP (fluorouracil, cyclophosphamide, prednisone)** *chemotherapy protocol*

**FD&C Red No. 2 (Food, Drug & Cosmetic Act)** [see: amaranth]

**FD&C Red No. 3 (Food, Drug & Cosmetic Act)** [see: erythrosine sodium]

**F-ddA (fluorodideoxyadenosine)** [see: lodenosine]

**FDDNP ([$^{18}$F] fluoroethyl [methyl] amino-2-naphthyl ethylidene malononitrile)** *PET scan contrast medium for detection of β-amyloid senile plaques and neurofibrillary tangles for early detection of Alzheimer disease*

**$^{18}$FDG (fludeoxyglucose)** [see: fludeoxyglucose F 18]

**FDh (2(3H) furanone di-hydro)** *a precursor to gamma hydroxybutyrate (GHB); a formerly legal alternative to GHB, now also illegal (Schedule I); also known as gamma butyrolactone (GBL)* [see: gamma hydroxybutyrate (GHB)]

**Fe$^{50}$ (or Fe50)** extended-release caplets OTC *hematinic* [ferrous sulfate, dried (source of iron)] 160 mg (50 mg)

$^{59}$**Fe** [see: ferric chloride Fe 59]

$^{59}$**Fe** [see: ferric citrate ($^{59}$Fe)]

$^{59}$**Fe** [see: ferrous citrate Fe 59]

$^{59}$**Fe** [see: ferrous sulfate Fe 59]

**febantel** USAN, INN, BAN *veterinary anthelmintic*

**febarbamate** INN

**febricides** *a class of agents that relieve or reduce fever* [also called: antifebriles; antipyretics; antithermics; febrifuges]

**febrifuges** *a class of agents that relieve or reduce fever* [also called: antifebriles; antipyretics; antithermics; febricides]

**febuprol** INN

**febuverine** INN

**FEC (fluorouracil, epirubicin, cyclophosphamide)** *chemotherapy protocol for breast cancer*

**feclemine** INN

**feclobuzone** INN

**FED (fluorouracil, etoposide, DDP)** *chemotherapy protocol for non–small cell lung cancer (NSCLC)*

**Fedahist** tablets (discontinued 2002) OTC *decongestant; antihistamine* [pseudoephedrine HCl; chlorpheniramine maleate] 60•4 mg

**Fedahist** Timecaps (timed-release capsules), Gyrocaps (extended-release capsules) (discontinued 2002) ℞ *decongestant; antihistamine* [pseudoephedrine HCl; chlorpheniramine maleate] 120•8 mg; 65•10 mg

**fedotozine** INN *investigational kappa selective opioid agonist for irritable bowel syndrome*

**fedrilate** INN

**Feen-A-Mint** enteric-coated tablets OTC *stimulant laxative* [bisacodyl] 5 mg

**Feiba VH Immuno** IV injection or drip ℞ *antihemophilic to correct factor VIII deficiency and coagulation deficiency* [anti-inhibitor coagulant complex, vapor heated and freeze-dried] (each bottle is labeled with dosage)

**felbamate** USAN, INN *anticonvulsant; adjunctive therapy for Lennox-Gastaut syndrome (orphan)*

**Felbatol** tablets, oral suspension (the FDA and the manufacturer strongly caution against its use due to adverse side effects) ℞ *anticonvulsant;*

adjunctive therapy for Lennox-Gastaut syndrome (orphan) [felbamate] 400, 600 mg; 600 mg/5 mL

**felbinac** USAN, INN, BAN anti-inflammatory

**Feldene** capsules ℞ antiarthritic; nonsteroidal anti-inflammatory drug (NSAID) [piroxicam] 10, 20 mg

**felipyrine** INN

**felodipine** USAN, INN, BAN vasodilator; antihypertensive; calcium channel blocker

**felonwood; felonwort** medicinal herb [see: bittersweet nightshade]

**felvizumab** USAN monoclonal antibody for prophylaxis and treatment of respiratory syncytial virus (RSV)

**felypressin** USAN, INN, BAN vasoconstrictor

**Fem pH** vaginal jelly OTC antibacterial; acidity modifier [acetic acid, glacial; oxyquinoline sulfate] 0.9%•0.025%

**Fem-1** tablets OTC analgesic; anti-inflammatory; diuretic [acetaminophen; pamabrom] 500•25 mg

**female fern (Polypodium vulgare)** root medicinal herb used as an anthelmintic, cholagogue, demulcent, and purgative

**female regulator** medicinal herb [see: life root]

**Femara** film-coated tablets ℞ aromatase inhibitor; estrogen antagonist; antineoplastic for advanced breast cancer in postmenopausal women [letrozole] 2.5 mg

**FemBack** caplets OTC analgesic; antihistaminic sleep aid [acetaminophen; salicylamide; phenyltoloxamine citrate] 150•150•44 mg

**FemCal** tablets (discontinued 2002) OTC dietary supplement [calcium carbonate; vitamin D; multiple minerals] 250 mg•100 IU•±

**Femcet** capsules (discontinued 2000) ℞ analgesic; barbiturate sedative [acetaminophen; caffeine; butalbital] 325•40•50 mg

**femhrt 1/5** tablets (in packs of 28) ℞ synthetic progestin/estrogen; hormone replacement therapy for postmenopausal symptoms [norethindrone acetate; ethinyl estradiol] 1 mg•5 μg

**femhrtLo** ℞ synthetic progestin/estrogen; investigational (NDA filed) low-dose version of **femhrt** for postmenopausal symptoms [norethindrone acetate; ethinyl estradiol]

**Feminique Disposable Douche** solution OTC antiseptic; antifungal; vaginal cleanser and deodorizer; acidity modifier [sodium benzoate; sorbic acid; lactic acid]

**Feminique Disposable Douche** solution OTC vaginal cleanser and deodorizer; acidity modifier [vinegar (acetic acid)]

**Femiron** tablets OTC hematinic [ferrous fumarate (source of iron)] 63 mg (20 mg) ⃝ Remeron

**Femiron Multi-Vitamins and Iron** tablets OTC vitamin/iron supplement [multiple vitamins; ferrous fumarate; folic acid] ±•20•0.4 mg

**Femizol-M** vaginal cream OTC antifungal [miconazole nitrate] 2%

**femoxetine** INN

**FemPatch** transdermal patch (discontinued 2003) ℞ estrogen replacement therapy for postmenopausal symptoms [estradiol] 25 μg/day

**Femring** vaginal ring ℞ synthetic estrogen; three-month hormone replacement for postmenopausal atrophic vaginitis [estradiol acetate] 12.4 mg (50 μg/day), 24.8 mg (100 μg day)

**FemSoft** urethral insert treatment for stress urinary incontinence [silicone plug]

**Femstat 3** vaginal cream in prefilled applicator (discontinued 2004) OTC antifungal [butoconazole nitrate] 2%

**FemStat One** vaginal cream (discontinued 2001) OTC antifungal [butoconazole nitrate] 2%

**Femtrace** tablets ℞ synthetic estrogen; hormone replacement for postmenopausal symptoms [estradiol acetate] 0.45, 0.9, 1.8 mg

**fenabutene** INN

**fenacetinol** INN

**fenaclon** INN
**fenadiazole** INN
**fenaftic acid** INN
**fenalamide** USAN, INN *smooth muscle relaxant*
**fenalcomine** INN
**fenamifuril** INN
**fenamisal** INN *antibacterial; tuberculostatic* [also: phenyl aminosalicylate]
**fenamole** USAN, INN *anti-inflammatory*
**fenaperone** INN
**fenarsone** [see: carbarsone]
**fenasprate** [see: benorilate]
**fenbendazole** USAN, INN, BAN *anthelmintic*
**fenbenicillin** INN [also: phenbenicillin]
**fenbufen** USAN, INN, BAN *anti-inflammatory*
**fenbutrazate** INN [also: phenbutrazate]
**fencamfamin** INN, BAN
**fencamfamin HCl** [see: fencamfamin]
**fencarbamide** INN *anticholinergic* [also: phencarbamide]
**fenchlorphos** BAN *systemic insecticide* [also: ronnel; fenclofos]
**fencilbutirol** USAN, INN *choleretic*
**fenclexonium metilsulfate** INN
**fenclofenac** USAN, INN, BAN *anti-inflammatory*
**fenclofos** INN *systemic insecticide* [also: ronnel; fenchlorphos]
**fenclonine** USAN, INN *serotonin inhibitor*
**fenclorac** USAN, INN *anti-inflammatory*
**fenclozic acid** INN, BAN
**fendiline** INN
**fendizoate** INN *combining name for radicals or groups*
**fendosal** USAN, INN, BAN *anti-inflammatory*
**feneritrol** INN
**Fenesin** sustained-release tablets (discontinued 2004) ℞ *expectorant* [guaifenesin] 600 mg
**Fenesin DM** tablets ℞ *antitussive; expectorant* [dextromethorphan hydrobromide; guaifenesin] 30•600 mg
**fenestrel** USAN, INN *estrogen*
**fenethazine** INN
**fenethylline** BAN *CNS stimulant* [also: fenethylline HCl; fenetylline]

**fenethylline HCl** USAN *CNS stimulant* [also: fenetylline; fenethylline]
**fenetradil** INN
**fenetylline** INN *CNS stimulant* [also: fenethylline HCl; fenethylline]
**fenflumizole** INN
**fenfluramine** INN, BAN *anorexiant; CNS depressant* [also: fenfluramine HCl]
**fenfluramine HCl** USAN *anorexiant; CNS depressant* [also: fenfluramine]
**fenfluthrin** INN, BAN
**fengabine** USAN, INN, BAN *mood regulator*
**fenharmane** INN
**fenimide** USAN, INN, BAN *antipsychotic*
**feniodium chloride** INN
**fenipentol** INN
**fenirofibrate** INN
**fenisorex** USAN, INN, BAN *anorectic*
**fenleuton** USAN *5-lipoxygenase inhibitor*
**fenmetozole** INN *antidepressant; narcotic antagonist* [also: fenmetozole HCl]
**fenmetozole HCl** USAN *antidepressant; narcotic antagonist* [also: fenmetozole]
**fenmetramide** USAN, INN, BAN *antidepressant*
**fennel (Anethum foeniculum; Foeniculum officinale; F. vulgare)** seeds *medicinal herb for colic, gas, intestinal problems, promoting expectoration, stimulating lactation and menses, and sedation in children*
**fennel oil** NF
**fenobam** USAN, INN *sedative*
**fenocinol** INN
**fenoctimine** INN *gastric antisecretory* [also: fenoctimine sulfate]
**fenoctimine sulfate** USAN *gastric antisecretory* [also: fenoctimine]
**fenofibrate** INN, BAN *antihyperlipidemic for primary hypercholesterolemia (types IIa and IIb hyperlipidemia), hypertriglyceridemia (types IV and V hyperlipidemia), and mixed dyslipidemia* 67, 134, 200 mg oral
**fenoldopam** INN, BAN *vasodilator for hypertensive emergencies; dopamine agonist* [also: fenoldopam mesylate]
**fenoldopam mesylate** USAN *vasodilator for hypertensive emergencies; dopa-*

*mine agonist* [also: fenoldopam] 10 mg/mL injection

**fenoprofen** USAN, INN, BAN *analgesic; antiarthritic; nonsteroidal anti-inflammatory drug (NSAID)*

**fenoprofen calcium** USAN, USP, BAN *analgesic; antiarthritic; nonsteroidal anti-inflammatory drug (NSAID)* 200, 300, 600 mg oral

**fenoterol** USAN, INN, BAN *bronchodilator; β-blocker* [also: fenoterol hydrobromide]

**fenoterol hydrobromide** JAN *investigational (NDA filed) bronchodilator; antiasthmatic; β-blocker* [also: fenoterol]

**fenoverine** INN

**fenoxazol** [see: pemoline]

**fenoxazoline** INN

**fenoxazoline HCl** [see: fenoxazoline]

**fenoxedil** INN

**fenoxypropazine** INN [also: phenoxypropazine]

**fenozolone** INN

**fenpentadiol** INN

**fenperate** INN

**fenpipalone** USAN, INN *anti-inflammatory*

**fenpipramide** INN, BAN

**fenpiprane** INN, BAN

**fenpiprane HCl** [see: fenpiprane]

**fenpiverinium bromide** INN

**fenprinast** INN *bronchodilator; antiallergic* [also: fenprinast HCl]

**fenprinast HCl** USAN *bronchodilator; antiallergic* [also: fenprinast]

**fenproporex** INN

**fenprostalene** USAN, INN, BAN *luteolysin*

**fenquizone** USAN, INN *diuretic*

**fenretinide** USAN, INN *synthetic retinoid; investigational (Phase III) chemopreventive for breast, bladder, oral, and skin cancers*

**fenspiride** INN *bronchodilator; antiadrenergic (α-receptor)* [also: fenspiride HCl]

**fenspiride HCl** USAN *bronchodilator; antiadrenergic (α-receptor)* [also: fenspiride]

**fentanyl** INN, BAN *narcotic analgesic; also abused as a street drug* [also: fentanyl citrate] ② Sentinel

**fentanyl citrate** USAN, USP, JAN *narcotic analgesic; also abused as a street drug* [also: fentanyl] 0.05 mg/mL injection

**Fentanyl Oralet** lozenges ℞ *oral transmucosal narcotic analgesic for anesthesia premedication* [fentanyl citrate] 100, 200, 300, 400 µg

**fenthion** BAN

**fentiazac** USAN, INN, BAN *anti-inflammatory*

**fenticlor** USAN, INN, BAN *topical anti-infective*

**fenticonazole** INN, BAN *antifungal* [also: fenticonazole nitrate]

**fenticonazole nitrate** USAN *antifungal* [also: fenticonazole]

**fentonium bromide** INN

**fenugreek (Trigonella foenum-graecum)** seeds *medicinal herb for boils, bronchial secretions, cellulitis, diabetes, hypercholesterolemia, kidney stones, lung infections, promoting expectoration, stomach irritation, and tuberculosis*

**fenyramidol** INN *analgesic; skeletal muscle relaxant* [also: phenyramidol HCl]

**fenyripol** INN *skeletal muscle relaxant* [also: fenyripol HCl]

**fenyripol HCl** USAN *skeletal muscle relaxant* [also: fenyripol]

**Feocyte** prolonged-action tablets ℞ *hematinic* [iron (as ferrous fumarate, ferrous gluconate, and ferrous sulfate); desiccated liver; vitamins $B_6$, $B_{12}$, and C; folic acid] 110•15•2•0.05•100•0.8 mg

**FeoGen** capsules ℞ *hematinic* [ferrous fumarate; cyanocobalamin; ascorbic acid; intrinsic factor concentrate] 66•0.01•250•100 mg

**FeoGen FA; FeoGen Forte** gelcaps ℞ *hematinic; vitamin/iron supplement* [iron; vitamins $B_{12}$ & C; folic acid] 66•0.01•250•1 mg; 151•0.01•60•1 mg

**Feosol** caplets OTC *hematinic; iron supplement* [carbonyl iron] 50 mg

**Feosol** elixir OTC *hematinic* [ferrous sulfate (source of iron)] 220 mg/5 mL (44 mg/5 mL) ⊉ Feostat; Fer-In-Sol; Festal

**Feosol** tablets OTC *hematinic* [ferrous sulfate, dried (source of iron)] 200 mg (65 mg)

**Feostat** chewable tablets, suspension, drops OTC *hematinic* [ferrous fumarate (source of iron)] 100 mg (33 mg); 100 mg/5 mL (33 mg/5 mL); 45 mg/0.6 mL (15 mg/0.6 mL) ⊉ Feosol

**fepentolic acid** INN

**fepitrizol** INN

**fepradinol** INN

**feprazone** INN, BAN

**fepromide** INN

**feprosidnine** INN

**Feratab** tablets OTC *hematinic* [ferrous sulfate, dried (source of iron)] 187 mg (60 mg)

**Fer-gen-sol** drops OTC *hematinic* [ferrous sulfate (source of iron)] 75 mg/0.6 mL (15 mg/0.6 mL)

**Fergon** tablets OTC *hematinic* [ferrous gluconate (source of iron)] 240 mg (27 mg)

**Feridex** IV injection ℞ *contrast agent for MRI of the liver* [ferumoxides] (11.2 mg iron)

**Fer-In-Sol** drops, syrup OTC *hematinic* [ferrous sulfate (source of iron)] 75 mg/0.6 mL (15 mg/0.6 mL); 90 mg/5 mL (18 mg/5 mL)

**Fer-Iron** drops OTC *hematinic* [ferrous sulfate (source of iron)] 75 mg/0.6 mL (15 mg/0.6 mL)

**fermium** *element (Fm)*

**fern; fern brake** *medicinal herb* [see: buckhorn brake; female fern]

**fern, flowering; king's fern; water fern** *medicinal herb* [see: buckhorn brake]

**fern-leaved foxglove** *medicinal herb* [see: feverweed]

**Fero-Folic-500** controlled-release Filmtabs (film-coated tablets) ℞ *hematinic* [ferrous sulfate; ascorbic acid; folic acid] 105•500•0.8 mg

**Fero-Grad-500** timed-release tablets OTC *hematinic; iron/vitamin C supplement* [iron (from ferrous sulfate); sodium ascorbate] 105•500 mg

**Ferotrinsic** capsules ℞ *hematinic* [ferrous fumarate; cyanocobalamin; ascorbic acid; intrinsic factor concentrate; folic acid] 110 mg•15 μg•75 mg•240 mg•0.5 mg

**Ferralet Plus** tablets OTC *hematinic* [ferrous gluconate; cyanocobalamin; ascorbic acid; folic acid] 46 mg•25 μg•400 mg•0.8 mg

**Ferretts** film-coated caplets OTC *hematinic; iron supplement* [ferrous fumarate] 325 mg (106 mg Fe)

**Ferrex 150** capsules OTC *iron supplement* [polysaccharide iron complex] 150 mg Fe

**Ferrex 150 Forte** capsules ℞ *hematinic* [polysaccharide iron complex; vitamin $B_{12}$; folic acid] 150 mg iron•25 μg•1 mg

**Ferrex 150 Forte Plus** capsules ℞ *hematinic* [polysaccharide iron complex; vitamins $B_{12}$ and C; folic acid] 150•0.025•60•1 mg

**Ferrex 150 Plus** capsules OTC *hematinic; vitamin/iron supplement* [polysaccharide iron complex; vitamin C] 150 mg iron•50 mg

**Ferrex PC; Ferrex PC Forte** film-coated tablets ℞ *vitamin/mineral/iron supplement for pregnancy and lactation* [multiple vitamins & minerals; polysaccharide iron complex; folic acid] ≛•60 mg Fe•1 mg

**ferric ammonium citrate** NF

**ferric ammonium sulfate**

**ferric cacodylate** NF

**ferric chloride**

**ferric chloride Fe 59** USAN *radioactive agent*

**ferric citrate ($^{59}$Fe)** INN

**ferric citrochloride** NF

**ferric fructose** USAN, INN *hematinic*

**ferric glycerophosphate** NF

**ferric hexacyanoferrate** *investigational (orphan) agent for internal contamination with radioactive or nonradioactive cesium or thallium*

**ferric hyaluronate** *adhesion barrier for open gynecological and lower GI surgery*

**ferric hydroxide sucrose complex** [see: iron sucrose; saccharated ferric oxide]

**ferric hypophosphite** NF

**ferric oxide** NF *coloring agent*

**ferric oxide, red** NF

**ferric oxide, yellow** NF

**ferric pyrophosphate, soluble** NF

**ferric subsulfate** NF *hemostatic used in a solution or paste to control superficial bleeding from skin biopsies, cervical biopsies, colposcopy, etc.*

**ferricholinate** [see: ferrocholinate]

**ferriclate calcium sodium** USAN *hematinic* [also: calcium sodium ferriclate]

**Ferriprox** R̟ *investigational (orphan) agent for chronic iron overload due to transfusion-dependent anemias* [deferiprone]

**ferristene** USAN *paramagnetic imaging agent for MRI*

**Ferrlecit** IV infusion R̟ *hematinic for iron deficiency of chronic hemodialysis with erythropoietin therapy* [sodium ferric gluconate (source of iron)] 62.5 mg Fe/5 mL

**ferrocholate** [see: ferrocholinate]

**ferrocholinate** INN

**Ferromar** sustained-release caplets OTC *hematinic* [ferrous fumarate; vitamin C] 201.5•200 mg

**ferropolimaler** INN

**Ferro-Sequels** timed-release tablets OTC *hematinic; iron supplement* [ferrous fumarate; docusate sodium] 50• ⸚ mg

**ferrotrenine** INN

**ferrous citrate Fe 59** USAN, USP *radioactive agent*

**ferrous fumarate** USP *hematinic (33% elemental iron)* 200, 325 mg oral

**ferrous gluconate** USP *hematinic (11.6% elemental iron)* 325 mg oral

**ferrous lactate** NF

**ferrous orotate** JAN

**ferrous sulfate** USP, JAN *hematinic (20% elemental iron)* 250, 325 mg oral; 220 mg/5 mL oral; 75 mg/0.6 mL oral

**ferrous sulfate, dried** USP *hematinic (30% elemental iron)*

**ferrous sulfate, exsiccated** [see: ferrous sulfate, dried]

**ferrous sulfate Fe 59** USAN *radioactive agent*

**Fertinex** subcu injection (discontinued 2003) R̟ *follicle-stimulating hormone (FSH); ovulation stimulant for polycystic ovary disease (orphan) and assisted reproductive technologies (ART); investigational (orphan) for spermatogenesis in hormone-deficient males* [urofollitropin] 75, 150 IU

**fertirelin** INN, BAN *veterinary gonadotropin-releasing hormone* [also: fertirelin acetate]

**fertirelin acetate** USAN *veterinary gonadotropin-releasing hormone* [also: fertirelin]

**ferucarbotran** USAN *superparamagnetic diagnostic aid*

**Ferula assafoetida; F. foetida; F. rubricaulis** *medicinal herb* [see: asafetida; asafoetida]

**ferumoxides** USAN *diagnostic aid for magnetic resonance imaging of the liver*

**ferumoxsil** USAN *oral MRI contrast medium for upper GI tract imaging*

**ferumoxtran-10** USAN *superparamagnetic diagnostic aid*

**FeSO$_4$ (ferrous sulfate)** [q.v.]

**Fetal Fibronectin Test** kit for professional use *in vitro diagnostic aid for fetal fibronectin in vaginal secretions at 24–34 weeks, a predictor of preterm delivery*

**fetal neural cells** [see: neural cells, porcine fetal]

**Fe-Tinic 150** capsules OTC *hematinic; iron supplement* [polysaccharide iron complex] 150 mg iron

**Fe-Tinic 150 Forte** capsules R̟ *hematinic* [polysaccharide iron complex; vitamin B$_{12}$; folic acid] 150 mg Fe• 25 μg•1 mg

**fetoxilate** INN *smooth muscle relaxant* [also: fetoxylate HCl; fetoxylate]

**fetoxylate** BAN *smooth muscle relaxant* [also: fetoxylate HCl; fetoxilate]

**fetoxylate HCl** USAN *smooth muscle relaxant* [also: fetoxilate; fetoxylate]

**fever root** *medicinal herb* [see: coral root]

**fever twig** *medicinal herb* [see: bittersweet nightshade]

**Feverall, Children's; Infant's Feverall; Junior Feverall** suppositories OTC *analgesic; antipyretic* [acetaminophen] 120 mg; 80 mg; 325 mg

**Feverall, Children's; Junior Feverall** Sprinkle Caps (powder) OTC *analgesic; antipyretic* [acetaminophen] 80 mg; 160 mg ☒ Fiberall

**feverbush** *medicinal herb* [see: winterberry]

**feverfew (Chrysanthemum parthenium; Leucanthemum parthenium; Pyrethrum parthenium; Tanacetum parthenium)** leaves and flowers *medicinal herb used as an aspirin substitute for chills, colds, fever, inflammation, and migraine and sinus headache*

**feverweed (Gerardia pedicularia)** plant *medicinal herb used as an antiseptic, diaphoretic, febrifuge, and sedative*

**fexicaine** INN, DCF

**Fexicam** ⒸⒶⓃ suppositories ℞ *nonsteroidal anti-inflammatory drug (NSAID) for rheumatoid arthritis, osteoarthritis, ankylosing spondylitis, and primary dysmenorrhea* [piroxicam] 20 mg

**fexinidazole** INN

**fexofenadine HCl** USAN *second-generation peripherally selective piperidine antihistamine for allergic rhinitis and chronic idiopathic urticaria*

**fezatione** INN

**fezolamine** INN *antidepressant* [also: fezolamine fumarate]

**fezolamine fumarate** USAN *antidepressant* [also: fezolamine]

**FGN-1** [now: exisulind]

**fiacitabine (FIAC)** USAN, INN *antiviral; investigational (Phase I/II) for HIV and AIDS*

**fialuridine (FIAU)** USAN, INN *antiviral; investigational (orphan) for chronic active hepatitis B*

**Fiberall** powder OTC *bulk laxative* [psyllium hydrophilic mucilloid] 3.5 g/tsp.

**FiberCon** tablets OTC *bulk laxative; antidiarrheal* [calcium polycarbophil] 500 mg

**Fiberlan** oral liquid OTC *enteral nutritional therapy* [lactose-free formula]

**Fiber-Lax** tablets OTC *bulk laxative; antidiarrheal* [calcium polycarbophil] 625 mg

**FiberNorm** tablets OTC *bulk laxative; antidiarrheal* [calcium polycarbophil] 625 mg

**fibracillin** INN

**Fibrillex** ℞ *investigational (orphan) agent for the treatment of secondary amyloidosis*

**Fibrimage** ℞ *investigational (Phase III) imaging agent for deep vein thrombosis* [technetium Tc 99m]

**fibrin** INN

**fibrinase** [see: factor XIII]

**fibrinogen ($^{125}$I)** INN [also: fibrinogen I 125]

**fibrinogen, human** USP *investigational (orphan)*

**fibrinogen I 125** USAN *vascular patency test; radioactive agent* [also: fibrinogen ($^{125}$I)]

**fibrinoligase** [see: factor XIII]

**fibrinolysin, human** INN [also: plasmin]

**fibrin-stabilizing factor (FSF)** [see: factor XIII]

**fibroblast growth factor, basic (bFGF)** [see: ersofermin]

**fibroblast interferon** [now: interferon beta]

**Fibrogammin P** ℞ *investigational (orphan) hemostatic for congenital factor XIII deficiency* [factor XIII, plasma-derived]

**fibronectin** *investigational (orphan) for nonhealing corneal ulcers or epithelial defects*

**Ficus carica** *medicinal herb* [see: fig]

**Fidelin** ℞ *natural hormone precursor; investigational (NDA filed, orphan) for systemic lupus erythematosus (SLE); investigational (orphan) replacement therapy for adrenal insufficiency* [dehydroepiandrosterone (DHEA)]

**fiduxosin HCl** USAN $\alpha_{1a}$-adrenoceptor antagonist for benign prostatic hyperplasia (BPH)

**50% Dextrose with Electrolyte Pattern A (or N)** IV infusion (discontinued 2001) ℞ intravenous nutritional/electrolyte therapy [combined electrolyte solution; dextrose]

**fig (Ficus carica)** fruit medicinal herb used as a demulcent, emollient, and laxative

**figwort (Scrophularia nodosa)** leaves, stems, and roots medicinal herb for abrasions, athlete's foot, cradle cap, fever, impetigo, restlessness, skin diseases, and skin tumors

**filaminast** USAN selective phosphodiesterase IV inhibitor for asthma

**filenadol** INN

**filgrastim** USAN, INN, BAN hematopoietic stimulant for severe chronic neutropenia (orphan); investigational (Phase III, orphan) cytokine for AIDS-related cytomegalovirus retinitis; investigational (orphan) for myelodysplastic syndrome

**Filipendula ulmaria** medicinal herb [see: meadowsweet]

**filipin** USAN, INN antifungal

**Filmix** ℞ investigational (orphan) neurosonographic contrast medium for intracranial tumors [microbubble contrast agent]

**Filmlok** (trademarked dosage form) film-coated tablet

**Filmseal** (trademarked dosage form) film-coated tablet

**Filmtabs** (trademarked dosage form) film-coated tablets

**FIME (fluorouracil, ICRF-159, MeCCNU)** chemotherapy protocol

**Finac** lotion OTC keratolytic for acne [salicylic acid; isopropyl alcohol] 2%•22.5%

**Finacea** gel ℞ antimicrobial and keratolytic for mild to moderate rosacea [azelaic acid] 15%

**Finajet; Finaplix** brand names for trenbolone acetate, a European veterinary anabolic steroid abused as a street drug

**finasteride** USAN, INN, BAN $\alpha$-reductase inhibitor; androgen hormone inhibitor for benign prostatic hyperplasia (BPH) and androgenic alopecia in men

**Finevin** cream ℞ antimicrobial and keratolytic for inflammatory acne vulgaris [azelaic acid] 20%

**finger leaf** medicinal herb [see: cinquefoil]

**Fioricet** tablets ℞ analgesic; barbiturate sedative [acetaminophen; caffeine; butalbital] 325•40•50 mg ☒ Lorcet

**Fioricet with Codeine** capsules ℞ narcotic antitussive; analgesic; barbiturate sedative [codeine phosphate; acetaminophen; caffeine; butalbital] 30•325•40•50 mg

**Fiorinal** capsules ℞ analgesic; barbiturate sedative [aspirin; caffeine; butalbital] 325•40•50 mg ☒ Florinef

**Fiorinal** tablets (discontinued 2000) ℞ analgesic; barbiturate sedative [aspirin; caffeine; butalbital] 325•40•50 mg ☒ Florinef

**Fiorinal with Codeine** capsules ℞ narcotic antitussive; analgesic; barbiturate sedative [codeine phosphate; aspirin; caffeine; butalbital] 30•325•40•50 mg

**Fiorinal-C ¼; Fiorinal-C ½** ⒸⒶⓃ capsules ℞ narcotic antitussive; analgesic; barbiturate sedative [codeine phosphate; aspirin; caffeine; butalbital] 15•330•40•50 mg; 30•330•40•50 mg

**Fiorpap** tablets (discontinued 2000) ℞ analgesic; barbiturate sedative [acetaminophen; caffeine; butalbital] 325•40•50 mg

**Fiortal** capsules (discontinued 2004) ℞ analgesic; barbiturate sedative [aspirin; caffeine; butalbital] 325•40•50 mg

**fipexide** INN

**fire ant venom allergenic extract** investigational (orphan) skin test and immunotherapy for fire ant reactions

**fireweed** medicinal herb [see: pilewort]

**First Choice** reagent strips for home use in vitro diagnostic aid for blood glucose

**First Response; First Response Early Result** test stick for home use *in vitro diagnostic aid; urine pregnancy test*

**First Response Ovulation Predictor** test kit for home use *in vitro diagnostic aid to predict ovulation time*

**fisalamine** [see: mesalamine]

**fit root (*Monotropa uniflora*)** *medicinal herb used as an antispasmodic, febrifuge, nervine, and sedative*

**FIV-ASA** suppositories ℞ *anti-inflammatory for active ulcerative colitis, proctosigmoiditis, and proctitis* [mesalamine (5-aminosalicylic acid)] 500 mg

**5 + 2 protocol (cytarabine, daunorubicin)** *chemotherapy protocol for acute myelocytic leukemia (AML)*

**5 + 2 protocol (cytarabine, mitoxantrone)** *chemotherapy protocol for acute myelocytic leukemia (AML)*

**5-ALA HCl; ALA** [see: aminolevulinic acid HCl]

**5% Alcohol and 5% Dextrose in Water; 10% Alcohol and 5% Dextrose in Water** IV infusion ℞ *for caloric replacement and rehydration* [dextrose; alcohol] 5%•5%; 10%•5%

**5 Benzagel; 10 Benzagel** gel ℞ *topical keratolytic for acne* [benzoyl peroxide] 5%; 10%

**5% Travert and Electrolyte No. 2; 10% Travert and Electrolyte No. 2** IV infusion ℞ *intravenous nutritional/electrolyte therapy* [combined electrolyte solution; invert sugar (50% dextrose + 50% fructose)]

**506U78** *investigational (orphan) for chronic lymphocytic leukemia*

**5-FC (5-fluorocytosine)** [see: flucytosine]

**five-finger grass; five fingers** *medicinal herb* [see: cinquefoil]

**five-fingers root** *medicinal herb* [see: ginseng]

**5-HT (5-hydroxytryptamine)** [see: serotonin]

**5-HT₃ (hydroxytryptamine) receptor antagonists** *a class of antiemetic and antinauseant agents used primarily after emetogenic cancer chemotherapy*

[also called: selective serotonin 5-HT₃ blockers]

**5-HTP (5-hydroxytryptophan)** [see: L-5 hydroxytryptophan]

**FK-463** *investigational (Phase III) treatment for AIDS-related fungal infections*

**FL (flutamide, leuprolide acetate)** *chemotherapy protocol for prostate cancer*

**FLAC (fluorouracil, leucovorin [rescue], Adriamycin, cyclophosphamide)** *chemotherapy protocol*

**flag, sweet; myrtle flag** *medicinal herb* [see: calamus]

**flag lily; poison flag; water flag** *medicinal herb* [see: blue flag]

**Flagyl** film-coated tablets, capsules ℞ *antibiotic; antiprotozoal; amebicide* [metronidazole] 250, 500 mg; 375 mg

**Flagyl ER** film-coated extended-release tablets ℞ *once-daily antibiotic for bacterial vaginosis* [metronidazole] 750 mg

**Flagyl IV** powder for injection ℞ *antibiotic; antiprotozoal; amebicide* [metronidazole HCl] 500 mg

**Flagyl IV RTU** (ready-to-use) injection ℞ *antibiotic; antiprotozoal; amebicide* [metronidazole] 500 mg/100 mL

**flamenol** INN

**Flanders Buttocks** ointment OTC *topical diaper rash treatment* [zinc oxide; peruvian balsam]

**flannel flower** *medicinal herb* [see: mullein]

**FLAP (fluorouracil, leucovorin [rescue], Adriamycin, Platinol)** *chemotherapy protocol*

**Flarex** Drop-Tainers (eye drop suspension) ℞ *topical ophthalmic corticosteroidal anti-inflammatory* [fluorometholone acetate] 0.1%

**FlashDose** (trademarked delivery system) *orally disintegrating tablets*

**Flatulex** drops OTC *antiflatulent* [simethicone] 40 mg/0.6 mL

**Flatulex** tablets OTC *adsorbent; detoxicant; antiflatulent* [activated charcoal; simethicone] 250•80 mg

**flavamine** INN

**flavine** [see: acriflavine HCl]

**flavocoxid** *natural flavonoids and flavins; natural COX-2 inhibitor; analgesic and anti-inflammatory for the dietary management of osteoarthritis*

**flavodic acid** INN

**flavodilol** INN *antihypertensive* [also: flavodilol maleate]

**flavodilol maleate** USAN *antihypertensive* [also: flavodilol]

**flavonoid** [see: troxerutin]

**Flavons** tablets OTC *dietary supplement* [mixed bioflavonoids] 500 mg

**Flavons-500** tablets OTC *dietary supplement* [citrus bioflavonoids] 500 mg

**flavopiridol** *investigational (Phase III) kinase inhibitor for lung cancer*

**flavoxate** INN, BAN *smooth muscle relaxant; urinary antispasmodic* [also: flavoxate HCl]

**flavoxate HCl** USAN *anticholinergic; smooth muscle relaxant; urinary antispasmodic* [also: flavoxate] 100 mg oral

**flaxseed (Linum usitatissimum)** *medicinal herb for arthritis, autoimmune diseases, colds, constipation, cough, heart disease, lowering cholesterol levels, skin disorders, and urinary tract infections*

**flazalone** USAN, INN, BAN *anti-inflammatory*

**FLe (fluorouracil, levamisole)** *chemotherapy protocol for colorectal cancer*

**flea seed; fleawort** *medicinal herb* [see: plantain]

**fleabane; horseweed (Erigeron canadensis)** *plant medicinal herb used as an astringent, diuretic, and hemostatic*

**fleawort; flea seed** *medicinal herb* [see: plantain]

**Flebogamma 5%** IV infusion ℞ *passive immunizing agent for primary (inherited) immunodeficiency disorders* [immune globulin] 5% (50 mg/mL)

**flecainide** INN, BAN *antiarrhythmic* [also: flecainide acetate]

**flecainide acetate** USAN *antiarrhythmic* [also: flecainide] 50, 100, 150 mg oral

**Fleet** disposable enema OTC *saline laxative* [sodium phosphate, monobasic; sodium phosphate, dibasic] 7•19 g/118 mL dose

**Fleet Babylax** rectal liquid OTC *hyperosmolar laxative* [glycerin] 4 mL/dose

**Fleet Bisacodyl** disposable enema OTC *stimulant laxative* [bisacodyl] 10 mg/30 mL dose

**Fleet Laxative** enteric-coated tablets, suppositories OTC *stimulant laxative* [bisacodyl] 5 mg; 10 mg

**Fleet Medicated Wipes** cleansing pads OTC *moisturizer and cleanser for external rectal/vaginal areas; astringent; antiseptic; antifungal* [hamamelis water; glycerin; alcohol] 50%•10%•7%

**Fleet Mineral Oil** disposable enema OTC *emollient laxative* [mineral oil] 118 mL dose

**Fleet Pain Relief** anorectal wipes OTC *topical local anesthetic* [pramoxine HCl; glycerin] 1%•12%

**Fleet Phospho-Soda** oral solution OTC *saline laxative* [sodium phosphate, monobasic; sodium phosphate, dibasic] 2.4•0.9 g/5 mL

**Fleet Prep Kits No. 1 to No. 3** OTC *pre-procedure bowel evacuant* [other Fleet products in combination kits]

**FLEP (fluorouracil, leucovorin, etoposide, Platinol)** *chemotherapy protocol*

**flerobuterol** INN

**fleroxacin** USAN, INN *antibacterial*

**flesinoxan** INN *investigational (Phase III) antidepressant and anxiolytic*

**flestolol** INN *antiadrenergic (β-receptor)* [also: flestolol sulfate]

**flestolol sulfate** USAN *antiadrenergic (β-receptor)* [also: flestolol]

**fletazepam** USAN, INN, BAN *skeletal muscle relaxant*

**Fletcher's Castoria** oral liquid OTC *stimulant laxative* [senna concentrate] 33.3 mg/mL

**fleur-de-lis** *medicinal herb* [see: blue flag]

**Flex-all 454** gel OTC *analgesic; antipruritic; counterirritant; topical local anesthetic* [methyl salicylate; menthol] ?•16%

**Flexaphen** capsules ℞ *skeletal muscle relaxant; analgesic* [chlorzoxazone; acetaminophen] 250•300 mg

**Flex-Care Especially for Sensitive Eyes** solution OTC *chemical disinfecting solution for soft contact lenses* [note: soft contact indication different from RGP contact indication for same product]

**Flex-Care Especially for Sensitive Eyes** solution OTC *disinfecting/wetting/soaking solution for rigid gas permeable contact lenses* [note: RGP contact indication different from soft contact indication for same product]

**Flexderm** sheets *absorbent wound dressing* [hydrogel polymer]

**Flexeril** film-coated tablets ℞ *skeletal muscle relaxant* [cyclobenzaprine HCl] 5, 10 mg ⊡ Flaxedil

**FlexiGel Strands** wound dressing OTC *absorbent dressing*

**Flexoject** IV or IM injection ℞ *skeletal muscle relaxant* [orphenadrine citrate] 30 mg/mL

**Flexon** IV or IM injection ℞ *skeletal muscle relaxant* [orphenadrine citrate] 30 mg/mL

**FlexPack HP** test for professional use *diagnostic aid for serum IgG antibodies to* H. pylori *(for peptic ulcers)*

**FlexPen** (trademarked form) *disposable prefilled self-injector for insulin*

**Flex-Power Performance Sports** cream OTC *analgesic* [trolamine salicylate] 10%

**Flextra-DS** tablets ℞ *analgesic; antipyretic; antihistaminic sleep aid* [acetaminophen; phenyltoloxamine citrate] 500•50 mg

**Flexzan; Flexzan Extra** adhesive sheets *absorbent, semi-occlusive wound dressing* [polyurethane foam]

**flibanserin** USAN *antidepressant*

**Flintstones Children's; Flintstones Plus Calcium; Flintstones Plus Extra C Children's** chewable tablets OTC *vitamin supplement* [multiple vitamins; folic acid] ≐•0.3 mg

**Flintstones Complete** chewable tablets OTC *vitamin/mineral/iron supplement* [multiple vitamins & minerals;

iron; folic acid; biotin] ≐•18 mg•0.4 mg•40 µg

**Flintstones Plus Iron** chewable tablets OTC *vitamin/iron supplement* [multiple vitamins; iron; folic acid] ≐•15•0.3 mg

**Flo-Coat** oral/rectal suspension ℞ *radiopaque contrast medium for gastrointestinal imaging* [barium sulfate] 100%

**Flocor** ℞ *investigational (Phase III, orphan) coagulation inhibitor for treatment of sickle cell vaso-occlusive crisis; investigational (orphan) for severe burns and for vasospasm following cerebral aneurysm repair* [poloxamer 188]

**floctafenine** USAN, INN, BAN *analgesic*

**Flolan** IV infusion ℞ *platelet aggregation inhibitor and vasodilator for primary pulmonary hypertension (orphan); investigational (orphan) heparin replacement for hemodialysis* [epoprostenol] 0.5, 1.5 mg

**Flomax** capsules ℞ $\alpha_1$-adrenergic *blocker for benign prostatic hyperplasia (BPH)* [tamsulosin HCl] 0.4 mg ⊡ Slow-Mag; Zomig

**flomoxef** INN

**Flonase** nasal spray ℞ *corticosteroidal anti-inflammatory for seasonal or perennial rhinitis* [fluticasone propionate] 50 µg/dose

**Flo-Pack** (trademarked packaging form) *vial for IV drip*

**flopropione** INN

**florantyrone** INN, BAN

**flordipine** USAN, INN *antihypertensive*

**floredil** INN

**Florentine iris** *medicinal herb* [see: orris root]

**floretione** [see: fluoresone]

**florfenicol** USAN, INN, BAN *veterinary antibacterial*

**Florical** capsules, tablets OTC *calcium/fluoride supplement* [calcium carbonate; sodium fluoride] 364•8.3 mg

**Florida Sunburn Relief** lotion OTC *topical analgesic; antipruritic; counterirritant* [phenol; camphor; menthol; benzyl alcohol] 0.4%•0.2%•0.15%•3%

**florifenine** INN

**Florinef Acetate** tablets ℞ *replacement therapy for adrenocortical insufficiency in Addison disease* [fludrocortisone acetate] 0.1 mg ⑫ Fiorinal

**Florone** cream, ointment ℞ *corticosteroidal anti-inflammatory* [diflorasone diacetate] 0.05%

**Florone E** cream ℞ *corticosteroidal anti-inflammatory; emollient* [diflorasone diacetate] 0.05%

**floropipamide** [now: pipamperone]

**floropipeton** [see: propyperone]

**Florvite** drops ℞ *pediatric vitamin supplement and dental caries preventative* [multiple vitamins; sodium fluoride] ≛•0.25, ≛•0.5 mg/mL

**Florvite; Florvite Half Strength** chewable tablets ℞ *pediatric vitamin supplement and dental caries preventative* [multiple vitamins; sodium fluoride; folic acid] ≛•1•0.3 mg; ≛•0.5•0.3 mg

**Florvite + Iron** drops ℞ *pediatric vitamin/iron supplement and dental caries preventative* [multiple vitamins & minerals; sodium fluoride; ferrous sulfate] ≛•0.25•10, ≛•0.5•10 mg/mL

**Florvite + Iron; Half Strength Florvite + Iron** chewable tablets ℞ *pediatric vitamin/iron supplement and dental caries preventative* [multiple vitamins & minerals; sodium fluoride; ferrous sulfate; folic acid] ≛•1•12•0.3 mg; ≛•0.5•12•0.3 mg

**flosequinan** USAN, INN, BAN *antihypertensive; vasodilator*

**flotrenizine** INN

**Flovent** metered dose inhaler, Rotadisk (inhalation powder), Diskus (inhalation powder) ℞ *corticosteroidal antiasthmatic* [fluticasone propionate] 44, 110, 220 μg/dose; 50, 100, 250 μg/dose; 50, 100, 250 μg/dose

**Flovent HFA** ⑯ inhalation aerosol in a metered-dose inhaler ℞ *corticosteroidal antiasthmatic* [fluticasone propionate] 50, 100, 250 μg/dose

**floverine** INN

**flower velure** *medicinal herb* [see: coltsfoot]

**flower-de-luce** *medicinal herb* [see: blue flag]

**floxacillin** USAN *antibacterial* [also: flucloxacillin]

**floxacrine** INN

**Floxin** film-coated tablets, UroPak (3-day supply) ℞ *broad-spectrum fluoroquinolone antibiotic* [ofloxacin] 200, 300, 400 mg; 6 tablets × 200 mg

**Floxin** IV injection (discontinued 2004) ℞ *broad-spectrum fluoroquinolone antibiotic* [ofloxacin] 200, 400 mg/vial

**Floxin Otic** ear drops ℞ *broad-spectrum fluoroquinolone antibiotic* [ofloxacin] 0.3% (3 mg/mL)

**Floxin Otic Singles** (premeasured containers) ℞ *broad-spectrum fluoroquinolone antibiotic* [ofloxacin] 0.3% (0.75 mg per 0.25 mL container)

**floxuridine** USAN, USP, INN *antimetabolic antineoplastic for GI adenocarcinoma metastatic to the liver* 500 mg injection

**Flu, Cold & Cough Medicine** powder for oral solution (discontinued 2002) OTC *antitussive; decongestant; antihistamine; analgesic* [dextromethorphan hydrobromide; pseudoephedrine HCl; chlorpheniramine maleate; acetaminophen] 20•60•4•500 mg/pkt.

**Flu OIA** (Optical ImmunoAssay) test for professional use *rapid (less than 20 minutes) diagnostic aid for influenza A and B in sputum, nasal aspirate, or nasopharyngeal swab*

**fluacizine** INN

**flualamide** INN

**fluanisone** INN, BAN

**fluazacort** USAN, INN *anti-inflammatory*

**flubanilate** INN *CNS stimulant* [also: flubanilate HCl]

**flubanilate HCl** USAN *CNS stimulant* [also: flubanilate]

**flubendazole** USAN, INN, BAN *antiprotozoal*

**flubenisolone** [see: betamethasone]

**flubepride** INN

**flubuperone** [see: melperone]

**flucarbril** INN
**flucetorex** INN
**flucindole** USAN, INN *antipsychotic*
**fluciprazine** INN
**fluclorolone acetonide** INN, BAN *corticosteroid; anti-inflammatory* [also: flucloronide]
**flucloronide** USAN *corticosteroid; anti-inflammatory* [also: fluclorolone acetonide]
**flucloxacillin** INN, BAN *antibacterial* [also: floxacillin]
**fluconazole** USAN, INN, BAN *systemic triazole antifungal* 50, 100, 150, 200 mg oral; 2 mg/mL injection
**flucrilate** INN *tissue adhesive* [also: flucrylate]
**flucrylate** USAN *tissue adhesive* [also: flucrilate]
**flucytosine** USAN, USP, INN, BAN *systemic antifungal*
**fludalanine** USAN, INN *antibacterial*
**Fludara** powder for IV injection ℞ *antineoplastic for chronic lymphocytic leukemia (CLL) and non-Hodgkin lymphoma (orphan)* [fludarabine phosphate] 50 mg
**fludarabine** INN *antimetabolite antineoplastic* [also: fludarabine phosphate]
**fludarabine phosphate** USAN *antimetabolite antineoplastic for chronic lymphocytic leukemia (CLL) and non-Hodgkin lymphoma (orphan)* [also: fludarabine]
**fludazonium chloride** USAN, INN *topical anti-infective*
**fludeoxyglucose (¹⁸F)** INN *diagnostic aid; radioactive agent* [also: fludeoxyglucose F 18]
**fludeoxyglucose F 18** USAN, USP *diagnostic aid; radioactive agent* [also: fludeoxyglucose (¹⁸F)]
**fludiazepam** INN
**fludorex** USAN, INN *anorectic; antiemetic*
**fludoxopone** INN
**fludrocortisone** INN, BAN *salt-regulating adrenocortical steroid; mineralocorticoid* [also: fludrocortisone acetate]
**fludrocortisone acetate** USP *salt-regulating adrenocortical steroid; mineralo-*

*corticoid; for adrenocortical insufficiency in Addison disease* [also: fludrocortisone] 0.1 mg oral
**fludroxicortide** [see: flurandrenolide]
**fludroxycortide** INN *topical corticosteroid* [also: flurandrenolide; flurandrenolone]
**flufenamic acid** USAN, INN, BAN *anti-inflammatory*
**flufenisal** USAN, INN *analgesic*
**flufosal** INN
**flufylline** INN
**flugestone** INN, BAN *progestin* [also: flurogestone acetate]
**flugestone acetate** [see: flurogestone acetate]
**fluindarol** INN
**fluindione** INN
**Flumadine** film-coated tablets, syrup ℞ *antiviral; prophylaxis and treatment for influenza A virus* [rimantadine HCl] 100 mg; 50 mg/5 mL
**flumazenil** USAN, INN, BAN *benzodiazepine antagonist/antidote*
**flumazepil** [see: flumazenil]
**flumecinol** INN *investigational (orphan) agent for neonatal hyperbilirubinemia*
**flumedroxone** INN, BAN
**flumequine** USAN, INN, BAN *antibacterial*
**flumeridone** USAN, INN, BAN *antiemetic*
**flumetasone** INN *corticosteroid; anti-inflammatory* [also: flumethasone]
**flumethasone** USAN, BAN *topical corticosteroidal anti-inflammatory* [also: flumetasone]
**flumethasone pivalate** USAN, USP, BAN *topical corticosteroidal anti-inflammatory*
**flumethiazide** INN, BAN
**flumethrin** BAN
**flumetramide** USAN, INN *skeletal muscle relaxant*
**flumexadol** INN
**flumezapine** USAN, INN, BAN *antipsychotic; neuroleptic*
**fluminorex** USAN, INN *anorectic*
**FluMist** prefilled single-use intranasal sprayers ℞ *flu vaccine* [influenza virus vaccine, live attenuated] 0.5 mL/dose
**flumizole** USAN, INN *anti-inflammatory*

**flumoxonide** USAN, INN *adrenocortical steroid*

**flunamine** INN

**flunarizine** INN, BAN *vasodilator* [also: flunarizine HCl]

**flunarizine HCl** USAN *vasodilator; investigational (orphan) for alternating hemiplegia* [also: flunarizine]

**flunidazole** USAN, INN *antiprotozoal*

**flunisolide** USAN, USP, INN, BAN *corticosteroidal anti-inflammatory for chronic asthma and rhinitis* 0.025% (25 μg/dose) nasal spray

**flunisolide acetate** USAN *anti-inflammatory*

**flunitrazepam** USAN, INN, BAN, JAN *benzodiazepine sedative and hypnotic; also abused as a "date rape" street drug*

**flunixin** USAN, INN, BAN *anti-inflammatory; analgesic*

**flunixin meglumine** USAN *anti-inflammatory; analgesic*

**flunoprost** INN

**flunoxaprofen** INN

**fluocinolide** [now: fluocinonide]

**fluocinolone** BAN *topical corticosteroidal anti-inflammatory* [also: fluocinolone acetonide]

**fluocinolone acetonide** USAN, USP, INN *topical corticosteroidal anti-inflammatory; investigational (orphan) for uveitis* [also: fluocinolone] 0.01%, 0.025% topical

**fluocinonide** USAN, USP, INN, BAN *topical corticosteroidal anti-inflammatory* 0.05% topical

**fluocortin** INN *anti-inflammatory* [also: fluocortin butyl]

**fluocortin butyl** USAN, BAN *anti-inflammatory* [also: fluocortin]

**fluocortolone** USAN, INN, BAN *corticosteroid; anti-inflammatory*

**fluocortolone caproate** USAN *corticosteroid; anti-inflammatory*

**Fluogen** IM injection, Steri-Vials, Steri-Dose (disposable syringes) (discontinued 2001) ℞ *flu vaccine* [influenza split-virus vaccine] 0.5 mL/dose

**Fluonex** cream ℞ *corticosteroidal anti-inflammatory* [fluocinonide] 0.05%

**Fluonid** topical solution ℞ *corticosteroidal anti-inflammatory* [fluocinolone acetonide] 0.01%

**fluopromazine** BAN *antipsychotic* [also: triflupromazine]

**Fluoracaine** eye drops ℞ *local anesthetic; corneal disclosing agent* [proparacaine HCl; fluorescein sodium] 0.5%•0.25%

**fluoracizine** [see: fluacizine]

**fluorescein** USP, BAN, JAN *ophthalmic diagnostic aid*

**fluorescein, soluble** [now: fluorescein sodium]

**fluorescein sodium** USP, BAN, JAN *ophthalmic diagnostic aid* 2% eye drops

**fluorescein sodium & proparacaine HCl** *corneal disclosing agent; topical ophthalmic anesthetic* 0.25%•0.5%

**Fluorescite** antecubital venous injection ℞ *ophthalmic diagnostic agent* [fluorescein sodium] 10%, 25%

**Fluoresoft** eye drops ℞ *diagnostic aid in fitting contact lenses* [fluorexon] 0.35%

**fluoresone** INN

**Fluorets** ophthalmic strips OTC *corneal disclosing agent* [fluorescein sodium] 1 mg

**fluorexon** *diagnosis and fitting aid for contact lenses*

**fluorhydrocortisone acetate** [see: fludrocortisone acetate]

**Fluoride** tablets OTC *dental caries preventative* [sodium fluoride] 2.21 mg

**Fluoride Loz** lozenges ℞ *topical dental caries preventative* [sodium fluoride] 2.21 mg

**Fluorigard** oral rinse OTC *topical dental caries preventative* [sodium fluoride; alcohol 6%] 0.05%

**Fluori-Methane** spray ℞ *topical vapocoolant anesthetic* [trichloromonofluoromethane; dichlorodifluoromethane] 85%•15%

**fluorine** *element (F)*

**fluorine F 18 fluorodeoxyglucose** [see: fludeoxyglucose F 18]

**Fluorinse** oral rinse ℞ *topical dental caries preventative* [sodium fluoride] 0.2%

**Fluor-I-Strip; Fluor-I-Strip A.T.** ophthalmic strips ℞ *corneal disclosing agent* [fluorescein sodium] 9 mg; 1 mg

**Fluoritab** chewable tablets, drops ℞ *dental caries preventative* [sodium fluoride] 1.1, 2.2 mg; 0.55 mg/drop

**fluormethylprednisolone** [see: dexamethasone]

**5-fluorocytosine (5-FC)** [see: flucytosine]

**fluorodeoxyglucose F 18** [see: fludeoxyglucose F 18]

**fluorodideoxyadenosine (F-ddA)** [see: lodenosine]

**fluorometholone** USP, INN, BAN *topical ophthalmic corticosteroidal anti-inflammatory* 0.1% eye drops

**fluorometholone acetate** USAN *topical ophthalmic corticosteroidal anti-inflammatory*

**fluoromethylene deoxycytidine (FMdC)** [now: tezacitabine]

**Fluor-Op** eye drop suspension ℞ *corticosteroidal anti-inflammatory* [fluorometholone] 0.1%

**Fluoroperm 32** ℞ *hydrophobic contact lens material* [paflufocon C]

**Fluoroperm 62** ℞ *hydrophobic contact lens material* [paflufocon B]

**Fluoroperm 92** ℞ *hydrophobic contact lens material* [paflufocon A]

**Fluoroperm 151** ℞ *hydrophobic contact lens material* [paflufocon D]

**Fluoroplex** cream, topical solution ℞ *antineoplastic for actinic keratoses and basal cell carcinomas* [fluorouracil] 1%

**fluoroquinolones** *a class of synthetic, broad-spectrum, antimicrobial, bactericidal antibiotics*

**fluorosalan** USAN *disinfectant* [also: flusalan]

**fluorouracil (5-FU)** USAN, USP, INN, BAN *antimetabolite antineoplastic for colorectal (orphan), esophageal (orphan), breast, stomach, and pancreatic cancers; topical antineoplastic for actinic keratoses and basal cell carcinoma; investigational (orphan) for glioblastoma multiforme* 50 mg/mL injection; 2%, 5% topical

**fluorouracil & cisplatin** *chemotherapy protocol for cervical cancer, used in conjunction with radiation therapy*

**fluorouracil & interferon alfa-2a** *investigational (orphan) for esophageal and advanced colorectal carcinoma*

**fluorouracil & leucovorin** *antineoplastic for metastatic colorectal cancer (orphan)*

**fluoruridine deoxyribose** [see: floxuridine]

**fluostigmine** [see: isoflurophate]

**Fluothane** liquid for vaporization ℞ *inhalation general anesthetic* [halothane]

**fluotracen** INN *antipsychotic; antidepressant* [also: fluotracen HCl]

**fluotracen HCl** USAN *antipsychotic; antidepressant* [also: fluotracen]

**fluoxetine** USAN, INN, BAN *selective serotonin reuptake inhibitor (SSRI) for depression, obsessive-compulsive disorder, bulimia nervosa, premenstrual dysphoric disorder, and panic disorder*

**fluoxetine HCl** USAN *selective serotonin reuptake inhibitor (SSRI) for major depression, obsessive-compulsive disorder, bulimia nervosa, premenstrual dysphoric disorder, and panic disorder; investigational (orphan) for autism* 10, 20, 40 mg oral; 20 mg/5 mL oral

**fluoximesterone** [see: fluoxymesterone]

**Flu-Oxinate** eye drops ℞ *topical ophthalmic anesthetic; corneal disclosing agent* [benoxinate HCl; fluorescein sodium] 0.4%•0.25%

**fluoxiprednisolone** [see: triamcinolone]

**fluoxymesterone** USP, INN, BAN *oral androgen for hypogonadism or testosterone deficiency in men, delayed puberty in boys, and metastatic breast cancer in women* 10 mg oral

**fluparoxan** INN, BAN *antidepressant* [also: fluparoxan HCl]

**fluparoxan HCl** USAN *antidepressant* [also: fluparoxan]

**flupenthixol** BAN *thioxanthene antipsychotic* [also: flupentixol]

**flupentixol** INN *thioxanthene antipsychotic* [also: flupenthixol]

**fluperamide** USAN, INN *antiperistaltic*

**fluperlapine** INN

**fluperolone** INN, BAN *corticosteroid; anti-inflammatory* [also: fluperolone acetate]

**fluperolone acetate** USAN *corticosteroid; anti-inflammatory* [also: fluperolone]

**fluphenazine** INN, BAN *phenothiazine antipsychotic* [also: fluphenazine enanthate]

**fluphenazine decanoate** *phenothiazine antipsychotic for prolonged parenteral neuroleptic therapy* 25 mg/mL injection

**fluphenazine enanthate** USP *phenothiazine antipsychotic for prolonged parenteral neuroleptic therapy* [also: fluphenazine]

**fluphenazine HCl** USP, BAN *phenothiazine antipsychotic* 1, 2.5, 5, 10 mg oral; 2.5 mg/5 mL oral; 2.5 mg/L injection

**flupimazine** INN

**flupirtine** INN, BAN *non-narcotic analgesic* [also: flupirtine maleate]

**flupirtine maleate** USAN *non-narcotic analgesic* [also: flupirtine]

**flupranone** INN

**fluprazine** INN

**fluprednidene** INN, BAN

**fluprednisolone** USAN, NF, INN, BAN *corticosteroid; anti-inflammatory*

**fluprednisolone valerate** USAN *corticosteroid; anti-inflammatory*

**fluprofen** INN, BAN

**fluprofylline** INN

**fluproquazone** USAN, INN, BAN *analgesic*

**fluprostenol** INN, BAN *prostaglandin* [also: fluprostenol sodium]

**fluprostenol sodium** USAN *prostaglandin* [also: fluprostenol]

**fluquazone** USAN, INN *anti-inflammatory*

**Flura** tablets ℞ *dental caries preventative* [sodium fluoride] 2.2 mg

**fluracil** [see: fluorouracil]

**fluradoline** INN *analgesic* [also: fluradoline HCl]

**fluradoline HCl** USAN *analgesic* [also: fluradoline]

**Flura-Drops** ℞ *dental caries preventative* [sodium fluoride] 0.55 mg/drop

**Flura-Loz** lozenges ℞ *topical dental caries preventative* [sodium fluoride] 2.2 mg

**flurandrenolide** USAN, USP *topical corticosteroid* [also: fludroxycortide; flurandrenolone] 0.05% topical

**flurandrenolone** BAN *topical corticosteroid* [also: flurandrenolide; fludroxycortide]

**flurantel** INN

**Flurate** eye drops ℞ *topical ophthalmic anesthetic; corneal disclosing agent* [benoxinate HCl; fluorescein sodium] 0.4%•0.25%

**flurazepam** INN, BAN *anticonvulsant; hypnotic; muscle relaxant; sedative; also abused as a street drug* [also: flurazepam HCl]

**flurazepam HCl** USAN, USP *anticonvulsant; hypnotic; muscle relaxant; sedative; also abused as a street drug* [also: flurazepam] 15, 30 mg oral

**flurbiprofen** USAN, USP, INN, BAN *antiarthritic; nonsteroidal anti-inflammatory drug (NSAID)* 50, 100 mg oral

**flurbiprofen sodium** USP *prostaglandin synthesis inhibitor; antimiotic; ophthalmic nonsteroidal anti-inflammatory drug (NSAID)* 0.03% eye drops

**Fluress** eye drops ℞ *topical ophthalmic anesthetic; corneal disclosing agent* [benoxinate HCl; fluorescein sodium] 0.4%•0.25%

**fluretofen** USAN, INN *anti-inflammatory; antithrombotic*

**flurfamide** [now: flurofamide]

**flurithromycin** INN

**flurocitabine** USAN, INN *antineoplastic*

**Fluro-Ethyl** aerosol spray ℞ *topical refrigerant anesthetic* [ethyl chloride; dichlorotetrafluoroethane] 25%•75%

**flurofamide** USAN, INN *urease enzyme inhibitor*

**flurogestone acetate** USAN *progestin* [also: flugestone]

**Flurosyn** ointment, cream ℞ *topical corticosteroidal anti-inflammatory* [fluocinolone acetonide] 0.025%; 0.01, 0.025%

**flurothyl** USAN, USP, BAN *CNS stimulant* [also: flurotyl]

**flurotyl** INN *CNS stimulant* [also: flurothyl]

**fluroxene** USAN, NF, INN *inhalation anesthetic*

**fluroxyspiramine** [see: spiramide]

**flusalan** INN *disinfectant* [also: fluorosalan]

**FluShield** IM injection, Tubex (cartridge-needle unit) (discontinued 2002) ℞ *flu vaccine* [influenza purified split-virus vaccine] 0.5 mL/dose

**flusoxolol** INN

**fluspiperone** USAN, INN *antipsychotic*

**fluspirilene** USAN, INN, BAN *diphenylbutylpiperidine antipsychotic*

**flutamide** USAN, INN, BAN *antiandrogen antineoplastic for prostatic carcinoma* 125 mg oral

**flutazolam** INN

**flutemazepam** INN

**Flutex** ointment, cream ℞ *topical corticosteroidal anti-inflammatory* [triamcinolone acetonide] 0.025%, 0.1%, 0.5%

**flutiazin** USAN, INN *veterinary anti-inflammatory*

**fluticasone** INN, BAN *corticosteroidal anti-inflammatory for chronic asthma or rhinitis* [also: fluticasone propionate]

**fluticasone propionate** USAN *corticosteroidal anti-inflammatory for chronic asthma or rhinitis; topical treatment for dermatoses* [also: fluticasone] 0.005%, 0.05% topical

**flutizenol** INN

**flutomidate** INN

**flutonidine** INN

**flutoprazepam** INN

**flutrimazole** INN

**flutroline** USAN, INN *antipsychotic*

**flutropium bromide** INN

**fluvastatin** INN, BAN *HMG-CoA reductase inhibitor for hypercholesterolemia and atherosclerosis* [also: fluvastatin sodium]

**fluvastatin sodium** USAN *HMG-CoA reductase inhibitor for hypercholesterolemia, hypertriglyceridemia, and atherosclerosis* [also: fluvastatin]

**Fluvirin** IM injection, prefilled syringes ℞ *flu vaccine* [influenza split-virus vaccine] 0.5 mL/dose

**fluvoxamine** INN, BAN *selective serotonin reuptake inhibitor (SSRI) for obsessive-compulsive disorder* [also: fluvoxamine maleate]

**fluvoxamine maleate** USAN *selective serotonin reuptake inhibitor (SSRI) for obsessive-compulsive disorder; investigational (Phase III) for depression and panic disorder* [also: fluvoxamine] 25, 50, 100 mg oral

**flux root** *medicinal herb* [see: pleurisy root]

**fluzinamide** USAN, INN *anticonvulsant*

**Fluzone** IM injection, prefilled syringes ℞ *flu vaccine* [influenza split-virus vaccine] 0.5 mL/dose

**Fluzone Preservative-Free: Pediatric Dose** prefilled syringes for IM injection ℞ *flu vaccine* [influenza split-virus or whole-virus vaccine] 0.25 mL/dose

**fluzoperine** INN

**flytrap** *medicinal herb* [see: dogbane]

**FMdC (fluoromethylene deoxycytidine)** [now: tezacitabine]

**FML; FML Forte** eye drop suspension ℞ *ophthalmic corticosteroidal anti-inflammatory* [fluorometholone] 0.1%; 0.25%

**FML S.O.P.** ophthalmic ointment ℞ *topical ophthalmic corticosteroidal anti-inflammatory* [fluorometholone] 0.1%

**FML-S** eye drop suspension ℞ *corticosteroidal anti-inflammatory; antibiotic* [fluorometholone; sulfacetamide sodium] 0.1%•10%

**FMS (fluorouracil, mitomycin, streptozocin)** *chemotherapy protocol*

**FMV (fluorouracil, MeCCNU, vincristine)** *chemotherapy protocol*

**FNC (fluorouracil, Novantrone, cyclophosphamide)** *chemotherapy protocol for breast cancer* [also: CFN; CNF]

**FNM (fluorouracil, Novantrone, methotrexate)** *chemotherapy protocol*

**foal's foot** *medicinal herb* [see: coltsfoot]

**FOAM (fluorouracil, Oncovin, Adriamycin, mitomycin)** *chemotherapy protocol*

**Foamicon** chewable tablets OTC *antacid* [aluminum hydroxide; magnesium trisilicate] 80•20 mg

**Focalin** tablets R *CNS stimulant for attention-deficit hyperactivity disorder (ADHD)* [dexmethylphenidate HCl] 2.5, 5, 10 mg

**focofilcon A** USAN *hydrophilic contact lens material*

**fodipir** USAN *excipient*

*Foeniculum officinale; F. vulgare medicinal herb* [see: fennel]

**Foille** spray OTC *local anesthetic; antiseptic* [benzocaine; chloroxylenol] 5%•0.63%

**Foille Medicated First Aid** ointment, aerosol spray OTC *local anesthetic; antiseptic* [benzocaine; chloroxylenol] 5%•0.1%; 5%•0.6%

**Foille Plus** aerosol spray OTC *local anesthetic; antiseptic* [benzocaine; chloroxylenol; alcohol 57.33%] 5%•0.6%

**folacin** [see: folic acid] ⑨ Fulvicin

**folate** [see: folic acid]

**folate sodium** USP

**Folergot-DF** tablets R *GI anticholinergic; sedative; analgesic* [belladonna alkaloids; phenobarbital; ergotamine tartrate] 0.2•40•0.6 mg

**folescutol** INN

**Folgard** tablets OTC *vitamin B supplement* [vitamins $B_6$ and $B_{12}$; folic acid] 10•0.115•0.8 mg

**Folgard RX 2.2** film-coated tablets R *vitamin B supplement* [vitamins $B_6$ and $B_{12}$; folic acid] 25•0.5•2.3 mg

**folic acid** USP, INN, BAN *vitamin $B_c$; vitamin M; hematopoietic; birth defect preventative* 0.4, 0.8, 1 mg oral; 5 mg/mL injection

**folinate-SF calcium** [see: leucovorin calcium]

**folinic acid** [see: leucovorin calcium]

**follicle-stimulating hormone (FSH)** BAN [also: menotropins]

**follidrin** [see: estradiol benzoate]

**Follistim** powder for subcu or IM injection R *recombinant follicle-stimulating hormone (FSH) for the induction of ovulation in women and spermatogenesis in men* [follitropin beta] 75 IU

**follitropin alfa** INN *recombinant follicle-stimulating hormone (FSH) for the induction of ovulation or spermatogenesis (orphan); adjunct to assisted reproductive technology (ART)*

**follitropin beta** INN *recombinant follicle-stimulating hormone (FSH) for the induction of ovulation in women and spermatogenesis in men*

**follotropin** [see: menotropins]

**Follow-Up** [see: Carnation Follow-Up]

**Folpace** tablets R *vitamin/magnesium supplement* [vitamins $B_6$ and $B_{12}$; folic acid; vitamin E; magnesium] 25 mg•425 μg•2.05 mg•100 IU•100 mg

**Foltrin** capsules R *hematinic* [ferrous fumarate; cyanocobalamin; ascorbic acid; intrinsic factor concentrate; folic acid] 110 mg•15 μg•75 mg•240 mg•0.5 mg

**Foltx** tablets R *vitamin B therapy for arteriosclerosis, cardiovascular and peripheral vascular disease, and neurological disorders* [vitamins $B_6$ and $B_{12}$; folic acid] 25•2•2.5 mg

**Folvite** IM injection R *hematinic* [folic acid] 5 mg/mL

**fomepizole** USAN, INN *antidote; alcohol dehydrogenase inhibitor for methanol or ethylene glycol poisoning (orphan)*

**FOMI; FOMi (fluorouracil, Oncovin, mitomycin)** *chemotherapy protocol*

**fomidacillin** INN, BAN

**fominoben** INN [also: fominoben HCl]

**fominoben HCl** JAN [also: fominoben]

**fomivirsen sodium** *antisense drug for AIDS-related CMV retinitis*

**fomocaine** INN, BAN

**fonatol** [see: diethylstilbestrol]

**fonazine mesylate** USAN *serotonin inhibitor* [also: dimetotiazine; dimethothiazine]

**fondaparinux sodium** *selective factor Xa inhibitor; antithrombotic for preven-*

tion of deep vein thrombosis (DVT) and acute pulmonary embolism following orthopedic surgery

**fontarsol** [see: dichlorophenarsine HCl]

**fopirtoline** INN

**Foradil** encapsulated powder for inhalation (used with an Aerolizer device) ℞ β₂ agonist; twice-daily bronchodilator for asthma, COPD, and emphysema [formoterol fumarate] 12 μg/dose

**Forane** liquid for vaporization ℞ inhalation general anesthetic [isoflurane]

**forasartan** USAN antihypertensive; CHF treatment; angiotensin II receptor antagonist

**Forcaltonin** nasal spray ℞ investigational (Phase III) agent for osteoporosis

**foreign colombo** medicinal herb [see: colombo]

**forfenimex** INN

**formaldehyde solution** USP disinfectant; anhidrotic

**Formalyde-10** spray ℞ for hyperhidrosis and bromhidrosis [formaldehyde] 10%

**formebolone** INN, BAN

**formetamide** [see: formetorex]

**formetorex** INN

**formidacillin** [see: fomidacillin]

**forminitrazole** INN, BAN

**formocortal** USAN, INN, BAN corticosteroid; anti-inflammatory

**formoterol** INN bronchodilator [also: eformoterol; formoterol fumarate]

**formoterol fumarate** USAN, JAN bronchodilator for asthma [also: formoterol; eformoterol fumarate]

**Formula 44 Cough Control Disks; Formula 44 Cough Silencers** lozenges (discontinued 2002) OTC antitussive; topical oral anesthetic [dextromethorphan hydrobromide; benzocaine] 5•1.25 mg; 2.5•1 mg

**Formula 405** cleansing bar OTC therapeutic skin cleanser

**Formula B** tablets ℞ vitamin supplement [multiple B vitamins; vitamin C; folic acid] ±•500•0.5 mg

**Formula B Plus** tablets ℞ vitamin/mineral/iron supplement [multiple vitamins

& minerals; ferrous fumarate; folic acid; biotin] ±•27•0.8•0.15 mg

**Formula EM** oral solution OTC antiemetic for nausea associated with influenza, morning sickness, motion sickness, inhalation anesthesia, or food and drink indiscretions [phosphorated carbohydrate solution (fructose; dextrose; phosphoric acid)] 1.87 g•1.87 g•21.5 mg per 5 mL

**Formula VM-2000** tablets OTC dietary supplement [multiple vitamins & minerals; multiple amino acids; iron; folic acid; biotin] ±•5 mg•0.2 mg•50 μg

**Formulation R** anorectal cream, anorectal ointment OTC temporary relief of hemorrhoidal symptoms [phenylephrine HCl] 0.25%

**4′-formylacetanilide thiosemicarbazone** [see: thioacetazone; thiacetazone]

**foropafant** INN

**forskolin** [see: colforsin]

**Forta Drink** powder OTC enteral nutritional therapy [lactose-free formula]

**Forta Shake** powder OTC enteral nutritional therapy [milk-based formula]

**Fortamet** extended-release film-coated tablets ℞ once-daily treatment for diabetes [metformin HCl] 500, 1000 mg

**Fortaz** powder or frozen premix for IV or IM injection ℞ cephalosporin antibiotic [ceftazidime] 0.5, 1, 2, 6 g

**Fortel Midstream** test stick for professional use in vitro diagnostic aid; urine pregnancy test

**Fortel Plus** test kit for home use in vitro diagnostic aid; urine pregnancy test

**Fortéo** subcu injection via prefilled self-injector ℞ parathyroid hormone for postmenopausal osteoporosis in women and primary or hypogonadal osteoporosis in men [teriparatide] 20 μg/day (750 μg/3 mL injector)

**Fortical** nasal delivery ℞ investigational (NDA filed) calcium regulator for hypercalcemia, Paget disease, and postmenopausal osteoporosis [calcitonin (salmon), recombinant]

**fortimicin A** [now: astromicin sulfate]

**Fortovase** capsules ℞ *antiretroviral protease inhibitor for HIV* [saquinavir] 200 mg

**40 winks** capsules OTC *antihistaminic sleep aid* [diphenhydramine HCl] 50 mg

**Forvade** gel ℞ *investigational (Phase I/II) nucleoside antiviral for AIDS-related genital herpes* [cidofovir]

**Forzest** (Indian name for U.S. product Cialis)

**Fosamax** tablets, oral solution ℞ *bisphosphonate bone resorption inhibitor for Paget disease and corticosteroid-induced or age-related osteoporosis in men and women; investigational (orphan) for bone manifestations of Gaucher disease and pediatric osteogenesis imperfecta* [alendronate sodium] 5, 10, 35, 40, 70 mg; 70 mg/75 mL bottle

**fosamprenavir calcium** USAN *antiretroviral; HIV-1 protease inhibitor; amprenavir prodrug*

**fosamprenavir sodium** USAN *antiviral; HIV protease inhibitor*

**fosarilate** USAN, INN *antiviral*

**fosazepam** USAN, INN, BAN *hypnotic*

**Foscan** ℞ *investigational (NDA filed) photodynamic therapy for head and neck cancer* [temoporfin]

**foscarnet sodium** USAN, INN, BAN *antiviral for cytomegalovirus (CMV) and various herpes viruses (HSV-1, HSV-2)*

**Foscavir** IV injection ℞ *antiviral for cytomegalovirus (CMV) retinitis and herpes simplex virus (HSV) infections in immunocompromised patients* [foscarnet sodium] 24 mg/mL

**foscolic acid** INN

**fosenazide** INN

**fosenopril sodium** [see: fosinopril sodium]

**fosfestrol** INN, BAN *antineoplastic; estrogen* [also: diethylstilbestrol diphosphate]

**fosfocreatinine** INN

**fosfomycin** USAN, INN, BAN *antibacterial* [also: fosfomycin calcium; fosfomycin sodium]

**fosfomycin calcium** JAN *antibacterial* [also: fosfomycin; fosfomycin sodium]

**fosfomycin sodium** JAN *antibacterial* [also: fosfomycin; fosfomycin calcium]

**fosfomycin tromethamine** USAN *broad-spectrum bactericidal antibiotic for urinary tract infections*

**fosfonet sodium** USAN, INN *antiviral*

**fosfosal** INN

**Fosfree** tablets OTC *vitamin/iron supplement* [multiple vitamins; iron] ≚ •29 mg

**fosfructose trisodium** USAN *investigational (Phase III) cardioprotective agent used in coronary artery bypass graft surgery; investigational (Phase II) for pain during sickle cell crisis*

**fosinopril** INN, BAN *antihypertensive; angiotensin-converting enzyme (ACE) inhibitor* [also: fosinopril sodium]

**fosinopril sodium** USAN *antihypertensive; angiotensin-converting enzyme (ACE) inhibitor; adjunctive treatment for CHF* [also: fosinopril] 10, 20, 40 mg oral

**fosinoprilat** USAN, INN *antihypertensive*

**fosmenic acid** INN

**fosmidomycin** INN

**fosphenytoin** INN *hydantoin anticonvulsant* [also: fosphenytoin sodium]

**fosphenytoin sodium** USAN *hydantoin anticonvulsant for grand mal status epilepticus (orphan)* [also: fosphenytoin]

**fospirate** USAN, INN *veterinary anthelmintic*

**fosquidone** USAN, INN, BAN *antineoplastic*

**fostedil** USAN, INN *vasodilator; calcium channel blocker*

**Fostex** cleansing bar (discontinued 2003) OTC *keratolytic for acne* [benzoyl peroxide] 10% ⌨ pHisoHex

**Fostex 10% BPO** gel (discontinued 2003) OTC *keratolytic for acne* [benzoyl peroxide] 10%

**Fostex 10% Wash** topical liquid (discontinued 2003) OTC *keratolytic for acne* [benzoyl peroxide] 10%

**Fostex Acne Cleansing** cream OTC *keratolytic for acne* [salicylic acid] 2%

**Fostex Acne Medication Cleansing**
bar OTC *medicated cleanser for acne*
[salicylic acid] 2%

**Fostex Medicated Cleansing Shampoo** OTC *antiseborrheic; keratolytic*
[sulfur; salicylic acid] 2%•2%

**fostriecin** INN *antineoplastic* [also: fostriecin sodium]

**fostriecin sodium** USAN *antineoplastic*
[also: fostriecin]

**Fostril** lotion OTC *acne treatment* [sulfur; zinc oxide]

**fosveset** USAN *ligant excipient*

**fotemustine** INN, BAN

**fo-ti; ho-shou-wu** *(Polygonum multiflorum)* root *medicinal herb for atherosclerosis, blood cleansing, constipation, improving liver and kidney function, insomnia, malaria, muscle aches, TB, and weak bones; also used to increase fertility, prevent aging, and promote longevity*

**Fototar** cream OTC *antipsoriatic; antiseborrheic* [coal tar] 2%

**fotretamine** INN

**Fouchet reagent (solution)**

**4 Hair** softgel capsules OTC *vitamin/mineral/iron supplement* [multiple vitamins & minerals; iron; folic acid; biotin] ±•2.5•33.3•0.25 mg

**4 Nails** softgel capsules OTC *vitamin/mineral/calcium/iron supplement* [multiple vitamins & minerals; calcium; iron; folic acid; biotin] ±•167•3•0.333•0.0083 mg

**4-Way Fast Acting** nasal spray OTC *nasal decongestant* [phenylephrine HCl] 1%

**4-Way Long Lasting** nasal spray (discontinued 2002) OTC *nasal decongestant* [oxymetazoline HCl] 0.05%

**40DS02** *investigational (orphan) for chronic iron overload due to transfusional treatments*

**4B5 antibody** *investigational (Phase I) fully human monoclonal antibody for immunotherapy in melanoma patients*

**Fourneau 309** (available only from the Centers for Disease Control) ℞

*antiparasitic for African trypanosomiasis and onchocerciasis* [suramin sodium]

**foxglove** *(Digitalis ambigua; D. ferriginea; D. grandiflora; D. lanata; D. lutea; D. purpurea)* leaves *medicinal herb for asthma, burns, congestive heart failure, edema, promoting wound healing, and sedation; not generally regarded as safe and effective for children as ingestion can be fatal*

**foxglove, American; false foxglove; fern-leaved foxglove** *medicinal herb*
[see: feverweed]

**foxtail** *medicinal herb* [see: club moss]

**frabuprofen** INN

**Fractar** (trademarked ingredient) OTC *antipsoriatic; antiseborrheic* [crude coal tar]

*Fragaria vesca* *medicinal herb* [see: strawberry]

**Fragmin** deep subcu injection, prefilled syringes ℞ *anticoagulant/antithrombotic for prevention of deep vein thrombosis (DVT) after abdominal or hip replacement surgery, unstable angina, and myocardial infarction* [dalteparin sodium] 10 000, 25 000 IU (64, 160 mg)/mL; 2500, 5000 IU (16, 32 mg)/0.2 mL, 7500 IU (48 mg)/0.3 mL, 10 000 IU (64 mg)/mL

**framycetin** INN, BAN *anti-infective wound dressing*

**francium** *element (Fr)*

*Frangula purshiana* *medicinal herb*
[see: cascara sagrada]

**frankincense** *(Boswellia serrata)* leaves and bark *medicinal herb for anaphylaxis, arthritis, asthma, blood cleansing, bronchial disorders, dysentery, rheumatism, skin ailments, ulcers, and wound healing*

**fraxinella** *(Dictamnus albus)* root, plant, and seed *medicinal herb used as an anthelmintic, diuretic, emmenagogue, expectorant, and febrifuge*

**Fraxiparine** Ⓒᴬᴺ subcu injection, prefilled syringes ℞ *anticoagulant/antithrombotic for prevention of deep vein thrombosis (DVT) after surgery, clotting during hemodialysis, unstable*

*angina, and myocardial infarction*
[nadroparin calcium] 9500 IU/mL;
0.2, 0.3, 0.4, 0.6, 0.8, 1 mL

**Fraxiparine Forte** ⓒᴬᴺ subcu injection,
prefilled syringes ℞ *anticoagulant/
antithrombotic for prevention of deep
vein thrombosis (DVT) after surgery,
clotting during hemodialysis, unstable
angina, and myocardial infarction*
[nadroparin calcium] 19 000 IU/mL;
0.6, 0.8, 1 mL

**FreAmine III 3% (8.5%) with Elec-
trolytes** IV infusion ℞ *total parenteral nutrition (8.5% only); peripheral
parenteral nutrition (both)* [multiple
essential and nonessential amino
acids; electrolytes]

**FreAmine III 8.5%; FreAmine III
10%** IV infusion ℞ *total parenteral
nutrition; peripheral parenteral nutrition* [multiple essential and nonessential amino acids]

**FreAmine HBC 6.9%** IV infusion ℞
*nutritional therapy for high metabolic
stress* [multiple branched-chain
essential and nonessential amino
acids; electrolytes]

**Free & Clear** shampoo OTC *soap-free
therapeutic cleanser*

**Freedavite** tablets OTC *vitamin/mineral/
iron supplement* [multiple vitamins &
minerals; ferrous fumarate6400.2] ≐
•10 mg

**Freedox** solution ℞ *investigational
(NDA filed) lazaroid for subarachnoid
hemorrhage (SAH), ischemic stroke,
spinal cord and head injury* [tirilazad
mesylate]

**Freezone** topical liquid OTC *keratolytic*
[salicylic acid in a collodion-like
vehicle] 13.6%

**frentizole** USAN, INN, BAN *immunoregulator*

**fringe tree** (*Chionanthus virginica*)
bark *medicinal herb used as an aperient, diuretic, febrifuge, and tonic*

**Frisium** (available in Canada as Alti-
Clobazam) ℞ *investigational benzodiazepine tranquilizer; anxiolytic* [clobazam]

**fronepidil** INN

**frost plant; frost weed; frostwort**
*medicinal herb* [see: rock rose]

**Frova** film-coated tablets ℞ *vascular
serotonin 5-HT$_{1B/1D}$ receptor agonist
for the acute treatment of migraine*
[frovatriptan succinate] 2.5 mg

**frovatriptan succinate** USAN *vascular
serotonin 5-HT$_{1B/1D}$ receptor agonist
for the acute treatment of migraine*

**froxiprost** INN

**β-fructofuranosidase** [see: sacrosidase]

**fructose (D-fructose)** USP *nutrient;
caloric replacement* [also: levulose]

**fructose-1,6-diphosphate (FDP)**
*investigational (Phase III) adjunct to
coronary artery bypass graft (CABG)
surgery; investigational (Phase III,
orphan) cytoprotective agent for vaso-
occlusive episodes of sickle cell disease*

**Fruit C 100; Fruit C 200; Fruit C
500** chewable tablets OTC *vitamin C
supplement* [ascorbic acid and calcium
ascorbate] 100 mg; 200 mg; 500 mg

**Fruity Chews** chewable tablets OTC
*vitamin supplement* [multiple vitamins; folic acid] ≐•0.3 mg

**Fruity Chews with Iron** chewable
tablets OTC *vitamin/iron supplement*
[multiple vitamins; iron; folic acid]
≐•12•0.3 mg

**frusemide** BAN *antihypertensive; loop
diuretic* [also: furosemide]

**FS Shampoo** (name changed to Capex
in 2003)

**FSF (fibrin-stabilizing factor)** [see:
factor XIII]

**FSH (follicle-stimulating hormone)**
[see: menotropins]

**ftalofyne** INN *veterinary anthelmintic*
[also: phthalofyne]

**ftaxilide** INN

**FTC** [see: emtricitabine]

**ftivazide** INN

**ftormetazine** INN

**ftorpropazine** INN

**FTY-720** *investigational (Phase II)
immunosuppressant for transplant
rejection and autoimmune disease*

**5-FU (5-fluorouracil)** [see: fluorouracil]

**fubrogonium iodide** INN

**fuchsin, basic** USP *topical antibacterial/ antifungal*

**Fucidin** ⓒⒶⓃ *cream, ointment* ℞ *topical antibiotic* [fusidic acid] 2%

**Fucidin H** ⓒⒶⓃ *cream* OTC *topical antibiotic and corticosteroidal anti-inflammatory* [fusidic acid; hydrocortisone] 2• 1 mg/g

*Fucus versiculosus medicinal herb* [see: kelp]

**FUDR** *powder for intra-arterial infusion* ℞ *antimetabolic antineoplastic for GI adenocarcinoma metastatic to the liver* [floxuridine] 500 mg

**FUDR; FUdR (5-fluorouracil deoxyribonucleoside)** [see: floxuridine]

**fuge, devil's** *medicinal herb* [see: mistletoe]

**Ful-Glo** *ophthalmic strips* ℞ *corneal disclosing agent* [fluorescein sodium] 0.6 mg

**Full Spectrum B** *tablets* OTC *vitamin supplement* [multiple B vitamins]

**fulmicoton** [see: pyroxylin]

**FU/LV (fluorouracil, leucovorin calcium [rescue])** *chemotherapy protocol for colorectal cancer* [also: F-CL]

**FU/LV/CPT-11 (fluorouracil, leucovorin calcium [rescue], CPT-11)** *chemotherapy protocol for metastatic colorectal cancer*

**fulvestrant** USAN *steroidal selective estrogen receptor down-regulator; antineoplastic for metastatic breast cancer in postmenopausal women*

**Fulvicin P/G** *tablets* (discontinued 2003) ℞ *systemic antifungal* [griseofulvin (ultramicrosize)] 125, 165, 250, 330 mg ☑ folacin; Furacin

**Fulvicin U/F** *tablets* (discontinued 2003) ℞ *systemic antifungal* [griseofulvin (microsize)] 250, 500 mg

**FUM (fluorouracil, methotrexate)** *chemotherapy protocol*

**fumagillin** INN, BAN

*Fumaria officinalis medicinal herb* [see: fumitory]

**fumaric acid** NF *acidifier*

**Fumatinic** *sustained-release capsules* ℞ *hematinic* [ferrous fumarate; cyanocobalamin; ascorbic acid] 200 mg (66 mg Fe)•5 μg•60 mg

**fumitory (*Fumaria officinalis*)** *plant medicinal herb for cardiovascular disorders, constipation, eczema, edema, and hepatobiliary disorders*

**fumoxicillin** USAN, INN *antibacterial*

**Funduscein-10; Funduscein-25** *antecubital venous injection* ℞ *ophthalmic diagnostic agent* [fluorescein sodium] 10%; 25%

**fungicidin** [see: nystatin]

**fungimycin** USAN *antifungal*

**Fungi-Nail** *topical liquid* OTC *antifungal; keratolytic; anesthetic* [resorcinol; salicylic acid; chloroxylenol; benzocaine; alcohol 50%] 1%•2%•2%•0.5%

**Fungizone** *cream, lotion* (discontinued 2003) ℞ *polyene antifungal* [amphotericin B] 3%

**Fungizone** *ointment* (discontinued 2001) ℞ *polyene antifungal* [amphotericin B] 3%

**Fungizone** *oral suspension* (discontinued 2004) ℞ *systemic polyene antifungal; "swish and swallow" treatment for oral candidiasis* [amphotericin B] 100 mg/mL

**Fungizone** *powder for IV infusion* ℞ *systemic polyene antifungal* [amphotericin B deoxycholate] 50 mg/vial

**Fung-O** *topical liquid* OTC *keratolytic* [salicylic acid] 17%

**Fungoid** *cream* (discontinued 2000) ℞ *antifungal* [clotrimazole] 1%

**Fungoid** *solution* (discontinued 2000) ℞ *antifungal* [clotrimazole] 1%

**Fungoid** *tincture* OTC *antifungal* [miconazole nitrate] 2%

**Fungoid AF** *topical solution* (discontinued 2000) OTC *antifungal* [undecylenic acid] 25%

**Fungoid-HC** *cream* ℞ *corticosteroidal anti-inflammatory; antipruritic; antifungal; antibacterial* [miconazole nitrate; hydrocortisone] 2%•1%

**FUP (fluorouracil, Platinol)** *chemotherapy protocol for gastric cancer*

**fuprazole** INN

**furacilin** [see: nitrofurazone]

**Furacin** topical solution, cream ℞ broad-spectrum antibacterial; adjunct to burn therapy and skin grafting [nitrofurazone] 0.2% ⧉ Fulvicin

**Furacin Soluble Dressing** ointment ℞ broad-spectrum antibacterial; adjunct to burn therapy and skin grafting [nitrofurazone] 0.2%

**furacrinic acid** INN, BAN

**Furadantin** oral suspension ℞ urinary antibiotic [nitrofurantoin] 25 mg/5 mL

**furafylline** INN

**Furalan** tablets ℞ urinary antibiotic [nitrofurantoin] 50, 100 mg

**furalazine** INN

**furaltadone** INN, BAN

**Furamide** (available only from the Centers for Disease Control) ℞ investigational anti-infective for amebiasis [diloxanide furoate]

**2(3H) furanone di-hydro (FDh)** a precursor to gamma hydroxybutyrate (GHB); a formerly legal alternative to GHB, now also illegal (Schedule I); also known as gamma butyrolactone (GBL) [see: gamma hydroxybutyrate (GHB)]

**furaprofen** USAN, INN anti-inflammatory

**furazabol** INN

**furazolidone** USP, INN, BAN bactericidal; antiprotozoal (Trichomonas); antidiarrheal

**furazolium chloride** USAN, INN antibacterial

**furazolium tartrate** USAN antibacterial

**furbucillin** INN

**furcloprofen** INN

**furegrelate** INN thromboxane synthetase inhibitor [also: furegrelate sodium]

**furegrelate sodium** USAN thromboxane synthetase inhibitor [also: furegrelate]

**furethidine** INN, BAN

**furfenorex** INN

**furfuryltrimethylammonium iodide** [see: furtrethonium iodide]

**furidarone** INN

**furmethoxadone** INN

**furobufen** USAN, INN anti-inflammatory

**furodazole** USAN, INN anthelmintic

**furofenac** INN

**furomazine** INN

**furomine** USAN ligand

**furosemide** USAN, USP, INN, JAN antihypertensive; loop diuretic [also: frusemide] 20, 40, 80 mg oral; 10 mg/mL oral; 40 mg/5 mL oral; 10 mg/mL injection

**furostilbestrol** INN

**furoxicillin** [see: fumoxicillin]

**Furoxone** tablets, oral liquid ℞ antibacterial [furazolidone] 100 mg; 50 mg/15 mL

**fursalan** USAN, INN disinfectant

**fursultiamine** INN

**furterene** INN

**furtrethonium iodide** INN

**furtrimethonium iodide** [see: furtrethonium iodide]

**fusafungine** INN, BAN

**fusidate sodium** USAN antibacterial

**fusidic acid** USAN, INN, BAN topical antibacterial

**fusidic acid, sodium salt** [see: fusidate sodium]

**FUVAC (5-FU, vinblastine, Adriamycin, cyclophosphamide)** chemotherapy protocol

**Fuzeon** powder for subcu injection ℞ fusion inhibitor for HIV infection [enfuvirtide] 90 mg/mL (108 mg/dose)

**fuzlocillin** INN, BAN

**fytic acid** INN

**FZ (flutamide, Zoladex)** chemotherapy protocol for prostate cancer

**G17DT immunogen** *investigational (orphan) agent for gastric cancer and adenocarcinoma of the pancreas*

**G-3139** *investigational (Phase III) adjunct used with docetaxel for malignant melanoma, breast cancer, and other malignancies; investigational (Phase I/II) for AIDS-related non-Hodgkin lymphoma*

**$^{67}$Ga** *[see: gallium citrate Ga 67]*

**GABA (gamma-aminobutyric acid)** *[see: γ-aminobutyric acid]*

**gabapentin** USAN, INN *anticonvulsant; treatment for postherpetic neuralgia; investigational (orphan) for amyotrophic lateral sclerosis* 100, 300, 400 mg oral

**Gabbromicina** *investigational (orphan) agent for tuberculosis and Mycobacterium avium complex (MAC) [aminosidine]*

**gabexate** INN

**Gabitril** Filmtabs (film-coated tablets) ℞ *anticonvulsant adjunct for partial seizures* [tiagabine HCl] 2, 4, 12, 16, 20 mg ⬚ Carbatrol

**gaboxadol** INN

**gadobenate dimeglumine** USAN *MRI diagnostic aid* [also: gadobenic acid]

**gadobenic acid** INN *MRI diagnostic aid* [also: gadobenate dimeglumine]

**gadobutrol** INN *investigational aid for MRI*

**gadodiamide** USAN, INN, BAN *parenteral MRI contrast medium*

**gadolinium** *element (Gd)*

**gadolinium texaphyrin (Gd-Tex)** *[now: motexafin gadolinium]*

**gadolinium-diethylenetriamine pentaacetic acid (Gd-DTPA)** *investigational MRI contrast media for cardiac imaging*

**gadopenamide** INN

**gadopentetate dimeglumine** USAN *parenteral MRI contrast medium* [also: gadopentetic acid]

**gadopentetic acid** INN, BAN *parenteral MRI contrast medium* [also: gadopentetate dimeglumine]

**gadoteric acid** INN

**gad**⬚
⬚

**gad**⬚
te⬚
*of the brain, head, and spine and liver structure and vascularity*

**gadoxanum** USAN *gadolinium-xanthan gum complex; diagnostic aid*

**gadozelite** USAN *gadolinium zeolite complex; diagnostic aid*

**GA-EPO (gene-activated erythropoietin)** *[see: erythropoietin, gene-activated]*

**gaiactamine** *[see: guaiactamine]*

**gaietamine** *[see: guaiactamine]*

**galactagogues** *a class of agents that promote or increase the flow of breast milk [also called: lactagogues]*

**galactochitosan** *investigational immune system stimulant and anticancer therapy*

**α-D-galactopyranose** *[see: galactose]*

**galactose** *ultrasound contrast medium*

**α-galactosidase** *[see: agalsidase alfa]*

**galamustine** INN

**galangal (Alpinia galanga; A. officinarum)** *rhizomes medicinal herb for diuresis, fungal infections, gas, hypertension, tumors, ulcers, and worms; also used as an antiplatelet agent*

**galantamine** USAN, INN *acetylcholinesterase inhibitor to increase cognition in Alzheimer disease*

**galantamine hydrobromide** USAN *acetylcholinesterase inhibitor to increase cognition in Alzheimer disease*

**galanthamine** *[see: galantamine]*

**Galardin** ℞ *investigational (orphan) matrix metalloproteinase (MMP) inhibitor for corneal ulcers [ilomastat]*

**galdansetron** INN, BAN *antiemetic [also: galdansetron HCl]*

**galdansetron HCl** USAN *antiemetic [also: galdansetron]*

**Galeopsis tetrahit** *medicinal herb [see: hemp nettle]*

**Galium aparine; G. verum** *medicinal herb [see: bedstraw]*

*Galium odoratum* medicinal herb [see: sweet woodruff]

**gallamine** BAN neuromuscular blocker [also: gallamine triethiodide]

**gallamine triethiodide** USP, INN neuromuscular blocker; muscle relaxant [also: gallamine]

**gallamone triethiodide** [see: gallamine triethiodide]

**gallic acid** NF

**gallic acid, bismuth basic salt** [see: bismuth subgallate]

**gallium** element (Ga)

**gallium ($^{67}$Ga) citrate** INN radiopaque contrast medium; radioactive agent [also: gallium citrate Ga 67]

**gallium citrate Ga 67** USAN, USP radiopaque contrast medium; radioactive agent [also: gallium ($^{67}$Ga) citrate]

**gallium nitrate** USAN bone resorption inhibitor for hypercalcemia of malignancy (orphan); investigational (Phase II) agent for AIDS-related non-Hodgkin lymphoma

**gallium nitrate nonahydrate** [see: gallium nitrate]

**gallopamil** INN, BAN

**gallotannic acid** [see: tannic acid]

**gallstone solubilizing agents** a class of drugs that dissolve gallstones

**galosemide** INN

**galtifenin** INN

**Galzin** capsules ℞ copper blocking/complexing agent for Wilson disease (orphan) [zinc acetate] 25, 50 mg

**gamfexine** USAN, INN antidepressant

**Gamimune N** IV infusion ℞ passive immunizing agent for HIV, ITP, and bone marrow transplantation; infection prophylaxis in pediatric HIV (orphan); investigational (orphan) for myocarditis and juvenile rheumatoid arthritis [immune globulin] 5%, 10%

**gamma benzene hexachloride** [now: lindane]

**gamma butyraldehyde (GHB-aldehyde)** a precursor to gamma hydroxybutyrate (GHB) [see: gamma hydroxybutyrate (GHB)]

**gamma butyrolactone (GBL)** precursor to gamma hydroxybutyrate (GHB); a formerly legal alternative to GHB, now also illegal (Schedule I); also known as 2(3H) furanone di-hydro (FDh) [see: gamma hydroxybutyrate (GHB)]

**gamma globulin** [see: globulin, immune]

**gamma hydroxybutyrate (GHB)** a CNS depressant used as an anesthetic in some countries, produced and abused as a "date rape" street drug in the U.S.; illegal in the U.S. (Schedule I); investigational (orphan) for narcolepsy, cataplexy, sleep paralysis, and hypnagogic hallucinations [the sodium salt is medically known as sodium oxybate]

**gamma oryzanol; gamma-oz** medicinal herb [see: rice bran oil]

**gamma-aminobutyric acid (GABA)** [see: γ-aminobutyric acid]

**Gammagard S/D** freeze-dried powder for IV infusion ℞ passive immunizing agent for HIV, idiopathic thrombocytopenic purpura (ITP), B-cell chronic lymphocytic leukemia, and Kawasaki syndrome [immune globulin, solvent/detergent treated] 50 mg/mL

**gamma-hydroxybutyrate sodium** [see: sodium oxybate]

**gamma-linolenic acid (GLA)** natural omega-6 fatty acid; investigational (orphan) for juvenile rheumatoid arthritis

**Gamma-OH** (banned in the U.S.; approved in Europe) ℞ sedative; hypnotic; antidepressant [gamma hydroxybutyrate (GHB)] 2.5 g

**gammaphos** [now: ethiofos]

**Gammar-P I.V.** (pasteurized) powder for IV infusion ℞ passive immunizing agent and immunomodulator for HIV; pediatric treatment of primary immune deficiency (PID) [immune globulin, heat treated] 5%

**gamma-vinyl GABA (gamma-aminobutyric acid)** [see: vigabatrin]

**gamolenic acid** INN, BAN

**Gamulin Rh** IM injection (discontinued 2001) ℞ obstetric Rh factor immunity suppressant [Rh$_O$(D) immune globulin] 300 μg

**Gamunex** IV infusion ℞ *passive immunizing agent for primary humoral immunodeficiency and idiopathic thrombocytopenic purpura* [immune globulin, chromatography purified] 10%

**ganaxolone** USAN *neuroactive steroid; investigational (orphan) for infantile spasms; investigational (Phase II) for migraine and adult epilepsy*

**ganciclovir** USAN, INN, BAN *antiviral for AIDS-related cytomegalovirus (CMV) infections (orphan) and CMV retinitis (orphan)* [also: ganciclovir sodium] 250, 500 mg oral

**ganciclovir sodium** USAN *antiviral for cytomegalovirus retinitis (orphan)* [also: ganciclovir]

**ganciclovir sodium & cytomegalovirus immune globulin intravenous (CMV-IGIV)** *investigational (orphan) for cytomegalovirus pneumonia in bone marrow transplant patients*

**ganglefene** INN

**gangliosides, sodium salts** *investigational (orphan) agent for retinitis pigmentosa*

**Ganidin NR** oral liquid ℞ *expectorant* [guaifenesin] 100 mg/5 mL

**ganirelix** INN *gonadotropin-releasing hormone (GnRH) antagonist for infertility* [also: ganirelix acetate]

**ganirelix acetate** USAN *gonadotropin-releasing hormone (GnRH) antagonist for infertility* [also: ganirelix]

**Ganite** IV infusion ℞ *bone resorption inhibitor for hypercalcemia of malignancy (orphan); investigational (Phase II) agent for AIDS-related non-Hodgkin lymphoma* [gallium nitrate] 25 mg/mL

**Gani-Tuss NR** oral liquid ℞ *narcotic antitussive; expectorant* [codeine phosphate; guaifenesin] 20•200 mg/10 mL

**Gani-Tuss-DM NR** oral liquid ℞ *antitussive; expectorant* [dextromethorphan hydrobromide; guaifenesin] 20•200 mg/10 mL

**Gantanol** tablets (discontinued 2001) ℞ *broad-spectrum sulfonamide bacteriostatic* [sulfamethoxazole] 500 mg

**Gantrisin** pediatric suspension ℞ *broad-spectrum sulfonamide antibiotic* [sulfisoxazole acetyl; alcohol 0.3%] 500 mg/5 mL

**gapicomine** INN

**gapromidine** INN

**Garamicina** (Mexican name for U.S. product Garamycin)

**Garamycin** cream, ointment (discontinued 2003) ℞ *antibiotic* [gentamicin sulfate] 0.1% �ⓓ Gamastan; kanamycin; Terramycin; Theramycin

**Garamycin** eye drops, ophthalmic ointment ℞ *ophthalmic antibiotic* [gentamicin sulfate] 3 mg/mL; 3 mg/g

**Garamycin** IV or IM injection ℞ *aminoglycoside antibiotic* [gentamicin sulfate] 40 mg/mL

**garcinia (Garcinia cambogia)** fruit *medicinal herb for appetite suppressant, thermogenesis, and weight control*

**garden nightshade** *medicinal herb* [see: bittersweet nightshade]

**garden patience** *medicinal herb* [see: yellow dock]

**Garfield; Garfield Plus Extra C** chewable tablets OTC *vitamin supplement* [multiple vitamins; folic acid] ≛•0.3 mg

**Garfield Complete with Minerals** chewable tablets OTC *vitamin/mineral/iron supplement* [multiple vitamins & minerals; iron; folic acid; biotin] ≛•18•0.4•0.04 mg

**Garfield Plus Iron** chewable tablets OTC *vitamin/iron supplement* [multiple vitamins; iron; folic acid] ≛•15•0.3 mg

**garget** *medicinal herb* [see: pokeweed]

**garlic (Allium sativum)** bulb *medicinal herb for asthma, cancer immunity, diabetes, digestive disorders, ear infections, flatulence, hypercholesterolemia, hypertension, and infectious diseases*

**Gas** chewable tablets OTC *antiflatulent* [simethicone] 125 mg

**GAS (group A streptococcal) vaccine** *investigational vaccine*

**gas gangrene antitoxin, pentavalent**

**gas gangrene antitoxin, polyvalent** [see: gas gangrene antitoxin, pentavalent]

**Gas Permeable Daily Cleaner** solution OTC *cleaning solution for rigid gas permeable contact lenses*

**Gas Relief** chewable tablets, drops OTC *antiflatulent* [simethicone] 80, 125 mg; 40 mg/0.6 mL

**Gas-Ban** tablets OTC *antacid; antiflatulent* [calcium carbonate; simethicone] 300•40 mg

**Gas-Ban DS** oral liquid OTC *antacid; antiflatulent* [aluminum hydroxide; magnesium hydroxide; simethicone] 400•400•40 mg/5 mL

**gastric acid inhibitors** [see: proton pump inhibitors]

**gastric mucin** BAN

**Gastrimmune** ℞ *investigational (Phase III) synthetic peptide vaccine for gastrointestinal cancers*

**Gastroccult** slide test for professional use *in vitro diagnostic aid for gastric occult blood*

**Gastrocrom** oral solution ℞ *mastocytosis treatment (orphan); investigational prophylactic treatment for food allergies* [cromolyn sodium] 100 mg/5 mL

**Gastrografin** oral solution ℞ *radiopaque contrast medium for gastrointestinal imaging* [diatrizoate meglumine; diatrizoate sodium (48.29% total iodine)] 660•100 mg/mL (367 mg/mL)

**GastroMARK** oral suspension ℞ *MRI contrast medium for upper GI tract imaging* [ferumoxsil] 175 µg iron/mL

**Gastrosed** drops, tablets (discontinued 2004) ℞ *GI/GU antispasmodic; antiparkinsonian; anticholinergic "drying agent" for allergic rhinitis and hyperhidrosis* [hyoscyamine sulfate] 0.125 mg/mL; 0.125 mg

**Gastro-Test** string capsules for professional use *in vitro diagnostic aid for GI disorders*

**Gastrozepine** (approved in Europe) ℞ *investigational (NDA filed) treatment for peptic ulcers* [pirenzepine HCl]

**Gas-X** chewable tablets, softgels OTC *antiflatulent* [simethicone] 80, 125 mg; 125 mg

**gatifloxacin** USAN *broad-spectrum fluoroquinolone antibiotic*

**gaultheria oil** [see: methyl salicylate]

**Gaultheria procumbens** *medicinal herb* [see: wintergreen]

**gauze, absorbent** USP *surgical aid*

**gauze, petrolatum** USP *surgical aid*

**gauze bandage** [see: bandage, gauze]

**gavestinel** USAN *N-methyl-D-aspartate (NMDA) receptor antagonist for stroke*

**gavilimomab** *investigational (orphan) agent for acute graft vs. host disease*

**Gaviscon** oral liquid OTC *antacid* [aluminum hydroxide; magnesium carbonate] 31.7•119.3 mg/5 mL

**Gaviscon; Gaviscon-2** chewable tablets OTC *antacid* [aluminum hydroxide; magnesium trisilicate] 80•20 mg; 160•40 mg

**Gaviscon Relief Formula** chewable tablets, oral liquid OTC *antacid* [aluminum hydroxide; magnesium carbonate] 160•105 mg; 254•237.5 mg/5 mL

**GBC-590** *investigational (Phase I/II) antineoplastic*

**GBH** *a mistaken acronym for gamma hydroxybutyrate (GHB)* [see: gamma hydroxybutyrate (GHB)]

**GBL (gamma butyrolactone)** *precursor to gamma hydroxybutyrate (GHB); a formerly legal alternative to GHB, now also illegal (Schedule I); also known as 2(3H) furanone di-hydro (FDh)* [see: gamma hydroxybutyrate (GHB)]

**G-CSF (granulocyte colony-stimulating factor)** [see: filgrastim]

**Gd texaphyrin** [see: motexafin gadolinum]

**Gd-DTPA (gadolinium-diethylene-triamine pentaacetic acid)** [q.v.]

**Gd-Tex** ℞ *investigational (Phase III) radiosensitizer for brain metastasis* [motexafin gadolinum]

**gedocarnil** INN *investigational treatment of central nervous system disorders*

**Gee-Gee** tablets (discontinued 2002) OTC *expectorant* [guaifenesin] 200 mg

**gefarnate** INN, BAN

**gefitinib** *epidermal growth factor receptor-tyrosine kinase inhibitor (EGFR-TKI); antineoplastic for advanced or metastatic non–small cell lung cancer (NSCLC); investigational (Phase III) for head and neck cancers*

**gelatin** NF *encapsulating, suspending, binding and coating agent*

**gelatin film, absorbable** USP *topical local hemostat for surgery*

**gelatin powder, absorbable** *topical local hemostat for surgery*

**gelatin solution, special intravenous** [see: polygeline]

**gelatin sponge, absorbable** USP *topical local hemostat for surgery*

**gelcaps** (dosage form) *soft gelatin capsules*

**Gelfilm; Gelfilm Ophthalmic** ℞ *topical local hemostat for surgery* [absorbable gelatin film]

**Gelfoam** powder ℞ *topical local hemostat for surgery* [absorbable gelatin powder] ⊡ Ger-O-Foam

**Gelfoam** sponge, packs, dental packs, prostatectomy cones ℞ *topical local hemostat for surgery* [absorbable gelatin sponge] ⊡ Ger-O-Foam

**Gelhist** pediatric oral suspension ℞ *decongestant; antihistamine* [phenylephrine tannate; chlorpheniramine tannate; pyrilamine tannate] 5•2•12.5 mg/5 mL

**Gel-Kam Rinse** dental gel OTC *topical caries preventative* [stannous fluoride] 0.4%

**Gelpirin** tablets (discontinued 2000) OTC *analgesic; antipyretic; anti-inflammatory* [acetaminophen; aspirin, buffered; caffeine] 125•240•32 mg

**Gelpirin-CCF** tablets (discontinued 2001) OTC *decongestant; antihistamine; analgesic; expectorant* [phenylpropanolamine HCl; chlorpheniramine maleate; acetaminophen; guaifenesin] 12.5•1•325•25 mg

**Gelseal** (trademarked dosage form) *soft gelatin capsule*

**gelsemium** *(Bignonia sempervirens; Gelsemium nitidum; G. sempervirens)* plant *medicinal herb for asthma, neuralgia, and respiratory disorders; not generally regarded as safe and effective as it is highly toxic*

**gelsolin, recombinant human** *investigational (orphan) for respiratory symptoms of cystic fibrosis and bronchiectasis*

**Gel-Tin** gel OTC *topical dental caries preventative* [stannous fluoride] 0.4%

**Gelusil** chewable tablets OTC *antacid; antiflatulent* [aluminum hydroxide; magnesium hydroxide; simethicone] 200•200•25 mg

**GEM 123** *investigational (Phase II) antisense oligonucleotide for AIDS-related cytomegalovirus retinitis*

**gemazocine** INN

**gemcadiol** USAN, INN *antihyperlipoproteinemic*

**gemcitabine** USAN, INN, BAN *antimetabolite antineoplastic*

**gemcitabine & carboplatin** *chemotherapy protocol for non–small cell lung cancer (NSCLC)*

**gemcitabine & cisplatin** *chemotherapy protocol for metastatic bladder cancer*

**gemcitabine HCl** USAN *antimetabolite antineoplastic for advanced or metastatic breast, pancreatic, and non–small cell lung cancers (NSCLC); investigational (Phase III) for cervical cancer*

**gemcitabine & vinorelbine** *chemotherapy protocol for non–small cell lung cancer (NSCLC)*

**gemcitabine-cis (gemcitabine, cisplatin)** *chemotherapy protocol for non–small cell lung cancer (NSCLC)*

**Gemcor** film-coated tablets ℞ *antihyperlipidemic for hypercholesterolemia* [gemfibrozil] 600 mg

**gemeprost** USAN, INN, BAN *prostaglandin*

**gemfibrozil** USAN, USP, INN, BAN *triglyceride-lowering antihyperlipidemic for hypertriglyceridemia (types IV and V hyperlipidemia) and coronary heart disease* 600 mg oral

**gemifloxacin mesylate** USAN *broad-spectrum fluoroquinolone antibiotic for respiratory tract infections*

**gemopatrilat** USAN *vasopeptidase inhibitor (VPI); angiotensin-converting enzyme (ACE) inhibitor for hypertension and congestive heart failure*

**gemtuzumab ozogamicin** USAN *antibody-targeted chemotherapy agent for acute myeloid leukemia (orphan)*

**Gemzar** powder for IV infusion R *antineoplastic for advanced or metastatic breast, pancreatic, and non–small cell lung cancers (NSCLC); investigational (Phase III) for cervical cancer* [gemcitabine HCl] 20 mg/mL

**Genac** tablets OTC *decongestant; antihistamine* [pseudoephedrine HCl; triprolidine HCl] 60●2.5 mg

**Gen-Acebutolol** ⒸⒶⓃ film-coated tablets R *antihypertensive; antianginal* [acebutolol HCl] 100, 200, 400 mg

**Genacol** tablets (discontinued 2001) OTC *antitussive; decongestant; antihistamine; analgesic* [dextromethorphan hydrobromide; phenylpropanolamine HCl; chlorpheniramine maleate; acetaminophen] 10●30●2●325 mg

**Genacol Cold & Flu Relief** tablets OTC *antitussive; decongestant; antihistamine; analgesic* [dextromethorphan hydrobromide; pseudoephedrine HCl; chlorpheniramine maleate; acetaminophen] 15●30●2●500 mg

**Genahist** capsules, tablets, oral liquid OTC *antihistamine* [diphenhydramine HCl] 25 mg; 25 mg; 12.5 mg/5 mL

**Gen-Allerate** tablets OTC *antihistamine* [chlorpheniramine maleate] 4 mg

**Genamin Cold** syrup (discontinued 2001) OTC *decongestant; antihistamine* [phenylpropanolamine HCl; chlorpheniramine maleate] 6.25●1 mg/5 mL

**Gen-Amiodarone** ⒸⒶⓃ tablets R *antiarrhythmic* [amiodarone HCl] 200 mg

**Gen-Amoxicillin** ⒸⒶⓃ capsules R *antibiotic* [amoxicillin trihydrate] 250, 500 mg

**Genapap** tablets, caplets OTC *analgesic; antipyretic* [acetaminophen] 325, 500 mg; 500 mg

**Genapap, Children's** chewable tablets, elixir OTC *analgesic; antipyretic* [acetaminophen] 80 mg; 160 mg/5 mL

**Genapap, Infants'** drops OTC *analgesic; antipyretic* [acetaminophen] 100 mg/mL

**Genaphed** tablets OTC *nasal decongestant* [pseudoephedrine HCl] 30 mg

**Genasal** nasal spray OTC *nasal decongestant* [oxymetazoline HCl] 0.05%

**Genasense** R *investigational (NDA filed, orphan) antineoplastic for malignant melanoma; investigational (Phase III, orphan) for multiple myeloma and chronic lymphocytic leukemia (CLL)* [augmerosen]

**Genasoft** softgels OTC *laxative; stool softener* [docusate sodium] 100 mg

**Genasoft Plus** softgels (discontinued 2003) OTC *stimulant laxative; stool softener* [casanthranol; docusate sodium] 30●100 mg

**Genaspor** cream OTC *topical antifungal* [tolnaftate] 1%

**Genatap** elixir (discontinued 2001) OTC *decongestant; antihistamine* [phenylpropanolamine HCl; brompheniramine maleate] 12.5●2 mg/5 mL Ⓓ Genapap

**Genaton** chewable tablets OTC *antacid* [aluminum hydroxide; magnesium trisilicate] 80●20 mg

**Genaton** oral liquid OTC *antacid* [aluminum hydroxide; magnesium carbonate] 31.7●137.3 mg/5 mL

**Genaton, Extra Strength** chewable tablets OTC *antacid* [aluminum hydroxide; magnesium carbonate] 160●105 mg

**Genatuss** syrup (discontinued 2002) OTC *expectorant* [guaifenesin; alcohol 3.5%] 100 mg/5 mL

**Genatuss DM** syrup OTC *antitussive; expectorant* [dextromethorphan hydrobromide; guaifenesin] 20●200 mg/10 mL

**Gen-bee with C** caplets OTC *vitamin supplement* [multiple B vitamins; vitamin C] ± •300 mg

**Gencalc 600** film-coated tablets (discontinued 2002) OTC *calcium supplement* [calcium carbonate] 1500 mg (600 mg Ca)

**Gen-Carbamazepine CR** (CAN) film-coated tablets ℞ *anticonvulsant; analgesic for trigeminal neuralgia; antimanic* [carbamazepine] 200, 400 mg

**Gencold** sustained-release capsules (discontinued 2001) OTC *decongestant; antihistamine* [phenylpropanolamine HCl; chlorpheniramine maleate] 75•8 mg

**Gen-Cyproterone** (CAN) tablets ℞ *antiandrogen* [cyproterone acetate] 50 mg

**Gendecon** tablets (discontinued 2002) OTC *decongestant; antihistamine; analgesic* [phenylephrine HCl; chlorpheniramine maleate; acetaminophen] 5•2•325 mg

**Gendex 75** IV infusion ℞ *plasma volume expander for shock due to hemorrhage, burns, or surgery* [dextran 75] 6%

**Gen-Doxazosin** (CAN) tablets ℞ *antihypertensive (α-blocker); treatment for benign prostatic hyperplasia* [doxazosin mesylate] 1, 2, 4, 8 mg

**Genebs** tablets, caplets OTC *analgesic; antipyretic* [acetaminophen] 325, 500 mg; 500 mg

**Generet-500** timed-release tablets OTC *hematinic* [ferrous sulfate; multiple B vitamins; sodium ascorbate] 105• ± •500 mg ⑨ Gentap

**Generix-T** tablets OTC *vitamin/mineral/iron supplement* [multiple vitamins & minerals; iron] ± •15 mg

**GenESA** computer-controlled IV infusion device ("GenESA System") ℞ *cardiac stressor for diagnosis of coronary artery disease* [arbutamine HCl] 0.05 mg/mL

**Gen-Etodolac** (CAN) capsules ℞ *analgesic; antiarthritic; nonsteroidal anti-inflammatory drug (NSAID)* [etodolac] 200, 300 mg

**Genevax-HIV** ℞ *investigational (Phase I/II) vaccine for HIV*

**Geneye** eye drops OTC *topical ophthalmic decongestant and vasoconstrictor* [tetrahydrozoline HCl] 0.05%

**Geneye Extra** eye drops OTC *topical ophthalmic decongestant, vasoconstrictor, and lubricant* [tetrahydrozoline HCl; polytheylene glycol 400] 0.05%•1%

**Gen-Fenofibrate Micro** (CAN) capsules ℞ *antihyperlipidemic* [fenofibrate, micronized] 200 mg

**Genfiber** powder OTC *bulk laxative* [psyllium hydrophilic mucilloid] 3.4 g/tsp.

**Gen-Fluoxetine** (CAN) capsules ℞ *selective serotonin reuptake inhibitor (SSRI) for depression and obsessive-compulsive disorder (OCD)* [fluoxetine HCl] 10, 20 mg

**Gen-Fluvoxamine** (CAN) film-coated tablets ℞ *selective serotonin reuptake inhibitor (SSRI) depression and obsessive-compulsive disorder (OCD)* [fluvoxamine maleate] 50, 100 mg

**Gen-Gliclazide** (CAN) tablets ℞ *antidiabetic* [gliclazide] 80 mg

**Gen-Glybe** (CAN) tablets ℞ *sulfonylurea antidiabetic* [glyburide] 2.5, 5 mg

**Gengraf** capsules, oral drops ℞ *immunosuppressant for allogenic kidney, liver, and heart transplants (orphan), rheumatoid arthritis (RA), and psoriasis* [cyclosporine] 25, 100 mg; 100 mg/mL

**Gen-Ipratropium** (CAN) inhalation solution ℞ *bronchodilator for asthma* [ipratropium bromide] 0.025%

*Genista tinctoria* medicinal herb [see: dyer's broom]

**genistein** *investigational antineoplastic for breast cancer; investigational for amyotrophic lateral sclerosis and stroke*

**Genite** oral liquid (discontinued 2002) OTC *antitussive; decongestant; antihistamine; analgesic* [dextromethorphan hydrobromide; pseudoephedrine HCl; doxylamine succinate; acetaminophen; alcohol 25%] 5•10• 1.25•167 mg/5 mL

**Gen-K** powder for oral solution ℞ *potassium supplement* [potassium chloride] 20 mEq K/pkt.

**Gen-Metformin** ⒸⒶⓃ film-coated tablets ℞ *biguanide antidiabetic* [metformin HCl] 500, 850 mg

**Gen-Metoprolol** ⒸⒶⓃ film-coated tablets ℞ *antihypertensive; antianginal* [metoprolol tartrate] 50, 100 mg

**Gen-Naproxen EC** ⒸⒶⓃ enteric-coated tablets ℞ *antiarthritic; nonsteroidal anti-inflammatory drug (NSAID)* [naproxen] 500 mg

**genophyllin** [see: aminophylline]

**Genoptic** eye drops ℞ *topical ophthalmic antibiotic* [gentamicin sulfate] 3 mg/mL

**Genoptic S.O.P.** ophthalmic ointment ℞ *topical ophthalmic antibiotic* [gentamicin sulfate] 3 mg/g

**Genotropin** MiniQuick (prefilled syringes in packs of 7) ℞ *growth hormone for children or adults with congenital or endogenous growth hormone deficiency, children with Turner syndrome or renal-induced growth failure, or AIDS-wasting syndrome (orphan)* [somatropin]

**Genotropin** powder for subcu injection ℞ *growth hormone for children or adults with congenital or endogenous growth hormone deficiency, children with Turner syndrome or renal-induced growth failure, or AIDS-wasting syndrome (orphan)* [somatropin] 1.5, 5.8 mg (4, 15 IU) per mL

**Genpril** film-coated tablets OTC *analgesic; antiarthritic; antipyretic; nonsteroidal anti-inflammatory drug (NSAID)* [ibuprofen] 200 mg

**Genprin** tablets OTC *analgesic; antipyretic; anti-inflammatory; antirheumatic* [aspirin] 325 mg

**Gen-Ranitidine** ⒸⒶⓃ film-coated tablets ℞ *histamine $H_2$ antagonist for gastric and duodenal ulcers* [ranitidine HCl] 150, 300 mg

**Gensan** tablets (discontinued 2000) OTC *analgesic; antipyretic; anti-inflammatory* [aspirin; caffeine] 400•32 mg

**Gentacidin** eye drops ℞ *ophthalmic antibiotic* [gentamicin sulfate] 3 mg/mL

**Gentacidin** ophthalmic ointment (discontinued 2001) ℞ *topical ophthalmic antibiotic* [gentamicin sulfate] 3 mg/g

**Gentak** eye drops, ophthalmic ointment ℞ *topical ophthalmic antibiotic* [gentamicin sulfate] 3 mg/mL; 3 mg/g

**gentamicin** BAN *aminoglycoside antibiotic* [also: gentamicin sulfate] 🅳 Jenamicin; kanamycin

**gentamicin sulfate** USAN, USP *aminoglycoside antibiotic* [also: gentamicin] 3 mg/mL eye drops; 3 mg/g ophthalmic; 0.1% topical; 10, 40 mg/mL injection

**gentamicin sulfate, liposomal** *investigational (orphan) agent for disseminated Mycobacterium avium-intracellulare infection*

**gentamicin-impregnated polymethyl methacrylate (PMMA) beads** *investigational (orphan) agent for chronic osteomyelitis*

**GenTeal** gel OTC *ophthalmic moisturizer/lubricant* [hydroxypropyl methylcellulose; carbopol 980]

**GenTeal; GenTeal Mild** eye drops OTC *ophthalmic moisturizer/lubricant* [hydroxypropyl methylcellulose]

**gentian (*Gentiana lutea*)** root *medicinal herb for aiding digestion, appetite stimulation, arthritis, hysteria, jaundice, liver disorders, and sore throat*

**gentian violet** USP *topical anti-infective/antifungal* [also: methylrosanilinium chloride] 1%, 2%

**Gen-Ticlodipine** ⒸⒶⓃ tablets ℞ *platelet aggregation inhibitor* [ticlodipine HCl] 250 mg

**gentisic acid ethanolamide** NF *complexing agent*

**Gentlax** tablets OTC *stimulant laxative* [bisacodyl] 5 mg

**Gentran 40** IV injection ℞ *plasma volume expander for shock due to hemorrhage, burns, or surgery* [dextran 40] 10%

**Gentran 70** IV infusion ℞ *plasma volume expander for shock due to hemor-*

*rhage, burns, or surgery* [dextran 70] 6%

**Gen-Verapamil** ⒸⒶⓃ film-coated tablets ℞ *antianginal; antiarrhythmic; antihypertensive* [verapamil HCl] 80, 120 mg

**Genvir** ℞ *investigational (Phase III) controlled-release form for acute genital herpes* [acyclovir]

**Gen-Xene** tablets (discontinued 2003) ℞ *benzodiazepine anxiolytic; minor tranquilizer; alcohol withdrawal aid; anticonvulsant adjunct* [chlorazepate dipotassium] 3.75, 7.5, 15 mg

**Gen-Zopiclone** ⒸⒶⓃ tablets ℞ *sedative; hypnotic* [zopiclone] 7.5 mg

**Geocillin** film-coated tablets ℞ *extended-spectrum penicillin antibiotic* [carbenicillin indanyl sodium] 382 mg

**Geodon** capsules ℞ *novel (atypical) antipsychotic* [ziprasidone HCl] 20, 40, 60, 80 mg

**Geodon** powder for IM injection ℞ *novel (atypical) antipsychotic; also used for rapid control of acute agitation* [ziprasidone mesylate] 20 mg/vial

**gepefrine** INN

**gepirone** INN *azapirone tranquilizer; anxiolytic; antidepressant* [also: gepirone HCl]

**gepirone HCl** USAN *investigational (NDA filed) azapirone tranquilizer; anxiolytic; antidepressant* [also: gepirone]

*Geranium maculatum medicinal herb* [see: alum root]

**2-geranylhydroquinone** [see: geroquinol]

*Gerardia pedicularia medicinal herb* [see: feverweed]

**Geravim** elixir OTC *vitamin/mineral supplement* [multiple B vitamins & minerals]

**Geravite** elixir OTC *geriatric vitamin supplement* [multiple B vitamins]

**Gerber Baby Low Iron Formula** oral liquid, powder for oral liquid OTC *total or supplementary infant feeding*

**Gerber Soy Formula** powder OTC *hypoallergenic infant formula* [soy protein formula]

**Geref** powder for IV injection ℞ *diagnostic aid for pituitary function; treatment for growth hormone deficiency (orphan), anovulation, and AIDS-related weight loss* [sermorelin acetate] 50 μg

**Gerimal** sublingual tablets, tablets ℞ *cognition adjuvant for age-related mental capacity decline* [ergoloid mesylates] 0.5, 1 mg; 1 mg

**Gerimed** film-coated tablets OTC *geriatric vitamin/mineral supplement* [multiple vitamins & minerals]

**Geriot** film-coated tablets OTC *hematinic; vitamin/mineral supplement* [carbonyl iron; multiple vitamins & minerals; folic acid; biotin] 50 mg•⅟•0.4 mg•45 μg

**Geritol Complete** tablets OTC *vitamin/mineral/iron supplement* [multiple vitamins & minerals; ferrous fumarate; folic acid; biotin] ⅟•18 mg•0.4 mg•45 μg

**Geritol Extend** caplets OTC *vitamin/mineral/iron supplement* [multiple vitamins & minerals; ferrous fumarate; folic acid] ⅟•10•0.2 mg

**Geritol Tonic** oral liquid OTC *hematinic* [ferric pyrophosphate; multiple B vitamins; alcohol 12%] 18•⅟ mg/15 mL

**Geritonic** oral liquid OTC *hematinic* [ferric ammonium citrate; liver fraction 1; multiple B vitamins & minerals; alcohol 20%] 105•375•⅟ mg/15 mL

**Gerivite** oral liquid OTC *geriatric vitamin/mineral supplement* [multiple B vitamins & minerals; alcohol 18%]

**Gerivites** tablets OTC *hematinic; vitamin/mineral supplement* [ferrous sulfate; multiple vitamins & minerals; folic acid] 50•⅟•0.4 mg

**German valerian** *medicinal herb* [see: valerian]

**Germanin** (available only from the Centers for Disease Control) ℞ *antiparasitic for African trypanosomiasis and onchocerciasis* [suramin sodium]

**germanium** *element (Ge)*

**germicides** *a class of agents that destroy micro-organisms* [see also: antiseptics; disinfectants]

**geroquinol** INN

**Geroton Forte** oral liquid OTC *geriatric vitamin/mineral supplement* [multiple B vitamins & minerals; alcohol 13.5%]

**gesarol** [see: chlorophenothane]

**gestaclone** USAN, INN *progestin*

**gestadienol** INN

**gestanin** [see: allyloestrenol]

**gestodene** USAN, INN, BAN *progestin*

**gestonorone caproate** USAN, INN *progestin* [also: gestronol]

**gestrinone** USAN, INN *progestin*

**gestronol** BAN *progestin* [also: gestonorone caproate]

**Get Better Bear Sore Throat Pops** OTC *throat emollient and protectant* [pectin] 19 mg

**Gets-It** topical liquid OTC *keratolytic* [salicylic acid; zinc chloride; alcohol 28%]

**gevotroline** INN *antipsychotic* [also: gevotroline HCl]

**gevotroline HCl** USAN *antipsychotic* [also: gevotroline]

**Gevrabon** oral liquid OTC *vitamin/mineral supplement* [multiple B vitamins & minerals; alcohol 18%]

**Gevral** tablets OTC *vitamin/mineral/iron supplement* [multiple vitamins & minerals; ferrous fumarate; folic acid] ±•18 mg•0.4 mg

**Gevral Protein** powder OTC *oral protein supplement* [calcium caseinate; sucrose]

**G-F 20** [see: hylan G-F 20]

**GFN (guaifenesin)** [q.v.]

**GFN 550/PSE 60/DM30** sustained-release tablets ℞ *expectorant; decongestant; antitussive* [guaifenesin; pseudoephedrine HCl; dextromethorphan hydrobromide] 550•60•30 mg

**GFN 600/Phenylephrine 20** tablets ℞ *decongestant; expectorant* [phenylephrine HCl; guaifenesin] 20•600 mg

**GFN 600/PSE 60/DM 30** sustained-release caplets ℞ *expectorant; decongestant; antitussive* [guaifenesin; pseudoephedrine HCl;

dextromethorphan hydrobromide] 600•60•30 mg

**GFN 1200/DM 60, GFN 1000/DM 50** sustained-release caplets ℞ *expectorant; antitussive* [guaifenesin; dextromethorphan hydrobromide] 1200•60 mg; 1000•50 mg

**GFN 1200/DM 60/PSE 120** sustained-release caplets ℞ *expectorant; antitussive; decongestant* [guaifenesin; dextromethorphan hydrobromide; pseudoephedrine HCl] 1200•60•120 mg

**GFN/PSE** sustained-release tablets ℞ *expectorant; decongestant* [guaifenesin; pseudoephedrine HCl] 1200•120 mg

**GG-Cen** capsules (discontinued 2000) OTC *expectorant* [guaifenesin] 200 mg

**GHB (gamma hydroxybutyrate)** *a CNS depressant used as an anesthetic in some countries, produced and abused as a "date rape" street drug in the U.S.; illegal in the U.S. (Schedule I)* [the sodium salt is medically known as sodium oxybate]

**GHB-aldehyde (gamma butyraldehyde)** *a precursor to gamma hydroxybutyrate (GHB)* [see: gamma hydroxybutyrate (GHB)]

**GHRF; GH-RF (growth hormone-releasing factor)** [q.v.]

**Gilead, balm of** *medicinal herb* [see: balm of Gilead]

**ginger (Zingiber officinale)** root *medicinal herb for childhood diseases, colds, colic, dizziness, fever, flu, gas pains, headache, indigestion, morning sickness, nausea, poor circulation, toothache, and vestibular disorders*

**ginger, wild** *medicinal herb* [see: wild ginger]

**ginkgo (Ginkgo biloba)** leaves *medicinal herb for Alzheimer disease, antioxidant, anxiety, asthma, attention-deficit disorder, chilblains, cerebral insufficiency, dementia, dizziness, memory loss, poor circulation, Raynaud disease, stroke, and tinnitus*

**ginseng (Panax spp.)** root *medicinal herb for age spots, blood diseases,*

depression, hemorrhage, increasing
endurance and longevity, and stress;
also used as an aphrodisiac [also see:
Siberian ginseng]

**ginseng, blue; yellow ginseng** medicinal herb [see: blue cohosh]

**giparmen** INN

**giractide** INN

**girisopam** INN

**gitalin** NF [also: gitalin amorphous]

**gitalin amorphous** INN [also: gitalin]

**gitaloxin** INN

**gitoformate** INN

**gitoxin 16-formate** [see: gitaloxin]

**gitoxin pentaacetate** [see: pengitoxin]

**GLA (gamma-linolenic acid)** [q.v.]

**glacial acetic acid** [see: acetic acid,
glacial]

**Gladase** ointment ℞ enzyme for wound
debridement; vulnerary [papain; urea]
830 000 U/g•10%

**glafenine** INN, DCF, JAN

**Glandosane** oral spray (discontinued
2000) OTC saliva substitute

**glaphenine** [see: glafenine]

**glatiramer acetate** USAN immunomodulator for relapsing-remitting multiple
sclerosis (orphan)

**Glauber salt** [see: sodium sulfate]

**glaucarubin**

**Glaucon** Drop-Tainers (eye drops)
(discontinued 2004) ℞ antiglaucoma
agent [epinephrine HCl] 1%, 2%

**GlaucTabs** tablets (discontinued 2003)
℞ carbonic anhydrase inhibitor for
glaucoma [methazolamide] 25, 50 mg

**glaze, pharmaceutical** NF tablet-coating agent

**glaziovine** INN

**Gleevec** film-coated tablets ℞ antineoplastic for chronic myeloid leukemia
(CML) (orphan) and gastrointestinal
stromal tumors (GIST) [imatinib
mesylate] 100, 400 mg

**glemanserin** USAN, INN anxiolytic

**gleptoferron** USAN, INN, BAN veterinary hematinic

**Gliadel** wafers ℞ nitrosourea-type alkylating antineoplastic cerebral implants

for excised brain tumors (orphan) [car-
mustine] 7.7 mg

**gliamilide** USAN, INN antidiabetic

**glibenclamide** INN, BAN sulfonylurea
antidiabetic [also: glyburide]

**glibornuride** USAN, INN, BAN antidiabetic

**glibutimine** INN

**glicaramide** INN

**glicetanile** INN antidiabetic [also: glicetanile sodium]

**glicetanile sodium** USAN antidiabetic
[also: glicetanile]

**gliclazide** INN, BAN sulfonylurea antidiabetic

**glicondamide** INN

**glidazamide** INN

**gliflumide** USAN, INN antidiabetic

**glimepiride** USAN, INN, BAN sulfonylurea antidiabetic

**glipentide** [see: glisentide]

**glipizide** USAN, INN, BAN sulfonylurea
antidiabetic 5, 10 mg oral

**Glipizide ER** extended-release tablets
℞ sulfonylurea antidiabetic [glipizide]
2.5, 5, 10 mg

**gliquidone** INN, BAN

**glisamuride** INN

**glisentide** INN

**glisindamide** INN

**glisolamide** INN

**glisoxepide** INN, BAN

**Glivec** (foreign name for U.S. product
Gleevec)

**globin zinc insulin** INN [also: insulin,
globin zinc]

**globulin, aerosolized pooled immune**
investigational (orphan) agent for respiratory syncytial virus lower respiratory
tract disease

**globulin, immune** USP passive immunizing agent for HIV, ITP, B-cell CLL,
and bone marrow transplantation;
infection prophylaxis in pediatric HIV
(orphan); investigational (orphan) for
myocarditis and juvenile rheumatoid
arthritis

**globulin, immune human serum**
[now: globulin, immune]

**Glofil-125** injection ℞ *radiopaque contrast medium* [iothalamate sodium I 125 (59.9% iodine)] 1 mg/mL

**Glossets** (trademarked form) *sublingual or rectal administration*

**gloxazone** USAN, INN, BAN *veterinary anaplasmodastat*

**gloximonam** USAN, INN *antibacterial*

**GlucaGen Diagnostic Kit** IV injection ℞ *agent to inhibit movement of the gastrointestinal tract during radiographic procedures* [glucagon, recombinant] 1 mg

**GlucaGen Emergency Kit** subcu, IV, or IM injection ℞ *emergency treatment of hypoglycemic crisis* [glucagon, recombinant] 1 mg

**glucagon** USP, INN, BAN *antidiabetic; glucose elevating agent; diagnostic aid for GI imaging*

**Glucagon Diagnostic Kit** IM or IV injection ℞ *to inhibit GI tract movement during radiographic procedures* [glucagon, recombinant] 1 mg (1 U)

**Glucagon Emergency Kit** subcu, IM, or IV injection ℞ *emergency treatment for hypoglycemic crisis* [glucagon, recombinant] 1 mg (1 U)

**glucalox** INN [also: glycalox]

**glucametacin** INN

**glucan synthesis inhibitors** *a class of antifungals* [also: echinocandins]

**D-glucaric acid, calcium salt tetrahydrate** [see: calcium saccharate]

**gluceptate** USAN, USP, INN, BAN *combining name for radicals or groups*

**gluceptate sodium** USAN *pharmaceutic aid*

**Glucerna; Glucerna Select; Glucerna Weight Loss Shake** ready-to-use oral liquid OTC *enteral nutritional therapy for abnormal glucose tolerance*

**D-glucitol** [see: sorbitol]

**D-glucitol hexanicotinate** [see: sorbinicate]

**β-glucocerebrosidase, macrophage-targeted** [see: alglucerase]

**glucocerebrosidase, recombinant retroviral vector** *investigational*

*(orphan) enzyme replacement for types I, II, or III Gaucher disease*

**glucocerebrosidase-β-glucosidase** [see: alglucerase]

**glucocorticoids** *a class of adrenal cortical steroids that modify the body's immune response*

**Glucofilm** reagent strips for home use *in vitro diagnostic aid for blood glucose*

**glucoheptonic acid, calcium salt** [see: calcium gluceptate]

**glucomannan (Amorphophallus konjac)** root *medicinal herb for constipation, diverticular disease, hemorrhoids, hypercholesterolemia, and obesity; it may produce altered insulin requirements or hypoglycemia in diabetics*

**Glucometer Encore; Glucometer Elite** reagent strips for home use *in vitro diagnostic aid for blood glucose*

**D-gluconic acid, calcium salt** [see: calcium gluconate]

**D-gluconic acid, magnesium salt** [see: magnesium gluconate]

**D-gluconic acid, monopotassium salt** [see: potassium gluconate]

**D-gluconic acid, monosodium salt** [see: sodium gluconate]

**GlucoNorm** ⒸⒶⓃ tablets ℞ *oral antidiabetic agent that stimulates release of insulin from the pancreas for type 2 diabetes* [repaglinide] 0.5, 1, 2 mg

**Glucophage** film-coated tablets ℞ *biguanide antidiabetic* [metformin HCl] 500, 850, 1000 mg

**Glucophage XR** extended-release tablets ℞ *once-daily biguanide antidiabetic* [metformin HCl] 500, 750 mg

**β-D-glucopyranuronamide** [see: glucuronamide]

**glucosamine** USAN, INN *pharmaceutic aid*

**glucosamine sulfate** *natural remedy for osteoarthritis*

**d-glucose** [see: dextrose]

**glucose, liquid** NF *tablet binder and coating agent; antihypoglycemic; diagnostic aid for diabetes* ⓢ Glutose

**d-glucose monohydrate** [see: dextrose]

**glucose oxidase**

**glucose polymers** *caloric replacement*

**Glucostix** reagent strips for home use *in vitro diagnostic aid for blood glucose*

**glucosulfamide** INN

**glucosulfone** INN

**glucosylceramidase** [see: alglucerase]

**Glucotrol** tablets ℞ *sulfonylurea antidiabetic* [glipizide] 5, 10 mg

**Glucotrol XL** extended-release tablets ℞ *sulfonylurea antidiabetic* [glipizide] 2.5, 5, 10 mg

**Glucovance** film-coated caplets ℞ *antidiabetic combination for type 2 diabetes* [glyburide; metformin HCl] 1.25•250, 2.5•500, 5•500 mg

**glucurolactone** INN

**glucuronamide** INN, BAN

**glunicate** INN

**gluside** [see: saccharin]

**gluside, soluble** [see: saccharin sodium]

**glusoferron** INN

**Glustat** ℞ *investigational α-glucosidase inhibitor for diabetes* [voglibose]

**glutamic acid (L-glutamic acid)** USAN, INN *nonessential amino acid; symbols: Glu, E 340, 500 mg oral*

**glutamic acid HCl** *gastric acidifier*

**glutamine (L-glutamine)** USAN, USP, JAN *nonessential amino acid that supplies energy to the brain to reduce fatigue and increase exercise endurance, combat hypoglycemia, and strengthen the GI tract; growth hormone secretagogue; investigational (orphan) for short bowel syndrome; symbols: Gln, Q*

**glutamine & somatropin** *investigational (orphan) for GI malabsorption due to short bowel syndrome*

**glutaral** USAN, USP, INN *disinfectant*

**glutaraldehyde** [see: glutaral]

**Glutarex-1** powder OTC *formula for infants with glutaric aciduria type I*

**Glutarex-2** powder OTC *enteral nutritional therapy for glutaric aciduria type I*

**glutasin** [see: glutamic acid HCl]

**glutathione** *endogenous antioxidant produced in the liver; unstable as an oral supplement, so levels are increased by using transdermal preparations, by supplementing its precursors, MSM*

*and NAC (q.v.), or by regenerating it with SAMe (q.v.)*

**L-glutathione, reduced** *investigational (orphan) for AIDS-related cachexia*

**glutaurine** INN

**glutethimide** USP, INN, BAN *sedative; sometimes abused as a street drug* 250, 500 mg oral

**Glutofac** tablets OTC *vitamin/mineral supplement* [multiple vitamins & minerals]

**Glutofac-ZX** caplets ℞ *vitamin/mineral supplement* [multiple vitamins & minerals; folic acid; biotin] ≛•1•0.2 mg

**Glutose** gel OTC *glucose elevating agent* [glucose] 40% ☑ glucose

**Glyate** syrup (discontinued 2002) OTC *expectorant* [guaifenesin; alcohol 3.5%] 100 mg/5 mL

**glyburide** USAN *sulfonylurea antidiabetic* [also: glibenclamide] 1.25, 1.5, 2.5, 3, 4.5, 5, 6 mg oral

**glyburide & metformin HCl** *sulfonylurea/biguanide antidiabetic combination for type 2 diabetes* 1.25•250, 2.5•500, 5•500 mg oral

**glybutamide** [see: carbutamide]

**glybuthiazol** INN

**glybuthizol** [see: glybuthiazol]

**glybuzole** INN

**glycalox** BAN [also: glucalox]

**glyceol** *investigational (orphan) agent for decreasing intracranial hypertension or cerebral edema*

**glycerides oleiques polyoxyethylenes** [see: peglicol 5 oleate]

**glycerin** USP *humectant; solvent; osmotic diuretic; hyperosmotic laxative; emollient/protectant; ophthalmic moisturizer* [also: glycerol]

**glycerol** INN *humectant; solvent; osmotic diuretic; hyperosmotic laxative; emollient/protectant; monoctanoin component D* [also: glycerin]

**glycerol, iodinated** USAN, BAN *(disapproved for use as an expectorant in 1991)*

**glycerol 1-decanoate** *monoctanoin component B* [see: monoctanoin]

**glycerol 1,2-dioctanoate** *monoctanoin component C* [see: monoctanoin]

**glycerol 1-octanoate** *monoctanoin component A* [see: monoctanoin]

**glycerol phosphate, manganese salt** [see: manganese glycerophosphate]

**glyceryl behenate** NF *tablet and capsule lubricant*

**glyceryl borate** [see: boroglycerin]

**glyceryl guaiacolate** [now: guaifenesin]

**glyceryl monostearate** NF *emulsifying agent*

**glyceryl triacetate** [now: triacetin]

**glyceryl trierucate** *investigational (orphan) agent for adrenoleukodystrophy* [also: glyceryl trioleate]

**glyceryl trinitrate** BAN *coronary vasodilator* [also: nitroglycerin]

**glyceryl trioleate** *investigational (orphan) agent for adrenoleukodystrophy* [also: glyceryl trierucate]

**glycerylaminophenaquine** [see: glafenine]

**Glyceryl-T** *capsules, oral liquid* ℞ *antiasthmatic; bronchodilator; expectorant* [theophylline; guaifenesin] 150•90 mg; 150•90 mg/15 mL

**glycinato dihydroxyaluminum hydrate** [see: dihydroxyaluminum aminoacetate]

**glycine** USP, INN *nonessential amino acid; urologic irrigant; symbols: Gly, G* [also: aminoacetic acid] 1.5%

**glycine aluminum-zirconium complex** [see: aluminum zirconium tetrachlorohydrex gly; aluminum zirconium trichlorohydrex gly]

*Glycine max medicinal herb* [see: soy]

**glyclopyramide** INN

**glycobiarsol** USP, INN [also: bismuth glycollylarsanilate]

**glycocholate sodium** [see: sodium glycocholate]

**glycocoll** [see: glycine]

**Glycofed** *tablets (discontinued 2002)* OTC *decongestant; expectorant* [pseudoephedrine HCl; guaifenesin] 30•100 mg

**glycol distearate** USAN *thickening agent*

**glycolic acid** *mild exfoliant and keratolytic*

**glycolipodipsipeptides** *a class of broadspectrum antibiotics that are bactericidal against gram-positive aerobic and anaerobic bacteria*

*p*-**glycolophenetidide** [see: fenacetinol]

**glycopeptides** *a class of antibiotic antineoplastics*

**glycophenylate** [see: mepenzolate bromide]

**glycoprotein (GP) IIb/IIIa receptor antagonists** *a class of platelet aggregation inhibitors for acute coronary syndrome, unstable angina, myocardial infarction, and cardiac surgery*

**glycopyrrolate** USAN, USP *GI antispasmodic; antisecretory; peptic ulcer adjunct* [also: glycopyrronium bromide] 0.2 mg/mL injection

**glycopyrrone bromide** [see: glycopyrrolate]

**glycopyrronium bromide** INN, BAN *GI antispasmodic; antisecretory; peptic ulcer adjunct* [also: glycopyrrolate]

**glycosaminoglycans** *a class of anticoagulants used for the prophylaxis of postoperative deep vein thrombosis (DVT)*

**glycosides, cardiac** *a class of cardiovascular drugs that increase the force of cardiac contractions* [also called: digitalis glycosides]

**Glycotuss** *tablets (discontinued 2002)* OTC *expectorant* [guaifenesin] 100 mg
🔊 Glytuss

**Glycotuss-DM** *tablets (discontinued 2002)* OTC *antitussive; expectorant* [dextromethorphan hydrobromide; guaifenesin] 10•100 mg

**glycyclamide** INN, BAN

**glycyrrhetinic acid** [see: enoxolone]

**glycyrrhiza** NF

*Glycyrrhiza glabra; G. palidiflora; G. uralensis medicinal herb* [see: licorice]

**glydanile sodium** [now: glicetanile sodium]

**glyhexamide** USAN, INN *antidiabetic*

**glyhexylamide** [see: metahexamide]

**Glylorin** ℞ *investigational (Phase III, orphan) for non-bullous congenital ichthyosiform erythroderma* [monolaurin]

**glymidine** BAN *antidiabetic* [also: glymidine sodium]

**glymidine sodium** USAN, INN *antidiabetic* [also: glymidine]

**glymol** [see: mineral oil]

**Glynase** PresTabs (micronized tablets) ℞ *sulfonylurea antidiabetic* [glyburide] 1.5, 3, 6 mg

**glyoctamide** USAN, INN *antidiabetic*

**Gly-Oxide** oral solution OTC *topical anti-inflammatory and anti-infective* [carbamide peroxide] 10%

**glyparamide** USAN *antidiabetic*

**glyphylline** [see: dyphylline]

**glypinamide** INN

**Glypressin** ℞ *investigational (orphan) for bleeding esophageal ulcers* [terlipressin]

**glyprothiazol** INN

**glyprothizol** [see: glyprothiazol]

**Glyquin** cream ℞ *hyperpigmentation bleaching agent* [hydroquinone (in a sunscreen base)] 4%

**Glyquin-XM** cream ℞ *hyperpigmentation bleaching agent* [hydroquinone (in a sunscreen base with vitamin E)] 4%

**Glyset** tablets ℞ *antidiabetic agent for type 2 diabetes; alpha-glucosidase inhibitor that delays the digestion of dietary carbohydrates* [miglitol] 25, 50, 100 mg

**glysobuzole** INN [also: isobuzole]

**Glytuss** film-coated tablets (discontinued 2002) OTC *expectorant* [guaifenesin] 200 mg ⊡ Glycotuss

**GM-CSF (granulocyte-macrophage colony-stimulating factor)** [see: regramostim; sargramostim; molgramostim]

**GMK** *investigational (Phase III) GM2 ganglioside protein vaccine for malignant melanoma*

**G-myticin** cream, ointment (discontinued 2003) ℞ *antibiotic* [gentamicin sulfate] 1 mg

*Gnaphalium polycephalum; G. uliginosum* medicinal herb [see: everlasting]

**Gn-RH, GnRH (gonadotropin-releasing hormone)** *an endogenous hormone, produced in the hypothalamus, which stimulates the release of luteinizing hormone (LH) and follicle-stimulating*

*hormone (FSH) from the pituitary* [also known as: luteinizing hormone–releasing hormone (LH-RH)]

**goatweed** *medicinal herb* [see: St. John wort]

**gold** *element (Au)*

**gold Au 198** USAN, USP *antineoplastic; liver imaging aid; radioactive agent*

**gold sodium thiomalate** USP *antirheumatic (50% gold)* [also: sodium aurothiomalate] 50 mg/mL injection

**gold sodium thiosulfate** NF [also: sodium aurotiosulfate]

**gold thioglucose** [see: aurothioglucose]

**gold thread (*Coptis trifolia*)** root *medicinal herb used as an antiphlogistic, bitter tonic, and sedative*

**golden senecio** *medicinal herb* [see: life root]

**goldenrod (*Solidago nemoralis; S. odora; S. virgaurea*)** leaves and flowering tops *medicinal herb used as an astringent, carminative, diaphoretic, diuretic, and stimulant*

**goldenseal (*Hydrastis canadensis*)** rhizome and root *medicinal herb used as an antibiotic and antiseptic and for internal bleeding, colon inflammation, eye infections, liver disorders, menorrhagia, mouth sores, muscular pain, sciatic pain, and vaginitis*

**GoLYTELY** powder for oral solution ℞ *pre-procedure bowel evacuant* [polyethylene glycol–electrolyte solution (PEG 3350)] 60 g/L

**gonacrine** [see: acriflavine]

**Gonadimmune** *investigational antigonadotropin-releasing hormone for prostate, breast, and endometrial cancer and endometriosis*

**gonadorelin** INN, BAN *gonad-stimulating principle* [also: gonadorelin acetate]

**gonadorelin acetate** USAN *gonad-stimulating principle for hypothalamic amenorrhea (orphan); diagnostic aid for fertility* [also: gonadorelin]

**gonadorelin HCl** USAN *gonad-stimulating principle; synthetic luteinizing hormone–releasing hormone (LH-RH);*

*in vivo diagnostic aid for anterior pituitary function*

**gonadotrophin, chorionic** INN, BAN *gonad-stimulating principle* [also: gonadotropin, chorionic]

**gonadotrophin, serum** INN

**gonadotropin, chorionic** USP *gonad-stimulating principle* [also: gonadotrophin, chorionic] 500, 1000, 2000 U/mL injection

**gonadotropin, serum** [see: gonadotrophin, serum]

**gonadotropin-releasing hormone (Gn-RH)** *an endogenous hormone, produced in the hypothalamus, which stimulates the release of luteinizing hormone (LH) and follicle-stimulating hormone (FSH) from the pituitary* [also known as: luteinizing hormone–releasing hormone (LH-RH)]

**gonadotropin-releasing hormone analogs** *a class of hormonal antineoplastics*

**gonadotropins** *a class of hormones that stimulate the ovaries, including follicle-stimulating hormone and luteinizing hormone*

**Gonak** ophthalmic solution OTC *gonioscopic examination aid* [hydroxypropyl methylcellulose] 2.5% ⑨ Gonic

**Gonal-f** subcu injection ℞ *recombinant follicle-stimulating hormone (FSH) for induction of ovulation or spermatogenesis (orphan); adjunct to assisted reproductive technology (ART)* [follitropin alfa] 75, 450, 1050 IU

**Gonal-f RFF Pen** (prefilled syringes) ℞ *recombinant follicle-stimulating hormone (FSH) for induction of ovulation or spermatogenesis; adjunct to assisted reproductive technology (ART)* [follitropin alfa] 300, 450, 900 IU

**Gonic** powder for IM injection ℞ *hormone for prepubertal cryptorchidism and hypogonadism; ovulation stimulant* [chorionic gonadotropin] 1000 U/mL ⑨ Gonak

*Goniopora* **spp.** *natural material* [see: coral]

**Gonioscopic Prism Solution** Drop-Tainers (eye drops) OTC *agent for bonding gonioscopic prisms to eye* [hydroxyethyl cellulose]

**Goniosol** ophthalmic solution OTC *gonioscopic examination aid* [hydroxypropyl methylcellulose] 2.5%

**Gonozyme Diagnostic** reagent kit for professional use *in vitro diagnostic aid for Neisseria gonorrhoeae*

**Good Sense Pain Relief Allergy Sinus** gelcaps OTC *decongestant; antihistamine; analgesic* [pseudoephedrine HCl; chlorpheniramine maleate; acetaminophen] 30•2•500 mg

**Good Sense Sinus** caplets OTC *decongestant; antihistamine; analgesic* [pseudoephedrine HCl; chlorpheniramine maleate; acetaminophen] 30•2•500 mg

**GoodStart** [see: Carnation Good Start]

**Goody's Body Pain** powder OTC *analgesic; antipyretic; anti-inflammatory* [acetaminophen; aspirin] 325•500 mg/dose

**Goody's Extra Strength Headache** powder OTC *analgesic; antipyretic; anti-inflammatory* [acetaminophen; aspirin; caffeine] 250•520•32.5 mg/dose

**Goody's PM** powder OTC *antihistaminic sleep aid; analgesic* [diphenhydramine citrate; acetaminophen] 38•500 mg

**goose grass** *medicinal herb* [see: bedstraw; cinquefoil]

**goose hair; gosling weed** *medicinal herb* [see: bedstraw]

**Gordobalm** OTC *analgesic; counterirritant; antiseptic* [methyl salicylate; menthol; camphor; alcohol 16%]

**Gordochom** topical solution OTC *antifungal; antiseptic* [undecylenic acid; chloroxylenol] 25%•3%

**Gordofilm** topical liquid ℞ *keratolytic* [salicylic acid in flexible collodion] 16.7%

**Gordogesic Creme** OTC *analgesic; counterirritant* [methyl salicylate] 10%

**Gordon's Urea 40%** cream ℞ *for removal of dystrophic nails* [urea] 40%

**Gormel Creme** OTC *moisturizer; emollient; keratolytic* [urea] 20%

**goserelin** USAN, INN, BAN *hormonal antineoplastic for prostate and breast cancer; luteinizing hormone-releasing hormone (LHRH) agonist* [also: goserelin acetate]

**goserelin acetate** JAN *hormonal antineoplastic for prostatic carcinoma, breast cancer, and endometriosis; luteinizing hormone-releasing hormone (LHRH) agonist* [also: goserelin]

**gosling weed; goose grass; goose hair** *medicinal herb* [see: bedstraw]

**gossypol (Gossypium spp.)** *seed oil medicinal herb for male and female contraception; not generally regarded as safe and effective as male sterility may be irreversible; investigational for metastatic endometrial carcinoma; investigational antiviral/interferon inducer for AIDS; investigational (orphan) for adrenal cortex cancer*

**gotu kola (Centella asiatica; Hydrocotyle asiatica)** *entire plant medicinal herb for abscesses, hypertension, contraception, leprosy, nervous breakdown, physical and mental fatigue, promoting wound healing, and rheumatism*

**goutberry** *medicinal herb* [see: blackberry]

**govafilcon A** USAN *hydrophilic contact lens material*

**G/P 1200/600** sustained-release tablets Ṟ *decongestant; expectorant* [pseudoephedrine HCl; guaifenesin] 60•1200 mg

**GP IIb/IIIa inhibitors** [see: glycoprotein (GP) IIb/IIIa receptor antagonists]

**gp100 adenoviral gene therapy** *investigational (Phase III, orphan) theraccine for metastatic melanoma*

**gp120 (glycoprotein 120) antigens** *investigational (Phase III) vaccine for HIV* [also: AIDS vaccine]

**gp160 (glycoprotein 160) antigens** *investigational (orphan) antiviral (therapeutic, Phase II) and vaccine (preventative, Phase I) for HIV and AIDS*

**GP-500** tablets Ṟ *decongestant; expectorant* [pseudoephedrine HCl; guaifenesin] 120•500 mg

**gp96 heat shock protein-peptide complex** *investigational (Phase III, orphan) antineoplastic for renal cell carcinoma and metastatic melanoma*

**grace, herb of** *medicinal herb* [see: rue]

**Gradumet** (trademarked dosage form) *controlled-release tablet*

**graftskin** *a living, bilayered skin construct for diabetic foot ulcers and pressure sores (the epidermal layer is living human keratinocytes; the dermal layer is living human fibroblasts)*

**gramicidin** USP, INN *antibacterial antibiotic*

**gramicidin & neomycin sulfate & polymyxin B sulfate** *topical antibiotic* 0.025 mg•1.75 mg•10 000 U per mL eye drops

**gramicidin S** INN

*Graminis rhizoma* *medicinal herb* [see: couch grass]

**granisetron** USAN, INN, BAN *serotonin 5-HT₃ receptor antagonist; antiemetic for nausea following chemotherapy, radiation, or surgery*

**granisetron HCl** USAN *serotonin 5-HT₃ receptor antagonist; antiemetic for nausea following chemotherapy, radiation, or surgery*

**Granulderm** aerosol spray Ṟ *topical enzyme for wound debridement* [trypsin; peruvian balsam] 0.1•72.5 mg/0.82 mL

**Granulex** aerosol spray Ṟ *topical enzymatic wound spray for decubitus ulcers* [trypsin; peruvian balsam] 0.1•72.5 mg/0.82 mL

**granulocyte colony-stimulating factor (G-CSF), recombinant** [see: filgrastim]

**granulocyte-macrophage colony-stimulating factor (GM-CSF)** [see: regramostim; sargramostim; molgramostim]

**GranuMed** aerosol spray Ṟ *topical enzyme for wound debridement* [trypsin; peruvian balsam] 0.1•72.5 mg/0.82 mL

**grape, bear's** *medicinal herb* [see: uva ursi]

**grape, Rocky Mountain; wild Oregon grape** *medicinal herb* [see: Oregon grape]

**grape seed (Vitis coigetiae; V. vinifera)** *oil medicinal herb for dental caries; also used as a dietary source of essential fatty acids and tocopherols*

**grape seed extract** *natural free radical scavenger for inflammatory collagen disease and peripheral vascular disease; contains 92%–95% procyanidolic oligomers (PCOs)*

**grapefruit (Citrus paradisi)** *medicinal herb for potassium replacement; the pectin is used to help reduce cholesterol and promote regression of atherosclerosis*

**grass burdock** *medicinal herb* [see: burdock]

**grass myrtle** *medicinal herb* [see: calamus]

**Gratiola officinalis** *medicinal herb* [see: hedge hyssop]

**gravelroot** *medicinal herb* [see: queen of the meadow]

**graybeard tree** *medicinal herb* [see: fringe tree]

**great wild valerian** *medicinal herb* [see: valerian]

**greater celandine** *medicinal herb* [see: celandine]

**green broom; greenweed** *medicinal herb* [see: dyer's broom]

**green hellebore (Veratrum viride)** *medicinal herb* [see: hellebore]

**green soap** [see: soap, green]

**green tea (Camellia sinensis)** *leaves medicinal herb used as an antihyperlipidemic, antimicrobial, antineoplastic, and antioxidant; also used to promote longevity by attenuating severe fatal diseases*

**Green Throat Spray; Red Throat Spray** OTC *topical antipruritic/counterirritant; mild local anesthetic* [phenol] 1.4%

**greenweed; green broom** *medicinal herb* [see: dyer's broom]

**grepafloxacin** INN *broad-spectrum fluoroquinolone antibiotic*

**grepafloxacin HCl** USAN *broad-spectrum fluoroquinolone antibiotic*

**Grifola frondosa** *medicinal herb* [see: maitake mushrooms]

**Grifulvin V** *tablets, oral suspension (discontinued 2003)* ℞ *systemic antifungal* [griseofulvin (microsize)] 250, 500 mg; 125 mg/5 mL

**Grindelia squarrosa** *medicinal herb* [see: gum weed]

**Grisactin 250** *capsules (discontinued 2004)* ℞ *systemic antifungal* [griseofulvin (microsize)] 250 mg

**Grisactin 500** *tablets (discontinued 2004)* ℞ *systemic antifungal* [griseofulvin (microsize)] 500 mg

**Grisactin Ultra** *tablets (discontinued 2004)* ℞ *systemic antifungal* [griseofulvin (ultramicrosize)] 250 mg

**griseofulvin** USP, INN, BAN *systemic antifungal*

**Gris-PEG** *film-coated tablets* ℞ *systemic antifungal* [griseofulvin (ultramicrosize)] 125, 250 mg

**ground apple** *medicinal herb* [see: chamomile]

**ground berry** *medicinal herb* [see: wintergreen]

**ground holly** *medicinal herb* [see: pipsissewa]

**ground lemon** *medicinal herb* [see: mandrake]

**ground lily** *medicinal herb* [see: birthroot]

**ground raspberry** *medicinal herb* [see: goldenseal]

**ground squirrel pea** *medicinal herb* [see: twin leaf]

**ground thistle** *medicinal herb* [see: carline thistle]

**group A streptococcal (GAS) vaccine** *investigational vaccine*

**group C meningococcal conjugate vaccine** *investigational vaccine*

**growth hormone, human (hGH)** [see: somatropin]

growth hormone-releasing factor
(GHRF; GH-RF) *investigational
(orphan) for inadequate endogenous
growth hormone in children*

G-strophanthin [see: ouabain]

GTI-2040 [see: antisense 20-mer
phosphorothiolate oligonucleotide]

guabenxan INN

guacetisal INN

guafecainol INN

guaiac

guaiacol NF

*p*-guaiacol [see: mequinol]

guaiacol carbonate NF

guaiacol glyceryl ether [see: guaifen-
esin]

guaiactamine INN

guaiapate USAN, INN *antitussive*

guaiazulene soluble [see: sodium gua-
lenate]

guaietolin INN

Guaifed sustained-release capsules ℞
*decongestant; expectorant* [phenyleph-
rine HCl; guaifenesin] 15•400 mg

Guaifed syrup OTC *decongestant; expectorant* [pseudoephedrine HCl; guai-
fenesin] 60•400 mg/10 mL

Guaifed-PD sustained-release capsules
℞ *decongestant; expectorant* [phenyl-
ephrine HCl; guaifenesin] 7.5•200 mg

guaifenesin USAN, USP, INN *expectorant* [also: guaiphenesin] 200 mg
oral; 100 mg/5 mL oral ⟲ guanfacine

guaifenesin & codeine phosphate
*expectorant; narcotic antitussive; nar-
cotic analgesic* 300•10 mg oral; 100•
10 mg/5 mL oral

Guaifenesin DAC oral liquid (discontinued 2002) OTC *narcotic antitussive; decongestant; expectorant*
[codeine phosphate; pseudoephedrine HCl; guaifenesin; alcohol 1.9%]
10•30•100 mg

guaifenesin & dextromethorphan
hydrobromide *expectorant; antitussive* 500•30, 1000•60 mg oral

guaifenesin & dyphylline *expectorant; antiasthmatic; bronchodilator*
200•200 mg oral

guaifenesin & hydrocodone bitartrate *expectorant; narcotic antitussive*
100•5 mg/5 mL oral

Guaifenesin NR oral liquid ℞ *expectorant* [guaifenesin] 100 mg/5 mL

guaifenesin & phenylephrine HCl
& phenylpropanolamine HCl
*expectorant; decongestant* PPA
banned in all OTC products in 2001

guaifenesin & pseudoephedrine
HCl *expectorant; decongestant* 595•
48, 600•60, 795•85 mg oral

Guaifenesin-DM extended-release
caplets ℞ *antitussive; expectorant*
[dextromethorphan hydrobromide;
guaifenesin] 30•600 mg

Guaifenesin-DM syrup OTC *antitussive; expectorant* [dextromethorphan
hydrobromide; guaifenesin] 20•200
mg/10 mL

Guaifenesin-DM NR oral liquid ℞
*antitussive; expectorant* [dextrometh-
orphan hydrobromide; guaifenesin]
20•200 mg/10 mL

Guaifenex oral liquid (discontinued
2002) ℞ *decongestant; expectorant*
[phenylpropanolamine HCl; phenylephrine HCl; guaifenesin] 20•5•
100 mg/5 mL

Guaifenex DM extended-release caplets ℞ *antitussive; expectorant* [dex-
tromethorphan hydrobromide; guai-
fenesin] 30•600 mg

Guaifenex G; Guaifenex LA
extended-release caplets (discontinued 2004) ℞ *expectorant* [guaifene-
sin] 1200 mg; 600 mg

Guaifenex GP extended-release film-
coated tablets ℞ *decongestant; expectorant* [pseudoephedrine HCl; guai-
fenesin] 120•1200 mg

Guaifenex PPA 75 extended-release
tablets (discontinued 2002) ℞ *decongestant; expectorant* [phenylpropanol-
amine HCl; guaifenesin] 75•600 mg

Guaifenex PSE 60; Guaifenex PSE
120 extended-release caplets ℞
*decongestant; expectorant* [pseudo-
ephedrine HCl; guaifenesin] 60•600
mg; 120•600 mg

**Guaifenex-Rx** extended-release tablets (AM and PM) (discontinued 2004) ℞ *decongestant; expectorant* [pseudo-ephedrine HCl + guaifenesin (AM); guaifenesin (PM)] 60•600 mg; 600 mg

**Guaifenex-Rx DM** extended-release tablets (AM and PM) (discontinued 2004) ℞ *decongestant + expectorant (AM); antitussive + expectorant (PM)* [pseudoephedrine HCl + guaifenesin (AM); dextromethorphan hydrobromide + guaifenesin (PM)] 60•600 mg; 30•600 mg

**guaifylline** INN *bronchodilator; expectorant* [also: guaithylline]

**GuaiMAX-D** extended-release caplets ℞ *decongestant; expectorant* [pseudoephedrine HCl; guaifenesin] 120•600 mg

**guaimesal** INN

**Guaipax** sustained-release tablets (discontinued 2002) ℞ *decongestant; expectorant* [phenylpropanolamine HCl; guaifenesin] 75•400 mg

**Guaipax PSE** sustained-release tablets ℞ *decongestant; expectorant* [pseudoephedrine HCl; guaifenesin] 120•600 mg

**guaiphenesin** BAN *expectorant* [also: guaifenesin]

**guaisteine** INN

**Guaitab** tablets (discontinued 2002) OTC *decongestant; expectorant* [pseudoephedrine HCl; guaifenesin] 60•400 mg

**Guaitex LA** sustained-release tablets (discontinued 2002) ℞ *decongestant; expectorant* [phenylpropanolamine HCl; guaifenesin] 75•400 mg

**Guaitex PSE** tablets ℞ *decongestant; expectorant* [pseudoephedrine HCl; guaifenesin] 120•500 mg

**guaithylline** USAN *bronchodilator; expectorant* [also: guaifylline]

**Guai-Vent/PSE** sustained-release tablets ℞ *decongestant; expectorant* [pseudoephedrine HCl; guaifenesin] 120•600 mg

**guamecycline** INN, BAN

**guanabenz** USAN, INN *centrally acting antiadrenergic antihypertensive*

**guanabenz acetate** USAN, USP, JAN *centrally acting antiadrenergic antihypertensive* 4, 8 mg oral

**guanacline** INN, BAN *antihypertensive* [also: guanacline sulfate]

**guanacline sulfate** USAN *antihypertensive* [also: guanacline]

**guanadrel** INN *antihypertensive* [also: guanadrel sulfate]

**guanadrel sulfate** USAN, USP *antihypertensive* [also: guanadrel]

**guanatol HCl** [see: chloroguanide HCl]

**guanazodine** INN

**guancidine** INN *antihypertensive* [also: guancydine]

**guancydine** USAN *antihypertensive* [also: guancidine]

**guanethidine** INN, BAN *antihypertensive* [also: guanethidine monosulfate] ⊡ guanidine

**guanethidine monosulfate** USAN, USP *antihypertensive; investigational (orphan) for reflex sympathetic dystrophy and causalgia* [also: guanethidine]

**guanethidine sulfate** USAN, USP, JAN *antihypertensive*

**guanfacine** INN, BAN *antihypertensive; antiadrenergic* [also: guanfacine HCl] ⊡ guaifenesin

**guanfacine HCl** USAN *antihypertensive; antiadrenergic* [also: guanfacine] 1, 2 mg oral

**guanidine HCl** *cholinergic muscle stimulant* 125 mg oral ⊡ guanethidine

**guanisoquin sulfate** USAN *antihypertensive* [also: guanisoquine]

**guanisoquine** INN *antihypertensive* [also: guanisoquin sulfate]

**guanoclor** INN, BAN *antihypertensive* [also: guanoclor sulfate]

**guanoclor sulfate** USAN *antihypertensive* [also: guanoclor]

**guanoctine** INN *antihypertensive* [also: guanoctine HCl]

**guanoctine HCl** USAN *antihypertensive* [also: guanoctine]

**guanoxabenz** USAN, INN *antihypertensive*

**guanoxan** INN, BAN *antihypertensive* [also: guanoxan sulfate]

**guanoxan sulfate** USAN *antihypertensive* [also: guanoxan]

**guanoxyfen** INN *antihypertensive; antidepressant* [also: guanoxyfen sulfate]

**guanoxyfen sulfate** USAN *antihypertensive; antidepressant* [also: guanoxyfen]

**guar gum** NF *dietary fiber supplement; tablet binder and disintegrant*

**guarana (*Paullinia cupana; P. sorbilis*)** seed paste *medicinal herb for dysentery, malaria, and weight reduction*

**guaranine** [see: caffeine]

**guggul (*Commiphora mukul*)** plant *medicinal herb for hypercholesterolemia and for arthritis and weight reduction in Ayurvedic medicine*

**GuiaCough CF** oral liquid (discontinued 2000) OTC *antitussive; decongestant; expectorant* [dextromethorphan hydrobromide; phenylpropanolamine HCl; guaifenesin; alcohol 4.75%] 10•12.5•100 mg/5 mL

**GuiaCough PE** syrup (discontinued 2000) OTC *decongestant; expectorant* [pseudoephedrine HCl; guaifenesin; alcohol 1.4%] 30•100 mg/5 mL

**Guiadrine DM** sustained-release caplets Ŗ *antitussive; expectorant* [dextromethorphan hydrobromide; guaifenesin] 30•600 mg

**Guiatex** capsules, oral liquid (discontinued 2002) Ŗ *decongestant; expectorant* [phenylephrine HCl; phenylpropanolamine HCl; guaifenesin] 5•45•200 mg; 5•20•100 mg/5 mL

**Guiatex LA** tablets (discontinued 2002) Ŗ *decongestant; expectorant* [phenylpropanolamine HCl; guaifenesin] 75•400 mg

**Guiatex PSE** tablets (discontinued 2002) Ŗ *decongestant; expectorant* [pseudoephedrine HCl; guaifenesin] 120•500 mg

**Guiatuss** syrup OTC *expectorant* [guaifenesin] 100 mg/5 mL ⏃ Guiatussin

**Guiatuss AC** syrup Ŗ *narcotic antitussive; expectorant* [codeine phosphate; guaifenesin; alcohol 3.5%] 20•200 mg/10 mL

**Guiatuss CF** oral liquid (discontinued 2002) OTC *antitussive; decongestant; expectorant* [dextromethorphan hydrobromide; phenylpropanolamine HCl; guaifenesin; alcohol 4.75%] 10•12.5•100 mg/5 mL

**Guiatuss DAC** oral liquid (discontinued 2002) Ŗ *narcotic antitussive; decongestant; expectorant* [codeine phosphate; pseudoephedrine HCl; guaifenesin; alcohol] 10•30•100 mg/5 mL

**Guiatuss DM** oral liquid OTC *antitussive; expectorant* [dextromethorphan hydrobromide; guaifenesin] 20•200 mg/10 mL

**Guiatuss PE** oral liquid OTC *decongestant; expectorant* [pseudoephedrine HCl; guaifenesin] 60•200 mg/10 mL

**Guiatussin DAC** syrup (discontinued 2002) Ŗ *narcotic antitussive; decongestant; expectorant* [codeine phosphate; pseudoephedrine HCl; guaifenesin; alcohol 1.6%] 10•30•100 mg/5 mL ⏃ Guiatuss

**Guiatussin with Codeine Expectorant** oral liquid (discontinued 2002) Ŗ *narcotic antitussive; expectorant* [codeine phosphate; guaifenesin; alcohol 3.5%] 10•100 mg/5 mL

**Guiatussin with Dextromethorphan** oral liquid (discontinued 2002) OTC *antitussive; expectorant* [dextromethorphan hydrobromide; guaifenesin; alcohol 1.4%] 15•100 mg/5 mL

**Guiavent** capsules (discontinued 2002) Ŗ *decongestant; expectorant* [pseudoephedrine HCl; guaifenesin] 120•250 mg

**Guiavent PD** pediatric capsules (discontinued 2002) Ŗ *decongestant; expectorant* [pseudoephedrine HCl; guaifenesin] 60•300 mg

**gum Arabic** *medicinal herb* [see: acacia]

**gum arabic** [see: acacia]

**gum ivy** *medicinal herb* [see: English ivy]

**gum myrrh tree** *medicinal herb* [see: myrrh]

**gum plant** *medicinal herb* [see: comfrey; yerba santa]

**gum senegal** [see: acacia]

**gum tree, hemlock** *medicinal herb* [see: hemlock]

**gum weed** *(Grindelia squarrosa)* flowering top and leaves *medicinal herb for asthma, bronchitis, bladder infection, poison ivy and oak, and psoriasis and other skin disorders*

**guncotton, soluble** [see: pyroxylin]

**gusperimus** INN *immunosuppressant; investigational (orphan) for acute renal graft rejection* [also: gusperimus trihydrochloride; gusperimus HCl]

**gusperimus HCl** JAN *immunosuppressant* [also: gusperimus trihydrochloride; gusperimus]

**gusperimus trihydrochloride** USAN *immunosuppressant* [also: gusperimus; gusperimus HCl]

**Gustase** tablets (discontinued 2002) OTC *digestive enzymes* [amylase; protease; cellulase] 30•6•2 mg

**Gustase Plus** tablet (discontinued 2002) ℞ *digestive enzymes; sedative* [amylase; protease; cellulase; homatropine methylbromide; phenobarbital] 30•6•2•2.5•8 mg

**gutta percha** USP *dental restoration agent*

**GW-2570** *investigational (Phase III) antidiabetic*

**GW275175** *investigational (Phase I) DNA maturation inhibitor for AIDS-related cytomegalovirus retinitis*

**GW433908** *investigational (Phase III) protease inhibitor for HIV infections*

**G-Well** lotion, shampoo (discontinued 2003) ℞ *pediculicide for lice; scabicide* [lindane] 1%

**gymnema** *(Gymnema melicida; G. sylvestre)* leaves and roots *medicinal herb for diabetes, hyperactivity, and hypoglycemia*

**Gynazole-1** vaginal cream in prefilled applicator OTC *antifungal for vulvovaginal candidiasis* [butoconazole nitrate] 2%

**Gynecort Female Creme** cream OTC *topical corticosteroidal anti-inflammatory* [hydrocortisone acetate] 1%

**Gyne-Lotrimin 3** vaginal inserts, combination pack (discontinued 2000 [replaced by 200 mg inserts]) OTC *antifungal* [clotrimazole] 100 mg; 100 mg + 1%

**Gyne-Lotrimin 3** vaginal inserts, vaginal cream, combination pack (inserts + cream) OTC *antifungal* [clotrimazole] 200 mg; 2%; 200 mg + 1%

**Gyne-Lotrimin 7** combination pack (name changed to Gyne-Lotrimin 3 in 2000 [with 200 mg inserts]) OTC *antifungal* [clotrimazole] 100 mg + 1%

**Gyne-Lotrimin 7** vaginal cream OTC *antifungal* [clotrimazole] 1%

**gynergon** [see: estradiol]

**Gyne-Sulf** vaginal cream (discontinued 2001) ℞ *broad-spectrum bacteriostatic* [sulfathiazole; sulfacetamide; sulfabenzamide] 3.42%•2.86%•3.7%

**Gynodiol** tablets ℞ *estrogen replacement therapy for the treatment of postmenopausal symptoms and prevention of postmenopausal osteoporosis; palliative therapy for prostate and metastatic breast cancers* [estradiol] 0.5, 1, 1.5, 2 mg

**gynoestryl** [see: estradiol]

**Gynogen L.A. 20** IM injection (discontinued 2003) ℞ *estrogen replacement therapy for the treatment of postmenopausal symptoms; hormonal antineoplastic for prostate cancer* [estradiol valerate in oil] 20 mg/mL

**Gynol II Contraceptive** vaginal gel, vaginal jelly OTC *spermicidal contraceptive (for use with a diaphragm)* [nonoxynol 9] 2%; 3%

**Gynostemma pentaphyllum** *medicinal herb* [see: jiaogulan]

**Gynovite Plus** tablets OTC *vitamin/mineral/calcium/iron supplement* [multiple vitamins & minerals; calcium; iron; folic acid; biotin] ≛•83•3•0.067•≛ mg

**Gy-Pak** (trademarked packaging form) *unit-of-issue package*

**gypsy weed** *medicinal herb* [see: speed-well]

**Gyrocap** (trademarked dosage form) *timed-release capsule*

**H 9600 SR** sustained-release caplets ℞ *decongestant; expectorant* [pseudo-ephedrine HCl; guaifenesin] 90•600 mg

**H₁ blockers** *a class of antihistamines* [also called: histamine H₁ antagonists]

**H₂ blockers** *a class of gastrointestinal antisecretory agents* [also called: histamine H₂ antagonists]

**²H (deuterium)** [see: deuterium oxide]

**H₂¹⁵O** [see: water O 15]

**³H (tritium)** [see: tritiated water]

**HAART (highly active antiretroviral therapy)** *multi-drug therapy given to HIV-positive patients to prevent progression to AIDS; a generic term applied to several different anti-HIV protocols*

**Habitrol** transdermal patch (discontinued 2003) ℞ *smoking deterrent; nicotine withdrawal aid* [nicotine] 17.5, 35, 52.5 mg

**hachimycin** INN, BAN

**HAD (hexamethylmelamine, Adriamycin, DDP)** *chemotherapy protocol*

**hafnium** *element (Hf)*

**Hair Booster Vitamin** tablets OTC *vitamin/mineral/iron supplement* [multiple B vitamins & minerals; iron; folic acid] ≛•18•0.4 mg

**halarsol** [see: dichlorophenarsine HCl]

**halazepam** USAN, USP, INN, BAN *benzodiazepine anxiolytic; sedative*

**halazone** USP, INN *disinfectant; water purifier*

**halcinonide** USAN, USP, INN, BAN *topical corticosteroidal anti-inflammatory*

**Halcion** tablets ℞ *benzodiazepine sedative; hypnotic* [triazolam] 0.125, 0.25 mg

**Haldol** IM injection ℞ *conventional (typical) antipsychotic; antidyskinetic for Tourette syndrome* [haloperidol lactate] 5 mg/mL ⊡ Halenol; Halog

**Haldol** oral concentrate (discontinued 2003) ℞ *conventional (typical) antipsychotic; antidyskinetic for Tourette syndrome* [haloperidol lactate] 2 mg/mL ⊡ Halenol; Halog

**Haldol** tablets (discontinued 2003) ℞ *conventional (typical) antipsychotic; antidyskinetic for Tourette syndrome* [haloperidol] 0.5, 1, 2, 5, 10, 20 mg

**Haldol Decanoate 50; Haldol Decanoate 100** long-acting IM injection ℞ *conventional (typical) antipsychotic* [haloperidol decanoate] 50 mg/mL; 100 mg/mL

**Halenol, Children's** oral liquid OTC *analgesic; antipyretic* [acetaminophen] 160 mg/5 mL

**haletazole** INN [also: halethazole]

**halethazole** BAN [also: haletazole]

**Haley's M-O** oral liquid OTC *saline/emollient laxative* [magnesium hydroxide; mineral oil] 900 mg•3.75 mL per 15 mL

**Halfan** tablets (discontinued 2003) ℞ *antimalarial (orphan)* [halofantrine HCl] 250 mg

**Halfprin; Halfprin 81** enteric-coated tablets OTC *analgesic; antipyretic; anti-inflammatory; antirheumatic* [aspirin] 165 mg; 81 mg

**Hall's Plus** lozenges OTC *topical oral analgesic; counterirritant; mild local anesthetic; antiseptic* [menthol] 10 mg

**Hall's Sugar Free Mentho-Lyptus** lozenges OTC *topical oral analgesic; counterirritant; mild local anesthetic; antiseptic* [menthol; eucalyptus oil] 5•2.8, 6•2.8 mg

**Halls Zinc Defense** lozenges OTC *topical anti-infective to relieve sore throat* [zinc acetate] 5 mg

**hallucinogens** *a class of agents that induce hallucinations*

**halobetasol propionate** USAN *topical corticosteroidal anti-inflammatory* [also: ulobetasol]

**halocarban** INN *disinfectant* [also: cloflucarban]

**halocortolone** INN

**halocrinic acid** [see: brocrinat]

**halofantrine** INN, BAN *antimalarial* [also: halofantrine HCl]

**halofantrine HCl** USAN *antimalarial (orphan)* [also: halofantrine]

**Halofed** tablets OTC *nasal decongestant* [pseudoephedrine HCl] 30, 60 mg

**halofenate** USAN, INN, BAN *antihyperlipoproteinemic; uricosuric*

**halofuginone** INN, BAN *antiprotozoal* [also: halofuginone hydrobromide]

**halofuginone hydrobromide** USAN *antiprotozoal; investigational (orphan) for scleroderma* [also: halofuginone]

**Halog** ointment, cream, solution ℞ *topical corticosteroidal anti-inflammatory* [halcinonide] 0.1%; 0.025%, 0.1%; 0.1% ⊘ Haldol

**Halog-E** cream ℞ *topical corticosteroidal anti-inflammatory; emollient* [halcinonide] 0.1%

**halometasone** INN

**halonamine** INN

**halopemide** USAN, INN *antipsychotic*

**halopenium chloride** INN, BAN

**haloperidol** USAN, USP, INN, BAN *butyrophenone antipsychotic; antidyskinetic for Tourette syndrome; treatment for children with behavioral disorders such as aggression, combativeness, explosive hyperexcitability, and poor impulse control* 0.5, 1, 2, 5, 10, 20 mg oral

**haloperidol decanoate** USAN, BAN *butyrophenone antipsychotic; antidyskinetic for Tourette syndrome; treatment for children with behavioral disorders such as aggression, combativeness, explosive hyperexcitability, and poor impulse control* 50, 100 mg/mL injection

**haloperidol lactate** *butyrophenone antipsychotic; antidyskinetic for Tourette syndrome; treatment for children with behavioral disorders such as aggression, combativeness, explosive hyperexcitability, and poor impulse control* 2 mg/mL oral; 5 mg/mL injection

**Haloperidol Long Acting** ⓒᴬᴺ *long-acting IM injection* ℞ *conventional (typical) antipsychotic* [haloperidol decanoate] 50, 100 mg/mL

**halopone chloride** [see: halopenium chloride]

**halopredone** INN *topical anti-inflammatory* [also: halopredone acetate]

**halopredone acetate** USAN *topical anti-inflammatory* [also: halopredone]

**haloprogesterone** USAN, INN *progestin*

**haloprogin** USAN, USP, INN, JAN *antibacterial; antifungal*

**halopyramine** BAN [also: chloropyramine]

**Halotestin** tablets (discontinued 2003) ℞ *androgen for hypogonadism or testosterone deficiency in men, delayed puberty in boys, and metastatic breast cancer in women* [fluoxymesterone] 2, 5, 10 mg ⊘ Halotex; Halotussin

**Halotex** cream, solution (discontinued 2004) ℞ *antifungal* [haloprogin] 1% ⊘ Halotestin

**halothane** USP, INN, BAN *inhalation general anesthetic*

**Halotussin** syrup OTC *expectorant* [guaifenesin; alcohol 3.5%] 100 mg/5 mL ⊘ Halotestin

**Halotussin AC** oral liquid ℞ *narcotic antitussive; expectorant* [codeine phosphate; guaifenesin] 20•200 mg/10 mL

**Halotussin DM** oral liquid, sugar-free oral liquid (discontinued 2002) OTC *antitussive; expectorant* [dextromethorphan hydrobromide; guaifenesin] 10•100 mg/5 mL

**haloxazolam** INN

**haloxon** INN, BAN

**halquinol** BAN *topical anti-infective* [also: halquinols]

**halquinols** USAN *topical anti-infective* [also: halquinol]

**Haltran** tablets OTC *analgesic; antiarthritic; antipyretic; nonsteroidal anti-inflammatory drug (NSAID)* [ibuprofen] 200 mg

**HAM (hexamethylmelamine, Adriamycin, melphalan)** *chemotherapy protocol*

**HAM (hexamethylmelamine, Adriamycin, methotrexate)** *chemotherapy protocol*

*Hamamelis virginiana medicinal herb* [see: witch hazel]

**hamamelis water** *medicinal herb* [see: witch hazel]

**hamycin** USAN, INN *antifungal*

**HandiHaler** (trademarked device) *inhalation powder dispenser*

**hard fat** [see: fat, hard]

**hardock** *medicinal herb* [see: burdock]

**hareburr** *medicinal herb* [see: burdock]

*Harpagophytum procumbens medicinal herb* [see: devil's claw]

**hashish** *(Cannabis sativa) euphoric/hallucinogenic street drug made from the resin of the flowering tops of the cannabis plant*

**Havrix** adult IM injection, pediatric IM injection ℞ *immunization against hepatitis A virus (HAV)* [hepatitis A vaccine, inactivated] 1440 ELISA units (EL.U.)/mL; 360, 720 EL.U./0.5 mL

**haw** *medicinal herb* [see: hawthorn]

**Hawaiian Tropic Cool Aloe with I.C.E.** gel OTC *topical local anesthetic; analgesic; counterirritant* [lidocaine; menthol] 2 • 2

**hawthorn** *(Crataegus laevigata; C. monogyna; C. oxyacantha)* flowers, leaves, and berries *medicinal herb for angina pectoris, arrhythmias, arteriosclerosis, enlarged heart, high or low blood pressure, hypoglycemia, palpitations, and tachycardia; also used as an antiseptic*

**Hayfebrol** oral liquid OTC *decongestant; antihistamine* [pseudoephedrine HCl; chlorpheniramine maleate] 60•4 mg/10 mL

**hazel, snapping; hazelnut** *medicinal herb* [see: witch hazel]

**H-BIG** IM injection (discontinued 2000) ℞ *hepatitis B immunizing agent* [hepatitis B immune globulin] 4, 5 mL

**H-BIG** IV injection *investigational (orphan) prophylaxis against hepatitis B reinfection in liver transplant patients* [hepatitis B immune globulin]

**HBIG (hepatitis B immune globulin)** [q.v.]

**hBNP (human B-type natriuretic peptide)** [see: nesiritide; nesiritide citrate]

**1% HC** ointment ℞ *topical corticosteroidal anti-inflammatory* [hydrocortisone] 1%

**HC (hydrocortisone)** [q.v.]

**4-HC (4-hydroperoxycyclophosphamide)** [q.v.]

**HC Derma-Pax** topical liquid OTC *corticosteroidal anti-inflammatory; antihistamine; antiseptic* [hydrocortisone; pyrilamine maleate; chlorpheniramine maleate; chlorobutanol] 0.5%•0.44%•0.06%•25%

**HCA (hydrocortisone acetate)** [q.v.]

**H-CAP (hexamethylmelamine, cyclophosphamide, Adriamycin, Platinol)** *chemotherapy protocol*

**hCG (human chorionic gonadotropin)** [see: gonadotropin, chorionic]

**HCT (hydrochlorothiazide)** [q.v.]

**HCTZ (hydrochlorothiazide)** [q.v.]

**HD 85** oral/rectal suspension ℞ *radiopaque contrast medium for gastrointestinal imaging* [barium sulfate] 85%

**HD 200 Plus** powder for oral suspension ℞ *radiopaque contrast medium for gastrointestinal imaging* [barium sulfate] 98%

**HDCV (human diploid cell vaccine)** [see: rabies vaccine]

**HDMTX (high-dose methotrexate [with leucovorin rescue])** *chemotherapy protocol for bone sarcoma*

**HDMTX-CF (high-dose methotrexate, citrovorum factor)** *chemotherapy protocol*

**HDMTX/LV (high-dose methotrex-ate, leucovorin [rescue])** *chemotherapy protocol*

**HDPEB (high-dose PEB protocol)** *chemotherapy protocol* [see: PEB]

**HD-VAC (high-dose [methotrex-ate], vinblastine, Adriamycin, cisplatin)** *chemotherapy protocol*

**HE-200** *investigational (Phase I/II) cellular energy regulator for HIV and AIDS*

**Head & Shoulders; Head & Shoulders Dry Scalp** shampoo OTC *antiseborrheic; antibacterial; antifungal* [pyrithione zinc] 1%

**Head & Shoulders Intensive Treatment** lotion/shampoo OTC *antiseborrheic; dandruff treatment* [selenium sulfide] 1%

**heal-all** *medicinal herb* [see: figwort; stone root; woundwort]

**healing herb** *medicinal herb* [see: comfrey]

**Healon; Healon GV** intraocular injection ℞ *viscoelastic agent for ophthalmic surgery* [hyaluronate sodium] 10 mg/mL; 14 mg/mL

**Healon Yellow** intraocular injection ℞ *viscoelastic agent for ophthalmic surgery; diagnostic agent* [hyaluronate sodium; fluorescein sodium] 10•0.005 mg/mL

**Healon5** ⓒⒶⓃ intraocular injection in preloaded syringes ℞ *viscoelastic agent for ophthalmic surgery* [hyaluronate sodium 5000] 23 mg/0.6 mL

**heart, mother's; shepherd's heart** *medicinal herb* [see: shepherd's purse]

**Heartline** enteric-coated tablets OTC *analgesic; antipyretic; anti-inflammatory; antirheumatic* [aspirin] 81 mg

**heather (Calluna vulgaris)** flowering shoots *medicinal herb used as an antiseptic, cholagogue, diaphoretic, diuretic, expectorant, and vasoconstrictor*

**heavy liquid petrolatum** [see: mineral oil]

**heavy water (D₂O)** [see: deuterium oxide]

**Hectorol** softgels ℞ *synthetic vitamin D analogue; calcium regulator for hyper-*parathyroidism secondary to chronic renal dialysis [doxercalciferol] 2.5, 5 μg

**hedaquinium chloride** INN, BAN

*Hedeoma pulegeoides* *medicinal herb* [see: pennyroyal]

*Hedera helix* *medicinal herb* [see: English ivy]

**hedge bindweed (Convolvulus sepium)** flowering plant and roots *medicinal herb used as a cholagogue, febrifuge, and purgative*

**hedge garlic (Sisymbrium alliaria)** *medicinal herb* [see: garlic]

**hedge hyssop (Gratiola officinalis)** plant *medicinal herb used as a cardiac, diuretic, purgative, and vermifuge*

**hedge-burs** *medicinal herb* [see: bedstraw]

**"hedgehog" proteins** *a class of novel human proteins that induce the formation of regenerative tissue*

**Heet Liniment** OTC *analgesic; counterirritant; antiseptic* [methyl salicylate; camphor; capsaicin; alcohol 70%] 15%•3.6%•0.025%

**hefilcon A** USAN *hydrophilic contact lens material*

**hefilcon B** USAN *hydrophilic contact lens material*

**hefilcon C** USAN *hydrophilic contact lens material*

**helenien** [see: xantofyl palmitate]

*Helianthemum canadense* *medicinal herb* [see: rock rose]

**Helicide** ℞ *investigational (Phase III) combination therapy for H. pylori infection*

**helicon** [see: aspirin]

**Helicosol** powder for oral solution ℞ *diagnostic aid for detection of H. pylori in the stomach* [carbon C 13 urea]

**Helidac** 14-day dose-pack ℞ *combination treatment for active duodenal ulcer with H. pylori infection* [bismuth subsalicylate (chewable tablets); metronidazole (tablets); tetracycline HCl (capsules)] 262.4 mg; 250 mg; 500 mg

**heliomycin** INN

**heliox** *helium-oxygen mixture used for respiratory distress (usually an 80%•20% mix)*

**Helistat** sponge ℞ *topical local hemostat for surgery* [absorbable collagen sponge]

**helium** USP *diluent for gases; element (He)*

**Helivax** ℞ *investigational (Phase II) H. pylori vaccine*

**Helixate FS** powder for IV injection ℞ *antihemophilic* [antihemophilic factor concentrate, recombinant, solvent/detergent-treated] 250, 500, 1000 IU

**hellebore (*Helleborus* spp.; *Veratrum* spp.)** rhizome *medicinal herb used as an antihypertensive; not generally regarded as safe and effective for internal consumption due to toxicity*

***Helleborus* spp.** *medicinal herb* [see: hellebore]

**helmet flower** *medicinal herb* [see: aconite; sandalwood; skullcap]

**helmet pod** *medicinal herb* [see: twin leaf]

**HEMA (2-hydroxyethyl methacrylate)** *contact lens material*

**Hemabate** IM injection ℞ *prostaglandin-type abortifacient; for postpartum uterine bleeding* [carboprost tromethamine] 250 μg/mL

**Hema-Check** slide tests for home use *in vitro diagnostic aid for fecal occult blood*

**Hema-Combistix** reagent strips *in vitro diagnostic aid for multiple urine products*

**Hemaspan** timed-release tablets OTC *hematinic; iron/vitamin C supplement* [iron (from ferrous fumarate); ascorbic acid; docusate sodium] 110•200•20 mg

**Hemastix** reagent strips for professional use *in vitro diagnostic aid for urine occult blood*

**Hematest** reagent tablets for professional use *in vitro diagnostic aid for fecal occult blood*

**hematin** [now: hemin]

**Hematinic** tablets ℞ *hematinic* [ferrous fumarate; folic acid] 106 mg Fe•1 mg

**Hematinic Plus** tablets ℞ *hematinic; vitamin/mineral supplement* [multiple vitamins & minerals; ferrous fumarate; folic acid] ≐ •106 mg Fe•1 mg

**hematinics** *a class of iron-containing agents for the prevention and treatment of iron-deficiency anemia*

**hematopoietics** *a class of antianemic agents that promote the formation of red blood cells*

**heme arginate** *investigational (orphan) for acute symptomatic porphyria and myelodysplastic syndrome*

**HemeSelect Collection** kit for home use *in vitro diagnostic aid for fecal occult blood* [for use with HemeSelect Reagent kit]

**HemeSelect Reagent** kit for professional use *in vitro diagnostic aid for fecal occult blood* [for use with HemeSelect Collection kit]

**Hemex** ℞ *investigational (orphan) for acute porphyric syndromes* [hemin; zinc mesoporphyrin]

**hemiacidrin** [see: citric acid, glucono-delta-lactone & magnesium carbonate]

**hemin** *enzyme inhibitor for acute intermittent porphyria (AIP), porphyria variegata, and hereditary coproporphyria (orphan)*

**hemin & zinc mesoporphyrin** *investigational (orphan) for acute porphyric syndromes*

**hemlock (*Tsuga canadensis*)** bark *medicinal herb used as an astringent, diaphoretic, and diuretic*

**Hemoccult** slide tests for professional use, test tape for professional use *in vitro diagnostic aid for fecal occult blood*

**Hemoccult II** slide tests for professional use *in vitro diagnostic aid for fecal occult blood*

**Hemoccult II Dispenserpak; Hemoccult II Dispenserpak Plus** slide tests for home use *in vitro diagnostic aid for fecal occult blood*

**Hemoccult SENSA; Hemoccult II SENSA** slide tests for professional use *in vitro diagnostic aid for fecal occult blood*

**Hemocitrate** *investigational (orphan) adjunct to leukapheresis procedures* [sodium citrate]

**Hemocyte** tablets OTC *hematinic* [ferrous fumarate (source of iron)] 324 mg (106 mg)

**Hemocyte Plus** elixir ℞ *hematinic* [polysaccharide-iron complex; multiple B vitamins & minerals; folic acid] 12•±•0.33 mg

**Hemocyte Plus** tablets ℞ *hematinic* [ferrous fumarate; multiple B vitamins & minerals; sodium ascorbate; folic acid] 106•±•200•1 mg

**Hemocyte-F** elixir ℞ *hematinic* [polysaccharide-iron complex; cyanocobalamin; folic acid] 100 mg Fe•25 μg•1 mg per 5 mL

**Hemocyte-F** tablets ℞ *hematinic* [ferrous fumarate; folic acid] 106•1 mg

**Hemofil M** IV injection ℞ *antihemophilic to correct coagulation deficiency* [antihemophilic factor concentrate] 10, 20, 30 mL

**hemoglobin, recombinant human (rHb1.1)** *investigational agent for chronic anemia*

**hemoglobin crosfumaril** USAN, INN *investigational (Phase III) blood substitute for perfusion deficit disorders and blood loss due to severe trauma*

**Hemokine** *investigational progenitor cell stimulator for neutropenia and thrombocytopenia* [muplestim]

**Hemolink** ℞ *investigational (Phase III) human blood substitute for surgery and chronic anemia associated with kidney failure*

**Hemonyne** IV infusion (discontinued 2001) ℞ *antihemophilic to correct factor IX deficiency (Christmas disease)* [coagulation factors II, VII, IX, and X, heat treated] 20, 40 mL

**Hemopad** fiber ℞ *topical hemostatic aid in surgery* [microfibrillar collagen hemostat]

**Hemophilus b conjugate vaccine** *active bacterin for* Haemophilus influenzae *type b*

**Hemopure** ℞ *investigational (Phase III) oxygen-carrier blood substitute* [hemoglobin glutamer 250 bovine]

**Hemorid for Women** cream OTC *topical local anesthetic and vasoconstrictor for hemorrhoids* [pramoxine HCl; phenylephrine HCl] 1%•0.25%

**Hemorid for Women** lotion OTC *topical emollient and protectant for hemorrhoids* [mineral oil; petrolatum; glycerin]

**Hemorid for Women** rectal suppositories OTC *vasoconstrictor and astringent for hemorrhoids* [zinc oxide; phenylephrine HCl] 11%•0.25%

**Hemorrhoidal HC** rectal suppositories ℞ *corticosteroidal anti-inflammatory for hemorrhoids* [hydrocortisone acetate] 25 mg

**hemostatics** *a class of therapeutic blood modifiers that arrest the flow of blood* [see also: astringents; styptics]

**Hemotene** fiber ℞ *topical hemostatic aid in surgery* [microfibrillar collagen hemostat] 1 g

**Hemovit** film-coated tablets ℞ *hematinic* [multiple B vitamins; vitamin C; folic acid; biotin] ±•60•1•0.3 mg

**hemp** *medicinal herb* [see: marijuana]

**hemp agrimony (Eupatorium cannabinum)** *plant medicinal herb used as a cholagogue, diaphoretic, diuretic, emetic, expectorant, and purgative*

**hemp nettle (Galeopsis tetrahit)** *plant medicinal herb used as an astringent, diuretic, and expectorant*

**Hem-Prep** anorectal ointment, rectal suppositories OTC *temporary relief of hemorrhoidal symptoms; topical vasoconstrictor; astringent* [phenylephrine HCl; zinc oxide] 0.025%•11%; 0.25%•11%

**Hemril** Uniserts (rectal suppositories) OTC *temporary relief of hemorrhoidal symptoms* [bismuth subgallate; bismuth resorcin compound; benzyl benzoate; peruvian balsam; zinc oxide] 2.25%•1.75%•1.2%•1.8%•11%

**Hemril-HC** Uniserts (suppositories) ℞ *corticosteroidal anti-inflammatory* for hemorrhoids [hydrocortisone acetate] 25 mg

**henbane (Hyoscyamus niger)** plant *medicinal herb used as an anodyne, antispasmodic, calmative, and narcotic; primarily used externally because of its high toxicity*

**heneicosafluorotripropylamine** [see: perfluamine]

**henna (Alkanna tinctoria)** root *medicinal herb used as an astringent, antibiotic, and cosmetic dye; not generally regarded as safe and effective*

**henna (Lawsonia inermis)** leaves *medicinal herb used as an astringent*

**HEOD (hexachloro-epoxy-octahy-dro-dimethanonaphthalene)** [see: dieldrin]

**Hepandrin** ℞ *anabolic steroid for weight gain; investigational (orphan) for muscular dystrophy, AIDS-wasting syndrome, and alcoholic hepatitis; also abused as a street drug* [oxandrolone]

**heparin** BAN *anticoagulant; antithrombotic* [also: heparin calcium]

**heparin, 2-0-desulfated** *investigational (orphan) for cystic fibrosis*

**heparin calcium** USP *anticoagulant; antithrombotic* [also: heparin]

**Heparin I.V. Flush** prefilled syringe ℞ *IV flush for catheter patency (not therapeutic)* [heparin sodium] 1 U/mL

**Heparin Lock Flush** solution ℞ *IV flush for catheter patency (not therapeutic)* [heparin sodium] 10, 100 U/mL

**heparin sodium** USP, INN, BAN *anticoagulant; antithrombotic* 1000, 2000, 2500, 5000, 7500, 10 000, 20 000, 40 000 U/mL injection

**heparin sodium & sodium chloride 0.45%** *anticoagulant; antithrombotic* 12 500 U•250 mL, 25 000 U•250 mL, 25 000 U•500 mL

**heparin sodium & sodium chloride 0.9%** *anticoagulant; antithrombotic* 1000 U•500 mL, 2000 U•1000 mL

**heparin sulfate** [see: danaparoid sodium]

**heparin whole blood** [see: blood, whole]

**heparinase 1** *investigational (Phase III) agent for the reversal of heparin-induced anticoagulation*

**heparinase III** *investigational cardio-protective agent*

**HepatAmine** IV infusion ℞ *nutritional therapy for hepatic failure and hepatic encephalopathy* [multiple branched-chain essential and nonessential amino acids; electrolytes]

**hepatica (Hepatica acutiloba; H. triloba)** leaves and flowers *medicinal herb used as a diuretic and pectoral*

**Hepatic-Aid II Instant Drink** powder OTC *enteral nutritional treatment for chronic liver disease* [multiple branched chain amino acids]

**hepatics** *a class of agents that affect the liver (a term used in folk medicine)*

**hepatitis A vaccine, inactivated** *active immunizing agent for the hepatitis A virus (HAV)*

**hepatitis B immune globulin (HBIG)** USP *passive immunizing agent; investigational (orphan) prophylaxis against hepatitis B reinfection in liver transplant patients*

**hepatitis B surface antigen (HBsAg)** [see: hepatitis B virus vaccine, inactivated]

**hepatitis B virus vaccine, inactivated** USP *active immunizing agent for hepatitis B and D*

**Hepflush-10** solution ℞ *IV flush for catheter patency (not therapeutic)* [heparin sodium] 10 U/mL

**Hep-Forte** capsules OTC *geriatric dietary supplement* [multiple vitamins & food products; folic acid; biotin] ≐• 60•≗ μg

**Hep-Lock; Hep-Lock U/P** solution ℞ *IV flush for catheter patency (not therapeutic)* [heparin sodium] 10, 100 U/mL

**HEPP (H-chain ε [IgE] pentapeptide)** [see: pentigetide]

**hepronicate** INN

**Hepsera** tablets ℞ *nucleotide analogue reverse transcriptase inhibitor for chronic hepatitis B virus (HBV) infection* [adefovir dipivoxil] 10 mg

**heptabarb** INN [also: heptabarbitone]

**heptabarbital** [see: heptabarb; hepta-barbitone]

**heptabarbitone** BAN [also: heptabarb]

**heptaminol** INN, BAN

**heptaminol HCl** [see: heptaminol]

**2-heptanamine** [see: tuaminoheptane]

**2-heptanamine sulfate** [see: tuami-noheptane sulfate]

**heptaverine** INN

**heptolamide** INN

**Heptovir** ⓒ tablets, oral solution ℞ antiviral nucleoside reverse transcriptase inhibitor for hepatitis B virus (HBV) [lamivudine] 100 mg; 5 mg/mL

**hepzidine** INN

**HER2 MAb (human epidermal growth factor receptor 2 mono-clonal antibodies)** [see: trastuzumab]

*Heracleum lanatum* medicinal herb [see: masterwort]

**herb of grace** medicinal herb [see: rue]

**HercepTest** test kit diagnostic aid for the HER2 protein, used to screen patients who may benefit from treatment with Herceptin

**Herceptin** powder for IV infusion ℞ anti-HER2 monoclonal antibody for metastatic breast cancer; investigational (NDA filed) for ovarian and female gen-ital tract cancers [trastuzumab] 440 mg

**Hercules woundwort** medicinal herb [see: woundwort]

**heroin** potent narcotic analgesic street drug which is highly addictive; banned in the U.S. [medically known as diamor-phine and diacetylmorphine HCl]

**heroin HCl** (banned in the U.S.) [see: diacetylmorphine HCl]

**Herpecin-L** lip balm OTC vulnerary; sunblock [allantoin; padimate O]

**herpes simplex virus gene** investiga-tional (orphan) for primary and meta-static brain tumors

**Herpetrol** tablets (discontinued 2001) OTC dietary supplement; claimed to pre-vent and treat herpes simplex infections [L-lysine; multiple vitamins; zinc]

**Herrick Lacrimal Plug** ℞ blocks the puncta and canaliculus to eliminate tear loss in keratitis sicca [silicone plug]

**HES (hydroxyethyl starch)** [see: hetastarch]

**Hespan** IV infusion ℞ plasma volume expander for shock due to hemorrhage, burns, surgery [hetastarch] 6 g/100 mL ② Histatan

**hesperidin** a bioflavonoid (q.v.)

**hesperidin methyl chalcone** [see: bioflavonoids]

**hetacillin** USAN, USP, INN, BAN anti-bacterial

**hetacillin potassium** USAN, USP anti-bacterial

**hetaflur** USAN, INN, BAN dental caries prophylactic

**hetastarch** USAN, BAN plasma volume extender [also: hydroxyethylstarch] 6% in normal saline

**heteronium bromide** USAN, INN, BAN anticholinergic

**Hetrazan** tablets (available for com-passionate use only) ℞ anthelmintic for Bancroft filariasis, onchocerciasis, tropical eosinophilia, and loiasis [diethylcarbamazine citrate] 50 mg

**hexaammonium molybdate tetra-hydrate** [see: ammonium molybdate]

**Hexabrix** injection ℞ radiopaque con-trast medium [ioxaglate meglumine; ioxaglate sodium (54.3% total iodine)] 393•196 mg/mL (320 mg/mL)

**HexaCAF; Hexa-CAF (hexameth-ylmelamine, cyclophosphamide, amethopterin, fluorouracil)** che-motherapy protocol for ovarian cancer

**hexacarbacholine bromide** INN [also: carbolonium bromide]

**hexachlorane** [see: lindane]

**hexachlorocyclohexane** [see: lindane]

**hexachlorophane** BAN topical anti-infec-tive; detergent [also: hexachlorophene]

**hexachlorophene** USP, INN topical anti-infective; detergent [also: hexa-chlorophane]

**hexacyclonate sodium** INN

**hexacyprone** INN

hexadecanoic acid, methylethyl ester [see: isopropyl palmitate]

hexadecanol [see: cetyl alcohol]

hexadecylamine hydrofluoride [see: hetaflur]

hexadecylpyridinium chloride [see: cetylpyridinium chloride]

hexadecyltrimethylammonium bromide [see: cetrimonium bromide]

hexadecyltrimethylammonium chloride [see: cetrimonium chloride]

2,4-hexadienoic acid, potassium salt [see: potassium sorbate]

hexadiline INN

hexadimethrine bromide INN, BAN

hexadiphane [see: prozapine]

Hexadrol tablets, elixir ℞ corticosteroid; anti-inflammatory [dexamethasone] 1.5, 4 mg; 0.5 mg/5 mL ② Hexalol

Hexadrol Phosphate intra-articular, intralesional, soft tissue, or IM injection ℞ corticosteroid; anti-inflammatory [dexamethasone sodium phosphate] 4, 10, 20 mg/mL

hexadylamine [see: hexadiline]

hexafluorenium bromide USAN, USP skeletal muscle relaxant; succinylcholine synergist [also: hexafluronium bromide]

hexafluorodiethyl ether [see: flurothyl]

hexaflurone bromide [see: hexafluorenium bromide]

hexafluronium bromide INN skeletal muscle relaxant; succinylcholine synergist [also: hexafluorenium bromide]

Hexalen capsules ℞ antineoplastic for advanced ovarian adenocarcinoma (orphan) [altretamine] 50 mg ② Hexalol

hexamarium bromide [see: distigmine bromide]

hexametazime BAN

hexamethone bromide [see: hexamethonium bromide]

hexamethonium bromide INN, BAN

hexamethylenamine [now: methenamine]

hexamethylenamine mandelate [see: methenamine mandelate]

hexamethylenetetramine [see: methenamine]

hexamethylmelamine (HMM; HXM) [see: altretamine]

hexamidine INN

hexamine hippurate BAN urinary antibacterial [also: methenamine hippurate]

hexamine mandelate [see: methenamine mandelate]

hexapradol INN

hexaprofen INN, BAN

hexapropymate INN, BAN

hexasonium iodide INN

hexavitamin USP

Hexavitamin tablets OTC vitamin supplement [multiple vitamins]

hexcarbacholine bromide INN [also: carbolonium bromide]

hexedine USAN, INN antibacterial

hexemal [see: cyclobarbital]

hexestrol NF, INN

hexetidine BAN

hexicide [see: lindane]

hexinol [see: cyclomenol]

hexobarbital USP, INN

hexobarbital sodium NF

hexobendine USAN, INN, BAN vasodilator

hexocyclium methylsulfate peptic ulcer adjunct [also: hexocyclium metilsulfate; hexocyclium methylsulphate]

hexocyclium methylsulphate BAN [also: hexocyclium methylsulfate; hexocyclium metilsulfate]

hexocyclium metilsulfate INN [also: hexocyclium methylsulfate; hexocyclium methylsulphate]

hexoprenaline INN, BAN tocolytic; bronchodilator [also: hexoprenaline sulfate]

hexoprenaline sulfate USAN, JAN investigational (NDA filed) tocolytic; bronchodilator [also: hexoprenaline]

hexopyrimidine [see: hexetidine]

hexopyrrolate [see: hexopyrronium bromide]

hexopyrronium bromide INN

hexydaline [see: methenamine mandelate]

**hexylcaine** INN *local anesthetic* [also: hexylcaine HCl]

**hexylcaine HCl** USP *local anesthetic* [also: hexylcaine]

**hexylene glycol** NF *humectant; solvent*

**hexylresorcinol** USP *anthelmintic; topical antiseptic*

**1-hexyltheobromine** [see: pentifylline]

**H-F Gel** ℞ *investigational (orphan) emergency treatment for hydrofluoric acid burns* [calcium gluconate]

**HFA-134a** *propellant used in CFC-free aerosol delivery systems*

**hFSH (human follicle-stimulating hormone)** [now: menotropins]

**HFZ (homofenazine)** [q.v.]

**¹⁹⁷Hg** [see: chlormerodrin Hg 197]

**¹⁹⁷Hg** [see: merisoprol acetate Hg 197]

**¹⁹⁷Hg** [see: merisoprol Hg 197]

**²⁰³Hg** [see: chlormerodrin Hg 203]

**²⁰³Hg** [see: merisoprol acetate Hg 203]

**hGH (human growth hormone)** [see: somatropin]

**HGP-30W** *investigational (Phase II) vaccine for HIV*

**HGP-30W & sargramostim** *investigational (Phase I) combination for HIV infection*

**HI-236** *investigational for multidrug-resistant HIV infection*

**hibenzate** INN *combining name for radicals or groups* [also: hybenzate]

**Hibiclens** sponge/brush OTC *broad-spectrum antimicrobial; germicidal* [chlorhexidine gluconate; alcohol 4%] 4%

**Hibiclens Antiseptic/AntiMicrobial Skin Cleanser** topical liquid OTC *broad-spectrum antimicrobial; germicidal* [chlorhexidine gluconate; alcohol 4%] 4%

**hibiscus (Hibiscus sabdariffa and other species)** flowers and leaves *medicinal herb for cancer, edema, heart problems and nervous disorders; also used topically as an emollient; not generally regarded as safe and effective*

**Hibistat Germicidal Hand Rinse** topical liquid OTC *broad-spectrum antimicrobial; germicidal* [chlorhexidine gluconate; alcohol 70%] 0.5%

**Hibistat Towelette** OTC *broad-spectrum antimicrobial; germicidal* [chlorhexidine gluconate; alcohol 70%] 0.5%

**HibTITER** IM injection ℞ *pediatric (2–71 months) vaccine for Haemophilus influenzae type b (HIB)* [Hemophilus b conjugate vaccine (with a diphtheria CRM₁₉₇ carrier)] 10• (25) µg/0.5 mL

**Hi-C DAZE (high-dose cytarabine, daunorubicin, azacitidine, etoposide)** *chemotherapy protocol for acute myelogenous leukemia (AML)*

**Hi-Cal VM** nutrition bar OTC *enteral nutritional therapy for HIV and AIDS*

**Hi-Cor 1.0; Hi-Cor 2.5** cream ℞ *topical corticosteroidal anti-inflammatory* [hydrocortisone] 1%; 2.5%

**HIDA (hepatoiminodiacetic acid)** [see: lidofenin]

**HiDAC (high-dose ara-C)** *chemotherapy protocol*

**Hieracium pilosella** *medicinal herb* [see: mouse ear]

**high angelica** *medicinal herb* [see: angelica]

**high molecular weight dextran** [see: dextran 70]

**high osmolar contrast media (HOCM)** *a class of older radiopaque agents that have a high osmolar concentration of iodine (the contrast agent), which corresponds to a higher incidence of adverse reactions* [also called: ionic contrast media]

**High Potency N-Vites** tablets OTC *vitamin supplement* [multiple B vitamins; vitamin C] ±•500 mg

**High Potency Tar** gel shampoo (discontinued 2003) OTC *antiseborrheic; antipsoriatic; antipruritic; antibacterial* [coal tar] 25%

**hilafilcon A** USAN *hydrophilic contact lens material*

**hilafilcon B** USAN *hydrophilic contact lens material*

**hillberry** *medicinal herb* [see: wintergreen]

**Himalayan ginseng (Panax pseudoginseng)** *medicinal herb* [see: ginseng]

**hindheel** *medicinal herb* [see: tansy]

**hini** *medicinal herb* [see: Culver root]

**hioxifilcon A** USAN *hydrophilic contact lens material*

**Hipotest** tablets OTC *dietary supplement* [multiple vitamins & minerals; multiple food products; calcium; iron; biotin] $\pm$•53.5•50•0.001 mg

**Hi-Po-Vites** tablets OTC *dietary supplement* [multiple vitamins & minerals; multiple food products; iron; folic acid; biotin] $\pm$•6•0.4•1 mg

**Hiprex** tablets ℞ *urinary antibiotic* [methenamine hippurate] 1 g

**Hirudo medicinalis** *natural treatment* [see: leeches]

**Histade** sustained-release capsules ℞ *decongestant; antihistamine* [pseudoephedrine HCl; chlorpheniramine maleate] 120•12 mg

**Histagesic Modified** tablets (discontinued 2002) OTC *decongestant; antihistamine; analgesic* [phenylephrine HCl; chlorpheniramine maleate; acetaminophen] 10•4•324 mg

**Histalet** syrup (discontinued 2002) ℞ *decongestant; antihistamine* [pseudoephedrine HCl; chlorpheniramine maleate] 45•3 mg/5 mL

**Histalet Forte** tablets (discontinued 2001) ℞ *decongestant; antihistamine* [phenylpropanolamine HCl; phenylephrine HCl; chlorpheniramine maleate; pyrilamine maleate] 50•10•4•25 mg

**Histalet X** tablets, syrup (discontinued 2002) ℞ *decongestant; expectorant* [pseudoephedrine HCl; guaifenesin] 120•400 mg; 45•200 mg/5 mL

**histamine dihydrochloride** USAN *investigational (Phase III) histamine $H_2$ receptor agonist for malignant melanoma and acute myeloid leukemia (AML); investigational (Phase II) for hepatitis C and renal cell carcinoma*

**histamine $H_1$ antagonists** *a class of antihistamines* [also called: $H_1$ blockers]

**histamine $H_2$ antagonists** *a class of gastrointestinal antisecretory agents* [also called: $H_2$ blockers]

**histamine phosphate** USP *gastric secretory stimulant; diagnostic aid for pheochromocytoma*

**histantin** [see: chlorcyclizine HCl]

**histapyrrodine** INN

**Histatab Plus** tablets OTC *decongestant; antihistamine* [phenylephrine HCl; chlorpheniramine maleate] 5•2 mg

**Hista-Vadrin** tablets (discontinued 2001) ℞ *decongestant; antihistamine* [phenylpropanolamine HCl; phenylephrine HCl; chlorpheniramine maleate] 40•5•6 mg

**Hista-Vent DA** sustained-release caplets ℞ *decongestant; antihistamine; anticholinergic to dry mucosal secretions* [phenylephrine HCl; chlorpheniramine maleate; methscopolamine nitrate] 20•8•2.5 mg

**Histenol-Forte** tablets OTC *antitussive; decongestant; analgesic* [dextromethorphan hydrobromide; pseudoephedrine HCl; acetaminophen] 10•30•325 mg

**Histerone 100** IM injection (discontinued 2001) ℞ *androgen replacement for delayed puberty or breast cancer* [testosterone] 100 mg/mL

**Histex** oral liquid ℞ *decongestant; antihistamine* [pseudoephedrine HCl; chlorpheniramine maleate] 60•4 mg/10 mL

**Histex CT** film-coated timed-release tablets ℞ *antihistamine for allergic rhinitis* [carbinoxamine maleate] 8 mg

**Histex HC** oral liquid ℞ *narcotic antitussive; decongestant; antihistamine* [hydrocodone bitartrate; pseudoephedrine HCl; carbinoxamine maleate] 5•30•2 mg/5 mL

**Histex Pd** oral liquid ℞ *antihistamine for allergic rhinitis* [carbinoxamine maleate] 4 mg/5 mL

**Histex SR** extended-release capsules ℞ *decongestant; antihistamine* [pseudoephedrine HCl; brompheniramine maleate] 120•10 mg

**Histex SR** film-coated, sustained-release tablets ℞ *decongestant; antihistamine; analgesic* [phenylephrine HCl; chlorpheniramine maleate; acetaminophen] 40•8•500 mg

**histidine (L-histidine)** USAN, USP, INN *amino acid (essential in infants and in renal failure, nonessential otherwise); symbols: His, H*

**histidine monohydrochloride** NF

**495-L-histidineglucosylceramidase** [see: imiglucerase]

**Histine DM; Histinex DM** syrup (discontinued 2002) ℞ *antitussive; decongestant; antihistamine* [dextromethorphan hydrobromide; phenylpropanolamine HCl; brompheniramine maleate] 10•12.5•2 mg/5 mL

**Histinex HC** syrup ℞ *narcotic antitussive; decongestant; antihistamine* [hydrocodone bitartrate; phenylephrine HCl; chlorpheniramine maleate] 5•10•4 mg/10 mL

**Histinex PV** syrup ℞ *narcotic antitussive; decongestant; antihistamine* [hydrocodone bitartrate; pseudoephedrine HCl; chlorpheniramine maleate] 5•60•4 mg/10 mL

**Histolyn-CYL** intradermal injection ℞ *diagnostic aid for histoplasmosis* [histoplasmin (mycelial derivative)] 1:100

**histoplasmin** USP *dermal histoplasmosis test; Histoplasma capsulatum cultures in mycelial or yeast lysate form* 1:100 injection (yeast lysate form)

**Histor-D** syrup (discontinued 2002) ℞ *decongestant; antihistamine* [phenylephrine HCl; chlorpheniramine maleate; alcohol 2%] 5•2 mg/5 mL

**Histosal** tablets (discontinued 2001) OTC *decongestant; antihistamine; analgesic* [phenylpropanolamine HCl; pyrilamine maleate; acetaminophen; caffeine] 20•12.5•324•30 mg

**histrelin** USAN, INN *LHRH agonist; investigational (orphan) for acute intermittent porphyria, hereditary coproporphyria, and variegate porphyria; investigational (Phase III) for prostate cancer*

**histrelin acetate** *LHRH agonist; central precocious puberty treatment (orphan)*

**Histussin D** oral liquid ℞ *narcotic antitussive; decongestant* [hydrocodone bitartrate; pseudoephedrine HCl] 5•60 mg/5 mL

**Histussin HC** syrup ℞ *narcotic antitussive; decongestant; antihistamine* [hydrocodone bitartrate; phenylephrine HCl; chlorpheniramine maleate] 2.5•5•2 mg/5 mL

**HIV immune globulin (HIVIG)** *investigational (Phase III, orphan) immunomodulator for AIDS and maternal/fetal HIV transfer*

**HIV immunotherapeutic (HIV-IT); HIV therapeutic** *investigational (Phase II) gene therapy for HIV; investigational (Phase I–III) antiviral for symptomatic HIV*

**HIV protease inhibitors** *a class of antivirals that block HIV replication*

**HIV vaccine** [see: AIDS vaccine]

**HIV-1 LA test** [see: Recombigen HIV-1 LA]

**HIV-1 peptide vaccine** *investigational (Phase I) vaccine for HIV*

**HIVAB HIV-1 EIA; HIVAB HIV-1/HIV-2 EIA; HIVAB HIV-2 EIA** reagent kit for professional use *in vitro diagnostic aid for HIV antibodies* [enzyme immunoassay (EIA)]

**HIVAG-1** reagent kit for professional use *in vitro diagnostic aid for HIV antibodies* [enzyme immunoassay (EIA)]

**hive vine** *medicinal herb* [see: squaw vine]

**Hi-Vegi-Lip** tablets (discontinued 2002) OTC *digestive enzymes* [pancreatin (lipase; protease; amylase)] 2400 mg (4800•60 000•60 000 USP units)

**Hivenyl** ℞ *investigational (Phase III) histamine $H_1$ antagonist for skin allergies*

**Hivid** film-coated tablets ℞ *antiviral for advanced HIV infection (orphan)* [zalcitabine] 0.375, 0.75 mg

**HIV-IG** ℞ *investigational (Phase III, orphan) immunomodulator for AIDS*

and maternal/fetal HIV transfer [HIV immune globulin]

**HK-Cardiosol** *investigational heart preservation solution*

**HMB (β-hydroxy-β-methylbutyrate)** [q.v.]

**HMB (homatropine methylbromide)** [q.v.]

**HMDP (hydroxymethylene diphosphonate)** [see: oxidronic acid]

**hMG (human menopausal gonadotropin)** [see: menotropins]

**HMG-CoA (3-hydroxy-3-methylglutaryl-coenzyme A) reductase inhibitors** *a class of antihyperlipidemics that reduce serum LDL, VLDL, and triglycerides, but increase HDL* [also called: "statins"]

**HMM (hexamethylmelamine)** [see: altretamine]

**HMR1964** *investigational (Phase III) for type 1 and type 2 diabetes*

**HMR-3647** *investigational (Phase III) ketolide antibiotic for community-acquired pneumonia (CAP)*

**HMR-4004** *investigational (Phase II) gene-modified T-lymphocytes for HIV and AIDS*

**HMS** *eye drop suspension* ℞ *steroidal anti-inflammatory* [medrysone] 1%

**HN₂ (nitrogen mustard)** [see: mechlorethamine HCl]

**HOAP-BLEO (hydroxydaunomycin, Oncovin, ara-C, prednisone, bleomycin)** *chemotherapy protocol*

**hoarhound** *medicinal herb* [see: horehound]

**hock heal** *medicinal herb* [see: woundwort]

**hog apple** *medicinal herb* [see: mandrake; noni]

**hogweed** *medicinal herb* [see: broom; masterwort]

**Hold, Children's** *lozenges (discontinued 2002)* OTC *antitussive* [dextromethorphan hydrobromide] 5 mg

**Hold DM** *lozenges* OTC *antitussive* [dextromethorphan hydrobromide] 5 mg

**holly** *(Ilex aquifolium; I. opaca; I. vomitoria) leaves and berries medici-*nal herb used as a CNS stimulant and emetic; not generally regarded as safe and effective

**holly, ground** *medicinal herb* [see: pipsissewa]

**holly bay** *medicinal herb* [see: magnolia]

**holly-leaved barberry; holly mahonia** *medicinal herb* [see: Oregon grape]

**holmium** *element (Ho)*

**holmium-166 DOTMP** *investigational (Phase III) skeletal targeted radiotherapy agent for treatment of multiple myeloma*

**holy thistle; blessed cardus** *medicinal herb* [see: blessed thistle]

**homarylamine** INN

**homatropine** BAN *ophthalmic anticholinergic* [also: homatropine hydrobromide]

**homatropine hydrobromide** USP *ophthalmic anticholinergic; cycloplegic; mydriatic* [also: homatropine] 5% eye drops

**homatropine methylbromide** USP, INN, BAN *anticholinergic*

**Home Access; Home Access Express** *test kit for home use in vitro diagnostic aid for HIV in the blood*

**Home Access Hepatitis C Check** *test kit for home use in vitro diagnostic aid for hepatitis C in the blood*

**homidium bromide** INN, BAN

**Hominex-1** *powder* OTC *formula for infants with homocystinuria or hypermethioninemia*

**Hominex-2** *powder* OTC *enteral nutritional therapy for homocystinuria or hypermethioninemia*

**homochlorcyclizine** INN, BAN

**homofenazine (HFZ)** INN

**homomenthyl salicylate** [see: homosalate]

**homopipramol** INN

**homosalate** USAN, INN *ultraviolet sunscreen*

**4-homosulfanilamide** [see: mafenide]

**homprenorphine** INN, BAN

**honey** *natural remedy used as an antibacterial and wound healing agent and as a gargle to promote expectoration; not generally regarded as safe and*

*effective for infants because of possible*
Clostridium botulinum *contamination*

**honeybee venom** *natural remedy* [see: bee venom]

**honeybloom** *medicinal herb* [see: dogbane]

**hoodwart** *medicinal herb* [see: skullcap]

**HOP (hydroxydaunomycin, Oncovin, prednisone)** *chemotherapy protocol*

**hopantenic acid** INN

**hops *(Humulus lupulus)*** flower *medicinal herb for aiding digestion, appetite stimulation, bronchitis, cystitis, delirium, edema, headache, hyperactivity, insomnia, intestinal cramps, menstrual disorders, nervousness, pain, excessive sexual desire, and TB*

**hoquizil** INN *bronchodilator* [also: hoquizil HCl]

**hoquizil HCl** USAN *bronchodilator* [also: hoquizil]

*Hordeum vulgare medicinal herb* [see: barley]

**horehound *(Marrubium vulgare)*** plant *medicinal herb for asthma, colds and cough, croup, inducing diaphoresis and diuresis, intestinal parasites, lung disorders, promoting expectoration, and respiratory disorders*

**horse chestnut *(Aesculus californica; A. glabra; A. hippocastanum)*** nuts and leaves *medicinal herb for arthritis, colds and congestion, hemorrhoids, rheumatism, and varicose veins; not generally regarded as safe and effective for internal use as it is highly toxic*

**horse-elder; horseheal** *medicinal herb* [see: elecampane]

**horsefoot; horsehoof** *medicinal herb* [see: coltsfoot]

**horsemint *(Monarda punctata)*** leaves and flowering tops *medicinal herb used as a cardiac, carminative, diaphoretic, diuretic, emmenagogue, stimulant, and sudorific*

**horseradish *(Armoracia lapathiofolia; A. rusticana)*** root *medicinal herb for appetite stimulation, colic, cough, edema, expelling afterbirth, hay*

*fever, poor circulation, sciatic pain, sinus disorders, and skin and internal tumors; also used as a vermifuge*

**horsetail *(Equisetum arvens)*** plant *medicinal herb for bladder disorders, brittle nails, glandular disorders, internal bleeding, nosebleeds, poor circulation, tuberculosis, and urinary disorders*

**horseweed; fleabane *(Erigeron canadensis)*** plant *medicinal herb used as an astringent, diuretic, and hemostatic*

**ho-shou-wu; fo-ti *(Polygonum multiflorum)*** root *medicinal herb for atherosclerosis, blood cleansing, constipation, improving liver and kidney function, insomnia, malaria, muscle aches, TB, and weak bones; also used to increase fertility, prevent aging, and promote longevity*

**H.P. Acthar Gel** IM or subcu injectable gel ℞ *corticosteroid; anti-inflammatory* [corticotropin repository] 80 U/mL

**HPMCP (hydroxypropyl methylcellulose phthalate)** [q.v.]

**HPMPC (3-hydroxy-2-phosphono-methoxypropyl cytosine [dihydrate])** [see: cidofovir]

**Hp-PAC** ⒸⒶⓌ blister packs for daily administration ℞ *multiple products for the eradication of* H. pylori [lansoprazole (delayed-release capsules); clarithromycin (tablets); amoxicillin trihydrate (capsules)] 30•500•500 mg

**H-R Lubricating** vaginal jelly OTC *lubricant* [hydroxypropyl methylcellulose]

**HspE7** *investigational (Phase III) agent for human papilloma virus–related anal dysplasia*

**5-HT (5-hydroxytryptamine)** [see: serotonin]

**HT (human thrombin)** [see: thrombin]

**HT; 3-HT (3-hydroxytyramine)** [see: dopamine]

**5-HTP (5-hydroxytryptophan)** [see: L-5 hydroxytryptophan]

**H-Tuss-D** oral liquid (discontinued 2002) ℞ *narcotic antitussive; decongestant* [hydrocodone bitartrate;

pseudoephedrine HCl; alcohol 5%] 5•60 mg/5 mL

**HU-1124** *investigational (Phase III) monoclonal antibody for the treatment for psoriasis; investigational (Phase I/II) for transplant rejection*

**Hu23F2G** [see: rovelizumab]

**huckleberry** *medicinal herb* [see: bilberry]

**HuM291 (human-mouse monoclonal antibody)** [now: visilizumab]

**Humalog** subcu injection, prefilled syringe cartridges, disposable pen injectors ℞ *insulin analogue for diabetes* [insulin lispro, human (rDNA)] 100 U/mL; 150 U/1.5 mL; 300 U/3 mL

**Humalog Mix 50/50** subcu injection, prefilled syringe cartridges, disposable pen injectors (discontinued 2002) ℞ *insulin analogue for diabetes* [insulin lispro protamine; insulin lispro, human (rDNA)] 50%•50% (100 U/mL total)

**Humalog Mix 75/25** vials, disposable pen injectors ℞ *insulin analogue for diabetes* [insulin lispro protamine; insulin lispro, human (rDNA)] 75%•25% (100 U/mL total)

**Humalog Mix25** Ⓐⓜ prefilled syringe cartridges, disposable pen injectors ℞ *insulin analogue for diabetes* [insulin lispro protamine; insulin lispro, human (rDNA)] 75%•25% (100 U/mL total)

**human acid alpha-glucosidase** *investigational (orphan) for glycogen storage disease type II*

**human albumin** [see: albumin, human]

**human amniotic fluid-derived surfactant** [see: surfactant, human amniotic fluid derived]

**human antihemophilic factor** [see: antihemophilic factor]

**human B-type natriuretic peptide (hBNP)** [see: nesiritide; nesiritide citrate]

**human chorionic gonadotropin (hCG)** [see: gonadotropin, chorionic]

**human complement receptor** [see: complement receptor type I, soluble recombinant human]

**human cytomegalovirus immune globulin** [see: cytomegalovirus immune globulin, human]

**human diploid cell vaccine (HDCV)** [see: rabies vaccine]

**human epidermal growth factor** [see: epidermal growth factor, human]

**human fibrinogen** [see: fibrinogen, human]

**human fibrinolysin** [see: fibrinolysin, human]

**human follicle-stimulating hormone (hFSH)** [now: menotropins]

**human growth hormone (hGH)** JAN *growth hormone* [also: somatropin]

**human growth hormone, recombinant (rhGH)** [see: somatropin]

**human growth hormone releasing factor (hGH-RF)** [see: growth hormone-releasing factor (GH-RF)]

**human immunodeficiency virus (HIV) immune globulin (HIVIG)** [see: HIV immune globulin]

**human insulin** [see: insulin, human; insulin aspart; insulin aspart protamine]

**human menopausal gonadotropin (hMG)** [see: menotropins]

**human respiratory syncytial virus immune globulin** [see: respiratory syncytial virus immune globulin, human]

**human retinal pigmented epithelial (RPE) cells on spherical cell-coated microcarriers (CCM)** *investigational (Phase II, orphan) dopamine-producing brain implants for stage 3 and 4 Parkinson disease*

**human serum albumin diethylenetriaminepentaacetic acid (DTPA) technetium ($^{99m}$Tc)** JAN *radioactive agent* [also: technetium Tc 99m pentetate]

**human superoxide dismutase (SOD)** [see: superoxide dismutase, human]

**human T-cell inhibitor** [see: muromonab-CD3]

**human T-cell lymphotrophic virus type III (HTLV-III)** [now: human immunodeficiency virus (HIV)]

**Human T-Lymphotropic Virus Type I EIA** reagent kit for professional use *in vitro diagnostic aid for HTLV I antibody in serum or plasma* [enzyme immunoassay (EIA)]

**Humate-P** IV injection ℞ *antihemophilic for von Willebrand disease (orphan)* [antihemophilic factor VIII; von Willebrand factor] 20–40 IU/mL

**Humatin** capsules ℞ *aminoglycoside antibiotic; amebicide* [paromomycin sulfate] 250 mg

**Humatrope** powder for subcu or IM injection; prefilled cartridges for HumatroPen (self-injection device) ℞ *growth hormone for adults or children with congenital or endogenous growth hormone deficiency, children with Turner syndrome or renal-induced growth failure, or AIDS-wasting syndrome (orphan)* [somatropin] 5 mg (15 IU) per vial; 6, 12, 24 mg

**HumatroPen** (trademarked device) *subcu self-injector for Humatrope*

**Humegon** powder for IM injection (discontinued 2002) ℞ *ovulation stimulant for women; spermatogenesis stimulant for men* [menotropins] 75, 150 IU

**Humibid DM** extended-release capsules ℞ *antitussive; expectorant* [dextromethorphan hydrobromide; guaifenesin; potassium guaiacolsulfonate] 50•400•200 mg

**Humibid DM** sustained-release caplets (discontinued 2004) ℞ *antitussive; expectorant* [dextromethorphan hydrobromide; guaifenesin] 30•600 mg

**Humibid DM Sprinkle** sustained-release capsules (discontinued 2002) ℞ *antitussive; expectorant* [dextromethorphan hydrobromide; guaifenesin] 15•300 mg

**Humibid L.A.** sustained-release caplets (discontinued 2004) ℞ *expectorant* [guaifenesin; potassium guaiacolsulfonate] 600•300 mg

**Humibid Pediatric** sustained-release capsules (discontinued 2004) ℞ *expectorant* [guaifenesin] 300 mg

**Humibid Sprinkle** (name changed to Humibid Pediatric in 2002)

**Humira** subcu injection in prefilled self-injectors ℞ *disease-modifying antirheumatic drug (DMARD) for moderate to severe rheumatoid arthritis (RA)* [adalimumab] 40 mg/0.8 mL dose

**HuMist Moisturizing** nasal mist OTC *nasal moisturizer* [sodium chloride (saline solution)] 0.65%

**Humorsol** Ocumeter (eye drops) (discontinued 2004) ℞ *antiglaucoma agent; reversible cholinesterase inhibitor miotic* [demecarium bromide] 0.125%, 0.25%

**Humulin 30/70** ⒸⒶⓃ subcu injection, prefilled syringe cartridges OTC *antidiabetic* [insulin; isophane insulin] 100 U/mL; 1.5 mL

**Humulin 50/50** subcu injection (prefilled cartridges available in Canada) OTC *antidiabetic* [isophane human insulin (rDNA); human insulin (rDNA)] 100 U/mL (150 U/1.5 mL in Canada)

**Humulin 70/30** subcu injection, prefilled syringe cartridges, disposable pen injectors OTC *antidiabetic* [isophane human insulin (rDNA); human insulin (rDNA)] 100 U/mL; 150 U/1.5 mL; 300 U/3 mL

**Humulin L** subcu injection OTC *antidiabetic* [insulin zinc, human (rDNA)] 100 U/mL

**Humulin N** subcu injection, prefilled syringe cartridges, disposable pen injectors OTC *antidiabetic* [isophane human insulin (rDNA)] 100 U/mL; 100 U/1.5 mL; 300 U/3 mL

**Humulin R** subcu injection OTC *antidiabetic* [human insulin (rDNA)] 100 U/mL; 1.5 mL

**Humulin R Regular U-500 (concentrated)** subcu injection ℞ *antidiabetic* [human insulin (rDNA)] 500 U/mL

**Humulin U** subcu injection OTC *antidiabetic* [insulin zinc, extended human (rDNA)] 100 U/mL

**Humulin-U** Ⓐ subcu injection OTC *antidiabetic* [extended insulin zinc] 100 U/mL

*Humulus lupulus medicinal herb* [see: hops]

**huperzine A** *natural extract from Chinese club moss that enhances memory, focus, and concentration; prevents the breakdown of the neurotransmitter acetylcholine*

**hurr-burr** *medicinal herb* [see: burdock]

**Hurricaine** spray liquid, topical liquid, gel OTC *mucous membrane anesthetic* [benzocaine] 20%

**HXM (hexamethylmelamine)** [see: altretamine]

**Hyacne** ℞ *investigational (Phase III) acne treatment*

**Hyalgan** intra-articular injection ℞ *viscoelastic lubricant and "shock absorber" for osteoarthritis and temporomandibular joint syndrome* [hyaluronate sodium] 20 mg/2 mL

**hyalosidase** INN, BAN

**hyaluronan** *viscoelastic lubricant and "shock absorber" for osteoarthritis of the knee*

**hyaluronate sodium** USAN, JAN *ophthalmic surgical aid; treatment for osteoarthritis and TMJ syndrome; veterinary synovitis agent* [also: hyaluronic acid]

**hyaluronic acid** BAN *ophthalmic surgical aid; treatment for osteoarthritis and TMJ syndrome; dermal filler for deep wrinkles and facial folds; veterinary synovitis agent* [also: hyaluronate sodium]

**hyaluronidase** USP, INN, BAN *dispersion aid; absorption facilitator; investigational (NDA filed) agent to clear vitreous hemorrhage*

**hyaluronoglucosaminidase** [see: hyalosidase]

**hyamate** [see: buramate]

**Hyate:C (Porcine)** powder for IV injection ℞ *antihemophilic for patients with antibodies to human factor VIII* [antihemophilic factor concentrate, porcine] 400–700 porcine units

**hybenzate** USAN *combining name for radicals or groups* [also: hibenzate]

**Hybolin Decanoate-50; Hybolin Decanoate-100** IM injection (discontinued 2000) ℞ *anabolic steroid for anemia of renal insufficiency* [nandrolone decanoate (in oil)] 50 mg/mL; 100 mg/mL

**Hybolin Improved** IM injection (discontinued 2000) ℞ *anabolic steroid for metastatic breast cancer in women* [nandrolone phenpropionate (in oil)] 50 mg/mL

**Hybrid Capture II Chlamydia Test** reagent kit for professional use *in vitro diagnostic aid for* Chlamydia trachomatis

**Hycamtin** powder for IV injection ℞ *topoisomerase I inhibitor; antineoplastic for ovarian and small cell lung cancers* [topotecan HCl] 4 mg/dose

**hycanthone** USAN, INN *antischistosomal*

**hycanthone mesylate** *antischistosomal*

**Hycet** oral liquid ℞ *narcotic analgesic* [hydrocodone bitartrate; acetaminophen; alcohol 7%] 2.5•108 mg/5 mL

**hyclate** INN *combining name for radicals or groups*

**HycoClear Tuss** syrup (discontinued 2002) ℞ *narcotic antitussive; expectorant* [hydrocodone bitartrate; guaifenesin] 5•100 mg/5 mL

**Hycodan** tablets, syrup ℞ *narcotic antitussive; anticholinergic* [hydrocodone bitartrate; homatropine methylbromide] 5•1.5 mg; 5•1.5 mg/5 mL ⑫ Hycomine; Vicodin

**Hycomine** syrup, pediatric syrup (discontinued 2002) ℞ *narcotic antitussive; decongestant* [hydrocodone bitartrate; phenylpropanolamine HCl] 5•25 mg/5 mL; 2.5•12.5 mg/5 mL ⑫ Byclomine; Hycodan; Vicodin

**Hycomine Compound** tablets (discontinued 2002) ℞ *narcotic antitussive; decongestant; antihistamine; analgesic* [hydrocodone bitartrate; phenylephrine HCl; chlorpheniramine maleate; acetaminophen; caffeine] 5•10•2•250•30 mg

**Hycort** cream, ointment ℞ *topical corticosteroidal anti-inflammatory* [hydrocortisone] 1%

**Hycosin Expectorant** syrup ℞ *narcotic antitussive; expectorant* [hydrocodone bitartrate; guaifenesin; alcohol 10%] 5•100 mg/5 mL

**Hycotuss Expectorant** syrup ℞ *narcotic antitussive; expectorant* [hydrocodone bitartrate; guaifenesin; alcohol 10%] 5•100 mg/5 mL

**hydantoins** *a class of anticonvulsants*

**Hydeltrasol** IV, IM injection ℞ *corticosteroid; anti-inflammatory* [prednisolone sodium phosphate] 20 mg/mL

**Hydergine** sublingual tablets, tablets, oral liquid ℞ *cognition adjuvant for age-related mental capacity decline* [ergoloid mesylates] 0.5, 1 mg; 1 mg; 1 mg/mL ② Hydramine

**Hydergine LC** liquid-filled capsules (discontinued 2004) ℞ *cognition adjuvant for age-related mental capacity decline* [ergoloid mesylates] 1 mg

**hydracarbazine** INN

**hydragogues** *a class of purgatives that produce abundant watery discharge from the bowels*

**hydralazine** INN, BAN *antihypertensive; peripheral vasodilator* [also: hydralazine HCl]

**hydralazine HCl** USP, JAN *antihypertensive; peripheral vasodilator* [also: hydralazine] 10, 25, 50, 100 mg oral; 20 mg/mL injection

**hydralazine polistirex** USAN *antihypertensive*

**Hydramine** syrup, elixir ℞ *antihistamine; antitussive* [diphenhydramine HCl] 12.5 mg/5 mL ② Bydramine; Hydergine; Hydramyn; Hytramyn

**hydrangea (*Hydrangea arborescens*)** leaves and root *medicinal herb for arthritis, bladder infections, gallstones, gonorrhea, gout, kidney stones, rheumatism, and urinary disorders*

**Hydrap-ES** tablets ℞ *antihypertensive; vasodilator; diuretic* [hydrochlorothia-zide; reserpine; hydralazine HCl] 15•0.1•25 mg

**hydrargaphen** INN, BAN

**hydrastine** USP

**hydrastine HCl** USP

**hydrastinine HCl** NF

*Hydrastis canadensis* *medicinal herb* [see: goldenseal]

**Hydrate** IV or IM injection ℞ *antinauseant; antiemetic; antivertigo; motion sickness preventative* [dimenhydrinate] 50 mg/mL

**hydrazinecarboximidamide monohydrochloride** [see: pimagedine HCl]

**hydrazinoxane** [see: domoxin]

**Hydrea** capsules ℞ *antineoplastic for melanoma, squamous cell carcinoma, myelocytic leukemia, and ovarian cancer; sickle cell anemia treatment (orphan)* [hydroxyurea] 500 mg

**Hydrisea** lotion OTC *moisturizer; emollient* [Dead Sea salts]

**Hydrisinol** cream, lotion OTC *moisturizer; emollient*

**Hydro Cobex** IM injection ℞ *hematinic; vitamin B$_{12}$ supplement* [hydroxocobalamin] 1000 μg/mL

**hydrobentizide** INN

**hydrobutamine** [see: butidrine]

**Hydrocare Cleaning and Disinfecting** solution OTC *chemical disinfecting solution for soft contact lenses*

**Hydrocare Preserved Saline** solution OTC *rinsing/storage solution for soft contact lenses* [sodium chloride (preserved saline solution)]

**Hydrocerin** cream base, lotion base OTC *nontherapeutic base for compounding various dermatological preparations*

**Hydrocet** capsules ℞ *narcotic analgesic* [hydrocodone bitartrate; acetaminophen] 5•500 mg

**hydrochloric acid** NF *acidifying agent*

**hydrochloric acid, diluted** NF *acidifying agent*

**hydrochlorothiazide (HCT; HCTZ)** USP, INN, BAN *antihypertensive; diuretic* 12.5, 25, 50, 100 mg oral; 50 mg/5 mL oral; 100 mg/mL oral

**hydrochlorothiazide & benazepril HCl** *antihypertensive; diuretic; angiotensin-converting enzyme (ACE) inhibitor* 6.25•5, 12.5•10, 12.5•20, 25•20 mg oral

**hydrochlorothiazide & bisoprolol fumarate** *antihypertensive; diuretic; β-blocker* 6.5•2.5, 6.5•5, 6.5•10 mg oral

**hydrochlorothiazide & captopril** *antihypertensive; diuretic; angiotensin-converting enzyme (ACE) inhibitor* 15•25, 25•25, 15•50, 25•50 mg oral

**hydrochlorothiazide & enalapril maleate** *antihypertensive; diuretic; angiotensin-converting enzyme (ACE) inhibitor* 12.5•5, 25•10 mg oral

**hydrochlorothiazide & lisinopril** *antihypertensive; diuretic; angiotensin-converting enzyme (ACE) inhibitor* 12.5•10, 12.5•20, 25•20 mg oral

**hydrochlorothiazide & triamterene** *antihypertensive; potassium-sparing diuretic* 25•37.5 mg oral

**hydrocholeretics** *a class of gastrointestinal drugs that exert laxative effects and increase volume and water content of bile actions*

**Hydrocil Instant** powder OTC *bulk laxative* [psyllium hydrophilic mucilloid] 3.5 g/scoop

**hydrocodone** INN, BAN *antitussive* [also: hydrocodone bitartrate]

**hydrocodone bitartrate** USAN, USP *narcotic antitussive* [also: hydrocodone]

**hydrocodone bitartrate & acetaminophen** *narcotic antitussive; analgesic* 5•325, 7.5•650, 7.5•750, 10•325, 10•500, 10•650, 10•750 mg oral; 2.5•167 mg/5 mL oral

**hydrocodone bitartrate & guaifenesin** *narcotic antitussive; expectorant* 5•100 mg/5 mL oral

**hydrocodone bitartrate & ibuprofen** *narcotic antitussive; analgesic* 7.5•200 mg oral

**hydrocodone bitartrate & pseudoephedrine HCl & carbinoxamine maleate** *narcotic antitussive; decongestant; antihistamine* 5•30•2 mg/5 mL oral

**Hydrocodone Compound** syrup (discontinued 2002) ℞ *narcotic antitussive; anticholinergic* [hydrocodone bitartrate; homatropine hydrobromide] 5•1.5 mg/5 mL

**Hydrocodone CP** syrup ℞ *narcotic antitussive; decongestant; antihistamine* [hydrocodone bitartrate; phenylephrine HCl; chlorpheniramine maleate] 2.5•5•2 mg/5 mL

**Hydrocodone GF** syrup ℞ *narcotic antitussive; expectorant* [hydrocodone bitartrate; guaifenesin] 5•100 mg/5 mL

**Hydrocodone HD** oral liquid ℞ *narcotic antitussive; decongestant; antihistamine* [hydrocodone bitartrate; phenylephrine HCl; chlorpheniramine maleate] 3.33•10•4 mg/10 mL

**Hydrocodone PA** syrup, pediatric syrup (discontinued 2002) ℞ *narcotic antitussive; decongestant* [hydrocodone bitartrate; phenylpropanolamine HCl] 5•25 mg/5 mL; 2.5•12.5 mg/5 mL

**hydrocodone polistirex** USAN *narcotic antitussive*

**Hydrocol** adhesive dressings *occlusive wound dressing* [hydrocolloid gel]

**hydrocolloid gel** *dressings for wet wounds*

**Hydrocort** cream ℞ *topical corticosteroidal anti-inflammatory* [hydrocortisone] 2.5%

**hydrocortamate** INN

**hydrocortamate HCl** [see: hydrocortamate]

**hydrocortisone (HC)** USP, INN, BAN *corticosteroid; anti-inflammatory* 5, 10, 20 mg oral; 0.5%, 1%, 2.5% topical

**hydrocortisone aceponate** INN *corticosteroid; anti-inflammatory*

**hydrocortisone acetate (HCA)** USP, BAN *corticosteroid; anti-inflammatory* 1% topical; 25 mg suppositories; 25, 50 mg/mL injection

**hydrocortisone buteprate** USAN [now: hydrocortisone probutate]

**hydrocortisone butyrate** BAN *topical corticosteroidal anti-inflammatory* [also: hydrocortisone probutate] 0.1% topical

**hydrocortisone cyclopentylpropionate** corticosteroid; anti-inflammatory [see: hydrocortisone cypionate]

**hydrocortisone cypionate** USP corticosteroid; anti-inflammatory

**hydrocortisone hemisuccinate** USP corticosteroid; anti-inflammatory

**hydrocortisone & iodoquinol** corticosteroidal anti-inflammatory; amebicide; antimicrobial 1%•1% topical

**hydrocortisone & neomycin sulfate & polymyxin B sulfate** topical ophthalmic corticosteroidal anti-inflammatory and antibiotic 1%•0.35%• 10 000 U/mL eye drops

**hydrocortisone probutate** USAN, USP topical corticosteroidal anti-inflammatory [previously known as: hydrocortisone buteprate]

**hydrocortisone sodium phosphate** USP, BAN corticosteroid; anti-inflammatory

**hydrocortisone sodium succinate** USP, BAN corticosteroid; anti-inflammatory

**hydrocortisone valerate** USAN, USP topical corticosteroidal anti-inflammatory 0.2% topical

**Hydrocortone** tablets ℞ corticosteroid; anti-inflammatory [hydrocortisone] 10, 20 mg

**Hydrocortone Acetate** intralesional, intra-articular, or soft tissue injection ℞ corticosteroid; anti-inflammatory [hydrocortisone acetate] 25, 50 mg/mL

**Hydrocortone Phosphate** IV, subcu, or IM injection ℞ corticosteroid; anti-inflammatory [hydrocortisone sodium phosphate] 50 mg/mL

*Hydrocotyle asiatica* medicinal herb [see: gotu kola]

**Hydrocream Base** OTC cream base

**Hydro-Crysti 12** IM injection ℞ hematinic; vitamin $B_{12}$ supplement [hydroxocobalamin] 1000 μg/mL

**HydroDIURIL** tablets ℞ antihypertensive; diuretic [hydrochlorothiazide] 25, 50, 100 mg

**Hydro-DP** syrup ℞ narcotic antitussive; decongestant; antihistamine [hydrocodone bitartrate; phenylephrine HCl; diphenhydramine HCl] 2•7.5•12.5 mg/5 mL

**hydrofilcon A** USAN hydrophilic contact lens material

**hydroflumethiazide** USP, INN, BAN antihypertensive; diuretic 50 mg oral

**hydrofluoric acid** dental caries prophylactic

**hydrofluoroalkane (HFA)** propellant used in CFC-free aerosol delivery systems [usually HFA-134a]

**hydrogen** element (H)

**hydrogen peroxide** USP topical anti-infective

**hydrogen tetrabromoaurate** [see: bromauric acid]

**hydrogenated ergot alkaloids** [now: ergoloid mesylates]

**hydrogenated vegetable oil** [see: vegetable oil, hydrogenated]

**Hydrogesic** capsules ℞ narcotic analgesic [hydrocodone bitartrate; acetaminophen] 5•500 mg

**hydromadinone** INN

**Hydromet** syrup ℞ narcotic antitussive; anticholinergic [hydrocodone bitartrate; homatropine methylbromide] 5•1.5 mg/5 mL

**Hydromide** syrup ℞ narcotic antitussive; anticholinergic [hydrocodone bitartrate; homatropine methylbromide] 5•1.5 mg/5 mL

**hydromorphinol** INN, BAN

**hydromorphone** INN, BAN narcotic analgesic; widely abused as a street drug [also: hydromorphone HCl]

**hydromorphone HCl** USP narcotic analgesic; widely abused as a street drug [also: hydromorphone] 2, 4, 8 mg oral; 5 mg/5 mL oral; 3 mg rectal; 1, 2, 4, 10 mg/mL injection

**hydromorphone sulfate**

**Hydromox** tablets (discontinued 2001) ℞ diuretic; antihypertensive [quinethazone] 50 mg

**Hydron CP** oral liquid ℞ narcotic antitussive; decongestant; antihistamine [hydrocodone bitartrate; phenyleph-rine HCl; chlorpheniramine male-ate] 5•10•2 mg/5 mL

**Hydron EX; Hydron KGS** oral liq-uid ℞ *narcotic antitussive; expectorant* [hydrocodone bitartrate; potassium guaiacolsulfonate] 2.5•120 mg/5 mL; 5•300 mg/5 mL

**Hydron PSC** oral liquid ℞ *narcotic antitussive; decongestant; antihistamine* [hydrocodone bitartrate; pseudo-ephedrine HCl; chlorpheniramine maleate] 5•30•2 mg/5 mL

**Hydropane** syrup ℞ *narcotic antitus-sive; anticholinergic* [hydrocodone bitartrate; homatropine methylbro-mide] 5•1.5 mg/5 mL

**Hydro-Par** tablets ℞ *antihypertensive; diuretic* [hydrochlorothiazide] 25, 50 mg

**Hydro-PC; Hydro-PC II** oral liquid ℞ *narcotic antitussive; decongestant; antihistamine* [hydrocodone bitar-trate; phenylephrine HCl; chlor-pheniramine maleate] 4•10•4 mg/10 mL; 4•15•4 mg/10 mL

**Hydropel** ointment OTC *skin protectant* [silicone; hydrophobic starch deriva-tive] 30%•10%

**Hydrophed** tablets ℞ *antiasthmatic; bronchodilator; decongestant; antihista-mine* [theophylline; ephedrine sulfate; hydroxyzine HCl] 130•25•10 mg

**Hydrophilic** OTC *ointment base*

**hydrophilic ointment** [see: ointment, hydrophilic]

**hydrophilic petrolatum** [see: petrola-tum, hydrophilic]

**Hydropres-50** tablets ℞ *antihyperten-sive; diuretic* [hydrochlorothiazide; reserpine] 50•0.125 mg

**hydroquinone** USP *hyperpigmentation bleaching agent* 3%, 4% topical

**hydroquinone methyl ether** [see: mequinol]

**Hydro-Serp** tablets ℞ *antihypertensive; diuretic* [hydrochlorothiazide; reser-pine] 50•0.125 mg

**Hydroserpine #1; Hydroserpine #2** tablets ℞ *antihypertensive; diuretic*

[hydrochlorothiazide; reserpine] 25•0.125 mg; 50•0.125 mg

**HydroSkin** cream, lotion, ointment OTC *corticosteroidal anti-inflammatory* [hydrocortisone] 1%

**hydrotalcite** INN, BAN

**HydroTex** cream (discontinued 2003) ℞ *corticosteroidal anti-inflammatory* [hydrocortisone] 0.5%

**Hydro-Tussin DM** oral liquid ℞ *anti-tussive; expectorant* [dextromethor-phan hydrobromide; guaifenesin] 20•200 mg/5 mL

**Hydro-Tussin HC** syrup ℞ *narcotic antitussive; decongestant; antihistamine* [hydrocodone bitartrate; pseudo-ephedrine HCl; chlorpheniramine maleate] 3•15•2 mg/5 mL

**Hydro-Tussin HD** oral liquid ℞ *nar-cotic antitussive; decongestant; expec-torant* [hydrocodone bitartrate; pseu-doephedrine HCl; guaifenesin] 5•60•200 mg/10 mL

**hydroxamethocaine** BAN [also: hydroxytetracaine]

**hydroxidione sodium succinate** [see: hydroxydione sodium succinate]

**hydroxindasate** INN

**hydroxindasol** INN

**hydroxizine chloride** [see: hydroxy-zine HCl]

**hydroxocobalamin** USAN, USP, INN, BAN, JAN *vitamin $B_{12}$; hematopoietic* [also: hydroxocobalamin acetate] 1 mg/mL injection

**hydroxocobalamin acetate** JAN *vita-min $B_{12}$; hematopoietic* [also: hydroxocobalamin]

**hydroxocobalamin & sodium thio-sulfate** *investigational (orphan) for severe acute cyanide poisoning*

**hydroxocobemine** [see: hydroxoco-balamin]

**3-hydroxy-2-phosphonomethoxy-propyl cytosine (HPMPC) dihy-drate** [see: cidofovir]

**N-hydroxyacetamide** [see: acetohy-droxamic acid]

**4′-hydroxyacetanilide** [see: acetamin-ophen]

**4'-hydroxyacetanilide salicylate**
[see: acetaminosalol]

**hydroxyamfetamine** INN *ophthalmic adrenergic; mydriatic* [also: hydroxyamphetamine hydrobromide; hydroxyamphetamine]

**hydroxyamphetamine** BAN *ophthalmic adrenergic; mydriatic* [also: hydroxyamphetamine hydrobromide; hydroxyamfetamine]

**hydroxyamphetamine hydrobromide** USP *ophthalmic adrenergic/vasoconstrictor; mydriatic* [also: hydroxyamfetamine; hydroxyamphetamine]

**4-hydroxyanisole (4HA); *p*-hydroxyanisole** [see: mequinol]

**hydroxyapatite** BAN *prosthetic aid* [also: durapatite; calcium phosphate, tribasic]

**2-hydroxybenzamide** [see: salicylamide]

**2-hydroxybenzoic acid** [see: salicylic acid]

***o*-hydroxybenzyl alcohol** [see: salicyl alcohol]

**hydroxybutanedioic acid** [see: malic acid]

**4-hydroxybutanoic acid** [see: gamma hydroxybutyrate (GHB)]

**4-hydroxybutanoic acid, sodium salt** [see: sodium oxybate]

**hydroxybutyrate sodium, gamma** [see: sodium oxybate]

**hydroxycarbamide** INN *antineoplastic* [also: hydroxyurea]

**hydroxychloroquine** INN, BAN *antimalarial; lupus erythematosus suppressant* [also: hydroxychloroquine sulfate]

**hydroxychloroquine sulfate** USP *antimalarial; antirheumatic; lupus erythematosus suppressant* (base=77.5%) [also: hydroxychloroquine] 200 mg oral

**25-hydroxycholecalciferol** [see: calcifediol]

**hydroxycincophene** [see: oxycinchophen]

**hydroxydaunomycin** [see: doxorubicin]

**14-hydroxydihydromorphine** [see: hydromorphinol]

**hydroxydione sodium succinate** INN, BAN

**1α-hydroxyergocalciferol** [see: doxercalciferol]

**hydroxyethyl cellulose** NF *suspending and viscosity-increasing agent; ophthalmic aid*

**2-hydroxyethyl methacrylate (HEMA)** *contact lens material*

**hydroxyethyl starch (HES)** [see: hetastarch]

**hydroxyethylstarch** JAN *plasma volume extender* [also: hetastarch]

**hydroxyhexamide**

**3-hydroxyisovalerate; β-hydroxyisovalerate** [see: β-hydroxy-β-methylbutyrate (HMB)]

**hydroxylapatite** [see: durapatite; calcium phosphate, tribasic]

**hydroxymagnesium aluminate** [see: magaldrate]

**hydroxymesterone** [see: medrysone]

**6-hydroxymethylacylfulvene** *investigational (orphan) for advanced or metastatic pancreatic cancer, ovarian cancer, or renal carcinoma*

**β-hydroxy-β-methylbutyrate (HMB)** *an endogenous metabolite of the amino acid L-leucine; a natural supplement taken to prevent exercise-induced muscle breakdown (proteolysis), resulting in larger muscle gains from resistance training; may have immunomodulatory effects*

**hydroxymethylene diphosphonate (HMDP)** [see: oxidronic acid]

**hydroxymethylgramicidin** [see: methocidin]

**N-hydroxynaphthalimide diethyl phosphate** [see: naftalofos]

**hydroxypethidine** INN, BAN

**hydroxyphenamate** USAN *minor tranquilizer* [also: oxyfenamate]

**N-4-hydroxyphenylretinamide** [see: fenretinide]

**hydroxyprocaine** INN, BAN

**hydroxyprogesterone** INN, BAN *synthetic progestin for amenorrhea, metrorrhagia, and dysfunctional uterine* *bleeding* [also: hydroxyprogesterone caproate]

**hydroxyprogesterone caproate** USP, INN, JAN *synthetic progestin for amenorrhea, metrorrhagia, and dysfunctional uterine bleeding* [also: hydroxyprogesterone] 125, 250 mg/mL IM injection (in oil)

**2-hydroxypropanoic acid, calcium salt, hydrate** [see: calcium lactate]

**hydroxypropyl cellulose** NF *topical protectant; emulsifying and coating agent* [also: hydroxypropylcellulose]

**hydroxypropyl methylcellulose** USP *suspending and viscosity-increasing agent; ophthalmic moisturizer and surgical aid* [also: hypromellose; hydroxypropylmethylcellulose]

**hydroxypropyl methylcellulose phthalate (HPMCP)** NF *tablet-coating agent* [also: hydroxypropylmethylcellulose phthalate]

**hydroxypropylcellulose** JAN *topical protectant; emulsifying and coating agent* [also: hydroxypropyl cellulose]

**hydroxypropylmethylcellulose** JAN *suspending and viscosity-increasing agent; ophthalmic surgical aid* [also: hydroxypropyl methylcellulose; hypromellose]

**hydroxypropylmethylcellulose phthalate** JAN *tablet-coating agent* [also: hydroxypropyl methylcellulose phthalate]

**hydroxypyridine tartrate** INN
**hydroxyquinoline** *topical antiseptic*
**4'-hydroxysalicylanilide** [see: osalmid]

**hydroxystearin sulfate** NF
**hydroxystenozole** INN
**hydroxystilbamidine** INN, BAN *antileishmanial* [also: hydroxystilbamidine isethionate]

**hydroxystilbamidine isethionate** USP *antileishmanial* [also: hydroxystilbamidine]

**hydroxysuccinic acid** [see: malic acid]
**hydroxytetracaine** INN [also: hydroxyamethocaine]
**hydroxytoluic acid** INN, BAN

**5-hydroxytryptamine$_1$ (5-HT$_1$)** [see: serotonin]

**5-hydroxytryptamine$_3$ (5-HT$_3$) receptor antagonists** *a class of antinauseant and antiemetic agents used primarily after emetogenic cancer chemotherapy*

**5-hydroxytryptophan (5-HTP)** [see: L-5 hydroxytryptophan]

**3-hydroxytyramine (HT; 3-HT)** [see: dopamine]

**hydroxyurea** USAN, USP, BAN *antimetabolite antineoplastic for melanoma, squamous cell carcinoma, myelocytic leukemia, and ovarian cancer; sickle cell anemia treatment (orphan); investigational adjunctive therapy for HIV* [also: hydroxycarbamide] 250, 500 mg oral

**1α-hydroxyvitamin D$_2$** [see: doxercalciferol]

**hydroxyzine** INN, BAN *anxiolytic; minor tranquilizer; antiemetic; piperazine antihistamine; antipruritic* [also: hydroxyzine HCl]

**hydroxyzine HCl** USP *anxiolytic; minor tranquilizer; antiemetic; piperazine antihistamine; antipruritic* [also: hydroxyzine] 10, 25, 50 mg oral; 10 mg/5 mL oral; 25, 50 mg/mL injection

**hydroxyzine pamoate** USP *anxiolytic; minor tranquilizer; antiemetic; piperazine antihistamine; antipruritic* 25, 50, 100 mg oral

**Hyflex-650** tablets ℞ *analgesic; antihistaminic sleep aid* [acetaminophen; phenyltoloxamine citrate] 650•60 mg

**Hygenic Cleansing** anorectal pads OTC *moisturizer and cleanser for external rectal/vaginal areas; astringent* [witch hazel] 50%

**Hygroton** tablets ℞ *antihypertensive; diuretic* [chlorthalidone] 25, 50, 100 mg ② Regroton

**Hylaform** gel for subcu injection ℞ *dermal filler for wrinkles and facial folds* [hylan B]

**hylan B** *hyaluronic acid gel–based dermal filler*

**hylan G-F 20** *hyaluronic acid gel-fluid polymer mixture for osteoarthritis and TMJ syndrome*

**Hylorel** tablets ℞ *antihypertensive* [guanadrel sulfate] 10, 25 mg

**Hylutin** IM injection (discontinued 2004) ℞ *synthetic progestin for amenorrhea, metrorrhagia, and dysfunctional uterine bleeding* [hydroxyprogesterone caproate in oil] 125, 250 mg/mL

**hymecromone** USAN, INN *choleretic*

**hyoscine hydrobromide** BAN *GI antispasmodic; prevent motion sickness; cycloplegic; mydriatic* [also: scopolamine hydrobromide]

**hyoscine methobromide** BAN *anticholinergic* [also: methscopolamine bromide]

**hyoscyamine (L-hyoscyamine)** USP, BAN *anticholinergic; urinary antispasmodic*

**hyoscyamine hydrobromide** USP *GI antispasmodic; anticholinergic*

**hyoscyamine sulfate** USP *GI/GU antispasmodic; antiparkinsonian; anticholinergic "drying agent" for allergic rhinitis and hyperhidrosis* [also: hyoscyamine sulphate] 0.375 mg oral; 0.125 mg/mL oral

**hyoscyamine sulphate** BAN *GI/GU antispasmodic; antiparkinsonian; anticholinergic "drying agent" for allergic rhinitis and hyperhidrosis* [also: hyoscyamine sulfate]

*Hyoscyamus niger medicinal herb* [see: henbane]

**Hyosophen** tablets, elixir ℞ *GI antispasmodic; anticholinergic; sedative* [atropine sulfate; scopolamine hydrobromide; hyoscyamine hydrobromide; phenobarbital] 0.0194•0.0065•0.1037•16.2 mg; 0.0194•0.0065•0.1037•16.2 mg/5 mL

**Hypaque Meglumine 30%** injection (discontinued 2001) ℞ *radiopaque contrast medium* [diatrizoate meglumine (46.67% iodine)] 300 mg/mL (141 mg/mL)

**Hypaque Meglumine 60%** injection ℞ *radiopaque contrast medium* [diatri-zoate meglumine (46.67% iodine)] 600 mg/mL (282 mg/mL)

**Hypaque Sodium** oral/rectal solution (discontinued 2001) ℞ *radiopaque contrast medium for gastrointestinal imaging* [diatrizoate sodium (59.87% iodine)] 416.7 mg (249 mg)

**Hypaque Sodium** powder for oral/rectal solution ℞ *radiopaque contrast medium for gastrointestinal imaging* [diatrizoate sodium (59.87% iodine)] 1002 mg (600 mg)

**Hypaque Sodium 20%** intracavitary instillation ℞ *radiopaque contrast medium for urological imaging* [diatrizoate sodium (59.87% iodine)] 200 mg/mL (120 mg/mL)

**Hypaque Sodium 25%** injection (discontinued 2001) ℞ *radiopaque contrast medium* [diatrizoate sodium (46.67% iodine)] 250 mg/mL (150 mg/mL)

**Hypaque Sodium 50%** injection ℞ *radiopaque contrast medium* [diatrizoate sodium (46.67% iodine)] 500 mg/mL (300 mg/mL)

**Hypaque-76** injection ℞ *radiopaque contrast medium* [diatrizoate meglumine; diatrizoate sodium (48.7% total iodine)] 660•100 mg/mL (370 mg/mL)

**Hypaque-Cysto** intracavitary instillation ℞ *radiopaque contrast medium for urological imaging* [diatrizoate meglumine (46.67% iodine)] 300 mg/mL (141 mg/mL)

**HyperHep** IM injection (name changed to BayHep B in 2000) ⃞ Hyper-Tet; Hyperstat

*Hypericum perforatum medicinal herb* [see: St. John wort]

**Hyperlyte; Hyperlyte R** IV admixture (discontinued 2001) ℞ *intravenous electrolyte therapy* [combined electrolyte solution]

**Hyperlyte CR** IV admixture ℞ *intravenous electrolyte therapy* [combined electrolyte solution]

**Hypermune RSV** ℞ *preventative for respiratory syncytial virus (RSV) infections in high-risk infants (orphan);*

*investigational (orphan) treatment for RSV* [respiratory syncytial virus immune globulin (RSV-IG)]

**hyperosmotic laxatives** *a subclass of laxatives that use the osmotic effect to retain water in the intestines, lowering colonic pH and increasing peristalsis* [see also: laxatives]

**HyperRab** IM injection (name changed to BayRab in 2000)

**Hyperstat** IV injection ℞ *vasodilator for hypertensive emergency* [diazoxide] 15 mg/mL ⓓ Hyper-Tet; HyperHep

**Hyper-Tet** IM injection (name changed to BayTet in 2000) ⓓ HyperHep; Hyperstat

**Hyphed** oral liquid ℞ *narcotic antitussive; decongestant; antihistamine* [hydrocodone bitartrate; pseudoephedrine HCl; chlorpheniramine maleate; alcohol 5%] 5•60•4 mg/10 mL

**Hy-Phen** tablets ℞ *narcotic analgesic* [hydrocodone bitartrate; acetaminophen] 5•500 mg

**hyphylline** [see: dyphylline]

**hypnogene** [see: barbital]

**hypnotics** *a class of agents that induce sleep*

**hypochlorous acid, sodium salt** [see: sodium hypochlorite]

**β-hypophamine** [see: vasopressin]

**α-hypophamine** [see: oxytocin]

**hypophosphorous acid** NF *antioxidant*

**Hyporet** (trademarked delivery system) *prefilled disposable syringe*

**HypoTears** ophthalmic ointment OTC *ocular moisturizer/lubricant* [white petrolatum; mineral oil]

**HypoTears; HypoTears PF** eye drops OTC *ophthalmic moisturizer/lubricant* [polyvinyl alcohol] 1%

**hyprolose** [see: hydroxypropyl cellulose]

**hypromellose** INN, BAN *suspending and viscosity-increasing agent* [also: hydroxypropyl methylcellulose; hydroxypropylmethylcellulose]

**Hyrexin-50** injection (discontinued 2002) ℞ *antihistamine; motion sickness preventative; sleep aid; antiparkinsonian* [diphenhydramine HCl] 50 mg/mL

**Hyskon** uterine infusion ℞ *hysteroscopy aid* [dextran 70; dextrose] 32%•10%

**Hysone** cream OTC *topical corticosteroidal anti-inflammatory; antifungal; antibacterial* [hydrocortisone; clioquinol] 10•30 mg/g

**hyssop** *(Hyssopus officinalis)* leaves *medicinal herb for chronic hay fever, congestion, cough, lung ailments, promoting expectoration, and sore throat*

**hyssop, hedge** *medicinal herb* [see: hedge hyssop]

**hyssop, Indian; wild hyssop** *medicinal herb* [see: blue vervain]

**hyssop, prairie** *medicinal herb* [see: wild hyssop]

**Hytakerol** capsules ℞ *vitamin D therapy for tetany and hypoparathyroidism* [dihydrotachysterol] 0.125 mg

**Hytinic** capsules, elixir OTC *hematinic; iron supplement* [polysaccharide-iron complex] 150 mg; 100 mg/5 mL

**Hytinic** IM injection ℞ *hematinic* [ferrous gluconate; multiple B vitamins; procaine HCl] 3 mg/mL • ± •2%

**Hytone** cream, lotion, ointment ℞ *topical corticosteroidal anti-inflammatory* [hydrocortisone] 1%, 2.5%; 1%, 2.5%; 2.5% ⓓ Vytone

**Hytone 1%** ointment, spray ℞ *topical corticosteroidal anti-inflammatory* [hydrocortisone] 1%

**Hytrin** soft capsules ℞ $\alpha_1$-*adrenergic blocker for hypertension and benign prostatic hyperplasia (BPH)* [terazosin HCl] 1, 2, 5, 10 mg

**Hytrin** ⓒⓐⓝ tablets, starter pack (1 mg × 7 + 2 mg × 7 + 5 mg × 14) ℞ $\alpha_1$-*adrenergic blocker for hypertension and benign prostatic hyperplasia (BPH)* [terazosin HCl] 1, 2, 5, 10 mg

**Hytuss** tablets OTC *expectorant* [guaifenesin] 100 mg

**Hytuss 2X** capsules OTC *expectorant* [guaifenesin] 200 mg

**Hyzaar** film-coated tablets ℞ *antihypertensive; angiotensin II receptor antagonist; diuretic* [losartan potassium; hydrochlorothiazide] 50•12.5, 100•25 mg

123]

**¹²⁵I** [see: diatrizoate sodium I 125]

¹²⁵I [see: diohippuric acid I 125]

¹²⁵I [see: diotyrosine I 125]

¹²⁵I [see: fibrinogen I 125]

¹²⁵I [see: insulin I 125]

¹²⁵I [see: iodohippurate sodium I 125]

¹²⁵I [see: iodopyracet I 125]

¹²⁵I [see: iomethin I 125]

¹²⁵I [see: iothalamate sodium I 125]

¹²⁵I [see: liothyronine I 125]

¹²⁵I [see: oleic acid I 125]

¹²⁵I [see: povidone I 125]

¹²⁵I [see: rose bengal sodium I 125]

¹²⁵I [see: sodium iodide I 125]

¹²⁵I [see: thyroxine I 125]

¹²⁵I [see: triolein I 125]

¹³¹I [see: albumin, aggregated iodinated I 131 serum]

¹³¹I [see: albumin, iodinated I 131 serum]

¹³¹I [see: diatrizoate sodium I 131]

¹³¹I [see: diohippuric acid I 131]

¹³¹I [see: diotyrosine I 131]

¹³¹I [see: ethiodized oil I 131]

¹³¹I [see: insulin I 131]

¹³¹I [see: iodipamide sodium I 131]

¹³¹I [see: iodoantipyrine I 131]

¹³¹I [see: iodocholesterol I 131]

¹³¹I [see: iodohippurate sodium I 131]

¹³¹I [see: iodopyracet I 131]

¹³¹I [see: iomethin I 131]

¹³¹I [see: iothalamate sodium I 131]

¹³¹I [see: iotyrosine I 131]

¹³¹I [see: liothyronine I 131]

¹³¹I [see: macrosalb (¹³¹I)]

¹³¹I [see: oleic acid I 131]

¹³¹I [see: povidone I 131]

¹³¹I [see: rose bengal sodium I 131]

¹³¹I [see: sodium iodide I 131]

¹³¹I [see: thyroxine I 131]

¹³¹I [see: tolpovidone I 131]

¹³¹I [see: triolein I 131]

**ibacitabine** INN

**ibafloxacin** USAN, INN, BAN *antibacterial*

**ibandronate sodium** USAN *bone resorption inhibitor for postmenopausal osteoporosis, metastatic bone disease, hypercalcemia of malignancy, and Paget disease*

**ibazocine** INN

**IBC (isobutyl cyanoacrylate)** [see: bucrylate]

**Iberet; Iberet-500** controlled-release Filmtabs (film-coated tablets) OTC *hematinic* [multiple B vitamins; ferrous sulfate; sodium ascorbate] ± • 105 • 150 mg; ± • 105 • 500 mg

**Iberet; Iberet-500** oral liquid (discontinued 2003) OTC *hematinic* [multiple B vitamins; ferrous sulfate] ± • 78.75 mg/15 mL

**Iberet-Folic-500** controlled-release Filmtabs (film-coated tablets) ℞ *hematinic* [ferrous sulfate; multiple B vitamins; sodium ascorbate; folic acid] 105 • ± • 500 • 0.8 mg

**iboga (*Tabernanthe iboga*)** *euphoric/ hallucinogenic street drug, the root of which is chewed or chopped into a fine powder and mixed with other drugs; doses high enough to induce hallucinations are also likely to cause death*

**ibopamine** USAN, INN, BAN *peripheral dopaminergic agent; vasodilator*

**ibritumomab tiuxetan** USAN *radioimmunotherapy carrier; radiolabeled with indium In 111 and yttrium Y 90 in the treatment protocol for non-Hodgkin B-cell lymphoma*

**ibrotal** [see: ibrotamide]

**ibrotamide** INN

**IB-Stat** oral spray ℞ *pediatric anticholinergic "drying agent" for allergic rhinitis and hyperhidrosis* [hyoscyamine sulfate] 0.125 mg/mL

**Ibu** film-coated tablets (discontinued 2000) ℞ *analgesic; antiarthritic; antipyretic; nonsteroidal anti-inflammatory drug (NSAID)* [ibuprofen] 400, 600, 800 mg

**ibudilast** INN

**ibufenac** USAN, INN, BAN *analgesic; anti-inflammatory*

**Ibuprin** tablets (discontinued 2000) OTC *analgesic; antiarthritic; antipyretic; nonsteroidal anti-inflammatory drug (NSAID)* [ibuprofen] 200 mg

**ibuprofen** USAN, USP, INN, BAN *analgesic; antiarthritic; antipyretic; nonsteroidal anti-inflammatory drug (NSAID); investigational (orphan) IV treatment for patent ductus arteriosus* 200, 400, 600, 800 mg oral; 100 mg/5 mL oral; 40 mg/mL oral

**ibuprofen aluminum** USAN *anti-inflammatory*

**ibuprofen & hydrocodone bitartrate** *analgesic; narcotic antitussive* 200•7.5 mg oral

**ibuprofen piconol** USAN *topical anti-inflammatory*

**Ibuprohm** caplets, tablets (discontinued 2000) OTC *analgesic; antiarthritic; antipyretic; nonsteroidal anti-inflammatory drug (NSAID)* [ibuprofen] 200 mg

**Ibuprohm** tablets ℞ *nonsteroidal anti-inflammatory drug (NSAID); antiarthritic; analgesic* [ibuprofen] 400 mg

**ibuproxam** INN

**Ibutab** tablets OTC *nonsteroidal anti-inflammatory drug (NSAID); antiarthritic; analgesic* [ibuprofen] 200 mg

**ibutamoren mesylate** USAN *growth hormone for congenital growth hormone deficiency, musculoskeletal impairment, and hip fractures*

**ibuterol** INN

**ibutilide** INN *antiarrhythmic* [also: ibutilide fumarate]

**ibutilide fumarate** USAN *antiarrhythmic for atrial fibrillation/flutter* [also: ibutilide]

**ibuverine** INN

**ibylcaine chloride** [see: butethamine HCl]

**IC-351** *investigational (NDA filed) PDE-5 (phosphodiesterase-5) inhibitor for erectile dysfunction*

**ICAPS** timed-release tablets OTC *vitamin/mineral supplement* [multiple vitamins & minerals]

**ICAPS Plus** tablets OTC *vitamin/mineral supplement* [multiple vitamins & minerals]

**Icar** pediatric suspension OTC *hematinic; iron supplement* [carbonyl iron] 15 mg/1.25 mL

**icatibant acetate** USAN *antiasthmatic*

**ICE (idarubicin, cytarabine, etoposide)** *chemotherapy protocol for acute myelogenous leukemia (AML)*

**ICE (ifosfamide [with mesna rescue], carboplatin, etoposide)** *chemotherapy protocol for osteosarcoma and lung cancer* [also: MICE]

**Iceland moss (Cetraria islandica)** plant *medicinal herb for anemia, bronchitis, hay fever, congestion, cough, digestive disorders, and lung disorders*

**ICE-T (ifosfamide [with mesna rescue], carboplatin, etoposide, Taxol)** *chemotherapy protocol for sarcoma, breast cancer, and non–small cell lung cancer (NSCLC)*

**IC-Green** powder for IV injection ℞ *in vivo diagnostic aid for cardiac output, hepatic function, and ophthalmic angiography* [indocyanine green] 25 mg

**ichthammol** USP, BAN *topical anti-infective* 10%, 20%

**iclazepam** INN

**icodextrin** INN, BAN *peritoneal dialysis solution for end-stage renal disease (orphan)*

**icopezil maleate** USAN *acetylcholinesterase inhibitor; cognition adjuvant for Alzheimer disease*

**icosapent** INN *omega-3 marine triglyceride* [also: eicosapentaenoic acid (EPA)]

**icospiramide** INN

**icotidine** USAN *antagonist to histamine $H_1$ and $H_2$ receptors*

**ictasol** USAN *disinfectant*

**Ictotest** reagent tablets for professional use *in vitro diagnostic aid for bilirubin in the urine*

**Icy Hot** balm, cream, stick OTC *analgesic; counterirritant* [methyl salicylate; menthol] 29%•7.6%; 30%•10%; 30%•10%

**IDA-based BF 12 (idarubicin, cytarabine, etoposide)** *chemotherapy protocol for acute myelogenous leukemia (AML)*

**Idamycin** powder for IV injection ℞ *anthracycline antibiotic antineoplastic for acute myeloid and other leukemias (orphan); investigational (orphan) for pediatric use* [idarubicin HCl] 5, 10, 20 mg

**Idamycin PFS** powder for IV injection ℞ *anthracycline antibiotic antineoplastic for acute myeloid and other leukemias (orphan); investigational (orphan) for pediatric use* [idarubicin HCl] 1 mg/mL

**idarubicin** INN, BAN *anthracycline antibiotic antineoplastic* [also: idarubicin HCl]

**idarubicin HCl** USAN, INN *anthracycline antibiotic antineoplastic for acute myeloid and other leukemias (orphan); investigational (orphan) for pediatric use* [also: idarubicin] 1 mg/mL injection

**idaverine** INN

**idazoxan** INN, BAN

**idebenone** INN, JAN *investigational treatment for Alzheimer disease*

**idenast** INN

**Identi-Dose** (trademarked dosage form) *unit dose package*

**idoxifene** USAN *antihormone antineoplastic; osteoporosis treatment; estrogen receptor antagonist for hormone replacement therapy*

**idoxuridine (IDU)** USAN, USP, INN, BAN, JAN *ophthalmic antiviral; investigational (orphan) for nonparenchymatous sarcomas*

**idralfidine** INN

**idremcinal** USAN *motilin agonist to stimulate gastrointestinal motility*

**idrobutamine** [see: butidrine]

**idrocilamide** INN

**idropranolol** INN

**IDU (idoxuridine)** [q.v.]

**iduronidase** [now: laronidase]

**IE (ifosfamide [with mesna rescue], etoposide)** *chemotherapy protocol for soft tissue sarcoma*

**ifenprodil** INN

**ifetroban** USAN *antithrombotic; anti-ischemic; antivasospastic*

**ifetroban sodium** USAN *antithrombotic; anti-ischemic; antivasospastic*

**Ifex** powder for IV injection ℞ *nitrogen mustard-type alkylating antineoplastic for testicular cancer (orphan); investigational (orphan) for bone and soft tissue sarcomas* [ifosfamide] 1, 3 g

**IFN (interferon)** [q.v.]

**IFN-alpha 2 (interferon alfa-2)** [see: interferon alfa-2b, recombinant]

**ifosfamide** USAN, USP, INN, BAN *nitrogen mustard-type alkylating antineoplastic for testicular cancer (orphan); investigational (orphan) for bone and soft tissue sarcomas* 1, 3 g injection

**IfoVP (ifosfamide [with mesna rescue], VePesid)** *chemotherapy protocol for osteosarcoma*

**ifoxetine** INN

**IG (immune globulin)** [see: globulin, immune]

**IgE pentapeptide** [see: pentigetide]

**Igel 56** *hydrophilic contact lens material* [hefilcon C]

**IGF-1 (insulin-like growth factor-1)** [now: mecasermin]

**IGF-1/BP3 complex** *investigational (Phase II) treatment for muscle degradation following severe burns and hip fracture surgery; investigational (Phase II) for type 1 diabetes*

**IgG1** [see: immunoglobulin G1]

**IGIM (immune globulin intramuscular)** [see: globulin, immune]

**IGIV (immune globulin intravenous)** [see: globulin, immune]

**igmesine HCl** USAN *sigma receptor ligand antidepressant*

**IL-1, IL-2, etc.** [see: interleukin-1, interleukin-2, etc.]

**IL-2 (interleukin-2)** [see: aldesleukin; teceleukin; celmoleukin]

**ilepcimide** USAN, INN *anticonvulsant; investigational (orphan) for drug-resistant generalized tonic-clonic epilepsy*

**Iletin** (U.S. products) [see under: Regular, NPH, and Lente]

**Iletin** Ⓒ subcu injection (discontinued 2001) OTC *antidiabetic* [insulin (beef-pork)] 100 U/mL

**Iletin** Ⓒ subcu injection (discontinued 2001) OTC *antidiabetic* [insulin zinc (beef-pork)] 100 U/mL

**Iletin NPH** Ⓒ subcu injection (discontinued 2001) OTC *antidiabetic* [insulin (beef-pork)] 100 U/mL

**Iletin II NPH** Ⓒ subcu injection OTC *antidiabetic* [insulin (pork)] 100 U/mL

**Iletin II Pork Lente** Ⓒ subcu injection OTC *antidiabetic* [insulin zinc (pork)] 100 U/mL

**Iletin II Pork NPH** Ⓒ subcu injection OTC *antidiabetic* [insulin (pork)] 100 U/mL

**Iletin II Pork Regular** Ⓒ subcu injection OTC *antidiabetic* [insulin (pork)] 100 U/mL

***Ilex aquifolium; I. opaca; I. vomitoria*** *medicinal herb* [see: holly]

***Ilex paraguariensis*** *medicinal herb* [see: yerba maté]

***Ilex verticillata*** *medicinal herb* [see: winterberry]

***Illicium anisatum; I. verum*** *medicinal herb* [see: star anise]

**ilmofosine** USAN, INN *antineoplastic*

**ilodecakin** USAN *interleukin 10, human clone; immunomodulator for Crohn disease, ulcerative colitis, rheumatoid arthritis (RA), and psoriasis*

**ilomastat** USAN *matrix metalloproteinase (MMP) inhibitor for corneal ulcers, inflammation, and cancers*

**ilonidap** USAN, INN *anti-inflammatory*

**Ilopan** IM injection, IV infusion ℞ *postoperative ileus prophylactic* [dexpanthenol] 250 mg/mL

**Ilopan-Choline** tablets (discontinued 2002) ℞ *antiflatulent for splenic flexure syndrome* [dexpanthenol; choline bitartrate] 50•25 mg

**iloperidone** USAN, INN *investigational (Phase III) selective serotonin and dopamine antagonist for schizophrenia*

**iloprost** INN, BAN *prostacyclin analogue for cardiovascular disorders; orphan status withdrawn 1996*

**Ilosone** tablets, Pulvules (capsules), oral suspension ℞ *macrolide antibiotic* [erythromycin estolate] 500 mg; 250 mg; 125, 250 mg/5 mL 🔲 inosine

**Ilotycin** ophthalmic ointment ℞ *antibiotic* [erythromycin] 0.5%

**Ilotycin Gluceptate** IV injection ℞ *macrolide antibiotic* [erythromycin gluceptate] 1 g/vial

**Ilozyme** tablets (discontinued 2002) ℞ *digestive enzymes* [lipase; protease; amylase] 11 000•30 000•30 000 USP units

**I-L-X** elixir OTC *hematinic* [ferrous gluconate; liver concentrate 1:20; multiple B vitamins] 70•98• ≜ mg/15 mL

**I-L-X B₁₂** caplets OTC *hematinic* [carbonyl iron; desiccated liver; multiple B vitamins; ascorbic acid] 37.5• 130• ≜ •120 mg

**I-L-X B₁₂** elixir OTC *hematinic* [ferric ammonium citrate; liver fraction 1; multiple B vitamins] 102•98• ≜ mg/15 mL

**imafen** INN *antidepressant* [also: imafen HCl]

**imafen HCl** USAN *antidepressant* [also: imafen]

**Imager ac** rectal suspension ℞ *radiopaque contrast medium for gastrointestinal imaging* [barium sulfate] 100%

**imanixil** INN

**imatinib mesylate** USAN *antineoplastic for chronic myeloid leukemia (CML) (orphan) and gastrointestinal stromal tumors (GIST)*

**imazodan** INN *cardiotonic* [also: imazodan HCl]

**imazodan HCl** USAN *cardiotonic* [also: imazodan]

**imcarbofos** USAN, INN *veterinary anthelmintic*

**imciromab** INN *antimyosin monoclonal antibody* [also: imciromab pentetate]

**imciromab pentetate** USAN, BAN *antimyosin monoclonal antibody; investigational (orphan) diagnostic aid for myocarditis and cardiac transplant rejection* [also: imciromab]

**Imdur** extended-release tablets ℞ *antianginal; vasodilator* [isosorbide mononitrate] 30, 60, 120 mg

**imexon** INN *investigational (orphan) for multiple myeloma*

**IMF (ifosfamide [with mesna rescue], methotrexate, fluorouracil)** *chemotherapy protocol*

**imiclopazine** INN

**imidapril** INN, BAN

**imidazole carboxamide** [see: dacarbazine

**imidazole salicylate** INN

**imidecyl iodine** USAN *topical anti-infective*

**imidocarb** INN, BAN *antiprotozoal (Babesia)* [also: imidocarb HCl]

**imidocarb HCl** USAN *antiprotozoal (Babesia)* [also: imidocarb]

**imidoline** INN *antipsychotic* [also: imidoline HCl]

**imidoline HCl** USAN *antipsychotic* [also: imidoline]

**imidurea** NF *antimicrobial*

**imiglucerase** USAN, INN *glucocerebrosidase enzyme replacement for types I, II, and III Gaucher disease (orphan)*

**Imigran** (foreign name for U.S. product Imitrex)

**imiloxan** INN *antidepressant* [also: imiloxan HCl]

**imiloxan HCl** USAN *antidepressant* [also: imiloxan]

**iminophenimide** INN

**iminostilbene** [see: carbamazepine]

**imipemide** [now: imipenem]

**imipenem** USAN, USP, INN, BAN, JAN *carbapenem antibiotic*

**imipramine** INN, BAN *tricyclic antidepressant* [also: imipramine HCl] ② Imferon; Norpramin; trimipramine

**imipramine HCl** USP *tricyclic antidepressant; treatment for childhood enuresis* [also: imipramine] 10, 25, 50 mg oral ② Imferon; Norpramin; trimipramine

**imipramine pamoate** *tricyclic antidepressant* ② Imferon; Norpramin; trimipramine

**imipraminoxide** INN

**imiquimod** USAN, INN *immunomodulator for external genital warts, perianal warts, actinic keratoses, and superficial basal cell carcinoma*

**imirestat** INN

**Imitrex** film-coated tablets ℞ *vascular serotonin 5-HT₁ receptor agonist for the acute treatment of migraine headaches* [sumatriptan succinate] 25, 50, 100 mg

**Imitrex** nasal spray ℞ *vascular serotonin 5-HT₁ receptor agonist for the acute treatment of migraine headaches* [sumatriptan] 5, 20 mg/dose

**Imitrex** subcu injection in vials, prefilled syringes, or STATdose self-injector kits (two prefilled syringes) ℞ *vascular serotonin 5-HT₁ receptor agonist for the acute treatment of migraine and cluster headaches* [sumatriptan succinate] 6 mg/0.5 mL dose

**ImmStat** ℞ *investigational gene therapy for HIV infection*

**ImmTher** ℞ *investigational (orphan) immunostimulant for pulmonary and hepatic metastases of colorectal adenocarcinoma* [disaccharide tripeptide glycerol dipalmitoyl]

**ImmuCyst** ⓒⁿ powder for intravesical instillation ℞ *antineoplastic for urinary bladder cancer* [BCG vaccine, live] 81 mg

**ImmuDyn** *investigational (orphan) agent to increase platelet count in immune thrombocytopenic purpura* [Pseudomonas aeruginosa purified extract]

**Immun-Aid** powder OTC *enteral nutritional therapy for immunocompromised patients*

**immune globulin (IG)** [see: globulin, immune]

**immune globulin intramuscular** [see: globulin, immune]

**immune globulin intravenous (IGIV)** [see: globulin, immune]

**immune globulin intravenous pentetate** USAN *radiodiagnostic imaging agent for inflammation and infection* [also: indium In 111 IGIV pentetate]

**immune serum globulin (ISG)** [see: globulin, immune]

**Immunex CRP** test kit for professional use *in vitro diagnostic aid for C-reactive protein (CRP) in blood to diagnose inflammatory conditions* [latex agglutination test]

**Immuno-C** ℞ *investigational (Phase II, orphan) treatment of cryptosporidiosis-induced diarrhea in immunocompromised patients* [*Cryptosporidium parvum* bovine colostrum IgG concentrate]

**Immunocal** powder for oral solution OTC *enteral nutritional therapy* [milk-based formula] 10 g/pkt.

**ImmunoCAP Specific IgE** blood test kit for professional use *in vitro diagnostic aid for IgE detection* [316 different allergens]

**immunoglobulin G1 (mouse monoclonal 7E11-C5.3 antihuman prostatic carcinoma cell) disulfide** [see: capromab pendetide]

**immunoglobulin G1 (mouse monoclonal ZCE025 antihuman antigen CEA) disulfide** [see: indium In 111 altumomab pentetate; altumomab]

**immunoglobulin G2 (human-mouse monoclonal HuM291 anti-CD3 antigen) disulfide** [now: visilizumab]

**immunosuppressants** *a class of drugs used to suppress the immune response, used primarily after organ transplantation surgery*

**ImmuRAID-AFP** ℞ *investigational (orphan) for diagnostic aid for AFP-producing tumors, hepatoblastoma, and hepatocellular carcinoma* [technetium Tc 99m murine monoclonal antibodies (MAb) to human alpha-fetoprotein (AFP)]

**ImmuRAID-hCG** ℞ *investigational (orphan) for diagnostic aid for hCG-producing tumors* [technetium Tc 99m murine monoclonal antibodies (MAb) to human chorionic gonadotropin (hCG)]

**ImmuRAIT-LL2** ℞ *investigational (orphan) treatment for B-cell leukemia*

*and lymphoma* [iodine I 131 murine monoclonal antibodies (MAb) IgG2a to B cell]

**Imodium** capsules ℞ *antidiarrheal* [loperamide HCl] 2 mg

**Imodium** ⒸⒶⓃ quick-dissolving lingual tablets OTC *antidiarrheal* [loperamide HCl] 2 mg

**Imodium A-D** caplets, oral liquid OTC *antidiarrheal* [loperamide HCl] 1 mg; 1 mg/5 mL

**Imodium Advanced** ⒸⒶⓃ chewable tablets OTC *antidiarrheal; antiflatulent* [loperamide HCl; simethicone] 2 • 125 mg

**Imogam** IM injection (discontinued 2001; replaced by Imogam Rabies-HT) ℞ *passive immunizing agent for rabies prophylaxis and treatment* [rabies immune globulin] 150 IU/mL

**Imogam Rabies-HT** IM injection ℞ *passive immunizing agent for rabies prophylaxis and treatment* [rabies immune globulin, heat treated] 150 IU/mL

**imolamine** INN

**Imovane** ⒸⒶⓃ tablets ℞ *sedative; hypnotic* [zopiclone] 7.5 mg

**Imovax** intradermal (ID) injection, IM injection ℞ *rabies prophylaxis* [rabies vaccine (HDCV)] 0.25 IU/0.1 mL; 2.5 IU/mL

**imoxiterol** INN

**impacarzine** INN

**Impact** ready-to-use oral liquid OTC *enteral nutritional therapy* [lactose-free formula]

**Impact Rubella** slide test for professional use *in vitro diagnostic aid for detection of rubella virus antibodies in serum* [latex agglutination test]

*Impatiens balsamina; I. biflora; I. capensis* medicinal herb [see: jewelweed]

**IMPE** [see: etipirium iodide]

**impromidine** INN, BAN *gastric secretion indicator* [also: impromidine HCl]

**impromidine HCl** USAN *gastric secretion indicator* [also: impromidine]

**improsulfan** INN

**Improved Analgesic** ointment OTC *analgesic; counterirritant* [methyl salicylate; menthol] 18.3% • 16%

**Improved Congestant** tablets (discontinued 2002) OTC *antihistamine; analgesic* [chlorpheniramine maleate; acetaminophen] 2 • 325 mg

**imuracetam** INN

**Imuran** IV injection ℞ *immunosuppressant for organ transplantation (orphan) and rheumatoid arthritis* [azathioprine sodium] 100 mg ⑨ Enduron; Imferon

**Imuran** tablets ℞ *immunosuppressant for organ transplantation (orphan) and rheumatoid arthritis* [azathioprine] 50 mg

**Imuthiol** ℞ *investigational (Phase II/III, orphan) immunomodulator for HIV and AIDS* [diethyldithiocarbamate]

**Imuvert** ℞ *investigational (orphan) for primary brain malignancies* [Serratia marcescens extract (polyribosomes)]

**¹¹¹In** [see: indium In 111 altumomab pentetate]

**¹¹¹In** [see: indium In 111 imciromab pentetate]

**¹¹¹In** [see: indium In 111 murine anti-CEA monoclonal antibody]

**¹¹¹In** [see: indium In 111 murine monoclonal antibody]

**¹¹¹In** [see: indium In 111 oxyquinoline]

**¹¹¹In** [see: indium In 111 pentetate]

**¹¹¹In** [see: indium In 111 pentetreotide]

**¹¹¹In** [see: indium In 111 satumomab pendetide]

**¹¹¹In** [see: pentetate indium disodium In 111]

**¹¹³ᵐIn** [see: indium chlorides In 113m]

**inactivated mumps vaccine** [see: mumps virus vaccine, inactivated]

**inactivated poliomyelitis vaccine (IPV)** [see: poliovirus vaccine, inactivated]

**inactivated poliovirus vaccine (IPV)** [see: poliovirus vaccine, inactivated]

**Inactivin** ℞ *investigational (Phase I/II) cellular energy regulator for HIV and AIDS* [HE-200 (code name—generic name not yet assigned)]

**inamrinone** USAN *cardiotonic* [also: amrinone]

**inamrinone lactate** *vasodilator for congestive heart failure* [previously known as amrinone lactate; name changed 2000]

**inaperisone** INN

**Inapsine** IV or IM injection ℞ *general anesthetic; antiemetic* [droperidol] 2.5 mg/mL

**incretin mimetic agents** *a class of antidiabetic drugs that improve the body's normal glucose-sensing mechanisms by activating the glucagon-like peptide-1 (GLP-1) receptors*

**indacrinic acid** [see: indacrinone]

**indacrinone** USAN, INN *antihypertensive; diuretic*

**indalpine** INN, BAN

**indanazoline** INN

**indanediones** *a class of anticoagulants that interfere with vitamin K–dependent clotting factors*

**indanidine** INN

**indanorex** INN

**indapamide** USAN, INN, BAN *antihypertensive; diuretic* 1.25, 2.5 mg oral

**indatraline** INN

**indecainide** INN *antiarrhythmic* [also: indecainide HCl]

**indecainide HCl** USAN *antiarrhythmic* [also: indecainide]

**indeloxazine** INN *antidepressant* [also: indeloxazine HCl]

**indeloxazine HCl** USAN *antidepressant* [also: indeloxazine]

**indenolol** INN, BAN

**Inderal** tablets, IV injection ℞ *antianginal; antihypertensive; antiarrhythmic; β-blocker; migraine preventative* [propranolol HCl] 10, 20, 40, 60, 80 mg; 1 mg/mL ⑨ Enduron; Enduronyl; Inderide

**Inderal LA** long-acting capsules ℞ *antianginal; antihypertensive; antiarrhythmic; β-blocker; migraine preventative* [propranolol HCl] 60, 80, 120, 160 mg

**Inderide 40/25; Inderide 80/25** tablets ℞ *antihypertensive; β-blocker; diuretic* [propranolol HCl; hydrochlorothiazide] 40•25 mg; 80•25 mg ℞ Inderal

**Inderide LA 80/50; Inderide LA 120/50; Inderide LA 160/50** long-acting capsules (discontinued 2004) ℞ *antihypertensive; β-blocker; diuretic* [propranolol HCl; hydrochlorothiazide] 80•50 mg; 120•50 mg; 160•50 mg

**Indian apple** *medicinal herb* [see: mandrake]

**Indian arrow; Indian arrow wood** *medicinal herb* [see: wahoo]

**Indian bark** *medicinal herb* [see: magnolia]

**Indian bay** *medicinal herb* [see: laurel]

**Indian corn (Zea mays)** styles (silk) *medicinal herb used as an analgesic, diuretic, demulcent, and litholytic*

**Indian cress (Tropaeolum majus)** flowers, leaves, and seeds *medicinal herb used as an antiseptic and expectorant*

**Indian elm** *medicinal herb* [see: slippery elm]

**Indian frankincense** *medicinal herb* [see: frankincense]

**Indian hemp** *medicinal herb* [see: marijuana]

**Indian hyssop** *medicinal herb* [see: blue vervain]

**Indian paint, red** *medicinal herb* [see: bloodroot]

**Indian paint, yellow** *medicinal herb* [see: goldenseal]

**Indian pipe** *medicinal herb* [see: fit root]

**Indian plant** *medicinal herb* [see: bloodroot; goldenseal]

**Indian poke (Veratrum viride)** *medicinal herb* [see: hellebore]

**Indian root** *medicinal herb* [see: spikenard; wahoo]

**Indian shamrock** *medicinal herb* [see: birthroot]

**Indian tobacco** *medicinal herb* [see: lobelia]

**Indiana protocol** *chemotherapy protocol for ovarian cancer* [see: PAC-I]

**indigo (Indigofera spp.)** plant *medicinal herb for fever, hemorrhoids, inducing emesis, inflammation, liver cleansing, ovarian and stomach cancer, pain, scorpion bites, and worms; not generally regarded as safe and effective*

**indigo, wild** *medicinal herb* [see: wild indigo]

**indigo carmine** BAN *cystoscopy aid* [also: indigotindisulfonate sodium]

**indigotindisulfonate sodium** USP *cystoscopy aid* [also: indigo carmine]

**indinavir** USAN *antiviral; HIV-1 protease inhibitor*

**indinavir sulfate** USAN *antiviral; HIV-1 protease inhibitor*

**indinavir sulfate & amprenavir** *investigational (Phase II) protease inhibitor combination for AIDS*

**indium** *element (In)*

**indium (¹¹¹In) diethylenetriamine pentaacetate** JAN *radionuclide cisternography aid; radioactive agent* [also: indium In 111 pentetate]

**indium chlorides In 113m** USAN, USP *radioactive agent*

**indium In 111 altumomab pentetate** USAN *radiodiagnostic monoclonal antibody for colorectal carcinoma; anticarcinoembryonic antigen* [also: altumomab]

**indium In 111 antimelanoma antibody XMMME-0001-DTPA** [see: antimelanoma antibody]

**indium In 111 CYT-103** [now: indium In 111 satumomab pendetide]

**indium In 111 ibritumomab tiuxetan** *radioimmunotherapy for non-Hodgkin B-cell lymphoma*

**indium In 111 IGIV pentetate** *radiodiagnostic imaging agent for inflammation and infection* [also: immune globulin intravenous pentetate]

**indium In 111 imciromab pentetate** *radioactive diagnostic aid for cardiac imaging*

**indium In 111 murine monoclonal antibodies (2B8-MXDTPA) & yttrium Y 90 murine MAb (2B8-MXDTPA)** *investigational (orphan) for non-Hodgkin B-cell lymphoma*

**indium In 111 murine monoclonal antibodies (MAb) Fab to myosin** [now: imciromab pentetate]

**indium In 111 oxyquinoline** USAN, USP *radioactive agent; diagnostic aid*

**indium In 111 pentetate** USP *radionuclide cisternography aid; radioactive agent* [also: indium ($^{111}$In) diethylenetriamine pentaacetate]

**indium In 111 pentetreotide** USAN *radioactive imaging agent for SPECT scans of neuroendocrine tumors; investigational (orphan) radiotherapeutic agent for somatostatin receptor–positive neuroendocrine tumors*

**indium In 111 satumomab pentetide** USAN *radiodiagnostic imaging aid for ovarian (orphan) and colorectal carcinoma* [also: satumomab]

**indobufen** INN

**indocate** INN

**Indochron E-R** extended-release tablets (discontinued 2000) ℞ *antiarthritic; nonsteroidal anti-inflammatory drug (NSAID) for ankylosing spondylitis and acute bursitis/tendinitis* [indomethacin] 75 mg

**Indocin** capsules, oral suspension, suppositories ℞ *antiarthritic; nonsteroidal anti-inflammatory drug (NSAID) for ankylosing spondylitis and acute bursitis/tendinitis* [indomethacin] 25, 50 mg; 25 mg/5 mL; 50 mg ⊡ Lincocin; Minocin

**Indocin I.V.** powder for IV injection ℞ *prostaglandin synthesis inhibitor for neonatal closure of patent ductus arteriosus* [indomethacin sodium trihydrate] 1 mg

**Indocin SR** sustained-release capsules ℞ *antiarthritic; nonsteroidal anti-inflammatory drug (NSAID) for ankylosing spondylitis and acute bursitis/tendinitis* [indomethacin] 75 mg

**indocyanine green** USP, JAN *in vivo diagnostic aid for cardiac output, hepatic function, and ophthalmic angiography*

**indolapril** INN *antihypertensive* [also: indolapril HCl]

**indolapril HCl** USAN *antihypertensive* [also: indolapril]

**indole 3-carbinol** *natural phytochemical found in cruciferous vegetables; antioxidant and estrogen blocker shown effective against hormone-related cancers of the prostate, the uterus, and especially the breast; restores the p21 tumor suppressor gene*

**indolidan** USAN, INN, BAN *cardiotonic*

**indolones** *a class of dopamine receptor antagonists with conventional (typical) antipsychotic activity* [also called: dihydroindolones]

**indometacin** INN, JAN *antiarthritic; nonsteroidal anti-inflammatory drug (NSAID)* [also: indomethacin]

**indometacin farnecil** JAN *antiarthritic; nonsteroidal anti-inflammatory drug (NSAID)* [also: indomethacin]

**indomethacin** USAN, USP, BAN *antiarthritic; nonsteroidal anti-inflammatory drug (NSAID) for ankylosing spondylitis and acute bursitis/tendinitis* [also: indometacin; indomethacin farnecil] 25, 50, 75 mg oral

**indomethacin sodium** USAN *anti-inflammatory*

**indomethacin sodium trihydrate** *neonatal closure of patent ductus arteriosus*

**indopanolol** INN

**indopine** INN

**indoprofen** USAN, INN, BAN *analgesic; anti-inflammatory*

**indoramin** USAN, INN, BAN *antihypertensive*

**indoramin HCl** USAN, BAN *antihypertensive*

**indorenate** INN *antihypertensive* [also: indorenate HCl]

**indorenate HCl** USAN *antihypertensive* [also: indorenate]

**indoxole** USAN, INN *antipyretic; anti-inflammatory*

**indriline** INN *CNS stimulant* [also: indriline HCl]

**indriline HCl** USAN *CNS stimulant* [also: indriline]

**inductin** [see: diphoxazide]

**Infalyte** oral solution OTC *electrolyte replacement* [sodium, potassium, and chloride electrolytes]

**Infanrix** IM injection ℞ *active immunizing agent for diphtheria, tetanus, and pertussis* [diphtheria & tetanus

**toxoids & acellular pertussis (DTaP) vaccine, adborbed]** 25 Lf•10 Lf•25 µg per 0.5 mL dose

**Infantaire** oral drops OTC *analgesic; antipyretic* [acetaminophen] 80 mg/0.8 mL

**Infasurf** intratracheal suspension ℞ *agent for prophylaxis and treatment of respiratory distress syndrome (RDS) in premature infants (orphan)* [calfactant] 6 mL

**Infatab** (trademarked dosage form) *pediatric chewable tablet*

**InFeD** IV or IM injection ℞ *hematinic* [iron dextran] 50 mg/mL ⚠ NSAID

**Infergen** subcu injection ℞ *consensus interferon for the treatment of chronic hepatitis C virus (HCV) infections* [interferon alfacon-1] 9, 15 µg/0.3 mL dose

**Inflamase Mild; Inflamase Forte** eye drops ℞ *corticosteroidal anti-inflammatory* [prednisolone sodium phosphate] 0.125%; 1%

**infliximab** *anti-inflammatory; anti-TNFα (tumor necrosis factor alpha) monoclonal antibody for Crohn disease (orphan) and rheumatoid arthritis (with methotrexate)*

**influenza purified surface antigen** [see: influenza split-virus vaccine]

**influenza split-virus vaccine** *subcategory of influenza virus vaccine*

**influenza subvirion vaccine** [see: influenza split-virus vaccine]

**influenza virus vaccine** USP *active immunizing agent for influenza* [virus strains for the 2004–2005 season: A/New Caledonia/20/99 (H1N1), A/Wyoming/03/2003 (H3N2), and B/Jiangsu/10/2003]

**influenza whole-virus vaccine** *subcategory of influenza virus vaccine*

**infraRUB** cream (discontinued 2004) OTC *analgesic; counterirritant* [methyl salicylate; menthol] 35%•10%

**Infumorph 200; Infumorph 500** concentrate for continuous microinfusion ℞ *narcotic analgesic; intraspinal microinfusion for intractable chronic pain (orphan)* [morphine sulfate] 10

mg/mL (200 mg/vial); 25 mg/mL (500 mg/vial)

**Infurfer** ⒸⒶⓃ IV or IM injection ℞ *hematinic* [iron dextran] 50 mg/mL

**Infuvite Adult** IV infusion ℞ *multivitamin adjunct for adults receiving parenteral nutrition* [multiple vitamins; folic acid; biotin] ±•600•60 µg

**Infuvite Pediatric** IV infusion ℞ *multivitamin adjunct for infants and children receiving parenteral nutrition* [multiple vitamins; folic acid; biotin] ±•140•20 µg

**INGN-201** *investigational (Phase III) gene therapy for head and neck cancers* [also: adenoviral p53 gene; p53 adenoviral gene]

**INH (isonicotinic acid hydrazide)** [see: isoniazid]

**Inhal-Aid** (trademarked form) *portable inhalation device*

**inhalants** *a class of street drugs that include nitrous oxide, volatile nitrites, and petroleum distillates* [see: nitrous oxide; volatile nitrites; petroleum distillate inhalants]

**inicarone** INN

**Inject-all** (trademarked delivery system) *prefilled disposable syringe*

**Inlay-Tabs** (trademarked dosage form) *tablets with contrasting inlay*

**InnoGel Plus** gel packs + comb (discontinued 2003) OTC *pediculicide for lice* [pyrethrins; piperonyl butoxide technical] 0.3%•3%

**Innohep** deep subcu injection ℞ *anticoagulant/antithrombotic for prevention of deep vein thrombosis (DVT)* [tinzaparin sodium] 20 000 IU anti–factor Xa/mL

**InnoLet** prefilled disposable syringe OTC *device for self-administration of insulin* (available prefilled with Novolin 70/30 or Novolin N) [insulin] 1–40 U/injection

**InnoPran XL** long-acting capsules ℞ *antihypertensive; β-blocker* [propranolol HCl] 80, 100 mg

**Innovar** injection (discontinued 2001) ℞ *narcotic analgesic; major*

*tranquilizer* [fentanyl citrate; droperidol] 0.05•2.5 mg/mL

**Inocor** IV injection (discontinued 2000) Ɍ *vasodilator for congestive heart failure* [inamrinone lactate] 5 mg/mL

**inocoterone** INN *anti-acne* [also: inocoterone acetate]

**inocoterone acetate** USAN *anti-acne* [also: inocoterone]

**INOmax** inhalation gas Ɍ *for neonatal hypoxic respiratory failure due to persistent pulmonary hypertension (orphan); investigational (orphan) for acute adult respiratory distress syndrome (ARDS)* [nitric oxide] 100, 800 ppm

**inosine** INN, JAN ② Ilosone

**inosine pranobex** BAN, JAN *investigational antiviral/immunomodulator for AIDS; investigational (orphan) for subacute sclerosing panencephalitis*

**inosiplex** [now: inosine pranobex]

**Inositech** capsules OTC *vitamin B supplement* [inositol] 324 mg

**inositol** NF *dietary lipotropic supplement* 250, 500, 650 mg oral

**inositol niacinate** USAN *peripheral vasodilator* [also: inositol nicotinate]

**inositol nicotinate** INN, BAN *peripheral vasodilator* [also: inositol niacinate]

**inotropes** *a class of drugs that affect the force or energy of muscle contractions*

**inprochone** [see: inproquone]

**inproquone** INN, BAN

**INSH (isonicotinoyl-salicylidene-hydrazine)** [see: salinazid]

**InspirEase** (trademarked form) *portable inhalation device*

**Inspra** film-coated tablets Ɍ *aldosterone receptor antagonist for hypertension and congestive heart failure (CHF); improves survival after a cardiovascular event* [eplerenone] 25, 50 mg

**Insta-Glucose** gel OTC *glucose elevating agent* [glucose] 40%

**insulin** USP, JAN *antidiabetic* ② inulin

**insulin, biphasic** INN, BAN *antidiabetic*

**insulin, biphasic isophane** BAN *antidiabetic*

**insulin, dalanated** USAN, INN *antidiabetic*

**insulin, globin zinc** USP [also: globin zinc insulin]

**insulin, isophane** USP, BAN, INN, JAN *antidiabetic*

**insulin, neutral** USAN, JAN *antidiabetic* [also: neutral insulin]

**insulin, NPH (neutral protamine Hagedorn)** [see: insulin, isophane]

**insulin, protamine zinc (PZI)** USP *antidiabetic* [also: insulin zinc protamine; protamine zinc insulin]

**insulin argine** INN *antidiabetic*

**insulin aspart** USAN, INN *antidiabetic; rapid-acting insulin analogue*

**insulin aspart protamine** *antidiabetic; intermediate-acting insulin analogue*

**insulin defalan** INN *antidiabetic*

**insulin detemir** USAN *antidiabetic; investigational (NDA filed) long-acting insulin formulation intended to provide continuous basal insulin levels through once- or twice-daily subcu injections*

**insulin glargine** INN *antidiabetic; long-acting, once-daily basal insulin analogue*

**insulin glulisine** *antidiabetic; rapid-onset, short-acting insulin analogue*

**insulin human** USAN, USP, INN, BAN, JAN *antidiabetic*

**insulin human, isophane** USP *antidiabetic*

**insulin human zinc** USP *antidiabetic*

**insulin human zinc, extended** USP *antidiabetic*

**insulin I 125** USAN *radioactive agent*

**insulin I 131** USAN *radioactive agent*

**insulin lispro** USAN, INN, BAN *antidiabetic*

**insulin lispro protamine** *antidiabetic*

**Insulin Reaction** gel OTC *glucose elevating agent* [glucose] 40%

**insulin zinc** USP, INN, BAN, JAN *antidiabetic*

**insulin zinc, extended** USP *antidiabetic* [also: insulin zinc suspension (crystalline)]

**insulin zinc, prompt** USP *antidiabetic* [also: insulin zinc suspension (amorphous)]

**insulin zinc protamine** JAN *antidia-betic* [also: insulin, protamine zinc; protamine zinc insulin]

**insulin zinc suspension (amorphous)** INN, BAN, JAN *antidiabetic* [also: insulin zinc, prompt]

**insulin zinc suspension (crystalline)** INN, BAN, JAN *antidiabetic* [also: insulin zinc, extended]

**insulin-like growth factor-1, recombinant human (rhIGF-1)** [now: mecasermin]

**Insuman** subcu injection OTC *investigational (Phase III) antidiabetic* [human insulin (rDNA)]

**Intal** solution for nebulization, aerosol spray Ṛ *anti-inflammatory; mast cell stabilizer for prophylactic treatment of allergy, asthma, and bronchospasm* [cromolyn sodium] 20 mg/2 mL ampule; 800 μg/dose ⧉ Endal

**Integra** (approved in 21 countries) *investigational artificial skin*

**Integrilin** IV injection Ṛ *GP IIb/IIIa platelet aggregation inhibitor for acute coronary syndrome, unstable angina, myocardial infarction, and cardiac surgery* [eptifibatide] 0.75, 2 mg/mL

**Intensol** (trademarked form) *concentrated oral solution*

**α-2-interferon** [see: interferon alfa-2b, recombinant]

**interferon, fibroblast** [now: interferon beta]

**interferon, leukocyte** [now: interferon alfa-n3]

**interferon α2b** [see: interferon alfa-2b]

**interferon αA** [see: interferon alfa-2a]

**interferon alfa** JAN *investigational (Phase III) oral treatment for Sjögren syndrome; investigational (Phase II) for AIDS-related xerostomia; investigational (orphan) for oral human papillomavirus (HPV) warts in HIV-infected patients*

**interferon alfa (BALL-1)** JAN

**interferon alfa-2 & interleukin-2 (aldesleukin)** *chemotherapy protocol for renal cell carcinoma*

**interferon alfa-2a (IFN-αA; rIFN-A)** USAN, INN, BAN, JAN *antineoplastic/antiviral for hairy cell leukemia, hepatitis C, Kaposi sarcoma (orphan), and chronic myelogenous leukemia (orphan); investigational (orphan) for renal cell carcinoma*

**interferon alfa-2a & fluorouracil** *investigational (orphan) for esophageal carcinoma and advanced colorectal cancer*

**interferon alfa-2a & teceleukin** *investigational (orphan) for metastatic renal cell carcinoma and metastatic malignant melanoma*

**interferon alfa-2b (IFN-α2)** USAN, INN, BAN *antineoplastic for hairy-cell leukemia, malignant melanoma, AIDS-related Kaposi sarcoma (orphan), and various other cancers; antiviral for condylomata acuminata and chronic hepatitis B and C; investigational (Phase I/II) cytokine for AIDS*

**interferon alfacon-1** USAN *bioengineered consensus interferon for the treatment of chronic hepatitis C virus (HCV) infections*

**interferon alfa-n1** USAN, INN, BAN *antineoplastic; biological response modifier for chronic hepatitis C (orphan); investigational (Phase III) cytokine for HIV; investigational (orphan) for human papillomavirus in severe respiratory papillomatosis*

**interferon alfa-n3** USAN *immunomodulator and antiviral for condyloma acuminata; investigational (Phase III) cytokine for HIV, AIDS, ARC, and hepatitis C*

**interferon & alitretinoin** *investigational (Phase I/II) combination treatment for AIDS-related Kaposi sarcoma*

**interferon beta (IFN-B)** BAN, JAN *antineoplastic; antiviral; immunomodulator*

**interferon beta-1a** USAN *immunomodulator for relapsing multiple sclerosis (orphan); investigational (orphan) for non-A, non-B hepatitis, Kaposi sarcoma, brain tumors, and various other cancers*

**interferon beta-1b** USAN *immunomodulator for relapsing-remitting multiple sclerosis (orphan)*

**interferon gamma-1a** JAN

**interferon gamma-1b** USAN, INN, BAN *antineoplastic; antiviral; immunoregulator for chronic granulomatous disease (orphan) and severe congenital osteopetrosis (orphan); investigational (orphan) for renal cell carcinoma*

**interferon gamma-2a** [see: interferon gamma-1b]

**α-interferons** [see: interferon alfa-n1 and -n3]

**Intergel** irrigating solution ℞ *adhesion barrier for open gynecological and lower GI surgical procedures* [ferric hyaluronate] 0.5%

**interleukin-1 beta** *investigational antineoplastic for melanoma; investigational liposome-encapsulated formulation for influenza A*

**interleukin-1 receptor antagonist, recombinant human** [now: anakinra]

**interleukin-2 (aldesleukin) & interferon alfa-2** *chemotherapy protocol for renal cell carcinoma*

**interleukin-2, liposome-encapsulated recombinant** *investigational (orphan) for brain, central nervous system, kidney, and pelvic cancers*

**interleukin-2, recombinant (IL-2)** [see: aldesleukin; teceleukin; celmoleukin]

**interleukin-2 receptor (IL-2R) fusion protein** *investigational (NDA filed) for cutaneous T-cell lymphoma (CTCL); investigational (Phase II) for other lymphomas and leukemias; investigational (Phase II) for squamous cell carcinoma of the head and neck*

**interleukin-4 (IL-4) Pseudomonas toxin fusion protein** *investigational (orphan) antineoplastic for astrocytic glioma* [also: NBI-3001]

**interleukin-10 (IL-10)** [see: ilodecakin]

**interleukin-11, recombinant human (rhIL-11)** *platelet growth factor for thrombocytopenia of chemotherapy or radiation (orphan)* [also: oprelvekin]

**interleukin-12 (IL-12)** [see: edodekin alfa]

**intermedine** INN

**intoplicine** INN *investigational (Phase I) antineoplastic and topoisomerase I and II inhibitor*

**Intrachol** ℞ *investigational (orphan) for choline deficiency of long-term parenteral nutrition* [choline chloride]

**IntraDose** injectable gel ℞ *investigational (NDA filed, orphan) alkylating antineoplastic for squamous cell carcinoma of the head and neck; investigational (orphan) for metastatic malignant melanoma* [cisplatin; epinephrine]

**Intralipid 10%; Intralipid 20%** IV infusion ℞ *nutritional therapy* [fat emulsion]

**IntraSite** gel OTC *wound dressing* [graft T starch copolymer] 2%

**intravascular perfluorochemical emulsion** *synthetic blood oxygen carrier for PTCA*

**intravenous fat emulsion** [see: fat emulsion, intravenous]

**intravenous immunoglobulin (IVIG)** *investigational IV solution of concentrated antibodies for AIDS*

**intrazole** USAN, INN *anti-inflammatory*

**Intrinsa** transdermal patch ℞ *investigational hormone replacement therapy for female sexual dysfunction (FSD) and hypoactive sexual desire disorder (HSDD) in women* [testosterone]

**intrinsic factor concentrate** *antianemic to enhance the body's utilization of vitamin $B_{12}$*

**intriptyline** INN *antidepressant* [also: intriptyline HCl]

**intriptyline HCl** USAN *antidepressant* [also: intriptyline]

**Introlan Half-Strength** oral liquid OTC *enteral nutritional therapy* [lactose-free formula]

**Introlite** oral liquid OTC *enteral nutritional therapy* [lactose-free formula]

**Intron A** subcu or IM injection ℞ *antineoplastic for hairy cell leukemia,* malignant melanoma, Kaposi sarcoma (orphan), and various other cancers; antiviral for condylomata acuminata and chronic hepatitis B and C; investigational (Phase I/II) cytokine for AIDS [interferon alfa-2b] 3, 5, 10, 18, 25, 50 million IU/vial

**Intropaste** oral paste ℞ radiopaque contrast medium for esophageal imaging [barium sulfate] 70%

**Intropin** IV injection (discontinued 2004) ℞ vasopressor for cardiac, pulmonary, traumatic, septic, or renal shock [dopamine HCl] 40, 80, 160 mg/mL ⊉ Ditropan; Isoptin

*Inula helenium* medicinal herb [see: elecampane]

**inulin** USP diagnostic aid for renal function 100 mg/mL injection ⊉ insulin

**Invanz** IV or IM injection ℞ broad-spectrum carbapenem antibiotic [ertapenem sodium] 1 g/vial

**invenol** [see: carbutamide]

**Inversine** tablets ℞ antiadrenergic; ganglionic blocker for severe hypertension [mecamylamine HCl] 2.5 mg

**invert sugar** [see: sugar, invert]

**Invirase** capsules (this product is being replaced by Fortovase) ℞ antiretroviral protease inhibitor for HIV [saquinavir mesylate] 200 mg

**iobenguane ($^{131}$I)** INN radioactive agent [also: iobenguane I 131]

**iobenguane I 123** USP radioactive agent

**iobenguane I 131** USAN radioactive agent [also: iobenguane ($^{131}$I)]

**iobenguane sulfate I 123** USAN radiopharmaceutical diagnostic aid for adrenomedullary disorders and neuroendocrine tumors

**iobenguane sulfate I 131** USAN diagnostic aid for pheochromocytoma (orphan)

**iobenzamic acid** USAN, INN, BAN radiopaque contrast medium for cholecystography

**Iobid DM** sustained-release tablets ℞ antitussive; expectorant [dextromethorphan hydrobromide; guaifenesin] 30•600 mg

**iobutoic acid** INN

**iocanlidic acid I 123** USAN cardiac diagnostic aid

**Iocare Balanced Salt** ophthalmic solution OTC intraocular irrigating solution [sodium chloride (balanced saline solution)]

**iocarmate meglumine** USAN radiopaque contrast medium [also: meglumine iocarmate]

**iocarmic acid** USAN, INN, BAN radiopaque contrast medium

**iocetamic acid** USAN, USP, INN, BAN oral radiopaque contrast medium for cholecystography (62% iodine)

**Iocon** shampoo (discontinued 2003) OTC antiseborrheic; antipsoriatic; antipruritic; antibacterial [coal tar; alcohol]

**Iodal HD** oral liquid (discontinued 2002) ℞ narcotic antitussive; decongestant; antihistamine [hydrocodone bitartrate; phenylephrine HCl; chlorpheniramine maleate] 1.67•5• 2 mg/5 mL

**iodamide** USAN, INN, BAN radiopaque contrast medium

**iodamide meglumine** USAN radiopaque contrast medium

**iodecimol** INN

**iodecol** [see: iodecimol]

**iodetryl** INN

**Iodex; Iodex-P** ointment OTC broad-spectrum antimicrobial [povidone-iodine] 4.7%; 10%

**Iodex with Methyl Salicylate** ointment OTC analgesic; counterirritant; anti-infective [methyl salicylate; iodine] 4.8%•4.7%

**iodinated ($^{125}$I) human serum albumin** INN radioactive agent; blood volume test [also: albumin, iodinated I 125 serum]

**iodinated ($^{131}$I) human serum albumin** INN, JAN radioactive agent; intrathecal imaging agent; blood volume test [also: albumin, iodinated I 131 serum]

**iodinated glycerol** [see: glycerol, iodinated]

**iodinated I 125 albumin** [see: albumin, iodinated I 125]

**iodinated I 131 aggregated albumin** [see: albumin, iodinated I 131 aggregated]

**iodinated I 131 albumin** [see: albumin, iodinated I 131]

**iodine** USP *broad-spectrum topical antiinfective; element (I)* 2% topical

**iodine I 123 murine monoclonal antibodies (MAb) to alpha-fetoprotein (AFP)** *investigational (orphan) diagnostic aid for AFP-producing tumors, hepatocellular carcinoma, and hepatoblastoma*

**iodine I 123 murine monoclonal antibodies (MAb) to human chorionic gonadotropin (hCG)** *investigational (orphan) diagnostic aid for hCG-producing tumors*

**iodine I 131 6B-iodomethyl-19-norcholesterol** *investigational (orphan) for adrenal cortical imaging*

**iodine I 131 metaiodobenzylguanidine sulfate** [now: iobenguane sulfate I 131]

**iodine I 131 murine monoclonal antibodies (MAb) to alpha-fetoprotein (AFP)** *investigational (orphan) treatment for AFP-producing tumors, hepatocellular carcinoma, and hepatoblastoma*

**iodine I 131 murine monoclonal antibodies (MAb) to human chorionic gonadotropin (hCG)** *investigational (orphan) treatment for hCG-producing tumors*

**iodine I 131 murine monoclonal antibodies (MAb) IgG₂a to B cell5** *investigational (orphan) for B-cell leukemia and lymphoma*

**iodine I 131 radiolabeled B1 monoclonal antibodies (MAb)** *investigational (orphan) for non-Hodgkin B-cell lymphoma*

**iodine I 131 tositumomab** *radiotherapy for non-Hodgkin lymphoma (NHL); radiotherapeutic agent bound to NHL monoclonal antibody for targeted delivery of radiation* [see also: tositumomab]

**iodipamide** USP, BAN *parenteral radiopaque contrast medium* [also: adipiodone]

**iodipamide meglumine** USP, BAN *parenteral radiopaque contrast medium (49.42% iodine)* [also: adipiodone meglumine]

**iodipamide methylglucamine** [see: iodipamide meglumine]

**iodipamide sodium** USP *parenteral radiopaque contrast medium*

**iodipamide sodium I 131** USAN *radioactive agent*

**iodisan** [see: prolonium iodide]

**iodixanol** USAN, INN, BAN *parenteral radiopaque contrast medium (49.1% iodine)*

**iodized oil** NF

**iodoalphionic acid** NF [also: pheniodol sodium]

**iodoantipyrine I 131** USAN *radioactive agent*

**iodobehenate calcium** NF

**m-iodobenzylguanidine sulfate I 123** [see: iobenguane sulfate I 123]

**iodocetylic acid (¹²³I)** INN *diagnostic aid* [also: iodocetylic acid I 123]

**iodocetylic acid I 123** USAN *diagnostic aid* [also: iodocetylic acid (¹²³I)]

**iodochlorhydroxyquin** [now: clioquinol]

**iodocholesterol (¹³¹I)** INN *radioactive agent* [also: iodocholesterol I 131]

**iodocholesterol I 131** USAN *radioactive agent* [also: iodocholesterol (¹³¹I)]

**iodoform** NF

**iodohippurate sodium I 123** USAN, USP *renal function test; radioactive agent*

**iodohippurate sodium I 125** USAN *radioactive agent*

**iodohippurate sodium I 131** USAN, USP *renal function test; radioactive agent* [also: sodium iodohippurate (¹³¹I)]

**iodohydroxyquin** [see: clioquinol]

**iodol** USP

**iodomethamate sodium** NF

**iodopanoic acid** [see: iopanoic acid]

**Iodopen** IV injection ℞ *iodine supplement* [sodium iodide (85% elemental iodine)] 118 μg/mL (100 μg I/mL)

**iodophthalein, soluble** [now: iodophthalein sodium]

**iodophthalein sodium** NF, INN

**iodopyracet** NF [also: diodone]

**iodopyracet I 125** USAN *radioactive agent*

**iodopyracet I 131** USAN *radioactive agent*

**iodoquinol** USAN, USP *amebicide; antimicrobial* [also: diiodohydroxyquinoline]

**iodoquinol & hydrocortisone** *amebicide; antimicrobial; corticosteroidal anti-inflammatory* 1%•1% topical

**Iodosorb** ⊛ paste, ointment OTC *antibacterial; antiulcerative wound dressing* [cadexomer iodine] 0.9%

**iodothiouracil** INN, BAN

**iodothymol** [see: thymol iodide]

**Iodotope** capsules, oral solution ℞ *radioactive agent for hyperthyroidism and thyroid carcinoma* [sodium iodide I 131] 1–50 mCi; 7.05 mCi/mL

**iodoxamate meglumine** USAN, BAN *radiopaque contrast medium*

**iodoxamic acid** USAN, INN, BAN *radiopaque contrast medium*

**iodoxyl** [see: iodomethamate sodium]

**Iofed** extended-release capsules (discontinued 2002) ℞ *decongestant; antihistamine* [pseudoephedrine HCl; brompheniramine maleate] 120•12 mg

**Iofed PD** extended-release capsules (discontinued 2002) ℞ *pediatric decongestant and antihistamine* [pseudoephedrine HCl; brompheniramine maleate] 60•6 mg

**iofendylate** INN *radiopaque contrast medium* [also: iophendylate]

**iofetamine ($^{123}$I)** INN *diagnostic aid; radioactive agent* [also: iofetamine HCl I 123]

**iofetamine HCl I 123** USAN *diagnostic aid; radioactive agent* [also: iofetamine ($^{123}$I)]

**Iofoam** (trademarked form) *foaming skin cleanser*

**ioglicic acid** USAN, INN, BAN *radiopaque contrast medium*

**ioglucol** USAN, INN *radiopaque contrast medium*

**ioglucomide** USAN, INN *radiopaque contrast medium*

**ioglunide** INN

**ioglycamic acid** USAN, INN, BAN *radiopaque contrast medium for cholecystography*

**iogulamide** USAN *radiopaque contrast medium*

**iohexol** USAN, INN, BAN *parenteral radiopaque contrast medium (46.36% iodine)*

**Iohist D** elixir (discontinued 2002) ℞ *decongestant; antihistamine* [phenylpropanolamine HCl; phenyltoloxamine citrate; pyrilamine maleate; pheniramine maleate] 25•4•4•4 mg/5 mL

**Iohist DM** syrup (discontinued 2002) ℞ *antitussive; decongestant; antihistamine* [dextromethorphan hydrobromide; phenylpropanolamine HCl; brompheniramine maleate] 10•12.5•2 mg/5 mL

**iolidonic acid** INN

**iolixanic acid** INN

**iomeglamic acid** INN

**iomeprol** USAN, INN, BAN *radiopaque contrast medium*

**iomethin I 125** USAN *neoplasm test; radioactive agent* [also: iometin ($^{125}$I)]

**iomethin I 131** USAN *neoplasm test; radioactive agent* [also: iometin ($^{131}$I)]

**iometin ($^{125}$I)** INN *neoplasm test; radioactive agent* [also: iomethin I 125]

**iometin ($^{131}$I)** INN *neoplasm test; radioactive agent* [also: iomethin I 131]

**iometopane I 123** USAN *diagnostic imaging aid for dopamine and serotonin transporter sites*

**iomorinic acid** INN

**Ionamin** capsules ℞ *anorexiant; CNS stimulant* [phentermine HCl resin complex] 15, 30 mg

**Ionax** foam OTC *medicated cleanser for acne* [benzalkonium chloride]

**Ionax Astringent Skin Cleanser** topical liquid OTC *keratolytic cleanser for acne* [salicylic acid; isopropyl alcohol]

**Ionax Scrub** OTC *abrasive medicated cleanser for acne* [benzalkonium chloride]

**ionic contrast media** *a class of older radiopaque agents that, in general, have a high osmolar concentration of iodine (the contrast agent), which corresponds to a higher incidence of adverse reactions* [also called: high osmolar contrast media (HOCM)]

**Ionil** shampoo OTC *antiseborrheic; keratolytic; antiseptic* [salicylic acid; benzalkonium chloride]

**Ionil Plus** shampoo OTC *antiseborrheic; keratolytic* [salicylic acid] 2%

**Ionil T** shampoo OTC *antiseborrheic; antipsoriatic; keratolytic; antiseptic* [coal tar; salicylic acid; benzalkonium chloride]

**Ionil-T Plus** shampoo OTC *antiseborrheic; antipsoriatic; antipruritic; antibacterial* [coal tar] 2%

**ionphylline** [see: aminophylline]

**iopamidol** USAN, USP, INN, BAN *parenteral radiopaque contrast medium (49% iodine)*

**iopanoic acid** USP, INN, BAN *oral radiopaque contrast medium for cholecystography (66.68% iodine)*

**iopentol** USAN, INN, BAN *radiopaque contrast medium*

**Iophen** tablets, elixir, drops Ŗ *expectorant* [iodinated glycerol] 30 mg; 60 mg/5 mL; 50 mg/mL

**Iophen-C** oral liquid (discontinued 2002) Ŗ *narcotic antitussive; expectorant* [codeine phosphate; iodinated glycerol] 10•30 mg/5 mL

**Iophen-DM** oral liquid (discontinued 2002) Ŗ *antitussive; expectorant* [dextromethorphan hydrobromide; iodinated glycerol] 10•30 mg/5 mL

**iophendylate** USP, BAN *radiopaque contrast medium* [also: iofendylate]

**iophenoic acid** INN [also: iophenoxic acid]

**iophenoxic acid** USP [also: iophenoic acid]

**Iophylline** elixir Ŗ *antiasthmatic; bronchodilator; expectorant* [theophylline; iodinated glycerol] 120•30 mg/15 mL

**Iopidine** Drop-Tainers (eye drops) Ŗ *topical sympathomimetic antiglaucoma agent* [apraclonidine HCl] 0.5%, 1%

**ioprocemic acid** USAN, INN *radiopaque contrast medium*

**iopromide** USAN, INN, BAN *parenteral radiopaque contrast medium (39% iodine)*

**iopronic acid** USAN, INN, BAN *radiopaque contrast medium for cholecystography*

**iopydol** USAN, INN, BAN *radiopaque contrast medium for bronchography*

**iopydone** USAN, INN, BAN *radiopaque contrast medium for bronchography*

**Iosal II** sustained-release tablets Ŗ *decongestant; expectorant* [pseudoephedrine HCl; guaifenesin] 60•600 mg

**iosarcol** INN

**iosefamic acid** USAN, INN *radiopaque contrast medium*

**ioseric acid** USAN, INN *radiopaque contrast medium*

**iosimide** INN

**iosulamide** INN *radiopaque contrast medium* [also: iosulamide meglumine]

**iosulamide meglumine** USAN *radiopaque contrast medium* [also: iosulamide]

**iosulfan blue** *parenteral radiopaque contrast medium for lymphography*

**iosumetic acid** USAN, INN *radiopaque contrast medium*

**iotalamic acid** INN *radiopaque contrast medium* [also: iothalamic acid]

**iotasul** USAN, INN *radiopaque contrast medium*

**iotetric acid** USAN, INN *radiopaque contrast medium*

**iothalamate meglumine** USP *parenteral radiopaque contrast medium (47% iodine)* [also: meglumine iothalamate]

**iothalamate sodium** USP *parenteral radiopaque contrast medium (59.9% iodine)* [also: sodium iothalamate]

**iothalamate sodium I 125** USAN *radioactive agent* [also: sodium iotalamate ($^{125}$I)]

**iothalamate sodium I 131** USAN *radioactive agent* [also: sodium iotalamate ($^{131}$I)]

**iothalamic acid** USP, BAN *radiopaque contrast medium* [also: iotalamic acid]

**iothiouracil sodium**

**iotranic acid** INN

**iotriside** INN

**iotrizoic acid** INN

**iotrol** [now: iotrolan]

**iotrolan** USAN, INN, BAN *parenteral radiopaque contrast medium*

**iotroxic acid** USAN, INN, BAN *radiopaque contrast medium*

**Iotussin HC** syrup (discontinued 2002) ℞ *narcotic antitussive; decongestant; antihistamine* [hydrocodone bitartrate; phenylephrine HCl; chlorpheniramine maleate] 2.5•5•2 mg/5 mL

**iotyrosine I 131** USAN *radioactive agent*

**ioversol** USAN, INN, BAN *parenteral radiopaque contrast medium (47.3% iodine)*

**ioxabrolic acid** INN

**ioxaglate meglumine** USAN *parenteral radiopaque contrast medium* [also: meglumine ioxaglate]

**ioxaglate sodium** USAN *parenteral radiopaque contrast medium* [also: sodium ioxaglate]

**ioxaglic acid** USAN, INN, BAN *radiopaque contrast medium*

**ioxilan** USAN, INN *diagnostic aid*

**ioxitalamic acid** INN

**ioxotrizoic acid** USAN, INN *radiopaque contrast medium*

**iozomic acid** INN

**IPA (ifosfamide, Platinol, Adriamycin)** *chemotherapy protocol for pediatric hepatoblastoma*

**ipazilide fumarate** USAN *antiarrhythmic*

**ipecac** USP *emetic*

**ipecac, milk** *medicinal herb* [see: birthroot; dogbane]

**ipecac, powdered** USP

**ipexidine** INN *dental caries prophylactic* [also: ipexidine mesylate]

**ipexidine mesylate** USAN, INN *dental caries prophylactic* [also: ipexidine]

**IPL-423** *investigational agent for rheumatoid arthritis*

**ipodate calcium** USP *oral radiopaque contrast medium for cholecystography (61.7% iodine)*

**ipodate sodium** USAN, USP *oral radiopaque contrast medium for cholecystography (61.4% iodine)* [also: sodium ipodate; sodium iopodate]

**IPOL** subcu injection ℞ *poliomyelitis vaccine* [poliovirus vaccine, inactivated] 0.5 mL

**Ipomoea pandurata** *medicinal herb* [see: wild jalap]

**Ipomoea violacea (morning glory)** seeds *contain lysergic acid amide, chemically similar to LSD, which produces hallucinations when ingested as a street drug* [see also: LSD]

**ipragratine** INN

**ipramidil** INN

**ipratropium bromide** USAN, INN, BAN *anticholinergic bronchodilator for bronchospasm; antisecretory for rhinorrhea* 0.02%, 0.03%, 0.06% inhalation; 0.03%, 0.06% nasal spray

**Ipravent** [see: Apo-Ipravent]

**iprazochrome** INN

**iprazone** [see: isoprazone]

**ipriflavone** INN

**iprindole** USAN, INN, BAN *antidepressant*

**Iprivasc** powder for subcu injection ℞ *anticoagulant; thrombin inhibitor for the prevention of deep vein thrombosis (DVT) in elective hip replacement surgery* [desirudin] 15 mg/dose

**iprocinodine HCl** USAN, BAN *veterinary antibacterial*

**iproclozide** INN, BAN

**iprocrolol** INN

**iprofenin** USAN *hepatic function test*

**iproheptine** INN

**iproniazid** INN, BAN

**ipronidazole** USAN, INN, BAN *antiprotozoal (Histomonas)*

**ipropethidine** [see: properidine]

**iproplatin** USAN, INN, BAN *antineoplastic*

**iprotiazem** INN

360    iproxamine

**iproxamine** INN *vasodilator* [also: iproxamine HCl]

**iproxamine HCl** USAN *vasodilator* [also: iproxamine]

**iprozilamine** INN

**ipsalazide** INN, BAN

**ipsapirone** INN, BAN *anxiolytic* [also: ipsapirone HCl]

**ipsapirone HCl** USAN *anxiolytic* [also: ipsapirone]

**Ipsatol Cough Formula for Children; Ipsatol Cough Formula for Adults** oral liquid (discontinued 2002) OTC *antitussive; decongestant; expectorant* [dextromethorphan hydrobromide; phenylpropanolamine HCl; guaifenesin] 10•9•100 mg/5 mL

**IPTD (isopropyl-thiadiazol)** [see: glyprothiazol]

**IPV (inactivated poliomyelitis vaccine)** [see: poliovirus vaccine, inactivated]

**IPV (inactivated poliovaccine)** [see: poliovirus vaccine, inactivated]

**iquindamine** INN

**Iquix** eye drops ℞ *fluoroquinolone antibiotic for corneal ulcers* [levofloxacin] 1.5%

**192Ir** [see: iridium Ir 192]

**irbesartan** USAN *angiotensin II receptor antagonist for hypertension; treatment to delay the progression of diabetic nephropathy*

**Ircon** tablets OTC *hematinic; iron supplement* [carbonyl iron] 66 mg iron

**Ircon-FA** tablets OTC *hematinic* [carbonyl iron; folic acid] 82 mg Fe•0.8 mg

**Iressa** film-coated tablets ℞ *antineoplastic for advanced or metastatic non–small cell lung cancer (NSCLC); investigational (Phase III) for head and neck cancers* [gefitinib] 250 mg

**irgasan** [see: triclosan]

**iridium** *element (Ir)*

**iridium Ir 192** USAN *radioactive agent*

**irindalone** INN

**irinotecan** INN *topoisomerase I inhibitor; antineoplastic for metastatic colon and rectal cancers* [also: irinotecan HCl]

**irinotecan HCl** USAN, JAN *topoisomerase I inhibitor; antineoplastic for metastatic colorectal cancer* [also: irinotecan]

**Iris florentina** *medicinal herb* [see: orris root]

**Iris versicolor** *medicinal herb* [see: blue flag]

**Irish broom** *medicinal herb* [see: broom]

**Irish moss (Chondrus crispus)** plant *medicinal herb used as a demulcent*

**irloxacin** INN

**irofulven** USAN *antineoplastic; DNA synthesis inhibitor; apoptosis inducer*

**irolapride** INN

**Iromin-G** tablets OTC *vitamin/iron supplement* [multiple vitamins; ferrous gluconate; folic acid] ±•30•0.8 mg

**iron** *element (Fe)*

**iron carbohydrate complex** [see: polyferose]

**iron dextran** USP *hematinic*

**iron heptonate** [see: gleptoferron]

**iron hydroxide sucrose complex** [see: iron sucrose; saccharated ferric oxide]

**iron oxide, saccharated** [see: iron sucrose; saccharated ferric oxide]

**iron perchloride** [see: ferric chloride]

**iron polymalether** [see: ferropolimaler]

**Iron Protein Plus** capsules OTC *hematinic; iron supplement* [iron protein succinylate] 300 mg (15 mg Fe)

**iron protein succinylate** *hematinic (5% elemental iron)*

**iron saccharate** [see: iron sucrose; saccharated ferric oxide]

**iron sorbitex** USAN, USP *hematinic*

**iron sucrose** USAN *hematinic for iron deficiency anemia in patients undergoing chronic dialysis* [also: saccharated ferric oxide]

**iron sugar** [see: iron sucrose; saccharated ferric oxide]

**Iron-Folic 500** timed-release tablets OTC *hematinic* [ferrous sulfate; multiple B vitamins; sodium ascorbate; folic acid] 105• ±•500•0.8 mg

**Irospan** timed-release tablets, timed-release capsules (name changed to Vitelle Irospan in 2000)

**Irrigate** eye wash (discontinued 2004) OTC *extraocular irrigating solution* [sterile isotonic solution]

**irritant laxatives** *a subclass of laxatives that work by direct action on the intestinal mucosa and nerve plexus to increase peristaltic action* [more commonly called stimulant laxatives]

**irsogladine** INN

**irtemazole** USAN, INN, BAN *uricosuric*

**IS 5-MN (isosorbide 5-mononitrate)** [see: isorbide mononitrate]

**isaglidole** INN

**isamfazone** INN

**isamoltan** INN

**isamoxole** USAN, INN, BAN *antiasthmatic*

**isatoribine** USAN *immunomodulator; cell growth regulator*

**isaxonine** INN

**isbogrel** INN

**iseganan** *antimicrobial* [also: iseganan HCl]

**iseganan HCl** USAN, INN *investigational (Phase III) antimicrobial rinse for oral mucositis, ventilator-associated pneumonia, and cystic fibrosis* [also: iseganan]

**isepamicin** USAN, INN, BAN *aminoglycoside antibiotic*

**isethionate** USAN, BAN *combining name for radicals or groups* [also: isetionate]

**isetionate** INN *combining name for radicals or groups* [also: isethionate]

**ISG (immune serum globulin)** [see: globulin, immune]

**ISIS 2503** *investigational (Phase II) Ha-ras selective antisense inhibitor for colon, breast, pancreatic, and non–small cell lung cancers (NSCLC)*

**ISIS 3521** *investigational (Phase III) antisense antineoplastic*

**ISIS 5132** *investigational (Phase II) anticancer agent for solid tumors*

**ISIS 13312** *investigational (Phase I/II) second-generation antisense agent for cytomegalovirus retinitis*

**ISIS-5132** *investigational (Phase III) antineoplastic*

**Ismelin** tablets R̥ *antihypertensive; investigational (orphan) for reflex sympathetic dystrophy and causalgia* [guanethidine monosulfate] 25 mg ⑫ Ritalin

**Ismo** film-coated tablets R̥ *antianginal; vasodilator* [isosorbide mononitrate] 20 mg

**Ismotic** solution R̥ *osmotic diuretic* [isosorbide] 45%

**iso-alcoholic elixir** NF

**isoaminile** INN, BAN

**isoamyl p-methoxycinnamate** [see: amiloxate]

**isoamyl nitrate** [see: amyl nitrite]

**Iso-B** capsules OTC *vitamin supplement* [multiple B vitamins; folic acid; biotin] ± • 200 • 100 μg

**isobromindione** INN

**isobucaine HCl** USP

**isobutamben** USAN, INN *topical anesthetic*

**isobutane** NF *aerosol propellant*

**isobutyl p-aminobenzoate** [see: isobutamben]

**isobutyl α-phenylcyclohexaneglycolate** [see: ibuverine]

**isobutyl 2-cyanoacrylate (IBC)** [see: bucrylate]

**isobutyl nitrite; butyl nitrite** *amyl nitrite substitutes, sold as euphoric street drugs, which produce a quick but short-lived "rush"* [see also: amyl nitrite; volatile nitrites]

**p-isobutylhydratropohydroxamic acid** [see: ibuproxam]

**isobutylhydrochlorothiazide** [see: buthiazide]

**isobutyramide** *investigational (orphan) for sickle cell disease, beta-thalassemia syndrome, and beta-hemoglobinopathies*

**isobuzole** BAN [also: glysobuzole]

**Isocaine HCl** injection (discontinued 2002) R̥ *injectable local anesthetic* [mepivacaine HCl] 3%

**Isocaine HCl** injection (discontinued 2002) R̥ *injectable local anesthetic* [mepivacaine HCl; levonordefrin] 2% • 1:20 000

**Isocal** oral liquid OTC *enteral nutritional therapy* [lactose-free formula]

**Isocal HCN** ready-to-use oral liquid OTC *enteral nutritional therapy* [lactose-free formula]

**Isocal HN** oral liquid OTC *enteral nutritional therapy* [lactose-free formula]

**isocarboxazid** USP, INN, BAN *antidepressant; MAO inhibitor*

**Isocet** tablets (discontinued 2000) R *analgesic; barbiturate sedative* [acetaminophen; caffeine; butalbital] 325•40•50 mg

**Isochron** extended-release tablets R *antianginal; vasodilator* [isosorbide dinitrate] 40 mg

**Isoclor Expectorant** oral liquid (discontinued 2002) R *narcotic antitussive; decongestant; expectorant* [codeine phosphate; pseudoephedrine HCl; guaifenesin; alcohol 5%] 10•30•100 mg/5 mL

**Isocom** capsules (discontinued 2002) R *cerebral vasoconstrictor and analgesic for vascular and tension headaches; "possibly effective" for migraine headaches* [isometheptene mucate; dichloralphenazone; acetaminophen] 65•100•325 mg

**isoconazole** USAN, INN, BAN *antibacterial; antifungal*

**isocromil** INN

**Isocult for Bacteriuria** culture paddles for professional use *in vitro diagnostic aid for nitrate, uropathogens, or bacteria in the urine*

**Isocult for Candida** culture paddles for professional use *in vitro diagnostic aid for* Candida albicans *in the vagina*

**Isocult for N. gonorrhoeae and Candida** culture test for professional use *in vitro diagnostic aid for gonorrhea and Candida in various specimens*

**Isocult for Neisseria gonorrhoeae** culture paddles for professional use *in vitro diagnostic aid for gonorrhea*

**Isocult for Staphylococcus aureus** culture paddles for professional use *in vitro diagnostic aid for* Staphylococcus aureus *in exudate*

**Isocult for Streptococcal pharyngitis** culture paddles for professional use *in vitro diagnostic test for streptococcal pharyngitis in throat swabs*

**Isocult for T. vaginalis and Candida** culture test for professional use *in vitro diagnostic aid for Trichomonas and Candida in vaginal or urethral cultures*

**isodapamide** [see: zidapamide]

**d-isoephedrine HCl** [see: pseudoephedrine HCl]

**isoetarine** INN *sympathomimetic bronchodilator* [also: isoetharine]

**isoethadione** [see: paramethadione]

**isoetharine** USAN, BAN *sympathomimetic bronchodilator* [also: isoetarine]

**isoetharine HCl** USP, BAN *sympathomimetic bronchodilator* 1% inhalation

**isoetharine mesylate** USP, BAN *sympathomimetic bronchodilator*

**isofezolac** INN

**isoflupredone** INN, BAN *anti-inflammatory* [also: isoflupredone acetate]

**isoflupredone acetate** USAN *anti-inflammatory* [also: isoflupredone]

**isoflurane** USAN, USP, INN, BAN *inhalation general anesthetic*

**isoflurophate** USP *antiglaucoma agent; irreversible cholinesterase inhibitor miotic* [also: dyflos]

**Isoject** (trademarked delivery system) *prefilled disposable syringe*

**Isolan** oral liquid OTC *enteral nutritional therapy* [lactose-free formula]

**isoleucine (L-isoleucine)** USAN, USP, INN, JAN *essential amino acid; symbols: Ile, I*

**isoleucine & leucine & valine** *investigational (orphan) for hyperphenylalaninemia*

**Isolyte E; Isolyte S; Isolyte S pH 7.4** IV infusion R *intravenous electrolyte therapy* [combined electrolyte solution]

**Isolyte E with 5% Dextrose** IV infusion (discontinued 2001) R *intravenous nutritional/electrolyte therapy* [combined electrolyte solution; dextrose]

**Isolyte G (H; M; P; R; S) with 5% Dextrose** IV infusion R *intravenous nutritional/electrolyte therapy* [combined electrolyte solution; dextrose]

**Isolyte S pH 7.4** IV infusion ℞ *intravenous electrolyte therapy* [combined electrolyte solution]

**isomazole** INN *cardiotonic* [also: isomazole HCl]

**isomazole HCl** USAN *cardiotonic* [also: isomazole]

**isomeprobamate** [see: carisoprodol]

**isomer** [def.] *One of a group of chemical compounds having the same molecular formula, but differing in either the arrangement of atoms or the bonds between atoms in the compound.* [see also: enantiomer]

**isomerol** USAN *antiseptic*

**isometamidium** BAN [also: isometamidium chloride]

**isometamidium chloride** INN [also: isometamidium]

**isomethadone** INN, BAN

**isomethepdrine chloride** [see: isometheptene]

**isometheptene** INN, BAN

**isometheptene HCl** [see: isometheptene]

**isometheptene mucate** USP *cerebral vasoconstrictor; "possibly effective" for migraine headaches*

**isometheptene mucate & dichloralphenazone & acetaminophen** *cerebral vasoconstrictor and analgesic for vascular and tension headaches; "possibly effective" for migraine headaches* 65•100•325 mg oral

**Isomil** oral liquid, powder for oral liquid OTC *hypoallergenic infant food* [soy protein formula] ⑤ Esimil

**Isomil DF** ready-to-use oral liquid OTC *hypoallergenic infant food for management of diarrhea* [soy protein formula]

**Isomil SF** oral liquid OTC *hypoallergenic infant food* [soy protein formula, sucrose free]

**isomylamine HCl** USAN *smooth muscle relaxant*

**isoniazid** USP, INN, BAN *bactericidal; primary tuberculostatic* 50, 100, 300 mg oral; 50 mg/5 mL oral

**isonicophen** [see: aconiazide]

**isonicotinic acid hydrazide (INH)** [see: isoniazid]

**isonicotinic acid vanillylidenehydrazide** [see: ftivazide]

**1-isonicotinoyl-2-salicylidenehydrazine (INSH)** [see: salinazid]

**isonicotinylhydrazine** [see: isoniazid]

**isonixin** INN

**isooctadecanol** [see: isostearyl alcohol]

**isooctadecyl alcohol** [see: isostearyl alcohol]

**Isopan** oral liquid OTC *antacid* [magaldrate] 540 mg/5 mL

**Isopan Plus** oral liquid OTC *antacid; antiflatulent* [magaldrate; simethicone] 540•40 mg/5 mL

**Isopap** capsules (discontinued 2002) ℞ *cerebral vasoconstrictor and analgesic for vascular and tension headaches; "possibly effective" for migraine headaches* [isometheptene mucate; dichloralphenazone; acetaminophen] 65•100•325 mg

**isopentyl *p*-methoxycinnamate** [see: amiloxate]

**isopentyl nitrite** [see: amyl nitrite]

**isophenethanol** [see: nifenalol]

**isoprazone** INN, BAN

**isoprednidene** INN, BAN

**isopregnenone** [see: dydrogesterone]

**isoprenaline** INN, BAN *sympathomimetic bronchodilator; vasopressor for shock* [also: isoproterenol HCl]

**L-isoprenaline** [see: levisoprenaline]

**isoprenaline HCl** [see: isoproterenol HCl]

**Isoprinosine** ℞ *investigational (NDA filed) antiviral/immunomodulator for AIDS; investigational (orphan) for subacute sclerosing panencephalitis* [inosine pranobex]

**isoprofen** INN

**isopropamide iodide** USP, INN, BAN *peptic ulcer adjunct*

**isopropanol** [see: isopropyl alcohol]

**isopropicillin** INN

**isoproponum iodide** [see: isopropamide iodide]

**7-isopropoxyisoflavone** [see: ipriflavone]

**isopropyl alcohol** USP *topical anti-infective/antiseptic; solvent*

**isopropyl alcohol, rubbing** USP *rubefacient*

**N-isopropyl meprobamate** [see: carisoprodol]

**isopropyl myristate** NF *emollient*

**isopropyl palmitate** NF *oleaginous vehicle*

**isopropyl sebacate**

**isopropyl unoprostone** [see: unoprostone isopropyl]

**isopropylantipyrine** [see: propyphenazone]

**isopropylarterenol HCl** [see: isoproterenol HCl]

**isopropylarterenol sulfate** [see: isoproterenol sulfate]

**isoproterenol HCl** USP *sympathomimetic bronchodilator; vasopressor for shock* [also: isoprenaline] 1:5000, 1:50 000 (0.2, 0.02 mg/mL) injection

**isoproterenol sulfate** USP *sympathomimetic bronchodilator*

**Isoptin** film-coated tablets (discontinued 2001) ℞ *antianginal; antiarrhythmic; antihypertensive; calcium channel blocker* [verapamil HCl] 40, 80, 120 mg ② Intropin

**Isoptin** IV injection (discontinued 2002) ℞ *antitachyarrhythmic; calcium channel blocker* [verapamil HCl] 5 mg/2 mL

**Isoptin SR** film-coated sustained-release tablets ℞ *antihypertensive; antianginal; antiarrhythmic; calcium channel blocker* [verapamil HCl] 120, 180, 240 mg

**Isopto Atropine** Drop-Tainers (eye drops) ℞ *cycloplegic; mydriatic* [atropine sulfate] 0.5%, 1%

**Isopto Carbachol** Drop-Tainers (eye drops) ℞ *antiglaucoma agent; direct-acting miotic* [carbachol] 0.75%, 1.5%, 3%

**Isopto Carpine** Drop-Tainers (eye drops) ℞ *topical antiglaucoma agent; direct-acting miotic* [pilocarpine HCl] 0.25%, 0.5%, 1%, 2%, 3%, 4%, 5%, 6%, 8%, 10% ② Isopto Eserine

**Isopto Cetamide** Drop-Tainers (eye drops) ℞ *antibiotic* [sulfacetamide sodium] 15%

**Isopto Cetapred** eye drop suspension (discontinued 2003) ℞ *corticosteroidal anti-inflammatory; antibiotic* [prednisolone acetate; sulfacetamide sodium] 0.25%•10%

**Isopto Homatropine** Drop-Tainers (eye drops) ℞ *cycloplegic; mydriatic* [homatropine hydrobromide] 2%, 5%

**Isopto Hyoscine** Drop-Tainers (eye drops) ℞ *cycloplegic; mydriatic* [scopolamine hydrobromide] 0.25%

**Isopto Plain; Isopto Tears** Drop-Tainers (eye drops) OTC *ophthalmic moisturizer/lubricant* [hydroxypropyl methylcellulose] 0.5%

**Isordil** Tembid (sustained-release capsules and tablets) (discontinued 2004) ℞ *antianginal; vasodilator* [isosorbide dinitrate] 40 mg ② Isuprel

**Isordil** Titradose (tablets), sublingual ℞ *antianginal; vasodilator* [isosorbide dinitrate] 5, 10, 20, 30, 40 mg; 2.5, 5, 10 mg ② Isuprel

**isosorbide** USAN, USP, INN, BAN *osmotic diuretic; investigational (orphan) agent for Fabry disease*

**isosorbide dinitrate** USAN, USP, INN, BAN *coronary vasodilator; antianginal* 2.5, 5, 10, 20, 30, 40 mg oral

**isosorbide mononitrate** USAN, INN, BAN *coronary vasodilator; antianginal* 10, 20, 30, 60, 120 mg oral

**Isosource; Isosource HN** oral liquid OTC *enteral nutritional therapy* [lactose-free formula]

**isospaglumic acid** INN

**isospirilene** [see: spirilene]

**isostearyl alcohol** USAN *emollient; solvent*

**isosulfamerazine** [see: sulfaperin]

**isosulfan blue** USAN *lymphangiography aid* [also: sulphan blue]

**isosulpride** INN

**Isotein HN** powder OTC *enteral nutritional therapy* [lactose-free formula]

**3-isothiocyanato-1-propene** [see: allyl isothiocyanate]

**isothiocyanic acid, allyl ester** [see: allyl isothiocyanate]

**isothipendyl** INN, BAN

**isothipendyl HCl** [see: isothipendyl]

**isotiquimide** USAN, INN, BAN *antiulcerative*

**Isotrate ER** extended-release tablets R *antianginal; vasodilator* [isosorbide dinitrate] 60 mg

**isotretinoin** USAN, USP, INN, BAN *systemic keratolytic for severe recalcitrant cystic acne; investigational (Phase III) for neuroblastoma*

**isotretinoin anisatil** USAN *keratolytic for acne vulgaris*

**Isovorin** R *chemotherapy "rescue" agent (orphan)* [L-leucovorin]

**Isovue-128** injection (discontinued 2001) R *radiopaque contrast medium* [iopamidol (49% iodine)] 261 mg/mL (128 mg/mL)

**Isovue-200; Isovue-250; Isovue-300; Isovue-370** injection R *radiopaque contrast medium* [iopamidol (49% iodine)] 408 mg/mL (200 mg/mL); 510 mg/mL (250 mg/mL); 612 mg/mL (300 mg/mL); 755 mg/mL (370 mg/mL)

**Isovue-M 200; Isovue-M 300** intrathecal injection R *radiopaque contrast medium for myelography* [iopamidol (49% iodine)] 408 mg/mL (200 mg/mL); 612 mg/mL (300 mg/mL)

**isoxaprolol** INN

**isoxepac** USAN, INN, BAN *anti-inflammatory*

**isoxicam** USAN, INN, BAN *nonsteroidal anti-inflammatory drug (NSAID); antiarthritic; analgesic; antipyretic*

**isoxsuprine** INN, BAN *peripheral vasodilator* [also: isoxsuprine HCl]

**isoxsuprine HCl** USP, JAN *peripheral vasodilator* [also: isoxsuprine] 10, 20 mg oral

**I-Soyalac** oral liquid OTC *hypoallergenic infant food* [soybean protein formula]

**isradipine** USAN, INN, BAN *antihypertensive; dihydropyridine calcium channel blocker*

**isrodipine** [see: isradipine]

**Istalol** eye drops R *topical antiglaucoma agent (β-blocker)* [timolol maleate] 0.5%

**Istin** (European name for U.S. product Norvasc)

**Isuprel** intracardiac, IV, IM, or subcu injection R *vasopressor for cardiac, hypovolemic, or septic shock; sympathomimetic bronchodilator* [isoproterenol HCl] 1:5000, 1:50 000 (0.2, 0.02 mg/mL) ⊡ Isordil

**Isuprel** Mistometer (metered-dose inhalation aerosol), solution for inhalation (discontinued 2001) R *sympathomimetic bronchodilator* [isoproterenol HCl] 103 μg/dose; 0.5% (1:200), 1% (1:100)

**itanoxone** INN

**itasetron** USAN *anxiolytic; antidepressant; antiemetic; serotonin 5-HT₃ receptor antagonist*

**itazigrel** USAN, INN *platelet antiaggregatory agent*

**itazogrel** [see: itazigrel]

**Itch Relief Gel Spritz** spray OTC *poison ivy treatment* [camphor] 0.5%

**itchweed (Veratrum viride)** *medicinal herb* [see: hellebore]

**Itch-X** spray, gel OTC *local anesthetic* [pramoxine HCl] 1%

**itobarbital** [see: butalbital]

**itraconazole** USAN, INN, BAN *systemic triazole antifungal* 100 mg oral

**itramin tosilate** INN [also: itramin tosylate]

**itramin tosylate** BAN [also: itramin tosilate]

**itrocainide** INN

**iturelix** USAN *gonadotropin releasing hormone antagonist; ovarian and testicular steroid suppressant*

**I-Valex-1** powder OTC *formula for infants with leucine catabolism disorder*

**I-Valex-2** powder OTC *enteral nutritional therapy for leucine catabolism disorder*

**Ivanaz** injection R *investigational (NDA filed) broad-spectrum carbapenem antibiotic* [MK-826 (code name—generic name not yet assigned)]

**Ivarest** cream OTC *poison ivy treatment* [calamine; diphenhydramine HCl] 14%•2%

**Ivarest** lotion (discontinued 2001) OTC *poison ivy treatment* [calamine; benzocaine] 14%•5%

**Iveegam** freeze-dried powder for IV infusion ℞ *passive immunizing agent for HIV and Kawasaki syndrome; investigational (orphan) for acute myocarditis and juvenile rheumatoid arthritis* [immune globulin] 50 mg/mL

**ivermectin** USAN, INN, BAN *antiparasitic; anthelmintic for strongyloidiasis and onchocerciasis*

**IVIG (intravenous immunoglobulin)** [q.v.]

**ivoqualine** INN

**ivy** *medicinal herb* [see: American ivy; English ivy; poison ivy]

**Ivy Block** lotion OTC *preventative for poison ivy, oak, or sumac; use before the risk of exposure* [bentoquatam] 5%

**Ivy Cleanse** medicated wipes OTC *to remove toxic oils from poison ivy, oak, or sumac* [isopropanol; cetyl alcohol]

**Ivy Soothe** cream OTC *poison ivy treatment; corticosteroidal anti-inflammatory* [hydrocortisone] 1%

**Ivy Stat** gel OTC *poison ivy treatment; corticosteroidal anti-inflammatory* [hydrocortisone] 1%

**Ivy Super Dry** topical liquid OTC *poison ivy treatment* [zinc acetate; isopropanol; benzyl alcohol] 2%•35%•10%

**Ivy-Chex** spray (discontinued 2003) OTC *poison ivy treatment* [polyvinylpyrrolidone-vinylacetate copolymers; methyl salicylate; benzalkonium chloride]

**Ivy-Dry** lotion OTC *poison ivy treatment* [zinc acetate; isopropanol] 2%•12.5%

**Ivy-Rid** spray (discontinued 2003) OTC *poison ivy treatment* [polyvinylpyrrolidone-vinylacetate copolymers; benzalkonium chloride]

**Ixel** ℞ *investigational (Phase III) serotonin and norepinephrine reuptake inhibitor for depression and fibromyalgia syndrome* [milnacipran]

**izonsteride** USAN *antineoplastic 5α-reductase inhibitor for prostate cancer*

...*erb*

...*rb*

...: allspice]

**Jamaica sarsaparilla** *medicinal herb* [see: sarsaparilla]

**Jamaica sorrel** *medicinal herb* [see: hibiscus]

**Jantoven** tablets ℞ *coumarin-derivative anticoagulant* [warfarin sodium] 1, 2, 2.5, 3, 4, 5, 6, 7.5, 10 mg

**Japanese encephalitis (JE) virus vaccine** *active immunization vaccine*

**jasmine (*Jasminum officinale*)** flowers *medicinal herb used as a calmative*

**jaundice berry** *medicinal herb* [see: barberry]

**jaundice root** *medicinal herb* [see: goldenseal]

**java pepper** *medicinal herb* [see: cubeb]

***Jeffersonia diphylla*** *medicinal herb* [see: twin leaf]

**Jenest-28** tablets (discontinued 2003) ℞ *biphasic oral contraceptive* [norethindrone; ethinyl estradiol]
Phase 1 (7 days): 500•35 μg;
Phase 2 (14 days): 1000•35 μg

**Jersey tea** *medicinal herb* [see: New Jersey tea]

**Jerusalem cowslip; Jerusalem sage** *medicinal herb* [see: lungwort]

**jessamine, yellow** *medicinal herb* [see: gelsemium]

**Jesuit's bark** *medicinal herb* [see: quinine]

**Jets** chewable tablets OTC *dietary supplement* [lysine; multiple vitamins] 300• ± mg

**JE-VAX** powder for subcu injection ℞ *active immunizing agent* [Japanese encephalitis virus vaccine] 0.5 mL

**Jevity; Jevity 1.5 Cal** ready-to-use oral liquid OTC *enteral nutritional therapy* [lactose-free formula] 237 mL cans

**Jevity Plus** ⒸⒶⓃ ready-to-use oral liquid OTC *enteral nutritional therapy* [lactose-free formula] 235 mL

**jewelweed (Impatiens balsamina; I. biflora; I. capensis)** juice *medicinal herb for prophylaxis and treatment of poison ivy rash*

**Jew's harp plant** *medicinal herb* [see: birthroot]

**jiaogulan (Gynostemma pentaphyllum)** leaves *medicinal herb used to regulate blood pressure and strengthen the immune system, and for its adaptogenic, antihyperlipidemic, antineoplastic, antioxidant, and cardio- and cerebrovascular protective effects*

**jimsonweed (Datura stramonium)** leaves and flowering tops *medicinal herb used as an analgesic, antiasthmatic, antispasmodic, hypnotic, and narcotic; also abused as a street drug*

**jodphthalein sodium** [see: iodophthalein sodium]

**joe-pye weed** *medicinal herb* [see: queen of the meadow]

**jofendylate** [see: iophendylate]

**Johnswort** *medicinal herb* [see: St. John's wort]

**Jolivette** tablets (in packs of 28) ℞ *oral contraceptive (progestin only)* [norethindrone] 0.35 mg

**jopanoic acid** [see: iopanoic acid]

**josamycin** USAN, INN *antibacterial*

**jotrizoic acid** [see: iotrizoic acid]

**Juglans cinerea** *medicinal herb* [see: butternut]

**Juglans nigra** *medicinal herb* [see: black walnut]

**Juglans regia** *medicinal herb* [see: English walnut]

**Junel Fe 1/20; Junel Fe 1.5/30** tablets (in packs of 28) ℞ *monophasic oral contraceptive; iron supplement* [norethindrone acetate; ethinyl estradiol; ferrous fumarate] 1 mg•20 μg•75 mg; 1.5 mg•30 μg•75 mg

**"Junior Strength"** products [see under product name]

**juniper (Juniperus communis)** berries *medicinal herb for arthritis, bleeding, bronchitis, colds, edema, infections, kidney infections, pancreatic disorders, uric acid build-up, urinary disorders, and water retention*

**juniper, prickly (Juniperus oxycedrus)** *medicinal herb* [see: juniper]

**juniper tar** USP *antieczematic*

**Just Tears** eye drops OTC *ophthalmic moisturizer/lubricant* [polyvinyl alcohol] 1.4%

**K+ 8; K+ 10** film-coated extended-release tablets ℞ *potassium supplement* [potassium chloride] 600 mg; 750 mg

**K+ Care** powder for oral solution ℞ *potassium supplement* [potassium chloride] 15, 20, 25 mEq K/pkt.

**K+ Care ET** effervescent tablets ℞ *potassium supplement* [potassium bicarbonate] 20, 25 mEq K

**⁴²K** [see: potassium chloride K 42]

**k82 ImmunoCap** test kit for professional use *in vitro diagnostic aid for specific latex allergies*

**KAb201** [see: anti-CEA sheep-human chimeric monoclonal antibodies (MAb) radiolabeled with iodine I 131]

**Kabikinase** powder for IV or intracoronary infusion (discontinued 2000) ℞ *thrombolytic enzyme for lysis of thrombi and catheter clearance* [streptokinase] 250 000, 600 000, 750 000, 1 500 000 IU

**Kadian** polymer-coated sustained-release pellets in capsules ℞ *narcotic analgesic* [morphine sulfate] 20, 30, 50, 60, 100 mg

**kainic acid** INN

**Kala** tablets OTC *dietary supplement; fever blister treatment; not generally regarded as safe and effective as an antidiarrheal* [*Lactobacillus acidophilus* (soy-based)] 200 million U

**kalafungin** USAN, INN *antifungal*

**Kaletra** gelcaps, oral solution ℞ *antiviral protease inhibitor for HIV infection* [lopinavir; ritonavir] 133.3•33.3 mg; 80•20 mg/mL

**kallidinogenase** INN, BAN

*Kalmia latifolia* medicinal herb [see: mountain laurel]

**kalmopyrin** [see: calcium acetylsalicylate]

**kalsetal** [see: calcium acetylsalicylate]

**Kaltostat; Kaltostat Fortex** pads OTC *wound dressing* [calcium alginate fiber]

**kalumb** *medicinal herb* [see: colombo]

**kanamycin** INN, BAN *aminoglycoside antibiotic; tuberculosis retreatment* [also: kanamycin sulfate] ② Garamycin; gentamicin

**kanamycin B** [see: bekanamycin]

**kanamycin sulfate** USP *aminoglycoside antibiotic; tuberculosis retreatment* [also: kanamycin] 75, 500, 1000 mg/ vial injection

**Kank-a** topical liquid/film OTC *mucous membrane anesthetic* [benzocaine] 20%

**kanna** (*Sceletium tortuosum*) *plant medicinal herb used as a antidepressant, anxiolytic, relaxant, and euphoriant*

**Kantrex** capsules, IV or IM injection, pediatric injection ℞ *aminoglycoside*

*antibiotic* [kanamycin sulfate] 500 mg; 500, 1000 mg; 75 mg

**Kao Lectrolyte** powder for oral solution OTC *pediatric electrolyte replenisher*

**Kaochlor 10%; Kaochlor S-F** oral liquid (discontinued 2003) ℞ *potassium supplement* [potassium chloride; alcohol 5%] 20 mEq K/15 mL ② K-Lor

**Kaodene Non-Narcotic** oral liquid OTC *antidiarrheal; GI adsorbent; antacid* [kaolin; pectin; bismuth subsalicylate] 130•6.48•² mg/mL

**kaolin** USP clay *natural material used topically as an emollient and drying agent and ingested for binding gastrointestinal toxins and controlling diarrhea* ② Calan; Kaon

**Kaon** elixir ℞ *potassium supplement* [potassium gluconate] 20 mEq K/15 mL ② Calan; kaolin

**Kaon-Cl; Kaon-Cl 10** extended-release tablets ℞ *potassium supplement* [potassium chloride] 500 mg (6.7 mEq K); 750 mg (10 mEq K) ② Calan; kaolin

**Kaon-Cl 20%** oral liquid ℞ *potassium supplement* [potassium chloride; alcohol 5%] 40 mEq K/15 mL ② Calan; kaolin

**Kaopectate** oral liquid OTC *antidiarrheal; antinauseant* [bismuth subsalicylate] 262, 575 mg/15 mL

**Kaopectate, Children's** oral liquid OTC *antidiarrheal; antinauseant* [bismuth subsalicylate] 261 mg/15 mL ② Kapectalin

**Kaopectate II** caplets (discontinued 2004) OTC *antidiarrheal* [loperamide HCl] 2 mg

**Kaopectate Advanced Formula** oral liquid (discontinued 2004) OTC *antidiarrheal; GI adsorbent* [attapulgite] 750 mg/15 mL

**Kaopectate Maximum Strength** caplets OTC *antidiarrheal; GI adsorbent* [attapulgite] 750 mg

**Kao-Spen** oral suspension OTC *GI adsorbent; antidiarrheal* [kaolin; pectin] 5.2 g•260 mg per 30 mL

**Kapectolin** oral liquid OTC *GI adsorbent; antidiarrheal* [kaolin; pectin] 90•2 g/30 mL ⑨ Kaopectate

**Kapseal** (trademarked dosage form) *capsules sealed with a band*

**karaya gum** *(Sterculia tragacantha; S. urens; S. villosa) medicinal herb used as a topical astringent and bulk laxative*

**Karidium** tablets, chewable tablets, drops ℞ *dental caries preventative* [sodium fluoride] 2.2 mg; 2.2 mg; 0.275 mg/drop

**Karigel; Karigel-N** gel ℞ *dental caries preventative* [sodium fluoride] 1.1%

**Kariva** tablets (in packs of 28) ℞ *biphasic oral contraceptive* [desogestrel; ethinyl estradiol]
Phase 1 (21 days): 150•20 μg;
Phase 2 (5 days): 0•10 μg

**karyocyte growth factor** [see: pegylated megakaryocyte growth and development factor, recombinant human]

**kasal** USAN *food additive*

**kaugoed; kougoed** *medicinal herb* [see: kanna]

**kava kava** *(Piper methysticum)* root *medicinal herb for insomnia and nervousness*

**Kay Ciel** oral liquid, powder for oral solution ℞ *potassium supplement* [potassium chloride] 20 mEq K/15 mL; 20 mEq K/pkt. ⑨ KCl

**Kayexalate** powder for oral or rectal suspension ℞ *potassium-removing agent for hyperkalemia* [sodium polystyrene sulfonate]

**Kaylixir** oral liquid ℞ *potassium supplement* [potassium gluconate; alcohol 5%] 20 mEq K/15 mL

**K-C** oral suspension OTC *antidiarrheal; GI adsorbent; antacid* [kaolin; pectin; bismuth subcarbonate] 5 g•260 mg•260 mg per 30 mL

**KCl (potassium chloride)** [q.v.] ⑨ Kay Ciel

**K-Dur 10; K-Dur 20** controlled-release tablets ℞ *potassium supplement* [potassium chloride] 750 mg (10 mEq K); 1500 mg (20 mEq K)

**kebuzone** INN

**Keflex** Pulvules (capsules), oral suspension ℞ *cephalosporin antibiotic* [cephalexin] 250, 500 mg; 125, 250 mg/5 mL ⑨ Keflet; Keflin

**Keftab** tablets ℞ *cephalosporin antibiotic* [cephalexin HCl] 500 mg

**Kefurox** powder for IV or IM injection (discontinued 2003) ℞ *cephalosporin antibiotic* [cefuroxime sodium] 0.75, 1.5, 7.5 g

**Kefzol** powder or frozen premix for IV or IM injection (discontinued 2003) ℞ *cephalosporin antibiotic* [cefazolin sodium] 0.5, 1, 10, 20 g ⑨ Cefzil

**kellofylline** [see: visnafylline]

**kelp** *(Fucus versiculosus)* plant *medicinal herb for brittle fingernails, cleaning arteries, colitis, eczema, goiter, obesity, and toning adrenal, pituitary, and thyroid glands*

**kelp** *(Laminaria digitata; L. japonica)* plant *medicinal herb for cervical dilation and cervical ripening*

**Kemadrin** tablets ℞ *anticholinergic; antiparkinsonian* [procyclidine HCl] 5 mg ⑨ Coumadin

**Kemsol** ⓒⒶⓃ solution for bladder instillation ℞ *anti-inflammatory for symptomatic relief of interstitial cystitis* [dimethyl sulfoxide (DMSO)] 70%

**Kemstro** orally disintegrating tablets ℞ *skeletal muscle relaxant* [baclofen] 10, 20 mg

**Kenacort** tablets, syrup (discontinued 2000) ℞ *corticosteroid; anti-inflammatory* [triamcinolone] 4, 8 mg; 4 mg/5 mL

**Kenaject-40** IM, intra-articular, intrabursal, intradermal injection ℞ *corticosteroid; anti-inflammatory* [triamcinolone acetonide] 40 mg/mL

**Kenalog** ointment, cream, lotion, aerosol spray ℞ *topical corticosteroidal anti-inflammatory* [triamcinolone acetonide] 0.025%, 0.1%, 0.5%; 0.025%, 0.1%, 0.5%; 0.025%, 0.1%; ≛ ⑨ Ketalar

**Kenalog in Orabase** oral paste ℞ *corticosteroidal anti-inflammatory* [triamcinolone acetonide] 0.1%

**Kenalog-10; Kenalog-40** IM, intra-articular, intrabursal, intradermal injection ℞ *corticosteroid; anti-inflammatory* [triamcinolone acetonide] 10 mg/mL; 40 mg/mL

**Kenalog-H** cream ℞ *corticosteroidal anti-inflammatory* [triamcinolone acetonide] 0.1%

**Kendall compound A** [see: dehydrocorticosterone]

**Kendall compound B** [see: corticosterone]

**Kendall compound E** [see: cortisone acetate]

**Kendall compound F** [see: hydrocortisone]

**Kendall desoxy compound B** [see: desoxycorticosterone acetate]

**Kenonel** cream ℞ *corticosteroidal anti-inflammatory* [triamcinolone acetonide] 1%

**Kenral-MPA** ⒸⒶⓃ [see: Alti-MPA]

**Kenwood Therapeutic** oral liquid OTC *vitamin/mineral supplement* [multiple vitamins & minerals]

**keoxifene HCl** [now: raloxifene HCl]

**Keppra** film-coated tablets, oral solution ℞ *anticonvulsant for partial-onset seizures* [levetiracetam] 250, 500, 750 mg; 100 mg/mL

**keracyanin** INN

**Keralac** cream ℞ *moisturizer; emollient; keratolytic* [urea] 50%

**Keralac** lotion ℞ *moisturizer; emollient; keratolytic* [urea; lactic acid; vitamin E] 35% • 2 • 2

**Keralac Nail Gel** ℞ *moisturizer; emollient; keratolytic* [urea] 50%

**Kerasal** ointment OTC *keratolytic for calloused feet* [salicylic acid; urea] 5% • 10%

**keratolytics** *a class of agents that cause sloughing of the horny layer of the epidermis and softening of the skin*

**Keri; Keri Light** lotion (discontinued 2004) OTC *moisturizer; emollient*

**Keri Creme** (discontinued 2004) OTC *moisturizer; emollient*

**KeriCort-10** cream OTC *topical corticosteroidal anti-inflammatory* [hydrocortisone] 1%

**Kerlone** tablets ℞ *antihypertensive; β-blocker* [betaxolol HCl] 10, 20 mg

**kernelwort** *medicinal herb* [see: figwort]

**Kerodex #51** cream OTC *skin protectant for dry or oily work*

**Kerodex #71** cream OTC *water repellant skin protectant for wet work*

**Kestrone 5** IM injection (discontinued 2003) ℞ *estrogen replacement therapy for postmenopausal symptoms; palliative therapy for inoperable prostatic and breast cancer* [estrone] 5 mg/mL

**Ketalar** IV or IM injection ℞ *rapid-acting general anesthetic; sometimes abused as a street drug due to its "dissociative state" effects* [ketamine HCl] 10, 50, 100 mg/mL ⓘ Kenalog

**ketamine** INN, BAN *a rapid-acting general anesthetic; sometimes abused as a street drug due to its "dissociative state" effects* [also: ketamine HCl]

**ketamine HCl** USAN, USP, JAN *a rapid-acting general anesthetic; sometimes abused as a street drug due to its "dissociative state" effects* [also: ketamine]

**ketanserin** USAN, INN, BAN *serotonin antagonist*

**ketazocine** USAN, INN *analgesic*

**ketazolam** USAN, INN, BAN *minor tranquilizer*

**Ketek** film-coated tablets ℞ *broad-spectrum ketolide antibiotic for respiratory tract infections* [telithromycin] 400 mg

**kethoxal** USAN *antiviral* [also: ketoxal]

**ketimipramine** INN *antidepressant* [also: ketipramine fumarate]

**ketimipramine fumarate** [see: ketipramine fumarate]

**ketipramine fumarate** USAN *antidepressant* [also: ketimipramine]

**7-KETO DHEA** *investigational dehydroepiandrosterone (DHEA) derivative for Alzheimer disease*

**ketobemidone** INN, BAN

**ketocaine** INN

**ketocainol** INN
**ketocholanic acid** [see: dehydrocholic acid]
**ketoconazole** USAN, USP, INN, BAN *broad-spectrum imidazole antifungal; investigational (Phase III) for seborrheic dermatitis* 200 mg oral; 2% topical
**Ketoderm** ⓒ cream ℞ *topical antifungal* [ketoconazole] 2%
**Keto-Diastix** reagent strips *in vitro diagnostic aid for multiple urine products*
**ketohexazine** [see: cetohexazine]
**ketolides** *a class of oral antibiotics*
**Ketonex-1** powder OTC *formula for infants with maple syrup urine disease*
**Ketonex-2** powder *enteral nutritional therapy for maple syrup urine disease (MSUD)*
**ketoprofen** USAN, INN, BAN, JAN *analgesic; antiarthritic; antipyretic; nonsteroidal anti-inflammatory drug (NSAID)* 50, 75, 100, 150, 200 mg oral
**ketorfanol** USAN, INN *analgesic*
**ketorolac** INN, BAN *analgesic; nonsteroidal anti-inflammatory drug (NSAID)* [also: ketorolac tromethamine]
**ketorolac tromethamine** USAN *analgesic; nonsteroidal anti-inflammatory drug (NSAID)* [also: ketorolac] 10 mg oral; 15, 30 mg/mL injection
**Ketostix** reagent strips for home use *in vitro diagnostic aid for acetone (ketones) in the urine*
**ketotifen** INN, BAN *antihistamine; mast cell stabilizer* [also: ketotifen fumarate]
**ketotifen fumarate** USAN, JAN *antihistamine; mast cell stabilizer* [also: ketotifen]
**ketotrexate** INN
**ketoxal** INN *antiviral* [also: kethoxal]
**Key-Plex** injection ℞ *parenteral vitamin therapy* [multiple B vitamins; vitamin C] ± • 50 mg/mL
**Key-Pred 25; Key-Pred 50** IM injection ℞ *corticosteroid; anti-inflammatory* [prednisolone acetate] 25 mg/mL; 50 mg/mL
**Key-Pred-SP** IV or IM injection ℞ *corticosteroid; anti-inflammatory* [prednisolone sodium phosphate] 20 mg/mL

**K-G Elixir** ℞ *potassium supplement* [potassium gluconate] 20 mEq K/15 mL
**KGHB (potassium gamma hydroxybutyrate)** [see: gamma hydroxybutyrate (GHB)]
**khellin** INN
**khelloside** INN
**Kid Kare Children's Cough/Cold** oral liquid OTC *antitussive; decongestant; antihistamine* [dextromethorphan hydrobromide; pseudoephedrine HCl; chlorpheniramine maleate] 10 • 30 • 2 mg/10 mL
**Kid Kare Nasal Decongestant** oral drops OTC *nasal decongestant* [pseudoephedrine HCl] 7.5 mg/0.8 mL
**kidney root** *medicinal herb* [see: queen of the meadow]
**KIE** syrup ℞ *bronchodilator; decongestant; expectorant* [ephedrine HCl; potassium iodide] 16 • 300 mg/10 mL
**Kindercal** oral liquid OTC *enteral nutritional therapy* [lactose-free formula]
**Kinerase** cream, lotion OTC *moisturizer; emollient* [N$^6$-furfuryladenine] 0.1%
**Kinerase Intensive Eye Cream** OTC *moisturizer; emollient* [kinetin; safflower oil] 0.125% • $\frac{?}{}$
**Kineret** prefilled syringe for subcu injection ℞ *interleukin-1 receptor antagonist (IL-1ra); nonsteroidal anti-inflammatory drug (NSAID) for rheumatoid arthritis (RA)* [anakinra] 100 mg/0.67 mL dose
**Kinevac** powder for IV injection ℞ *diagnostic aid for gallbladder function* [sincalide] 1 µg/mL
**king's clover** *medicinal herb* [see: melilot]
**king's cure** *medicinal herb* [see: pipsissewa]
**king's fern** *medicinal herb* [see: buckhorn brake]
**kininase II inhibitors** [see: angiotensin-converting enzyme inhibitors]
**kinnikinnik** *medicinal herb* [see: uva ursi]
**Kionex** powder for oral suspension ℞ *potassium-removing agent for hyper-*

*kalemia* [sodium polystyrene sulfonate] 15 g/dose

**kitasamycin** USAN, INN, BAN, JAN *antibacterial* [also: acetylkitasamycin; kitasamycin tartrate]

**kitasamycin tartrate** JAN *antibacterial* [also: kitasamycin; acetylkitasamycin]

**KL4 surfactant** *investigational (Phase II/III, orphan) for respiratory distress syndrome in adults and premature infants and meconium aspiration in newborn infants* [also: lucinactant]

**Klamath weed** *medicinal herb* [see: St. John's wort]

**Klaron** lotion ℞ *antibiotic for acne* [sulfacetamide sodium] 10%

**KLB6; Ultra KLB6** softgels OTC *dietary supplement* [vitamin B$_6$; multiple food supplements] 3.5• ± mg; 16.7• ± mg

**K-Lease** extended-release capsules (discontinued 2004) ℞ *potassium supplement* [potassium chloride] 750 mg (10 mEq K)

**Kleen-Handz** solution OTC *topical antiseptic* [ethyl alcohol] 62%

**Klerist-D** tablets, sustained-release capsules (discontinued 2002) ℞ *decongestant; antihistamine* [pseudoephedrine HCl; chlorpheniramine maleate] 60•4 mg; 120•8 mg

**Klonopin** tablets, Rx Pak (prescription package), Tel-E-Dose (unit dose package), Wafers (orally disintegrating tablets) ℞ *anticonvulsant; anxiolytic for panic disorder; investigational (orphan) for hyperexplexia (startle disease)* [clonazepam] 0.5, 1, 2 mg; 0.5, 1, 2 mg; 0.5, 1, 2 mg; 0.125, 0.25, 0.5, 1, 2 mg ⧆ clonidine

**K-Lor** powder for oral solution ℞ *potassium supplement* [potassium chloride] 15, 20 mEq K/pkt. ⧆ Kaochlor

**Klor-Con; Klor-Con/25** powder for oral solution ℞ *potassium supplement* [potassium chloride] 20 mEq K/pkt.; 25 mEq K/pkt.

**Klor-Con 8; Klor-Con 10** film-coated extended-release tablets ℞ *potassium supplement* [potassium chloride] 600 mg (8 mEq K); 750 mg (10 mEq K)

**Klor-Con M10; Klor-Con M15; Klor-Con M20** extended-release tablets ℞ *potassium supplement* [potassium chloride] 750 mg (10 mEq K); 1125 mg (15 mEq K); 1500 mg (20 mEq K)

**Klor-Con/EF** effervescent tablets ℞ *potassium supplement* [potassium bicarbonate; potassium citrate] 25 mEq K

**Klorvess** oral liquid, effervescent granules, effervescent tablets ℞ *potassium supplement* [potassium chloride] 20 mEq K/15 mL; 20 mEq K/pkt.; 20 mEq K

**Klotrix** film-coated controlled-release tablets ℞ *potassium supplement* [potassium chloride] 750 mg (10 mEq K) ⧆ Liotrix

**Klout** topical liquid OTC *pesticide-free lice removal agent* [acetic acid; isopropanol; sodium laureth sulfate]

**K-Lyte** ⑬ effervescent tablets ℞ *urinary alkalizer for hypocitruria* [potassium citrate] 2.5 g

**K-Lyte; K-Lyte DS** effervescent tablets ℞ *potassium supplement* [potassium bicarbonate; potassium citrate] 25 mEq K; 50 mEq K

**K-Lyte/Cl** powder for oral solution ℞ *potassium supplement* [potassium chloride] 25 mEq K/dose

**K-Lyte/Cl; K-Lyte/Cl 50** effervescent tablets ℞ *potassium supplement* [potassium chloride] 25 mEq K; 50 mEq K

**knitback; knitbone** *medicinal herb* [see: comfrey]

**knob grass; knob root** *medicinal herb* [see: stone root]

**K-Norm** controlled-release capsules (discontinued 2004) ℞ *potassium supplement* [potassium chloride] 750 mg (10 mEq K)

**knotted marjoram** *medicinal herb* [see: marjoram]

**knotweed** *(Polygonum aviculare; P. hydropiper; P. persicaria; P. punctatum)* plant *medicinal herb used as an antiseptic, astringent, diaphoretic,* *diuretic, emmenagogue, rubefacient, and stimulant*

**Koāte-DVI** (double viral inactivation) powder for IV injection ℞ *antihemophilic to correct coagulation deficiency* [antihemophilic factor concentrate, solvent/detergent and dry heat treated]

**Koāte-HP** powder for IV injection (discontinued 2001) ℞ *antihemophilic to correct coagulation deficiency* [antihemophilic factor VIII] 250, 500, 1000, 1500 IU

**Kof-Eze** lozenges OTC *topical analgesic; counterirritant; mild local anesthetic* [menthol] 6 mg

**Kogenate** powder for IV injection ℞ *antihemophilic for treatment of hemophilia A and presurgical prophylaxis of hemophiliacs (orphan)* [antihemophilic factor concentrate, recombinant]

**Kogenate FS** powder for IV injection ℞ *antihemophilic for treatment of hemophilia A* [antihemophilic factor concentrate, recombinant; sucrose] 500 IU•28 mg

**KOH (potassium hydroxide)** [q.v.]

**kola nut** *(Cola acuminata)* seed *medicinal herb used as a stimulant; natural source of caffeine*

**Kolephrin** caplets OTC *decongestant; antihistamine; analgesic* [pseudoephedrine HCl; chlorpheniramine maleate; acetaminophen] 30•2•325 mg

**Kolephrin GG/DM** oral liquid OTC *antitussive; expectorant* [dextromethorphan hydrobromide; guaifenesin] 20•300 mg/10 mL

**Kolephrin/DM** caplets OTC *antitussive; decongestant; antihistamine; analgesic* [dextromethorphan hydrobromide; pseudoephedrine HCl; chlorpheniramine maleate; acetaminophen] 10•30•2•325 mg

**kolfocon A** USAN *hydrophobic contact lens material*

**kolfocon B** USAN *hydrophobic contact lens material*

**kolfocon C** USAN *hydrophobic contact lens material*

**kolfocon D** USAN *hydrophobic contact lens material*

**Kolyum** oral liquid ℞ *potassium supplement* [potassium gluconate; potassium chloride] 20 mEq K/15 mL

**kombucha (yeast/bacteria/fungus symbiont)** fermented tea *natural treatment for aging, cancer, intestinal disorders, and rheumatism*

**Kondon's Nasal** jelly (discontinued 2002) OTC *nasal decongestant* [ephedrine] 1%

**Kondremul Plain** emulsion OTC *emollient laxative* [mineral oil]

**Konsyl** powder for oral solution OTC *bulk laxative* [psyllium] 6 g/tsp. or pkt.

**Konsyl Easy Mix Formula** powder for oral solution OTC *bulk laxative with electrolytes* [psyllium; electrolytes] 6•≚ g/tsp. or pkt.

**Konsyl Fiber** tablets OTC *bulk laxative; antidiarrheal* [calcium polycarbophil] 625 mg

**Konsyl Orange** powder for oral solution OTC *bulk laxative* [psyllium] 3.4 g/tbsp. or pkt.

**Konsyl-D** powder OTC *bulk laxative* [psyllium] 3.4 g/tsp.

**Konyne 80** IV infusion (discontinued 2001) ℞ *antihemophilic to correct factor VIII (hemophilia A) and factor IX (hemophilia B; Christmas disease) deficiencies* [coagulation factors II, VII, IX, and X, heat treated] 20, 40 mL

**Kophane Cough & Cold Formula** oral liquid (discontinued 2002) OTC *antitussive; decongestant; antihistamine* [dextromethorphan hydrobromide; phenylpropanolamine HCl; chlorpheniramine maleate] 10•12.5•2 mg/5 mL

**Korean ginseng** *(Panax ginseng; P. shin-seng)* medicinal herb [see: ginseng]

**Koromex** vaginal cream (discontinued 2002) OTC *spermicidal contraceptive (for use with a diaphragm)* [octoxynol 9] 3%

**Koromex** vaginal foam, vaginal jelly (discontinued 2002) OTC *spermicidal*

*contraceptive* [nonoxynol 9] 12.5%; 3% ⑨ Komex

**Koromex Crystal Clear** vaginal gel (discontinued 2002) OTC *spermicidal contraceptive (for use with a diaphragm)* [nonoxynol 9] 2%

**kougoed; kaugoed** *medicinal herb* [see: kanna]

**Kovitonic** oral liquid OTC *hematinic* [ferric pyrophosphate; multiple B vitamins; lysine; folic acid] 42•±• 10•0.1 mg/15 mL

**K-Pek** oral suspension OTC *antidiarrheal; GI adsorbent* [attapulgite] 750 mg/15 mL

**K-Pek II** caplets OTC *antidiarrheal* [loperamide HCl] 2 mg

**K-Phos M.F.** tablets ℞ *urinary acidifier* [potassium acid phosphate; sodium acid phosphate] 155•350 mg (1.1 mEq K, 2.9 mEq Na)

**K-Phos Neutral** film-coated caplets ℞ *urinary acidifier; phosphorus supplement* [sodium phosphate, dibasic; potassium phosphate, monobasic; sodium phosphate, monobasic] 250 mg P

**K-Phos No. 2** tablets ℞ *urinary acidifier* [potassium acid phosphate; sodium acid phosphate] 305•700 mg (2.3 mEq K, 5.8 mEq Na)

**K-Phos Original** tablets ℞ *urinary acidifier* [potassium acid phosphate] 500 mg (3.7 mEq K)

**K.P.N.** tablets OTC *vitamin/mineral/calcium/iron supplement* [multiple vitamins & minerals; calcium; iron; folic acid] ±•333•11•0.27 mg

**81mKr** [see: krypton Kr 81m]

**85Kr** [see: krypton clathrate Kr 85]

**Kredex** (European name for U.S. product Coreg)

**Kristalose** powder for oral solution ℞ *hyperosmotic laxative* [lactulose] 10, 20 g/pkt.

**Kronocap** (trademarked dosage form) *sustained-release capsule*

**Kronofed-A** sustained-release capsules ℞ *decongestant; antihistamine* [pseudoephedrine HCl; chlorpheniramine maleate] 120•8 mg

**Kronofed-A Jr.** sustained-release pediatric capsules ℞ *decongestant; antihistamine* [pseudoephedrine HCl; chlorpheniramine maleate] 60•4 mg

**krypton** *element (Kr)*

**krypton clathrate Kr 85** USAN *radioactive agent*

**krypton Kr 81m** USAN, USP *radioactive agent*

**K-Tab** film-coated extended-release tablets ℞ *potassium supplement* [potassium chloride] 750 mg (10 mEq K)

**Kudrox** oral suspension (discontinued 2004) OTC *antacid* [aluminum hydroxide; magnesium hydroxide; simethicone] 500•450•40 mg/5 mL

**kudzu (Pueraria lobata; P. thunbergiana)** *root medicinal herb for the management of alcoholism*

**Kutapressin** subcu or IM injection (discontinued 2004) ℞ *claimed to be an anti-inflammatory for multiple dermatoses* [liver derivative complex] 25.5 mg/mL

**Kutrase** capsules ℞ *porcine-derived digestive enzymes* [lipase; protease; amylase] 2400•30 000•30 000 USP units

**Ku-Zyme** capsules ℞ *porcine-derived digestive enzymes* [lipase; protease; amylase] 1200•15 000•15 000 USP units

**Ku-Zyme HP** capsules ℞ *porcine-derived digestive enzymes* [lipase; protease; amylase] 8000•30 000•30 000 USP units

**K-vescent** effervescent powder ℞ *potassium supplement* [potassium chloride] 20 mEq K/pkt.

**Kwelcof** oral liquid ℞ *narcotic antitussive; expectorant* [hydrocodone bitartrate; guaifenesin] 5•100 mg/5 mL

**Kwellada-P** ⒸⒶⓃ creme rinse OTC *pediculicide for lice; scabicide* [permethrin] 1%

**Kwellada-P** ⒸⒶⓃ lotion OTC *pediculicide for lice; scabicide* [permethrin] 5%

**K-Y** vaginal jelly OTC *lubricant* [glycerin; hydroxyethyl cellulose]

**K-Y Plus** vaginal gel OTC *spermicidal contraceptive (for use with a diaphragm)* [nonoxynol 9] 2.2%

**kyamepromazin** [see: cyamemazine]

**Kytril** film-coated tablets, oral solution, IV infusion ℞ *serotonin 5-HT₃ receptor antagonist; antiemetic for nausea following chemotherapy, radiation, or surgery* [granisetron HCl] 1 mg; 1 mg/5 mL; 1 mg/mL

**L-5 hydroxytryptophan (L-5HTP)** *natural precursor to serotonin; investigational (orphan) for postanoxic intention myoclonus; investigational for depression and prophylaxis of migraine headaches*

**LA-12** IM injection ℞ *hematinic; vitamin B₁₂ supplement* [hydroxocobalamin] 1000 μg/mL

**LAAM (l-acetyl-α-methadol [or] l-alpha-acetyl-methadol)** [see: levomethadyl acetate]

**labetalol** INN, BAN *antihypertensive; antiadrenergic (α- and β-receptor)* [also: labetalol HCl]

**labetalol HCl** USAN, USP *antihypertensive; antiadrenergic (α- and β-receptor)* [also: labetalol] 100, 200, 300 mg oral; 5 mg/mL injection

**labetuzumab** *monoclonal antibody to CEA; investigational (orphan) for colorectal, pancreatic, ovarian, and small cell lung cancer*

**Labrador tea (Ledum groenlandicum; L. latifolium; L. palustre)** leaves *medicinal herb for bronchial infections, cough, diarrhea, headache, kidney disorders, lung infections, malignancies, rheumatism, and sore throat*

**Labstix** reagent strips *in vitro diagnostic aid for multiple urine products*

**Lac-Hydrin** cream, lotion ℞ *moisturizer; emollient* [ammonium lactate] 12%

**Lac-Hydrin Five** lotion OTC *moisturizer; emollient* [lactic acid]

**LACI (lipoprotein-associated coagulation inhibitor)** [see: tifacogin]

**lacidipine** USAN, INN, BAN *investigational antihypertensive; calcium channel blocker*

**Lacipil** (approved in Europe) ℞ *investigational antihypertensive; calcium channel blocker* [lacidipine]

**LAC-Lotion** ℞ *moisturizer; emollient* [ammonium lactate] 12%

**Lacril** eye drops OTC *ophthalmic moisturizer/lubricant* [hydroxypropyl methylcellulose] 0.5%

**Lacri-Lube NP; Lacri-Lube S.O.P.** ophthalmic ointment OTC *ocular moisturizer/lubricant* [white petrolatum; mineral oil; lanolin]

**Lacrisert** ophthalmic insert OTC *ophthalmic moisturizer/lubricant* [hydroxypropyl cellulose] 5 mg

**lactagogues** *a class of agents that promote or increase the flow of breast milk* [also called: galactagogues]

**LactAid** oral liquid, tablets OTC *digestive aid for lactose intolerance* [lactase enzyme] 250 U/drop; 3000 U

**lactalfate** INN

**lactase enzyme** *digestive enzyme for lactose intolerance*

**lactated potassic saline** [see: potassic saline, lactated]

**lactated Ringer (LR) injection** [see: Ringer injection, lactated]

**lactated Ringer (LR) solution** [see: Ringer injection, lactated]

**lactic acid** USP *pH adjusting agent*

**LactiCare** lotion OTC *emollient; moisturizer* [lactic acid]

**LactiCare-HC** lotion ℞ *topical corticosteroidal anti-inflammatory* [hydrocortisone] 1%, 2.5%

**Lactinex** granules, chewable tablets OTC *dietary supplement; fever blister treatment; not generally regarded as safe and effective as an antidiarrheal* [Lactobacillus acidophilus; L. bulgaricus]

**Lactinol** lotion ℞ *emollient; moisturizer* [lactic acid] 10%

**Lactinol-E** cream ℞ *emollient; moisturizer* [lactic acid; vitamin E] 10%• 116.67 IU/g

**lactitol** INN, BAN

*Lactobacillus acidophilus* natural bacteria [see: acidophilus]

*Lactobacillus bulgaricus* dietary supplement; not generally regarded as safe and effective as an antidiarrheal

**lactobin** investigational (orphan) for AIDS-related diarrhea

**lactobionic acid, calcium salt, dihydrate** [see: calcium lactobionate]

**Lactocal-F** film-coated tablets ℞ *vitamin/mineral/calcium/iron supplement* [multiple vitamins & minerals; calcium; iron; folic acid] ≜ •200•65• 1 mg

**lactoflavin** [see: riboflavin]

**LactoFree** oral liquid, powder for oral liquid OTC *hypoallergenic infant formula* [milk-based formula, lactose free]

**LactoFree LIPIL** oral liquid, powder for oral liquid OTC *hypoallergenic infant formula fortified with omega-3 fatty acids* [milk-based formula, lactose free]

**β-lactone** [see: propiolactone]

**γ-lactone D-glucofuranuronic acid** [see: glucurolactone]

**lactose** NF *tablet and capsule diluent; dietary supplement*

**Lactrase** capsules OTC *digestive aid for lactose intolerance* [lactase enzyme] 250 mg

**Lactrex 12%** cream ℞ *emollient; moisturizer* [lactic acid] 12%

*Lactuca sativa* medicinal herb [see: lettuce]

*Lactuca virosa* medicinal herb [see: wild lettuce]

**lactulose** USAN, USP, INN, BAN *hyperosmotic laxative; synthetic disaccharide used to prevent and treat portal-systemic encephalopathy* 10 g/15 mL oral or rectal

**ladakamycin** [now: azacitidine]

**Lady Esther** cream OTC *moisturizer; emollient* [mineral oil]

**lady's mantle (*Alchemilla xanthochlora; A. vulgaris*)** plant *medicinal herb for diarrhea and other digestive disorders; also used as an astringent, anti-inflammatory agent, menstrual cycle regulator, and muscle relaxant*

**lady's slipper (*Cypripedium pubescens*)** root *medicinal herb for chorea, hysteria, insomnia, nervousness, and restlessness*

**laidlomycin** INN *veterinary growth stimulant* [also: laidlomycin propionate potassium]

**laidlomycin propionate potassium** USAN *veterinary growth stimulant* [also: laidlomycin]

**Laki-Lorand factor** [see: factor XIII]

**lamb mint** *medicinal herb* [see: peppermint; spearmint]

**Lambda** ℞ *investigational (Phase III) treatment for hyperphosphatemia in chronic renal failure* [lanthanum carbonate]

**lamb's quarter** *medicinal herb* [see: birthroot]

**Lamictal** tablets, chewable/dispersible tablets ℞ *phenyltriazine anticonvulsant; adjunctive treatment for Lennox-Gastaut syndrome (orphan) and bipolar disorder* [lamotrigine] 25, 100, 150, 200 mg; 2, 5, 25 mg

**lamifiban** USAN, INN *glycoprotein (GP) IIb/IIIa receptor inhibitor; antiplatelet/ antithrombotic agent for unstable angina*

**lamifiban HCl** USAN *glycoprotein (GP) IIb/IIIa receptor inhibitor; antiplatelet/ antithrombotic agent for unstable angina*

*Laminaria digitata; L. japonica* medicinal herb [see: kelp]

**Lamisil** spray (became OTC and name changed to Lamisil AT in 2000)

**Lamisil** tablets ℞ *systemic allylamine antifungal for onychomycosis* [terbinafine HCl] 250 mg

**Lamisil AT** cream, spray, drops OTC *allylamine antifungal* [terbinafine HCl] 1%

**Lamisil DermGel** gel (discontinued 2002) ℞ *topical allylamine antifungal* [terbinafine HCl] 1%

**Lamium album** *medicinal herb* [see: blind nettle]

**lamivudine** USAN, INN, BAN *nucleoside reverse transcriptase inhibitor; antiviral for HIV and chronic hepatitis B infections*

**lamivudine & saquinavir mesylate & ritonavir** *investigational (Phase II) reverse transcriptase inhibitor and protease inhibitor combination for HIV infection*

**lamivudine & zidovudine & amprenavir** *investigational (Phase III) second-generation protease inhibitor combination for AIDS*

**lamivudine & zidovudine & efavirenz** *investigational (Phase III) antiviral combination for HIV and AIDS*

**lamotrigine** USAN, INN, BAN *phenyltriazine anticonvulsant; adjunctive treatment for Lennox-Gastaut syndrome (orphan) and bipolar disorder*

**Lampit** (available only from the Centers for Disease Control) ℞ *investigational anti-infective for Chagas disease* [nifurtimox]

**Lamprene** capsules ℞ *bactericidal; tuberculostatic; leprostatic (orphan)* [clofazimine] 50 mg

**lamtidine** INN, BAN

**Lanabiotic** ointment OTC *antibiotic; local anesthetic* [polymyxin B sulfate; neomycin sulfate; bacitracin zinc; lidocaine] 10 000 U•3.5 mg•500 U•40 mg per g

**Lanacane** spray, cream OTC *topical local anesthetic; antiseptic* [benzocaine; benzethonium chloride] 20%•0.1%; 6%•0.1%

**Lanacaps** (dosage form) *timed-release capsules*

**Lanacort 5** cream, ointment OTC *topical corticosteroidal anti-inflammatory* [hydrocortisone acetate] 0.5%

**Lanacort 10** cream, ointment OTC *topical corticosteroidal anti-inflammatory* [hydrocortisone acetate] 1%

**Lanaphilic** cream OTC *moisturizer; emollient; keratolytic* [urea] 20%

**Lanaphilic** OTC *ointment base*

**Lanaphilic with Urea** OTC *ointment base* [urea] 10%

**Lanatabs** (dosage form) *sustained-release tablets*

**lanatoside** NF, INN, BAN

**Laniazid** tablets ℞ *tuberculostatic* [isoniazid] 50 mg

**Laniazid C.T.** tablets ℞ *tuberculostatic* [isoniazid] 300 mg

**lanolin** USP *ointment base; water-in-oil emulsion; emollient/protectant*

**lanolin, anhydrous** USP *absorbent ointment base*

**lanolin alcohols** *ointment base ingredient*

**Lanolor** cream OTC *moisturizer; emollient*

**Lanophyllin** elixir ℞ *antiasthmatic; bronchodilator* [theophylline] 80 mg/15 mL

**Lanorinal** tablets, capsules (discontinued 2000) ℞ *analgesic; barbiturate sedative* [aspirin; caffeine; butalbital] 325•40•50 mg

**lanoteplase** USAN *investigational (Phase III) thrombolytic and tissue plasminogen activator (tPA)*

**Lanoxicaps** capsules ℞ *cardiac glycoside to increase cardiac output; antiarrhythmic* [digoxin] 0.05, 0.1, 0.2 mg

**Lanoxin** tablets, pediatric elixir, IV or IM injection ℞ *cardiac glycoside to increase cardiac output; antiarrhythmic* [digoxin] 0.125, 0.25 mg; 0.05 mg/mL; 0.1, 0.25 mg/mL

**lanreotide acetate** USAN *antineoplastic*

**lansoprazole** USAN, INN, BAN *proton pump inhibitor for gastric and duodenal ulcers, erosive esophagitis, GERD, and other gastroesophageal disorders*

**lanthanum** *element (La)*

**lanthanum carbonate** *investigational (Phase III) treatment for hyperphosphatemia in chronic renal failure*

**Lantus** prefilled cartridges for OptiPen One device (discontinued 2003) ℞ *human insulin analogue; long-acting, once-daily antidiabetic* [insulin glargine (rDNA)] 300 IU/3 mL

**Lantus** subcu injection ℞ *human insulin analogue; long-acting, once-daily antidiabetic* [insulin glargine (rDNA)] 100 IU/mL

*Lapacho colorado; L. morado* medicinal herb [see: pau d'arco]

**lapirium chloride** INN *surfactant* [also: lapyrium chloride]

**LAPOCA (L-asparaginase, Oncovin, cytarabine, Adriamycin)** *chemotherapy protocol*

**laprafylline** INN

**lapyrium chloride** USAN *surfactant* [also: lapirium chloride]

**laramycin** [see: zorbamycin]

**larch (*Larix americana; L. europaea*)** bark, resin, young shoots, and needles *medicinal herb used as an anthelmintic, diuretic, laxative, and vulnerary; powdered bark is 98% arabinogalactans* [see also: arabinogalactans]

**Largon** IV or IM injection (discontinued 2004) ℞ *sedative; analgesic adjunct* [propiomazine HCl] 20 mg/mL

**Lariam** tablets ℞ *antimalarial for acute chloroquine-resistant malaria (orphan)* [mefloquine HCl] 250 mg

*Larix americana; L. europaea* medicinal herb [see: larch]

**Larodopa** capsules ℞ *dopamine precursor; antiparkinsonian* [levodopa] 100, 250, 500 mg

**Larodopa** tablets ℞ *dopamine precursor; antiparkinsonian* [levodopa] 100, 250, 500 mg

**laronidase** *enzyme replacement therapy for mucopolysaccharidosis I (MPS I) (orphan)*

**laroxyl** [see: amitriptyline]

*Larrea divaricata; L. glutinosa; L. tridentata* medicinal herb [see: chaparral]

**lasalocid** USAN, INN, BAN *coccidiostat for poultry*

**Lasan** cream, ointment ℞ *topical antipsoriatic* [anthralin] 0.1%, 0.2%, 0.4%; 0.4%

**Lasan HP-1** cream ℞ *topical antipsoriatic* [anthralin] 1%

**Lasix** tablets, oral solution, IM or IV injection ℞ *antihypertensive; loop diuretic* [furosemide] 20, 40, 80 mg; 10 mg/mL; 10 mg/mL ☑ Esidrix; Lidex

**lasofoxifene tartrate** USAN *selective estrogen receptor modulator (SERM) for osteoporosis and the reduction of cardiovascular risk; investigational (Phase III) for breast cancer*

**Lassar paste** [betanaphthol (q.v.) + zinc oxide (q.v.)]

**latamoxef** INN, BAN *anti-infective* [also: moxalactam disodium]

**latamoxef disodium** [see: moxalactam disodium]

**latanoprost** USAN, INN *topical prostaglandin agonist for glaucoma and ocular hypertension*

**latex agglutination test** *in vitro diagnostic aid*

**laudexium methylsulfate** [see: laudexium metilsulfate; laudexium methylsulphate]

**laudexium methylsulphate** BAN [also: laudexium metilsulfate]

**laudexium metilsulfate** INN [also: laudexium methylsulphate]

**lauralkonium chloride** INN

**laurel (*Laurus nobilis*)** leaves and fruit *medicinal herb used as an aromatic, astringent, carminative, and stomachic*

**laurel, mountain; rose laurel; sheep laurel** *medicinal herb* [see: mountain laurel]

**laurel, red; swamp laurel** *medicinal herb* [see: magnolia]

**laurel, spurge; spurge olive** *medicinal herb* [see: mezereon]

**laureth 4** USAN *surfactant*

**laureth 9** USAN *spermaticide; surfactant*

**laureth 10S** USAN *spermaticide*

**lauril** INN *combining name for radicals or groups*

**laurilsulfate** INN *combining name for radicals or groups* [also: sodium lauryl sulfate]

**laurixamine** INN

**laurocapram** USAN, INN *excipient*

**laurocapram & methotrexate** *investigational (orphan) for topical treatment of Mycosis fungoides*

**lauroguadine** INN
**laurolinium acetate** INN, BAN
**lauromacrogol 400** INN
*Laurus nobilis medicinal herb* [see: laurel]
*Laurus persea medicinal herb* [see: avocado]
**lauryl isoquinolinium bromide** USAN *anti-infective*
**lavender (*Lavandula* spp.)** flowers, leaves, and oil *medicinal herb for acne, bile flow stimulation, diabetes, edema, flatulence, hyperactivity, insomnia, intestinal spasms, migraine headache, and stimulating menstrual flow*
**lavender oil** NF
**lavoltidine** INN *antiulcerative; histamine $H_2$-receptor blocker* [also: lavoltidine succinate; loxtidine]
**lavoltidine succinate** USAN *antiulcerative; histamine $H_2$-receptor blocker* [also: lavoltidine; loxtidine]
**lawrencium** *element (Lr)*
*Lawsonia inermis medicinal herb* [see: henna]
**Laxative & Stool Softener** softgels OTC *stimulant laxative; stool softener* [casanthranol; docusate sodium] 30•100 mg
**laxatives** *a class of agents that promote evacuation of the bowels or have a mild purgative effect; subclasses: saline, stimulant, bulk-producing, emollient, stool-softening, and hyperosmotic* [see also: cathartics; purgatives; various subclasses]
**Lax-Pills** tablets OTC *stimulant laxative* [sennosides] 15, 25 mg
**lazabemide** USAN, INN *antiparkinsonian*
**lazabemide HCl** USAN *investigational treatment for Alzheimer disease*
**lazaroids** *a class of potent antioxidants that can protect against oxygen radical–mediated lipid peroxidation and progressive neuronal degeneration following brain or spinal trauma, subarachnoid hemorrhage, or stroke* [also called: 21-aminosteroids]
**Lazer Creme** OTC *moisturizer; emollient* [vitamins A and E] 3333.3•116.67 U/g

**Lazer Formalyde** solution ℞ *for hyperhidrosis and bromhidrosis* [formaldehyde] 10%
**LazerSporin-C** ear drops ℞ *topical corticosteroidal anti-inflammatory; antibiotic* [hydrocortisone; neomycin sulfate; polymyxin B sulfate] 1%•5 mg•10 000 U per mL
**LC-65** solution OTC *cleaning solution for hard, soft, or rigid gas permeable contact lenses*
**L-Carnitine** tablets, capsules OTC *dietary amino acid* [levocarnitine] 500 mg; 250 mg
**LCD (liquor carbonis detergens)** [see: coal tar]
**LCR (leurocristine)** [see: vincristine]
**LCx *Neisseria gonorrhoeae* Assay** reagent kit for professional use *in vitro diagnostic aid for* Neisseria gonorrhoeae
**lead** *element (Pb)*
**lecimibide** USAN *hypocholesterolemic; antihyperlipidemic*
**lecithin** NF *emulsifier; surfactant; natural phospholipid mixture of various phosphatidylcholines used as an antihypercholesterolemic and cognition enhancer for Alzheimer and other dementias* 420, 1200 mg oral
**lecithol** *natural remedy* [see: lecithin]
**LED (liposome-encapsulated doxorubicin)** [see: doxorubicin HCl, liposome-encapsulated]
**Lederject** (trademarked delivery system) *prefilled disposable syringe*
**ledoxantrone trihydrochloride** USAN *antineoplastic; topoisomerase II inhibitor* [previously: sedoxantrone trihydrochloride]
*Ledum groenlandicum; L. latifolium; L. palustre medicinal herb* [see: Labrador tea]
**leeches (*Hirudo medicinalis*)** *natural adjunct to postsurgical wound management*
**leek (*Allium porrum*)** bulb, lower stem, and leaves *medicinal herb used as an appetite stimulant, decongestant, and diuretic*
**lefetamine** INN

**leflunomide** USAN, INN *anti-inflammatory for rheumatoid arthritis; investigational (orphan) for malignant glioma, ovarian cancer, and prevention of rejection of organ transplants; investigational (Phase II) for prostate and non–small cell lung cancers; investigational (Phase III) for first relapse glioblastoma multiforme*

**Legalon** *investigational (orphan) antitoxin for Amanita phalloides (mushroom) intoxication* [disodium silibinin dihemisuccinate]

**Legatrin PM** caplets OTC *prevention and treatment of nocturnal leg cramps* [diphenhydramine HCl; acetaminophen] 50•500 mg

**legs, red** *medicinal herb* [see: bistort]

**leiopyrrole** INN

**lemidosul** INN

**lemon (Citrus limon)** *fruit and peel medicinal herb used as an astringent, refrigerant, and source of vitamin C*

**lemon, ground; wild lemon** *medicinal herb* [see: mandrake]

**lemon balm (Melissa officinalis)** plant *medicinal herb used as an antispasmodic and sedative; also used for Graves disease and cold sores*

**lemon oil** NF

**lemon verbena (Aloysiatriphylla spp.)** leaves and flowers *medicinal herb for fever, flatulence, gastrointestinal spasms and other disorders, and sedation*

**lemon walnut** *medicinal herb* [see: butternut]

**lemongrass (Andropogon citratus; Cymbopogon citratus)** leaves *medicinal herb for colds, cough, fever, gastrointestinal spasm and other disorders, nervousness, pain, and rheumatism; also used as an antiemetic*

**Lemotussin-DM** oral liquid ℞ *antitussive; decongestant; antihistamine; expectorant* [dextromethorphan hydrobromide; pseudoephedrine HCl; chlorpheniramine maleate; guaifenesin; potassium giaiacolsulfonate] 7.5•10•2•50•50 mg

**lenampicillin** INN

**lenercept** USAN *tumor necrosis factor (TNF) receptor antagonist for septic shock, multiple sclerosis, inflammatory bowel disease, and rheumatoid arthritis*

**leniquinsin** USAN, INN *antihypertensive*

**lenitzol** [see: amitriptyline]

**lenograstim** USAN, INN, BAN *immunomodulator; antineutropenic; hematopoietic stimulant*

**lenperone** USAN, INN *antipsychotic*

**Lens Drops** solution OTC *rewetting solution for hard or soft contact lenses*

**Lens Lubricant** solution OTC *rewetting solution for hard or soft contact lenses*

**Lens Plus Daily Cleaner** solution OTC *surfactant cleaning solution for soft contact lenses*

**Lens Plus Oxysept** products [see: Oxysept]

**Lens Plus Rewetting Drops** OTC *rewetting solution for soft contact lenses*

**Lens Plus Sterile Saline** aerosol solution OTC *rinsing/storage solution for soft contact lenses* [sodium chloride (saline solution)]

**Lente Iletin II** subcu injection OTC *antidiabetic* [insulin zinc (pork)] 100 U/mL

**Lente L** subcu injection (discontinued 2000) OTC *antidiabetic* [insulin zinc (pork)] 100 U/mL

**lentin** [see: carbachol]

**lentinan** JAN *investigational (Phase II/III) immunomodulator for HIV and AIDS*

**Lentinula edodes** *medicinal herb* [see: shiitake mushrooms]

**Leontodon taraxacum** *medicinal herb* [see: dandelion]

**Leonurus cardiaca** *medicinal herb* [see: motherwort]

**leopard's bane** *medicinal herb* [see: arnica]

**Lepidium meyenii** *medicinal herb* [see: maca]

**lepirudin** *anticoagulant for heparin-associated thrombocytopenia (HAT) (orphan)*

**leprostatics** *a class of drugs effective against leprosy*

**leptacline** INN

**leptandra; purple leptandra** *medicinal herb* [see: Culver root]

**lercanidipine** *investigational calcium channel blocker*

**lergotrile** USAN, INN *prolactin enzyme inhibitor*

**lergotrile mesylate** USAN *prolactin enzyme inhibitor*

**leridistim** USAN *interleukin-3 and granulocyte colony-stimulating factor receptor agonist for chemotherapy-induced neutropenia and thrombocytopenia*

**Lescol** capsules ℞ *HMG-CoA reductase inhibitor for hypercholesterolemia, hypertriglyceridemia, and atherosclerosis* [fluvastatin sodium] 20, 40 mg

**Lescol XL** film-coated extended-release tablets ℞ *HMG-CoA reductase inhibitor for hypercholesterolemia, hypertriglyceridemia, and atherosclerosis* [fluvastatin sodium] 80 mg

**lesopitron** INN *investigational anxiolytic*

**lesser centaury** *medicinal herb* [see: centaury]

**Lessina** film-coated tablets (in packs of 21 or 28) ℞ *monophasic oral contraceptive; emergency postcoital contraceptive* [levonorgestrel; ethinyl estradiol] 0.1 mg•20 μg

**leteprinim potassium** USAN *investigational (Phase II) nerve growth factor for Alzheimer disease, spinal cord injury, and stroke*

**letimide** INN *analgesic* [also: letimide HCl]

**letimide HCl** USAN *analgesic* [also: letimide]

**letosteine** INN

**letrazuril** INN *investigational (Phase II) treatment for AIDS-related cryptosporidial diarrhea*

**letrozole** USAN, INN *aromatase inhibitor; estrogen antagonist; antineoplastic for advanced breast cancer in postmenopausal women*

**lettuce (Lactuca sativa)** juice and leaves *medicinal herb used as an anodyne, antispasmodic, expectorant, and sedative (for herbal medical use, common garden lettuce is harvested after it has gone to seed, and a milky juice is extracted)*

**Leucanthemum parthenium** *medicinal herb* [see: feverfew]

**leucarsone** [see: carbarsone]

**leucine (L-leucine)** USAN, USP, INN, JAN *essential amino acid; symbols: Leu, L*

**leucine & isoleucine & valine** *investigational (orphan) for hyperphenylalaninemia*

**leucinocaine** INN

**leucocianidol** INN

**leucomycin** [see: kitasamycin; spiramycin]

**Leucotropin** ℞ *investigational (Phase III) granulocyte-macrophage colony-stimulating factor (GM-CSF) for white cell rescue following chemotherapy (trial discontinued 2000)* [regramostim]

**L-leucovorin** *chemotherapy "rescue" agent (orphan)*

**leucovorin calcium** USP *antianemic; folate replenisher; antidote to folic acid antagonist; chemotherapy "rescue" agent (orphan)* [also: calcium folinate] 5, 15, 25 mg oral; 3, 10 mg injection; 50, 100, 350 mg/vial injection

**leucovorin & fluorouracil** *antineoplastic for metastatic colorectal cancer (orphan)*

**leucovorin & methotrexate** *antineoplastic for osteosarcoma (orphan)*

**LeukArrest** ℞ *investigational (Phase III) treatment for acute ischemic stroke (trial discontinued 2000)* [rovelizumab]

**Leukeran** tablets ℞ *nitrogen mustard-type alkylating antineoplastic for multiple leukemias, lymphomas, and neoplasms* [chlorambucil] 2 mg

**Leukine** IV infusion ℞ *myeloid reconstitution after autologous bone marrow transplant (orphan); investigational (Phase III) cytokine for HIV infection* [sargramostim] 250, 500 μg

**leukocyte interferon** [now: interferon alfa-n3]

**leukocyte protease inhibitor** [see: secretory leukocyte protease inhibitor]

**leukocyte typing serum** USP *in vitro blood test*

**leukopoietin** [see: sargramostim]

**LeukoScan** *investigational (Phase III) diagnostic aid for osteomyelitis; investigational (NDA filed) diagnostic aid for infectious lesions* [technetium Tc 99m sulesomab]

**leukotriene receptor antagonists (LTRAs); leukotriene receptor inhibitors** *a class of antiasthmatics that inhibit bronchoconstriction when used prophylactically (will not reverse bronchospasm)*

**LeukoVAX** ℞ *investigational (Phase I/II) white blood cell formulation for treatment of rheumatoid arthritis*

**leupeptin** *investigational (orphan) aid to microsurgical peripheral nerve repair*

**Leuprogel** *sustained-release subcu injection* ℞ *investigational (Phase III) antihormonal antineoplastic for advanced prostate cancer* [leuprolide acetate]

**leuprolide acetate** USAN *testosterone suppressant; antihormonal antineoplastic for various cancers; LHRH agonist for central precocious puberty (orphan)* [also: leuprorelin] *5 mg/mL injection*

**leuprorelin** INN, BAN *testosterone suppressant; antihormonal antineoplastic for various cancers* [also: leuprolide acetate]

**leurocristine (LCR)** [see: vincristine]

**leurocristine sulfate** [see: vincristine sulfate]

**Leustatin** IV infusion ℞ *antineoplastic for hairy-cell leukemia (orphan); investigational (orphan) for chronic lymphocytic leukemia, myeloid leukemia, multiple sclerosis, and non-Hodgkin lymphoma* [cladribine] *1 mg/mL*

**LeuTech** *investigational (NDA filed) radiolabeled infection imaging agent for equivocal appendicitis*

**Leuvectin** ℞ *investigational (Phase I/II, orphan) gene-based therapy for advanced metastatic renal cell carcinoma*

**Levacet** *caplets* OTC *analgesic; antihistaminic sleep aid* [aspirin; acetaminophen; salicylamide; phenyltolox-amine citrate; caffeine] 400•400•150•50•40 mg

**levacetylmethadol** INN *narcotic analgesic* [also: levomethadyl acetate]

**levalbuterol** *sympathomimetic bronchodilator; single-isomer albuterol*

**levalbuterol HCl** USAN *sympathomimetic bronchodilator; single-isomer albuterol*

**levalbuterol sulfate** USAN *sympathomimetic bronchodilator; single-isomer albuterol*

**Levall 5.0** *oral liquid* ℞ *narcotic antitussive; decongestant; expectorant* [hydrocodone bitartrate; phenylephrine HCl; guaifenesin] 5•15•100 mg/5 mL

**levallorphan** INN, BAN [also: levallorphan tartrate] ☑ levorphanol

**levallorphan tartrate** USP [also: levallorphan]

**levamfetamine** INN *anorectic* [also: levamfetamine succinate; levamphetamine]

**levamfetamine succinate** USAN *anorectic* [also: levamfetamine; levamphetamine]

**levamisole** INN, BAN *biological response modifier; antineoplastic; veterinary anthelmintic* [also: levamisole HCl]

**levamisole HCl** USAN, USP *biological response modifier; antineoplastic; veterinary anthelmintic* [also: levamisole]

**levamphetamine** BAN *anorectic* [also: levamfetamine succinate; levamfetamine]

**levant berry (Anamirta cocculus; A. paniculata)** *leaves and berries medicinal herb for epilepsy, lice, malaria, morphine poisoning, and worms; not generally regarded as safe and effective for ingestion or topical application on abraded skin*

**Levaquin** *film-coated tablets, IV infusion* ℞ *broad-spectrum fluoroquinolone antibiotic* [levofloxacin] 250, 500, 750 mg; 250, 500, 750 mg

**levarterenol** [see: norepinephrine bitartrate]

**levarterenol bitartrate** [now: norepinephrine bitartrate]

**Levatol** tablets ℞ *antihypertensive; β-blocker* [penbutolol sulfate] 20 mg

**Levbid** extended-release tablets ℞ *GI/GU antispasmodic; antiparkinsonian; anticholinergic "drying agent" for allergic rhinitis or hyperhidrosis* [hyoscyamine sulfate] 0.375 mg

**levcromakalim** USAN, INN, BAN *antiasthmatic; antihypertensive*

**levcycloserine** USAN, INN *enzyme inhibitor*

**levdobutamine** INN *cardiotonic* [also: levdobutamine lactobionate]

**levdobutamine lactobionate** USAN *cardiotonic* [also: levdobutamine]

**levdropropizine** INN

**Levemir** (approved in Europe) ℞ *antidiabetic; investigational (NDA filed) long-acting insulin formulation intended to provide continuous basal insulin levels through once- or twice-daily subcu injections* [insulin detemir]

**levemopamil** INN *investigational treatment for stroke*

**levetiracetam** USAN, INN *anticonvulsant for partial-onset seizures*

**levisoprenaline** INN

*Levisticum officinale* medicinal herb [see: lovage]

**Levitra** film-coated tablets ℞ *phosphodiesterase type 5 (PDE5) inhibitor; selective vasodilator for erectile dysfunction (ED)* [vardenafil HCl] 2.5, 5, 10, 20 mg

**Levlen** tablets (in Slidecases of 28) ℞ *monophasic oral contraceptive; emergency postcoital contraceptive* [levonorgestrel; ethinyl estradiol] 0.15 mg•30 μg

**Levlite** tablets (in Slidecases of 28) ℞ *monophasic oral contraceptive* [levonorgestrel; ethinyl estradiol] 0.1 mg•20 μg

**levlofexidine** INN

**levmetamfetamine** USAN *nasal decongestant*

**levobetaxolol** INN *topical antiglaucoma agent (β-blocker)* [also: levobetaxolol HCl]

**levobetaxolol HCl** USAN *topical antiglaucoma agent (β-blocker)* [also: levobetaxolol]

**levobunolol** INN, BAN *topical antiglaucoma agent (β-blocker)* [also: levobunolol HCl]

**levobunolol HCl** USAN, USP *topical antiglaucoma agent (β-blocker)* [also: levobunolol] 0.25%, 0.5% eye drops

**levobupivacaine HCl** USAN *long-acting local anesthetic*

**levocabastine** INN, BAN *antihistamine* [also: levocabastine HCl]

**levocabastine HCl** USAN *antihistamine* [also: levocabastine]

**levocarbinoxamine tartrate** [see: rotoxamine tartrate]

**levocarnitine** USAN, USP, INN *dietary amino acid for primary and secondary genetic carnitine deficiency (orphan) and end-stage renal disease (orphan); investigational (orphan) for pediatric cardiomyopathy* 200 mg/mL injection

**levocetirizine** *investigational second-generation piperazine antihistamine for allergic rhinitis; isomer of cetirizine*

**levodopa** USAN, USP, INN, BAN, JAN *antiparkinsonian; dopamine precursor* ② methyldopa

**levodopa & carbidopa** *antiparkinsonian; dopamine precursor plus synergist* 100•10, 100•25, 200•50, 250•25 mg oral

**Levo-Dromoran** subcu or IV injection (discontinued 2001) ℞ *narcotic analgesic* [levorphanol tartrate] 2 mg/mL

**Levo-Dromoran** tablets ℞ *narcotic analgesic* [levorphanol tartrate] 2 mg

**levofacetoperane** INN

**levofenfluramine** INN

**levofloxacin** USAN, INN, JAN *broad-spectrum fluoroquinolone antibiotic*

**levofuraltadone** USAN, INN *antibacterial; antiprotozoal*

**levoglutamide** INN, DCF [now: glutamine]

**Levolet** tablets ℞ *synthetic thyroid hormone (T$_4$ fraction only)* [levothyroxine sodium]

**levoleucovorin calcium** USAN *antidote to folic acid antagonists*

**levomenol** INN

**levomepate** [see: atromepine]

**levomepromazine** INN *analgesic* [also: methotrimeprazine]

**levomethadone** INN

**levomethadyl acetate** USAN *narcotic analgesic* [also: levacetylmethadol]

**levomethadyl acetate HCl** USAN *narcotic analgesic for management of opiate addiction (orphan)*

**levomethorphan** INN, BAN

**levometiomeprazine** INN

**levomoprolol** INN

**levomoramide** INN, BAN

**levonantradol** INN, BAN *analgesic* [also: levonantradol HCl]

**levonantradol HCl** USAN *analgesic* [also: levonantradol]

**levonordefrin** USP *adrenergic; vasoconstrictor* [also: corbadrine]

**levonorgestrel** USAN, USP, INN, BAN *progestin; contraceptive implant; emergency "morning after" oral contraceptive*

**Levophed** IV infusion ℞ *vasopressor for acute hypotensive shock* [norepinephrine bitartrate] 1 mg/mL

**levophenacylmorphan** INN, BAN

**Levoprome** IM injection (discontinued 2003) ℞ *central analgesic; CNS depressant* [methotrimeprazine HCl] 20 mg/mL

**levopropicillin** INN *antibacterial* [also: levopropylcillin potassium]

**levopropicillin potassium** [see: levopropylcillin potassium]

**levopropoxyphene** INN, BAN *antitussive* [also: levopropoxyphene napsylate]

**levopropoxyphene napsylate** USAN *antitussive* [also: levopropoxyphene]

**levopropylcillin potassium** USAN *antibacterial* [also: levopropicillin]

**levopropylhexedrine** INN

**levoprotiline** INN

**Levora** tablets (packs of 28) ℞ *monophasic oral contraceptive* [levonorgestrel; ethinyl estradiol] 0.15 mg•30 µg

**levorin** INN

**levorphanol** INN, BAN *narcotic analgesic* [also: levorphanol tartrate] ② levallorphan

**levorphanol tartrate** USP *narcotic analgesic* [also: levorphanol] 2 mg oral

**levosimendan** USAN *investigational (Phase III) calcium sensitizer and vasodilator for decompensated heart failure*

**Levo-T** tablets (discontinued 2003) ℞ *synthetic thyroid hormone (T$_4$ fraction only)* [levothyroxine sodium] 25, 50, 75, 100, 125, 150, 200, 300 µg

**Levothroid** ⒶⓃ tablets ℞ *synthetic thyroid hormone (T$_4$ fraction only)* [levothyroxine sodium] 25, 50, 75, 100, 112, 125, 150, 175, 200, 300 µg

**Levothroid** caplets, powder for injection ℞ *synthetic thyroid hormone (T$_4$ fraction only)* [levothyroxine sodium] 25, 50, 75, 88, 100, 112, 125, 150, 175, 200, 300 µg; 200 µg

**levothyroxine sodium** USP, INN *synthetic thyroid hormone (T$_4$ fraction only)* [also: thyroxine] 25, 50, 75, 88, 100, 112, 125, 150, 175, 200, 300 µg oral; 200, 500 µg injection ② liothyronine

**levothyroxine sodium & tiratricol** *investigational (orphan) to suppress thyroid-stimulating hormone (TSH) in thyroid cancer*

**Levovist** ⒶⓃ powder for IV injection ℞ *ultrasound contrast medium for echocardiography* [galactose; palmitic acid]

**levoxadrol** INN *local anesthetic; smooth muscle relaxant* [also: levoxadrol HCl]

**levoxadrol HCl** USAN *local anesthetic; smooth muscle relaxant* [also: levoxadrol]

**Levoxyl** tablets ℞ *synthetic thyroid hormone (T$_4$ fraction only)* [levothyroxine sodium] 25, 50, 75, 88, 100, 112, 125, 137, 150, 175, 200, 300 µg

**Levsin** IV, IM, or subcu injection ℞ *GI/GU antispasmodic to reduce motility during radiologic imaging; preoperative antimuscarinic to reduce salivary*

and gastric secretions [hyoscyamine sulfate] 0.5 mg/mL

**Levsin** tablets, drops, elixir ℞ *GI/GU antispasmodic; antiparkinsonian; anticholinergic "drying agent" for allergic rhinitis and hyperhidrosis* [hyoscyamine sulfate] 0.125 mg; 0.125 mg/mL; 0.125 mg/5 mL

**Levsin PB** drops ℞ *GI/GU antispasmodic; anticholinergic; sedative* [hyoscyamine sulfate; phenobarbital; alcohol 5%] 0.125•15 mg/mL

**Levsin with Phenobarbital** tablets ℞ *GI/GU antispasmodic; anticholinergic; sedative* [hyoscyamine sulfate; phenobarbital] 0.125•15 mg

**Levsinex** Timecaps (timed-release capsules) ℞ *GI/GU antispasmodic; antiparkinsonian; anticholinergic "drying agent" for allergic rhinitis or hyperhidrosis* [hyoscyamine sulfate] 0.375 mg

**Levsin/SL** sublingual tablets (also may be chewed or swallowed) ℞ *GI/GU antispasmodic; anticholinergic* [hyoscyamine sulfate] 0.125 mg

**Levulan Kerastick** topical solution ℞ *photosensitizer for photodynamic therapy of precancerous actinic keratoses of the face and scalp (for use with the BLU-U Blue Light Photodynamic Therapy Illuminator)* [aminolevulinic acid HCl] 20%

**levulose** BAN *nutrient; caloric replacement* [also: fructose]

**Lexapro** film-coated tablets, oral solution ℞ *selective serotonin reuptake inhibitor (SSRI) for major depression and generalized anxiety disorder* [escitalopram oxalate] 5, 10, 20 mg; 5 mg/5 mL

**lexipafant** USAN *platelet activating factor (PAF) antagonist; investigational (Phase III) treatment for acute pancreatitis*

**lexithromycin** USAN, INN *antibacterial*

**Lexiva** film-coated caplets ℞ *antiretroviral; HIV-1 protease inhibitor* [fosamprenavir calcium] 700 mg (=600 mg base)

**lexofenac** INN

**Lexxel** film-coated combination-release tablets ℞ *antihypertensive; angiotensin-converting enzyme (ACE) inhibitor; calcium channel blocker* [enalapril maleate (immediate release); felodipine (extended release)] 5•5, 5•2.5 mg

**LH·RF (luteinizing hormone–releasing factor) acetate hydrate** [see: gonadorelin acetate]

**LH·RF diacetate tetrahydrate** [now: gonadorelin acetate]

**LH·RF dihydrochloride** [now: gonadorelin HCl]

**LH·RF HCl** [see: gonadorelin HCl]

**LH·RH (luteinizing hormone–releasing hormone)** *an endogenous hormone, produced in the hypothalamus, which stimulates the release of luteinizing hormone (LH) and follicle-stimulating hormone (FSH) from the pituitary* [also known as: gonadotropin-releasing hormone (Gn-RH)]

**liarozole** INN, BAN *antipsoriatic; aromatase inhibitor* [also: liarozole fumarate]

**liarozole fumarate** USAN *antipsoriatic; aromatase inhibitor; investigational (orphan) for congenital ichthyosis* [also: liarozole]

**liarozole HCl** USAN *antineoplastic for prostate cancer; aromatase inhibitor*

**liatermin** USAN *dopaminergic neuronal growth stimulator for Parkinson disease*

*Liatris scariosa; L. spicata; L. squarrosa* *medicinal herb* [see: blazing star]

**libecillide** INN

**libenzapril** USAN, INN *angiotensin-converting enzyme (ACE) inhibitor*

**Librax** capsules ℞ *GI anticholinergic; anxiolytic* [clidinium bromide; chlordiazepoxide HCl] 2.5•5 mg

**Librel** tablets ℞ *investigational (Phase III) continuous-use oral contraceptive* [levonorgestrel; ethinyl estradiol]

**Libritabs** film-coated tablets (discontinued 2003) ℞ *benzodiazepine anxiolytic; sedative* [chlordiazepoxide] 10, 25 mg

**Librium** capsules, powder for injection ℞ *benzodiazepine anxiolytic; sedative; alcohol withdrawal aid; sometimes*

*abused as a street drug* [chlordiazepoxide HCl] 5, 10, 25 mg; 100 mg

**Lice-Enz** foam shampoo (discontinued 2003) OTC *pediculicide for lice* [pyrethrins; piperonyl butoxide] 0.3%•3%

**licofelone** *investigational (Phase III) analgesic/antiarthritic/nonsteroidal antiinflammatory drug (NSAID) with low gastric side effects*

**licorice (*Glycyrrhiza glabra; G. pallidiflora; G. uralensis*)** *root medicinal herb for Addison disease, blood cleansing, colds, cough, drug withdrawal, female disorders, hoarseness, hypoglycemia, lung disorders, sore throat, and stomach ulcers; also used as an expectorant and to increase energy*

**licostinel** USAN *investigational (Phase I) NMDA receptor antagonist for stroke*

**licryfilcon A** USAN *hydrophilic contact lens material*

**licryfilcon B** USAN *hydrophilic contact lens material*

**Lid Wipes-SPF** solution, pads (discontinued 2003) OTC *eyelid cleansing wipes for blepharitis or contact lenses*

**Lidakol** cream ℞ *investigational (Phase II) antiviral lipase inhibitor for HIV infection and AIDS-related Kaposi sarcoma* [docosanol] 10%

**LidaMantle** cream ℞ *local anesthetic* [lidocaine HCl] 3%

**LidaMantle HC** cream ℞ *corticosteroidal anti-inflammatory; local anesthetic* [hydrocortisone acetate; lidocaine] 0.5%•3%

**lidamidine** INN *antiperistaltic* [also: lidamidine HCl]

**lidamidine HCl** USAN *antiperistaltic* [also: lidamidine]

**Lidex** cream, ointment, topical solution ℞ *topical corticosteroidal anti-inflammatory* [fluocinonide] 0.05% ☒ Lasix; Lidox; Wydase

**Lidex** gel (discontinued 2000) ℞ *topical corticosteroidal anti-inflammatory* [fluocinonide] 0.05% ☒ Lasix; Lidox; Wydase

**Lidex-E** cream ℞ *corticosteroidal anti-inflammatory; emollient* [fluocinonide] 0.05%

**lidimycin** INN *antifungal* [also: lydimycin]

**lidocaine** USP, INN *topical local anesthetic; investigational (orphan) transdermal delivery for post-herpetic neuralgia* [also: lignocaine]

**lidocaine benzyl benzoate** [see: denatonium benzoate]

**lidocaine HCl** USP *local anesthetic; antiarrhythmic* [also: lignocaine HCl] 2%, 4%, 5% topical; 1%, 1.5%, 2% injection; 4%, 10%, 20% IV admixture

**lidocaine HCl in dextrose** *local anesthetic for obstetrical use* 1.5%•7.5%, 5%•7.5% injection

**lidocaine HCl & epinephrine** *injectable local anesthetic; vasoconstrictor* 0.5%•1:200 000, 1%•1:100 000, 1%•1:200 000, 1.5%•1:200 000, 2%•1:50 000, 2%•1:100 000, 2%•1:200 000 injection

**Lidoderm** transdermal patch ℞ *local anesthetic for post-herpetic neuralgia (orphan)* [lidocaine] 5%

**lidofenin** USAN, INN *hepatic function test*

**lidofilcon A** USAN *hydrophilic contact lens material*

**lidofilcon B** USAN *hydrophilic contact lens material*

**lidoflazine** USAN, INN, BAN *coronary vasodilator*

**Lidoject-1; Lidoject-2** injection (discontinued 2002) ℞ *injectable local anesthetic* [lidocaine HCl] 1%; 2%

**LidoPen** auto-injector (automatic IM injection device) (discontinued 2002) ℞ *emergency injection for cardiac arrhythmias* [lidocaine HCl] 10%

**Lidosense 4** cream OTC *local anesthetic* [lidocaine] 4%

**Lidosite Topical System** transdermal patch ℞ *local anesthetic* [lidocaine HCl; epinephrine] 10%•0.1%

**LID-Pack** ⓒ *ophthalmic ointment + towelettes* OTC *antibiotic* [polymyxin B sulfate; bacitracin zinc] 10 000•500 U/g

**lifarizine** USAN, INN, BAN *platelet aggregation inhibitor*

**life everlasting** *medicinal herb* [see: everlasting]

**Life Extension Booster; Life Extension Super Booster** softgels OTC *vitamin/mineral supplement* [multiple vitamins & minerals]

**Life Extension Herbal Mix** powder for oral solution OTC *dietary supplement*

**Life Extension Mix; Life Extension Mix with Niacin; Life Extension Mix without Copper** caplets, capsules, powder for oral solution OTC *vitamin/mineral supplement* [multiple vitamins & minerals]

**Life Extension Two-Per-Day** tablets OTC *vitamin/mineral supplement* [multiple vitamins & minerals]

**life root (Senecio aureus; S. jacoboea; S. vulgaris)** *medicinal herb for childbirth pain, diaphoresis, edema, fever, and stimulation of labor and menses; not generally regarded as safe and effective for ingestion because of hepatotoxicity*

**LifeCare** bags (packaging form) *premixed IV infusion bags*

**life-of-man** *medicinal herb* [see: spikenard]

**lifibrate** USAN, INN *antihyperlipoproteinemic*

**lifibrol** USAN, INN *antihyperlipidemic*

**LIG (lymphocyte immune globulin)** [q.v.]

**light mineral oil** [see: mineral oil, light]

**lignocaine** BAN *topical local anesthetic* [also: lidocaine]

**lignocaine HCl** BAN *local anesthetic; antiarrhythmic* [also: lidocaine HCl]

**lignosulfonic acid, sodium salt** [see: polignate sodium]

**lilopristone** INN

**lily, conval; May lily** *medicinal herb* [see: lily of the valley]

**lily, ground** *medicinal herb* [see: birthroot]

**lily, white pond; sweet water lily; sweet-scented pond lily; sweet-scented water lily; white water**

**lily; toad lily** *medicinal herb* [see: white pond lily]

**lily of the valley (Convallaria majalis)** flower, leaves, and rhizome *medicinal herb for arrhythmia, edema, epilepsy, and heart disorders*

**limaprost** INN

**limarsol** [see: acetarsone]

**Limbitrol DS 10-25** tablets ℞ *antidepressant; anxiolytic* [chlordiazepoxide; amitriptyline HCl] 10•25 mg

**Limbrel** capsules ℞ *natural COX-2 inhibitor; analgesic and anti-inflammatory for the dietary management of osteoarthritis* [flavocoxid] 250 mg

**lime** USP *pharmaceutic necessity*

**lime, sulfurated (calcium polysulfide, calcium thiosulfate)** USP *wet dressing/soak for cystic acne and seborrhea*

**lime tree** *medicinal herb* [see: linden tree]

**Lin-Amox** ⒸⒶⓃ capsules, oral suspension ℞ *antibiotic* [amoxicillin trihydrate] 250, 500 mg; 125, 250 mg/5 mL

**linarotene** USAN, INN *antikeratinizing agent*

**Lin-Buspirone** ⒸⒶⓃ tablets ℞ *azaspirone anxiolytic* [buspirone HCl] 10 mg

**Lincocin** capsules, IV or IM injection ℞ *lincosamide antibiotic* [lincomycin HCl] 500 mg; 300 mg/mL ⑨ Cleocin; Indocin

**lincomycin** USAN, INN, BAN *lincosamide antibiotic*

**lincomycin HCl** USP *lincosamide antibiotic* 300 mg/mL injection

**Lincorex** IV or IM injection ℞ *lincosamide antibiotic* [lincomycin HCl] 300 mg/mL

**lincosamides** *a class of antimicrobial antibiotics with potentially serious side effects, to which bacterial resistance has been shown*

**lindane** USAN, USP, INN, BAN *pediculicide for lice; scabicide* 1% topical

**linden tree (Tilia americana; T. cordata; T. europaea; T. platyphyllos)** flowers *medicinal herb for diaphoresis, diarrhea, headache, hypertension, indigestion, nasal congestion, nervousness,* skin moisturizer, stomach disorders, and throat irritation

**linezolid** USAN *oxazolidinone antibiotic for gram-positive bacterial infections*

**Linguets** (trademarked form) *buccal tablets*

**Linker protocol (daunorubicin, vincristine, prednisone, asparaginase, teniposide, cytarabine, methotrexate [with leucovorin rescue])** *chemotherapy protocol for acute lymphocytic leukemia (ALL)*

**Lin-Megestrol** ⓒᴬᴺ *tablets* ℞ *progestin; hormonal antineoplastic for advanced carcinoma of the breast or endometrium* [megestrol acetate] 40, 160 mg

**linogliride** USAN, INN *antidiabetic*

**linogliride fumarate** USAN *antidiabetic*

**linolexamide** [see: clinolamide]

**linopiridine** USAN, INN *cognition enhancer for Alzheimer disease*

**Lin-Pravastatin** ⓒᴬᴺ *tablets* ℞ *HMG-CoA reductase inhibitor for hyperlipidemia and hypertriglyceridemia* [pravastatin sodium] 10, 20, 40 mg

**linseed** *medicinal herb* [see: flaxseed]

**linsidomine** INN

**lint bells** *medicinal herb* [see: flaxseed]

**lintopride** INN

**Linum usitatissimum** *medicinal herb* [see: flaxseed]

**lion's ear; lion's tail** *medicinal herb* [see: motherwort]

**lion's tooth** *medicinal herb* [see: dandelion]

**Lioresal** *caplets* ℞ *skeletal muscle relaxant* [baclofen] 10, 20 mg

**Lioresal** *intrathecal injection* ℞ *skeletal muscle relaxant for intractable spasticity due to spinal cord injury or disease (orphan); investigational (orphan) for dystonia* [baclofen] 0.05 mg/0.5 mL (50 μg/mL), 10 mg/20 mL (500 μg/mL), 10 mg/5 mL (2000 μg/mL)

**liothyronine** INN, BAN *radioactive agent* [also: liothyronine I 125] ⓢ levothyroxine

**liothyronine I 125** USAN *radioactive agent* [also: liothyronine]

**liothyronine I 131** USAN *radioactive agent*

**liothyronine sodium** USP, BAN *synthetic thyroid hormone ($T_3$ fraction only); treatment of myxedema coma or precoma (orphan)*

**liotrix** USAN, USP *synthetic thyroid hormone (a 4:1 mixture of $T_4$ and $T_3$)* ⓢ Klotrix

**Lip Medex** *ointment* OTC *topical antipruritic/counterirritant; mild local anesthetic* [camphor; phenol] 1%•0.54%

**lipancreatin** [see: pancrelipase]

**lipase** *digestive enzyme* [24 IU/mg in pancrelipase; 2 IU/mg in pancreatin]

**lipase of pancreas** [see: pancrelipase]

**lipase triacylglycerol** [see: pancrelipase]

**Lipidil Supra** ⓒᴬᴺ *film-coated tables* ℞ *antihyperlipidemic for hypercholesterolemia and hypertriglyceridemia* [fenofibrate] 100, 160 mg

**Lipil** [see: Enfamil LIPIL; LactoFree LIPIL; ProSobee LIPIL]

**Lipisorb** *powder* OTC *enteral nutritional therapy* [lactose-free formula]

**Lipitor** *film-coated tablets* ℞ *HMG-CoA reductase inhibitor for hypercholesterolemia, dysbetalipoproteinemia, and hypertriglyceridemia* [atorvastatin calcium] 10, 20, 40, 80 mg

**Lipoflavonoid** *capsules* OTC *dietary lipotropic with vitamin supplementation* [choline; inositol; multiple B vitamins; vitamin C; lemon bioflavonoids] 111.3•111.3•≜•100•100 mg

**Lipogen** *capsules, caplets* OTC *dietary lipotropic with vitamin supplementation* [choline; inositol; multiple vitamins] 111•111•≜ mg

**α-lipoic acid; lipoicin** *natural antioxidant* [see: alpha lipoic acid]

**Lipomul** *oral liquid* OTC *dietary fat supplement* [corn oil] 10 g/15 mL

**Liponol** *capsules* OTC *dietary lipotropic with vitamin supplementation* [choline; inositol; methionine; multiple B vitamins] 115•83•110•≜ mg

**lipopeptides** [see: cyclic lipopeptides]

**lipoprotein OspA, recombinant** discontinued 2002) *active immunizing agent against Lyme disease*

**lipoprotein-associated coagulation inhibitor (LACI)** [see: tifacogin]

**liposomal gentamicin** [see: gentamicin liposome]

**liposome-encapsulated doxorubicin HCl (LED)** [see: doxorubicin HCl, liposome-encapsulated]

**liposome-encapsulated recombinant interleukin-2** [see: interleukin-2, liposome-encapsulated recombinant]

**liposome-encapsulated T4 endonuclease V** [see: T4 endonuclease V, liposome encapsulated]

**Liposyn II 20%; Liposyn III 20%** IV infusion ℞ *nutritional therapy* [fat emulsion]

**Lipotriad** caplets OTC *dietary lipotropic with vitamin supplementation* [choline; inositol; multiple vitamins] 111 • ² • ² mg

**lipotropics** *a class of oral nutritional supplements*

**Lipram 4500** delayed-release capsules containing enteric-coated microspheres ℞ *porcine-derived digestive enzymes* [lipase; protease; amylase] 4500 • 25 000 • 20 000 USP units

**Lipram-CR5; Lipram-CR10; Lipram-CR20** delayed-release capsules containing enteric-coated microspheres ℞ *porcine-derived digestive enzymes* [lipase; protease; amylase] 5000 • 18 750 • 16 600 USP units; 10 000 • 37 500 • 33 200 USP units; 20 000 • 75 000 • 66 400 USP units

**Lipram-PN10; Lipram-PN16; Lipram-PN20** delayed-release capsules containing enteric-coated microspheres ℞ *porcine-derived digestive enzymes* [lipase; protease; amylase] 10 000 • 30 000 • 30 000 USP units; 16 000 • 48 000 • 48 000 USP units; 20 000 • 44 000 • 56 000 USP units

**Lipram-UL12; Lipram-UL18; Lipram-UL20** delayed-release capsules containing enteric-coated microspheres ℞ *porcine-derived diges-*

*tive enzymes* [lipase; protease; amylase] 12 000 • 39 000 • 39 000 USP units; 18 000 • 58 500 • 58 500 USP units; 20 000 • 65 000 • 65 000 USP units

**liquefied phenol** [see: phenol, liquefied]

**Liquibid; Liquibid 1200** sustained-release tablet (discontinued 2004) ℞ *expectorant* [guaifenesin] 600 mg; 1200 mg

**Liquibid-D; Liquibid-D 1200** sustained-release tablets ℞ *decongestant; expectorant* [phenylephrine HCl; guaifenesin] 40 • 600 mg; 40 • 1200 mg

**Liquibid-PD** sustained-release tablets ℞ *decongestant; expectorant* [phenylephrine HCl; guaifenesin] 25 • 275 mg

**LiquiCaps** (dosage form) *soft liquid-filled gelcaps*

**Liqui-Char** oral liquid OTC *adsorbent antidote for poisoning* [activated charcoal] 12.5 g/60 mL, 15 g/75 mL, 25 g/120 mL, 30 g/120 mL, 50 g/240 mL

**Liqui-Coat HD** concentrated oral suspension ℞ *radiopaque contrast medium for gastrointestinal imaging* [barium sulfate] 210%

**Liquid Caps** (dosage form) *soft liquid-filled gelcaps*

**liquid glucose** [see: glucose, liquid]

**liquid petrolatum** [see: mineral oil]

**Liquid Pred** syrup ℞ *corticosteroid; anti-inflammatory* [prednisone; alcohol 5%] 5 mg/5 mL

**Liquid Tabs** (dosage form) *liquid-filled tablets*

**Liquidambar orientalis; L. styraciflua** *medicinal herb* [see: storax]

**Liqui-Doss** emulsion OTC *emollient laxative* [mineral oil]

**Liquifilm Tears; Liquifilm Forte** eye drops OTC *ophthalmic moisturizer/lubricant* [polyvinyl alcohol] 1.4%; 3%

**Liquifilm Wetting** solution OTC *wetting solution for hard contact lenses*

**Liqui-Gels** (trademarked dosage form) *soft liquid-filled gelcaps*

**Liqui-Histine DM** syrup (discontinued 2002) ℞ *antitussive; decongestant; antihistamine* [dextromethorphan hydrobromide; phenylpropanolamine

HCl; brompheniramine maleate] 10•12.5•2 mg/5 mL

**Liqui-Histine-D** elixir (discontinued 2001) ℞ *decongestant; antihistamine* [phenylpropanolamine HCl; phenyltoloxamine citrate; pyrilamine maleate; pheniramine maleate] 12.5•4•4•4 mg/5 mL

**Liquimat** lotion OTC *antibacterial and exfoliant for acne* [sulfur] 4%

**Liquiprin Drops for Children** OTC *analgesic; antipyretic* [acetaminophen] 80 mg/1.66 mL

**Liquitab** (trademarked dosage form) *chewable tablet*

**LiquiVent** ℞ *investigational (Phase III) blood substitute; investigational (Phase III) treatment for pediatric acute respiratory distress syndrome (ARDS); investigational (Phase II/III) agent for adults with acute lung injury or ARDS* [perflubron]

**liquor carbonis detergens (LCD)** [see: coal tar]

**liroldine** INN

**lisadimate** USAN, INN *sunscreen*

**lisinopril** USAN, INN, BAN *antihypertensive; angiotensin-converting enzyme (ACE) inhibitor; adjunctive treatment for CHF* 2.5, 5, 10, 20, 30, 40 mg oral

**lisinopril & hydrochlorothiazide** *antihypertensive; angiotensin-converting enzyme (ACE) inhibitor; diuretic* 10•12.5, 20•12.5, 20•25 mg oral

**lisofylline (LSF)** USAN *acetyltransferase inhibitor; investigational (Phase III) immunomodulator and cytokine inhibitor for acute myeloid leukemia and bone marrow transplants; investigational agent for prevention of GI tract damage during chemotherapy; investigational (Phase II/III) for ARDS and acute lung injury*

**Listerine; Cool-Mint Listerine; FreshBurst Listerine; Natural Citrus Listerine; Tartar Control Listerine** mouthwash/gargle OTC *topical oral antiseptic; analgesic* [thymol; eucalyptol; methyl salicylate; menthol; alcohol 22%–26%] 0.06%•0.09%•0.06%•0.04%

**Listermint Arctic Mint** mouthwash/gargle OTC

**lisuride** INN [also: lysuride]

**Lithane** CAN capsules ℞ *antipsychotic for manic episodes* [lithium carbonate] 150, 300 mg

**lithium** *element (Li)*

**lithium benzoate** NF

**lithium carbonate** USAN, USP *antimanic; immunity booster in chemotherapy and AIDS* 150, 300, 450, 600 mg oral

**lithium citrate** USP *antimanic; immunity booster in chemotherapy and AIDS* 300 mg/5 mL oral

**lithium hydroxide** USP *antimanic*

**lithium hydroxide monohydrate** [see: lithium hydroxide]

**lithium salicylate** NF

**Lithobid** slow-release tablets ℞ *antipsychotic for manic episodes* [lithium carbonate] 300 mg

**litholytics** *a class of agents that dissolve stones or calculi* [see also: antilithics]

**Lithonate** capsules ℞ *antipsychotic for manic episodes* [lithium carbonate] 300 mg

**Lithostat** tablets ℞ *adjunctive therapy in chronic urea-splitting urinary tract infections* [acetohydroxamic acid] 250 mg

**Lithotabs** film-coated tablets ℞ *antipsychotic for manic episodes* [lithium carbonate] 300 mg

**litracen** INN

**Little Colds for Infants and Children** oral drops OTC *nasal decongestant* [phenylephrine HCl] 0.25%

**Little Noses Gentle Formula, Infants and Children** nose drops OTC *nasal decongestant* [phenylephrine HCl] 0.125%

**liver, desiccated; liver extracts** *source of vitamin $B_{12}$*

**Liver Combo No. 5** IM injection (discontinued 2004) ℞ *hematinic; vitamin B supplement* [liver extracts; vitamin $B_{12}$; folic acid] 10 μg•100 μg•0.4 mg per mL

**liver derivative complex** *claimed to be an anti-inflammatory for various dermatological conditions*
**liver lily** *medicinal herb* [see: blue flag]
**liverleaf; liverwort** *medicinal herb* [see: hepatica]
**Livial** (approved in Europe, Asia, and South America) ℞ *investigational (NDA filed) synthetic steroid for osteoporosis and other postmenopausal symptoms* [tibolone]
**lividomycin** INN
**Livitrinsic-f** capsules ℞ *hematinic* [ferrous fumarate; cyanocobalamin; ascorbic acid; intrinsic factor concentrate; folic acid] 110 mg•15 μg•75 mg•240 mg•0.5 mg
**Livostin** eye drop suspension ℞ *antihistamine for allergic conjunctivitis* [levocabastine HCl] 0.05%
**Livostin** ⓒ nasal spray ℞ *antihistamine for seasonal allergic rhinitis* [levocabastine HCl] 0.05%
**lixazinone sulfate** USAN *cardiotonic; phosphodiesterase inhibitor*
**lixivaptan** USAN *selective V2-receptor antagonist for nonhypovolemic hyponatremia*
**LKV Infant Drops** powder + liquid OTC *vitamin supplement* [multiple vitamins; biotin] ±•75 μg/0.6 mL
**LLD factor** [see: cyanocobalamin]
**10% LMD** IV injection ℞ *plasma volume expander for shock due to hemorrhage, burns, or surgery* [dextran 40] 10%
**LMD (low molecular weight dextran)** [see: dextran 40]
**LMF (Leukeran, methotrexate, fluorouracil)** *chemotherapy protocol*
**LMWD (low molecular weight dextran)** [see: dextran 40]
**L·M·X4** cream OTC *local anesthetic* [lidocaine, liposome-encapsulated] 4%
**L·M·X5** anorectal cream OTC *local anesthetic* [lidocaine, liposome-encapsulated] 5%
**Lobac** capsules ℞ *skeletal muscle relaxant; analgesic* [salicylamide; phenyl-

toloxamine; acetaminophen] 200•20•300 mg
**Lobana Body** lotion OTC *moisturizer; emollient*
**Lobana Body Shampoo; Lobana Liquid Lather** topical liquid OTC *soap-free therapeutic skin cleanser* [chloroxylenol]
**Lobana Derm-Ade** cream OTC *moisturizer; emollient* [vitamins A, D, and E]
**Lobana Peri-Garde** ointment OTC *moisturizer; emollient; antiseptic* [vitamins A, D, and E; chloroxylenol]
**lobelia (Lobelia inflata)** plant (tincture) *medicinal herb for arthritis, asthma, bronchitis, hay fever, colds, cough, ear infections, epilepsy, fever, food poisoning, lockjaw, nervousness, pain, pneumonia, preventing miscarriage, whooping cough, and worms*
**lobeline** INN *nicotine withdrawal aid* [also: lobeline HCl]
**lobeline HCl** JAN *nicotine withdrawal aid* [also: lobeline]
**lobendazole** USAN, INN *veterinary anthelmintic*
**lobenzarit** INN *antirheumatic* [also: lobenzarit sodium]
**lobenzarit sodium** USAN *antirheumatic* [also: lobenzarit]
**lobradimil** USAN *receptor-mediated permeabilizer; investigational (Phase III) blood-brain barrier permeability-enhancing agent for carrying carboplatin to brain tumors*
**lobucavir** USAN, INN *antiviral; investigational (Phase III) for AIDS-related asymptomatic cytomegalovirus (clinical trials discontinued 1999)*
**lobuprofen** INN
**LoCholest; LoCholest Light** powder for oral suspension ℞ *cholesterol-lowering antihyperlipidemic; also used for biliary obstruction* [cholestyramine resin] 4 g/dose
**locicortolone dicibate** INN
**locicortone** [see: locicortolone dicibate]
**Locoid** cream, ointment, solution ℞ *corticosteroidal anti-inflammatory* [hydrocortisone butyrate] 0.1%

**Locoid Lipocream** R *corticosteroidal anti-inflammatory* [hydrocortisone butyrate (in an oil-in-water emulsion)] 0.1% (70% oil•30% water)

**locust plant** *medicinal herb* [see: senna]

**lodaxaprine** INN

**lodazecar** INN

**lodelaben** USAN, INN *antiarthritic; emphysema therapy adjunct*

**lodenosine** USAN *investigational (Phase II) reverse transcriptase antiviral for HIV infection*

**Lodine** film-coated tablets, capsules R *analgesic; antiarthritic; nonsteroidal anti-inflammatory drug (NSAID)* [etodolac] 400, 500 mg; 200, 300 mg

**Lodine XL** film-coated extended-release tablets R *once-daily analgesic and antiarthritic; nonsteroidal anti-inflammatory drug (NSAID)* [etodolac] 400, 500, 600 mg

**lodinixil** INN

**lodiperone** INN

**Lodosyn** tablets R *decarboxylase inhibitor; antiparkinsonian adjunct (used with levodopa; no effect when given alone)* [carbidopa] 25 mg

**lodoxamide** INN, BAN *antiallergic; antiasthmatic* [also: lodoxamide ethyl]

**lodoxamide ethyl** USAN *antiallergic; antiasthmatic* [also: lodoxamide]

**lodoxamide trometamol** BAN *antiallergic; antiasthmatic* [also: lodoxamide tromethamine]

**lodoxamide tromethamine** USAN *antiasthmatic; antiallergic for vernal keratoconjunctivitis (orphan)* [also: lodoxamide trometamol]

**Lodrane** oral liquid R *decongestant; antihistamine* [pseudoephedrine HCl; brompheniramine maleate] 60•4 mg/5 mL

**Lodrane 12 D** sustained-release tablets R *decongestant; antihistamine* [pseudoephedrine HCl; brompheniramine maleate] 45•6 mg

**Lodrane LD** sustained-release capsules R *decongestant; antihistamine* [pseudoephedrine HCl; brompheniramine maleate] 60•6 mg

**Loestrin 21 1/20; Loestrin 21 1.5/30** tablets (in packs of 21) R *monophasic oral contraceptive* [norethindrone acetate; ethinyl estradiol] 1 mg•20 μg; 1.5 mg•30 μg

**Loestrin Fe 1/20; Loestrin Fe 1.5/30** tablets (in packs of 28) R *monophasic oral contraceptive; iron supplement* [norethindrone acetate; ethinyl estradiol; ferrous fumarate] 1 mg•20 μg•75 mg; 1.5 mg•30 μg•75 mg

**lofemizole** INN *anti-inflammatory; analgesic; antipyretic* [also: lofemizole HCl]

**lofemizole HCl** USAN *anti-inflammatory; analgesic; antipyretic* [also: lofemizole]

**Lofenalac** powder for oral solution (name changed to Phenyl-Free in 2003)

**lofendazam** INN, BAN

**lofentanil** INN, BAN *narcotic analgesic* [also: lofentanil oxalate]

**lofentanil oxalate** USAN *narcotic analgesic* [also: lofentanil]

**lofepramine** INN, BAN *antidepressant* [also: lofepramine HCl]

**lofepramine HCl** USAN *antidepressant* [also: lofepramine]

**lofexidine** INN, BAN *antihypertensive* [also: lofexidine HCl]

**lofexidine HCl** USAN *centrally acting antiadrenergic antihypertensive; investigational (Phase III) treatment for opiate withdrawal syndrome* [also: lofexidine]

**Lofibra** capsules R *antihyperlipidemic for primary hypercholesterolemia (types IIa and IIb hyperlipidemia), hypertriglyceridemia (types IV and V hyperlipidemia), and mixed dyslipidemia* [fenofibrate] 67, 134, 200 mg

**loflucarban** INN

**Logen** tablets R *antidiarrheal* [diphenoxylate HCl; atropine sulfate] 2.5• 0.025 mg

**LoKara** lotion R *corticosteroidal anti-inflammatory* [desonide] 0.05%

**LOMAC (leucovorin, Oncovin, methotrexate, Adriamycin, cyclophosphamide)** *chemotherapy protocol*

**Lomanate** oral liquid ℞ *antidiarrheal* [diphenoxylate HCl; atropine sulfate] 2.5•0.025 mg/5 mL

**lombazole** INN, BAN

**lomefloxacin** USAN, INN, BAN *broad-spectrum fluoroquinolone antibiotic*

**lomefloxacin HCl** USAN *broad-spectrum fluoroquinolone antibiotic*

**lomefloxacin mesylate** USAN *antibacterial*

**lometraline** INN *antipsychotic; antiparkinsonian* [also: lometraline HCl]

**lometraline HCl** USAN *antipsychotic; antiparkinsonian* [also: lometraline]

**lometrexol** INN *antineoplastic* [also: lometrexol sodium]

**lometrexol sodium** USAN *antineoplastic* [also: lometrexol]

**lomevactone** INN

**lomifylline** INN

**lomofungin** USAN *antifungal*

**Lomotil** tablets, oral liquid ℞ *antidiarrheal* [diphenoxylate HCl; atropine sulfate] 2.5•0.025 mg; 2.5•0.025 mg/5 mL

**lomustine** USAN, INN, BAN *nitrosourea-type alkylating antineoplastic for brain tumors and Hodgkin disease*

**lonafarnib** *investigational (Phase III) antineoplastic for lung cancer*

**Lonalac** powder OTC *enteral nutritional therapy* [milk-based formula]

**lonapalene** USAN *antipsoriatic*

**lonaprofen** INN

**lonazolac** INN

**lonidamine** INN

**Loniten** tablets ℞ *antihypertensive; vasodilator* [minoxidil] 2.5, 10 mg ⊘ clonidine

**Lonox** tablets ℞ *antidiarrheal* [diphenoxylate HCl; atropine sulfate] 2.5•0.025 mg ⊘ Lovenox

**loop diuretics** *a class of diuretic agents that inhibit the reabsorption of sodium and chloride*

**Lo/Ovral** tablets (in Pilpaks of 21 or 28) ℞ *monophasic oral contraceptive; emergency postcoital contraceptive* [norgestrel; ethinyl estradiol] 0.3 mg•30 μg

**loperamide** INN, BAN *antiperistaltic; antidiarrheal* [also: loperamide HCl]

**loperamide HCl** USAN, USP, JAN *antiperistaltic; antidiarrheal* [also: loperamide] 2 mg oral; 1 mg/5 mL oral

**loperamide oxide** INN, BAN *antiperistaltic; antidiarrheal*

***Lophophora williamsii*** *a flowering Mexican cactus whose heads (mescal buttons) are used to produce mescaline, a hallucinogenic street drug*

**Lopid** film-coated tablets ℞ *triglyceride-lowering antihyperlipidemic for hypertriglyceridemia (types IV and V hyperlipidemia) and coronary heart disease* [gemfibrozil] 600 mg (300 mg capsules available in Canada)

**lopinavir** USAN *antiviral protease inhibitor for HIV infection*

**lopirazepam** INN

**loprazolam** INN, BAN

**lopremone** [now: protirelin]

**Lopressor** tablets, IV injection ℞ *antianginal; antihypertensive; β-blocker* [metoprolol tartrate] 50, 100 mg; 1 mg/mL

**Lopressor HCT 50/25; Lopressor HCT 100/25; Lopressor HCT 100/50** tablets ℞ *antihypertensive; β-blocker; diuretic* [metoprolol tartrate; hydrochlorothiazide] 50•25 mg; 100•25 mg; 100•50 mg

**loprodiol** INN

**Loprox** cream, gel, topical suspension, shampoo ℞ *antifungal for tinea pedis, tinea cruris, tinea corporis, tinea versicolor, candidiasis, and seborrheic dermatitis* [ciclopirox olamine] 1%

**Loprox** lotion (discontinued 2003) ℞ *antifungal* [ciclopirox olamine] 1%

**Lorabid** Pulvules (capsules), powder for oral suspension ℞ *carbacephem antibiotic* [loracarbef] 200, 400 mg; 100, 200 mg/5 mL

**loracarbef** USAN, INN *carbacephem antibiotic*

**lorajmine** INN *antiarrhythmic* [also: lorajmine HCl]

**lorajmine HCl** USAN *antiarrhythmic* [also: lorajmine]

**lorapride** INN

**loratadine** USAN, INN, BAN *second-generation peripherally selective piperidine antihistamine for allergic rhinitis and chronic idiopathic urticaria* 10 mg oral

**lorazepam** USAN, USP, INN, BAN *benzodiazepine anxiolytic; preanesthetic sedative; anticonvulsant* 0.5, 1, 2 mg oral; 2, 4 mg/mL injection

**Lorazepam Intensol** oral drops ℞ *benzodiazepine anxiolytic; sedative; anticonvulsant* [lorazepam] 2 mg/mL

**lorbamate** USAN, INN *muscle relaxant*

**lorcainide** INN, BAN *antiarrhythmic* [also: lorcainide HCl]

**lorcainide HCl** USAN *antiarrhythmic* [also: lorcainide]

**Lorcet Plus; Lorcet 10/650** tablets ℞ *narcotic analgesic* [hydrocodone bitartrate; acetaminophen] 7.5•650 mg; 10•650 mg

**Lorcet-HD** capsules ℞ *narcotic analgesic* [hydrocodone bitartrate; acetaminophen] 5•500 mg ☑ Fioricet

**lorcinadol** INN, INN, BAN *analgesic*

**loreclezole** USAN, INN, BAN *antiepileptic*

**Lorenzo oil (erucic acid and oleic acid)** *natural treatment for childhood adrenoleukodystrophy and adrenomyeloneuropathy in adults*

**lorglumide** INN

**lormetazepam** USAN, INN, BAN *sedative; hypnotic*

**lornoxicam** USAN, INN, BAN *analgesic; anti-inflammatory*

**Lorothidol** (available only from the Centers for Disease Control) ℞ *investigational anti-infective for paragonimiasis and fascioliasis* [bithionol]

**Loroxide** lotion (discontinued 2003) OTC *keratolytic for acne* [benzoyl peroxide] 5.5%

**lorpiprazole** INN

**Lortab** elixir ℞ *narcotic analgesic* [hydrocodone bitartrate; acetaminophen] 2.5•167 mg/5 mL

**Lortab 2.5/500; Lortab 5/500; Lortab 7.5/500; Lortab 10/500** tablets ℞ *narcotic analgesic* [hydrocodone bitartrate; acetaminophen] 2.5•500 mg; 5•500 mg; 7.5•500 mg; 10•500 mg

**Lortab ASA** tablets ℞ *narcotic analgesic* [hydrocodone bitartrate; aspirin] 5•500 mg

**lortalamine** USAN, INN *antidepressant*

**Lortuss DM** oral liquid OTC *antitussive; decongestant; antihistamine* [dextromethorphan hydrobromide; phenylephrine HCl; brompheniramine maleate] 15•7.5•2 mg/5 mL

**Lortuss HC** oral liquid ℞ *narcotic antitussive; decongestant* [hydrocodone bitartrate; phenylephrine HCl] 3.5•7.5 mg/5 mL

**lorzafone** USAN, INN *minor tranquilizer*

**losartan** INN *angiotensin II receptor antagonist for hypertension; treatment to delay the progression of diabetic nephropathy* [also: losartan potassium]

**losartan potassium** USAN *angiotensin II receptor antagonist for hypertension; treatment to delay the progression of diabetic nephropathy* [also: losartan]

**Losec** CAN delayed-release tablets ℞ *proton pump inhibitor for gastric and duodenal ulcers and other gastroesophageal disorders* [omeprazole] 10, 20 mg

**Losec 1-2-3 A** CAN ℞ *7-day regimen for eradication of H. pylori–associated peptic ulcer disease* [Losec, 20 mg b.i.d; amoxicillin, 1000 mg b.i.d; clarithromycin, 500 mg b.i.d.]

**Losec 1-2-3 M** CAN ℞ *7-day regimen for eradication of H. pylori–associated peptic ulcer disease* [Losec, 20 mg b.i.d; metronidazole, 500 mg b.i.d; clarithromycin, 250 mg b.i.d.]

**losigamone** INN

**losindole** INN

**losmiprofen** INN

**losoxantrone** INN *antineoplastic* [also: losoxantrone HCl]

**losoxantrone HCl** USAN *antineoplastic* [also: losoxantrone]

**losulazine** INN *antihypertensive* [also: losulazine HCl]

**losulazine HCl** USAN *antihypertensive* [also: losulazine]

**Lotemax** eye drop suspension ℞ *corti-costeroidal anti-inflammatory* [loteprednol etabonate] 0.5%

**Lotensin** tablets ℞ *antihypertensive; angiotensin-converting enzyme (ACE) inhibitor* [benazepril HCl] 5, 10, 20, 40 mg

**Lotensin HCT 5/6.25; Lotensin HCT 10/12.5; Lotensin HCT 20/12.5; Lotensin HCT 20/25** tablets ℞ *antihypertensive; angiotensin-converting enzyme (ACE) inhibitor; diuretic* [benazepril HCl; hydrochlorothiazide] 5•6.25 mg; 10•12.5 mg; 20•12.5 mg; 20•25 mg

**loteprednol** INN *corticosteroidal anti-inflammatory* [also: loteprednol etabonate]

**loteprednol etabonate** USAN *ophthalmic corticosteroidal anti-inflammatory* [also: loteprednol]

**lotifazole** INN

**lotrafiban HCl** USAN *platelet aggregation inhibitor; GP IIb/IIIa receptor antagonist*

**Lotrel** capsules ℞ *antihypertensive; angiotensin-converting enzyme (ACE) inhibitor; calcium channel blocker* [amlodipine besylate; benazepril HCl] 2.5•10, 5•10, 5•20, 10•20 mg

**lotrifen** INN

**Lotrimin** cream, solution, lotion (discontinued 2003) ℞ *antifungal* [clotrimazole] 1% ② Otrivin

**Lotrimin AF** cream, topical solution, lotion OTC *antifungal* [clotrimazole] 1%

**Lotrimin AF** powder, spray powder, spray liquid OTC *antifungal* [miconazole nitrate] 2%

**Lotrimin Ultra** cream OTC *antifungal* [butenafine HCl] 1%

**Lotrisone** cream, lotion ℞ *corticosteroidal anti-inflammatory; antifungal* [betamethasone dipropionate; clotrimazole] 0.05%•1%

**Lotronex** film-coated tablets ℞ *serotonin 5-HT₃ receptor antagonist for irritable bowel syndrome (IBS)* [alosetron HCl] 0.562, 1.124 mg (=0.5, 1 mg base)

**lotucaine** INN

**lousewort** *medicinal herb* [see: betony; feverweed]

**lovage** *(Angelica levisticum; Levisticum officinale)* leaves and roots *medicinal herb for bad breath, boils, edema, flatulence, and sore throat; also used topically as a skin emollient*

**lovastatin** USAN, INN, BAN *HMG-CoA reductase inhibitor for hypercholesterolemia, hyperlipidemia, and atherosclerosis; also for primary prevention of coronary heart disease* 10, 20, 40 mg oral

**Lovenox** deep subcu injection in pre-filled syringes ℞ *anticoagulant/antithrombotic for prevention of deep vein thrombosis (DVT) following knee, hip, or abdominal surgery, unstable angina, and myocardial infarction* [enoxaparin sodium] 30 mg/0.3 mL, 40 mg/0.4 mL, 60 mg/0.6 mL, 80, 120 mg/0.8 mL, 100, 150 mg/mL, 300 mg/3 mL ② Lonox

**loviride** USAN, INN *investigational non-nucleoside reverse transcriptase inhibitor (NNRTI) antiviral for HIV*

**low molecular weight dextran (LMD; LMWD)** [see: dextran 40]

**low molecular weight heparins** *a class of anticoagulants used for the prophylaxis or treatment of thromboembolic complications of surgery and ischemic complications of unstable angina or myocardial infarction*

**low osmolar contrast media (LOCM)** *a class of newer radiopaque agents that have a low osmolar concentration of iodine (the contrast agent), which corresponds to a lower incidence of adverse reactions* [also called: nonionic contrast media]

**Lowila Cake** bar OTC *soap-free therapeutic skin cleanser*

**Low-Ogestrel** tablets (in packs of 28) ℞ *monophasic oral contraceptive; emergency postcoital contraceptive* [norgestrel; ethinyl estradiol] 0.3 mg•30 µg

**Lowsium Plus** oral suspension OTC *antacid; antiflatulent* [magaldrate; simethicone] 540•40 mg/5 mL

**loxanast** INN

**Loxapac** ⒸⒶⓃ oral concentrate, IM injection (discontinued 2001) ℞ *conventional (typical) antipsychotic* [loxapine HCl] 25 mg/mL; 50 mg/mL

**Loxapac** ⒸⒶⓃ tablets (discontinued 2001) ℞ *conventional (typical) antipsychotic* [loxapine] 5, 10, 25, 50 mg

**loxapine** USAN, INN, BAN *minor tranquilizer; dibenzoxazepine antipsychotic*

**loxapine HCl** *minor tranquilizer; dibenzoxazepine antipsychotic*

**loxapine succinate** USAN *minor tranquilizer; dibenzoxazepine antipsychotic* 5, 10, 25, 50 mg oral

**loxiglumide** INN

**Loxitane** capsules ℞ *conventional (typical) antipsychotic* [loxapine succinate] 5, 10, 25, 50 mg ⑨ doxepin

**Loxitane C** oral concentrate (discontinued 2003) ℞ *conventional (typical) antipsychotic* [loxapine HCl] 25 mg/mL

**Loxitane IM** injection (discontinued 2002) ℞ *conventional (typical) antipsychotic* [loxapine HCl] 50 mg/mL

**loxoprofen** INN

**loxoribine** USAN, INN *immunostimulant; vaccine adjuvant; orphan status withdrawn 1996*

**loxotidine** [now: lavoltidine succinate]

**loxtidine** BAN *antiulcerative; histamine $H_2$-receptor blocker* [also: lavoltidine succinate; lavoltidine]

**lozilurea** INN

**Lozi-Tabs** (trademarked form) *lozenges*

**Lozol** film-coated tablets ℞ *antihypertensive; diuretic* [indapamide] 1.25, 2.5 mg

**L-PAM** (L-phenylalanine mustard) [see: melphalan]

**LR (lactated Ringer) solution** [see: Ringer injection, lactated]

**LSD (lysergic acid diethylamide)** *hallucinogenic street drug associated with disorders of sensory and temporal perception, depersonalization, and ataxia* [medically known as lysergide]

**LSF (lisofylline)** [q.v.]

**LTRAs (leukotriene receptor antagonists)** *a class of antiasthmatics*

**Lu texaphyrin** [see: motexafin lutetium]

**lubeluzole** USAN, INN *investigational neural protective for ischemic stroke*

**LubraSol Bath Oil** (discontinued 2003) OTC *bath emollient*

**Lubricating Jelly** OTC *vaginal lubricant* [glycerin; propylene glycol]

**Lubricoat** (trademarked ingredient) *surgical aid* [ferric hyaluronate]

**Lubriderm** cream, lotion (discontinued 2004) OTC *moisturizer; emollient*

**Lubriderm Bath Oil** (discontinued 2004) OTC *bath emollient*

**Lubrin** vaginal inserts OTC *lubricant for sexual intercourse* [glycerin; caprylic triglyceride]

**LubriTears** eye drops OTC *ophthalmic moisturizer/lubricant* [hydroxypropyl methylcellulose] 0.3%

**LubriTears** ophthalmic ointment OTC *ocular moisturizer/lubricant* [white petrolatum; mineral oil; lanolin]

**lucanthone** INN, BAN *antischistosomal* [also: lucanthone HCl]

**lucanthone HCl** USAN, USP *antischistosomal* [also: lucanthone]

**lucartamide** INN

**lucensomycin** [see: lucimycin]

**Lucidex** enteric-coated tablets OTC *CNS stimulant; analeptic* [caffeine] 100 mg

**Lucilia caesar** *natural treatment* [see: maggots]

**lucimycin** INN

**lucinactant** *investigational (Phase II/III, orphan) for respiratory distress syndrome in adults and premature infants and meconium aspiration in newborn infants* [also: KL4 surfactant]

**Ludiomil** coated tablets (discontinued 2001) ℞ *tetracyclic antidepressant* [maprotiline HCl] 25, 50, 75 mg

**Luer-lock** (trademarked delivery device) *prefilled self-injection syringe*

**lufironil** USAN, INN *collagen inhibitor*

**lufuradom** INN

**Lufyllin** tablets, elixir, IM injection ℞ *antiasthmatic; bronchodilator* [dyphylline] 200 mg; 100 mg/15 mL; 250 mg/mL

**Lufyllin 400** tablets ℞ *antiasthmatic; bronchodilator* [dyphylline] 400 mg

**Lufyllin-EPG** tablets, elixir ℞ *antiasthmatic; bronchodilator; decongestant; expectorant; sedative* [dyphylline; ephedrine HCl; guaifenesin; phenobarbital] 100•16•200•16 mg; 150•24•300•24 mg/15 mL

**Lufyllin-GG** tablets, elixir ℞ *antiasthmatic; bronchodilator; expectorant* [dyphylline; guaifenesin] 200•200 mg; 100•100 mg/15 mL

**Lugol** solution ℞ *thyroid-blocking therapy; topical antimicrobial* [iodine; potassium iodide] 5%•10%

**Lumenax** (name changed to Xifaxan upon marketing release in 2004)

**Lumigan** eye drops ℞ *synthetic prostamide analogue for glaucoma and ocular hypertension* [bimatoprost] 0.03%

**Luminal Sodium** IV or IM injection ℞ *long-acting barbiturate sedative, hypnotic, and anticonvulsant; also abused as a street drug* [phenobarbital sodium] 130 mg/mL ⊡ Tuinal

**lumiracoxib** *investigational (Phase III) antiarthritic for osteoarthritis; analgesic for acute pain; COX-2 inhibitor; nonsteroidal anti-inflammatory drug (NSAID)*

**Lunelle** IM injection ℞ *once-monthly injectable contraceptive* [estradiol cypionate; medroxyprogesterone acetate] 5•25 mg/0.5 mL

**lung surfactant, synthetic** [see: colfosceril palmitate]

**lungwort (*Pulmonaria officinalis*)** flowering plant *medicinal herb used as an astringent, demulcent, emollient, expectorant, and pectoral*

**2,6-lupetidine** [see: nanofin]

**lupitidine** INN *veterinary antagonist to histamine H$_2$ receptors* [also: lupitidine HCl]

**lupitidine HCl** USAN *veterinary antagonist to histamine H$_2$ receptors* [also: lupitidine]

**Lupron; Lupron Pediatric** subcu injection (daily) ℞ *hormonal antineoplastic for prostatic cancer and central precocious puberty (orphan)* [leuprolide acetate] 5 mg/mL ⊡ Mepron; Napron

**Lupron Depot** microspheres for IM injection (monthly) ℞ *hormonal antineoplastic for prostatic cancer, endometriosis, and uterine fibroids* [leuprolide acetate] 3.75, 7.5 mg ⊡ Mepron; Napron

**Lupron Depot–3 month; Lupron Depot–4 month** microspheres for IM injection ℞ *hormonal antineoplastic for prostatic cancer* [leuprolide acetate] 11.5, 22.5 mg; 30 mg ⊡ Mepron; Napron

**Lupron Depot-Ped** microspheres for IM injection (monthly) ℞ *hormonal antineoplastic for central precocious puberty (orphan)* [leuprolide acetate] 7.5, 11.25, 15 mg ⊡ Mepron; Napron

**luprostiol** INN, BAN

**Luride** Lozi-Tabs (chewable tablets), drops, gel ℞ *dental caries preventative* [sodium fluoride] 0.25, 1.1, 2.2 mg; 1.1 mg/mL; 1.2%

**Luride SF** Lozi-Tabs (lozenges) ℞ *topical dental caries preventative* [sodium fluoride] 2.2 mg

**Lurline PMS** tablets (name changed to Vitelle Lurline PMS in 2000)

**lurosetron mesylate** USAN *antiemetic*

**lurtotecan dihydrochloride** USAN *antineoplastic; topoisomerase I inhibitor*

**Lustra; Lustra-AF** cream ℞ *hyperpigmentation bleaching agent* [hydroquinone] 4%

**lutein** *natural carotenoid used to prevent and treat age-related macular degeneration (AMD), retinitis pigmentosa (RP), and other retinal dysfunction*

**luteinizing hormone–releasing factor acetate hydrate** [see: gonadorelin acetate]

**luteinizing hormone–releasing factor diacetate tetrahydrate** [now: gonadorelin acetate]

**luteinizing hormone–releasing factor dihydrochloride** [now: gonadorelin HCl]

**luteinizing hormone–releasing factor HCl** [see: gonadorelin HCl]

**luteinizing hormone–releasing hormone (LH·RH)** *an endogenous hormone, produced in the hypothalamus, which stimulates the release of luteinizing hormone (LH) and follicle-stimulating hormone (FSH) from the pituitary* [also known as: gonadotropin-releasing hormone (Gn-RH)]

**lutetium** *element (Lu)*

**lutetium texaphyrin** [now: motexafin lutetium]

**Lu-Tex** ℞ *investigational for the photodynamic treatment of cancer; investigational (Phase I/II) photosensitizer for ophthalmologic indications including age-related macular degeneration* [motexafin lutetium]

**lutrelin** INN *luteinizing hormone-releasing hormone (LHRH) agonist* [also: lutrelin acetate]

**lutrelin acetate** USAN *luteinizing hormone-releasing hormone (LHRH) agonist* [also: lutrelin]

**Lutrepulse** powder for continuous ambulatory infusion ℞ *gonadotropin-releasing hormone for hypothalamic amenorrhea (orphan)* [gonadorelin acetate] 0.8, 3.2 mg

**Lutrin** ℞ *investigational photodynamic therapy for recurrent breast cancer*

**lutropin alfa** USAN *gonadotropin; investigational treatment for chronic anovulation due to hypogonadism*

**Luveris** ℞ *investigational treatment for chronic anovulation due to hypogonadism* [lutropin alfa]

**Luvox** film-coated tablets (discontinued 2004) ℞ *selective serotonin reuptake inhibitor (SSRI) for obsessive-compulsive disorder (OCD)* [fluvoxamine maleate] 25, 50, 100 mg

**luxabendazole** INN, BAN

**Luxiq** foam ℞ *topical corticosteroidal anti-inflammatory for scalp dermatoses* [betamethasone valerate] 0.12%

**L-VAM (leuprolide acetate, vinblastine, Adriamycin, mitomycin)** *chemotherapy protocol*

**lyapolate sodium** USAN *anticoagulant* [also: sodium apolate]

**lycetamine** USAN *topical antimicrobial*

**lycine HCl** [see: betaine HCl]

**lycopene** *natural substance found in high concentration in ripe tomatoes; a member of the carotene family; used as an antineoplastic and antioxidant*

**Lycopodium clavatum** *medicinal herb* [see: club moss]

**Lycopus virginicus** *medicinal herb* [see: bugleweed]

**Lyderm** ⒸⒶⓃ cream, ointment, gel ℞ *topical corticosteroidal anti-inflammatory* [fluocinonide] 0.05%

**lydimycin** USAN *antifungal* [also: lidimycin]

**Lyme borreliosis vaccine** [see: lipoprotein OspA, recombinant]

**lymecycline** INN, BAN

**LYMErix** IM injection (discontinued 2002) ℞ *active immunizing agent against Lyme disease* [lipoprotein OspA, recombinant] 30 μg/0.5 mL

**Lymphazurin 1%** subcu injection ℞ *radiopaque contrast medium for lymphography* [isosulfan blue] 10 mg/mL (1%)

**LymphoCide** ℞ *investigational (Phase III, orphan) monoclonal antibodies for AIDS-related non-Hodgkin lymphoma* [yttrium Y 90–labeled epratuzumab]

**lymphocyte immune globulin (LIG)** *passive immunizing agent to prevent allograft rejection of renal transplants; treatment for aplastic anemia; investigational (orphan) for organ and bone marrow transplants* [also: antithymocyte globulin (ATG)]

**lymphogranuloma venereum antigen** USP

**LymphoScan** ℞ *investigational (Phase III, orphan) for diagnostic aid for non-Hodgkin B-cell lymphoma, AIDS-related lymphomas, and other acute and chronic B-cell leukemias* [technetium Tc 99m bectumomab]

**lynestrenol** USAN, INN *progestin* [also: lynoestrenol]

**lynoestrenol** BAN *progestin* [also: lynestrenol]

**Lyo-Ject** (trademarked delivery system) *prefilled dual-chambered syringe with lyophilized powder and diluent*

**Lypholized Vitamin B Complex & Vitamin C with B₁₂** injection ℞ *parenteral vitamin therapy* [multiple B vitamins; vitamin C] ≛ • 50 mg/mL

**Lypholyte; Lypholyte II** IV admixture ℞ *intravenous electrolyte therapy* [combined electrolyte solution]

**lypressin** USAN, USP, INN, BAN *posterior pituitary hormone; antidiuretic; vasoconstrictor*

**Lyrica** (approved in Europe) ℞ *investigational (NDA filed) agent for neuropathic pain from diabetic neuropathy, peripheral neuropathy, and postherpetic neuropathy; investigational (Phase III) for generalized anxiety disorder (GAD)* [pregabalin]

**lysergic acid diethylamide (LSD)** *street drug* [see: LSD; lysergide]

**lysergide** INN, BAN, DCF

**lysine (L-lysine)** USAN, INN *essential amino acid; symbols: Lys, K; natural remedy for the prophylaxis and treatment of recurrent oral and genital herpes simplex outbreaks; inhibits HSV replication* 312, 500, 1000 mg oral

**lysine acetate** USP *amino acid*

**DL-lysine acetylsalicylate** [see: aspirin DL-lysine]

**lysine HCl** USAN, USP *amino acid*

**L-lysine monoacetate** [see: lysine acetate]

**L-lysine monohydrochloride** [see: lysine HCl]

**8-L-lysine vasopressin** [see: lypressin]

**Lysodase** ℞ *investigational (orphan) chronic enzyme replacement therapy for Gaucher disease* [PEG-glucocerebrosidase]

**Lysodren** tablets ℞ *antibiotic antineoplastic for inoperable adrenal cortical carcinoma and Cushing syndrome* [mitotane] 500 mg

**lysostaphin** USAN *antibacterial enzyme; investigational agent for methicillin-resistant* Staphylococcus aureus *(MRSA) endocarditis*

**lysuride** BAN [also: lisuride]

**M-CSF (macrophage colony-stimulating factor)** [now: cilmostim]

**M-2 protocol (vincristine, carmustine, cyclophosphamide, prednisone, melphalan)** *chemotherapy protocol for multiple myeloma*

**MAA (macroaggregated albumin)** [see: albumin, aggregated]

**Maalox** chewable tablets (discontinued 2001) OTC *antacid* [aluminum hydroxide; magnesium hydroxide] 200 • 200, 350 • 350 mg ⊡ Marax

**Maalox** oral suspension OTC *antacid* [aluminum hydroxide; magnesium hydroxide] 225 • 200 mg/5 mL ⊡ Marax

**Maalo[x]** ... ued ... bona...

**Maalo[x]** ... men ... *calcium supplement* [calcium carbonate] 600 mg

**Maalox Anti-Diarrheal** caplets (discontinued 2001) OTC *antidiarrheal* [loperamide HCl] 2 mg

**Maalox Anti-Gas** chewable tablets OTC *antiflatulent* [simethicone] 80 mg

**Maalox Anti-Gas, Extra Strength** oral suspension OTC *antacid; antiflatulent* [aluminum hydroxide; magnesium hydroxide; simethicone] 500 • 450 • 40 mg/5 mL

**Maalox H2 Acid Controller** ⓐ film-coated tablets OTC *histamine $H_2$ antagonist for heartburn and acid indigestion* [famotidine] 10 mg

**Maalox HRF** (Heartburn Relief Formula) oral liquid (discontinued 2001) OTC *antacid* [aluminum hydroxide; magnesium carbonate] 140•175 mg/5 mL

**Maalox Plus** chewable tablets, oral suspension (discontinued 2001) OTC *antacid; antiflatulent* [aluminum hydroxide; magnesium hydroxide; simethicone] 200•200•25 mg; 500•450•40 mg/5 mL

**Maalox Quick Dissolve** chewable tablets OTC *antacid; calcium supplement* [calcium carbonate] 600, 1000 mg

**Maalox TC** oral suspension OTC *antacid* [aluminum hydroxide; magnesium hydroxide] 600•300 mg/5 mL

**Maalox Therapeutic Concentrate** oral suspension (renamed Maalox TC in 2003)

**MAb; MAB** (monoclonal antibodies)

**MABOP** (Mustargen, Adriamycin, bleomycin, Oncovin, prednisone) *chemotherapy protocol*

**mabuterol** INN

**MAC** (methotrexate, actinomycin D, chlorambucil) *chemotherapy protocol*

**MAC; MAC III** (methotrexate, actinomycin D, cyclophosphamide) *chemotherapy protocol for gestational trophoblastic neoplasm*

**MAC** (mitomycin, Adriamycin, cyclophosphamide) *chemotherapy protocol*

**maca** (*Lepidium meyenii*) root *medicinal herb used as an adaptogen, aphrodisiac in males, fertility aid in females, and to relieve stress*

**MACC** (methotrexate, Adriamycin, cyclophosphamide, CCNU) *chemotherapy protocol for non–small cell lung cancer (NSCLC)*

**mace** (*Myristica fragrans*) dried nutmeg aril (the fleshy network surrounding the seed) *medicinal herb* [see: nutmeg]

**MACHO** (methotrexate, asparaginase, cyclophosphamide, hydroxydaunomycin, Oncovin) *chemotherapy protocol*

**MACOP-B** (methotrexate, Adriamycin, cyclophosphamide, Oncovin, prednisone, bleomycin) *chemotherapy protocol for non-Hodgkin lymphoma*

**macroaggregated albumin (MAA)** [see: albumin, aggregated]

**macroaggregated iodinated ($^{131}$I) human albumin** [see: macrosalb ($^{131}$I)]

**Macrobid** capsules ℞ *urinary antibiotic* [nitrofurantoin (macrocrystals); nitrofurantoin monohydrate] 25•75 mg

**Macrodantin** capsules ℞ *urinary antibiotic* [nitrofurantoin (macrocrystals)] 25, 50, 100 mg

**Macrodex** IV infusion ℞ *plasma volume expander for shock due to hemorrhage, burns, or surgery* [dextran 70] 6%

**macrogol 4000** INN, BAN [also: polyethylene glycol 4000]

**macrogol ester 2000** INN *surfactant* [also: polyoxyl 40 stearate]

**macrogol ester 400** INN *surfactant* [also: polyoxyl 8 stearate]

**macrolides** *a class of antibiotics that are bacteriostatic or bactericidal, depending on drug concentration*

**macrophage colony-stimulating factor (M-CSF)** [now: cilmostim]

**macrophage-targeted β-glucocerebrosidase** [now: alglucerase]

**macrosalb ($^{131}$I)** INN, BAN

**macrosalb ($^{99m}$Tc)** INN, BAN [also: technetium ($^{99m}$Tc) labeled macroaggregated human ...]

**Macroscint** ℞ *investigational inflammation and infection imaging aid* [indium In 111 IGIV pentetate]

**Macrotys actaeoides** *medicinal herb* [see: black cohosh]

**Macrulin** *investigational (Phase I) oral agent for type 2 diabetes* [insulin]

**Macugen** injection ℞ *investigational (NDA filed) pegylated anti-VEGF (vascular endothelial growth factor) agent for wet age-related macular degeneration* [pegaptanib sodium]

**MAD (MeCCNU, Adriamycin)** *chemotherapy protocol*

**mad-dog weed; mad weed** *medicinal herb* [see: skullcap]

**MADDOC (mechlorethamine, Adriamycin, dacarbazine, DDP, Oncovin, cyclophosphamide)** *chemotherapy protocol*

**madnep; madness** *medicinal herb* [see: masterwort]

**maduramicin** USAN, INN *anticoccidal*

**mafenide** USAN, INN, BAN *bacteriostatic; adjunct to burn therapy*

**mafenide acetate** USP *broad-spectrum bacteriostatic to prevent meshed autograft loss on second- and third-degree burns (orphan)*

**mafenide HCl**

**mafilcon A** USAN *hydrophilic contact lens material*

**mafoprazine** INN

**mafosfamide** INN

**Mag-200** tablets OTC *magnesium supplement* [magnesium oxide] 200 mg Mg

**magaldrate** USAN, USP, INN *antacid* 540 mg/5 mL oral

**Magaldrate Plus** oral suspension OTC *antacid; antiflatulent* [magaldrate; simethicone] 540•40 mg/5 mL

**Magalox Plus** chewable tablets OTC *antacid; antiflatulent* [aluminum hydroxide; magnesium hydroxide; simethicone] 200•200•25 mg

**Magan** tablets ℞ *analgesic; antirheumatic* [magnesium salicylate] 545 mg

**Mag-Cal** tablets OTC *dietary supplement* [calcium carbonate; vitamin D; multiple minerals] 416.7 mg•66.7 IU•≛

**Mag-Cal Mega** tablets OTC *mineral supplement* [magnesium; calcium] 800•400 mg

**Mag-G** tablets OTC *magnesium supplement* [magnesium gluconate dihydrate] 500 mg (27 mg Mg)

**maggots (Lucilia caesar; Phaenicia sericata; Pharmia regina)** *natural treatment for debriding necrotic tissue in abscesses, burns, cellulitis, gangrene, osteomyelitis, and ulcers*

**magic mouthwash** *a slang term for a combination of a local anesthetic plus one or more of the following: an antihistamine, a corticosteroid, an antifungal, an antibiotic—with or without an antacid used as a carrier*

**Maginex** enteric-coated tablets (discontinued 2004) OTC *magnesium supplement* [magnesium-L-aspartate HCl] 615 mg (61 mg Mg)

**Maginex DS** powder for oral liquid (discontinued 2004) OTC *magnesium supplement* [magnesium-L-aspartate HCl] 1230 mg (122 mg Mg)/pkt.

**Magnacal** ready-to-use oral liquid OTC *enteral nutritional therapy* [lactose-free formula]

**Magnalox** oral liquid (discontinued 2000) OTC *antacid* [aluminum hydroxide; magnesium hydroxide] 225•220 mg/5 mL

**Magnaprin; Magnaprin Arthritis Strength Captabs** film-coated tablets OTC *analgesic; antipyretic; anti-inflammatory; antirheumatic* [aspirin (buffered with aluminum hydroxide, magnesium hydroxide, and calcium carbonate)] 325 mg

**MagneBind 200; MagneBind 300** tablets OTC *calcium/magnesium supplement that binds dietary phosphate* [magnesium carbonate; calcium carbonate] 200•400 mg; 300•250 mg

**MagneBind 400 Rx** tablets ℞ *calcium/magnesium supplement that binds dietary phosphate* [magnesium carbonate; calcium carbonate; folic acid] 400•200•1 mg

**magnesia, milk of** USP *antacid; saline laxative* [also: magnesium hydroxide] 400 mg/5 mL oral

**magnesia magma** [now: magnesia, milk of]

**magnesium** *element* (Mg)

**magnesium aluminosilicate hydrate** [see: almasilate]

**magnesium aluminum silicate** NF *suspending agent*

**magnesium amino acid chelate** *dietary magnesium supplement*

**magnesium aspartate** [see: potassium aspartate & magnesium aspartate]

**magnesium carbonate** USP *antacid; dietary magnesium supplement*

**magnesium carbonate hydrate** [see: magnesium carbonate]

**magnesium chloride** USP *electrolyte replenisher* 1.97 mEq/mL (20%) injection

**magnesium chloride hexahydrate** [see: magnesium chloride]

**magnesium citrate** USP *dietary magnesium supplement; saline laxative* 100 mg Mg oral; 1.75 g/30 mL oral

**magnesium clofibrate** INN

**magnesium D-gluconate dihydrate** [see: magnesium gluconate]

**magnesium D-gluconate hydrate** [see: magnesium gluconate]

**magnesium EDTA (ethylene diamine tetraacetic acid)** [see: edetate magnesium disodium]

**magnesium gluconate** USP *dietary magnesium supplement* 12.7 mg Mg oral

**magnesium glycinate** USAN

**magnesium hydroxide** USP *antacid; saline laxative* [also: magnesia, milk of]

**magnesium hydroxycarbonate** *antiurolithic*

**magnesium oxide** USP *antacid; sorbent; magnesium supplement* 400 mg oral

**magnesium phosphate** USP *antacid*

**magnesium phosphate pentahydrate** [see: magnesium phosphate]

**magnesium salicylate** USP *analgesic; antipyretic; anti-inflammatory; antirheumatic*

**magnesium salicylate tetrahydrate** [see: magnesium salicylate]

**magnesium silicate** NF *tablet excipient*

**magnesium silicate hydrate** [see: magnesium trisilicate]

**magnesium stearate** NF *tablet and capsule lubricant*

**magnesium sulfate** USP, JAN *anticonvulsant; saline laxative; electrolyte replenisher* 4%, 8%, 12.5%, 50% (0.325, 0.65, 1, 4 mEq/mL) injection

**magnesium sulfate heptahydrate** [see: magnesium sulfate]

**magnesium trisilicate** USP *antacid*

**magnesium-L-aspartate HCl** *dietary magnesium supplement*

**Magnevist** IV injection, prefilled syringes ℞ *MRI contrast medium* [gadopentetate dimeglumine] 469 mg/mL

**magnolia (*Magnolia glauca*)** bark *medicinal herb used as an antiperiodic, aromatic, astringent, diaphoretic, febrifuge, stimulant, and tonic*

**Magnox** oral suspension OTC *antacid* [aluminum hydroxide; magnesium hydroxide] 225•200 mg/5 mL

**Magonate** tablets, oral liquid OTC *magnesium supplement* [magnesium gluconate dihydrate] 500 mg (27 mg Mg); 1 g (54 mg Mg)/5 mL

**Magonate Natal** oral drops OTC *pediatric magnesium supplement* [magnesium gluconate] 3.52 mg Mg/mL

**Mag-Ox 400** tablets OTC *antacid; magnesium supplement* [magnesium oxide] 400 mg (241 mg Mg)

**Magsal** tablets ℞ *analgesic; antipyretic; anti-inflammatory; antihistaminic sleep aid* [magnesium salicylate; phenyltoloxamine citrate] 600•25 mg

**Mag-Tab SR** sustained-release caplets OTC *magnesium supplement* [magnesium lactate dihydrate] 84 mg Mg

**Magtrate** tablets OTC *magnesium supplement* [magnesium gluconate] 500 mg (29 mg Mg)

**mahogany birch; mountain mahogany** *medicinal herb* [see: birch]

**Mahonia aquifolium** *medicinal herb* [see: Oregon grape]

**ma-huang** *medicinal herb* [see: ephedra]

**MAID (mesna [rescue], Adriamycin, ifosfamide, dacarbazine)** *chemotherapy protocol for soft tissue and bone sarcomas*

**maitake mushrooms** (*Grifola fron-dosa*) cap and stem *medicinal herb for cancer, diabetes, hypercholesterolemia, hypertension, obesity, and stimulation of the immune system*

**maitansine** INN *antineoplastic* [also: maytansine]

**Maitec** injection ℞ *investigational (orphan) agent for disseminated* Myco-bacterium avium-*intracellulare infection* [gentamicin sulfate, liposomal]

*Majorana hortensis medicinal herb* [see: marjoram]

**Major-Con** chewable tablets OTC *anti-flatulent* [simethicone] 80 mg

**Major-gesic** tablets OTC *antihistamine; analgesic* [phenyltoloxamine citrate; acetaminophen] 30•325 mg

**malaleuca** *medicinal herb* [see: tea tree oil]

**Malarone; Malarone Pediatric** film-coated tablets ℞ *malaria prophylaxis and treatment* [atovaquone; proguanil HCl (chloroguanide HCl)] 250•100 mg; 62.5•25 mg

**malathion** USP, BAN *pediculicide for lice*

**maletamer** INN *antiperistaltic* [also: malethamer]

**malethamer** USAN *antiperistaltic* [also: maletamer]

**maleylsulfathiazole** INN

**malic acid** NF *acidifying agent*

**malidone** [see: aloxidone]

**Mallamint** chewable tablets OTC *ant-acid* [calcium carbonate] 420 mg

**Mallazine** eye drops OTC *topical oph-thalmic decongestant and vasoconstric-tor* [tetrahydrozoline HCl] 0.05%

**mallow** (*Malva rotundifolia; M. syl-vestris*) plant *medicinal herb used as an astringent, demulcent, emollient, and expectorant*

**mallow, marsh** (*Althaea officinalis*) *medicinal herb* [see: marsh mallow]

**malonal** [see: barbital]

**malotilate** USAN, INN *liver disorder treatment*

*Malpighia glabra; M. punicifolia medicinal herb* [see: acerola]

**Maltsupex** coated tablets, powder, oral liquid OTC *bulk laxative* [barley malt soup extract] 750 mg; 8 g/scoop; 16 g/tbsp.

*Malva rotundifolia; M. sylvestris medicinal herb* [see: mallow]

**Mammol** ointment OTC *emollient for nipples of nursing mothers* [bismuth subnitrate] 40%

*m*-**AMSA (acridinylamine methane-sulphon anisidide)** [see: amsacrine]

**Mandameth** enteric-coated tablets ℞ *urinary antibiotic* [methenamine man-delate] 0.5, 1 g

**Mandelamine** film-coated tablets ℞ *urinary antibiotic* [methenamine man-delate] 0.5, 1 g

**mandelic acid** NF

**Mandol** powder for IV or IM injection (discontinued 2003) ℞ *cephalosporin antibiotic* [cefamandole nafate] 1 g ⚕ nadolol

**mandrake** (*Mandragora officinarium; Podophyllum peltatum*) root and resin *medicinal herb for cancer, condy-lomata, constipation, fever, indigestion, liver disorders, lower bowel disorders, warts, and worms; not generally regarded as safe and effective for chil-dren or pregnant women*

**Manerex** ⒸⒶⓃ film-coated tablets ℞ *antidepressant; MAO inhibitor* [moclo-bemide] 100, 150 mg

**mangafodipir trisodium** USAN *para-magnetic contrast agent for MRI of the liver*

**manganese** *element* (Mn)

**manganese chloride** USP *dietary man-ganese supplement* 0.1 mg/mL injection

**manganese chloride tetrahydrate** [see: manganese chloride]

**manganese citrate** *dietary manganese supplement* (30% elemental manganese)

**manganese gluconate (manganese D-gluconate)** USP *dietary manganese supplement*

**manganese glycerophosphate** NF

**manganese hypophosphite** NF

**manganese phosphinate** [see: man-ganese hypophosphite]

**manganese sulfate** USP *dietary manganese supplement* 0.1 mg/mL injection

**manganese sulfate monohydrate** [see: manganese sulfate]

**mangofodipir trisodium** *MRI contrast medium for liver imaging*

**manidipine 6300** INN

**manna sugar** [see: mannitol]

**mannite** [see: mannitol]

**mannitol (D-mannitol)** USP *renal function test aid; antihypertensive; osmotic diuretic; urologic irrigant* 10%, 15%, 20%, 25% injection

**mannitol hexanitrate** INN

**mannityl nitrate** [see: mannitol hexanitrate]

**D-mannoheptulose** *the active principle in avocado that suppresses excess insulin production by the pancreas; investigational treatment for obesity and type 2 diabetes* [also: avocado sugar extract]

**mannomustine** INN, BAN

**mannosulfan** INN

**manozodil** INN

**Mantoux test** [see: tuberculin]

**MAO inhibitors (monoamine oxidase inhibitors)** [q.v.]

**Maolate** tablets ℞ *skeletal muscle relaxant* [chlorphenesin carbamate] 400 mg

**Maox 420** tablets OTC *antacid* [magnesium oxide] 420 mg

**MAP (mitomycin, Adriamycin, Platinol)** *chemotherapy protocol*

**Mapap** tablets OTC *analgesic; antipyretic* [acetaminophen] 325, 500 mg

**Mapap, Children's** oral liquid OTC *analgesic; antipyretic* [acetaminophen] 160 mg/5 mL

**Mapap Cold Formula** tablets OTC *antitussive; decongestant; antihistamine; analgesic* [dextromethorphan hydrobromide; pseudoephedrine HCl; chlorpheniramine maleate; acetaminophen] 15•30•2•325 mg

**Mapap Infant Drops** OTC *analgesic; antipyretic* [acetaminophen] 100 mg/mL

**Mapap Sinus** geltabs OTC *decongestant; analgesic; antipyretic* [pseudo-

ephedrine HCl; acetaminophen] 30•500 mg

**maple lungwort** *medicinal herb* [see: lungwort]

**maprotiline** USAN, INN *tetracyclic antidepressant*

**maprotiline HCl** USP *tetracyclic antidepressant* 25, 50, 75 mg oral

**Maranox** tablets OTC *analgesic; antipyretic* [acetaminophen] 325 mg

**Marax** tablets ℞ *antiasthmatic; bronchodilator; decongestant* [theophylline; ephedrine sulfate] 130•25 mg ⊘ Atarax; Maalox

**Marax-DF** pediatric syrup ℞ *antiasthmatic; bronchodilator; decongestant; antihistamine* [theophylline; ephedrine sulfate; hydroxyzine HCl] 97.5•18.75•7.5 mg/15 mL

**Marblen** tablets, oral liquid OTC *antacid* [calcium carbonate; magnesium carbonate] 520•400 mg; 540•400 mg/5 mL

**Marcaine HCl** injection ℞ *injectable local anesthetic* [bupivacaine HCl] 0.25%, 0.5%, 0.75%

**Marcaine HCl** injection ℞ *injectable local anesthetic* [bupivacaine HCl; epinephrine bitartrate] 0.25%•1:200 000, 0.5%•1:200 000, 0.75%•1:200 000 ⊘ Narcan

**Marcaine Spinal** injection (discontinued 2002) ℞ *injectable local anesthetic* [bupivacaine HCl] 0.75%

**Marcillin** capsules (discontinued 2002) ℞ *aminopenicillin antibiotic* [ampicillin] 500 mg

**Marcof Expectorant** syrup ℞ *narcotic antitussive; expectorant* [hydrocodone bitartrate; potassium guaiacolsulfonate] 5•300 mg/5 mL

**mare's tail** *medicinal herb* [see: fleabane; horseweed]

**Marezine** tablets OTC *antiemetic; anticholinergic; antihistamine; motion sickness preventative* [cyclizine HCl] 50 mg

**Margesic** capsules ℞ *analgesic; barbiturate sedative* [acetaminophen; caffeine; butalbital] 325•40•50 mg

**Margesic H** capsules ℞ *narcotic analgesic* [hydrocodone bitartrate; acetaminophen] 5•500 mg

**maribavir** USAN *antiviral for cytomegalovirus infections*

**maridomycin** INN

**marigold (Calendula officinalis)** *florets medicinal herb for bruises, cuts, dysmenorrhea, eye infections, fever, and skin diseases; not generally regarded as safe and effective*

**marijuana** ⒸⒶⓃ *approved for compassionate use in terminally ill patients*

**marijuana; marihuana (Cannabis sativa)** *euphoric/hallucinogenic street drug made from the dried leaves and flowering tops of the cannabis plant; medicinal herb for asthma, analgesia, leprosy, and loss of appetite; investigational for HIV*

**marimastat** USAN *investigational (Phase III) antineoplastic; matrix metalloproteinase (MMP) inhibitor*

**Marine Lipid Concentrate** softgels OTC *dietary supplement* [omega-3 fatty acids] 1200 mg

**Marinol** oil-filled gelcaps ℞ *antiemetic for chemotherapy; appetite stimulant for AIDS patients (orphan)* [dronabinol] 2.5, 5, 10 mg

**mariptiline** INN

**marjoram (Majorana hortensis; Origanum vulgare)** plant *medicinal herb for abdominal cramps, colic, headache, indigestion, respiratory problems, and violent cough*

**Marlin Salt System** tablets OTC *rinsing/storage solution for soft contact lenses* [sodium chloride (normal saline solution)] 250 mg

**Marlin Salt System II** tablets OTC *rinsing/storage solution for soft contact lenses* [sodium chloride (normal saline solution)] 250 mg

**Marmine** IV or IM injection ℞ *antinauseant; antiemetic; antivertigo; motion sickness preventative* [dimenhydrinate] 50 mg/mL

**Marmine** tablets OTC *antinauseant; antiemetic; antivertigo; motion sickness preventative* [dimenhydrinate] 50 mg

**Marnatal-F** film-coated tablets ℞ *vitamin/mineral/calcium/iron supplement* [multiple vitamins & minerals; calcium; iron; folic acid] ≛•250•60•1 mg

**Marogen** ℞ *investigational (orphan) hematinic for anemia of end-stage renal disease* [epoetin beta]

**maroxepin** INN

**Marplan** tablets ℞ *antidepressant; monoamine oxidase (MAO) inhibitor* [isocarboxazid] 10 mg

**Marpres** tablets ℞ *antihypertensive; vasodilator; diuretic* [hydrochlorothiazide; reserpine; hydralazine HCl] 15•0.1•25 mg

**Marrubium vulgare** *medicinal herb* [see: horehound]

**marsh clover; marsh trefoil** *medicinal herb* [see: buckbean]

**marsh mallow (Althaea officinalis)** root *medicinal herb for asthma, boils, bronchial infections, cough, emphysema, infected wounds, kidney disorders, lung congestion, sore throat, and urinary bleeding*

**MARstem** ℞ *investigational (orphan) agent for myelodysplastic syndrome and neutropenia due to bone marrow transplantation* [angiotensin 1-7]

**MART-1 adenoviral gene therapy** *investigational (orphan) for metastatic malignant melanoma*

**Marten-Tab** caplets ℞ *analgesic; barbiturate sedative* [acetaminophen; butalbital] 325•50 mg

**Marthritic** tablets ℞ *analgesic; antipyretic; anti-inflammatory; antirheumatic* [salsalate] 750 mg

**Marvelon** ⒸⒶⓃ tablets (in packs of 21 or 28) ℞ *monophasic oral contraceptive* [desogestrel; ethinyl estradiol] 0.15 mg•30 μg

**masoprocol** USAN, INN *antineoplastic for actinic keratoses (AK)*

**Massé Breast** cream OTC *moisturizer and emollient for nipples of nursing women*

**Massengill Baking Soda Freshness**
solution OTC *vaginal cleanser and deodorizer; acidity modifier* [sodium bicarbonate]

**Massengill Disposable Douche** solution OTC *antiseptic/germicidal; vaginal cleanser and deodorizer; acidity modifier* [cetylpyridinium chloride; lactic acid; sodium lactate]

**Massengill Disposable Douche; Massengill Vinegar & Water Extra Mild** solution OTC *vaginal cleanser and deodorizer; acidity modifier* [vinegar (acetic acid)]

**Massengill Douche** powder OTC *astringent; analgesic; counterirritant; vaginal cleanser and deodorizer* [ammonium alum; phenol; methyl salicylate; menthol; thymol]

**Massengill Douche** solution concentrate OTC *vaginal cleanser and deodorizer; acidity modifier* [lactic acid; sodium lactate; sodium bicarbonate]

**Massengill Feminine Cleansing Wash** topical liquid OTC *for external perivaginal cleansing*

**Massengill Medicated** towelettes OTC *topical corticosteroidal anti-inflammatory* [hydrocortisone] 0.5%

**Massengill Medicated Douche with Cepticin; Massengill Medicated Disposable Douche with Cepticin** solution OTC *antiseptic/germicidal; vaginal cleanser and deodorizer* [povidone-iodine] 12%; 10%

**Massengill Vinegar & Water Extra Cleansing with Puraclean** solution OTC *antiseptic/germicidal; vaginal cleanser and deodorizer; acidity modifier* [cetylpyridinium chloride; vinegar (acetic acid)]

**mast cell stabilizers** *a class of topical agents that inhibit the antigen-induced release of inflammatory mediators (e.g., various histamines and leukotrienes) from human mast cells; used on nasal, ophthalmological, and gastrointestinal mucosa* [also known as: mediator release inhibitors]

**masterwort** *(Heracleum lanatum)* root and seed *medicinal herb used as an antispasmodic, carminative, and stimulant*

**Mastisol** topical liquid OTC *adhesive for securing dressings, IV lines, etc. on the skin*

**maté** *medicinal herb* [see: yerba maté]

**Matricaria chamomilla** *medicinal herb* [see: chamomile]

**matrix metalloproteinase (MMP) inhibitors** *a class of investigational (Phase III) antineoplastics and investigational (orphan) agents to treat corneal ulcers*

**Matulane** capsules ℞ *antineoplastic for Hodgkin disease; investigational for other lymphomas, melanoma, brain tumors, and lung cancer* [procarbazine HCl] 50 mg

**Mavik** Ⓒᴬᴺ capsules ℞ *antihypertensive; angiotensin-converting enzyme (ACE) inhibitor* [trandolapril] 0.5, 1, 2 mg

**Mavik** tablets ℞ *antihypertensive; angiotensin-converting enzyme (ACE) inhibitor; treatment for CHF* [trandolapril] 1, 2, 4 mg

**maxacalcitol** USAN *investigational vitamin $D_3$ analogue for the topical treatment of psoriasis*

**Maxair** Autohaler (breath-activated metered-dose inhaler) ℞ *sympathomimetic bronchodilator* [pirbuterol acetate] 0.2 mg/dose

**Maxalt** caplets ℞ *vascular serotonin 5-$HT_{1B/1D}$ receptor agonist for the acute treatment of migraine* [rizatriptan benzoate] 5, 10 mg

**Maxalt-MLT** orally disintegrating tablets ℞ *vascular serotonin 5-$HT_{1B/1D}$ receptor agonist for the acute treatment of migraine* [rizatriptan benzoate] 5, 10 mg

**Maxalt-RPD** Ⓒᴬᴺ orally disintegrating tablets ℞ *vascular serotonin 5-$HT_{1B/1D}$ receptor agonist for the acute treatment of migraine* [rizatriptan benzoate] 5, 10 mg

**Maxamine** ℞ *investigational (NDA filed, orphan) adjuvant to interleukin-2 for*

stage IV malignant melanoma and acute myelogenous leukemia; investigational (Phase II) adjunct to interferon alfa-2b for chronic hepatitis C [aldesleukin]

**Maxaquin** film-coated tablets ℞ *broad-spectrum fluoroquinolone antibiotic* [lomefloxacin HCl] 400 mg

**MaxEPA** soft capsules OTC *dietary supplement* [omega-3 fatty acids; multiple vitamins & minerals] 1000• ≐ mg

**Maxibolin** *an anabolic steroid abused as a street drug* [see: ethylestrenol]

**Maxicam** ℞ *investigational (NDA filed) nonsteroidal anti-inflammatory drug (NSAID); antiarthritic; analgesic; antipyretic* [isoxicam]

**Maxidex** Drop-Tainers (eye drop suspension) ℞ *topical ophthalmic corticosteroidal anti-inflammatory* [dexamethasone] 0.1%

**Maxidone** caplets ℞ *narcotic analgesic* [hydrocodone bitartrate; acetaminophen] 10•750 mg

**Maxifed** caplets ℞ *decongestant; expectorant* [pseudoephedrine HCl; guaifenesin] 80•700 mg

**Maxifed DM; Maxifed DMX** sustained-release caplets OTC *antitussive; decongestant; expectorant* [dextromethorphan hydrobromide; pseudoephedrine HCl; guaifenesin] 30•60•580 mg; 40•80•700 mg

**Maxifed-G** sustained-release caplets OTC *decongestant; expectorant* [pseudoephedrine HCl; guaifenesin] 60•580 mg

**Maxiflor** cream, ointment ℞ *corticosteroidal anti-inflammatory* [diflorasone diacetate] 0.05%

**Maxilube** jelly OTC *vaginal lubricant*

**Maximum Blue Label; Maximum Green Label** tablets OTC *vitamin/mineral supplement* [multiple vitamins & minerals; folic acid; biotin] ≐•130•50 μg

**Maximum Red Label** tablets OTC *vitamin/mineral/iron supplement* [multiple vitamins & minerals; iron; folic acid; biotin] ≐•3.3 mg•0.13 mg•50 μg

**"Maximum Strength"** products [see under product name]

**Maxiphen DM** extended-release caplets ℞ *antitussive; decongestant; expectorant* [dextromethorphan hydrobromide; phenylephrine HCl; guaifenesin] 60•40•1000 mg

**Maxipime** powder for IV or IM injection ℞ *cephalosporin antibiotic* [cefepime HCl] 0.5, 1, 2 g

**Maxitrol** eye drop suspension, ophthalmic ointment ℞ *topical ophthalmic corticosteroidal anti-inflammatory; antibiotic* [dexamethasone; neomycin sulfate; polymyxin B sulfate] 0.1%•0.35%•10 000 U/mL; 0.1%•0.35%•10 000 U/g

**Maxi-Tuss DM** oral liquid ℞ *antitussive; expectorant* [dextromethorphan hydrobromide; guaifenesin] 20•200 mg/5 mL

**Maxi-Tuss HC; Maxi-Tuss HCX** oral liquid ℞ *narcotic antitussive; decongestant; antihistamine* [hydrocodone bitartrate; phenylephrine HCl; chlorpheniramine maleate] 2.5•10•4 mg/5 mL; 6•12•2 mg/5 mL

**Maxi-Tuss HCG** oral liquid ℞ *narcotic antitussive; expectorant* [hydrocodone bitartrate; guaifenesin] 6•200 mg/5 mL

**Maxivate** lotion (discontinued 2004) ℞ *corticosteroidal anti-inflammatory* [betamethasone dipropionate] 0.05%

**Maxivate** ointment, cream ℞ *corticosteroidal anti-inflammatory* [betamethasone dipropionate] 0.05%

**Maxi-Vite** tablets OTC *vitamin/mineral/calcium/iron supplement* [multiple vitamins & minerals; calcium; iron; folic acid; biotin] ≐•53.5•1.5•0.4•0.001 mg

**Maxolon** tablets ℞ *antidopaminergic; antiemetic for chemotherapy; peristaltic* [metoclopramide HCl] 10 mg

**Maxovite** sustained-release tablets OTC *vitamin/mineral supplement* [multiple vitamins & minerals; folic acid; biotin] ≐•330•11.7 μg

**Maxzide** tablets ℞ *antihypertensive; diuretic* [triamterene; hydrochlorothiazide] 37.5•25, 75•50 mg ⑦ Microzide

**May apple** *medicinal herb* [see: mandrake]

**May bells; May lily** *medicinal herb* [see: lily of the valley]

**May bush; May tree** *medicinal herb* [see: hawthorn]

**May lily** *medicinal herb* [see: lily of the valley]

**maytansine** USAN *antineoplastic* [also: maitansine]

**May-Vita** elixir (discontinued 2003) ℞ *vitamin supplement* [multiple B vitamins; folic acid] ≛•0.1 mg

**Mazanor** tablets (discontinued 2001) ℞ *anorexiant; CNS stimulant* [mazindol] 1 mg

**mazapertine succinate** USAN *antipsychotic; dopamine receptor antagonist*

**mazaticol** INN

**MAZE (m-AMSA, azacitidine, etoposide)** *chemotherapy protocol*

**mazindol** USAN, USP, INN, BAN *anorexiant; CNS stimulant; investigational (orphan) treatment for Duchenne muscular dystrophy* ⑦ mebendazole

**mazipredone** INN

**MB (methylene blue)** [q.v.]

**m-BACOD; M-BACOD (methotrexate, bleomycin, Adriamycin, cyclophosphamide, Oncovin, dexamethasone)** *chemotherapy protocol for non-Hodgkin lymphoma* ("m" is 200 mg/m²; "M" is 3 g/m²)

**m-BACOD reduced dose (methotrexate, bleomycin, Adriamycin, cyclophosphamide, Oncovin, dexamethasone)** *chemotherapy protocol for HIV-associated non-Hodgkin lymphoma*

**M-BACOS (methotrexate, bleomycin, Adriamycin, cyclophosphamide, Oncovin, Solu-Medrol)** *chemotherapy protocol*

**MBC (methotrexate, bleomycin, cisplatin)** *chemotherapy protocol for head and neck cancer*

**MBD (methotrexate, bleomycin, DDP)** *chemotherapy protocol*

**MBR (methylene blue, reduced)** [see: methylene blue]

**MC (mitoxantrone, cytarabine)** *chemotherapy protocol for acute myelocytic leukemia (AML)*

**M-Caps** capsules ℞ *urinary acidifier to control ammonia production* [racemethionine] 200 mg

**MCBP (melphalan, cyclophosphamide, BCNU, prednisone)** *chemotherapy protocol*

**MCC (mycobacterial cell wall complex)** [see: urocidin]

**MCH (microfibrillar collagen hemostat)** [q.v.]

**MCK-442** *investigational (Phase III) non-nucleoside reverse transcriptase inhibitor (NNRTI) for AIDS*

**MCP (melphalan, cyclophosphamide, prednisone)** *chemotherapy protocol*

**M-CSF (macrophage colony-stimulating factor)** [now: cilmostim]

**MCT** oil OTC *dietary fat supplement* [medium chain triglycerides from coconut oil]

**MCT (medium chain triglycerides)** [q.v.]

**MCV (methotrexate, cisplatin, vinblastine)** *chemotherapy protocol*

**MD-76 R** injection ℞ *radiopaque contrast medium* [diatrizoate meglumine; diatrizoate sodium (48.7% total iodine)] 660•100 mg/mL (370 mg/mL)

**MDA (methylenedioxyamphetamine)** [see: MDMA, MDEA]

**MDEA (3,4-methylenedioxyethamphetamine)** *a hallucinogenic amphetamine derivative closely related to MDMA, abused as a street drug, which causes dependence* [also see: amphetamines; MDMA]

**MD-Gastroview** oral solution ℞ *radiopaque contrast medium for gastrointestinal imaging* [diatrizoate meglumine; diatrizoate sodium (48.29%

total iodine)] 660•100 mg/mL (367 mg/mL)

**MDI** (dosage form) *metered-dose inhaler*

**MDMA (3,4-methylenedioxymeth- amphetamine)** *widely abused hallu- cinogenic street drug that is chemically related to amphetamines and mescaline and causes dependence* [see also: amphetamines; mescaline; MDEA]

**MDP (methylene diphosphonate)** [now: medronate disodium]

**MDX-240** *investigational (Phase II) virus-specific antibody for AIDS*

**MDX-447** *investigational (Phase I/II) anticancer antibody*

**MEA (mercaptoethylamine)** [see: mercaptamine]

**meadow cabbage** *medicinal herb* [see: skunk cabbage]

**meadow sorrel** *medicinal herb* [see: sorrel]

**meadowsweet (Filipendula ulmaria)** plant *medicinal herb used for ulcers and upper respiratory problems; also used as an astringent, diaphoretic, and diuretic*

**mealberry** *medicinal herb* [see: uva ursi]

**mealy starwort** *medicinal herb* [see: star grass]

**measles, mumps & rubella virus vaccine, live** USP *active immunizing agent for measles (rubeola), mumps and rubella*

**measles immune globulin** USP

**measles & rubella virus vaccine, live** USP *active immunizing agent for measles (rubeola) and rubella*

**measles virus vaccine, live** USP *active immunizing agent for measles (rubeola)*

**Mebadin** (available only from the Cen- ters for Disease Control) ℞ *investiga- tional anti-infective for amebiasis and amebic dysentery* [dehydroemetine]

**meballymal** [see: secobarbital]

**mebamoxine** [see: benmoxin]

**mebanazine** INN, BAN

**Mebaral** tablets ℞ *long-acting barbitur- ate sedative, hypnotic and anticonvul- sant* [mephobarbital] 32, 50, 100 mg ⊡ Medrol

**mebendazole** USAN, USP, INN *anthel- mintic for trichuriasis, enterobiasis, ascariasis, and uncinariasis* 100 mg oral ⊡ mazindol

**mebenoside** INN

**mebeverine** INN *smooth muscle relax- ant* [also: mebeverine HCl]

**mebeverine HCl** USAN *smooth muscle relaxant* [also: mebeverine]

**mebezonium iodide** INN, BAN

**mebhydrolin** INN, BAN

**mebiquine** INN

**mebolazine** INN

**mebrofenin** USAN, INN *hepatobiliary function test*

**mebrophenhydramine HCl** [see: embramine HCl]

**mebubarbital** [see: pentobarbital]

**mebumal** [see: pentobarbital]

**mebutamate** USAN, INN *antihypertensive*

**mebutizide** INN

**mecamylamine** INN *antiadrenergic; ganglionic blocker for severe hyperten- sion* [also: mecamylamine HCl]

**mecamylamine HCl** USP *antiadrener- gic; ganglionic blocker for severe hyper- tension* [also: mecamylamine]

**mecamylamine HCl & nicotine** *investigational (Phase III) transdermal patch for smoking cessation*

**mecarbinate** INN

**mecarbine** [see: mecarbinate]

**mecasermin** USAN, INN, BAN *investiga- tional (NDA filed, orphan) for amyo- trophic lateral sclerosis, type 1 and type 2 diabetes, growth hormone insuffi- ciency, and post-poliomyelitis syndrome* [previously known as insulin-like growth factor 1 (IGF-1)]

**MeCCNU (methyl chloroethyl- cyclohexyl-nitrosourea)** [see: semustine]

**mecetronium ethylsulfate** USAN *anti- septic* [also: mecetronium etilsulfate]

**mecetronium etilsulfate** INN *antisep- tic* [also: mecetronium ethylsulfate]

**mechlorethamine HCl** USP *nitrogen mustard-type alkylating antineoplastic* [also: chlormethine; mustine; nitro- gen mustard N-oxide HCl]

**meciadanol** INN

**mecillinam** INN, BAN *antibacterial* [also: amdinocillin]

**mecinarone** INN

**Meclan** cream (discontinued 2003) ℞ *antibiotic for acne* [meclocycline sulfosalicylate] 1% ② Meclomen; Mezlin

**meclizine HCl** USP *antiemetic; antihistamine; anticholinergic; motion sickness relief* [also: meclozine] 12.5, 25, 50 mg oral ② mescaline

**meclocycline** USAN, INN, BAN *topical antibiotic*

**meclocycline sulfosalicylate** USAN, USP *topical antibiotic*

**meclofenamate sodium** USAN, USP *analgesic; antiarthritic; nonsteroidal anti-inflammatory drug (NSAID)* 50, 100 mg oral

**meclofenamic acid** USAN, INN *nonsteroidal anti-inflammatory drug (NSAID)*

**meclofenoxate** INN, BAN

**meclonazepam** INN

**mecloqualone** USAN, INN *sedative; hypnotic*

**mecloralurea** INN

**meclorisone** INN, BAN *topical anti-inflammatory* [also: meclorisone dibutyrate]

**meclorisone dibutyrate** USAN *topical anti-inflammatory* [also: meclorisone]

**mecloxamine** INN

**meclozine** INN, BAN *antiemetic; antihistamine; anticholinergic; motion sickness relief* [also: meclizine HCl] ② mescaline

**mecobalamin** USAN, INN *vitamin; hematopoietic*

**mecrilate** INN *tissue adhesive* [also: mecrylate]

**mecrylate** USAN *tissue adhesive* [also: mecrilate]

**MECY (methotrexate, cyclophosphamide)** *chemotherapy protocol*

**mecysteine** INN

**Meda Cap** capsules OTC *analgesic; antipyretic* [acetaminophen] 500 mg

**Meda Tab** tablets OTC *analgesic; antipyretic* [acetaminophen] 325 mg

**Medacote** lotion OTC *topical antihistamine; astringent; antipruritic* [pyrilamine maleate; zinc oxide] 1% • ²

**Medalone 40; Medalone 80** [see: depMedalone 40; depMedalone 80]

**medazepam** INN *minor tranquilizer* [also: medazepam HCl]

**medazepam HCl** USAN *minor tranquilizer* [also: medazepam]

**medazomide** INN

**medazonamide** [see: medazomide]

**Medebar Plus** rectal suspension ℞ *radiopaque contrast medium for gastrointestinal imaging* [barium sulfate] 100%

**Medent-DM** sustained-release tablets ℞ *antitussive; decongestant; expectorant* [dextromethorphan hydrobromide; pseudoephedrine HCl; guaifenesin] 30 • 60 • 800 mg

**Mederma** gel OTC *moisturizer and emollient for scars* [PEG-4; onion extract; xanthan gum; allantoin]

**Medescan** oral suspension ℞ *radiopaque contrast medium for gastrointestinal imaging* [barium sulfate] 2.3%

**medetomidine** INN, BAN *veterinary analgesic; veterinary sedative* [also: medetomidine HCl]

**medetomidine HCl** USAN *veterinary analgesic; veterinary sedative* [also: medetomidine]

**mediator release inhibitors** *a class of topical agents that inhibit the antigen-induced release of inflammatory mediators (e.g., various histamines and leukotrienes) from human mast cells; used on nasal, ophthalmological, and gastrointestinal mucosa* [also known as: mast cell stabilizers]

**medibazine** INN

**Medicago sativa** *medicinal herb* [see: alfalfa]

**medical air** [see: air, medical]

**Medicated Acne Cleanser** OTC *topical acne treatment* [colloidal sulfur; resorcinol] 4% • 2%

**medicinal zinc peroxide** [see: zinc peroxide, medicinal]

**Medicone** anorectal ointment OTC *topical local anesthetic* [benzocaine] 20%

**Medicone** rectal suppositories (discontinued 2004) OTC *topical vasoconstrictor for hemorrhoids* [phenylephrine HCl] 0.25%

**Medi-First Sinus Decongestant** tablets OTC *nasal decongestant* [pseudoephedrine HCl] 30 mg

**medifoxamine** INN

**Medigesic** capsules ℞ *analgesic; barbiturate sedative* [acetaminophen; caffeine; butalbital] 325•40•50 mg

**Medihaler-Iso** inhalation aerosol (discontinued 2001) ℞ *sympathomimetic bronchodilator* [isoproterenol sulfate] 80 μg/dose

**medinal** [see: barbital sodium]

**Mediplast** plaster OTC *keratolytic* [salicylic acid] 40%

**Mediplex** Tabules (tablets) OTC *vitamin/mineral supplement* [multiple vitamins & minerals]

**Mediplex Plus** tablets OTC *vitamin/mineral supplement* [multiple vitamins & minerals; folic acid] ≛•0.4 mg

**Medi-Quik** ointment (discontinued 2001) OTC *topical antibiotic* [polymyxin B sulfate; neomycin; bacitracin] 5000 U•3.5 mg•400 U per g

**Medi-Quik** spray OTC *topical local anesthetic; antiseptic* [lidocaine; benzalkonium chloride] 2%•0.13%

**medium chain triglycerides (MCT)** *dietary lipid supplement*

**medorinone** USAN, INN *cardiotonic*

**medorubicin** INN

**Medotar** ointment OTC *antipsoriatic; antiseborrheic; astringent; antiseptic* [coal tar; zinc oxide] 1%• ≛

**Medralone 40; Medralone 80** intralesional, soft tissue, and IM injection (discontinued 2002) ℞ *corticosteroid; anti-inflammatory; immunosuppressant* [methylprednisolone acetate] 40 mg/mL; 80 mg/mL

**medrogestone** USAN, INN, BAN *progestin*

**Medrol** tablets, Dosepak (unit of use package) ℞ *corticosteroid; anti-inflammatory; immunosuppressant* [methylprednisolone] 2, 4, 8, 16, 24, 32 mg
⧉ Mebaral

**medronate disodium** USAN *pharmaceutic aid*

**medronic acid** USAN, INN, BAN *pharmaceutic aid*

**medroxalol** USAN, INN, BAN *antihypertensive*

**medroxalol HCl** USAN *antihypertensive*

**medroxiprogesterone acetate** [see: medroxyprogesterone acetate]

**medroxyprogesterone** INN, BAN *synthetic progestin for secondary amenorrhea or abnormal uterine bleeding; hormonal antineoplastic* [also: medroxyprogesterone acetate]

**medroxyprogesterone acetate** USP *synthetic progestin for secondary amenorrhea, abnormal uterine bleeding, and endometrial hyperplasia; hormonal antineoplastic* [also: medroxyprogesterone] 2.5, 5, 10 mg oral; 150 mg/mL depot injection

**MED-Rx** controlled-release tablets (14-day, 56-tablet regimen) (discontinued 2002) ℞ *decongestant; expectorant* [pseudoephedrine HCl + guaifenesin (blue tablets); guaifenesin (white tablets)] 60•600 mg; 600 mg

**MED-Rx DM** controlled-release tablets (14-day, 56-tablet regimen) ℞ *decongestant + expectorant (AM); antitussive + expectorant (PM)* [pseudoephedrine HCl + guaifenesin (AM); dextromethorphan hydrobromide + guaifenesin (PM)] 60•600 mg; 30•600 mg

**medrylamine** INN

**medrysone** USAN, USP, INN *ophthalmic corticosteroidal anti-inflammatory*

**mefeclorazine** INN

**mefenamic acid** USAN, USP, INN, BAN *analgesic; nonsteroidal anti-inflammatory drug (NSAID)*

**mefenidil** USAN, INN *cerebral vasodilator*

**mefenidil fumarate** USAN *cerebral vasodilator*

**mefenidramium metilsulfate** INN

**mefenorex** INN *anorectic* [also: mefenorex HCl]

**mefenorex HCl** USAN *anorectic* [also: mefenorex]

**mefeserpine** INN

**mefexamide** USAN, INN *CNS stimulant*

**mefloquine** USAN, INN, BAN *antimalarial*

**mefloquine HCl** USAN *antimalarial for acute chloroquine-resistant malaria (orphan)* 250 mg oral

**Mefoxin** powder or frozen premix for IV or IM injection R *cephamycin antibiotic* [cefoxitin sodium] 1, 2, 10 g

**mefruside** USAN, INN *diuretic*

**Mega AO** Ⓐ tablets OTC *antioxidant/ vitamin supplement* [multiple vitamins; coenzyme Q10; folic acid; biotin] ≝•4•0.333•0.167 mg

**Mega VM-80** tablets OTC *geriatric vitamin/mineral supplement* [multiple vitamins & minerals; folic acid; biotin] ≝•400•80 μg

**Mega-B** tablets OTC *vitamin supplement* [multiple B vitamins; folic acid; biotin] ≝•100•100 μg

**Megace** oral suspension R *treatment for AIDS-related anorexia and cachexia (orphan)* [megestrol acetate] 40 mg/mL

**Megace** tablets R *hormonal antineoplastic for advanced carcinoma of the breast or endometrium* [megestrol acetate] 40 mg

**Megagen** R *investigational (orphan) adjunct to hematopoietic stem cell transplantation* [megakaryocyte growth and development factor, pegylated, recombinant human]

**megakaryocyte growth and development factor, pegylated, recombinant human** *investigational (orphan) adjunct to hematopoietic stem cell transplantation*

**megallate** INN *combining name for radicals or groups*

**megalomicin** INN *antibacterial* [also: megalomicin potassium phosphate]

**megalomicin potassium phosphate** USAN *antibacterial* [also: megalomicin]

**Megaton** elixir R *vitamin/mineral supplement* [multiple B vitamins & minerals; folic acid] ≝•0.1 mg

**megestrol** INN, BAN *hormonal antineoplastic for breast or endometrial cancer; investigational (Phase III) for liver cancer* [also: megestrol acetate]

**megestrol acetate** USAN, USP *hormonal antineoplastic for breast or endometrial cancer; therapy for AIDS-related anorexia and cachexia (orphan)* [also: megestrol] 20, 40 mg oral; 40 mg/mL oral

**meglitinide** INN

**meglucycline** INN

**meglumine** USP, INN *radiopaque contrast medium*

**meglumine diatrizoate** BAN *oral/ parenteral radiopaque contrast medium (46.67% iodine)* [also: diatrizoate meglumine]

**meglumine iocarmate** BAN *radiopaque contrast medium* [also: iocarmate meglumine]

**meglumine iothalamate** BAN *parenteral radiopaque contrast medium (47% iodine)* [also: iothalamate meglumine]

**meglumine ioxaglate** BAN *radiopaque contrast medium* [also: ioxaglate meglumine]

**meglutol** USAN, INN *antihyperlipoproteinemic*

**mel B** [see: melarsoprol]

**mel W** [see: melarsonyl potassium]

**Melacine** R *investigational (NDA filed, orphan) theraccine for invasive stage III–IV melanoma; investigational (Phase III) for early-stage melanoma* [melanoma vaccine]

**meladrazine** INN, BAN

**melafocon A** USAN *hydrophobic contact lens material*

**melagatran** *parenteral anticoagulant and direct thrombin inhibitor*

***Melaleuca alternifolia*** *medicinal herb* [see: tea tree oil]

**Melanex** solution (discontinued 2003) R *hyperpigmentation bleaching agent* [hydroquinone] 3%

**melanoma vaccine** *investigational (NDA filed, orphan) therapeutic vaccine for invasive stage III–IV melanoma; investigational (Phase III) for early-stage melanoma*

**melarsonyl potassium** INN, BAN

**melarsoprol** INN, BAN, DCF *investigational anti-infective for trypanosomiasis*

**melatonin** *natural sleep aid; investigational (orphan) for circadian rhythm sleep disorders in blind people with no light perception*

**melengestrol** INN *antineoplastic; progestin* [also: melengestrol acetate]

**melengestrol acetate** USAN *antineoplastic; progestin* [also: melengestrol]

**meletimide** INN

**melfalan** [see: melphalan]

**Melfiat-105** Unicelles (sustained-release capsules) ℞ *anorexiant; CNS stimulant* [phendimetrazine tartrate] 105 mg

*Melia azedarach* *medicinal herb* [see: pride of China]

**melilot (*Melilotus alba; M. officinalis*)** *flowering plant medicinal herb used as an antispasmodic, diuretic, emollient, expectorant, and vulnerary*

**Melimmune** *investigational (orphan) for non-Hodgkin B-cell lymphoma* [indium In 111 murine monoclonal antibodies (MAb) (2B8-MXDTPA); yttrium Y 90 murine MAb (2B8-MXDTPA)]

**melinamide** INN

*Melissa officinalis* *medicinal herb* [see: lemon balm]

**melitracen** INN *antidepressant* [also: melitracen HCl]

**melitracen HCl** USAN *antidepressant* [also: melitracen]

**melizame** USAN, INN *sweetener*

**Mellaril** tablets, concentrate for oral solution (discontinued 2004) ℞ *conventional (typical) antipsychotic* [thioridazine HCl] 15, 100, 200 mg; 30 mg/mL ⊘ Aldoril; Elavil; Eldepryl; Enovil; Equanil; Moderil

**Mellaril-S** oral suspension (discontinued 2003) ℞ *conventional (typical) antipsychotic* [thioridazine HCl] 25, 100 mg/5 mL

**meloxicam** USAN, INN, BAN *analgesic; antiarthritic; antipyretic; COX-2 inhibitor; nonsteroidal anti-inflammatory drug (NSAID)*

**Melpaque HP** cream ℞ *hyperpigmentation bleaching agent* [hydroquinone (in a sunscreen base)] 4%

**melperone** INN, BAN

**melphalan (MPL)** USAN, USP, INN, BAN, JAN *nitrogen mustard-type alkylating antineoplastic for multiple myeloma (orphan) and ovarian cancer; investigational (orphan) for metastatic melanoma*

**Melquin HP** cream ℞ *hyperpigmentation bleaching agent* [hydroquinone] 4%

**memantine** INN *NMDA (N-methyl-D-aspartate) antagonist; neuroprotective agent* [also: memantine HCl]

**memantine HCl** *NMDA (N-methyl-D-aspartate) antagonist for Alzheimer disease; investigational (Phase III) neuroprotective agent for diabetic neuropathy, vascular dementia, Parkinson disease, and AIDS dementia* [also: memantine]

**Memorette** (trademarked packaging form) *patient compliance package*

**memotine** INN *antiviral* [also: memotine HCl]

**memotine HCl** USAN *antiviral* [also: memotine]

**menabitan** INN *analgesic* [also: menabitan HCl]

**menabitan HCl** USAN *analgesic* [also: menabitan]

**Menactra** ℞ *investigational (Phase III) vaccine for meningitis*

**menadiol** BAN *vitamin $K_4$; prothrombogenic* [also: menadiol sodium diphosphate]

**menadiol sodium diphosphate** USP *vitamin $K_4$; prothrombogenic* [also: menadiol]

**menadiol sodium sulfate** INN

**menadione** USP *vitamin $K_3$; prothrombogenic*

**menadione sodium bisulfite** USP, INN

**Menadol** captabs OTC *analgesic; antiarthritic; antipyretic; nonsteroidal anti-inflammatory drug (NSAID)* [ibuprofen] 200 mg

**menaphthene** [see: menadione]

**menaphthone** [see: menadione]

**menaphthone sodium bisulfite** [see: menadione sodium bisulfite]

**menaquinone** *vitamin $K_2$; prothrombogenic*

**menatetrenone** INN
**menbutone** INN, BAN
**mendelevium** *element (Md)*
**Menest** film-coated tablets ℞ *a mixture of equine estrogens; hormone replacement therapy for the treatment of postmenopausal symptoms; palliative therapy for prostate and breast cancers* [esterified estrogens] 0.3, 0.625, 1.25, 2.5 mg
**menfegol** INN
**menglytate** INN
**menichlopholan** [see: niclofolan]
**Meni-D** capsules ℞ *anticholinergic; antivertigo agent; motion sickness preventative* [meclizine HCl] 25 mg
**meningococcal polysaccharide vaccine, group A** USP *active bacterin for meningitis (Neisseria meningitidis)*
**meningococcal polysaccharide vaccine, group C** USP *active bacterin for meningitis (Neisseria meningitidis)*
**meningococcal polysaccharide vaccine, group W-135** *active bacterin for meningitis (Neisseria meningitidis)*
**meningococcal polysaccharide vaccine, group Y** *active bacterin for meningitis (Neisseria meningitidis)*
*Menispermum cocculus; M. lacunosum medicinal herb* [see: levant berry]
**menitrazepam** INN
**menoctone** USAN, INN *antimalarial*
**menogaril** USAN, INN *antibiotic antineoplastic*
**Menomune-A/C/Y/W-135** powder for subcu injection ℞ *meningitis vaccine* [meningococcal polysaccharide vaccine, groups A, C, Y, and W-135] 50 μg of each group per 0.5 mL dose
**Menoplex** tablets (discontinued 2000) OTC *analgesic; antipyretic; antihistaminic sleep aid* [acetaminophen; phenyltoloxamine citrate] 325•30 mg
**Menostar** transdermal patch ℞ *estrogen replacement therapy for postmenopausal symptoms* [17β-estradiol] 14 μg/day
**menotropins** USAN, USP *gonadotropin; gonad-stimulating principle for the induction of ovulation in women and the stimulation of spermatogenesis in men*

**Mentax** cream ℞ *benzylamine antifungal* [butenafine HCl] 1%
*Mentha piperita medicinal herb* [see: peppermint]
*Mentha pulegium medicinal herb* [see: pennyroyal]
*Mentha spicata medicinal herb* [see: spearmint]
**menthol** USP *topical analgesic and antipruritic; counterirritant; mild local anesthetic*
**Mentholatum** vaporizing ointment OTC *counterirritant; cough suppressant* [menthol; camphor] 9%•1.3%
**Mentholatum Cherry Chest Rub for Kids** vaporizing ointment OTC *counterirritant; cough suppressant* [menthol; camphor; eucalyptus oil] 4.7%•2.6%•1.2%
**MenthoRub** vaporizing ointment (discontinued 2000) OTC *counterirritant; cough suppressant* [menthol; camphor; eucalyptus oil; oil of turpentine] 2.6%•4.73%• ? • ?
**menthyl anthranilate** [see: meradimate]
*Menyanthes trifoliata medicinal herb* [see: buckbean]
**meobentine** INN *antiarrhythmic* [also: meobentine sulfate]
**meobentine sulfate** USAN *antiarrhythmic* [also: meobentine]
**mepacrine** INN *anthelmintic; antimalarial* [also: quinacrine HCl]
**mepacrine HCl** [see: quinacrine HCl]
**meparfynol** [see: methylpentynol]
**mepartricin** USAN, INN *antifungal; antiprotozoal*
**mepazine acetate** [see: pecazine]
**mepenzolate bromide** USP, INN *GI antispasmodic; anticholinergic; peptic ulcer adjunct*
**mepenzolate methylbromide** [see: mepenzolate bromide]
**mepenzolone bromide** [see: mepenzolate bromide]
**Mepergan** injection (discontinued 2004) ℞ *narcotic analgesic; sedative* [meperidine HCl; promethazine HCl] 25•25 mg/mL

**Mepergan Fortis** capsules (discontinued 2004) ℞ *narcotic analgesic; sedative* [meperidine HCl; promethazine HCl] 50•25 mg

**meperidine HCl** USP *narcotic analgesic; also abused as a street drug* [also: pethidine] 50, 100 mg oral; 50 mg/5 mL oral; 25, 50, 75, 100 mg/mL injection ⊘ meprobamate

**Mephaquin** ℞ *antimalarial for acute chloroquine-resistant malaria (orphan)* [mefloquine HCl]

**mephenesin** NF, INN

**mephenhydramine** [see: moxastine]

**mephenoxalone** INN

**mephentermine** INN *adrenergic; vasoconstrictor; vasopressor for hypotensive shock* [also: mephentermine sulfate]

**mephentermine sulfate** USP *adrenergic; vasoconstrictor; vasopressor for hypotensive shock* [also: mephentermine]

**mephenytoin** USAN, USP, INN *hydantoin anticonvulsant* [also: methoin] ⊘ Mephyton; Mesantoin

**mephobarbital** USP, JAN *anticonvulsant; sedative* [also: methylphenobarbital; methylphenobarbitone]

**Mephyton** tablets ℞ *coagulant to correct anticoagulant-induced prothrombin deficiency; vitamin K supplement* [phytonadione] 5 mg ⊘ mephenytoin; methadone

**mepicycline** [see: pipacycline]

**MEPIG (mucoid exopolysaccharide *Pseudomonas* [hyper]immune globulin)** [q.v.]

**mepindolol** INN, BAN

**mepiperphenidol bromide**

**mepiprazole** INN, BAN

**mepirizole** [see: epirizole]

**mepiroxol** INN

**mepitiostane** INN

**mepivacaine** INN *local anesthetic* [also: mepivacaine HCl]

**mepivacaine HCl** USP *local anesthetic* [also: mepivacaine] 3% injection

**mepivacaine HCl & levonordefrin** *injectable local anesthetic; vasoconstrictor* 2%•1:20 000 injection

**mepixanox** INN

**mepolizumab** USAN *immunomodulator*

**mepramidil** INN

**meprednisone** USAN, USP, INN

**meprobamate** USP, INN, BAN, JAN *anxiolytic; sedative; hypnotic; minor tranquilizer; also abused as a street drug* 200, 400 mg oral ⊘ meperidine

**Mepron** oral suspension ℞ *antiprotozoal for AIDS-related* Pneumocystis carinii *pneumonia (orphan); investigational (orphan) for AIDS-related* Toxoplasma gondii *encephalitis* [atovaquone] 750 mg/5 mL ⊘ Lupron; Napron

**meproscillarin** INN, BAN

**meprothixol** BAN [also: meprotixol]

**meprotixol** INN [also: meprothixol]

**meprylcaine** INN *local anesthetic* [also: meprylcaine HCl]

**meprylcaine HCl** USP *local anesthetic* [also: meprylcaine]

**meptazinol** INN, BAN *analgesic* [also: meptazinol HCl]

**meptazinol HCl** USAN *analgesic* [also: meptazinol]

**mepyramine** INN, BAN *antihistamine* [also: pyrilamine maleate]

**mepyramine maleate** [see: pyrilamine maleate]

**mepyrium** [see: amprolium]

**mepyrrotazine** [see: dimelazine]

**mequidox** USAN, INN *antibacterial*

**mequinol** USAN, INN *hyperpigmentation bleaching agent*

**mequitamium iodide** INN

**mequitazine** INN, BAN

**mequitazium iodide** [see: mequitamium iodide]

**meradimate** USAN *ultraviolet A sunscreen*

**meragidone sodium**

**meralein sodium** USAN, INN *topical anti-infective*

**meralluride** NF, INN

**merbaphen** USP

**merbromin** NF, INN *general antiseptic*

**mercaptamine** INN *antiurolithic* [also: cysteamine]

**mercaptoarsenical** [see: arsthinol]

**mercaptoarsenol** [see: arsthinol]

**mercaptoethylamine (MEA)** [see: mercaptamine]

**mercaptomerin (MT6)** INN [also: mercaptomerin sodium]

**mercaptomerin sodium** USP [also: mercaptomerin]

**mercaptopurine (6-MP)** USP, INN *antimetabolite antineoplastic*

**mercuderamide** INN

**mercufenol chloride** USAN *topical anti-infective*

**mercumatilin sodium** INN

**mercuric oxide, yellow** NF *ophthalmic antiseptic (FDA ruled it "not safe and effective" in 1992)*

**mercuric salicylate** NF

**mercuric succinimide** NF

**mercurobutol** INN

**Mercurochrome** solution (discontinued 2000) OTC *antiseptic* [merbromin] 2%

**mercurophylline** NF, INN

**mercurous chloride** [see: calomel]

**mercury** *element (Hg)*

**mercury, ammoniated** USP *topical anti-infective; antipsoriatic*

**mercury amide chloride** [see: mercury, ammoniated]

**mercury oleate** NF

**merethoxylline procaine**

**mergocriptine** INN

**Meridia** capsules ℞ *anorexiant for the treatment of obesity* [sibutramine HCl] 5, 10, 15 mg

**merisoprol acetate Hg 197** USAN *radioactive agent*

**merisoprol acetate Hg 203** USAN *radioactive agent*

**merisoprol Hg 197** USAN *renal function test; radioactive agent*

**Meritene** powder OTC *enteral nutritional therapy* [milk-based formula]

**meropenem** USAN, INN, BAN *broad-spectrum carbapenem antibiotic for intra-abdominal infections and bacterial meningitis*

**Merrem** powder for IV infusion ℞ *broad-spectrum carbapenem antibiotic for intra-abdominal infections and bacterial meningitis* [meropenem] 500, 1000 mg

**mersalyl** INN

**mersalyl sodium** [see: mersalyl]

**Mersol** solution, tincture OTC *antiseptic; antibacterial; antifungal* [thimerosal] 1:1000

**mertiatide** INN

**Meruvax II** powder for subcu injection ℞ *rubella vaccine* [rubella virus vaccine, live] 0.5 mL

**mesabolone** INN

**mesalamine** USAN *anti-inflammatory; treatment of ulcerative colitis and proctitis* [also: mesalazine]

**mesalazine** INN, BAN *anti-inflammatory; treatment of ulcerative colitis and proctitis* [also: mesalamine]

**Mesantoin** tablets (discontinued 2000) ℞ *hydantoin anticonvulsant* [mephenytoin] 100 mg ② mephenytoin; Mestinon; Metatensin

**mescaline** *hallucinogenic street drug derived from the flowering heads (mescal buttons) of a Mexican cactus* ② meclizine

**Mescolor** sustained-release film-coated tablets ℞ *decongestant; antihistamine; anticholinergic to dry mucosal secretions* [pseudoephedrine HCl; chlorpheniramine maleate; methscopolamine nitrate] 120•8•2.5 mg

**meseclazone** USAN, INN *anti-inflammatory*

**mesembryanthemum** *medicinal herb* [see: kanna]

**mesifilcon A** USAN *hydrophilic contact lens material*

**mesilate** INN *combining name for radicals or groups* [also: mesylate]

**mesna** USAN, INN, BAN *prophylaxis for ifosfamide-induced hemorrhagic cystitis (orphan); investigational (orphan) treatment for cyclophosphamide-induced hemorrhagic cystitis* 100 mg/mL injection

**Mesnex** film-coated caplets, IV injection ℞ *prophylaxis for ifosfamide-induced hemorrhagic cystitis (orphan); investigational (orphan) treatment for cyclophosphamide-induced hemorrhagic cystitis* [mesna] 400 mg; 100 mg/mL

mesocarb INN
meso-inositol [see: inositol]
meso-NDGA (nordihydroguaiaretic acid) [see: masoprocol]
meso-nordihydroguaiaretic acid (NDGA) [see: masoprocol]
mesoridazine USAN, INN *phenothiazine antipsychotic*
mesoridazine besylate USP *phenothiazine antipsychotic*
mespiperone C 11 USAN *radiopharmaceutical imaging aid for PET scans of the brain (produced at bedside for immediate administration)*
mespirenone INN
mestanolone INN, BAN
mestenediol [see: methandriol]
mesterolone USAN, INN, BAN *androgen; also abused as a street drug*
**Mestinon** tablets, Timespan (extended-release tablets), syrup, IM or IV injection R *cholinergic/anticholinesterase muscle stimulant; muscle relaxant reversal; treatment for myasthenia gravis* [pyridostigmine bromide] 60 mg; 180 mg; 60 mg/5 mL; 5 mg/mL ⚕ Mesantoin; Metatensin
mestranol USAN, USP, INN *estrogen*
mesudipine INN
mesulergine INN
mesulfamide INN
mesulfen INN [also: mesulphen]
mesulphen BAN [also: mesulfen]
mesuprine INN *vasodilator; smooth muscle relaxant* [also: mesuprine HCl]
mesuprine HCl USAN *vasodilator; smooth muscle relaxant* [also: mesuprine]
mesuximide INN *succinimide anticonvulsant* [also: methsuximide]
mesylate USAN, USP, BAN *combining name for radicals or groups* [also: mesilate]
metabromsalan USAN, INN *disinfectant*
metabutethamine HCl NF
metabutoxycaine HCl NF
metacetamol INN, BAN
metaclazepam INN
metacycline INN *antibacterial* [also: methacycline]

**Metadate CD** dual-release capsules, sprinkle caps R *CNS stimulant; once-daily treatment for attention-deficit hyperactivity disorder (ADHD)* [methylphenidate HCl] 10, 20, 30 mg (30% immediate release; 70% extended release)
**Metadate ER** extended-release tablets R *CNS stimulant for attention-deficit hyperactivity disorder (ADHD) and narcolepsy* [methylphenidate HCl] 10, 20 mg
**Metadol** ⓒ oral liquid R *narcotic analgesic; treatment for opioid dependence* [methadone HCl] 10 mg/mL
**Metaglip** film-coated tablets R *antidiabetic combination for type 2 diabetes* [glipizide; metformin HCl] 2.5•250, 2.5•500, 5•500 mg
metaglycodol INN
metahexamide INN
metahexanamide [see: metahexamide]
**Metahydrin** tablets R *diuretic; antihypertensive* [trichlormethiazide] 4 mg ⚕ Metandren
metalkonium chloride INN
metallibure INN *anterior pituitary activator for swine* [also: methallibure]
metalol HCl USAN *antiadrenergic (β-receptor)*
metamelfalan INN
metamfazone INN [also: methamphazone]
metamfepramone INN [also: dimepropion]
metamfetamine INN *CNS stimulant; widely abused as a street drug* [also: methamphetamine HCl]
metamizole sodium INN *analgesic; antipyretic* [also: dipyrone]
metampicillin INN
**Metamucil** capsules OTC *bulk laxative* [psyllium husk] 520 mg
**Metamucil** effervescent powder OTC *bulk laxative; antacid* [psyllium hydrophilic mucilloid; sodium bicarbonate; potassium bicarbonate] 3.4• ? • ? g/pkt.
**Metamucil** wafers OTC *bulk laxative* [psyllium husk] 3.4 g

**Metamucil Original Texture; Metamucil Smooth Texture** powder OTC *bulk laxative* [psyllium husk] 3.4 g/dose

**metandienone** INN [also: methandrostenolone; methandienone]

**metanixin** INN

**metaoxedrine chloride** [see: phenylephrine HCl]

**metaphosphoric acid, potassium salt** [see: potassium metaphosphate]

**metaphosphoric acid, trisodium salt** [see: sodium trimetaphosphate]

**metaphyllin** [see: aminophylline]

**metapramine** INN

**metaproterenol polistirex** USAN *sympathomimetic bronchodilator* [also: orciprenaline] ☑ metoprolol

**metaproterenol sulfate** USAN, USP *sympathomimetic bronchodilator* 10, 20 mg oral; 0.4%, 0.6%, 5% inhalation

**metaradrine bitartrate** [see: metaraminol bitartrate]

**metaraminol** INN *adrenergic; vasopressor for acute hypotensive shock, anaphylaxis, or traumatic shock* [also: metaraminol bitartrate]

**metaraminol bitartrate** USP *adrenergic; vasopressor for acute hypotensive shock, anaphylaxis, or traumatic shock* [also: metaraminol]

**Metastat** (name changed to Metadol upon marketing release in 2001)

**Metastron** IV injection R *analgesic for metastatic bone pain* [strontium chloride Sr 89] 10.9–22.6 mg/mL (4 mCi)

**Metatensin #2; Metatensin #4** tablets R *antihypertensive* [trichlormethiazide; reserpine] 2•0.1 mg; 4•0.1 mg ☑ Mesantoin; Mestinon

**metaterol** INN

**metaxalone** USAN, INN, BAN *skeletal muscle relaxant* ☑ metolazone

**metazamide** INN

**metazepium iodide** [see: buzepide metiodide]

**metazide** INN

**metazocine** INN, BAN

**metbufen** INN

**metcaraphen HCl**

**metembonate** INN *combining name for radicals or groups*

**meteneprost** USAN, INN *oxytocic; prostaglandin*

**metenolone** INN *anabolic steroid; also abused as a street drug* [also: methenolone acetate; methenolone; metenolone acetate]

**metenolone acetate** JAN *anabolic steroid; also abused as a street drug* [also: methenolone acetate; metenolone; methenolone]

**metenolone enanthate** JAN *anabolic steroid; also abused as a street drug* [also: methenolone enanthate]

**metergoline** INN, BAN

**metergotamine** INN

**metescufylline** INN

**metesculetol** INN

**metesind glucuronate** USAN *specific thymidylate synthase (TS) inhibitor antineoplastic* ☑ medicine

**metethoheptazine** INN

**metetoin** INN *anticonvulsant* [also: methetoin]

**metformin** USAN, INN, BAN *biguanide antidiabetic* [also: metformin HCl]

**Metformin ER** extended-release tablets R *once-daily treatment for diabetes* [metformin HCl] 500 mg

**metformin HCl** USAN, JAN *biguanide antidiabetic* [also: metformin] 500, 625, 750, 850, 1000 mg oral

**metformin HCl & glyburide** *biguanide/sulfonylurea antidiabetic combination for type 2 diabetes* 250•1.25, 500•2.5, 500•5 mg oral

**methacholine bromide** NF

**methacholine chloride** USP, INN *cholinergic; bronchoconstrictor for in vivo pulmonary challenge tests*

**methacrylic acid copolymer** NF *tablet-coating agent*

**methacycline** USAN *antibacterial* [also: metacycline]

**methacycline HCl** USP *gram-negative and gram-positive bacteriostatic; antirickettsial*

**methadol** [see: dimepheptanol]

**methadone** INN *narcotic analgesic; narcotic addiction detoxicant; often abused as a street drug* [also: methadone HCl] ☒ Mephyton

**methadone HCl** USP *narcotic analgesic; narcotic addiction detoxicant; often abused as a street drug* [also: methadone] 5, 10, 40 mg oral; 5, 10 mg/5 mL oral; 10 mg/mL oral; 10 mg/mL injection

**methadonium chloride** [see: methadone HCl]

**Methadose** tablets, oral concentrate, powder ℞ *narcotic analgesic; narcotic addiction detoxicant; often abused as a street drug* [methadone HCl] 5, 10, 40 mg; 10 mg/mL; 50, 100, 500, 1000 g

**methadyl acetate** USAN *narcotic analgesic* [also: acetylmethadol]

**methafilcon B** USAN *hydrophilic contact lens material*

**Methagual** OTC *analgesic; counterirritant* [methyl salicylate; guaiacol] 8%•2%

**Methalgen** cream OTC *analgesic; counterirritant* [methyl salicylate; menthol; camphor; mustard oil]

**methallenestril** INN

**methallenestrol** [see: methallenestril]

**methallibure** USAN *anterior pituitary activator for swine* [also: metallibure]

**methalthiazide** USAN *diuretic; antihypertensive*

**methamoctol**

**methamphazone** BAN [also: metamfazone]

**methamphetamine HCl** USP *CNS stimulant; widely abused as a street drug* [also: metamfetamine] 5 mg oral

**methampyrone** [now: dipyrone]

**methanabol** [see: methandriol]

**methandienone** BAN [also: methandrostenolone; metandienone]

**methandriol**

**methandrostenolone** USP *steroid; discontinued for human use, but the veterinary product is still available and sometimes abused as a street drug* [also: metandienone; methandienone]

**methaniazide** INN

**methanol** [see: methyl alcohol]

**methantheline bromide** USP *peptic ulcer adjunct* [also: methanthelinium bromide]

**methanthelinium bromide** INN, BAN *anticholinergic* [also: methantheline bromide]

**methaphenilene** INN, BAN [also: methaphenilene HCl]

**methaphenilene HCl** NF [also: methaphenilene]

**methapyrilene** INN [also: methapyrilene fumarate]

**methapyrilene fumarate** USP [also: methapyrilene]

**methapyrilene HCl** USP

**methaqualone** USAN, USP, INN, BAN *hypnotic; sedative; widely abused as a street drug, which leads to dependence*

**methaqualone HCl** USP

**metharbital** USP, INN, JAN *anticonvulsant* [also: metharbitone]

**metharbitone** BAN *anticonvulsant* [also: metharbital]

**methastyridone** INN

**Methatropic** capsules OTC *dietary lipotropic with vitamin supplementation* [choline; inositol; methionine; multiple B vitamins] 115•83•110• ☀ mg

**methazolamide** USP, INN *carbonic anhydrase inhibitor for glaucoma* 25, 50 mg oral

**Methblue 65** tablets ℞ *urinary anti-infective and antiseptic; antidote to cyanide poisoning* [methylene blue] 65 mg

**methcathinone** *a highly addictive manufactured street drug similar to cathinone, with amphetamine-like effects* [see also: cathinone; *Catha edulis*]

**methdilazine** USP, INN *phenothiazine antihistamine; antipruritic*

**methdilazine HCl** USP *phenothiazine antihistamine; antipruritic*

**methenamine** USP, INN *urinary antibiotic* ☒ methionine

**methenamine hippurate** USAN, USP *urinary antibiotic* [also: hexamine hippurate]

**methenamine mandelate** USP *urinary antibiotic* 0.5, 1 g oral; 0.5 g/5 mL oral

**methenamine sulfosalicylate** *topical antipsoriatic*

**methenolone** BAN *anabolic steroid; also abused as a street drug* [also: methenolone acetate; metenolone; metenolone acetate]

**methenolone acetate** USAN *anabolic steroid; also abused as a street drug* [also: metenolone; methenolone; metenolone acetate]

**methenolone enanthate** USAN *anabolic steroid; also abused as a street drug* [also: metenolone enanthate]

**metheptazine** INN

**Methergine** coated tablets, IV or IM injection R̥ *oxytocic for induction of labor, control of postpartum uterine atony, and postpartum hemorrhage* [methylergonovine maleate] 0.2 mg; 0.2 mg/mL

**methestrol** INN

**methetharimide** [see: bemegride]

**methetoin** USAN *anticonvulsant* [also: metetoin]

**methicillin sodium** USAN, USP *penicillinase-resistant penicillin antibiotic* [also: meticillin]

**methimazole** USP *thyroid inhibitor* [also: thiamazole] 5, 10 mg oral

**methindizate** BAN [also: metindizate]

**methiodal sodium** USP, INN

**methiomeprazine** INN

**methiomeprazine HCl** [see: methiomeprazine]

**methionine (DL-methionine)** NF, JAN *urinary acidifier* [also: racemethionine] 500 mg oral

**methionine (L-methionine)** USAN, USP, INN, JAN *essential amino acid; symbols: Met, M; investigational (orphan) for AIDS myelopathy* ② methenamine

**methionyl neurotropic factor, brain-derived, recombinant** *investigational (orphan) for amyotrophic lateral sclerosis*

**methionyl stem cell factor, recombinant human** *investigational (orphan) for progressive bone marrow failure*

**N-methionylleptin (human)** [see: metreleptin]

**methiothepin** [see: metitepine]

**methisazone** USAN *antiviral* [also: metisazone]

**methisoprinol** [now: inosine pranobex]

**Methitest** tablets R̥ *androgen for hypogonadism or testosterone deficiency in men, delayed puberty in boys, and metastatic breast cancer in women; also abused as a street drug* [methyltestosterone] 10, 25 mg

**methitural** INN

**methixene HCl** USAN *smooth muscle relaxant* [also: metixene] ② methoxsalen

**methocamphone methylsulfate** [see: trimethidinium methosulfate]

**methocarbamol** USP, INN, BAN, JAN *skeletal muscle relaxant* 500, 750 mg oral; 100 mg/mL injection

**methocidin** INN

**methohexital** USP, INN *barbiturate general anesthetic* [also: methohexitone]

**methohexital sodium** USP *barbiturate general anesthetic*

**methohexitone** BAN *barbiturate general anesthetic* [also: methohexital]

**methoin** BAN *anticonvulsant* [also: mephenytoin]

**methonaphthone** [see: menbutone]

**methophedrine** [see: methoxyphedrine]

**methophenazine** [see: metofenazate]

**methopholine** USAN *analgesic* [also: metofoline]

**methoprene** INN

**methopromazine** INN

**methopromazine maleate** [see: methopromazine]

**methopyrimazole** [see: epirizole]

**d-methorphan** [see: dextromethorphan]

**d-methorphan hydrobromide** [see: dextromethorphan hydrobromide]

**methoserpidine** INN, BAN

**methotrexate (MTX)** USAN, USP, INN, BAN, JAN *antimetabolite antineoplastic for leukemia, lymphoma, and various solid tumors; systemic antipsoriatic; antirheumatic for juvenile rheumatoid arthritis (orphan)* 2.5 mg oral

**methotrexate & laurocapram** *investigational (orphan) for topical treatment of Mycosis fungoides*

**methotrexate & leucovorin** *antineoplastic for osteosarcoma (orphan)*

**Methotrexate LPF Sodium** preservative-free injection ℞ *antimetabolite antineoplastic for leukemia, lymphoma, and various solid tumors; systemic antipsoriatic; antirheumatic* [methotrexate sodium] 2.5 mg/mL

**methotrexate sodium** USP *antirheumatic; systemic antipsoriatic; antimetabolite antineoplastic for leukemia, lymphoma, various solid tumors, and osteogenic sarcoma (orphan)* 20, 1000 mg/vial injection; 2.5 mg/mL injection

**methotrimeprazine** USAN, USP *central analgesic; CNS depressant* [also: levomepromazine]

**methotrimeprazine maleate** *CNS depressant; neuroleptic*

**methoxamine** INN *adrenergic; vasoconstrictor; vasopressor for hypotensive shock during surgery* [also: methoxamine HCl]

**methoxamine HCl** USP *adrenergic; vasoconstrictor; vasopressor for hypotensive shock during surgery* [also: methoxamine]

**methoxiflurane** [see: methoxyflurane]

**methoxsalen (8-methoxsalen)** USP *repigmentation agent for vitiligo; antipsoriatic; palliative treatment for cutaneous T-cell lymphoma (CTCL); investigational (orphan) for diffuse systemic sclerosis and cardiac allografts* ⊡ methixene

**methoxy polyethylene glycol** [see: polyethylene glycol monomethyl ether]

**2-methoxyestradiol** *investigational (orphan) for multiple myeloma*

**methoxyfenoserpin** [see: mefeserpine]

**methoxyflurane** USAN, USP, INN, BAN *inhalation general anesthetic*

**methoxyphedrine** INN

**p-methoxyphenacyl** [see: anisatil]

**methoxyphenamine** INN [also: methoxyphenamine HCl]

**methoxyphenamine HCl** USP [also: methoxyphenamine]

**4-methoxyphenol** [see: mequinol]

**o-methoxyphenyl salicylate acetate** [see: guacetisal]

**methoxypromazine maleate** [see: methopromazine]

**8-methoxypsoralen (8-MOP)** [see: methoxsalen]

**5-methoxyresorcinol** [see: flamenol]

**methphenoxydiol** [see: guaifenesin]

**methscopolamine bromide** USP *GI antispasmodic; peptic ulcer adjunct* [also: hyoscine methobromide]

**methscopolamine nitrate** *anticholinergic*

**methsuximide** USP, BAN *succinimide anticonvulsant for absence (petit mal) seizures* [also: mesuximide]

**methyclothiazide** USAN, USP, INN *diuretic; antihypertensive* 2.5, 5 mg oral

**methydromorphine** [see: methyldihydromorphine]

**methyl alcohol** NF *solvent*

**methyl benzoquate** BAN *coccidiostat for poultry* [also: nequinate]

**methyl cresol** [see: cresol]

**methyl cysteine** [see: mecysteine]

**methyl p-hydroxybenzoate** [see: methylparaben]

**methyl isobutyl ketone** NF *alcohol denaturant*

**methyl nicotinate** USAN

**methyl palmoxirate** USAN *antidiabetic*

**methyl phthalate** [see: dimethyl phthalate]

**methyl salicylate** NF *flavoring agent; counterirritant; topical anesthetic*

**methyl sulfoxide** [see: dimethyl sulfoxide]

**methyl violet** [see: gentian violet]

**l-methylaminoethanolcatechol** [see: epinephrine]

**methylaminopterin** [see: methotrexate]

**methylandrostenediol** [see: methandriol]

**methylatropine nitrate** USAN *anticholinergic* [also: atropine methonitrate]

**methylbenactyzium bromide** INN

**methylbenzethonium chloride** USP, INN *topical anti-infective/antiseptic*

**α-methylbenzylhydrazine** [see: mebanazine]

**methylcarbamate of salicylanilide** [see: anilamate]

**methyl-CCNU (chloroethyl-cyclo-hexyl-nitrosourea)** [see: semustine]

**methylcellulose** USP, INN *ophthalmic moisturizer; suspending and viscosity-increasing agent; bulk laxative*

**methylcellulose, propylene glycol ether of** [see: hydroxypropyl methylcellulose]

**methylchromone** INN, BAN

**N-methyl-D-aspartate (NMDA)** *an endogenous neurotransmitter similar to glutamate; an NMDA inhibitor blocks the action of glutamate, which can over-stimulate the receptors and become neurotoxic in excessive amounts, causing various dementias and CNS disorders*

**methyldesorphine** INN, BAN

**methyldigoxin** [see: metildigoxin]

**methyldihydromorphine** INN

**methyldihydromorphinone HCl** [see: metopon]

**methyldinitrobenzamide** [see: dinitolmide]

**methyldioxatrine** [see: meletimide]

**N-methyldiphenethylamine** [see: demelverine]

**α-methyl-DL-thyroxine ethyl ester** [see: etiroxate]

**methyldopa** USAN, USP, INN, BAN, JAN *centrally acting antiadrenergic antihypertensive* 250, 500 mg oral ⑨ levodopa

**α-methyldopa** [now: methyldopa]

**methyldopate** BAN *centrally acting antiadrenergic antihypertensive* [also: methyldopate HCl]

**methyldopate HCl** USAN, USP *centrally acting antiadrenergic antihypertensive* [also: methyldopate] 50 mg/mL injection

**methylene blue (MB)** USP *antimethemoglobinemic; GU antiseptic; antidote to cyanide poisoning; diagnostic aid for gastric secretions* [also: methylthio-ninium chloride] 65 mg oral; 10 mg/mL injection

**methylene chloride** NF *solvent*

**methylene diphosphonate (MDP)** [now: medronate disodium]

**methylenedioxyamphetamine (MDA)** [see: MDMA, MDEA]

**3,4-methylenedioxyethamphet-amine (MDEA)** [q.v.]

**3,4-methylenedioxymethamphet-amine (MDMA)** [q.v.]

**6-methyleneoxytetracycline (MOTC)** [see: methacycline]

**methylenprednisolone** [see: prednylidene]

**methylergometrine** INN *oxytocic* [also: methylergonovine maleate]

**methylergometrine maleate** [see: methylergonovine maleate]

**methylergonovine maleate** USP *oxytocic for induction of labor, control of postpartum uterine atony, and postpartum hemorrhage* [also: methylergometrine]

**methylergonovinium bimaleate** [see: methylergonovine maleate]

**methylergotamine** [see: metergotamine]

**methylestrenolone** [see: normethandrone]

**methyl-GAG (methylglyoxal-*bis*-guanylhydrazone)** [see: mitoguazone]

**methylglyoxal-*bis*-guanylhydrazone (methyl-GAG; MGBG)** [see: mitoguazone]

**1-methylhexylamine** [see: tuaminoheptane]

**1-methylhexylamine sulfate** [see: tuaminoheptane sulfate]

**N-methylhydrazine** [see: procarbazine]

**Methylin** tablets, chewable tablets ℞ *CNS stimulant for attention-deficit hyperactivity disorder (ADHD) and narcolepsy* [methylphenidate HCl] 5, 10, 20 mg; 2.5, 5, 10 mg

**Methylin ER** extended-release tablets ℞ *CNS stimulant for attention-deficit hyperactivity disorder (ADHD) and narcolepsy* [methylphenidate HCl] 10, 20 mg

**methylmorphine** [see: codeine]
**methyl-nitro-imidazole** [see: carnidazole]
**methylnortestosterone** [see: normethandrone]
**methylparaben** USAN, NF *antifungal agent; preservative*
**methylparaben sodium** USAN, NF *antimicrobial preservative*
**methylparafynol** [see: meparfynol]
**methylpentynol** INN, BAN
**methylperidol** [see: moperone]
**(+)-methylphenethylamine** [see: dextroamphetamine]
**(−)-methylphenethylamine** [see: levamphetamine]
**methylphenethylamine HCl** [see: amphetamine HCl]
**methylphenethylamine phosphate** [see: amphetamine phosphate]
**(−)-methylphenethylamine succinate** [see: levamfetamine succinate]
**methylphenethylamine sulfate** [see: amphetamine sulfate]
**(+)-methylphenethylamine sulfate** [see: dextroamphetamine sulfate]
**methylphenidate** INN, BAN *CNS stimulant for attention-deficit hyperactivity disorder (ADHD) and narcolepsy; also abused as a street drug* [also: methylphenidate HCl]
**methylphenidate HCl (MPH)** USP, JAN *CNS stimulant for attention-deficit hyperactivity disorder (ADHD) and narcolepsy; also abused as a street drug* [also: methylphenidate] 5, 10, 20 mg oral
**methylphenobarbital** INN *anticonvulsant; sedative* [also: mephobarbital; methylphenobarbitone]
**methylphenobarbitone** BAN *anticonvulsant; sedative* [also: mephobarbital; methylphenobarbital]
*d*-**methylphenylamine sulfate** [see: dextroamphetamine sulfate]
**methylphytyl napthoquinone** [see: phytonadione]
**methylprednisolone** USP, INN, BAN, JAN *corticosteroid; anti-inflammatory; immunosuppressant* 4, 16 mg oral

**methylprednisolone aceponate** INN
**methylprednisolone acetate** USP, JAN *corticosteroid; anti-inflammatory; immunosuppressant* 20, 40, 80 mg/mL injection
**methylprednisolone hemisuccinate** USP *corticosteroid; anti-inflammatory*
**methylprednisolone sodium phosphate** USAN *corticosteroid; anti-inflammatory* 40, 125, 500, 1000 mg/vial injection
**methylprednisolone sodium succinate** USP, JAN *corticosteroid; anti-inflammatory; immunosuppressant*
**methylprednisolone suleptanate** USAN, INN *corticosteroid; anti-inflammatory*
**methylpromazine**
**4-methylpyrazole (4-MP)** [see: fomepizole]
**methylrosaniline chloride** [now: gentian violet]
**methylrosanilinium chloride** INN *topical anti-infective* [also: gentian violet]
**methylscopolamine bromide** [see: methscopolamine bromide]
**methylsulfate** USP *combining name for radicals or groups* [also: metilsulfate]
**methylsulfonylmethane (MSM)** *natural source of sulfur; promotes an increase in collagen and the endogenous antioxidant glutathione*
**methyltestosterone** USP, INN, BAN *oral/parenteral androgen for hypogonadism or testosterone deficiency in men, delayed puberty in boys, and metastatic breast cancer in women; also abused as a street drug* 10, 25 mg oral
**methyltheobromine** [see: caffeine]
**methylthionine chloride** [see: methylene blue]
**methylthionine HCl** [see: methylene blue]
**methylthioninium chloride** INN *antimethemoglobinemic; antidote to cyanide poisoning* [also: methylene blue]
**methylthiouracil** USP, INN
**methyltrienolone** [see: metribolone]
**methynodiol diacetate** USAN *progestin* [also: metynodiol]

**methyprylon** USP, INN *sedative; hypnotic* [also: methprylone]

**methyprylone** BAN *sedative* [also: methyprylon]

**methyridene** BAN [also: metyridine]

**methysergide** USAN, INN, BAN *migraine-specific vasoconstrictor and peripheral serotonin antagonist for the prophylaxis of vascular headaches*

**methysergide maleate** USP *migraine-specific vasoconstrictor and peripheral serotonin antagonist for the prophylaxis of vascular headaches*

**metiamide** USAN, INN *antagonist to histamine H$_2$ receptors*

**metiapine** USAN, INN *antipsychotic*

**metiazinic acid** INN

**metibride** INN

**meticillin** INN *penicillinase-resistant penicillin antibiotic* [also: methicillin sodium]

**meticillin sodium** *penicillinase-resistant penicillin antibiotic* [see: methicillin sodium]

**Meticorten** tablets ℞ *corticosteroid; anti-inflammatory; immunosuppressant* [prednisone] 1 mg

**meticrane** INN

**metildigoxin** INN

**metilsulfate** INN *combining name for radicals or groups* [also: methylsulfate]

**Metimyd** eye drop suspension, ophthalmic ointment ℞ *corticosteroidal anti-inflammatory; antibiotic* [prednisolone acetate; sulfacetamide sodium] 0.5%•10%

**metindizate** INN [also: methindizate]

**metioprim** USAN, INN, BAN *antibacterial*

**metioxate** INN

**metipirox** INN

**metipranolol** USAN, INN, BAN *topical antiglaucoma agent (β-blocker)*

**metipranolol HCl** *topical antiglaucoma agent (β-blocker)* 0.3% eye drops

**metiprenaline** INN

**metirosine** INN *antihypertensive* [also: metyrosine]

**metisazone** INN *antiviral* [also: methisazone]

**metitepine** INN

**metixene** INN *smooth muscle relaxant* [also: methixene HCl]

**metixene HCl** [see: methixene HCl]

**metizoline** INN *adrenergic; vasoconstrictor* [also: metizoline HCl]

**metizoline HCl** USAN *adrenergic; vasoconstrictor* [also: metizoline]

**metkefamide** INN *analgesic* [also: metkephamid acetate]

**metkefamide acetate** [see: metkephamid acetate]

**metkephamid acetate** USAN *analgesic* [also: metkefamide]

**metochalcone** INN

**metocinium iodide** INN

**metoclopramide** INN, BAN, JAN *antiemetic for chemotherapy; GI stimulant; antidopaminergic; radiosensitizer* [also: metoclopramide HCl]

**metoclopramide HCl** USAN, USP, JAN *antiemetic for chemotherapy; GI stimulant; antidopaminergic; radiosensitizer* [also: metoclopramide] 5, 10 mg oral; 5, 10 mg/5 mL oral; 5 mg/mL injection

**metoclopramide monohydrochloride monohydrate** [see: metoclopramide HCl]

**metocurine iodide** USAN, USP *neuromuscular blocker; muscle relaxant* 2 mg/mL injection

**metofenazate** INN

**metofoline** INN *analgesic* [also: methopholine]

**metogest** USAN, INN *hormone*

**metolazone** USAN, INN *antihypertensive; diuretic* 2.5, 5, 10 mg oral ② metaxalone

**metomidate** INN, BAN

**metopimazine** USAN, INN *antiemetic*

**Metopirone** softgels ℞ *diagnostic aid for pituitary function* [metyrapone] 250 mg ② metyrapone

**metopon** INN

**metopon HCl** [see: metopon]

**metoprine** USAN *antineoplastic*

**metoprolol** USAN, INN, BAN *antihypertensive; antiadrenergic (β-receptor)* ② metaproterenol

**metoprolol fumarate** USAN *antihypertensive; antiadrenergic (β-receptor)*

**metoprolol succinate** USAN *antianginal; antihypertensive; antiadrenergic (β-receptor)*

**metoprolol tartrate** USAN, USP *antihypertensive; antiadrenergic (β-receptor)* 25, 50, 100 mg oral; 1 mg/mL injection

**metoquizine** USAN, INN *anticholinergic*

**metoserpate** INN *veterinary sedative* [also: metoserpate HCl]

**metoserpate HCl** USAN *veterinary sedative* [also: metoserpate]

**metostilenol** INN

**metoxepin** INN

**metoxiestrol** [see: moxestrol]

**metrafazoline** INN

**metralindole** INN

**metrazifone** INN

**metreleptin** USAN *metabolic regulator for obesity*

**metrenperone** USAN, INN, BAN *veterinary myopathic*

**metribolone** INN

**metrifonate** USAN, INN *veterinary anthelmintic; investigational (NDA filed) acetylcholinesterase inhibitor for Alzheimer dementia* [also: trichlorfon; metriphonate]

**metrifudil** INN

**metriphonate** BAN *veterinary anthelmintic* [also: trichlorfon; metrifonate]

**metrizamide** USAN, INN *parenteral radiopaque contrast medium (48.25% iodine)*

**metrizoate sodium** USAN *radiopaque contrast medium* [also: sodium metrizoate]

**Metro I.V.** ready-to-use injection ℞ *antibiotic; antiprotozoal; amebicide* [metronidazole] 500 mg/100 mL

**MetroCream; MetroGel; MetroLotion** ℞ *antibiotic for rosacea (orphan); investigational (orphan) for decubitus ulcers and perioral dermatitis* [metronidazole] 0.75%

**MetroGel Vaginal** gel ℞ *antibacterial for bacterial vaginosis* [metronidazole] 0.75%

**metronidazole** USAN, USP, INN, BAN *antibiotic; antiprotozoal/amebicide; acne rosacea treatment (orphan); investigational (orphan) for decubitus ulcers and perioral dermatitis* 250, 375, 500, 750 mg oral; 500 mg/100 mL injection; 0.75% topical

**metronidazole benzoate** *antiprotozoal (Trichomonas)*

**metronidazole HCl** USAN *antibiotic; antiprotozoal; amebicide*

**metronidazole phosphate** USAN *antibacterial; antiprotozoal*

**MET-Rx** food bar, powder for drink OTC *enteral nutritional therapy* 100 g; 72 g

**Metubine Iodide** IV injection (discontinued 2004) ℞ *neuromuscular blocker; anesthesia adjunct* [metocurine iodide] 2 mg/mL

**metuclazepam** [see: metaclazepam]

**meturedepa** USAN, INN *antineoplastic*

**metynodiol** INN *progestin* [also: methynodiol diacetate]

**metynodiol diacetate** [see: methynodiol diacetate]

**metyrapone** USAN, USP, INN *diagnostic aid for pituitary function* Ⓓ Metopirone; metyrosine

**metyrapone tartrate** USAN *pituitary function test*

**metyridine** INN [also: methyridene]

**metyrosine** USAN, USP *antihypertensive; pheochromocytomic agent* Ⓓ metyrapone

**Mevacor** tablets ℞ *HMG-CoA reductase inhibitor for hypercholesterolemia and atherosclerosis; also for primary prevention of coronary heart disease* [lovastatin] 10, 20, 40 mg

**mevastatin** INN

**mevinolin** [now: lovastatin]

**mexafylline** INN

**mexazolam** INN

**mexenone** INN, BAN

**mexiletine** INN, BAN *antiarrhythmic* [also: mexiletine HCl]

**mexiletine HCl** USAN, USP *antiarrhythmic* [also: mexiletine]

**mexiprostil** INN

**Mexitil** capsules ℞ *antiarrhythmic* [mexiletine HCl] 150, 200, 250 mg

**mexoprofen** INN

**mexrenoate potassium** USAN, INN *aldosterone antagonist*

**Mexsana Medicated** powder OTC *topical diaper rash treatment* [kaolin; zinc oxide; eucalyptus oil; camphor; corn starch]

**mezacopride** INN

**mezepine** INN

**mezereon** *(Daphne mezereum)* bark *medicinal herb used as a cathartic, diuretic, emetic, and rubefacient; eating the berries can be fatal, and people have been poisoned by eating birds that ate the berries*

**mezilamine** INN

**Mezlin** powder for IV or IM injection (discontinued 2004) ℞ *extended-spectrum penicillin antibiotic* [mezlocillin sodium] 1, 2, 3, 4, 20 g/vial ⊡ Meclan

**mezlocillin** USAN, INN *extended-spectrum penicillin antibiotic*

**mezlocillin sodium** USP *extended-spectrum penicillin antibiotic*

**MF (methotrexate [with leucovorin rescue], fluorouracil)** *chemotherapy protocol for breast cancer*

**MF (mitomycin, fluorouracil)** *chemotherapy protocol*

**MFP (melphalan, fluorouracil, medroxyprogesterone acetate)** *chemotherapy protocol*

**MG Cold Sore Formula** solution OTC *topical oral anesthetic; antipruritic/counterirritant* [lidocaine; menthol] ⨪ •1%

**MG217 Dual Treatment** lotion (name changed to MG217 Medicated Tar in 2000)

**MG217 Medicated** conditioner (discontinued 2003) OTC *antipsoriatic; antiseborrheic* [coal tar solution] 2%

**MG217 Medicated** ointment OTC *antipsoriatic; antiseborrheic; antifungal; keratolytic* [coal tar solution; colloidal sulfur; salicylic acid] 2%•1.1%•1.5%

**MG217 Medicated** shampoo (discontinued 2003) OTC *antipsoriatic; antiseborrheic; antifungal; keratolytic* [coal tar solution; salicylic acid] 5%•2%

**MG217 Medicated Tar** lotion, ointment OTC *antipsoriatic; antiseborrheic* [coal tar solution] 1%; 2%

**MG217 Medicated Tar** shampoo OTC *antiseborrheic; antipsoriatic; antipruritic; antibacterial* [coal tar] 3%

**MG217 Medicated Tar-Free** shampoo OTC *antiseborrheic; keratolytic* [sulfur; salicylic acid] 5%•3%

**MG217 Sal-Acid** ointment OTC *antipsoriatic; keratolytic* [salicylic acid] 3%

**MG400** shampoo OTC *antiseborrheic; keratolytic* [salicylic acid; sulfur] 3%•5%

**MGA (melengestrol acetate)** [q.v.]

**MGBG (methylglyoxal-*bis*-guanyl-hydrazone)** [see: mitoguazone]

**MGI-114** *investigational (Phase II) antineoplastic for hormone-refractory prostate and ovarian cancers*

**MGW (magnesium sulfate + glycerin + water) enema** [q.v.]

**MHP-A** tablets ℞ *urinary antibiotic; antiseptic; analgesic; antispasmodic* [methenamine; phenyl salicylate; methylene blue; benzoic acid; atropine sulfate; hyoscyamine sulfate] 40.8•18.1•5.4•4.5•0.03•0.03 mg

**Miacalcin** nasal spray ℞ *calcium regulator for postmenopausal osteoporosis (only)* [calcitonin (salmon)] 200 IU/0.09 mL dose

**Miacalcin** subcu or IM injection ℞ *calcium regulator for Paget disease (orphan), hypercalcemia, and postmenopausal osteoporosis* [calcitonin (salmon)] 200 IU/mL

**Mi-Acid** gelcaps OTC *antacid* [calcium carbonate; magnesium carbonate] 311•232 mg

**Mi-Acid; Mi-Acid II** oral liquid OTC *antacid; antiflatulent* [aluminum hydroxide; magnesium hydroxide; simethicone] 200•200•20 mg/5 mL; 400•400•40 mg/5 mL

**mianserin** INN, BAN *serotonin inhibitor; antihistamine* [also: mianserin HCl]

**mianserin HCl** USAN, JAN *serotonin inhibitor; antihistamine* [also: mianserin]

**mibefradil** INN *vasodilator and calcium channel blocker for hypertension and chronic stable angina* [also: mibefradil dihydrochloride]

**mibefradil dihydrochloride** USAN *vasodilator and calcium channel blocker for hypertension and chronic stable angina* [also: mibefradil]

**M$^{131}$IBG** [now: iobenguane sulfate I 131]

**MIBG-I-123** [see: iobenguane sulfate I 123]

**mibolerone** USAN, INN *anabolic; androgen*

**micafungin** *investigational (Phase III) echinocandin antifungal agent*

**Micanol** Ⓒᴬᴺ cream OTC *antipsoriatic* [anthralin] 1%, 3%

**Micardis** tablets ℞ *long-acting antihypertensive; angiotensin II receptor antagonist* [telmisartan] 20, 40, 80 mg

**Micardis HCT** tablets ℞ *long-acting antihypertensive; angiotensin II receptor antagonist; diuretic* [telmisartan; hydrochlorothiazide] 40•12.5, 80•12.5 mg

**Micardis Plus** Ⓒᴬᴺ tablets ℞ *long-acting antihypertensive; angiotensin II receptor antagonist; diuretic* [telmisartan; hydrochlorothiazide] 80•12.5 mg

**Micatin** cream, powder, spray powder, spray liquid OTC *antifungal* [miconazole nitrate] 2%

**MICE (mesna [rescue], ifosfamide, carboplatin, etoposide)** *chemotherapy protocol for osteosarcoma and lung cancer* [also: ICE]

**micinicate** INN

**Miconal** cream ℞ *topical antipsoriatic* [anthralin] 1%

**miconazole** USP, INN, BAN, JAN *fungicidal*

**Miconazole 7** vaginal suppositories OTC *antifungal* [miconazole nitrate] 100 mg

**miconazole nitrate** USAN, USP, JAN *antifungal* 2% topical

**Micrainin** tablets ℞ *analgesic; antipyretic; anti-inflammatory; anxiolytic;*

*sedative* [aspirin; meprobamate] 325• 200 mg

**MICRhoGAM** IM injection, prefilled syringes ℞ *obstetric Rh factor immunity suppressant* [Rh$_O$(D) immune globulin (gamma globulin)] 50 μg (5%) ⍰ microgram

**microbubble contrast agent** *investigational (orphan) neurosonographic diagnostic aid for intracranial tumors*

**Microcaps** (trademarked dosage form) *fast-melting tablets*

**microcrystalline cellulose** [see: cellulose, microcrystalline]

**microcrystalline wax** [see: wax, microcrystalline]

**microfibrillar collagen hemostat (MCH)** *topical local hemostatic*

**Microgestin Fe 1/20; Microgestin Fe 1.5/30** tablets (in packs of 28) ℞ *monophasic oral contraceptive; iron supplement* [norethindrone acetate; ethinyl estradiol; ferrous fumarate] 1 mg• 20 μg•75 mg; 1.5 mg•30 μg•75 mg

**Micro-K; Micro-K 10** Extencaps (controlled-release capsules) ℞ *potassium supplement* [potassium chloride] 600 mg (8 mEq K); 750 mg (10 mEq K)

**Micro-K LS** extended-release powder for oral solution ℞ *potassium supplement* [potassium chloride] 20 mEq K/ pkt.

**MicroKlenz** topical liqid OTC *antiseptic wound cleanser* [acemannan]

**Microlipid** emulsion OTC *dietary fat supplement* [safflower oil] 50%

**Micronase** tablets ℞ *sulfonylurea antidiabetic* [glyburide] 1.25, 2.5, 5 mg

**microNefrin** solution for inhalation OTC *sympathomimetic bronchodilator for bronchial asthma and COPD* [racepinephrine HCl] 2.25%

**micronized aluminum** *astringent*

**Micronized Glyburide** tablets ℞ *sulfonylurea antidiabetic* [glyburide] 1.5, 3 mg

**micronomicin** INN

**Micronor** [see: Ortho Micronor]

**Microstix-3** reagent strips for professional use *in vitro diagnostic aid for nitrate, uropathogens, or bacteria in the urine*

**MicroTrak** *Chlamydia trachomatis* slide test for professional use *in vitro diagnostic aid for* Chlamydia trachomatis

**MicroTrak HSV 1/HSV 2 Culture Identification/Typing Test** culture test for professional use *in vitro diagnostic aid for herpes simplex virus in tissue cultures*

**MicroTrak HSV 1/HSV 2 Direct Specimen Identification/Typing Test** slide test for professional use *in vitro diagnostic aid for herpes simplex virus in external lesions*

**MicroTrak** *Neisseria gonorrhoeae* **Culture Confirmation Test** reagent kit for professional use *in vitro diagnostic aid for* Neisseria gonorrhoeae

**Microzide** capsules ℞ *once-daily antihypertensive; thiazide diuretic* [hydrochlorothiazide] 12.5 mg ⃞ Maxzide

**mictine** [see: aminometradine]

**midaflur** USAN, INN *sedative*

**midaglizole** INN

**midalcipran** [see: milnacipran]

**midamaline** INN

**Midamor** tablets ℞ *antihypertensive; potassium-sparing diuretic* [amiloride HCl] 5 mg

**midazogrel** INN

**midazolam** INN, BAN, JAN *short-acting benzodiazepine general anesthetic* [also: midazolam HCl]

**midazolam HCl** USAN *short-acting benzodiazepine general anesthetic* [also: midazolam] 1, 5 mg/mL injection

**midazolam maleate** USAN *intravenous anesthetic*

**Midchlor** capsules (discontinued 2000) ℞ *cerebral vasoconstrictor and analgesic for vascular and tension headaches; "possibly effective" for migraine headaches* [isometheptene mucate; dichloralphenazone; acetaminophen] 65•100•325 mg

**midecamycin** INN

**midodrine** INN, BAN *antihypotensive; vasoconstrictor; vasopressor for orthostatic hypotension (OH)* [also: midodrine HCl]

**midodrine HCl** USAN, JAN *antihypotensive; vasoconstrictor; vasopressor for orthostatic hypotension (orphan)* [also: midodrine] 2.5, 5, 10 mg oral

**Midol, Maximum Strength Cramp Formula** tablets OTC *analgesic; antiarthritic; antipyretic; nonsteroidal anti-inflammatory drug (NSAID)* [ibuprofen] 200 mg

**Midol Maximum Strength Menstrual** caplets, gelcaps OTC *analgesic; anti-inflammatory; antihistaminic sleep aid* [acetaminophen; caffeine; pyrilamine maleate] 500•60•15 mg

**Midol Multi-Symptom Formula** caplets (discontinued 2000) OTC *analgesic; anti-inflammatory; antihistaminic sleep aid* [acetaminophen; pyrilamine maleate] 325•12.5 mg

**Midol Multi-Symptom Menstrual** caplets (name changed to Midol Maximum Strength Menstrual in 2000)

**Midol PM** caplets OTC *analgesic; antipyretic; antihistaminic sleep aid* [acetaminophen; diphenhydramine] 500•25 mg

**Midol PMS** caplets, gelcaps OTC *analgesic; anti-inflammatory; diuretic; antihistaminic sleep aid* [acetaminophen; pamabrom; pyrilamine maleate] 500•25•15 mg

**Midol Teen** caplets OTC *analgesic; anti-inflammatory; diuretic* [acetaminophen; pamabrom] 500•25 mg

**Midrin** capsules ℞ *cerebral vasoconstrictor and analgesic for vascular and tension headaches; "possibly effective" for migraine headaches* [isometheptene mucate; dichloralphenazone; acetaminophen] 65•100•325 mg ⃞ Mydfrin

**Midstream Pregnancy Test** kit for home use *in vitro diagnostic aid; urine pregnancy test*

**MIFA (mitomycin, fluorouracil, Adriamycin)** *chemotherapy protocol*

**mifarmonab** [see: imciromab pentetate]

**Mifegyne** (European name for U.S. product Mifeprex)

**mifentidine** INN

**Mifeprex** tablets ℞ *abortifacient; postcoital contraceptive; progesterone antagonist investigational for meningioma, endometriosis, and Cushing syndrome* [mifepristone] 200 mg (note: not available to pharmacies; must be obtained from a physician in an office, clinic, or hospital setting)

**mifepristone** USAN, INN, BAN *abortifacient; postcoital contraceptive; progesterone antagonist investigational for meningioma, endometriosis, and Cushing syndrome*

**mifobate** USAN, INN *antiatherosclerotic*

**miglitol** USAN, INN, BAN *antidiabetic agent for type 2 diabetes; alpha-glucosidase inhibitor that delays the digestion of dietary carbohydrates*

**miglustat** *glucosylceramide synthase inhibitor; substrate reduction therapy (SRT) to reduce the glycosphingolipid (GSL) production in type I Gaucher disease*

**mignonette, Jamaica** *medicinal herb* [see: henna *(Lawsonia)*]

**Migranal** nasal spray ℞ *rapid-acting antimigraine agent* [dihydroergotamine mesylate] 0.05 mg/spray

**Migratine** capsules ℞ *cerebral vasoconstrictor and analgesic for vascular and tension headaches; "possibly effective" for migraine headaches* [isomethepptene mucate; dichloralphenazone; acetaminophen] 65•100•325 mg

**mikamycin** INN, BAN

**MiKasome** ℞ *investigational (Phase II) antibiotic liposomal formulation for complicated urinary tract infections and AIDS-related mycobacterial infections* [amikacin]

**milacemide** INN *anticonvulsant; antidepressant* [also: milacemide HCl]

**milacemide HCl** USAN *anticonvulsant; antidepressant* [also: milacemide]

**milameline HCl** USAN *partial muscarinic agonist for Alzheimer disease*

**mild silver protein** [see: silver protein, mild]

**milenperone** USAN, INN, BAN *antipsychotic*

**Miles Nervine** caplets OTC *antihistaminic sleep aid* [diphenhydramine HCl] 25 mg

**milfoil** *medicinal herb* [see: yarrow]

**milipertine** USAN, INN *antipsychotic*

**milk ipecac** *medicinal herb* [see: birthroot; dogbane]

**milk of bismuth** [see: bismuth, milk of]

**milk of magnesia** [see: magnesia, milk of]

**Milk of Magnesia-Cascara, Concentrated** oral suspension OTC *antacid; saline/stimulant laxative* [milk of magnesia; aromatic cascara fluidextract; alcohol 7%] 30•5 mL/15 mL

**milk thistle (Silybum marianum)** seeds *medicinal herb for Amanita mushroom poisoning, bronchitis, gallbladder disorders, hemorrhage, liver damage, peritonitis, spleen disorders, stomach disorders, and varicose veins*

**Milkinol** emulsion (discontinued 2000) OTC *emollient laxative* [mineral oil]

**milkweed (Asclepias syriaca)** roots *medicinal herb used as a diuretic, emetic, purgative, and tonic*

**milnacipran** INN *investigational (Phase III) serotonin and norepinephrine reuptake inhibitor for depression and fibromyalgia syndrome*

**milodistim** USAN *antineutropenic; hematopoietic stimulant; granulocyte macrophage colony-stimulating factor (GM-CSF) + interleukin 3*

**Milontin** Kapseals (capsules) (discontinued 2002) ℞ *succinimide anticonvulsant* [phensuximide] 500 mg ⊇ Dilantin; Miltown; Mylanta

**miloxacin** INN

**milrinone** USAN, INN, BAN *cardiotonic*

**milrinone lactate** *vasodilator for congestive heart failure* 1 mg/mL injection

**miltefosine** INN

**Miltown** tablets ℞ *anxiolytic; also abused as a street drug* [meprobamate] 200, 400 mg ⊇ Milontin

**Miltown-600** tablets (discontinued 2001) ℞ *anxiolytic; also abused as a*

*street drug* [meprobamate] 600 mg ⑨
Milontin

**milverine** INN

**mimbane** INN *analgesic* [also: mimbane HCl]

**mimbane HCl** USAN *analgesic* [also: mimbane]

**minalrestat** USAN *aldose reductase inhibitor for diabetic neuropathy and other long-term diabetic complications*

**minaprine** USAN, INN, BAN *psychotropic*

**minaprine HCl** USAN *antidepressant*

**minaxolone** USAN, INN *anesthetic*

**mindodilol** INN

**mindolic acid** [see: clometacin]

**mindoperone** INN

**MINE (mesna [rescue], ifosfamide, Novantrone, etoposide)** *chemotherapy protocol for non-Hodgkin lymphoma*

**MINE-ESHAP (alternating cycles of MINE and ESHAP)** *chemotherapy protocol for non-Hodgkin lymphoma*

**minepentate** INN, BAN

**Mineral Ice** [see: Therapeutic Mineral Ice]

**mineral oil** USP *emollient/protectant; laxative; solvent*

**mineral oil, light** NF *tablet and capsule lubricant; vehicle*

**mineralocorticoids** *a class of adrenal cortical steroids that are used for partial replacement therapy in adrenocortical insufficiency*

**Mini Thin Asthma Relief** tablets (discontinued 2000) OTC *decongestant; expectorant* [ephedrine HCl; guaifenesin] 25•100, 25•200 mg

**Mini Thin Pseudo** tablets (discontinued 2000) OTC *nasal decongestant* [pseudoephedrine HCl] 60 mg

**Mini Two-Way Action** tablets OTC *bronchodilator; decongestant; expectorant* [ephedrine HCl; guaifenesin] 12.5•200, 25•200 mg

**MiniAdFVIII** ℞ *investigational (orphan) agent for hemophilia A* [adenovirus-based vector Factor VIII complementary DNA to somatic cells]

**mini-BEAM (BCNU, etoposide, ara-C, melphalan)** *chemotherapy protocol for Hodgkin lymphoma*

**mini-COAP (cyclophosphamide, Oncovin, ara-C, prednisone)** *chemotherapy protocol*

**Minidyne** solution OTC *broad-spectrum antimicrobial* [povidone-iodine] 10%

**Mini-Gamulin Rh** IM injection (discontinued 2000) ℞ *obstetric Rh factor immunity suppressant* [Rh$_O$(D) immune globulin] 50 μg

**Min-I-Mix** (delivery system) *dual-chambered prefilled syringe*

**Minipress** capsules ℞ *antihypertensive; α$_1$-adrenergic blocker* [prazosin HCl] 1, 2, 5 mg

**Minirin** nasal spray ℞ *posterior pituitary hormone for hemophilia A (orphan), von Willebrand disease (orphan), central diabetes insipidus, and nocturnal enuresis* [desmopressin acetate; chlorobutanol] 10•500 μg/dose

**Minitran** transdermal patch ℞ *antianginal; vasodilator* [nitroglycerin] 9, 18, 36, 54 mg (0.1, 0.2, 0.4, 0.6 mg/hr.)

**Minit-Rub** OTC *analgesic; counterirritant* [methyl salicylate; menthol; camphor] 15%•3.5%•2.3%

**Minizide 1; Minizide 2; Minizide 5** capsules ℞ *antihypertensive; α-blocker; diuretic* [prazosin HCl; polythiazide] 1•0.5 mg; 2•0.5 mg; 5•0.5 mg

**Minocin** pellet-filled capsules, oral suspension ℞ *tetracycline antibiotic* [minocycline HCl] 50, 100 mg; 50 mg/5 mL ⑨ Indocin; Mithracin; niacin

**Minocin** powder for IV injection ℞ *tetracycline antibiotic* [minocycline] 100 mg/vial ⑨ Indocin; Mithracin; niacin

**minocromil** USAN, INN, BAN *prophylactic antiallergic*

**minocycline** USAN, INN, BAN *gram-negative and gram-positive bacteriostatic; antirickettsial*

**minocycline HCl** USP *gram-negative and gram-positive bacteriostatic; antirickettsial; adjunct to scaling and root planing for periodontitis* 50, 75, 100 mg oral

**Minox** ⓒ topical solution OTC *hair growth stimulant* [minoxidil] 2%

**minoxidil** USAN, USP, INN, BAN *antihypertensive; peripheral vasodilator; hair growth stimulant* 2.5, 10 mg oral

**Minoxidil for Men** topical solution OTC *hair growth stimulant* [minoxidil; alcohol 60%] 2%, 5%

**mint; lamb mint; mackerel mint; Our Lady's mint** *medicinal herb* [see: spearmint]

**mint, brandy; lamb mint** *medicinal herb* [see: peppermint]

**mint, mountain** *medicinal herb* [see: marjoram; Oswego tea]

**mint, squaw** *medicinal herb* [see: pennyroyal]

**Mintezol** chewable tablets, oral suspension Ŗ *anthelmintic for strongyloidiasis (threadworm), larva migrans, and trichinosis* [thiabendazole] 500 mg; 500 mg/5 mL

**Mintox** chewable tablets, oral suspension OTC *antacid* [aluminum hydroxide; magnesium hydroxide] 200•200 mg; 225•200 mg/5 mL

**Mintox Plus** oral liquid OTC *antacid; antiflatulent* [aluminum hydroxide; magnesium hydroxide; simethicone] 500•450•40 mg/5 mL

**Minute-Gel** Ŗ *topical dental caries preventative* [acidulated phosphate fluoride] 1.23%

**Miochol-E** solution Ŗ *direct-acting miotic for ophthalmic surgery* [acetylcholine chloride] 1:100

**mioflazine** INN, BAN *coronary vasodilator* [also: mioflazine HCl]

**mioflazine HCl** USAN *coronary vasodilator* [also: mioflazine]

**Miostat** solution Ŗ *direct-acting miotic for ophthalmic surgery* [carbachol] 0.01%

**miotics** *a class of drugs that cause the pupil of the eye to contract*

**mipafilcon A** USAN *hydrophilic contact lens material*

**mipimazole** INN

**Miradon** tablets (discontinued 2003) Ŗ *indanedione-derivative anticoagulant* [anisindione] 50 mg

**MiraFlow** solution OTC *cleaning solution for hard or soft contact lenses*

**MiraForte** [see: Super MiraForte with Chrysin]

**MiraLax** powder for oral solution Ŗ *hyperosmotic laxative; pre-procedure bowel evacuant* [polyethylene glycol 3350] 17 g/dose

**Mirapex** tablets Ŗ *dopamine agonist; antiparkinsonian* [pramipexole dihydrochloride] 0.125, 0.25, 0.5, 1, 1.5 mg

**Miraphen PSE** extended-release tablets Ŗ *decongestant; expectorant* [pseudoephedrine HCl; guaifenesin] 120•600 mg

**MiraSept Step 2** solution OTC *rinsing/storage solution for soft contact lenses* [sodium chloride (preserved saline solution)]

**MiraSept System** solutions OTC *two-step chemical disinfecting system for soft contact lenses* [hydrogen peroxide based] 3%

**Mircette** tablets (in packs of 28) Ŗ *biphasic oral contraceptive* [desogestrel; ethinyl estradiol]
Phase 1 (21 days): 150•20 μg;
Phase 2 (5 days): 0•10 μg

**Mirena** intrauterine device (IUD) Ŗ *long-term (5 year) contraceptive insert* [levonorgestrel] 20 μg/day

**Mireze** ⓒ eye drops (name changed to Alocril in 2001)

**mirfentanil** INN *analgesic* [also: mirfentanil HCl]

**mirfentanil HCl** USAN *analgesic* [also: mirfentanil]

**mirincamycin** INN *antibacterial; antimalarial* [also: mirincamycin HCl]

**mirincamycin HCl** USAN *antibacterial; antimalarial* [also: mirincamycin]

**mirisetron maleate** USAN *anxiolytic*

**miristalkonium chloride** INN

**miroprofen** INN

**mirosamicin** INN

**mirostipen** USAN *myeloprotectant*

**mirtazapine** USAN, INN *tetracyclic antidepressant; serotonin 5-HT$_{1A}$ agonist* 15, 30, 45 mg oral

**misonidazole** USAN, INN *antiprotozoal (Trichomonas)*

**misoprostol** USAN, INN, BAN *prevents NSAID-induced gastric ulcers; has been used for cervical ripening and induction of labor; use by pregnant women can cause abortion, premature birth, or birth defects* 100, 200 μg oral

**Mission Prenatal; Mission Prenatal F.A.; Mission Prenatal H.P.** tablets OTC *vitamin/iron supplement* [multiple vitamins; ferrous gluconate; folic acid] ≟•30•0.4 mg; ≟• 30•0.8 mg; ≟•30•0.8 mg

**Mission Prenatal Rx** tablets R *vitamin/calcium/iron supplement* [multiple vitamins; calcium; iron; folic acid] ≟•175•29.5•1 mg

**Mission Surgical Supplement** tablets OTC *vitamin/iron supplement* [multiple vitamins; ferrous gluconate] ≟•27 mg

**mistletoe (Phoradendron flavescens; P. serotinum; P. tomentosum; Viscum album)** plant *medicinal herb for cancer, chorea, epilepsy, hypertension, internal hemorrhages, menstrual disorders, nervousness, poor circulation, and spleen disorders; not generally regarded as safe and effective for ingestion as it is highly toxic*

**Mistometer** (trademarked form) *metered-dose inhalation aerosol*

**Mitchella repens** *medicinal herb* [see: squaw vine]

**Mithracin** powder for IV infusion (discontinued 2002) R *antibiotic antineoplastic for testicular cancer* [plicamycin] 2.5 mg ⸰ Minocin

**mithramycin** [now: plicamycin] ⸰ mitomycin

**mitindomide** USAN, INN *antineoplastic*

**mitobronitol** INN, BAN

**mitocarcin** USAN, INN *antineoplastic*

**mitoclomine** INN, BAN

**mitocromin** USAN *antineoplastic*

**mitoflaxone** INN

**mitogillin** USAN, INN *antineoplastic*

**mitoguazone** INN *investigational antineoplastic for multiple myeloma and head, esophagus, and prostate cancer;* *investigational (orphan) for non-Hodgkin lymphoma*

**mitolactol** INN *investigational (orphan) antineoplastic for brain tumors and recurrent or metastatic cervical squamous cell carcinoma*

**mitomalcin** USAN, INN *antineoplastic*

**mitomycin** USAN, USP, INN, BAN *antibiotic antineoplastic; investigational (orphan) for refractory glaucoma and glaucoma surgery* 5, 20, 40 mg injection ⸰ mithramycin; Mutamycin

**mitomycin C (MTC)** [see: mitomycin]

**mitonafide** INN

**mitopodozide** INN, BAN

**mitoquidone** INN, BAN

**mitosper** USAN, INN *antineoplastic*

**mitotane** USAN, USP, INN *antibiotic antineoplastic for inoperable adrenal cortical carcinoma and Cushing syndrome*

**mitotenamine** INN, BAN

**mitotic inhibitors** *a class of antineoplastics that inhibit cell division (mitosis)*

**mitoxantrone** INN *antibiotic antineoplastic* [also: mitoxantrone HCl; mitozantrone]

**mitoxantrone HCl** USAN *antibiotic antineoplastic for prostate cancer and acute nonlymphocytic leukemia (ANLL) (orphan); immunomodulator for progressive and relapsing-remitting multiple sclerosis* [also: mitoxantrone; mitozantrone]

**mitozantrone** BAN *antineoplastic* [also: mitoxantrone HCl; mitoxantrone]

**mitozolomide** INN, BAN

**Mitran** capsules (discontinued 2003) R *benzodiazepine anxiolytic; sedative* [chlordiazepoxide HCl] 10 mg

**Mitrolan** chewable tablets (discontinued 2004) OTC *bulk laxative; antidiarrheal* [calcium polycarbophil] 625 mg

**mitronal** [see: cinnarizine]

**mitumomab** USAN *antineoplastic monoclonal antibody for $G_{D3}$ ganglioside-expressing tumors; investigational (Phase III) for small cell lung cancer*

**MIV (mitoxantrone, ifosfamide, VePesid)** *chemotherapy protocol*

**Mivacron** IV infusion ℞ *muscle relaxant; adjunct to anesthesia* [mivacurium chloride] 0.5, 2 mg/mL

**mivacurium chloride** USAN, INN, BAN *neuromuscular blocking agent*

**mivobulin isethionate** USAN *antineoplastic; mitotic inhibitor; tubulin binder*

**Mixed E 400; Mixed E 1000** softgels OTC *vitamin supplement* [vitamin E] 400 IU; 1000 IU

**mixed respiratory vaccine (MRV)** *active bacterin for respiratory tract infections*

**mixed tocopherols** [see: vitamin E]

**mixidine** USAN, INN *coronary vasodilator*

**Mix-O-Vial** (trademarked packaging form) *two-compartment vial*

**mizoribine** INN

**MK-663** *investigational (Phase III) agent for osteoarthritis*

**MK-826** *investigational (NDA filed) broad-spectrum carbapenem antibiotic*

**MKC-442** *investigational (Phase III) non-nucleoside reverse transcriptase inhibitor (NNRTI) for HIV and AIDS*

**ML-3000** *investigational (Phase II) anti-inflammatory and analgesic*

**MM (mercaptopurine, methotrexate)** *chemotherapy protocol*

**MMOPP (methotrexate, mechlorethamine, Oncovin, procarbazine, prednisone)** *chemotherapy protocol*

**MMP (matrix metalloproteinase) inhibitors** [q.v.]

**MMR (measles, mumps & rubella vaccines)** [q.v.]

**M-M-R II** powder for subcu injection ℞ *measles, mumps and rubella vaccine* [measles, mumps, and rubella virus vaccine, live] 0.5 mL

**MOB (mechlorethamine, Oncovin, bleomycin)** *chemotherapy protocol*

**MOB-III (mitomycin, Oncovin, bleomycin, cisplatin)** *chemotherapy protocol*

**Moban** oral concentrate (discontinued 2003) ℞ *conventional (typical) antipsychotic* [molindone HCl] 20 mg/mL ② Mobidin; Modane

**Moban** tablets ℞ *conventional (typical) antipsychotic* [molindone HCl] 5, 10, 25, 50 mg ② Mobidin; Modane

**mobecarb** INN

**mobenzoxamine** INN

**Mobic** tablets ℞ *once-daily analgesic, antiarthritic, and antipyretic; COX-2 inhibitor; nonsteroidal anti-inflammatory drug (NSAID)* [meloxicam] 7.5, 15 mg

**Mobicox** ⓒ tablets ℞ *once-daily analgesic, antiarthritic, and antipyretic; COX-2 inhibitor; nonsteroidal anti-inflammatory drug (NSAID)* [meloxicam] 7.5, 15 mg

**Mobidin** tablets ℞ *analgesic; antipyretic; anti-inflammatory; antirheumatic* [magnesium salicylate] 600 mg ② Moban

**Mobigesic** tablets OTC *analgesic; antipyretic; anti-inflammatory; antihistaminic sleep aid* [magnesium salicylate; phenyltoloxamine citrate] 325•30 mg

**Mobist** ℞ *investigational neuroprotectant*

**Mobisyl Creme** OTC *topical analgesic* [trolamine salicylate] 10%

**MOBP (mitomycin, Oncovin, bleomycin, Platinol)** *chemotherapy protocol for cervical cancer*

**moccasin snake antivenin** [see: antivenin (Crotalidae) polyvalent]

**mocimycin** INN

**mociprazine** INN

**mock pennyroyal** *medicinal herb* [see: pennyroyal]

**moclobemide** USAN, INN, BAN *antidepressant; MAO inhibitor*

**moctamide** INN

**Moctanin** biliary infusion ℞ *anticholelithogenic for dissolution of cholesterol gallstones (orphan)* [monoctanoin]

**modafinil** USAN, INN *analeptic for excessive daytime sleepiness (orphan); investigational for fatigue associated with multiple sclerosis*

**modaline** INN *antidepressant* [also: modaline sulfate]

**modaline sulfate** USAN *antidepressant* [also: modaline]

**Modane** enteric-coated tablets OTC *stimulant laxative* [bisacodyl] 5 mg ② Moban; Mudrane

**Modane Bulk** powder (discontinued 2003) OTC *bulk laxative* [psyllium husk] 3.4 g/tsp.

**Modane Soft** capsules (discontinued 2003) OTC *laxative; stool softener* [docusate sodium] 100 mg

**modecainide** USAN, INN *antiarrhythmic*

**Modecate** ⒸⒶⓃ subcu or IM injection ℞ *conventional (typical) antipsychotic* [fluphenazine decanoate] 25, 100 mg/mL

**Modicon** tablets (in Dialpaks and Veridates of 28) ℞ *monophasic oral contraceptive* [norethindrone; ethinyl estradiol] 0.5 mg•35 μg Ⓘ Mylicon

**modified Bagshawe protocol** *chemotherapy protocol* [see: CHAMOCA]

**modified bovine lung surfactant extract** [see: beractant]

**modified Burow solution** [see: aluminum acetate solution]

**modified cellulose gum** [now: croscarmellose sodium]

**modified Shohl solution (sodium citrate & citric acid)** *urinary alkalinizer; compounding agent*

**Modiodal** (foreign name for U.S. product Provigil)

**Moditen Enanthate** ⒸⒶⓃ subcu or IM injection ℞ *conventional (typical) antipsychotic* [fluphenazine enanthate] 25 mg/mL

**Moditen HCl** ⒸⒶⓃ tablets ℞ *conventional (typical) antipsychotic* [fluphenazine HCl] 10 mg

**Moducal** powder OTC *carbohydrate caloric supplement* [glucose polymers]

**Moduretic** tablets ℞ *antihypertensive; diuretic* [amiloride HCl; hydrochlorothiazide] 5•50 mg

**moexipril** INN, BAN *antihypertensive; angiotensin-converting enzyme (ACE) inhibitor*

**moexipril HCl** USAN *antihypertensive; angiotensin-converting enzyme (ACE) inhibitor* 7.5, 15 mg oral

**moexiprilat** INN

**MOF (MeCCNU, Oncovin, fluorouracil)** *chemotherapy protocol*

**mofebutazone** INN

**mofedione** [see: oxazidione]

**mofegiline** INN *antiparkinsonian* [also: mofegiline HCl]

**mofegiline HCl** USAN *antiparkinsonian* [also: mofegiline]

**mofetil** USAN, INN *combining name for radicals or groups*

**mofloverine** INN

**mofoxime** INN

**MOF-STREP; MOF-Strep (MeCCNU, Oncovin, fluorouracil, streptozocin)** *chemotherapy protocol*

**Mogadon** (approved in Canada and Europe) ℞ *investigational benzodiazepine tranquilizer; anxiolytic; anticonvulsant; hypnotic* [nitrazepam]

**moguisteine** INN

**Moist Again** vaginal gel OTC *lubricant* [glycerin; aloe vera]

**Moi-Stir** oral spray, Swabsticks OTC *saliva substitute* Ⓘ moisture

**Moisture Drops** eye drops OTC *ophthalmic moisturizer/lubricant* [hydroxypropyl methylcellulose] 0.5%

**Moisture Eyes** eye drops OTC *ocular moisturizer/lubricant* [propylene glycol] 0.95%

**molfarnate** INN

**molgramostim** USAN, INN, BAN *antineutropenic; hematopoietic stimulant; investigational (Phase II/III) cytokine to AIDS*

**molinazone** USAN, INN *analgesic*

**molindone** INN *dihydroindolone antipsychotic* [also: molindone HCl]

**molindone HCl** USAN *dihydroindolone antipsychotic* [also: molindone]

**Mollifene Ear Wax Removing Formula** drops OTC *agent to emulsify and disperse ear wax* [carbamide peroxide] 6.5%

**molracetam** INN

**molsidomine** USAN, INN *antianginal; coronary vasodilator*

**molybdenum** *element (Mo)*

**Molypen** IV injection ℞ *intravenous nutritional therapy* [ammonium molybdate tetrahydrate] 25 μg/mL

**Momentum** caplets OTC *analgesic; antipyretic; anti-inflammatory; antihis-*

*tamine* [aspirin; phenyltoloxamine citrate] 500•15 mg

**Momentum Muscular Backache Formula** caplets OTC *analgesic; antipyretic; anti-inflammatory* [magnesium salicylate] 580 mg

**mometasone** INN, BAN *topical corticosteroidal anti-inflammatory* [also: mometasone furoate]

**mometasone furoate** USAN *topical corticosteroidal anti-inflammatory; inhalation aerosol for allergic rhinitis* [also: mometasone]

*Momordica charantia* medicinal herb [see: bitter melon]

**MOMP (mechlorethamine, Oncovin, methotrexate, prednisone)** *chemotherapy protocol*

**Monafed** sustained-release tablets (discontinued 2002) ℞ *expectorant* [guaifenesin] 600 mg

**Monafed DM** tablets (discontinued 2002) ℞ *antitussive; expectorant* [dextromethorphan hydrobromide; guaifenesin] 30•600 mg

**monalazone disodium** INN

**monalium hydrate** [see: magaldrate]

**Monarc-M** powder for IV injection ℞ *antihemophilic* [antihemophilic factor VIII, solvent/detergent-treated and monoclonal purified] 10–15 IU

*Monarda didyma* medicinal herb [see: Oswego tea]

*Monarda fistulosa* medicinal herb [see: wild bergamot]

*Monarda punctata* medicinal herb [see: horsemint]

**monascus yeast (Monascus purpureus)** *natural remedy for gastric disorders, indigestion, lowering cholesterol, and poor circulation*

**monatepil** INN *antianginal; antihypertensive* [also: monatepil maleate]

**monatepil maleate** USAN *antianginal; antihypertensive* [also: monatepil]

**monensin** USAN, INN *antiprotozoal; antibacterial; antifungal*

**Monistat** cream OTC *antifungal* [miconazole nitrate] 2%

**Monistat 1** vaginal ointment in prefilled applicator OTC *antifungal* [tioconazole] 6.5%

**Monistat 1 Combination Pack** vaginal inserts + cream OTC *antifungal* [miconazole nitrate] 200 mg + 2%

**Monistat 1-Day** vaginal ointment in prefilled applicator OTC *antifungal* [tioconazole] 6.5%

**Monistat 3** vaginal cream, combination pack (vaginal inserts + cream), cream combination pak (vaginal cream in prefilled applicators + external cream) OTC *antifungal* [miconazole nitrate] 2%; 200 mg + 2%; 4% + 2%

**Monistat 3** vaginal inserts (discontinued 2001) OTC *antifungal* [miconazole nitrate] 200 mg

**Monistat 7** vaginal inserts, vaginal cream, combination pack (inserts + cream) OTC *antifungal* [miconazole nitrate] 100 mg; 2%; 100 mg + 2%

**Monistat Dual-Pak** vaginal inserts + cream (name changed to Monistat 1 Combination Pack in 2001)

**Monistat-Derm** cream ℞ *antifungal* [miconazole nitrate] 2%

**mono- & di-acetylated monoglycerides** NF *plasticizer*

**mono- & di-glycerides** NF *emulsifying agent*

**monoamine oxidase inhibitors (MAOIs)** *a class of antidepressants that increase CNS monoamine neurotransmitters (epinephrine, norepinephrine, and serotonin)*

**monobactams** *a class of bactericidal antibiotics effective against gram-negative aerobic pathogens*

**monobasic potassium phosphate** [see: potassium phosphate, monobasic]

**monobasic sodium phosphate** [see: sodium phosphate, monobasic]

**monobenzone** USP, INN *depigmenting agent for vitiligo*

**monobenzyl ether of hydroquinone** [see: monobenzone]

**monobromated camphor** [see: camphor, monobromated]

**Monocal** tablets OTC *calcium/fluoride supplement* [calcium; fluoride] 250• 3 mg

**monocalcium phosphate** [see: calcium phosphate, dibasic]

**Monocaps** tablets OTC *vitamin/mineral/ iron supplement* [multiple vitamins & minerals; ferrous fumerate; folic acid; biotin] ±•14 mg•0.1 mg•15 µg ⊠ Monoclate; Monoket

**Mono-Chlor** topical liquid ℞ *cauterant; keratolytic* [monochloroacetic acid] 80%

**monochloroacetic acid** *strong keratolytic/cauterant*

**monochlorothymol** [see: chlorothymol]

**monochlorphenamide** [see: clofenamide]

**Monocid** powder for IV or IM injection (discontinued 2004) ℞ *cephalosporin antibiotic* [cefonicid sodium] 1, 10 g ⊠ Monocete

**Monoclate P** powder for IV injection ℞ *antihemophilic to correct coagulation deficiency* [antihemophilic factor concentrate, recombinant] ⊠ Monocaps; Monoket

**monoclonal antibody 5A8 to CD4** *investigational (orphan) for post-exposure prophylaxis to occupational HIV exposure*

**monoclonal antibody 5G1.1, humanized** *investigational (orphan) C5 complement inhibitor for dermatomyositis*

**monoclonal antibody 7E3** [see: abciximab]

**monoclonal antibody B43.13** *investigational (orphan) for epithelial ovarian cancer*

**monoclonal antibody to CD22 antigen on B-cells, radiolabeled** [now: epratuzumab]

**monoclonal antibody to CEA, humanized** [now: labetuzumab]

**monoclonal antibody to cytomegalovirus, human** *investigational (orphan) prophylaxis for CMV retinitis and CMV disease in solid organ transplants*

**monoclonal antibody E5** [now: edobacomab]

**monoclonal antibody to hepatitis B virus, human** *investigational (orphan) hepatitis B prophylaxis for liver transplant*

**monoclonal antibody LL2, humanized** [now: epratuzumab]

**monoclonal antibody to lupus nephritis** *investigational (orphan) for immunization against lupus nephritis*

**monoclonal antibody PM-81** *investigational (orphan) for acute myelogenous leukemia*

**monoclonal antibody PM-81 & AML-2-23** *investigational (orphan) for bone marrow transplant for acute myelogenous leukemia*

**monoclonal antibody to CD147, murine** *investigational (Phase III, orphan) monoclonal antibody for steroid-resistant graft vs. host disease that reverses unwanted immune response without general immune system suppression* [also: ABX-CBL]

**monoclonal factor IX** [see: factor IX complex]

**Monocor** ⓒᴬᴺ film-coated tablets ℞ *antihypertensive; antiadrenergic (β-blocker)* [bisoprolol fumarate] 5, 10 mg

**monoctanoin** USAN, BAN *anticholelithogenic for dissolution of cholesterol gallstones (orphan)*

**monoctanoin component A**
**monoctanoin component B**
**monoctanoin component C**
**monoctanoin component D**

**Mono-Diff** reagent kit for professional use *in vitro diagnostic aid for mononucleosis*

**Monodox** capsules ℞ *tetracycline antibiotic* [doxycycline monohydrate] 50, 100 mg

**Mono-Drop** (trademarked delivery system) *prefilled eye drop dispenser*

**monoethanolamine** NF *surfactant*

**monoethanolamine oleate** INN *sclerosing agent* [also: ethanolamine oleate]

**Mono-Gesic** film-coated tablets (discontinued 2004) ℞ *analgesic; antipy-*

retic; anti-inflammatory; antirheumatic [salsalate] 750 mg

**Monoket** tablets ℞ antianginal; vasodilator [isosorbide mononitrate] 10, 20 mg ⧉ Monocete

**Mono-Latex** reagent kit for professional use in vitro diagnostic aid for mononucleosis

**monolaurin** investigational (Phase III, orphan) for nonbullous congenital ichthyosiform erythroderma

**monometacrine** INN

**Mononessa** tablets (in packs of 28) ℞ monophasic oral contraceptive [norgestimate; ethinyl estradiol] 0.25 mg• 35 µg

**Mononine** powder for IV infusion ℞ antihemophilic for factor IX deficiency (hemophilia B; Christmas disease) (orphan) [factor IX concentrate] 100 IU/mL

**monooctanoin** [see: monoctanoin]

**monophenylbutazone** [see: mofebutazone]

**monophosphothiamine** INN

**Mono-Plus** reagent kit for professional use in vitro diagnostic aid for mononucleosis

**monopotassium 4-aminosalicylate** [see: aminosalicylate potassium]

**monopotassium carbonate** [see: potassium bicarbonate]

**monopotassium D-gluconate** [see: potassium gluconate]

**monopotassium monosodium tartrate tetrahydrate** [see: potassium sodium tartrate]

**monopotassium phosphate** [see: potassium phosphate, monobasic]

**Monopril** tablets ℞ antihypertensive; angiotensin-converting enzyme (ACE) inhibitor; adjunctive treatment for CHF [fosinopril sodium] 10, 20, 40 mg

**Monopril-HCT** tablets ℞ antihypertensive; angiotensin-converting enzyme (ACE) inhibitor; diuretic [fosinopril sodium; hydrochlorothiazide] 10• 12.5, 20•12.5 mg

**monosodium p-aminohippurate** [see: aminohippurate sodium]

**monosodium 4-aminosalicylate dihydrate** [see: aminosalicylate sodium]

**monosodium carbonate** [see: sodium bicarbonate]

**monosodium D-gluconate** [see: sodium gluconate]

**monosodium D-thyroxine hydrate** [see: dextrothyroxine sodium]

**monosodium glutamate** NF flavoring agent; perfume

**monosodium L-ascorbate** [see: sodium ascorbate]

**monosodium L-thyroxine hydrate** [see: levothyroxine sodium]

**monosodium phosphate dihydrate** [see: sodium phosphate, monobasic]

**monosodium phosphate monohydrate** [see: sodium phosphate, monobasic]

**monosodium salicylate** [see: sodium salicylate]

**monosodium sulfite** [see: sodium bisulfite]

**Monospot** slide test for professional use in vitro diagnostic aid for mononucleosis

**monostearin** [see: glyceryl monostearate]

**Monosticon Dri-Dot** slide test for professional use in vitro diagnostic aid for mononucleosis

**monosulfiram** BAN [also: sulfiram]

**Mono-Sure** slide test for professional use in vitro diagnostic aid for mononucleosis

**Mono-Test** slide test for professional use in vitro diagnostic aid for mononucleosis

**monothioglycerol** NF preservative

*Monotropa uniflora* medicinal herb [see: fit root]

**Mono-Vacc Test (O.T.)** single-use intradermal puncture test device (discontinued 2002) tuberculosis skin test [old tuberculin] 5 U

**Monovial** (trademarked delivery system) single-use vial with transfer needle set

**monoxerutin** INN

**Monsel solution** [see: ferric subsulfate]

**montelukast sodium** USAN *leukotriene receptor inhibitor for allergic rhinitis and the prophylaxis and chronic treatment of asthma*

**monteplase** INN

**montirelin** INN

**montmorillonite (redmond clay)** *natural remedy for bug bites and stings and other skin problems*

**Monuril** (foreign name for U.S. product Monurol)

**Monurol** granules for oral solution ℞ *broad-spectrum bactericidal antibiotic for urinary tract infections* [fosfomycin tromethamine] 3 g/pkt.

**moose elm** *medicinal herb* [see: slippery elm]

**8-MOP** capsules ℞ *systemic psoralens for psoriasis, repigmentation of idiopathic vitiligo, and cutaneous T-cell lymphoma (CTCL); used to increase tolerance to sunlight and enhance pigmentation* [methoxsalen] 10 mg

**MOP (mechlorethamine, Oncovin, prednisone)** *chemotherapy protocol*

**MOP (mechlorethamine, Oncovin, procarbazine)** *chemotherapy protocol for pediatric brain tumors*

**8-MOP (8-methoxypsoralen)** [see: methoxsalen]

**MOP-BAP (mechlorethamine, Oncovin, procarbazine, bleomycin, Adriamycin, prednisone)** *chemotherapy protocol*

**moperone** INN

**mopidamol** INN

**mopidralazine** INN

**MOPP (mechlorethamine, Oncovin, procarbazine, prednisone)** *chemotherapy protocol for Hodgkin lymphoma and brain cancer (medulloblastoma)*

**MOPP (mustine HCl, Oncovin, procarbazine, prednisone)** *chemotherapy protocol*

**MOPP/ABV (mechlorethamine, Oncovin, procarbazine, prednisone, Adriamycin, bleomycin, vinblastine)** *chemotherapy protocol for Hodgkin lymphoma*

**MOPP/ABVD (alternating cycles of MOPP and ABVD)** *chemotherapy protocol for Hodgkin lymphoma*

**MOPP-BLEO; MOPP-Bleo (mechlorethamine, Oncovin, procarbazine, prednisone, bleomycin)** *chemotherapy protocol*

**MOPPHDB (mechlorethamine, Oncovin, procarbazine, prednisone, high-dose bleomycin)** *chemotherapy protocol*

**MOPPLDB (mechlorethamine, Oncovin, procarbazine, prednisone, low-dose bleomycin)** *chemotherapy protocol*

**MOPr (mechlorethamine, Oncovin, procarbazine)** *chemotherapy protocol*

**moprolol** INN

**moquizone** INN

**moracizine** INN, BAN *antiarrhythmic* [also: moricizine]

**morantel** INN *anthelmintic* [also: morantel tartrate]

**morantel tartrate** USAN *anthelmintic* [also: morantel]

**Moranyl** (available only from the Centers for Disease Control) ℞ *antiparasitic for African trypanosomiasis and onchocerciasis* [suramin sodium]

**morazone** INN, BAN

**morclofone** INN

**More-Dophilus** powder OTC *dietary supplement; fever blister treatment; not generally regarded as safe and effective as an antidiarrheal* [Lactobacillus acidophilus] 4 billion U/g

**morforex** INN

**moricizine** USAN *antiarrhythmic* [also: moracizine]

**moricizine HCl** *antiarrhythmic*

**morinamide** INN

**Morinda citrifolia** *medicinal herb* [see: noni]

**Mormon tea** *medicinal herb* [see: ephedra]

**morniflumate** USAN, INN *anti-inflammatory*

**morning glory (Ipomoea violacea)** *seeds contain lysergic acid amide, chemically similar to LSD, which pro-*

duce hallucinations when ingested as a street drug [see also: LSD]

**morocromen** INN

**moroxydine** INN, BAN

**morphazinamide** [see: morinamide]

**Morphelan** (name changed to Avinza upon marketing release in 2002)

**morpheridine** INN, BAN

**morphine** BAN narcotic analgesic; widely abused as a street drug, which leads to dependence [also: morphine sulfate]

**morphine dinicotinate ester** [see: nicomorphine]

**morphine HCl** USP narcotic analgesic preferred in Germany and England; widely abused as a street drug, which leads to dependence

**Morphine LP** ⒸⒶⓃ epidural injection ℞ narcotic analgesic [morphine sulfate] 0.5, 1 mg/mL

**morphine sulfate (MS)** USP narcotic analgesic preferred in the U.S.; intraspinal microinfusion for intractable chronic pain (orphan); widely abused as a street drug, which leads to dependence [also: morphine] 10, 15, 30, 60 mg oral; 10, 20 mg/5 mL oral; 0.5, 1, 2, 4, 5, 10, 15, 25, 50 mg/mL injection; 5, 10, 20, 30 mg rectal

**4-morpholinecarboximidoylguanidine** [see: moroxydine]

**2-morpholinoethylrutin** [see: ethoxazorutoside]

**3-morpholinosydnoneimine** [see: linsidomine]

**morpholinyl succinimide** [see: morsuximide]

**morpholinylethyl morphine** [see: pholcodine]

**morrhuate sodium** USP sclerosing agent [also: sodium morrhuate] 50 mg/mL injection

**morsuximide** INN

**morsydomine** [see: molsidomine]

**mortification root** medicinal herb [see: marsh mallow]

**Morton Salt Substitute; Morton Seasoned Salt Substitute** OTC salt substitute [potassium chloride] 64 mEq K/5 g; 56 mEq K/5 g

*Morus nigra; M. rubra* medicinal herb [see: mulberry]

*Moschus moschiferus* natural remedy [see: deer musk]

**Mosco** topical liquid OTC keratolytic [salicylic acid in flexible collodion] 17.6%

**mosquito plant** medicinal herb [see: pennyroyal]

**motapizone** INN

**MOTC (methyleneoxytetracycline)** [see: methacycline]

**motexafin gadolinium** USAN investigational (Phase III) radiosensitizer for brain metastases

**motexafin lutetium** USAN investigational photo-antineoplastic for recurrent breast cancer; investigational photoangioplastic for atherosclerosis; investigational (Phase I/II) photosensitizer for ophthalmic therapy and imaging

**mother of thyme** medicinal herb [see: thyme]

**motherwort (Leonurus cardiaca)** flowering tops and leaves medicinal herb used as an antispasmodic, astringent, calmative, cardiac, emmenagogue, hepatic, laxative, nervine, and stomachic

**Motilium** ⒸⒶⓃ film-coated tablets ℞ antiemetic for diabetic gastroparesis and chronic gastritis (investigational (NDA filed) in the U.S.) [domperidone maleate] 10 mg

**Motofen** tablets ℞ antidiarrheal [difenoxin HCl; atropine sulfate] 1•0.025 mg

**motrazepam** INN

**motretinide** USAN, INN keratolytic

**Motrin** tablets ℞ analgesic; antiarthritic; antipyretic; nonsteroidal anti-inflammatory drug (NSAID) [ibuprofen] 400, 600, 800 mg

**Motrin, Children's** chewable tablets, oral suspension OTC analgesic; antiarthritic; antipyretic; nonsteroidal anti-inflammatory drug (NSAID) [ibuprofen] 50 mg; 100 mg/5 mL

**Motrin, Infants'** oral drops OTC analgesic; antipyretic; nonsteroidal anti-

*inflammatory drug (NSAID)* [ibuprofen] 40 mg/mL

**Motrin, Junior Strength** tablets, chewable tablets OTC *analgesic; antiarthritic; antipyretic; nonsteroidal antiinflammatory drug (NSAID)* [ibuprofen] 100 mg

**Motrin Children's Cold** oral suspension OTC *decongestant; analgesic; antipyretic* [pseudoephedrine HCl; ibuprofen] 15•100 mg/5 mL

**Motrin IB** tablets, gelcaps OTC *analgesic, antiarthritic; antipyretic; nonsteroidal anti-inflammatory drug (NSAID)* [ibuprofen] 200 mg

**Motrin IB Sinus** caplets (name changed to Motrin Sinus Headache in 2002)

**Motrin Migraine Pain** caplets OTC *analgesic; nonsteroidal anti-inflammatory drug (NSAID)* [ibuprofen] 200 mg

**Motrin Sinus Headache** caplets OTC *decongestant; analgesic* [pseudoephedrine HCl; ibuprofen] 30•200 mg

**mountain ash *(Sorbus americana; S. aucuparia)*** fruit *medicinal herb used as an aperient, astringent, and diuretic*

**mountain balm** *medicinal herb* [see: yerba santa]

**mountain box; mountain cranberry** *medicinal herb* [see: uva ursi]

**mountain laurel *(Kalmia latifolia)*** leaves *medicinal herb used as an astringent and sedative*

**mountain mahogany** *medicinal herb* [see: birch]

**mountain mint** *medicinal herb* [see: marjoram; Oswego tea]

**mountain snuff; mountain tobacco** *medicinal herb* [see: arnica]

**mountain sorrel** *medicinal herb* [see: wood sorrel]

**mountain strawberry** *medicinal herb* [see: strawberry]

**mountain sumach** *medicinal herb* [see: sumach]

**mountain sweet** *medicinal herb* [see: New Jersey tea]

**mountain tea** *medicinal herb* [see: wintergreen]

**mouse ear *(Hieracium pilosella)*** plant *medicinal herb used as an astringent, cholagogue, and diuretic*

**MouthKote** oral spray OTC *saliva substitute*

**MouthKote O/R** mouthwash OTC *anesthetic and antimicrobial throat irrigation* [benzyl alcohol; menthol]

**MouthKote O/R** oral solution OTC *topical antihistamine* [diphenhydramine] 1.25%

**MouthKote P/R** oral solution, ointment (discontinued 2004) OTC *topical antihistamine* [diphenhydramine HCl] 1.25%; 25%

**mouthroot** *medicinal herb* [see: gold thread]

**moveltipril** INN

**moxadolen** INN

**moxalactam disodium** USAN, USP *bactericidal antibiotic* [also: latamoxef]

**moxantrazole** [now: teloxantrone HCl]

**moxaprindine** INN

**moxastine** INN

**moxaverine** INN, BAN

**moxazocine** USAN, INN *analgesic; antitussive*

**moxestrol** INN

**moxicoumone** INN

**moxidectin** USAN, INN *veterinary antiparasitic*

**moxifloxacin HCl** USAN *broad-spectrum fluoroquinolone antibiotic*

**moxilubant maleate** USAN *leukotriene $B_4$ receptor antagonist for rheumatoid arthritis and psoriasis*

**moxipraquine** INN, BAN

**moxiraprine** INN

**moxisylyte** INN [also: thymoxamine]

**moxnidazole** USAN, INN *antiprotozoal (Trichomonas)*

**moxonidine** USAN, INN *centrally acting sympatholytic for hypertension, congestive heart failure, and type 2 diabetes*

**M-oxy** tablets ℞ *narcotic analgesic* [oxycodone HCl] 5 mg

**MP (melphalan, prednisone)** *chemotherapy protocol for multiple myeloma*

**MP (mitoxantrone, prednisone)** *chemotherapy protocol for prostate cancer*

**4-MP (4-methylpyrazole)** [see: fomepizole]

**6-MP (6-mercaptopurine)** [see: mercaptopurine]

**MPA (medroxyprogesterone acetate)** [q.v.]

**MPA (mycophenolic acid)** [q.v.]

**MPF** [see: Mucoprotective Factor]

**m-PFL (methotrexate, Platinol, fluorouracil, leucovorin [rescue])** *chemotherapy protocol*

**MPH (methylphenidate HCl)** [q.v.]

**MPL (melphalan)** [q.v.]

**MPL + PRED (melphalan, prednisone)** *chemotherapy protocol*

**M-Prednisol-40; M-Prednisol-80** intralesional, soft tissue, and IM injection (discontinued 2004) ℞ *corticosteroid; anti-inflammatory; immunosuppressant* [methylprednisolone acetate] 40 mg/mL; 80 mg/mL

**MPTS (minocycline periodontal therapeutic system)** ℞ *investigational (NDA filed) system used in conjunction with scaling and root planing for periodontitis* [minocycline]

**MRV** subcu injection (discontinued 2000) ℞ *active respiratory bacteria immunizing agent* [mixed respiratory vaccine]

**MRV (mixed respiratory vaccine)** [q.v.]

**M-R-Vax II** powder for subcu injection (discontinued 2004) ℞ *measles and rubella vaccine* [measles and rubella virus vaccine, live] 0.5 mL

**MS (magnesium salicylate)** [q.v.]

**MS (morphine sulfate)** [q.v.]

**MS Contin** controlled-release tablets ℞ *narcotic analgesic; preoperative sedative and anxiolytic* [morphine sulfate] 15, 30, 60, 100, 200 mg

**MSD Enteric-Coated ASA** ⒸⒶⓃ tablets OTC *analgesic; antipyretic; anti-inflammatory; antirheumatic* [aspirin] 325, 650 mg

**MSIR** capsules (discontinued 2003) ℞ *narcotic analgesic; preoperative sedative and anxiolytic* [morphine sulfate] 15, 30 mg

**MSIR** tablets, oral solution, oral concentrate ℞ *narcotic analgesic; preoperative sedative and anxiolytic* [morphine sulfate] 15, 30 mg; 10, 20 mg/5 mL; 20 mg/mL

**MSM (methylsulfonylmethane)** *natural source of sulfur; promotes an increase in collagen and the endogenous antioxidant glutathione*

**MSTA (Mumps Skin Test Antigen)** intradermal injection ℞ *diagnostic aid to assess immune system competency (not effective in testing immunity to mumps virus)* [mumps skin test antigen] 0.1 mL (4 U/0.1 mL)

**MT6 (mercaptomerin)** [q.v.]

**M-Tabs** (trademarked form) *orally disintegrating tablets*

**MTC (mitomycin C)** [see: mitomycin]

**MTC-DOX** (trademarked delivery system) *investigational (Phase I/II) magnetic targeted carrier for the treatment of primary liver cancer* [doxorubicin]

**MTC-DOX (magnetically targeted carrier with doxorubicin)** *investigational (orphan) delivery method for liver cancer chemotherapy*

**M.T.E.-4; M.T.E.-5; M.T.E.-6; M.T.E.-7; M.T.E.-4 Concentrated; M.T.E.-5 Concentrated; M.T.E.-6 Concentrated** IV injection ℞ *intravenous nutritional therapy* [multiple trace elements (metals)]

**mTHPC** [see: temoporfin]

**MTX (methotrexate)** [q.v.]

**MTX + MP + CTX (methotrexate, mercaptopurine, cyclophosphamide)** *chemotherapy protocol*

**MTX/6-MP (methotrexate, mercaptopurine)** *chemotherapy protocol for acute lymphocytic leukemia (ALL); the ongoing continuation protocol* [also: 1DMTX/6-MP (the first-day initiation protocol)]

**MTX/6-MP/VP (methotrexate, mercaptopurine, vincristine, prednisone)** *chemotherapy protocol for acute lymphocytic leukemia (ALL)*

**MTX-CDDPAdr (methotrexate [with leucovorin rescue], CDDP,**

**Adriamycin)** *chemotherapy protocol for pediatric osteosarcoma*

**Mucinex** dual-release tablets OTC *expectorant* [guaifenesin] 600 (100 mg immediate release, 500 mg extended release)

**Muco-Fen; Muco-Fen 800; Muco-Fen 1200** timed-release tablets (discontinued 2004) ℞ *expectorant* [guaifenesin] 1000 mg; 800 mg; 1200 mg

**Muco-Fen DM** sustained-release tablets ℞ *antitussive; expectorant* [dextromethorphan hydrobromide; guaifenesin] 60●1000 mg

**Muco-Fen LA** timed-release tablets (discontinued 2002) ℞ *expectorant* [guaifenesin] 600 mg

**mucoid exopolysaccharide** *Pseudomonas* **hyperimmune globulin (MEPIG)** *investigational (orphan) for pulmonary infections of cystic fibrosis*

**mucolytics** *a class of respiratory inhalant drugs that destroy or inhibit mucin*

**Mucomyst** solution for nebulization or intratracheal instillation ℞ *mucolytic* [acetylcysteine sodium] 10%, 20%

**Mucomyst 10** IV ℞ *investigational (orphan) for severe acetaminophen overdose* [acetylcysteine]

**Mucoprotective Factor (MPF)** (trademarked ingredient) *aromatic flavored syrup* [eriodictyon]

**Mucosil-10; Mucosil-20** solution for nebulization or intratracheal instillation (discontinued 2004) ℞ *mucolytic* [acetylcysteine sodium] 10%; 20%

**Mudrane** tablets ℞ *antiasthmatic; bronchodilator; decongestant; expectorant; sedative* [aminophylline; ephedrine HCl; potassium iodide; phenobarbital] 111●16●195●8 mg ⧉ Modane

**Mudrane GG** tablets ℞ *antiasthmatic; decongestant; expectorant; sedative* [theophylline; ephedrine HCl; guaifenesin; phenobarbital] 111●16●100●8 mg

**Mudrane GG-2** tablets ℞ *antiasthmatic; bronchodilator; expectorant* [theophylline; guaifenesin] 111●100 mg

**mugwort (Artemisia vulgaris)** root and plant *medicinal herb used as a diaphoretic, emmenagogue, and laxative*

**muira puama (Ptychopetalum olacoides)** stem *medicinal herb used as an aphrodisiac and treatment for impotence in South America; clinical trials in France confirm these effects*

**mulberry (Morus nigra; M. rubra)** bark *medicinal herb used as an anthelmintic and cathartic*

**mullein (Verbascum nigrum; V. phlomoides; V. thapsiforme; V. thapsus)** plant *medicinal herb for asthma, bleeding in bowel and lungs, bronchitis, bruises, cough, croup, diarrhea, earache, gout, hemorrhoids, insomnia, lymphatic system, nervousness, pain, pleurisy, sinus congestion, and tuberculosis*

**MulTE-Pak-4; MulTE-Pak-5** IV injection ℞ *intravenous nutritional therapy* [multiple trace elements (metals)]

**Multi 75** timed-release tablets OTC *vitamin/mineral supplement* [multiple vitamins & minerals; folic acid; biotin] ≛●0.4●⅔ mg

**Multi Vit with Iron** drops OTC *vitamin/iron supplement* [multiple vitamins; iron] ≛●10 mg/mL

**Multi Vitamin Concentrate** injection ℞ *parenteral vitamin supplement* [multiple vitamins]

**Multi-12; Multi-12 Pediatric** ⒸⒶⓃ IV infusion ℞ *vitamin supplement* [multiple vitamins]

**Multi-Day** tablets OTC *vitamin supplement* [multiple vitamins; folic acid] ≛●0.4 mg

**Multi-Day Plus Iron** tablets OTC *vitamin/iron supplement* [multiple vitamins; iron; folic acid] ≛●18●0.4 mg

**Multi-Day Plus Minerals** tablets OTC *vitamin/mineral/iron supplement* [multiple vitamins & minerals; iron; folic acid; biotin] ≛●18 mg●0.4 mg●30 μg

**Multi-Day with Calcium and Extra Iron** tablets OTC *vitamin/calcium/iron supplement* [multiple vitamins; calcium; iron; folic acid] ≛•≛•27•0.4 mg

**Multifol** caplets ℞ *vitamin/calcium/iron supplement* [multiple vitamins; calcium; iron (as ferrous fumarate); folic acid] ≛•125•65•1 mg

**MultiKine** injection ℞ *investigational (Phase III) antineoplastic for prostate cancer; investigational (Phase I) immunotherapeutic agent for HIV infection; investigational for cancer of the oral cavity* [multiple leukocytes and interleukins]

**Multilex; Multilex-T & M** tablets OTC *vitamin/mineral/iron supplement* [multiple vitamins & minerals; iron] ≛•15 mg

**Multilyte-20; Multilyte-40** IV admixture ℞ *intravenous electrolyte therapy* [combined electrolyte solution]

**Multi-Mineral** tablets OTC *mineral supplement* [multiple minerals]

**Multiple Trace Element; Multiple Trace Element Concentrated; Multiple Trace Element Pediatric** IV injection (discontinued 2003) ℞ *intravenous nutritional therapy* [multiple trace elements (metals)]

**Multiple Trace Element Neonatal; Multiple Trace Element with Selenium; Multiple Trace Element with Selenium Concentrated** IV injection ℞ *intravenous nutritional therapy* [multiple trace elements (metals)]

**Multistix; Multistix 2; Multistix 7; Multistix 8 SG; Multistix 9; Multistix 9 SG; Multistix 10 SG; Multistix SG** reagent strips OTC *in vitro diagnostic aid for multiple urine products*

**Multistix PRO** reagent strips for professional use ℞ *in vitro diagnostic aid for urine protein/creatinine ratio*

**Multitest CMI** single-use intradermal skin test device (discontinued 2004) ℞ *skin test for multiple allergen sensitivity* [skin test antigens (seven different); glycerin (one for test control)]

**Multitrace-5 Concentrate** IV injection ℞ *intravenous nutritional therapy* [multiple trace elements (metals)]

**multivitamin infusion, neonatal formula** *investigational (orphan) total parenteral nutrition for very low birth-weight infants*

**Multi-Vitamin Mineral with Beta-Carotene** tablets OTC *vitamin/mineral/iron supplement* [multiple vitamins & minerals; ferrous fumarate; folic acid; biotin] ≛•27•0.4•0.45 mg

**Multivitamin with Fluoride** drops ℞ *pediatric vitamin supplement and dental caries preventative* [multiple vitamins; fluoride] ≛•0.25, ≛•0.5 mg/mL

**Multivitamins** capsules OTC *vitamin supplement* [multiple vitamins]

**Mulvidren-F** Softabs (chewable tablets) ℞ *pediatric vitamin supplement and dental caries preventative* [multiple vitamins; fluoride] ≛•1 mg

**mumps skin test antigen (MSTA)** USP *diagnostic aid to assess immune system competency*

**mumps vaccine** [see: mumps virus vaccine, inactivated]

**mumps virus vaccine, inactivated** NF

**mumps virus vaccine, live** USP *active immunizing agent for mumps*

**Mumpsvax** powder for subcu injection ℞ *mumps vaccine* [mumps virus vaccine, live] 0.5 mL

**mupirocin** USAN, INN, BAN *topical antibiotic* 2% topical

**mupirocin calcium** USAN *topical antibiotic* (base=93%)

**muplestim** USAN *progenitor cell stimulator for neutropenia and thrombocytopenia*

**murabutide** INN

**Murine** eye drops OTC *ophthalmic moisturizer/lubricant* [polyvinyl alcohol] 0.5%

**Murine Ear Drops** OTC *agent to emulsify and disperse ear wax* [carbamide peroxide; alcohol] 6.5%•6.3%

**Murine Plus** eye drops OTC *topical ophthalmic decongestant and vasoconstrictor* [tetrahydrozoline HCl] 0.05%

**Muro 128** eye drops, ophthalmic ointment OTC *corneal edema-reducing agent* [sodium chloride (hypertonic saline solution)] 2%, 5%; 5%

**murocainide** INN

**Murocel** eye drops OTC *ophthalmic moisturizer/lubricant* [methylcellulose] 1%

**Murocoll-2** eye drops ℞ *cycloplegic; mydriatic* [scopolamine hydrobromide; phenylephrine HCl] 0.3%•10%

**murodermin** INN

**muromonab-CD3** USAN, INN *immunosuppressive monoclonal antibody (MAb) for renal, hepatic, and cardiac transplants*

**Muroptic-5** eye drops OTC *corneal edema-reducing agent* [sodium chloride (hypertonic saline solution)] 5%

**muscarinic agonists** *a class of investigational analgesics*

**MuscleRub** ointment (discontinued 2000) OTC *analgesic; counterirritant* [methyl salicylate; menthol] 15%•10%

**Muse** single-use intraurethral suppository ℞ *vasodilator for erectile dysfunction* [alprostadil] 125, 150, 500, 1000 μg

**musk** *natural remedy* [see: deer musk]

**mustaral oil** [see: allyl isothiocyanate]

**mustard (Brassica alba; Sinapis alba)** seeds and oil *medicinal herb for indigestion and liver and lung disorders; also used as an appetizer, diuretic, emetic, and soak for aching feet, arthritis, and rheumatism*

**mustard oil** [see: allyl isothiocyanate]

**Mustargen** powder for IV or intracavitary injection ℞ *nitrogen mustard-type alkylating antineoplastic for multiple carcinomas, lymphomas and leukemias, mycosis fungoides, and polycythemia vera* [mechlorethamine HCl] 10 mg

**Musterole Deep Strength Rub** OTC *analgesic; counterirritant* [methyl salicylate; methyl nicotinate; menthol] 30%•0.5%•3%

**Musterole Extra Strength** OTC *topical analgesic; counterirritant* [camphor; menthol] 5%•3%

**mustine** BAN *nitrogen mustard-type alkylating antineoplastic* [also: mechlorethamine HCl; chlormethine; nitrogen mustard N-oxide HCl]

**mustine HCl** [see: mechlorethamine HCl]

**Mutamycin** powder for IV injection ℞ *antibiotic antineoplastic for stomach, pancreatic, breast, colon, head, neck, and lung cancers* [mitomycin] 5, 20, 40 mg ⊡ mitomycin

**muzolimine** USAN, INN *diuretic; antihypertensive*

**MV (mitomycin, vinblastine)** *chemotherapy protocol for breast cancer*

**MV (mitoxantrone, VePesid)** *chemotherapy protocol for acute myelocytic leukemia (ALL)*

**MVAC; M-VAC (methotrexate, vinblastine, Adriamycin, cisplatin)** *chemotherapy protocol for bladder cancer*

**M-Vax** ℞ *investigational (Phase III, orphan) theraccine for postsurgical stage III malignant melanoma* [DNP-conjugated tumor vaccine]

**MVF (mitoxantrone, vincristine, fluorouracil)** *chemotherapy protocol*

**M.V.I. Neonatal** IV infusion ℞ *investigational (orphan) total parenteral nutrition for very low birthweight infants* [multiple vitamins]

**M.V.I. Pediatric** injection ℞ *parenteral vitamin supplement* [multiple vitamins; folic acid; biotin] ±•140•20 μg/5 mL

**M.V.I.-12** injection ℞ *parenteral vitamin supplement* [multiple vitamins; folic acid; biotin] ±•400•60 μg/5 mL

**M.V.M.** capsules OTC *vitamin/mineral/ iron supplement* [multiple vitamins & minerals; iron; folic acid; biotin] ±•3.6 mg•0.08 mg•160 μg

**MVP (mitomycin, vinblastine, Platinol)** *chemotherapy protocol for non–small cell lung cancer (NSCLC)*

**MVPP (mechlorethamine, vinblastine, procarbazine, prednisone)** *chemotherapy protocol for Hodgkin lymphoma*

**MVT (mitoxantrone, VePesid, thiotepa)** *chemotherapy protocol*

**MVVPP (mechlorethamine, vincristine, vinblastine, procarbazine, prednisone)** *chemotherapy protocol*

**Myadec** tablets OTC *vitamin/mineral/iron supplement* [multiple vitamins & minerals; iron; folic acid; biotin] ± • 18 mg•0.4 mg•30 μg

**Myambutol** film-coated tablets ℞ *tuberculostatic* [ethambutol HCl] 100, 400 mg ⌧ Nembutal

**Mycelex** cream, solution (discontinued 2000) ℞ *topical antifungal* [clotrimazole] 1%

**Mycelex** troches ℞ *antifungal; oral candidiasis prophylaxis or treatment* [clotrimazole] 10 mg

**Mycelex OTC** cream, solution (discontinued 2000) OTC *topical antifungal* [clotrimazole] 1%

**Mycelex Twin Pack** vaginal inserts + cream (discontinued 2001) ℞ *antifungal* [clotrimazole] 500 mg; 1%

**Mycelex-3** vaginal cream in prefilled applicator OTC *antifungal* [butoconazole nitrate] 2%

**Mycelex-7** vaginal cream, combination pack (vaginal inserts + cream) OTC *antifungal* [clotrimazole] 1%; 100 mg + 1%

**Mycelex-7** vaginal inserts (discontinued 2001) OTC *antifungal* [clotrimazole] 100 mg

**Mycelex-G** vaginal inserts (discontinued 2001) ℞ *antifungal* [clotrimazole] 500 mg

**Mycifradin Sulfate** oral solution ℞ *aminoglycoside antibiotic* [neomycin sulfate] 125 mg/5 mL

**Myciguent** ointment, cream (discontinued 2003) OTC *antibiotic* [neomycin sulfate] 3.5 mg/g

**Mycinaire Saline Mist** nasal spray OTC *nasal moisturizer* [sodium chloride (saline solution)] 0.65%

**Mycinette** throat spray OTC *topical anesthetic; oral antiseptic; astringent* [phenol; alum] 1.4%•0.3%

**Mycinettes** lozenges OTC *topical oral anesthetic* [benzocaine] 15 mg

**"mycins"** *brief term for a class of antibiotics derived from various strains of the fungus-like bacteria* Streptomyces, *or their synthetic analogues, whose generic names end in "mycin," such as lincomycin* [properly called: aminoglycosides]

**Myci-Spray** nasal spray OTC *nasal decongestant; antihistamine* [phenylephrine HCl; pyrilamine maleate] 0.25%•0.15%

**Mycitracin Plus** ointment (discontinued 2001) OTC *topical antibiotic; local anesthetic* [polymyxin B sulfate; neomycin sulfate; bacitracin; lidocaine] 5000 U•3.5 mg•500 U•40 mg per g

**Mycitracin Triple Antibiotic** ointment (discontinued 2001) OTC *topical antibiotic* [polymyxin B sulfate; neomycin sulfate; bacitracin] 5000 U•3.5 mg•500 U per g

**mycobacterial cell wall complex (MCC)** [see: urocidin]

*Mycobacterium avium* **sensitin RS-10** *investigational (orphan) diagnostic aid for* Mycobacterium avium *infection in immunocompromised patients*

**Myco-Biotic II** cream ℞ *topical corticosteroidal anti-inflammatory; antifungal* [triamcinolone acetonide; neomycin sulfate; nystatin] 0.1%• 0.5%•100 000 U per g

**Mycobutin** capsules ℞ *antiviral/antibacterial for prevention of* Mycobacterium avium *complex (MAC) in advanced HIV patients (orphan)* [rifabutin] 150 mg

**Mycocide NS** solution OTC *topical antiseptic* [benzalkonium chloride]

**Mycogen II** cream, ointment ℞ *topical corticosteroidal anti-inflammatory; antifungal* [triamcinolone acetonide; nystatin] 0.1%•100 000 U per g

**Mycolog-II** cream, ointment ℞ *topical corticosteroidal anti-inflammatory; antifungal* [triamcinolone acetonide; nystatin] 0.1%•100 000 U per g

**Myconel** cream ℞ *topical corticosteroidal anti-inflammatory; antifungal*

[triamcinolone acetonide; nystatin] 0.1%•100 000 U per g

**mycophenolate mofetil** USAN *immunosuppressant for allogenic renal, hepatic, or cardiac transplants; purine biosynthesis inhibitor*

**mycophenolate mofetil HCl** USAN *immunosuppressant for allogenic renal, hepatic, or cardiac transplants; purine biosynthesis inhibitor*

**mycophenolic acid (MPA)** USAN, INN *antineoplastic; immunosuppressant to prevent organ rejection of kidney transplants*

**Mycostatin** cream, ointment, powder ℞ *antifungal* [nystatin] 100 000 U/g; 100 000 U/g; 100 000 U/g

**Mycostatin** film-coated tablets ℞ *systemic antifungal* [nystatin] 500 000 U

**Mycostatin** oral suspension (discontinued 2004) ℞ *antifungal; oral candidiasis treatment* [nystatin] 100 000 U/mL

**Mycostatin** Pastilles (troches) ℞ *antifungal; oral candidiasis treatment* [nystatin] 200 000 U

**Mycostatin** vaginal inserts (discontinued 2001) ℞ *topical antifungal* [nystatin] 100 000 U

**Myco-Triacet II** cream, ointment ℞ *topical corticosteroidal anti-inflammatory; antifungal* [triamcinolone acetonide; nystatin] 0.1%•100 000 U per g

**mydeton** [see: tolperisone]

**Mydfrin 2.5%** eye drops ℞ *topical ophthalmic decongestant and vasoconstrictor; mydriatic* [phenylephrine HCl] 2.5% ⊡ Midrin; Myfedrine

**Mydriacyl** Drop-Tainers (eye drops) ℞ *cycloplegic; mydriatic* [tropicamide] 0.5%, 1%

**mydriatics** *a class of drugs that cause the pupil of the eye to dilate*

**myelin** *investigational (orphan) for multiple sclerosis*

**myeloid progenitor inhibitory factor 1 (MPIF-1)** [see: mirostipen]

**myelosan** [see: busulfan]

**myfadol** INN

**Myfortic** film-coated delayed-release tablets ℞ *immunosuppressant for allo-*

*genic renal, hepatic, or cardiac transplants* [mycophenolic acid] 180, 360 mg

**Mygel; Mygel II** oral suspension OTC *antacid; antiflatulent* [aluminum hydroxide; magnesium hydroxide; simethicone] 200•200•20 mg/5 mL; 400•400•40 mg/5 mL

**Mykrox** tablets ℞ *antihypertensive; diuretic* [metolazone] 0.5 mg

**Mylagen** gelcaps OTC *antacid* [calcium carbonate; magnesium carbonate] 311•232 mg

**Mylagen; Mylagen II** oral liquid OTC *antacid; antiflatulent* [aluminum hydroxide; magnesium hydroxide; simethicone] 200•200•20 mg/5 mL; 400•400•40 mg/5 mL

**Mylanta** chewable tablets, oral liquid OTC *antacid; antiflatulent* [aluminum hydroxide; magnesium hydroxide; simethicone] 200•200•20, 400•400•40 mg; 200•200•20, 400•400•40 mg/5 mL ⊡ Dilantin; Milontin

**Mylanta** gelcaps OTC *antacid* [calcium carbonate; magnesium carbonate] 311•232 mg

**Mylanta** lozenges OTC *antacid* [calcium carbonate] 600 mg

**Mylanta, Children's** oral liquid, chewable tablets OTC *antacid* [calcium carbonate] 400 mg/5 mL; 400 mg

**Mylanta AR** ("acid reducer") tablets OTC *histamine $H_2$ antagonist for heartburn and acid indigestion* [famotidine] 10 mg

**Mylanta Gas** chewable tablets OTC *antiflatulent* [simethicone] 40, 80, 125 mg

**Mylanta Supreme** oral liquid OTC *antacid* [calcium carbonate; magnesium hydroxide] 400•135 mg/5 mL

**Myleran** tablets ℞ *alkylating antineoplastic for chronic myelogenous leukemia (CML)* [busulfan] 2 mg ⊡ Mylicon

**Mylicon** drops OTC *antiflatulent* [simethicone] 40 mg/0.6 mL ⊡ Modicon; Myleran

**Mylinax** ℞ *investigational (orphan) agent for chronic progressive multiple sclerosis* [cladribine]

**Mylocel** film-coated caplets ℞ *antineoplastic for melanoma, squamous cell carcinoma, myelocytic leukemia, and ovarian cancer* [hydroxyurea] 1000 mg

**Myloral** ℞ *investigational (Phase III) oral treatment for multiple sclerosis* [bovine myelin]

**Mylotarg** powder for IV injection ℞ *antibody-targeted chemotherapy agent for acute myeloid leukemia (orphan)* [gemtuzumab ozogamicin] 5 mg/vial

**Mylovenge** ℞ *investigational (orphan) agent for multiple myeloma* [antigen-presenting cells pulsed with tumor immunoglobulin idiotype]

**Myminic Expectorant** oral liquid (discontinued 2002) OTC *decongestant; expectorant* [phenylpropanolamine HCl; guaifenesin; alcohol 5%] 12.5•100 mg/5 mL

**Myminicol** oral liquid (discontinued 2002) OTC *antitussive; decongestant; antihistamine* [dextromethorphan hydrobromide; phenylpropanolamine HCl; chlorpheniramine maleate] 10•12.5•2 mg/5 mL

**Mynatal** capsules ℞ *vitamin/mineral/calcium/iron supplement* [multiple vitamins & minerals; calcium; iron; folic acid; biotin] ≝•300•65•1•0.03 mg

**Mynatal FC** caplets ℞ *vitamin/mineral/calcium/iron supplement* [multiple vitamins & minerals; calcium; iron; folic acid; biotin] ≝•250•60•1•0.03 mg

**Mynatal P.N.** captabs ℞ *vitamin/calcium/iron supplement* [multiple vitamins; calcium; iron; folic acid] ≝•125•60•1 mg

**Mynatal P.N. Forte** caplets ℞ *vitamin/mineral/calcium/iron supplement* [multiple vitamins & minerals; calcium; iron; folic acid] ≝•250•60•1 mg

**Mynatal Rx** caplets ℞ *vitamin/mineral/calcium/iron supplement* [multiple vitamins & minerals; calcium; iron; folic acid; biotin] ≝•200•60•1•0.03 mg

**Mynate 90 Plus** delayed-release caplets ℞ *vitamin/calcium/iron supplement* [multiple vitamins; calcium; iron; folic acid] ≝•250•90•1 mg

**Myobloc** injection ℞ *neurotoxin complex for symptomatic treatment of cervical dystonia (orphan)* [botulinum toxin, type B] 5000 U/mL

**Myochrysine** IM injection ℞ *antirheumatic* [gold sodium thiomalate] 50 mg/mL

**Myocide NS** solution OTC *topical antiseptic* [benzalkonium chloride]

**Myoflex Creme** OTC *topical analgesic* [trolamine salicylate] 10%

**Myolin** IV or IM injection ℞ *skeletal muscle relaxant* [orphenadrine citrate] 30 mg/mL

**Myoscint** (approved in Europe) *investigational (orphan) imaging agent for cardiac necrosis and myocarditis* [imciromab pentetate]

**Myotonachol** tablets (discontinued 2001) ℞ *cholinergic urinary stimulant for postsurgical and postpartum urinary retention* [bethanechol chloride] 10, 25 mg

**Myotrophin** injection ℞ *investigational (NDA filed, orphan) for amyotrophic lateral sclerosis, type 1 and type 2 diabetes, growth hormone insufficiency, and post-poliomyelitis syndrome* [mecasermin]

**Myoview** ℞ *cardiovascular imaging aid* [technetium Tc 99m tetrofosmin]

**Myphetane DC Cough** syrup (discontinued 2002) ℞ *narcotic antitussive; decongestant; antihistamine* [codeine phosphate; phenylpropanolamine HCl; brompheniramine maleate; alcohol 1.2%] 10•12.5•2 mg/5 mL

**Myphetane DX Cough** syrup (discontinued 2002) ℞ *antitussive; decongestant; antihistamine* [dextromethorphan hydrobromide; pseudoephedrine HCl; brompheniramine maleate; alcohol 1%] 10•30•2 mg/5 mL

**myralact** INN, BAN

*Myrica cerifera* medicinal herb [see: bayberry]

**myricodine** [see: myrophine]

*Myristica fragrans* medicinal herb [see: nutmeg; mace]

**myristica oil** [see: nutmeg oil]
**myristyl alcohol** NF *stiffening agent*
**myristyltrimethylammonium bromide** *antiseborrheic*
**myrophine** INN, BAN
*Myroxylon balsamum; M. pereirae medicinal herb* [see: Peruvian balsam]
**myrrh *(Commiphora abssynica; C. molmol; C. myrrha)*** *seeds medicinal herb for bad breath, bronchitis, cancer, constipation, hay fever, hemorrhoids, leprosy, lung diseases, mouth and skin sores, sore throat, syphilis, and stimulating menses; also used as an antiseptic and astringent*
**myrtecaine** INN
*Myrtilli fructus medicinal herb* [see: bilberry]
**myrtle** *medicinal herb* [see: periwinkle]
**myrtle, bog** *medicinal herb* [see: buckbean]
**myrtle, wax** *medicinal herb* [see: bayberry]
**myrtle flag; grass myrtle; sweet myrtle** *medicinal herb* [see: calamus]
**Mysoline** oral suspension (discontinued 2004) ℞ *anticonvulsant for grand mal, psychomotor, or focal epileptic seizures* [primidone] 250 mg/5 mL
**Mysoline** tablets ℞ *anticonvulsant for grand mal, psychomotor, or focal epileptic seizures* [primidone] 50, 250 mg
**myspamol** [see: proquamezine]
**Mytelase** caplets ℞ *anticholinesterase muscle stimulant; myasthenia gravis treatment* [ambenonium chloride] 10 mg

**Mytrex** cream, ointment (discontinued 2004) ℞ *corticosteroidal anti-inflammatory; antifungal* [triamcinolone acetonide; nystatin] 0.1%• 100 000 U/g
**Mytussin** syrup (discontinued 2002) OTC *expectorant* [guaifenesin; alcohol 3.5%] 100 mg/5 mL
**Mytussin AC Cough** syrup ℞ *narcotic antitussive; expectorant* [codeine phosphate; guaifenesin; alcohol 3.5%] 10•100 mg/5 mL
**Mytussin DAC** syrup (discontinued 2002) ℞ *narcotic antitussive; decongestant; expectorant* [codeine phosphate; pseudoephedrine HCl; guaifenesin; alcohol 1.7%] 10•30•100 mg/5 mL
**Mytussin DM** syrup OTC *antitussive; expectorant* [dextromethorphan hydrobromide; guaifenesin] 10•100 mg/5 mL
**myuizone** [see: thioacetazone; thiacetazone]
**My-Vitalife** capsules OTC *vitamin/mineral/calcium/iron supplement* [multiple vitamins & minerals; calcium; iron; folic acid; biotin] ±•130•27•0.4• 0.03 mg
**MZM** tablets ℞ *carbonic anhydrase inhibitor for glaucoma* [methazolamide] 25, 50 mg
**MZM (methazolamide)** [q.v.]
**M-Zole 3 Combination Pack** vaginal suppositories + cream OTC *antifungal* [miconazole nitrate] 200 mg; 2%
**M-Zole 7 Dual Pack** vaginal suppositories + cream OTC *antifungal* [miconazole nitrate] 100 mg; 2%

**N₂ (nitrogen)** [q.v.]
**N-3 polyunsaturated fatty acids** [see: doconexent; icosapent; omega-3 marine triglycerides]
**Na PCA; sodium PCA (sodium pyrrolidone carboxylic acid)** [q.v.]

**²²Na** [see: sodium chloride Na 22]
**nabazenil** USAN, INN *anticonvulsant*
**Nabi-HB** IM injection ℞ *immunizing agent following exposure to hepatitis B surface antigen* [hepatitis B immune globulin] 1, 5 mL

**nabilone** USAN, INN, BAN *minor tranquilizer*

**nabitan** INN *analgesic* [also: nabitan HCl]

**nabitan HCl** USAN *analgesic* [also: nabitan]

**naboctate** INN *antiglaucoma agent; antinauseant* [also: naboctate HCl]

**naboctate HCl** USAN *antiglaucoma agent; antinauseant* [also: naboctate]

**nabumetone** USAN, INN, BAN *antiarthritic; nonsteroidal anti-inflammatory drug (NSAID)* 500, 750 mg oral

**nabutan HCl** [now: nabitan HCl]

**NAC (N-acetyl cysteine)** *natural source of cysteine; promotes an increase in the endogenous antioxidant glutathione* [also see: acetylcysteine]

**NAC (nitrogen mustard, Adriamycin, CCNU)** *chemotherapy protocol*

**nacartocin** INN

**NaCl (sodium chloride)** [q.v.]

**NAD (nicotinamide-adenine dinucleotide)** [see: nadide]

**nadide** USAN, INN *antagonist to alcohol and narcotics*

**nadisan** [see: carbutamide]

**nadolol** USAN, USP, INN, BAN *antianginal; antihypertensive; antiadrenergic (β-receptor)* 20, 40, 80, 120, 160 mg oral ⌖ Nandol

**nadoxolol** INN

**nadroparin calcium** INN, BAN *anticoagulant; low molecular weight heparin*

**naepaine HCl** NF

**nafamostat** INN *anticoagulant; antifibrinolytic* [also: nafamostat mesylate; nafamostat mesilate]

**nafamostat mesilate** JAN *anticoagulant; antifibrinolytic* [also: nafamostat mesylate; nafamostat]

**nafamostat mesylate** USAN *anticoagulant; antifibrinolytic* [also: nafamostat; nafamostat mesilate]

**nafarelin** INN, BAN *luteinizing hormone-releasing hormone (LHRH) agonist* [also: nafarelin acetate]

**nafarelin acetate** USAN *luteinizing hormone-releasing hormone (LHRH) agonist for central precocious puberty*

*(orphan) and endometriosis* [also: nafarelin]

**Nafazair** eye drops R *topical ophthalmic decongestant and vasoconstrictor* [naphazoline HCl] 0.1%

**nafazatrom** INN, BAN

**nafcaproic acid** INN

**nafcillin** INN *penicillinase-resistant penicillin antibiotic* [also: nafcillin sodium]

**nafcillin sodium** USAN, USP *penicillinase-resistant penicillin antibiotic* [also: nafcillin] 1, 2 g IV infusion

**nafenodone** INN

**nafenopin** USAN, INN *antihyperlipoproteinemic*

**nafetolol** INN

**nafimidone** INN *anticonvulsant* [also: nafimidone HCl]

**nafimidone HCl** USAN *anticonvulsant* [also: nafimidone]

**nafiverine** INN

**naflocort** USAN, INN *topical adrenocortical steroid*

**nafomine** INN *muscle relaxant* [also: nafomine malate]

**nafomine malate** USAN *muscle relaxant* [also: nafomine]

**nafoxadol** INN

**nafoxidine HCl** USAN, INN *antiestrogen*

**nafronyl oxalate** USAN *vasodilator* [also: naftidrofuryl]

**naftalofos** USAN, INN *veterinary anthelmintic*

**naftazone** INN, BAN

**naftidrofuryl** INN *vasodilator* [also: nafronyl oxalate]

**naftifine** INN, BAN *broad-spectrum antifungal* [also: naftifine HCl]

**naftifine HCl** USAN *broad-spectrum antifungal* [also: naftifine]

**Naftin** cream, gel R *topical antifungal* [naftifine HCl] 1%

**naftopidil** INN

**naftoxate** INN

**naftypramide** INN *antibacterial*

**Naganol** (available only from the Centers for Disease Control) R *antiparasitic for African trypanosomiasis and onchocerciasis* [suramin sodium]

**naganol** [see: suramin sodium]

**NaGHB (sodium gamma hydroxy-butyrate)** [see: gamma hydroxybutyrate (GHB); sodium oxybate]

**nagrestipen** USAN *stem cell inhibitory protein*

**nalazosulfamide** [see: salazosulfamide]

**nalbuphine** INN, BAN *narcotic agonist-antagonist analgesic; narcotic antagonist* [also: nalbuphine HCl]

**nalbuphine HCl** USAN *narcotic agonist-antagonist analgesic; narcotic antagonist* [also: nalbuphine] 10, 20 mg/mL injection

**Naldecon** sustained-release tablets, syrup, pediatric syrup, pediatric drops (discontinued 2001) ℞ *decongestant; antihistamine* [phenylpropanolamine HCl; phenylephrine HCl; chlorpheniramine maleate; phenyltoloxamine citrate] 40•10•5•15 mg; 20•5•2.5•7.5 mg/5 mL; 5•1.25•0.5•2 mg/5 mL; 5•1.25•0.5•2 mg/mL ⊡ Nalfon

**Naldecon CX Adult** oral liquid (discontinued 2002) ℞ *narcotic antitussive; decongestant; expectorant* [codeine phosphate; phenylpropanolamine HCl; guaifenesin] 10•12.5•200 mg/5 mL

**Naldecon DX** children's syrup, pediatric drops (discontinued 2002) OTC *pediatric antitussive, decongestant, and expectorant* [dextromethorphan hydrobromide; phenylpropanolamine HCl; guaifenesin] 5•6.25•100 mg/5 mL; 5•6.25•50 mg/mL

**Naldecon DX Adult** oral liquid (discontinued 2002) OTC *antitussive; decongestant; expectorant* [dextromethorphan hydrobromide; phenylpropanolamine HCl; guaifenesin] 10•12.5•200 mg/5 mL

**Naldecon EX** children's syrup, pediatric drops (discontinued 2002) OTC *decongestant; expectorant* [phenylpropanolamine HCl; guaifenesin] 6.25•100 mg/5 mL; 6.25•50 mg/mL

**Naldecon Senior DX** oral liquid (discontinued 2003) OTC *antitussive; expectorant* [dextromethorphan hydrobromide; guaifenesin] 20•400 mg/10 mL

**Naldecon Senior EX** oral liquid OTC *expectorant* [guaifenesin] 200 mg/5 mL

**Naldelate** syrup, pediatric syrup (discontinued 2001) ℞ *decongestant; antihistamine* [phenylpropanolamine HCl; phenylephrine HCl; chlorpheniramine maleate; phenyltoloxamine citrate] 20•5•2.5•7.5 mg/5 mL; 5•1.25•0.5•2 mg/5 mL

**Naldelate DX Adult** oral liquid (discontinued 2002) OTC *antitussive; decongestant; expectorant* [dextromethorphan hydrobromide; phenylpropanolamine HCl; guaifenesin] 10•12.5•200 mg/5 mL

**Nalfon** Pulvules (capsules) ℞ *analgesic; antiarthritic; nonsteroidal anti-inflammatory drug (NSAID)* [fenoprofen calcium] 200, 300 mg ⊡ Naldecon

**Nalgest** sustained-release tablets, syrup, pediatric syrup, pediatric drops (discontinued 2001) ℞ *decongestant; antihistamine* [phenylpropanolamine HCl; phenylephrine HCl; chlorpheniramine maleate; phenyltoloxamine citrate] 40•10•5•15 mg; 20•5•2.5•7.5 mg/5 mL; 5•1.25•0.5•2 mg/5 mL; 5•1.25•0.5•2 mg/mL

**nalidixane** [see: nalidixic acid]

**nalidixate sodium** USAN *antibacterial*

**nalidixic acid** USAN, USP, INN *urinary antibiotic*

**Nallpen** powder for IV or IM injection (discontinued 2002) ℞ *penicillinase-resistant penicillin antibiotic* [nafcillin sodium] 0.5, 1, 2, 10 g

**nalmefene** USAN, INN, BAN *narcotic antagonist; antidote to opioid overdose*

**nalmefene HCl** *narcotic antagonist; postanesthesia "stir-up"; antidote to opioid overdose*

**nalmetrene** [now: nalmefene]

**nalmexone** INN *analgesic; narcotic antagonist* [also: nalmexone HCl]

**nalmexone HCl** USAN *analgesic; narcotic antagonist* [also: nalmexone]

**nalorphine** INN [also: nalorphine HCl]

**nalorphine HCl** USP [also: nalorphine]

**naloxiphane tartrate** [see: levallorphan tartrate]

**naloxone** INN, BAN *narcotic antagonist* [also: naloxone HCl]

**naloxone HCl** USAN, USP, JAN *narcotic antagonist* [also: naloxone] 0.02, 0.4 mg/mL injection

**naloxone HCl & buprenorphine HCl** *investigational (orphan) for opiate addictions*

**naloxone HCl & pentazocine** *narcotic agonist-antagonist analgesic* 0.5•50 mg oral

**naltrexone** USAN, INN, BAN *narcotic antagonist*

**naltrexone HCl** *opiate blockage and maintenance in formerly opiate-dependent individuals (orphan); investigational (Phase III) treatment for alcoholism* 50 mg oral

**Namenda** film-coated caplets *NMDA (N-methyl-D-aspartate) antagonist for Alzheimer disease; investigational (Phase III) neuroprotective agent for diabetic neuropathy, vascular dementia, Parkinson disease, and AIDS dementia* [memantine HCl] 5, 10 mg

**naminterol** INN

**[¹³N]ammonia** [see: ammonia N 13]

**namoxyrate** USAN, INN *analgesic*

**namuron** [see: cyclobarbitone]

**nanafrocin** INN

**nandrolone** BAN *anabolic* [also: nandrolone cyclotate]

**nandrolone cyclotate** USAN *anabolic* [also: nandrolone]

**nandrolone decanoate** USAN, USP *androgen/anabolic steroid for anemia of renal insufficiency; sometimes abused as a street drug* 100, 200 mg/mL injection (in oil)

**nandrolone phenpropionate** USP *androgen/anabolic steroid for metastatic breast cancer in women; sometimes abused as a street drug*

**naniopine** [see: nanofin]

**NanobacTEST-S** for professional use *blood serum test for the presence of nanobacterial antigens and antibodies*

**NanobacTEST-U/A** for professional use *rapid screening urine test for the presence of live, uncalcified nanobacteria by visual color comparison* [ELISA test]

**nanofin** INN

**nanterinone** INN, BAN

**nantradol** INN *analgesic* [also: nantradol HCl]

**nantradol HCl** USAN *analgesic* [also: nantradol]

**NAPA (N-acetyl-*p*-aminophenol)** [see: acetaminophen]

**NAPA (N-acetyl-procainamide)** [q.v.]

**napactadine** INN *antidepressant* [also: napactadine HCl]

**napactadine HCl** USAN *antidepressant* [also: napactadine]

**napadisilate** INN *combining name for radicals or groups* [also: napadisylate]

**napadisylate** BAN *combining name for radicals or groups* [also: napadisilate]

**napamezole** INN *antidepressant* [also: napamezole HCl]

**napamezole HCl** USAN *antidepressant* [also: napamezole]

**Na-PCA** topical spray OTC *natural skin moisturizing factor; humectant* [sodium pyrrolidone carboxylic acid; aloe vera]

**naphazoline** INN, BAN *topical ophthalmic decongestant and vasoconstrictor; nasal decongestant* [also: naphazoline HCl; naphazoline nitrate]

**naphazoline HCl** USP *topical ophthalmic decongestant and vasoconstrictor; nasal decongestant* [also: naphazoline; naphazoline nitrate] 0.1% eye drops

**naphazoline HCl & antazoline phosphate** *topical ocular decongestant and antihistamine* 0.05%•0.5%

**naphazoline HCl & pheniramine maleate** *topical ocular decongestant and antihistamine* 0.025%•0.3% eye drops

**naphazoline nitrate** JAN *topical ocular vasoconstrictor; nasal decongestant* [also: naphazoline HCl; naphazoline]

**Naphazoline Plus** eye drops OTC *topical ophthalmic decongestant and antihistamine* [naphazoline HCl; pheniramine maleate] 0.025%•0.3%

**Naphcon** eye drops OTC *topical ophthalmic decongestant and vasoconstrictor* [naphazoline HCl] 0.012%

**Naphcon Forte** Drop-Tainers (eye drops) Ŗ *topical ophthalmic decongestant and vasoconstrictor* [naphazoline HCl] 0.1%

**Naphcon-A** Drop-Tainers (eye drops) OTC *topical ophthalmic decongestant and antihistamine* [naphazoline HCl; pheniramine maleate] 0.025%•0.3%

**Naphoptic-A** eye drops Ŗ *topical ophthalmic decongestant and antihistamine* [naphazoline HCl; pheniramine maleate] 0.025%•0.3%

**2-naphthol** [see: betanaphthol]

**naphthonone** INN

**naphthypramide** [see: naftypramide]

**Naphuride** (available only from the Centers for Disease Control) Ŗ *antiparasitic for African trypanosomiasis and onchocerciasis* [suramin sodium]

**napirimus** INN

**napitane mesylate** USAN *antidepressant; α-adrenergic blocker; norepinephrine uptake antagonist*

**Naprelan** controlled-release tablets Ŗ *once-daily analgesic and antiarthritic; nonsteroidal anti-inflammatory drug (NSAID)* [naproxen sodium] 412.5, 550 mg (=375, 500 mg base)

**naprodoxime** INN

**Napron X** tablets (discontinued 2000) Ŗ *analgesic; antiarthritic; nonsteroidal anti-inflammatory drug* [naproxen] 500 mg ⊗ Lupron; Mepron

**Naprosyn** tablets, oral suspension Ŗ *analgesic; antiarthritic; nonsteroidal anti-inflammatory drug (NSAID)* [naproxen] 250, 375, 500 mg; 125 mg/5 mL ⊗ Meprospan; Natacyn

**Naprosyn EC** [see: EC-Naprosyn]

**naproxen** USAN, USP, INN, BAN, JAN *analgesic; antiarthritic; nonsteroidal anti-inflammatory drug (NSAID)* 250, 375, 500 mg oral; 125 mg/5 mL oral

**naproxen sodium** USAN, USP *analgesic; antiarthritic; antipyretic; nonsteroidal anti-inflammatory drug (NSAID)* (base=91%) 220, 275, 550 mg oral

**naproxol** USAN, INN *anti-inflammatory; analgesic; antipyretic*

**napsagatran** USAN, INN *antithrombotic*

**napsilate** INN *combining name for radicals or groups* [also: napsylate]

**napsylate** USAN, BAN *combining name for radicals or groups* [also: napsilate]

**Naqua** tablets Ŗ *diuretic; antihypertensive* [trichlormethiazide] 2, 4 mg

**naranol** INN *antipsychotic* [also: naranol HCl]

**naranol HCl** USAN *antipsychotic* [also: naranol]

**narasin** USAN, INN, BAN *coccidiostat; veterinary growth stimulant*

**naratriptan** INN, BAN *vascular serotonin 5-HT$_{1D}$ receptor agonist for the acute treatment of migraine* [also: naratriptan HCl]

**naratriptan HCl** USAN *vascular serotonin 5-HT$_{1D}$ receptor agonist for the acute treatment of migraine* [also: naratriptan]

**Narcan** IV, IM, or subcu injection Ŗ *narcotic antagonist for opiate dependence or overdose; hypotension treatment* [naloxone HCl] 0.4, 1 mg/mL ⊗ Marcaine

**Narcan** neonatal injection (discontinued 2003) Ŗ *narcotic antagonist for opiate dependence* [naloxone HCl] 0.02 mg/mL ⊗ Marcaine

**narcotic agonist-antagonists** *a class of opioid or morphine-like analgesics with lower abuse potential than pure narcotic agonist analgesics*

**narcotic agonists; narcotics** *a class of opioid or morphine-like analgesics that relieve pain and induce sleep*

**narcotine** [see: noscapine]

**narcotine HCl** [see: noscapine HCl]

**nard** *medicinal herb* [see: spikenard]

**Nardil** sugar-coated tablets Ŗ *antipsychotic; monoamine oxidase inhibitor (MAOI) for treatment-resistant atypical depression* [phenelzine sulfate] 15 mg ⊗ Norinyl

**Naropin** injection Ŗ *long-acting local anesthetic* [ropivacaine HCl] 2, 5, 7.5, 10 mg/mL

**narrow dock** *medicinal herb* [see: yellow dock]

**Nasabid** prolonged-action capsules (discontinued 2002) ℞ *decongestant; expectorant* [pseudoephedrine HCl; guaifenesin] 90•250 mg

**Nasabid SR** long-acting tablets ℞ *decongestant; expectorant* [pseudoephedrine HCl; guaifenesin] 90•600 mg

**Nasacort** nasal spray (discontinued 2003) ℞ *corticosteroidal anti-inflammatory for seasonal or perennial rhinitis* [triamcinolone acetonide] 55 μg/dose

**Nasacort AQ** metered-dose aerosol ℞ *corticosteroidal anti-inflammatory for seasonal or perennial rhinitis* [triamcinolone acetonide] 55 μg/dose

**NāSal** nasal spray, nose drops OTC *nasal moisturizer* [sodium chloride (saline solution)] 0.65%

**Nasal Decongestant** pediatric oral drops OTC *nasal decongestant* [pseudoephedrine HCl] 7.5 mg/0.8 mL

**Nasal Decongestant** spray OTC *nasal decongestant* [oxymetazoline HCl] 0.05%

**Nasal Decongestant, Children's Non-Drowsy** oral liquid OTC *nasal decongestant* [pseudoephedrine HCl] 15 mg/5 mL

**Nasal Decongestant Sinus Non-Drowsy** tablets OTC *decongestant; analgesic; antipyretic* [pseudoephedrine HCl; acetaminophen] 30•500 mg

**Nasal Jelly** ointment (discontinued 2002) OTC *nasal moisturizer* [phenol; camphor; menthol; eucalyptus oil; oil of lavender]

**Nasal Moist** nasal spray OTC *nasal moisturizer* [sodium chloride (saline solution)] 0.65%

**Nasal Relief** nasal spray OTC *nasal decongestant* [oxymetazoline HCl] 0.05%

**Nasal Spray** OTC *nasal moisturizer* [sodium chloride (saline solution)]

**NasalCrom** nasal spray OTC *anti-inflammatory/mast cell stabilizer for the prophylaxis of allergic rhinitis; treatment for mastocytosis (orphan)* [cromolyn sodium] 4% (5.2 mg/dose)

**NasalCrom, Children's** nasal spray (discontinued 2003) OTC *anti-inflammatory/mast cell stabilizer for the prophylaxis of allergic rhinitis* [cromolyn sodium] 4% (5.2 mg/dose)

**NasalCrom A** nasal spray + tablets OTC *anti-inflammatory/mast cell stabilizer for the prophylaxis of allergic rhinitis; antihistamine* [cromolyn sodium; chlorpheniramine maleate] 4% (5.2 mg/dose); 4 mg

**NasalCrom CA** nasal spray + tablets OTC *anti-inflammatory/mast cell stabilizer for the prophylaxis of allergic rhinitis; decongestant; analgesic* [cromolyn sodium; pseudoephedrine HCl; acetaminophen] 4% (5.2 mg/dose); 30 mg•500 mg

**Nasal-Ease with Zinc** nasal gel OTC *nasal moisturizer and anti-infective* [zinc acetate]

**Nasal-Ease with Zinc Gluconate** nasal spray OTC *nasal moisturizer and anti-infective* [zinc gluconate]

**Nasalide** nasal spray (discontinued 2004) ℞ *corticosteroidal anti-inflammatory for seasonal or perennial rhinitis* [flunisolide] 0.025% (25 μg/dose)

**Nasarel** metered dose nasal spray ℞ *corticosteroidal anti-inflammatory for seasonal or perennial rhinitis* [flunisolide] 0.025% (29 μg/dose)

**Nasatab LA** long-acting film-coated caplets ℞ *decongestant; expectorant* [pseudoephedrine HCl; guaifenesin] 120•500 mg

**Nascobal** nasal gel in metered-dose applicator ℞ *maintenance administration following intramuscular vitamin $B_{12}$ therapy* [cyanocobalamin] 500 μg/0.1 mL dose

**NASHA (non-animal stabilized hyaluronic acid)** [see: hyaluronic acid]

**Nashville rabbit antithymocyte serum** [see: lymphocyte immune globulin, antithymocyte]

**Nashville Rabbit Antithymocyte Serum** ℞ *investigational (orphan)*

passive immunizing agent to prevent allograft rejection of solid organ and bone marrow transplants [antithymocyte globulin, rabbit]

**Nasonex** nasal spray ℞ corticosteroid for the prophylaxis and treatment of seasonal and perennial allergic rhinitis [mometasone furoate] 0.05% (50 μg/dose)

**Nasturtium officinale** medicinal herb [see: watercress]

**NataChew** chewable tablets ℞ prenatal vitamin/mineral supplement [multiple vitamins & minerals; ferrous fumarate; folic acid] ± • 29 • 1 mg

**Natacyn** eye drop suspension ℞ ophthalmic antifungal agent [natamycin] 5% ☑ Naprosyn

**NataFort** film-coated tablets ℞ prenatal vitamin/iron supplement [multiple vitamins; ferrous sulfate; folic acid] ± • 60 • 1 mg

**NatalCare Plus; NatalCare Three** film-coated tablets ℞ vitamin/mineral/calcium/iron supplement [multiple vitamins & minerals; calcium; iron; folic acid] ± • 200 • 27 • 1 mg

**Natalins** tablets (discontinued 2001) OTC vitamin/calcium/iron supplement [multiple vitamins; calcium; iron; folic acid] ± • 200 • 30 • 0.5 mg

**Natalins Rx** tablets (name changed to Enfamil Natalins Rx in 2001)

**natalizumab** investigational (NDA filed) humanized monoclonal antibody (huMAb) for treatment of multiple sclerosis and Crohn disease

**natamycin** USAN, USP, INN, BAN ophthalmic fungicidal antibiotic [also: pimaricin]

**Natarex Prenatal** tablets ℞ vitamin/calcium/iron supplement [multiple vitamins; calcium; iron; folic acid; biotin] ± • 200 • 60 • 1 • 0.03 mg

**NataTab CFe; NataTab FA; NataTab Rx** film-coated tablets ℞ prenatal vitamin/mineral supplement [multiple vitamins & minerals]

**nateglinide** USAN amino acid–derivative; oral antidiabetic agent that stimu-

lates the release of insulin from the pancreas for type 2 diabetes

**Natelle-EZ** caplets ℞ vitamin/mineral/calcium/iron supplement [multiple vitamins & minerals; calcium; iron; folic acid biotin] ± • 100 • 25 • 1 • 0.3 mg

**Natrecor** powder for IV injection ℞ human B-type natriuretic peptide (hBNP); vasodilator for acute congestive heart failure [nesiritide citrate] 1.58 mg/vial

**Natru-Vent** nasal spray OTC nasal decongestant [xylometazoline HCl] 0.05%, 0.1%

**Natural Fiber Laxative** powder OTC bulk laxative [psyllium hydrophilic mucilloid] 3.4 g/dose

**natural killer cell stimulatory factor** [see: edodekin alfa]

**Naturalyte** oral solution OTC electrolyte replacement [sodium, potassium, and chloride electrolytes] 240 mL, 1 L

**Nature Throid** tablets ℞ thyroid replacement therapy for hypothyroidism or thyroid cancer [thyroid, desiccated (porcine)] 32.4, 64.8, 129.6, 194.4 mg

**Nature's Choice** ⓐ powder for oral solution OTC vitamin/mineral/calcium/iron supplement [multiple vitamins & minerals; calcium; iron; folic acid; biotin] ± • 500 • 4 • 0.08 • 0.06 mg

**Nature's Remedy** tablets OTC stimulant laxative [cascara sagrada; aloe] 150 • 100 mg

**Nature's Tears** eye drops OTC ophthalmic moisturizer/lubricant [hydroxypropyl methylcellulose] 0.4%

**Naturetin** tablets ℞ antihypertensive; diuretic [bendroflumethiazide] 5 mg

**Naturvus** hydrophilic contact lens material [hefilcon B]

**Nausea Relief** oral solution OTC antiemetic for nausea associated with influenza, morning sickness, motion sickness, inhalation anesthesia, or food and drink indiscretions [phosphorated carbohydrate solution (dextrose, fructose, and phosphoric acid)] 1.87 g • 1.87 g • 21.5 mg per dose

**Nausetrol** oral solution OTC *antiemetic for nausea associated with influenza, morning sickness, motion sickness, inhalation anesthesia, or food and drink indiscretions* [phosphorated carbohydrate solution (fructose, dextrose, and orthophosphoric acid)]

**Navane** capsules ℞ *conventional (typical) antipsychotic* [thiothixene] 1, 2, 5, 10, 20 mg

**Navane** oral concentrate ℞ *conventional (typical) antipsychotic* [thiothixene HCl] 5 mg/mL

**Navelbine** IV injection ℞ *antineoplastic for Hodgkin disease and lung, breast and ovarian cancer* [vinorelbine tartrate] 10 mg/mL

**naxagolide** INN *antiparkinsonian; dopamine agonist* [also: naxagolide HCl]

**naxagolide HCl** USAN *antiparkinsonian; dopamine agonist* [also: naxagolide]

**naxaprostene** INN

**naxifylline** USAN *treatment of edema due to congestive heart failure*

**NBI-3001** *investigational (Phase I/II, orphan) for glioblastoma or astrocytic glioma* [also: interleukin-4 Pseudomonas toxin fusion protein]

**9-NC (9-nitrocamptothecin)** [see: rubitecan]

**ND Clear** sustained-release capsules ℞ *decongestant; antihistamine* [pseudoephedrine HCl; chlorpheniramine maleate] 120•8 mg

**ND-Gesic** tablets (discontinued 2002) OTC *decongestant; antihistamine; analgesic* [phenylephrine HCl; chlorpheniramine maleate; pyrilamine maleate; acetaminophen] 5•2•12.5•300 mg

**NE-1530** *investigational (Phase II) agent for the prevention of otitis media (clinical trials discontinued 1999)*

**nealbarbital** INN [also: nealbarbitone]

**nealbarbitone** BAN [also: nealbarbital]

**nebacumab** USAN, INN, BAN *antiendotoxin monoclonal antibody; investigational (orphan) for gram-negative bacteremia in endotoxin shock*

**Nebcin** IV or IM injection, pediatric injection, powder for injection ℞ *aminoglycoside antibiotic* [tobramycin sulfate] 10, 40 mg/mL; 10 mg/mL; 1.2 g

**nebidrazine** INN

**nebivolol** USAN, INN *investigational (NDA filed) antihypertensive (selective $\beta_1$-blocker)*

**nebracetam** INN

**nebramycin** USAN, INN *antibacterial*

**nebramycin factor 6** [see: tobramycin]

**NebuPent** inhalation aerosol ℞ *antiprotozoal; treatment and prophylaxis of Pneumocystis carinii pneumonia (orphan)* [pentamidine isethionate] 300 mg

**Necon 0.5/35; Necon 1/35** tablets (in packs of 21 or 28) ℞ *monophasic oral contraceptive* [norethindrone; ethinyl estradiol] 0.5 mg•35 μg; 1 mg•35 μg

**Necon 1/50** tablets (in packs of 21 or 28) ℞ *monophasic oral contraceptive* [norethindrone; mestranol] 1 mg• 50 μg

**Necon 10/11** tablets (in packs of 21 or 28) ℞ *biphasic oral contraceptive* [norethindrone; ethinyl estradiol] Phase 1 (10 days): 500•35 μg; Phase 2 (11 days): 1000•35 μg

**Necon 7/7/7** tablets (in packs of 28) ℞ *triphasic oral contraceptive* [norethindrone; ethinyl estradiol] Phase 1 (7 days): 500•35 μg; Phase 2 (7 days): 750•35 μg; Phase 3 (7 days): 1000•35 μg

**nedocromil** USAN, INN, BAN *anti-inflammatory; prophylactic antiallergic; mast cell stabilizer*

**nedocromil calcium** USAN *anti-inflammatory; prophylactic antiallergic; mast cell stabilizer*

**nedocromil sodium** USAN *anti-inflammatory; mast cell stabilizer; antiasthmatic; prophylactic antiallergic*

**neem tree (Azadirachta indica)** fruit, leaves, root, and oil *medicinal herb for contraception, diabetes, heart disease, malaria, skin diseases, ulcers, and worms; also used as a pesticide and insect repellent; not generally regarded* *as safe and effective for infants as it may cause death*

**nefazodone** INN *antidepressant; selective serotonin and norepinephrine reuptake inhibitor (SSNRI)* [also: nefazodone HCl]

**nefazodone HCl** USAN *antidepressant; selective serotonin and norepinephrine reuptake inhibitor (SSNRI); discontinued 2004 due to safety concerns* [also: nefazodone] 50, 100, 150, 200, 250 mg oral

**neflumozide** INN *antipsychotic* [also: neflumozide HCl]

**neflumozide HCl** USAN *antipsychotic* [also: neflumozide]

**nefocon A** USAN *hydrophobic contact lens material*

**nefopam** INN *analgesic* [also: nefopam HCl]

**nefopam HCl** USAN *analgesic* [also: nefopam]

**nefrolan** [see: clorexolone]

**NegGram** caplets, oral suspension ℞ *urinary antibiotic* [nalidixic acid] 250, 500, 1000 mg; 250 mg/5 mL

**nelarabine** USAN *antineoplastic for T-cell and B-cell lymphomas*

**neldazosin** INN

**nelezaprine** INN *muscle relaxant* [also: nelezaprine maleate]

**nelezaprine maleate** USAN *muscle relaxant* [also: nelezaprine]

**nelfilcon A** USAN *hydrophilic contact lens material*

**nelfinavir mesylate** USAN *antiretroviral; protease inhibitor for HIV-1 infection*

**nelfinavir mesylate & amprenavir** *investigational (Phase II) protease inhibitor combination for AIDS*

**Nelova 0.5/35E; Nelova 1/35E** tablets (in packs of 21 or 28) (discontinued 2001) ℞ *monophasic oral contraceptive* [norethindrone; ethinyl estradiol] 0.5 mg•35 μg; 1 mg•35 μg

**Nelova 1/50M** tablets (in packs of 21 or 28) (discontinued 2001) ℞ *monophasic oral contraceptive* [norethindrone; mestranol] 1 mg•50 μg

**Nelova 10/11** tablets (in packs of 21 and 28) (discontinued 2001) ℞ *biphasic oral contraceptive* [norethindrone; ethinyl estradiol]
Phase 1 (10 days): 0.5 mg•35 μg;
Phase 2 (11 days): 1 mg•35 μg

**nemadectin** USAN, INN *veterinary antiparasitic*

**nemazoline** INN *nasal decongestant* [also: nemazoline HCl]

**nemazoline HCl** USAN *nasal decongestant* [also: nemazoline]

**Nembutal** elixir ℞ *sedative; hypnotic; also abused as a street drug* [pentobarbital] 20 mg/5 mL ⚇ Myambutal

**Nembutal Sodium** capsules, IV or IM injection, suppositories ℞ *sedative; hypnotic; also abused as a street drug* [pentobarbital sodium] 50, 100 mg; 50 mg/mL; 30, 60, 120, 200 mg

**neoarsphenamine** NF, INN

**Neocaf** ℞ *investigational (orphan) for apnea of prematurity* [caffeine]

**Neo-Calglucon** syrup (discontinued 2002) OTC *calcium supplement* [calcium glubionate] 1.8 g/5 mL

**neocarzinostatin** [now: zinostatin]

**Neocate One +** ready-to-use oral liquid OTC *pediatric enteral nutritional therapy* [lactose-free formula] 237 mL

**Neocera** (trademarked ingredient) *suppository base* [polyethylent glycol 400, 1450, and 8000; polysorbate 60]

**neocid** [see: chlorophenothane]

**neocinchophen** NF, INN

**NeoDecadron** Ocumeter (eye drops), ophthalmic ointment ℞ *topical ophthalmic corticosteroidal anti-inflammatory; antibiotic* [dexamethasone sodium phosphate; neomycin sulfate] 0.1%•0.35%; 0.05%•0.35%

**Neo-Dexair** eye drops ℞ *topical ophthalmic corticosteroidal anti-inflammatory; antibiotic* [dexamethasone sodium phosphate; neomycin sulfate] 0.1%•0.35%

**Neo-Dexameth** eye drops ℞ *topical ophthalmic corticosteroidal anti-inflammatory; antibiotic* [dexamethasone sodium phosphate; neomycin sulfate] 0.1%•0.35%

**Neo-Diaral** capsules OTC *antidiarrheal* [loperamide] 2 mg

**Neo-Durabolic** IM injection (discontinued 2000) ℞ *anabolic steroid for anemia of renal insufficiency* [nandrolone decanoate (in oil)] 50, 200 mg/mL

**neodymium** *element (Nd)*

**Neo-fradin** oral solution ℞ *aminoglycoside antibiotic* [neomycin sulfate] 125 mg/5 mL

**Neoloid** oral emulsion OTC *stimulant laxative* [castor oil] 36.4%

**Neomark** ℞ *investigational (NDA filed, orphan) radiosensitizer for primary brain tumors* [broxuridine]

**neo-mercazole** [see: carbimazole]

**Neomixin** ointment (discontinued 2001) OTC *topical antibiotic* [polymyxin B sulfate; neomycin sulfate; bacitracin zinc] 5000 U•3.5 mg•400 U per g ② neomycin

**neomycin** INN, BAN *antibacterial* [also: neomycin palmitate] ② Neomixin

**neomycin B** [see: framycetin]

**neomycin palmitate** USAN *antibacterial* [also: neomycin]

**neomycin sulfate** USP *aminoglycoside antibiotic* 500 mg oral

**neomycin sulfate & polymyxin B sulfate & bacitracin zinc** *topical antibiotic* 5 mg•10 000 U•400 U per g ophthalmic

**neomycin sulfate & polymyxin B sulfate & dexamethasone** *topical ophthalmic antibiotic and corticosteroidal anti-inflammatory* 0.35%•10 000 U/mL•0.1% eye drops

**neomycin sulfate & polymyxin B sulfate & gramicidin** *topical antibiotic* 1.75 mg•10 000 U•0.025 mg per mL eye drops

**neomycin sulfate & polymyxin B sulfate & hydrocortisone** *topical ophthalmic antibiotic and corticosteroidal anti-inflammatory* 0.35%•10 000 U/mL•1% eye drops

**neomycin undecenoate** [see: neomycin undecylenate]

**neomycin undecylenate** USAN *antibacterial; antifungal*

**neon** *element (Ne)*

**Neopap** suppositories OTC *analgesic; antipyretic* [acetaminophen] 125 mg

**neopenyl** [see: clemizole penicillin]

**neoquate** [see: nequinate]

**Neoral** gelcaps, oral solution ℞ *immunosuppressant for allogenic kidney, liver, and heart transplants (orphan), rheumatoid arthritis, and psoriasis* [cyclosporine; alcohol 11.9%] 25, 100 mg; 100 mg/mL

**Neosar** powder for IV injection ℞ *nitrogen mustard-type alkylating antineoplastic for multiple leukemias, lymphomas, blastomas, sarcomas and organ cancers* [cyclophosphamide] 100 mg

**Neosol** orally disintegrating tablets ℞ *GI/GU antispasmodic; antiparkinsonian; anticholinergic "drying agent" for allergic rhinitis and hyperhidrosis* [hyoscyamine sulfate] 0.125 mg

**Neosporin** cream (discontinued 2001) OTC *antibiotic* [polymyxin B sulfate; neomycin sulfate] 10 000 U•3.5 mg per g

**Neosporin** Drop Dose (eye drops) ℞ *antibiotic* [polymyxin B sulfate; neomycin sulfate; gramicidin] 10 000 U•1.75 mg•0.025 mg per mL

**Neosporin** ointment (discontinued 2001) OTC *antibiotic* [polymyxin B sulfate; neomycin sulfate; bacitracin] 10 000 U•3.5 mg•500 U per g

**Neosporin** ophthalmic ointment ℞ *antibiotic* [polymyxin B sulfate; neomycin sulfate; bacitracin zinc] 10 000 U•5 mg•400 U per g

**Neosporin G.U. Irrigant** solution ℞ *antibiotic* [neomycin sulfate; polymyxin B sulfate] 40 mg•200 000 U per mL

**Neosporin Original** ointment OTC *antibiotic* [polymyxin B sulfate; neomycin sulfate; bacitracin zinc] 5000 U•3.5 mg•400 U per g

**Neosporin Plus** cream (discontinued 2001) OTC *antibiotic; local anesthetic* [polymyxin B sulfate; neomycin; lidocaine] 10 000 U•3.5 mg•40 mg per g

**Neosporin Plus** ointment (discontinued 2001) OTC *antibiotic; local anesthetic* [polymyxin B sulfate; bacitracin zinc; neomycin; lidocaine] 10 000 U•500 U•3.5 mg•40 mg per g

**Neosporin Plus Pain Relief** cream OTC *antibiotic; local anesthetic* [polymyxin B sulfate; neomycin sulfate; pramoxine HCl] 10 000 U•3.5 mg•10 mg per g

**Neosporin Plus Pain Relief** ointment OTC *antibiotic; local anesthetic* [polymyxin B sulfate; neomycon sulfate; bacitracin zinc; pramoxine HCl] 10 000 U•3.5 mg•500 U•10 mg per g

**Neosten** timed-release tablets ℞ *investigational (NDA filed) agent for osteoporosis* [sodium fluoride]

**neostigmine** BAN *cholinergic/anticholinesterase muscle stimulant* [also: neostigmine bromide]

**neostigmine bromide** USP, INN, BAN *cholinergic/anticholinesterase muscle stimulant* [also: neostigmine] 15 mg oral

**neostigmine methylsulfate** USP *cholinergic/anticholinesterase muscle stimulant; urinary stimulant for postsurgical urinary retention; treatment for myasthenia gravis; antidote to neuromuscular blockers* 1:1000 (1 mg/mL), 1:2000 (0.5 mg/mL) injection

**Neostrata Skin Lightening** gel OTC *hyperpigmentation bleaching agent* [hydroquinone] 2%

**Neo-Synephrine** eye drops, viscous solution ℞ *topical ophthalmic decongestant and vasoconstrictor; mydriatic* [phenylephrine HCl] 2.5%, 10%; 10%

**Neo-Synephrine** IV, IM, or subcu injection ℞ *vasopressor for hypotensive or cardiac shock* [phenylephrine HCl] 1% (10 mg/mL)

**Neo-Synephrine** nasal spray, nose drops (multiple name changes in 2002) OTC *nasal decongestant* [phenylephrine HCl] 0.25%, 0.5%, 1%; 0.125%, 0.25%, 0.5%, 1%

**Neo-Synephrine 4-Hour Mild Formula** nasal spray OTC *nasal decongestant* [phenylephrine HCl] 0.25%

**Neo-Synephrine 4-Hour Regular Strength; Neo-Synephrine 4-Hour Extra Strength** nasal spray, nose drops OTC *nasal decongestant* [phenylephrine HCl] 0.5%; 1%

**Neo-Synephrine 12-Hour; Neo-Synephrine 12-Hour Extra Moisturizing** nasal spray OTC *nasal decongestant* [oxymetazoline HCl] 0.05%

**Neo-Tabs** tablets ℞ *aminoglycoside antibiotic* [neomycin sulfate] 500 mg

**NeoTect** kit for injection preparation ℞ *radiopharmaceutical imaging agent for lung cancer; investigational (NDA filed) for malignant melanoma and neuroendocrine disorders* [depreotide]

**Neotrace-4** IV injection ℞ *intravenous nutritional therapy* [multiple trace elements (metals)]

**Neotricin HC** ophthalmic ointment ℞ *topical ophthalmic corticosteroidal anti-inflammatory; antibiotic* [hydrocortisone acetate; neomycin sulfate; bacitracin zinc; polymyxin B sulfate] 1%•3.5%•400 U/g•10 000 U/g

**Neotrofin** ℞ *investigational (Phase II/III) nerve growth factor for Alzheimer disease, spinal cord injuries, and stroke* [leteprinim potassium]

**Neovastat** ℞ *investigational (Phase III) shark cartilage–based angiogenesis inhibitor for osteoarthritis, rheumatoid arthritis, and various cancers; investigational (orphan) for renal cell carcinoma* [AE-941 (code name—generic name not yet assigned)] ☑ Novastan

**nepafenac** USAN *topical ophthalmic anti-inflammatory and analgesic*

**Nepeta cataria** *medicinal herb* [see: catnip]

**Nephplex Rx** tablets ℞ *vitamin/zinc supplement* [multiple B vitamins; ascorbic acid; folic acid; biotin; zinc] ≛•60•1•0.3•12.5 mg

**NephrAmine 5.4%** IV infusion ℞ *nutritional therapy for renal failure*

[multiple essential amino acids; electrolytes]

**nephritics** *a class of agents that affect the kidney (a term used in folk medicine)*

**Nephro-Calci** tablets OTC *calcium supplement* [calcium carbonate] 1500 mg (600 mg Ca)

**Nephrocaps** capsules ℞ *vitamin supplement* [multiple B vitamins; vitamin C; folic acid; biotin] ± •100 mg•1 mg•150 μg

**Nephro-Fer** tablets OTC *hematinic* [ferrous fumarate (source of iron)] 350 mg (115 mg)

**Nephro-Fer Rx** film-coated tablets ℞ *hematinic* [ferrous fumarate; folic acid] 106.9•1 mg

**Nephron** solution for inhalation OTC *sympathomimetic bronchodilator* [racepinephrine HCl] 2.25%

**Nephron FA** tablets ℞ *hematinic* [ferrous fumarate; multiple B vitamins; ascorbic acid; folic acid; biotin; docusate sodium] 66.6• ± •40•1•0.3• 75 mg

**Nephro-Vite Rx** film-coated tablets ℞ *vitamin supplement* [multiple B vitamins; vitamin C; folic acid; biotin] ± •60 mg•1 mg•300 μg

**Nephro-Vite Rx + Fe** film-coated tablets ℞ *hematinic* [ferrous fumarate; multiple B vitamins; ascorbic acid; folic acid; biotin] 100• ± •60• 1•0.3 mg

**Nephro-Vite Vitamin B Complex and C Supplement** tablets OTC *vitamin supplement* [multiple B vitamins; vitamin C; folic acid; biotin] ± •60•0.8•0.3 mg

**Nephrox** oral suspension OTC *antacid; laxative* [aluminum hydroxide; mineral oil 10%] 320 mg/5 mL

**nepicastat HCl** USAN *dopamine β-hydroxylase inhibitor for congestive heart failure*

**Nepro** oral liquid OTC *enteral nutritional therapy for acute or chronic renal failure* [lactose-free formula] 240 mL

**neptamustine** INN *antineoplastic* [also: pentamustine]

**Neptazane** tablets (discontinued 2004) ℞ *carbonic anhydrase inhibitor for glaucoma* [methazolamide] 25, 50 mg

**neptunium** *element (Np)*

**nequinate** USAN, INN *coccidiostat for poultry* [also: methyl benzoquate]

**neramexane** *investigational (Phase III) NMDA (N-methyl-D-aspartate)-receptor antagonist for Alzheimer disease*

**neraminol** INN

**nerbacadol** INN

**nerelimomab** USAN *monoclonal antibody; investigational (Phase III) cytokine modulator for septic shock*

**neridronic acid** INN

***Nerium indicum; N. oleander*** *medicinal herb* [see: oleander]

**nervines** *a class of agents that have a calming or soothing effect on the nerves (a term used in folk medicine)*

**Nervocaine 1%** injection (discontinued 2002) ℞ *injectable local anesthetic* [lidocaine HCl] 1%

**Nesacaine; Nesacaine MPF** injection ℞ *injectable local anesthetic* [chloroprocaine HCl] 1%, 2%; 2%, 3%

**nesapidil** INN

**nesiritide** USAN *human B-type natriuretic peptide (hBNP); vasodilator for acute congestive heart failure*

**nesiritide citrate** *human B-type natriuretic peptide (hBNP); vasodilator for acute congestive heart failure*

**nesosteine** INN

**Nestabs** tablets (name changed to Vitelle Nestabs OTC in 2000)

**Nestabs CBF; Nestabs FA** tablets ℞ *vitamin/calcium/iron supplement for pregnancy and lactation* [multiple vitamins; calcium; iron; folic acid] ± •200•50•1 mg; ± •200•29•1 mg

**Nestle VHC 2.25** oral liquid OTC *enteral nutritional therapy* [lactose-free formula]

**Nestrex** tablets (name changed to Vitelle Nestrex in 2001)

**nethalide** [see: pronetalol]

**netilmicin** INN, BAN *aminoglycoside antibiotic* [also: netilmicin sulfate]

**netilmicin sulfate** USAN, USP *amino-glycoside antibiotic* [also: netilmicin]

**netobimin** USAN, INN, BAN *veterinary anthelmintic*

**netrafilcon A** USAN *hydrophilic contact lens material*

**Netromicina** (Mexican name for U.S. product Netromycin)

**Netromycin** IV or IM injection (discontinued 2003) ℞ *aminoglycoside antibiotic* [netilmicin sulfate] 100 mg/mL

**nettle** *(Urtica dioica; U. urens)* leaves and root *medicinal herb for blood cleansing, bronchitis, diarrhea, edema, hypertension, bleeding, and rheumatism; competitively binds to sex hormone–binding globulin (SHBG) to increase the level of free testosterone*

**nettle, hemp; bee nettle; dog nettle; hemp dead nettle** *medicinal herb* [see: hemp nettle]

**nettle flowers; dead nettle; stingless nettle; white nettle** *medicinal herb* [see: blind nettle]

**Neulasta** subcu injection in prefilled syringe ℞ *hematopoietic stimulant for severe chronic neutropenia following cancer chemotherapy* [pegfilgrastim] 6 mg/0.6 mL

**Neumega** subcu injection ℞ *platelet growth factor for prevention of thrombocytopenia following chemotherapy or radiation (orphan)* [oprelvekin] 5 mg

**Neupogen** IV or subcu injection, pre-filled syringes ℞ *hematopoietic stimulant for severe chronic neutropenia (orphan); investigational (Phase III, orphan) cytokine for AIDS-related cytomegalovirus retinitis; investigational (orphan) for myelodysplastic syndrome* [filgrastim] 300 μg/mL; 300, 480 μg

**Neuprex** injection ℞ *investigational (Phase III, orphan) agent for gram-negative sepsis, hemorrhagic shock, and meningococcemia; investigational agent for lung infection in cystic fibrosis* [bactericidal and permeability-increasing protein, recombinant (rBPI-21)]

**neural dopaminergic cells (or precursors), porcine fetal** *investigational (orphan) intracerebral implant for stage 4 and 5 Parkinson disease*

**neural gabaergic cells (or precursors), porcine fetal** *investigational (orphan) intracerebral implant for Huntington disease*

**Neuramate** tablets (discontinued 2001) ℞ *anxiolytic* [meprobamate] 400 mg

**NeuRecover-DA; NeuRecover-SA** capsules OTC *dietary supplement* [multiple vitamins & minerals; multiple amino acids; folic acid] ± •0.067 mg; ± •0.067 mg

**NeuRecover-LT** capsules (discontinued 2001) OTC *dietary supplement* [multiple vitamins & minerals; multiple amino acids; folic acid] ± •0.03 mg

**Neurelan** *investigational (orphan) agent for multiple sclerosis and spinal cord injury* [fampridine]

**Neurobloc** (name changed to Myobloc upon marketing release in 2001)

**NeuroCell-HD** ℞ *investigational (orphan) intracerebral implant for patients with Huntington disease* [neural gabaergic cells, porcine fetal]

**NeuroCell-PD** ℞ *investigational (Phase II/III, orphan) intracerebral implant for patients with advanced Parkinson disease* [neural dopaminergic cells, porcine fetal]

**Neurodep** injection ℞ *parenteral vitamin therapy* [multiple B vitamins; vitamin C] ± •50 mg/mL

**Neurodep-Caps** capsules OTC *vitamin supplement* [vitamins $B_1$, $B_6$, and $B_{12}$] 125•125•1 mg

**Neurolite** injection ℞ *imaging aid for SPECT brain scans* [technetium Tc 99m bicisate]

**Neurontin** capsules, film-coated caplets, oral solution ℞ *anticonvulsant for partial-onset seizures; treatment for postherpetic neuralgia; investigational (orphan) for amyotrophic lateral sclerosis* [gabapentin] 100, 300, 400 mg; 600, 800 mg; 250 mg/5 mL

**neurosin** [see: calcium glycerophosphate]

**NeuroSlim** capsules OTC *dietary supplement* [multiple vitamins & minerals; multiple amino acids; folic acid; biotin] ≚•0.066•0.05 mg

**neurotrophic growth factor** [see: methionyl neurotrophic factor]

**neurotrophin-1** *investigational (orphan) for motor neuron disease and amyotrophic lateral sclerosis*

**neurotrophin-3 (NT-3)** *investigational agent for treating peripheral neuropathies; investigational for constipation*

**neustab** [see: thioacetazone; thiacetazone]

**Neut** IV or subcu injection ℞ *pH buffer for metabolic acidosis; urinary alkalinizer* [sodium bicarbonate] 4% (0.48 mEq Na/mL)

**Neutra-Caine** liquid ℞ *mixed with injectable local anesthetics to reduce stinging pain at the injection site* [sodium bicarbonate] 7.5%

**NeutraGard Advanced** dental gel ℞ *topical caries preventative* [sodium fluoride] 1.1%

**neutral acriflavine** [see: acriflavine]

**Neutral C** Ⓒᴬᴺ capsules OTC *vitamin C supplement* [calcium polyascorbate; lemon bioflavonoids; echinacea] 600•≚•≚ mg

**Neutral C + CoEnzyme Q10** Ⓒᴬᴺ capsules OTC *vitamin/mineral supplement* [multiple vitamins; multiple minerals; calcium ascorbate; coenzyme Q10; folic acid] ≚•≚•320•10•0.5 mg

**neutral insulin** INN, BAN, JAN *antidiabetic* [also: insulin, neutral]

**Neutralca-S** Ⓒᴬᴺ oral suspension OTC *antacid* [aluminum hydroxide; magnesium hydroxide] 200•200 mg/5 mL

**neutramycin** USAN, INN *antibacterial*

**Neutra-Phos** powder for oral solution OTC *phosphorus supplement* [monobasic sodium phosphate; monobasic potassium phosphate; dibasic sodium phosphate; dibasic potassium phosphate] 250 mg P/pkt.

**Neutra-Phos-K** powder for oral solution OTC *phosphorus supplement* [monobasic potassium phosphate; dibasic potassium phosphate] 250 mg P/pkt.

**NeuTrexin** powder for IV injection ℞ *antiprotozoal for AIDS-related Pneumocystis carinii pneumonia (orphan); investigational (orphan) antineoplastic for multiple cancers* [trimetrexate glucuronate] 25 mg

**neutroflavine** [see: acriflavine]

**Neutrogena Acne Mask** (discontinued 2003) OTC *keratolytic cleansing mask for acne* [benzoyl peroxide] 5%

**Neutrogena Antiseptic Cleanser for Acne-Prone Skin** topical liquid OTC *cleanser for acne* [benzethonium chloride]

**Neutrogena Body** lotion, oil OTC *moisturizer; emollient*

**Neutrogena Clear Pore** topical liquid OTC *keratolytic cleansing mask for acne* [benzoyl peroxide] 3.5%

**Neutrogena Drying** gel OTC *topical astringent and antiseptic for acne* [hamamelis water; isopropyl alcohol]

**Neutrogena Moisture** lotion OTC *moisturizer; emollient*

**Neutrogena Non-Drying Cleansing** lotion OTC *soap-free therapeutic skin cleanser*

**Neutrogena Norwegian Formula Hand** cream OTC *moisturizer; emollient*

**Neutrogena Oil-Free Acne Wash** topical liquid OTC *keratolytic cleanser for acne* [salicylic acid] 2%

**Neutrogena Soap; Neutrogena Cleansing for Acne-Prone Skin; Neutrogena Baby Cleansing Formula Soap; Neutrogena Dry Skin Soap; Neutrogena Oily Skin Soap** bar OTC *therapeutic skin cleanser*

**Neutrogena T/Derm** topical oil (discontinued 2003) OTC *antipsoriatic; antiseborrheic* [coal tar] 5%

**Neutrogena T/Gel** shampoo, conditioner (discontinued 2003) OTC *anti-*

*seborrheic; antipsoriatic; antipruritic; antibacterial* [coal tar] 2%; 1.5%

**Neutrogena T/Gel Original** shampoo OTC *antiseborrheic; antipsoriatic; antipruritic; antibacterial* [coal tar extract] 2%

**Neutrogena T/Sal** shampoo OTC *antiseborrheic; antipsoriatic; antipruritic; antibacterial* [salicylic acid; coal tar] 2%•2%

**nevirapine** USAN, INN *antiviral nonnucleoside reverse transcriptase inhibitor (NNRTI) for HIV-1*

**nevirapine & zidovudine & didanosine** *investigational (Phase III) antiviral combination for HIV infection*

**New Jersey tea (Ceanothus americanus)** *root bark medicinal herb used as an astringent, expectorant, and sedative*

**New Zealand green-lipped mussel (Perna canaliculus)** *freeze-dried body or gonads natural treatment for osteoarthritis and rheumatoid arthritis*

**new-estranol 1** [see: diethylstilbestrol]

**new-oestranol 1** [see: diethylstilbestrol]

**new-oestranol 11** [see: diethylstilbestrol dipropionate]

**NewPaks** (trademarked delivery form) *ready-to-use closed system containers*

**New-Skin** topical liquid, spray OTC *skin protectant; antiseptic* [hydroxyquinoline]

**nexeridine** INN *analgesic* [also: nexeridine HCl]

**nexeridine HCl** USAN *analgesic* [also: nexeridine]

**Nexium** delayed-release capsules containing enteric-coated pellets Ɍ *proton pump inhibitor for gastric and duodenal ulcers, erosive esophagitis, GERD, and other gastroesophageal disorders* [esomeprazole magnesium] 20, 40 mg

**Nexium IV** Ɍ *investigational (NDA filed) intravenous delivery of the proton pump inhibitor for patients who cannot take the drug orally* [esomeprazole magnesium]

**Nexrutine** capsules OTC *dietary supplement; selective COX-2 inhibitor; anti-*

*inflammatory; antipyretic* [Phellodendron amurense extract] 250 mg

**NFL (Novantrone, fluorouracil, leucovorin [rescue])** *chemotherapy protocol for breast cancer*

**NG-29** *investigational (orphan) diagnostic aid for pituitary release of growth hormone*

**N-Graft** Ɍ *investigational (orphan) intracerebral implant for patients with advanced Parkinson disease (for co-implantation with fetal neural cells)* [Sertoli cells, porcine]

**N.G.T.** cream Ɍ *topical corticosteroidal anti-inflammatory; antifungal* [triamcinolone acetonide; nystatin] 0.1%• 100 000 U per g

**niacin (vitamin B$_3$)** USP *water-soluble vitamin; peripheral vasodilator; antihyperlipidemic* [also: nicotinic acid] 50, 100, 125, 250, 400, 500 mg oral ⑨ Minocin

**niacinamide (vitamin B$_3$)** USP *water-soluble vitamin; enzyme cofactor* [also: nicotinamide] 100, 500 mg oral

**niacinamide hydroiodide** *expectorant*

**Niacor** immediate-release tablets Ɍ *vitamin B$_3$ therapy; peripheral vasodilator; antihyperlipidemic for hypertriglyceridemia (types IV and V hyperlipidemia)* [niacin] 500 mg

**nialamide** NF, INN

**niaprazine** INN

**Niaspan** extended-release caplets Ɍ *peripheral vasodilator; antihyperlipidemic; vitamin B$_3$* [niacin] 500, 750, 1000 mg

**NiaStase** ⒸⒶⓃ powder for IV injection Ɍ *recombinant coagulation Factor VII for hemophilia A and B* [eptacog alfa (activated)] 1.2, 2.4, 4.8 mg/vial

**nibroxane** USAN, INN *topical antimicrobial*

**Nicabate** (European name for U.S. product Nicoderm)

**nicafenine** INN

**nicainoprol** INN

**nicametate** INN, BAN

**nicaraven** INN

**nicarbazin** BAN

**nicardipine** INN, BAN *vasodilator; calcium channel blocker* [also: nicardipine HCl]

**nicardipine HCl** USAN *antianginal; antihypertensive; vasodilator; calcium channel blocker* [also: nicardipine] 20, 30 mg oral

**NicCheck I** reagent strips *in vitro diagnostic aid for urine nicotine, used to determine the smoking status of the subject*

**NicCheck II** reagent strips *investigational in vitro diagnostic aid for urine nicotine, used to determine exposure to passive cigarette smoke*

**N'Ice** throat spray OTC *topical analgesic; counterirritant; mild local anesthetic* [menthol] 0.12%

**N'Ice; N'Ice 'n Clear** lozenges OTC *topical oral analgesic; counterirritant; mild local anesthetic* [menthol] 5 mg

**N'Ice Vitamin C Drops** (lozenges) OTC *vitamin C supplement* [ascorbic acid; menthol] 60•⅔ mg

**nicergoline** USAN, INN *vasodilator*

**niceritrol** INN, BAN

**nicethamide** BAN [also: nikethamide]

**niceverine** INN

**nickel** *element (Ni)*

**niclofolan** INN, BAN

**niclosamide** USAN, INN *anthelmintic for cestodiasis (tapeworm)*

**nicoboxil** INN

**nicoclonate** INN

**nicocodine** INN, BAN

**nicocortonide** INN

**Nicoderm CQ Step 1; Nicoderm CQ Step 2; Nicoderm CQ Step 3** transdermal patch OTC *smoking deterrent; nicotine withdrawal aid* [nicotine] 21 mg/day; 14 mg/day; 7 mg/day

**nicodicodine** INN, BAN

**nicoduozide (isoniazid + nicothiazone)**

**nicofibrate** INN

**nicofuranose** INN

**nicofurate** INN

**nicogrelate** INN

**Nicomide** tablets ℞ *vitamin/mineral supplement* [nicotinamide; zinc oxide; cupric oxide; folic acid] 750•25•1.5•0.5 mg

**nicomol** INN

**nicomorphine** INN, BAN

**nicopholine** INN

**nicorandil** USAN, INN *coronary vasodilator*

**Nicorette** chewing gum OTC *smoking deterrent; nicotine withdrawal aid* [nicotine polacrilex] 2, 4 mg

**Nicorette Plus** ⓒᴬᴺ chewing pieces OTC *smoking deterrent; nicotine withdrawal aid* [nicotine polacrilex] 4 mg

**Nicosyn** lotion ℞ *antibiotic for acne* [sulfacetamide sodium; sulfur] 10%•5%

**nicothiazone** INN

**nicotinaldehyde thiosemicarbazone** [see: nicothiazone]

**nicotinamide (vitamin B₃)** INN, BAN, JAN *water-soluble vitamin; enzyme cofactor* [also: niacinamide]

**nicotinamide-adenine dinucleotide (NAD)** [now: nadide]

**nicotine** *a very poisonous alkaloid used as an insecticide and external parasiticide; the active principle in tobacco; smoking cessation aid* [also see: tobacco] 7, 14, 21 mg/day transdermal

**nicotine bitartrate** USAN *smoking cessation aid*

**nicotine & mecamylamine HCl** *investigational (Phase III) transdermal patch for smoking cessation*

**nicotine polacrilex** USAN *smoking deterrent; nicotine withdrawal aid* 2, 4 mg oral

**nicotine resin complex** [see: nicotine polacrilex]

**Nicotinex** elixir (discontinued 2004) OTC *vitamin B₃ supplement; antihyperlipidemic* [niacin] 50 mg/5 mL

**nicotinic acid (vitamin B₃)** INN, BAN, JAN *water-soluble vitamin; peripheral vasodilator; antihyperlipidemic* [also: niacin]

**nicotinic acid amide** [see: niacinamide]

**nicotinic acid 1-oxide** [see: oxiniacic acid]

**nicotinohydroxamic acid** [see: nicoxamat]

**6-nicotinoyl dihydrocodeine** [see: nicodicodine]
**6-nicotinoylcodeine** [see: nicocodine]
**4-nicotinoylmorpholine** [see: nicopholine]
**nicotinyl alcohol** USAN, BAN *peripheral vasodilator*
**nicotinyl tartrate**
**Nicotrol** oral inhaler ℞ *smoking deterrent; nicotine withdrawal aid* [nicotine] 10 mg (4 mg delivered) per cartridge
**Nicotrol NS** nasal spray ℞ *smoking deterrent; nicotine withdrawal aid* [nicotine] 0.5 mg/spray
**Nicotrol Step 1; Nicotrol Step 2; Nicotrol Step 3** transdermal patch OTC *smoking deterrent; nicotine withdrawal aid* [nicotine] 15 mg/day; 10 mg/day; 5 mg/day
**nicotylamide** [see: niacinamide]
**nicoumalone** BAN [also: acenocoumarol]
**nicoxamat** INN
**nictiazem** INN
**nictindole** INN
**Nidagel** ⊛ vaginal gel ℞ *antibacterial for bacterial vaginosis* [metronidazole] 0.75%
**Nidran** ℞ *alkylating antineoplastic* [nimustin HCl]
**nidroxyzone** INN
**Nifediac CC** film-coated extended-release tablets ℞ *antianginal; antihypertensive; calcium channel blocker* [nifedipine] 30, 60, 90 mg
**Nifedical XL** film-coated sustained-release tablets ℞ *antianginal; antihypertensive; calcium channel blocker* [nifedipine] 30, 60 mg
**nifedipine** USAN, USP, INN, BAN *antianginal; antihypertensive; coronary vasodilator; calcium channel blocker; investigational (orphan) for interstitial cystitis* 10, 20, 30, 60, 90 mg oral
**nifenalol** INN
**nifenazone** INN, BAN
**Niferex** tablets, elixir OTC *hematinic; iron supplement* [polysaccharide-iron complex] 50 mg; 100 mg/5 mL

**Niferex-150** capsules OTC *hematinic; iron supplement* [polysaccharide-iron complex] 150 mg
**Niferex-150 Forte** capsules ℞ *hematinic* [polysaccharide-iron complex; cyanocobalamin; folic acid] 150 mg Fe•25 µg•1 mg
**Niferex-PN** film-coated tablets ℞ *prenatal vitamin/iron supplement* [polysaccharide-iron complex; multiple vitamins & minerals; folic acid] 60• ±•1 mg
**Niferex-PN Forte** film-coated tablets ℞ *prenatal vitamin/mineral/calcium/iron supplement* [multiple vitamins & minerals; calcium; polysaccharide-iron complex; folic acid] ±•250• 60•1 mg
**niflumic acid** INN
**nifluridide** USAN *ectoparasiticide*
**nifungin** USAN, INN
**nifuradene** USAN, INN *antibacterial*
**nifuralazine** [see: furalazine]
**nifuraldezone** USAN, INN *antibacterial*
**nifuralide** INN
**nifuramizone** [see: nifurethazone]
**nifuratel** USAN, INN *antibacterial; antifungal; antiprotozoal (Trichomonas)*
**nifuratrone** USAN, INN *antibacterial*
**nifurazolidone** [see: furazolidone]
**nifurdazil** USAN, INN *antibacterial*
**nifurethazone** INN
**nifurfoline** INN
**nifurhydrazone** [see: nihydrazone]
**nifurimide** USAN, INN *antibacterial*
**nifurizone** INN
**nifurmazole** INN
**nifurmerone** USAN, INN *antifungal*
**nifuroquine** INN
**nifuroxazide** INN
**nifuroxime** NF, INN
**nifurpipone (NP)** INN
**nifurpirinol** USAN, INN *antibacterial*
**nifurprazine** INN
**nifurquinazol** USAN, INN *antibacterial*
**nifursemizone** USAN, INN *antiprotozoal for poultry (Histomonas)*
**nifursol** USAN, INN *antiprotozoal for poultry (Histomonas)*
**nifurthiazole** USAN, INN *antibacterial*

**nifurthiline** [see: thiofuradene]

**nifurtimox** INN, BAN (available only from Centers for Disease Control and Prevention) *investigational anti-infective for Chagas disease*

**nifurtoinol** INN

**nifurvidine** INN

**nifurzide** INN

**Night Time Cold/Flu Relief** oral liquid (discontinued 2002) OTC *antitussive; decongestant; antihistamine; analgesic* [dextromethorphan hydrobromide; pseudoephedrine HCl; doxylamine succinate; acetaminophen; alcohol 10%] 30•60•12.5•1000 mg/30 mL

**nightshade; nightshade vine** *medicinal herb* [see: bittersweet nightshade]

**nightshade, American** *medicinal herb* [see: pokeweed]

**nightshade, deadly** *medicinal herb* [see: belladonna]

**nightshade, fetid; stinking nightshade** *medicinal herb* [see: henbane]

**nightshade, three-leaved** *medicinal herb* [see: birthroot]

**Night-Time Effervescent Cold** tablets for oral solution (discontinued 2002) OTC *decongestant; antihistamine; analgesic; antipyretic* [phenylpropanolamine HCl; diphenhydramine citrate; aspirin] 15•38.33•325 mg

**Nighttime Sleep Aid** tablets (discontinued 2002) OTC *antihistaminic sleep aid* [diphenhydramine HCl] 50 mg

**NightTime TheraFlu** powder for oral solution (discontinued 2002) OTC *antitussive; decongestant; antihistamine; analgesic* [dextromethorphan hydrobromide; pseudoephedrine HCl; chlorpheniramine maleate; acetaminophen] 30•60•4•1000 mg/pkt. ℞ Thera-Flur

**niguldipine** INN

**nihydrazone** INN

**nikethamide** NF, INN [also: nicethamide]

**Nilandron** tablets ℞ *antiandrogen antineoplastic for metastatic prostate cancer* [nilutamide] 50, 150 mg

**nileprost** INN

**nilestriol** INN *estrogen* [also: nylestriol]

**nilprazole** INN

**Nilstat** cream, ointment ℞ *antifungal* [nystatin] 100 000 U/g ℞ Nitrostat; nystatin

**Nilstat** film-coated tablets (discontinued 2000) ℞ *systemic antifungal* [nystatin] 500 000 U

**Nilstat** oral suspension, powder for oral suspension ℞ *antifungal; oral candidiasis treatment* [nystatin] 100 000 U/mL; 150 million, 500 million, 1 billion, 2 billion U

**niludipine** INN

**nilutamide** USAN, INN, BAN *antiandrogen antineoplastic adjunct to surgical or chemical castration for metastatic prostate cancer*

**nilvadipine** USAN, INN, JAN *calcium channel antagonist*

**nimazone** USAN, INN *anti-inflammatory*

**Nimbex** IV infusion ℞ *nondepolarizing neuromuscular blocking agent for anesthesia* [cisatracurium besylate] 2, 10 mg/mL

**Nimbus; Nimbus Quick Strip** test kit for home use *in vitro diagnostic aid; urine pregnancy test* [monoclonal antibody-based enzyme immunoassay]

**Nimbus Plus** test kit for professional use *in vitro diagnostic aid; urine pregnancy test*

**nimesulide** INN, BAN

**nimetazepam** INN

**nimidane** USAN, INN *veterinary acaricide*

**nimodipine** USAN, INN, BAN *vasodilator; calcium channel blocker for subarachnoid hemorrhage (SAH)*

**nimorazole** INN

**Nimotop** soft liquid-filled capsules ℞ *calcium channel blocker for subarachnoid hemorrhage (SAH)* [nimodipine] 30 mg

**nimustine** INN *alkylating neoplastic*

**nimustine HCl** *alkylating neoplastic*

**niobium** *element (Nb)*

**niometacin** INN

**Nion B Plus C** caplets OTC *vitamin supplement* [multiple B vitamins; vitamin C] ±•300 mg

**Nipent** powder for IV injection ℞ *antibiotic antineoplastic for hairy cell leukemia (orphan); investigational (orphan) for chronic lymphocytic leukemia and cutaneous T-cell lymphoma; investigational (Phase III) for AIDS-related non-Hodgkin lymphoma* [pentostatin] 10 mg

**niperotidine** INN

**nipradilol** INN

**Nipride** *brand discontinued 1992* [see: sodium nitroprusside]

**niprofazone** INN

**niridazole** USAN, INN *antischistosomal*

**nisbuterol** INN *bronchodilator* [also: nisbuterol mesylate]

**nisbuterol mesylate** USAN *bronchodilator* [also: nisbuterol]

**nisin** *investigational agent for severe colonic bacterial infections*

**nisobamate** USAN, INN *minor tranquilizer*

**nisoldipine** USAN, INN, BAN, JAN *coronary vasodilator; calcium channel blocker for hypertension*

**nisoxetine** USAN, INN *antidepressant*

**nisterime** INN *androgen* [also: nisterime acetate]

**nisterime acetate** USAN *androgen* [also: nisterime]

**nitarsone** USAN, INN *antiprotozoal (Histomonas)*

**nitazoxanide (NTZ)** INN *antiprotozoal for pediatric diarrhea due to Cryptosporidium parvum and Giardia lamblia infections; investigational (orphan) for AIDS-related diarrhea*

**Nite Time Children's Liquid** OTC *antitussive; decongestant; antihistamine* [dextromethorphan hydrobromide; pseudoephedrine HCl; chlorpheniramine maleate] 15•30•2 mg/15 mL

**Nite Time Cold Formula for Adults** oral liquid OTC *antitussive; decongestant; antihistamine; analgesic* [dextromethorphan hydrobromide; pseudoephedrine HCl; doxylamine succinate; acetaminophen; alcohol 10%] 30•60•12.5•1000 mg/30 mL

**nithiamide** USAN *veterinary antibacterial* [also: aminitrozole; acinitrazole]

**nitisinone** *adjunctive treatment for hereditary tyrosinemia type 1 (HT-1), a pediatric liver disease (orphan)*

**nitracrine** INN

**nitrafudam** INN *antidepressant* [also: nitrafudam HCl]

**nitrafudam HCl** USAN *antidepressant* [also: nitrafudam]

**nitralamine HCl** USAN *antifungal*

**nitramisole** INN *anthelmintic* [also: nitramisole HCl]

**nitramisole HCl** USAN *anthelmintic* [also: nitramisole]

**nitraquazone** INN

**nitrates** *a class of antianginal agents that cause the relaxation of vascular smooth muscles*

**nitratophenylmercury** [see: phenylmercuric nitrate]

**nitrazepam** USAN, INN, BAN, JAN *investigational benzodiazepine sedative; anxiolytic; anticonvulsant; hypnotic*

**Nitrazine** paper for professional use (discontinued 2002) *in vitro diagnostic aid for urine pH determination*

**nitre, sweet spirit of** [see: ethyl nitrite]

**nitrefazole** INN, BAN

**Nitrek** transdermal patch ℞ *antianginal; vasodilator* [nitroglycerin] 22.4, 44.8, 67.2 mg (0.2, 0.4, 0.6 mg/hr.)

**nitrendipine** USAN, INN, BAN, JAN *investigational (NDA filed) antihypertensive; calcium channel blocker*

**nitric acid** NF *acidifying agent*

**nitric oxide** *inhalation gas for neonatal hypoxic respiratory failure due to persistent pulmonary hypertension (orphan); investigational (orphan) for acute adult respiratory distress syndrome; investigational to prevent reperfusion injury following lung transplants*

**nitricholine perchlorate** INN

**p-nitrobenzenearsonic acid** [see: nitarsone]

**Nitro-Bid** ointment ℞ *antianginal; vasodilator* [nitroglycerin] 2% (15 mg/inch) ⊡ Nicobid

**Nitro-Bid IV** infusion ℞ *antianginal; vasodilator; perioperative antihyperten-*

*sive; for congestive heart failure with myocardial infarction* [nitroglycerin] 5 mg/mL

**9-nitrocamptothecin (9-NC)** [now: rubitecan]

**nitroclofene** INN

**nitrocycline** USAN, INN *antibacterial*

**nitrodan** USAN, INN *anthelmintic*

**Nitro-Derm** transdermal patch (discontinued 2000) ℞ *antianginal; vasodilator* [nitroglycerin] 160 mg (0.8 mg/hr.)

**Nitrodisc** transdermal patch ℞ *antianginal; vasodilator* [nitroglycerin] 16, 24, 32 mg (0.2, 0.3, 0.4 mg/hr.)

**Nitro-Dur** transdermal patch ℞ *antianginal; vasodilator* [nitroglycerin] 20, 40, 60, 80, 120, 160 mg (0.1, 0.2, 0.3, 0.4, 0.6, 0.8 mg/hr.)

**nitroethanolamine** [see: aminoethyl nitrate]

**nitrofuradoxadone** [see: furmethoxadone]

**nitrofural** INN *broad-spectrum bactericidal; adjunct to burn treatment* [also: nitrofurazone]

**nitrofurantoin** USP, INN *urinary antibiotic* 50, 100 mg oral

**nitrofurantoin sodium** *urinary antibiotic*

**nitrofurazone** USP, BAN *broad-spectrum bactericidal; adjunct to burn treatment and skin grafting* [also: nitrofural] 0.2% topical

**nitrofurmethone** [see: furaltadone]

**nitrofuroxizone** [see: nidroxyzone]

**Nitrogard** transmucosal extended-release tablets ℞ *antianginal; vasodilator* [nitroglycerin] 2, 3 mg

**nitrogen ($N_2$)** NF *air displacement agent; element (N)*

**nitrogen monoxide** [see: nitrous oxide]

**nitrogen mustard N-oxide HCl** JAN *alkylating antineoplastic* [also: mechlorethamine HCl; chlormethine; mustine]

**nitrogen mustards** *a class of alkylating antineoplastics*

**nitrogen oxide ($N_2O$)** [see: nitrous oxide]

**nitroglycerin** USP *coronary vasodilator; antianginal; antihypertensive* [also: glyceryl trinitrate] 0.3, 0.4, 0.6 mg sublingual; 2.5, 6.5, 9 mg oral; 5 mg/mL injection; 0.2, 0.4, 0.6 mg/hr. transdermal; 2% topical ⊠ Nitroglyn

**Nitroglyn** extended-release capsules (discontinued 2004) ℞ *antianginal; vasodilator* [nitroglycerin] 2.5, 6.5, 9, 13 mg ⊠ nitroglycerin

**nitrohydroxyquinoline** [see: nitroxoline]

**Nitrol** ointment, Appli-Kit (ointment & adhesive dosage covers) (discontinued 2003) ℞ *antianginal; vasodilator* [nitroglycerin] 2% (15 mg/inch)

**Nitrolan** oral liquid OTC *enteral nutritional therapy* [lactose-free formula]

**Nitrolingual Pumpspray** CFC-free translingual aerosol ℞ *antianginal; vasodilator* [nitroglycerin] 0.4 mg/spray

**nitromannitol** [see: mannitol hexanitrate]

**nitromersol** USP *topical anti-infective*

**nitromide** USAN *coccidiostat for poultry; antibacterial*

**nitromifene** INN

**nitromifene citrate** USAN *antiestrogen*

**Nitrong** sustained-release tablets (discontinued 2004) ℞ *antianginal; vasodilator* [nitroglycerin] 2.6, 6.5, 9 mg

**Nitropress** powder for IV injection, flip-top vials ℞ *vasodilator for hypertensive emergency* [sodium nitroprusside] 50 mg/dose

**nitroprusside sodium** [see: sodium nitroprusside]

**NitroQuick** sublingual tablets ℞ *antianginal; vasodilator* [nitroglycerin] 0.3, 0.4, 0.6 mg (1/200, 1/150, 1/100 gr.)

**nitroscanate** USAN, INN *veterinary anthelmintic*

**nitrosoureas** *a class of alkylating antineoplastics*

**Nitrostat** sublingual tablets ℞ *antianginal; vasodilator* [nitroglycerin] 0.3, 0.4, 0.6 mg (1/200, 1/150, 1/100 gr.)

**nitrosulfathiazole** INN [also: para-nitrosulfathiazole]

**NitroTab** sublingual tablets ℞ *antianginal; vasodilator* [nitroglycerin] 0.3, 0.4, 0.6 mg (1/200, 1/150, 1/100 gr.)

**Nitro-Time** extended-release capsules ℞ *antianginal; vasodilator* [nitroglycerin] 2.5, 6.5, 9 mg

**nitrous acid, sodium salt** [see: sodium nitrite]

**nitrous oxide (N₂O)** USP *a weak inhalation general anesthetic; sometimes abused as a street drug to create a dreamy or floating sensation*

**nitroxinil** INN

**nitroxoline** INN, BAN

**nivacortol** INN *corticosteroid; anti-inflammatory* [also: nivazol]

**nivadipine** [see: nilvadipine]

**nivaquine** [see: chloroquine phosphate]

**nivazol** USAN *corticosteroid; anti-inflammatory* [also: nivacortol]

**Nivea After Tan; Nivea Moisturizing; Nivea Moisturizing Extra Enriched** lotion OTC *moisturizer; emollient*

**Nivea Moisturizing; Nivea Skin** oil OTC *moisturizer; emollient*

**Nivea Moisturizing Creme Soap** bar OTC *therapeutic skin cleanser*

**Nivea Ultra Moisturizing Creme** OTC *moisturizer; emollient*

**nivimedone sodium** USAN *antiallergic*

**Nix** creme rinse OTC *pediculicide for lice; scabicide* [permethrin; alcohol 20%] 1%

**nixylic acid** INN

**nizatidine** USAN, USP, INN, BAN, JAN *histamine H₂ antagonist for gastric and duodenal ulcers* 150, 300 mg oral

**nizofenone** INN

**Nizoral** cream (discontinued 2003) ℞ *antifungal* [ketoconazole] 2%

**Nizoral** shampoo ℞ *antifungal* [ketoconazole] 2%

**Nizoral** tablets ℞ *systemic imidazole antifungal* [ketoconazole] 200 mg

**Nizoral A-D** shampoo OTC *antifungal for dandruff* [ketoconazole] 1%

**NMDA (N-methyl-D-aspartate)** [q.v.]

**N-Multistix; N-Multistix SG** reagent strips *in vitro diagnostic aid for multiple urine products*

**NN-622** *investigational (Phase III) dual-acting insulin sensitizer for type 2 diabetes*

**NNRTIs (non-nucleoside reverse transcriptase inhibitors)** [see: reverse transcriptase inhibitors]

**No Pain-HP** roll-on OTC *topical analgesic* [capsaicin] 0.075%

**nobelium** *element (No)*

**noberastine** USAN, INN, BAN *antihistamine*

**noble yarrow** *medicinal herb* [see: yarrow]

**nocebo effect** [L. I will harm] *a perceived adverse effect from an inert substance* [compare to: placebo effect]

**nocloprost** INN

**nocodazole** USAN, INN *antineoplastic*

**nodding wakerobin** *medicinal herb* [see: birthroot]

**NōDōz** chewable tablets (discontinued 2001) OTC *CNS stimulant; analeptic* [caffeine] 100 mg

**NōDōz** coated caplets OTC *CNS stimulant; analeptic* [caffeine] 200 mg

**nofecainide** INN

**nofetumomab merpentan** *monoclonal antibody imaging agent for small cell lung cancer*

**nogalamycin** USAN, INN *antineoplastic*

**No-Hist** capsules (discontinued 2002) ℞ *nasal decongestant* [phenylephrine HCl; phenylpropanolamine HCl; pseudoephedrine HCl] 5•40•40 mg

**Nolahist** tablets OTC *nonselective piperidine antihistamine for allergic rhinitis* [phenindamine tartrate] 25 mg

**Nolamine** timed-release tablets (discontinued 2001) ℞ *decongestant; antihistamine* [phenylpropanolamine HCl; chlorpheniramine maleate; phenindamine tartrate] 50•4•24 mg

**nolatrexed dihydrochloride** *investigational (Phase III) thymidylate synthase inhibitor for liver cancer*

**nolinium bromide** USAN, INN *antisecretory; antiulcerative*

**Nolvadex** tablets ℞ *antiestrogen anti-neoplastic for advanced postmenopausal breast cancer; also for breast cancer prevention in high-risk patients* [tamoxifen citrate] 10, 20 mg

**nomegestrol** INN

**nomelidine** INN

**nomifensine** INN *antidepressant* [also: nomifensine maleate]

**nomifensine maleate** USAN *antidepressant* [also: nomifensine]

**nonabine** INN, BAN

**nonabsorbable surgical suture** [see: suture, nonabsorbable surgical]

**nonachlazine** [now: azaclorzine HCl]

**nonacog alfa** USAN, INN *synthetic human blood coagulation factor IX; antihemophilic for hemophilia B and Christmas disease (orphan)* [also: factor IX complex]

**nonanedioic acid** [see: azelaic acid]

**nonaperone** INN

**nonapyrimine** INN

**nonathymulin** INN

**nondestearinated cod liver oil** [see: cod liver oil, nondestearinated]

**Non-Habit Forming Stool Softener** capsules OTC *laxative; stool softener* [docusate sodium] 100 mg

**noni** *(Morinda citrifolia)* berries *medicinal herb for arthritis, bacterial infections, diabetes, drug addiction, headache, hypertension, liver and skin disorders, pain, and slowing aging; also used as an antioxidant*

**nonionic contrast media** *a class of newer radiopaque agents that, in general, have a low osmolar concentration of iodine (the contrast agent), which corresponds to a lower incidence of adverse reactions* [also called: low osmolar contrast media (LOCM)]

**nonivamide** INN

**non-nucleoside reverse transcriptase inhibitors (NNRTIs)** [see: reverse transcriptase inhibitors]

**nonoxinol 4** INN *surfactant* [also: nonoxynol 4]

**nonoxinol 9** INN *wetting and solubilizing agent; spermaticide* [also: nonoxynol 9]

**nonoxinol 15** INN *surfactant* [also: nonoxynol 15]

**nonoxinol 30** INN *surfactant* [also: nonoxynol 30]

**nonoxynol 4** USAN *surfactant* [also: nonoxinol 4]

**nonoxynol 9** USAN, USP *wetting and solubilizing agent; spermicide* [also: nonoxinol 9]

**nonoxynol 10** NF *surfactant*

**nonoxynol 15** USAN *surfactant* [also: nonoxinol 15]

**nonoxynol 30** USAN *surfactant* [also: nonoxinol 30]

**nonsteroidal anti-inflammatory drugs (NSAIDs)** *a class of anti-inflammatory drugs that have analgesic and antipyretic effects*

**nonylphenoxypolyethoxyethanol** [see: nonoxynol 4, 9, 15, & 30]

**Nootropil** ℞ *cognition adjuvant; investigational (orphan) for myoclonus* [piracetam]

**nopal** plant *medicinal herb for cleansing the lymphatic system, diabetes, digestion, obesity, neutralizing toxins, and preventing arteriosclerosis*

**Nora-BE** tablets (in packs of 28) ℞ *oral contraceptive (progestin only)* [norethindrone] 0.35 mg

**noracymethadol** INN *analgesic* [also: noracymethadol HCl]

**noracymethadol HCl** USAN *analgesic* [also: noracymethadol]

**noradrenaline bitartrate** [see: norepinephrine bitartrate]

**noramidopyrine methanesulfonate sodium** [see: dipyrone]

**norandrostenolone phenylpropionate** [see: nandrolone phenpropionate]

**norastemizole** *investigational (Phase III) third generation, nonsedating antihistamine for allergy*

**norbolethone** USAN *anabolic* [also: norboletone]

**norboletone** INN *anabolic* [also: norbolethone]

**norbudrine** INN [also: norbutrine]

**norbutrine** BAN [also: norbudrine]

**norclostebol** INN

**Norco** tablets ℞ *narcotic analgesic and antitussive* [hydrocodone bitartrate; acetaminophen] 5•325, 7.5•325, 10•325 mg

**norcodeine** INN, BAN

**Norcuron** powder for IV injection ℞ *nondepolarizing neuromuscular blocker; adjunct to anesthesia* [vecuronium bromide] 10, 20 mg/vial

**norcycline** [see: sancycline]

**nordazepam** INN

**nordefrin HCl** NF

**Nordette** tablets (in Pilpaks of 21 or 28) ℞ *monophasic oral contraceptive; emergency postcoital contraceptive* [levonorgestrel; ethinyl estradiol] 0.15 mg•30 μg

**nordinone** INN

**NordiPen** (trademarked device) *subcu self-injector for Norditropin*

**Norditropin** powder for subcu injection, prefilled cartridges for Nordi-Pen (self-injection device) ℞ *growth hormone for adults or children with congenital or endogenous growth hormone deficiency, children with Turner syndrome or renal-induced growth failure* [somatropin] 4, 8 mg (12, 24 IU) per vial; 5, 10, 15 mg (15, 30, 45 IU) per 1.5 mL cartridge

**Norel** capsules (discontinued 2001) ℞ *decongestant; expectorant* [phenylephrine HCl; phenylpropanolamine HCl; guaifenesin] 5•45•200 mg

**Norel DM** oral liquid ℞ *pediatric decongestant, antihistamine, and expectorant* [phenylephrine HCl; chlorpheniramine maleate; dextromethorphan hydrobromide] 10•4•15 mg/5 mL

**Norel Plus** capsules (discontinued 2002) ℞ *decongestant; antihistamine; analgesic* [phenylpropanolamine HCl; chlorpheniramine maleate; phenyltoloxamine dihydrogen citrate; acetaminophen] 25•4•25•325 mg

**norelgestromin** USAN *investigational progestin-type contraceptive*

**norephedrine HCl** [see: phenylpropanolamine HCl]

**norepinephrine** INN *adrenergic; vasoconstrictor; vasopressor for shock* [also: norepinephrine bitartrate]

**norepinephrine bitartrate** USAN, USP *adrenergic; vasoconstrictor; vasopressor for acute hypotensive shock* [also: norepinephrine] 1 mg/mL injection

**norethandrolone** NF, INN

**norethindrone** USP *progestin for amenorrhea, abnormal uterine bleeding, and endometriosis* [also: norethisterone]

**norethindrone acetate** USP *progestin for amenorrhea, abnormal uterine bleeding, and endometriosis*

**norethisterone** INN, BAN, JAN *progestin* [also: norethindrone]

**norethynodrel** USAN, USP *progestin* [also: noretynodrel]

**noretynodrel** INN *progestin* [also: norethynodrel]

**noreximide** INN

**norfenefrine** INN

**Norflex** sustained-release tablets, IV or IM injection ℞ *skeletal muscle relaxant* [orphenadrine citrate] 100 mg; 30 mg/mL

**norfloxacin** USAN, USP, INN, BAN, JAN *broad-spectrum fluoroquinolone antibiotic*

**norfloxacin succinil** INN

**norflurane** USAN, INN *inhalation anesthetic*

**Norforms** vaginal suppositories OTC *feminine deodorant* [polyethylene glycol]

**Norgesic; Norgesic Forte** tablets ℞ *skeletal muscle relaxant; analgesic* [orphenadrine citrate; aspirin; caffeine] 25•385•30 mg; 50•770•60 mg

**norgesterone** INN

**norgestimate** USAN, INN, BAN *progestin*

**norgestomet** USAN, INN *progestin*

**norgestrel** USAN, USP, INN *progestin*

**d-norgestrel** *(incorrect enantiomer designation)* [now: levonorgestrel]

**D-norgestrel** [see: levonorgestrel]

**norgestrienone** INN

**Norinyl 1 + 35** tablets (in Wallettes of 28) ℞ *monophasic oral contracep-*

*tive* [norethindrone; ethinyl estradiol] 1 mg•35 μg ⊇ Nardil

**Norinyl 1 + 50** tablets (in Wallettes of 28) ℞ *monophasic oral contraceptive* [norethindrone; mestranol] 1 mg•50 μg

**Norisodrine with Calcium Iodide** syrup (discontinued 2002) ℞ *bronchodilator; expectorant* [isoproterenol sulfate; calcium iodide; alcohol 6%] 3•150 mg

**Noritate** cream ℞ *antibiotic for rosacea* [metronidazole] 1%

**norletimol** INN

**norleusactide** INN [also: pentacosactride]

**norlevorphanol** INN, BAN

**norlupinanes** *a class of antibiotics* [also called: quinolizidines]

**½ normal saline (½ NS; 0.45% sodium chloride)** *electrolyte replacement*

**normal saline (NS; 0.9% sodium chloride)** *electrolyte replacement* [also: saline solution]

**normal serum albumin** [see: albumin, human]

**Normaline** tablets OTC *sodium chloride replacement; dehydration preventative* [sodium chloride] 250 mg

**normethadone** INN, BAN

**normethandrolone** [see: normethandrone]

**normethandrone**

**normethisterone** [see: normethandrone]

**Normiflo** deep subcu injection in pre-filled syringes (discontinued 2000) ℞ *a low molecular weight heparin–type anticoagulant for the prevention of deep vein thrombosis (DVT) following knee replacement surgery* [ardeparin sodium] 5000, 10 000 U/0.5 mL

**Normix** ℞ *investigational (orphan) antibacterial for hepatic encephalopathy* [rifaximin]

**Normodyne** film-coated tablets, IV infusion ℞ *antihypertensive; α- and β-blocker* [labetalol HCl] 100, 200, 300 mg; 5 mg/mL

**normorphine** INN, BAN

**Normosang** ℞ *investigational (orphan) for acute symptomatic porphyria and myelodysplastic syndrome* [heme arginate]

**Normosol-M** IV infusion ℞ *intravenous electrolyte therapy* [combined electrolyte solution] 1000 mL

**Normosol-M and 5% Dextrose; Normosol-R and 5% Dextrose** IV infusion ℞ *intravenous nutritional/electrolyte therapy* [combined electrolyte solution; dextrose]

**Normosol-R; Normosol-R pH 7.4** IV infusion ℞ *intravenous electrolyte therapy* [combined electrolyte solution]

**Noroxin** film-coated tablets ℞ *broad-spectrum fluoroquinolone antibiotic* [norfloxacin] 400 mg

**Norpace** capsules ℞ *antiarrhythmic* [disopyramide phosphate] 100, 150 mg

**Norpace CR** controlled-release capsules ℞ *antiarrhythmic* [disopyramide phosphate] 100, 150 mg

**norpipanone** INN, BAN

**Norplant** implantable Silastic capsules (discontinued 2003) ℞ *long-term (5-year) contraceptive system* [levonorgestrel] 216 mg (6 capsules × 36 mg)

**Norpramin** film-coated tablets ℞ *tricyclic antidepressant* [desipramine HCl] 10, 25, 50, 75, 100, 150 mg ⊇ imipramine

**norpseudoephedrine** [see: cathine]

**Nor-QD** tablets (in packs of 28) ℞ *oral contraceptive (progestin only)* [norethindrone] 0.35 mg

**nortestosterone phenylpropionate** [see: nandrolone phenpropionate]

**Nor-Tet** capsules ℞ *broad-spectrum antibiotic* [tetracycline HCl] 250, 500 mg

**nortetrazepam** INN

**Nortrel 0.5/35; Nortrel 1/35** tablets (in packs of 21 or 28) ℞ *monophasic oral contraceptive* [norethindrone; ethinyl estradiol] 0.5 mg•35 μg; 1 mg•35 μg

**nortriptyline HCl** USAN, USP, INN *tricyclic antidepressant* [10, 25, 50, 75 mg oral; 10 mg/5 mL oral] ⊇ amitriptyline

472   Norvasc

**Norvasc** tablets ℞ *antianginal; antihypertensive; calcium channel blocker* [amlodipine] 2.5, 5, 10 mg

**norvinisterone** INN

**norvinodrel** [see: norgesterone]

**Norvir** soft capsules, oral solution ℞ *antiviral protease inhibitor for HIV infection* [ritonavir] 100 mg; 80 mg/mL

**Norway pine; Norway spruce** *medicinal herb* [see: spruce]

**Norwich** tablets OTC *analgesic; antipyretic; anti-inflammatory; antirheumatic* [aspirin] 325, 500 mg

**Norzine** IM injection, suppositories, tablets ℞ *antiemetic* [thiethylperazine maleate] 5 mg/mL; 10 mg; 10 mg

**nosantine** INN, BAN

**noscapine** USP, INN *antitussive*

**noscapine HCl** NF

**Nose Better** gel OTC *emollient; moisturizer; protectant; counterirritant* [allantoin; camphor; menthol] 0.5%•0.75%•0.5%

**nosebleed** *medicinal herb* [see: yarrow]

**nosiheptide** USAN, INN *veterinary growth stimulant*

**Nōstril; Children's Nōstril** nasal spray (discontinued 2002) OTC *nasal decongestant* [phenylephrine HCl] 0.5%; 0.25%

**Nōstrilla 12-Hour** nasal spray OTC *nasal decongestant* [oxymetazoline HCl] 0.05%

**notensil maleate** [see: acepromazine]

**Notuss PD** oral liquid ℞ *narcotic antitussive; decongestant; antihistamine* [hydrocodone bitartrate; phenylephrine HCl; dexchlorpheniramine maleate] 4•5•2 mg/5 mL

**Nouriva Repair** cream OTC *emollient/protectant* [petrolatum; paraffin; mineral oil]

**NovaCare** film-coated tablets ℞ *prenatal vitamin/mineral/calcium/iron supplement* [multiple vitamins & minerals; calcium; iron; folic acid] ± • 250•40•1 mg

**Novacet** lotion ℞ *acne treatment* [sulfacetamide sodium; sulfur] 10%•5%

**Novacort** gel ℞ *corticosteroidal anti-inflammatory; local anesthetic* [hydrocortisone acetate; pramoxine] 2%•1%

**Nova-Dec** tablets OTC *vitamin/mineral/iron supplement* [multiple vitamins & minerals; iron; folic acid; biotin] ± • 30 mg•0.4 mg•30 µg

**Novafed A** sustained-release capsules (discontinued 2002) ℞ *decongestant; antihistamine* [pseudoephedrine HCl; chlorpheniramine maleate] 120•8 mg

**Novagest Expectorant with Codeine** oral liquid (discontinued 2002) ℞ *narcotic antitussive; decongestant; expectorant* [codeine phosphate; pseudoephedrine HCl; guaifenesin; alcohol 1.4%] 10•30•100 mg/5 mL

**Novahistine DH** syrup ℞ *narcotic antitussive; decongestant; antihistamine* [codeine phosphate; pseudoephedrine HCl; chlorpheniramine maleate; alcohol 5%] 10•30•2 mg/5 mL

**Novahistine DMX** oral liquid OTC *antitussive; decongestant; expectorant* [dextromethorphan hydrobromide; pseudoephedrine HCl; guaifenesin; alcohol 5%] 10•30•100 mg/5 mL

**novamidon** [see: aminopyrine]

**Novamine; Novamine 15%** IV infusion ℞ *total parenteral nutrition; peripheral parenteral nutrition* [multiple essential and nonessential amino acids]

**Novamoxin** CAN capsules, chewable tablets, oral suspension ℞ *aminopenicillin antibiotic* [amoxicillin trihydrate] 250, 500 mg; 125, 250 mg; 125, 250 mg/5 mL

**Novantrone** IV infusion ℞ *antibiotic antineoplastic for prostate cancer and acute nonlymphocytic leukemia (ANLL) (orphan); immunomodulator for progressive and relapsing-remitting multiple sclerosis* [mitoxantrone HCl] 2 mg/mL

**Novarel** powder for IM injection ℞ *hormone for prepubertal cryptorchidism and hypogonadism; ovulation stimulant; testosterone stimulant* [chorionic gonadotropin] 1000 U/mL

**Novasal** film-coated tablets ℞ *analgesic; antipyretic; anti-inflammatory* [magnesium salicylate tetrahydrate] 600 mg

**Novasen** ⓒᴬᴺ enteric-coated tablets OTC *analgesic; antipyretic; anti-inflammatory; antirheumatic* [aspirin] 325, 650 mg

**NovaSource Renal** oral liquid OTC *nutritional therapy for renal failure* [multiple vitamins & minerals] 237 mL/pkt.

**Novastan** (name changed to Acova upon marketing release in 2000) ⑨ Neovastat; Ovastat

**novel (atypical) antipsychotics** *a class of agents with a high affinity to the serotonin receptors and varying degrees of affinity to other neurotransmitter receptors; "atypical" due to the low incidence of extrapyramidal side effects (EPS)* [compare to: conventional (typical) antipsychotics]

**Novo-Amiodarone** ⓒᴬᴺ tablets ℞ *antiarrhythmic* [amiodarone HCl] 200 mg

**novobiocin** INN, BAN *bacteriostatic antibiotic* [also: novobiocin calcium]

**novobiocin calcium** USP *bacteriostatic antibiotic* [also: novobiocin]

**novobiocin sodium** USP *bacteriostatic antibiotic*

**Novocain** injection ℞ *injectable local anesthetic* [procaine HCl] 1%, 2%, 10%

**Novo-Cefaclor** ⓒᴬᴺ capsules ℞ *cephalosporin antibiotic* [cefaclor] 250, 500 mg

**Novo-Cefadroxil** ⓒᴬᴺ capsules ℞ *cephalosporin antibiotic* [cefadroxil] 500 mg

**Novo-Clonazepam** ⓒᴬᴺ tablets ℞ *anticonvulsant* [clonazepam] 0.5, 2 mg

**Novo-Cyproterone** ⓒᴬᴺ tablets ℞ *antiandrogen antineoplastic for advanced prostatic carcinoma* [cyproterone acetate] 50 mg

**Novo-Difenac-K** ⓒᴬᴺ tablets ℞ *analgesic; antiarthritic; nonsteroidal anti-inflammatory drug (NSAID)* [diclofenac potassium] 50 mg

**Novo-Diltiazem CD** ⓒᴬᴺ (once daily) controlled-delivery capsules ℞ *antihypertensive; antianginal; antiarrhyth-mic; calcium channel blocker* [diltiazem HCl] 120, 180, 240, 300 mg

**Novo-Divalproex** ⓒᴬᴺ enteric-coated tablets ℞ *anticonvulsant* [divalproex sodium] 125, 250, 500 mg

**Novo-Domperidone** ⓒᴬᴺ film-coated tablets ℞ *antiemetic for diabetic gastroparesis and chronic gastritis* [domperidone maleate] 10 mg

**Novo-Fluvoxamine** ⓒᴬᴺ tablets ℞ *selective serotonin reuptake inhibitor (SSRI) for depression and obsessive-compulsive disorder (OCD)* [fluvoxamine maleate] 50, 100 mg

**Novo-Gemfibrozil** ⓒᴬᴺ capsules, tablets ℞ *antihyperlipidemic for hypertriglyceridemia and coronary heart disease* [gemfibrozil] 300 mg; 600 mg

**Novo-Glyburide** ⓒᴬᴺ tablets ℞ *sulfonylurea antidiabetic* [glyburide] 2.5, 5 mg

**Novo-Hydrazide** ⓒᴬᴺ tablets ℞ *antihypertensive; diuretic* [hydrochlorothiazide] 25, 50 mg

**Novo-Ketoconazole** ⓒᴬᴺ tablets ℞ *broad-spectrum antifungal* [ketoconazole] 200 mg

**Novolin 70/30** subcu injection OTC *antidiabetic* [isophane human insulin (rDNA); human insulin (rDNA)] 100 U/mL

**Novolin 70/30 PenFill** NovoPen cartridge OTC *antidiabetic* [isophane human insulin (rDNA); human insulin (rDNA)] 150 U/1.5 mL, 300 U/3 mL

**Novolin 70/30 Prefilled** syringes OTC *antidiabetic* [isophane human insulin (rDNA); human insulin (rDNA)] 150 U/1.5 mL

**Novolin ge 10/90 PenFill** ⓒᴬᴺ NovoPen cartridges OTC *antidiabetic* [human insulin (rDNA); isophane human insulin (rDNA)] 3 mL

**Novolin ge 20/80 PenFill** ⓒᴬᴺ NovoPen cartridges OTC *antidiabetic* [human insulin (rDNA); isophane human insulin (rDNA)] 3 mL

**Novolin ge 30/70** ⓒᴬᴺ vials for subcu injection OTC *antidiabetic* [human insulin (rDNA); isophane human insulin (rDNA)] 100 U/mL; 1.5, 3 mL

**Novolin ge 30/70 PenFill** Ⓒ Novo-Pen cartridges OTC *antidiabetic* [human insulin (rDNA); isophane human insulin (rDNA)] 100 U/mL; 1.5, 3 mL

**Novolin ge 40/60 PenFill** Ⓒ Novo-Pen cartridges OTC *antidiabetic* [human insulin (rDNA); isophane human insulin (rDNA)] 3 mL

**Novolin ge 50/50 PenFill** Ⓒ Novo-Pen cartridges OTC *antidiabetic* [human insulin (rDNA); isophane human insulin (rDNA)] 3 mL

**Novolin ge Lente** Ⓒ vials for subcu injection OTC *antidiabetic* [human insulin zinc (rDNA)] 100 U/mL

**Novolin ge NPH** Ⓒ vials for subcu injection OTC *antidiabetic* [isophane human insulin (rDNA)] 100 U/mL; 1.5, 3 mL

**Novolin ge NPH PenFill** Ⓒ Novo-Pen cartridges OTC *antidiabetic* [isophane human insulin (rDNA)] 100 U/mL; 1.5, 3 mL

**Novolin ge Toronto** Ⓒ vials for subcu injection OTC *antidiabetic* [human insulin (rDNA)] 100 U/mL; 1.5, 3 mL

**Novolin ge Toronto PenFill** Ⓒ NovoPen cartridges OTC *antidiabetic* [human insulin (rDNA)] 100 U/mL; 1.5, 3 mL

**Novolin ge Ultralente** Ⓒ vials for subcu injection OTC *antidiabetic* [human insulin zinc (rDNA)] 100 U/mL

**Novolin L** vials for subcu injection (discontinued 2003) OTC *antidiabetic* [insulin zinc, human (rDNA)] 100 U/mL

**Novolin N** vials for subcu injection OTC *antidiabetic* [isophane human insulin (rDNA)] 100 U/mL

**Novolin N PenFill** NovoPen cartridge OTC *antidiabetic* [isophane human insulin (rDNA)] 150 U/1.5 mL, 300 U/3 mL

**Novolin N Prefilled** syringes OTC *antidiabetic* [isophane human insulin (rDNA)] 150 U/1.5 mL

**Novolin R** vials for subcu injection OTC *antidiabetic* [human insulin (rDNA)] 100 U/mL

**Novolin R PenFill** NovoPen cartridges OTC *antidiabetic* [human insulin (rDNA)] 150 U/1.5 mL, 300 U/3 mL

**Novolin R Prefilled** syringes OTC *antidiabetic* [human insulin (rDNA)] 150 U/1.5 mL

**NovoLog** vials for subcu injection ℞ *rapid-acting insulin analogue for diabetes* [human insulin aspart (rDNA)] 100 U/mL

**NovoLog FlexPen** self-injector ℞ *rapid-acting insulin analogue for diabetes* [human insulin aspart (rDNA)] 300 U/3 mL

**NovoLog Mix 70/30 FlexPen** self-injector ℞ *insulin analogue for diabetes with rapid onset and intermediate duration of action* [insulin aspart protamine; insulin aspart] 70%•30%

**NovoLog Mix 70/30 PenFill** Novo-Pen cartridges ℞ *insulin analogue for diabetes with rapid onset and intermediate duration of action* [insulin aspart protamine; insulin aspart] 70%•30%

**NovoLog PenFill** NovoPen cartridges ℞ *rapid-acting insulin analogue for diabetes* [human insulin aspart (rDNA)] 300 U/3 mL

**Novo-Lorazem** Ⓒ tablets ℞ *benzodiazepine anxiolytic* [lorazepam] 0.5, 1, 2 mg

**Novo-Medrone** Ⓒ tablets ℞ *progestin for secondary amenorrhea, abnormal uterine bleeding, and endometrial hyperplasia* [medroxyprogesterone acetate] 2.5, 5, 10 mg

**Novo-Metformin** Ⓒ film-coated tablets ℞ *biguanide antidiabetic* [metformin HCl] 500, 850 mg

**Novo-Metoprol** Ⓒ tablets, film-coated caplets ℞ *antihypertensive; antianginal; antiadrenergic (β-blocker)* [metoprolol tartrate] 50, 100 mg

**Novo-Moclobemide** ⓒ tablets ℞ *antidepressant* [moclobemide] 100, 150, 300 mg

**Novo-Naprox** ⓒ tablets ℞ *analgesic; antiarthritic; nonsteroidal anti-inflammatory drug (NSAID)* [naproxen] 125, 250, 375, 500 mg

**Novo-Naprox SR** ⓒ sustained-release tablets ℞ *analgesic; antiarthritic; nonsteroidal anti-inflammatory drug (NSAID)* [naproxen] 750 mg

**Novo-Naprox-EC** ⓒ enteric-coated tablets ℞ *analgesic; antiarthritic; nonsteroidal anti-inflammatory drug (NSAID)* [naproxen] 250, 375, 500 mg

**Novo-Nizatidine** ⓒ capsules ℞ *histamine $H_2$ antagonist for treatment of gastric and duodenal ulcers* [nizatidine] 150, 300 mg

**Novo-Norfloxacin** ⓒ tablets ℞ *broad-spectrum fluoroquinolone antibiotic* [norfloxacin] 400 mg

**NovoNorm** (European name for U.S. product Prandin)

**Novopaque** oral/rectal suspension (discontinued 2001) ℞ *radiopaque contrast medium for gastrointestinal imaging* [barium sulfate] 60%

**NovoPen 1.5; NovoPen Junior** prefilled reusable syringe *uses Novolin PenFill cartridges and NovoFine 30-gauge disposable needles* [insulin (several types available)] 1–40 U/injection

**Novo-Ranidine** ⓒ film-coated tablets ℞ *histamine $H_2$ antagonist for gastric and duodenal ulcers* [ranitidine HCl] 150, 300 mg

**NovoRapid** (U.S. name changed to NovoLog upon marketing release in 2000)

**NovoRapid** ⓒ vials for subcu injection ℞ *rapid-acting insulin analogue for diabetes* [insulin aspart, human (rDNA)] 100 U/mL

**Novo-Salmol** ⓒ tablets ℞ *sympathomimetic bronchodilator* [salbutamol sulfate] 2, 4 mg

**Novo-Semide** ⓒ tablets ℞ *antihypertensive; loop diuretic* [furosemide] 20, 40, 80 mg

**Novo-Sertraline** ⓒ capsules ℞ *selective serotonin reuptake inhibitor (SSRI) for depression* [sertraline HCl] 25, 50, 100 mg

**NovoSeven** powder for IV injection ℞ *coagulant for hemophilia A and B (orphan)* [factor VIIa, recombinant] 1.2, 2.4, 4.8 mg/vial

**Novo-Terazosin** ⓒ tablets ℞ *antihypertensive (α-blocker); treatment for benign prostatic hyperplasia (BPH)* [terazosin HCl] 1, 2, 5, 10 mg

**Novo-Timol** ⓒ eye drops (discontinued 2001) ℞ *topical antiglaucoma agent (β-blocker)* [timolol maleate] 0.25%, 0.5%

**Novo-Triptyn** ⓒ tablets ℞ *tricyclic antidepressant* [amitriptyline HCl] 10, 25, 50 mg

**NovoVac** ℞ *investigational (Phase I/II) antibody vaccine for melanoma*

**Novoxapam** ⓒ tablets ℞ *benzodiazepine anxiolytic* [oxazepam] 10, 15, 30 mg

**NOVP (Novantrone, Oncovin, vinblastine, prednisone)** *chemotherapy protocol for Hodgkin lymphoma*

**noxiptiline** INN [also: noxiptyline]

**noxiptyline** BAN [also: noxiptiline]

**noxythiolin** BAN [also: noxytiolin]

**noxytiolin** INN [also: noxythiolin]

**NP (nifurpipone)** [q.v.]

**NPH (neutral protamine Hagedorn) insulin** [see: insulin, isophane]

**NPH Iletin II** subcu injection OTC *antidiabetic* [isophane insulin (pork)] 100 U/mL

**NPH-N** subcu injection (discontinued 2000) OTC *antidiabetic* [isophane insulin (pork)] 100 U/mL

**NRTIs (nucleoside reverse transcriptase inhibitors)** [see: reverse transcriptase inhibitors]

**NS (normal saline)** [q.v.]

**NSAIDs (nonsteroidal anti-inflammatory drugs)** [q.v.] ⃝ InFeD

**NTBC** *investigational (orphan) for tyrosinemia type I*

**NTZ (nitazoxanide)** [q.v.]

**NTZ Long Acting** nasal spray, nose drops (discontinued 2002) OTC *nasal decongestant* [oxymetazoline HCl] 0.05%

**Nubain** IV, subcu or IM injection ℞ *narcotic agonist-antagonist analgesic* [nalbuphine HCl] 10, 20 mg/mL

**Nu-Beclomethasone** Ⓒ nasal spray ℞ *corticosteroidal anti-inflammatory for chronic asthma and rhinitis* [beclomethasone dipropionate] 50 µg/ metered dose

**nucleoside reverse transcriptase inhibitors (NRTI)** *a class of antiretroviral drugs that inhibits the activity of reverse transcriptase (polymerase) in viral cells, causing a termination of DNA chain elongation, which prevents replication of the cells* [see: reverse transcriptase inhibitors]

**nuclomedone** INN

**nuclotixene** INN

**Nucofed** capsules, syrup ℞ *narcotic antitussive; decongestant* [codeine phosphate; pseudoephedrine HCl] 20•60 mg; 20•60 mg/5 mL

**Nucofed Expectorant** syrup (discontinued 2002) ℞ *narcotic antitussive; decongestant; expectorant* [codeine phosphate; pseudoephedrine HCl; guaifenesin; alcohol 12.5%] 20•60• 200 mg/5 mL

**Nucofed Pediatric Expectorant** syrup ℞ *narcotic antitussive; decongestant; expectorant* [codeine phosphate; pseudoephedrine HCl; guaifenesin; alcohol 6%] 10•30•100 mg/5 mL

**Nucotuss Expectorant** oral liquid (discontinued 2002) ℞ *narcotic antitussive; decongestant; expectorant* [codeine phosphate; pseudoephedrine HCl; guaifenesin; alcohol 12.5%] 20•60•200 mg/5 mL

**Nucotuss Pediatric Expectorant** oral liquid ℞ *narcotic antitussive; decongestant; expectorant* [codeine phosphate; pseudoephedrine HCl; guaifenesin; alcohol 6%] 10•30•100 mg/5 mL

**Nu-Diltiaz-CD** Ⓒ capsules ℞ *antihypertensive; antianginal* [diltiazem HCl] 120, 180, 240 mg

**Nu-Divalproex** Ⓒ tablets ℞ *anticonvulsant* [divalproex sodium] 125, 250, 500 mg

**Nu-Enalapril** Ⓒ tablets ℞ *antihypertensive; angiotensin-converting enzyme (ACE) inhibitor* [enalapril maleate]

**nufenoxole** USAN, INN *antiperistaltic*

**Nu-Fluvoxamine** Ⓒ tablets ℞ *selective serotonin reuptake inhibitor (SSRI) for depression and obsessive-compulsive disorder (OCD)* [fluvoxamine maleate]

**Nuhist** pediatric oral suspension ℞ *decongestant; antihistamine* [phenylephrine tannate; chlorpheniramine tannate] 5•4.5 mg/5 mL

**Nu-Iron** elixir OTC *hematinic; iron supplement* [polysaccharide-iron complex] 100 mg/5 mL

**Nu-Iron 150** capsules OTC *hematinic; iron supplement* [polysaccharide-iron complex] 150 mg

**Nu-Iron Plus** elixir ℞ *hematinic* [polysaccharide-iron complex; cyanocobalamin; folic acid] 300 mg•75 µg• 3 mg per 15 mL

**Nu-Iron V** film-coated tablets ℞ *vitamin/iron supplement* [polysaccharide-iron complex; multiple vitamins; folic acid] 60•≚•1 mg

**Nu-knit** (trademarked form) *oxidized cellulose hemostatic pad*

**NuLev** orally disintegrating tablets ℞ *GI/GU antispasmodic; antiparkinsonian; anticholinergic "drying agent" for allergic rhinitis* [hyoscyamine sulfate] 0.125 mg

**NuLytely** powder for oral solution ℞ *pre-procedure bowel evacuant* [polyethylene glycol–electrolyte solution (PEG 3350)] 60, 105 g/L

**Nu-Moclobemide** Ⓒ tablets ℞ *antidepressant* [moclobemide] 100, 150 mg

**Numorphan** IV, IM, or subcu injection, suppositories ℞ *narcotic analgesic; preoperative support of anesthesia; investigational (orphan) for intractable*

pain in narcotic-tolerant patients [oxymorphone HCl] 1, 1.5 mg/mL; 5 mg

**Numzident** gel OTC *topical oral anesthetic* [benzocaine] 10%

**Numzit Teething** gel OTC *topical oral anesthetic* [benzocaine] 7.5%

**Numzit Teething** lotion OTC *topical oral anesthetic* [benzocaine; alcohol 12.1%] 0.2%

**Nupercainal** ointment, cream OTC *topical local anesthetic* [dibucaine] 1%; 0.5%

**Nupercainal** rectal suppositories OTC *emollient; astringent* [cocoa butter; zinc oxide] 2.1•0.25 g

**Nuprin** tablets, caplets OTC *analgesic; antiarthritic; antipyretic; nonsteroidal anti-inflammatory drug (NSAID)* [ibuprofen] 200 mg

**Nuprin Backache** caplets OTC *analgesic; antipyretic; anti-inflammatory* [magnesium salicylate] 580 mg

**Nu-Prochlor** ⊛ film-coated tablets ℞ *conventional (typical) antipsychotic; antiemetic* [prochlorperazine bimaleate] 5, 10 mg

**Nuquin HP** cream ℞ *hyperpigmentation bleaching agent* [hydroquinone (in a sunscreen base)] 4%

**Nuquin HP** gel (discontinued 2003) ℞ *hyperpigmentation bleaching agent* [hydroquinone (in a sunscreen base)] 4%

**Nuromax** IV injection ℞ *nondepolarizing neuromuscular blocker; adjunct to anesthesia* [doxacurium chloride] 1 mg/mL

**Nursette** (trademarked form) *prefilled disposable bottle*

**Nu-Salt** OTC *salt substitute* [potassium chloride] 68 mEq K/5 g

**nut, oil** *medicinal herb* [see: butternut]

**Nu-Tears** eye drops OTC *ophthalmic moisturizer/lubricant* [polyvinyl alcohol] 1.4%

**Nu-Tears II** eye drops OTC *ophthalmic moisturizer/lubricant* [polyvinyl alcohol; polyethylene glycol 400] 1%•1%

**Nu-Timolol** ⊛ tablets ℞ *antihypertensive; antiadrenergic (β-blocker);*

*migraine prophylaxis* [timolol maleate] 5, 10, 20 mg

**nutmeg (Myristica fragrans)** seed and aril *medicinal herb for diarrhea, flatulence, inducing expectorant, insomnia, mouth sores, rheumatism, salivary stimulation, and stimulating menstruation*

**nutmeg oil** NF

**Nutracort** cream ℞ *topical corticosteroidal anti-inflammatory* [hydrocortisone] 1%

**Nutraderm** cream, lotion OTC *moisturizer; emollient*

**Nutraderm** OTC *lotion base*

**Nutraderm Bath Oil** OTC *bath emollient*

**Nutraloric** powder OTC *enteral nutritional therapy* [milk-based formula]

**Nutrament** oral liquid OTC *enteral nutritional therapy* 12 oz. cans

**Nutramigen** oral liquid, powder for oral liquid OTC *hypoallergenic infant food* [enzymatically hydrolyzed protein formula]

**Nutraplus** cream, lotion OTC *moisturizer; emollient; keratolytic* [urea] 10%

**Nutra-Soothe** bath oil OTC *bath emollient* [colloidal oatmeal; light mineral oil]

**Nutren 1.0** oral liquid OTC *enteral nutritional therapy* [lactose-free formula]

**Nutren 1.5** oral liquid OTC *enteral nutritional therapy* [lactose-free formula]

**Nutren 2.0** ready-to-use oral liquid OTC *enteral nutritional therapy* [lactose-free formula]

**Nutr-E-Sol** oral liquid OTC *vitamin supplement* [vitamin E] 133 IU/5 mL

**Nutricon** tablets OTC *vitamin/mineral/calcium/iron supplement* [multiple vitamins & minerals; calcium; iron; folic acid; biotin] ±•200•20•0.4•0.15 mg

**Nutrifac ZX** caplets ℞ *vitamin/mineral supplement* [multiple vitamins & minerals; folic acid; biotin] ±•1•0.2 mg

**NutriFocus** ready-to-use oral liquid OTC *enteral nutritional therapy* [milk-based formula] 237 mL cans

**NutriHeal** ready-to-use oral liquid OTC *enteral nutritional therapy* [milk-based formula] 250 mL cans

**Nutrilan** ready-to-use oral liquid OTC *enteral nutritional therapy* [lactose-free formula]

**Nutrilyte; Nutrilyte II** IV admixture ℞ *intravenous electrolyte therapy* [combined electrolyte solution]

**Nutrineal Peritoneal Dialysis Solution with 1.1% Amino Acid** ℞ *investigational (orphan) nutritional supplement for continuous ambulatory peritoneal dialysis patients*

**Nutropin** powder for subcu injection ℞ *growth hormone for adults or children with congenital or endogenous growth hormone deficiency, children with Turner syndrome or renal-induced growth failure, or AIDS-wasting syndrome (orphan)* [somatropin] 5, 10 mg (13, 26 IU)/vial

**Nutropin AQ** subcu injection, Pen (prefilled syringe) ℞ *growth hormone for congenital or renal-induced growth failure and Turner syndrome (orphan); investigational (orphan) for severe burns* [somatropin] 10 mg (30 IU)/vial, 10 mg (30 IU)/2 mL cartridge

**Nutropin Depot** sustained-release injection (discontinued 2004) ℞ *once- or twice-monthly doseform* [somatropin] 13.5, 18, 22.5 mg

**Nutrox** capsules OTC *dietary supplement* [multiple vitamins & minerals; multiple amino acids]

**Nu-Valproic** ⓒ capsules ℞ *anticonvulsant* [valproic acid] 250 mg

**NuvaRing** vaginal ring ℞ *self-administered one-month contraceptive insert* [ethinyl estradiol; etonogestrel] 15• 120 µg/day

**nuvenzepine** INN

**Nuvion** ℞ *investigational monoclonal antibody for organ transplants, autoimmune diseases, and other T-lymphocyte disorders* [visilizumab]

**nyctal** [see: carbromal]

**nydrane** [see: benzchlorpropamid]

**Nydrazid** IM injection ℞ *tuberculostatic* [isoniazid] 100 mg/mL

**nylestriol** USAN *estrogen* [also: nilestriol]

**nylidrin HCl** USP *peripheral vasodilator* [also: buphenine]

*Nymphaea odorata* medicinal herb [see: white pond lilly]

**Nyotran** ℞ *investigational (NDA filed) systemic antifungal for Aspergillus fumigatus infections; investigational (Phase III) for cryptococcal meningitis* [nystatin, liposomal]

**NyQuil Cold/Cough Relief, Children's** oral liquid OTC *antitussive; decongestant; antihistamine* [dextromethorphan hydrobromide; pseudoephedrine HCl; chlorpheniramine maleate] 15•30•2 mg/15 mL

**NyQuil Cough** syrup OTC *antitussive; antihistamine* [dextromethorphan hydrobromide; doxylamine succinate] 30•12.5 mg/30 mL

**NyQuil Hot Therapy** powder for oral solution (discontinued 2002) OTC *antitussive; decongestant; antihistamine; analgesic* [dextromethorphan hydrobromide; pseudoephedrine HCl; doxylamine succinate; acetaminophen] 30•60•12.5•1000 mg/pkt.

**NyQuil LiquiCaps** (name changed to NyQuil Multi-Symptom Cold & Flu Relief in 2002)

**NyQuil Multi-Symptom Cold & Flu Relief** LiquiCaps (liquid-filled capsules) OTC *antitussive; decongestant; antihistamine; analgesic* [dextromethorphan hydrobromide; pseudoephedrine HCl; doxylamine succinate; acetaminophen] 10•30• 6.25•250 mg

**NyQuil Multisymptom Cold/Flu Relief** oral liquid OTC *antitussive; decongestant; antihistamine; analgesic* [dextromethorphan hydrobromide; pseudoephedrine HCl; doxylamine succinate; acetaminophen; alcohol 10%] 30•60•12.5•1000 mg/30 mL

**NyQuil Nighttime Cold/Flu Medicine** oral liquid (discontinued 2002) OTC *antitussive; decongestant; antihistamine; analgesic* [dextromethorphan hydrobromide; pseudoephedrine HCl; doxylamine succinate; aceta-

minophen; alcohol 25%] 5•10•
1.25•167 mg/5 mL

**nystatin** USP, INN, BAN, JAN *polyene
antifungal* 500 000 U/mL oral;
100 000 mg vaginal; 100 000 U/g
topical ⌕ Nilstat; Nitrostat

**Nystex** cream, ointment (discontinued 2003) ℞ *antifungal* [nystatin]
100 000 U/g

**Nystex** oral suspension (discontinued
2003) ℞ *antifungal; oral candidiasis
treatment* [nystatin] 100 000 U/mL

**Nystop** powder ℞ *topical antifungal*
[nystatin] 100 000 U/g

**Nytcold Medicine** oral liquid (discontinued 2002) OTC *antitussive;
decongestant; antihistamine; analgesic*
[dextromethorphan hydrobromide;
pseudoephedrine HCl; doxylamine
succinate; acetaminophen; alcohol
25%] 5•10•1.25•167 mg/5 mL

**Nytol** tablets OTC *antihistaminic sleep aid*
[diphenhydramine HCl] 25, 50 mg

**NZ-1001** *investigational (orphan) phosphorylated enzyme replacement therapy
for Pompe disease*

**NZGLM (New Zealand green-
lipped mussel)** [q.v.]

**O₂ (oxygen)** [q.v.]

**oak** *medicinal herb* [see: white oak]

**OAP (Oncovin, ara-C, prednisone)**
*chemotherapy protocol*

**oatmeal, colloidal** *demulcent*

**oats (Avena sativa)** grain and straw
*medicinal herb for dry itchy skin, hyperlipidemia, indigestion, insomnia, nervousness, opium addiction, reducing
the desire to smoke, and strengthening
the heart*

**obecalp** *placebo (spelled backward)* [q.v.]

**Obenix** capsules (discontinued 2001)
℞ *anorexiant; CNS stimulant* [phentermine HCl] 37.5 mg

**obidoxime chloride** USAN, INN *cholinesterase reactivator*

**oblimersen** *investigational (Phase III)
antisense therapy for lung cancer and
lymphoma*

**Obstetrix-100** tablets ℞ *prenatal vitamin/mineral/calcium/iron supplement;
stool softener* [multiple vitamins; calcium; iron; folic acid; zinc; docusate
sodium] ±•250•100•1•25•50 mg

**Obtrex** tablets ℞ *prenatal vitamin/mineral supplement; stool softener* [multiple vitamins and minerals; docusate
sodium] ±•50 mg

...uoride] — ...

**O-Cal Prenatal** tablets ℞ *vitamin/mineral/calcium/iron supplement* [multiple
vitamins & minerals; calcium; iron;
folic acid] ±•200•15•1 mg

**ocaperidone** USAN, INN, BAN *antipsychotic*

**Occlusal-HP** topical liquid OTC *keratolytic* [salicylic acid in polyacrylic
vehicle] 17%

**Occucoat** ophthalmic solution ℞ *ophthalmic surgical aid* [hydroxypropyl
methylcellulose] 2%

**Ocean** nasal spray OTC *nasal moisturizer* [sodium chloride (saline solution)] 0.65%

**ocfentanil** INN *narcotic analgesic* [also:
ocfentanil HCl]

**ocfentanil HCl** USAN *narcotic analgesic*
[also: ocfentanil]

**ociltide** INN

**Ocimum basilicum** *medicinal herb* [see:
basil]

**ocinaplon** USAN *anxiolytic*

**OCL** oral solution ℞ *pre-procedure bowel evacuant* [polyethylene glycol–electrolyte solution (PEG 3350)] 60 g/L

**ocrase** INN

**ocrilate** INN *tissue adhesive* [also: ocrylate]

**ocrylate** USAN *tissue adhesive* [also: ocrilate]

**OCT (22-oxacalcitriol)** [see: maxacalcitol]

**octabenzone** USAN, INN *ultraviolet screen*

**octacaine** INN

**octacosactrin** BAN [also: tosactide]

**octacosanol** *natural extract of wheat germ used to treat hypercholesterolemia; effective for lowering LDL-cholesterol, raising HDL-cholesterol, stopping the formation of arterial lesions and plaque deposits, and inhibiting clot formation*

**octadecafluorodecehydronaphthalene** [see: perflunafene]

**octadecanoic acid, calcium salt** [see: calcium stearate]

**octadecanoic acid, sodium salt** [see: sodium stearate]

**octadecanoic acid, zinc salt** [see: zinc stearate]

**1-octadecanol** [see: stearyl alcohol]

**9-octadecenylamine hydrofluoride** [see: dectaflur]

**octafonium chloride** INN

**Octagam** IV infusion ℞ *passive immunizing agent for primary immune deficient diseases and severe combined immunodeficiencies* [immune globulin, solvent/detergent treated] 5% in 1, 2.5, 5, 10 g bottles

**Octamide PFS** IV or IM injection ℞ *antiemetic for chemotherapy; GI stimulant; peristaltic* [metoclopramide HCl] 5 mg/mL

**octamoxin** INN

**octamylamine** INN

**octanoic acid** USAN, INN *antifungal*

**octapinol** INN

**octastine** INN

**octatropine methylbromide** INN, BAN *anticholinergic; peptic ulcer adjunct* [also: anisotropine methylbromide]

**octatropone bromide** [see: anisotropine methylbromide]

**octaverine** INN, BAN

**octazamide** USAN, INN *analgesic*

**octenidine** INN, BAN *topical anti-infective* [also: octenidine HCl]

**octenidine HCl** USAN *topical anti-infective* [also: octenidine]

**octenidine saccharin** USAN *dental plaque inhibitor*

**Octicare** ear drops, ear drop suspension ℞ *topical corticosteroidal anti-inflammatory; antibiotic* [hydrocortisone; neomycin sulfate; polymyxin B sulfate] 1%•5 mg•10 000 U per mL

**octicizer** USAN *plasticizer*

**octil** INN *combining name for radicals or groups*

**octimibate** INN

**octinoxate** USAN *ultraviolet B sunscreen*

**octisalate** USAN *ultraviolet sunscreen*

**octisamyl** [see: octamylamine]

**Octocaine HCl** injection ℞ *injectable local anesthetic* [lidocaine HCl; epinephrine] 2%•1:50 000, 2%• 1:100 000

**octoclothepine** [see: clorotepine]

**octocrilene** INN *ultraviolet screen* [also: octocrylene]

**octocrylene** USAN *ultraviolet screen* [also: octocrilene]

**octodecactide** [see: codactide]

**octodrine** USAN, INN *adrenergic; vasoconstrictor; local anesthetic*

**octopamine** INN

**octotiamine** INN

**octoxinol** INN *surfactant/wetting agent* [also: octoxynol 9]

**octoxynol 9** USAN, NF *surfactant/wetting agent; spermicide* [also: octoxinol]

**OctreoScan** powder for injection ℞ *radiopaque contrast medium* [oxidronate sodium] 2 mg

**OctreoScan 111** injection ℞ *radioactive imaging agent for SPECT scans of neuroendocrine tumors* [indium In 111 pentetreotide] 10 µg/vial

**octreotide** USAN, INN, BAN *gastric antisecretory*

**octreotide acetate** USAN *gastric antisecretory for acromegaly and severe diarrhea due to VIPomas and other tumors (orphan)*

**octreotide pamoate** USAN *antineoplastic*

**octriptyline** INN *antidepressant* [also: octriptyline phosphate]

**octriptyline phosphate** USAN *antidepressant* [also: octriptyline]

**octrizole** USAN, INN *ultraviolet screen*

**octyl methoxycinnamate** [see: octinoxate]

**octyl salicylate** [see: octisalate]

**S-octyl thiobenzoate** [see: tioctilate]

**octyl-2-cyanoacrylate** [see: ocrylate]

**octyldodecanol** NF *oleaginous vehicle*

**OcuCaps** caplets OTC *vitamin/mineral supplement* [vitamins A, C, and E; multiple minerals] 5000 IU•400 mg•182 mg•≛

**OcuClear** eye drops OTC *topical ophthalmic decongestant and vasoconstrictor* [oxymetazoline HCl] 0.025%

**OcuCoat** prefilled syringe OTC *ophthalmic surgical aid* [hydroxypropyl methylcellulose] 2%

**OcuCoat; OcuCoat PF** eye drops OTC *ophthalmic moisturizer/lubricant* [hydroxypropyl methylcellulose] 0.8%

**Ocudose** (trademarked delivery device) *single-use eye drop dispenser*

**Ocufen** eye drops ℞ *topical ophthalmic nonsteroidal anti-inflammatory drug (NSAID); intraoperative miosis inhibitor* [flurbiprofen sodium] 0.03%

**ocufilcon A** USAN *hydrophilic contact lens material*

**ocufilcon B** USAN *hydrophilic contact lens material*

**ocufilcon C** USAN *hydrophilic contact lens material*

**ocufilcon D** USAN *hydrophilic contact lens material*

**ocufilcon F** USAN *hydrophilic contact lens material*

**Ocuflox** eye drops ℞ *topical fluoroquinolone antibiotic for bacterial conjunctivitis and corneal ulcers (orphan)* [ofloxacin] 0.3%

**Ocumeter** (trademarked delivery device) *prefilled eye drop dispenser*

**Ocupress** eye drops ℞ *antiglaucoma agent (β-blocker)* [carteolol HCl] 1%

**Ocusert Pilo-20; Ocusert Pilo-40** continuous-release ocular wafer ℞ *topical antiglaucoma agent; direct-acting miotic* [pilocarpine] 20 μg/hr.; 40 μg/hr.

**OCuSOFT** solution, pads OTC *eyelid cleanser for blepharitis or contact lenses*

**OCuSoft VMS** film-coated tablets OTC *vitamin/mineral supplement* [vitamins A, C, and E; multiple minerals] 5000 IU•60 mg•30 mg•≛

**Ocusulf-10** eye drops ℞ *antibiotic* [sulfacetamide sodium] 10%

**Ocutricin** ophthalmic ointment ℞ *topical ophthalmic antibiotic* [polymyxin B sulfate; neomycin sulfate; bacitracin zinc] 10 000 U•3.5 mg•400 U per g

**Ocuvite; Ocuvite PreserVision** film-coated tablets OTC *vitamin/mineral supplement* [vitamins A, C, and E; multiple minerals] 5000 IU•60 mg•30 IU•≛; 7160 IU•113 mg•100 IU•≛

**Ocuvite Extra** tablets OTC *vitamin/mineral supplement* [vitamins A, C, and E; multiple B vitamins; multiple minerals; lutein] 1000 IU•300 mg•100 IU•≛•≛•2 mg

**Ocuvite Lutein** capsules OTC *vitamin/mineral supplement* [vitamins C and E; multiple minerals; lutein] 60 mg•30 IU•≛•6 mg

**Odor Free ArthriCare** [see: ArthriCare, Odor Free]

*Oenothera biennis* medicinal herb [see: evening primrose]

**OEP (oil of evening primrose)** [see: evening primrose]

**Oesclim** Ⓒ transdermal patch ℞ *estrogen replacement therapy for postmenopausal symptoms* [estradiol-17β hemihydrate] 25, 50 μg/day

**Oesto-Mins** powder OTC *vitamin/mineral supplement* [vitamins C and D; calcium; magnesium; potassium] 500

mg•100 IU•250 mg•250 mg•45 mg per 4.5 g

**oestradiol** BAN *estrogen replacement therapy for the treatment of postmenopausal disorders and prevention of postmenopausal osteoporosis; palliative therapy for prostatic and breast cancers* [also: estradiol]

**oestradiol benzoate** BAN [also: estradiol benzoate]

**oestradiol valerate** BAN *estrogen* [also: estradiol valerate]

**oestriol succinate** BAN *estrogen* [also: estriol; estriol succinate]

**oestrogenine** [see: diethylstilbestrol]

**oestromenin** [see: diethylstilbestrol]

**oestrone** BAN *estrogen replacement therapy for postmenopausal disorders; palliative therapy for prostatic and breast cancers* [also: estrone]

**Off-Ezy Corn & Callus Remover** kit (topical liquid + cushion pads) OTC *keratolytic* [salicylic acid in a collodion-like vehicle] 17%

**Off-Ezy Wart Remover** topical liquid OTC *keratolytic* [salicylic acid in a collodion-like vehicle] 17%

**ofloxacin** USAN, INN, BAN, JAN *broad-spectrum fluoroquinolone antibiotic; topical corneal ulcer treatment (orphan)* 200, 300, 400 mg oral; 0.3% eye drops

**ofornine** USAN, INN *antihypertensive*

**oftasceine** INN

**Ogen** tablets ℞ *natural estrogen replacement therapy for the treatment of postmenopausal symptoms and prevention of postmenopausal osteoporosis* [estrone (from estropipate)] 0.625 (0.75), 1.25 (1.5), 2.5 (3) mg

**Ogen Vaginal** cream ℞ *natural estrogen replacement for postmenopausal atrophic vaginitis* [estropipate] 1.5 mg/g

**Ogestrel 0.5/50** tablets (in packs of 28) ℞ *monophasic oral contraceptive; emergency postcoital contraceptive* [norgestrel; ethinyl estradiol] 0.5 mg•50 μg

**oglufanide disodium** USAN *immunomodulator; investigational (Phase III)* *angiogenesis inhibitor antineoplastic for Kaposi sarcoma and solid tumor cancers*

**oidiomycin** *diagnostic aid for cell-mediated immunity; extract of the Oidiomycetes fungus family*

**oil nut** *medicinal herb* [see: butternut]

**oil of evening primrose (OEP)** [see: evening primrose]

**oil of mustard** [see: allyl isothiocyanate]

**Oil of Olay Foaming Face Wash** topical liquid OTC *cleanser for acne*

**oil ricini** [see: castor oil]

**Oilatum Soap** bar OTC *therapeutic skin cleanser*

**ointment, hydrophilic** USP *ointment base; oil-in-water emulsion*

**ointment, white** USP *oleaginous ointment base*

**ointment, yellow** USP *ointment base*

**olaflur** USAN, INN, BAN *dental caries prophylactic*

**olamine** USAN, INN *combining name for radicals or groups*

**olanexidine HCl** USAN *topical antibiotic for nosocomial or wound infections*

**olanzapine** USAN, INN *thienobenzodiazepine antipsychotic for schizophrenia and manic episodes of a bipolar disorder*

**olaquindox** INN, BAN

**old man's beard** *medicinal herb* [see: fringe tree; woodbine]

**old tuberculin (OT)** [see: tuberculin]

*Olea europaea* *medicinal herb* [see: olive]

**oleander (Nerium indicum; N. oleander)** plant *medicinal herb for asthma, cancer, corns, epilepsy, and heart disease; not generally regarded as safe and effective in any form as it is very toxic*

**oleandomycin** INN [also: oleandomycin phosphate]

**oleandomycin, triacetate ester** [see: troleandomycin]

**oleandomycin phosphate** NF [also: oleandomycin]

**oleic acid** NF *emulsion adjunct*

**oleic acid I 125** USAN *radioactive agent*

**oleic acid I 131** USAN *radioactive agent*

**oleovitamin A** [now: vitamin A]

**oleovitamin A & D** USP *source of vitamins A and D*

**oleovitamin D, synthetic** [now: ergocalciferol]

**olethytan 20** [see: polysorbate 80]

**oletimol** INN

**oleum caryophylii** [see: clove oil]

**oleum gossypii seminis** [see: cottonseed oil]

**oleum maydis** [see: corn oil]

**oleum ricini** [see: castor oil]

**oleyl alcohol** NF *emulsifying agent; emollient*

**oligomycin D** [see: rutamycin]

**olive (Olea europaea)** leaves, bark, and fruit *medicinal herb used as an antiseptic, astringent, cholagogue, demulcent, emollient, febrifuge, hypoglycemic, laxative, and tranquilizer*

**olive, spurge; spurge laurel** *medicinal herb* [see: mezereon]

**olive oil** NF *pharmaceutic aid*

**olivomycin** INN

**olizumab** *investigational (Phase III) recombinant humanized monoclonal antibody for asthma*

**olmesartan** USAN *antihypertensive; angiotensin II receptor antagonist*

**olmesartan medoxomil** USAN, INN *antihypertensive; angiotensin II receptor antagonist*

**olmidine** INN

**olopatadine** INN *antiallergic; antiasthmatic*

**olopatadine HCl** USAN *antiallergic; antiasthmatic; ophthalmic antihistamine and mast cell stabilizer*

**olpimedone** INN

**olsalazine** INN, BAN *GI anti-inflammatory* [also: olsalazine sodium]

**olsalazine sodium** USAN *GI anti-inflammatory; treatment of ulcerative colitis* [also: olsalazine]

**oltipraz** INN

**Olux** topical foam ℞ *corticosteroidal anti-inflammatory for scalp dermatoses and plaque psoriasis* [clobetasol propionate; alcohol 60%] 0.05%

**olvanil** USAN, INN *analgesic*

**OM 401** *investigational (orphan) for sickle cell disease*

**omaciclovir** USAN *antiviral DNA polymerase inhibitor for herpes zoster*

**OMAD (Oncovin, methotrexate/ citrovorum factor, Adriamycin, dactinomycin)** *chemotherapy protocol*

**omalizumab** *recombinant humanized monoclonal antibody (rhuMAb) to immunoglobulin E (anti-IgE) for treatment of moderate to severe asthma*

**omapatrilat** *vasopeptidase inhibitor (VPI); investigational (NDA filed) endopeptidase and angiotensin-converting enzyme (ACE) inhibitor for hypertension and congestive heart failure*

**omega-3 fatty acids** [see: doconexent; icosapent; omega-3 marine triglycerides]

**omega-3 fatty acids with all double bonds in the *cis* configuration** *investigational (orphan) preventative for organ graft rejection*

**omega-3 marine triglycerides** BAN [12% doconexent (q.v.) + 18% icosapent (q.v.)]

**omeprazole** USAN, INN, BAN, JAN *proton pump inhibitor for gastric and duodenal ulcers, erosive esophagitis, GERD, and other gastroesophageal disorders; investigational (Phase III) to prevent upper GI bleeding* 10, 20 mg oral

**omeprazole magnesium** USAN *proton pump inhibitor for gastric and duodenal ulcers, erosive esophagitis, GERD, and other gastroesophageal disorders* (base= 97%)

**omeprazole sodium** USAN *gastric antisecretory*

**omidoline** INN

**Omnicef** capsules, oral suspension ℞ *cephalosporin antibiotic* [cefdinir] 300 mg; 125 mg/5 mL

**OmniHIB** powder for IM injection, prefilled syringes ℞ *Haemophilus influenzae type b (HIB) vaccine* [Hemophilus b conjugate vaccine; tetanus toxoid] 10•24 μg/0.5 mL

**OMNIhist L.A.** long-acting tablets ℞ *decongestant; antihistamine; anticholinergic to dry mucosal secretions* [phenylephrine HCl; chlorpheniramine maleate; methscopolamine nitrate] 20•8•2.5 mg

**Omnipaque** injection ℞ *radiopaque contrast medium* [iohexol (46.36% iodine)] 302, 388, 518, 647, 755 mg/mL (140, 180, 240, 300, 350 mg/mL)

**Omnipaque** injection (discontinued 2001) ℞ *radiopaque contrast medium* [iohexol (46.36% iodine)] 453 mg/mL (210 mg/mL)

**Omnipen** capsules, powder for oral suspension (discontinued 2002) ℞ *aminopenicillin antibiotic* [ampicillin] 250, 500 mg; 125, 250 mg/5 mL ⑨ Unipen

**Omnipen-N** powder for IV or IM injection (discontinued 2002) ℞ *aminopenicillin antibiotic* [ampicillin sodium] 125, 250, 500 mg, 1, 2, 10 g

**Omniscan** IV injection ℞ *MRI contrast medium* [gadodiamide] 287 mg/mL

**omoconazole** INN *antifungal*

**omoconazole nitrate** USAN *antifungal*

**omonasteine** INN

**OMS Concentrate** drops (discontinued 2001) ℞ *narcotic analgesic* [morphine sulfate] 20 mg/mL

**onapristone** INN *investigational antineoplastic for hormone-dependent cancers*

**Oncaspar** IV or IM injection ℞ *antineoplastic for acute lymphocytic leukemia (orphan) and acute lymphoblastic leukemia* [pegaspargase] 750 IU/mL

**Oncet** capsules (discontinued 2002) ℞ *narcotic antitussive; analgesic* [hydrocodone bitartrate; acetaminophen] 5•500 mg

**Oncocine-HspE7** ℞ *investigational (Phase I) agent for cervical cancer*

**Onconase** ℞ *investigational (Phase III) treatment for pancreatic, breast, colorectal, prostate, and small cell lung cancers* [ranpirnase]

**Oncophage** ℞ *investigational (Phase III, orphan) antineoplastic for renal cell carcinoma and metastatic melanoma* [gp96 heat shock protein-peptide complex]

**OncoRad OV103** ℞ *investigational (orphan) antineoplastic for ovarian cancer* [CYT-103-Y-90 (code name —generic name not yet assigned)]

**OncoScint CR/OV** ℞ *radiodiagnostic imaging aid for ovarian (orphan) and colorectal cancer* [indium In 111 satumomab pendetide]

**Onco-TCS** *investigational (Phase III) antineoplastic for advanced non-Hodgkin lymphoma* [vincristine liposomal]

**OncoTICE** ⒸⒶⓃ powder for intravesical instillation ℞ *antineoplastic for urinary bladder cancer* [BCG vaccine, Tice strain] 50 mg

**OncoTrac** imaging kit ℞ *investigational (orphan) for diagnostic imaging agent for metastasis of malignant melanoma* [technetium Tc 99m antimelanoma murine monoclonal antibodies (MAb)]

**Oncovin** IV injection, Hyporets (prefilled syringes) ℞ *antineoplastic for lung and breast cancers, various leukemias, lymphomas, and sarcomas* [vincristine sulfate] 1 mg/mL ⑨ Ancobon

**Oncovite** tablets OTC *vitamin supplement* [multiple vitamins]

**ondansetron** INN, BAN *serotonin 5-HT$_3$ receptor antagonist; antiemetic for nausea following chemotherapy, radiation, or surgery* [also: ondansetron HCl]

**ondansetron HCl** USAN *serotonin 5-HT$_3$ receptor antagonist; antiemetic for nausea following chemotherapy, radiation, or surgery* [also: ondansetron]

**Ondrox** sustained-release tablets OTC *vitamin/mineral/calcium supplement* [multiple vitamins & minerals; multiple amino acids; calcium; folic acid; biotin] ±•±•50•0.2•0.015 mg

**1+1-F Creme** ℞ *topical corticosteroidal anti-inflammatory; antifungal; antibacterial; local anesthetic* [hydrocortisone; clioquinol; pramoxine] 1%•3%•1%

**1% HC** ointment ℞ *topical corticosteroidal anti-inflammatory* [hydrocortisone] 1%

**One Touch** reagent strips for home use *in vitro diagnostic aid for blood glucose*

**109.881** *investigational (Phase III) taxoid for breast cancer*

**166Ho-DOTMP** *investigational (orphan) for multiple myeloma*

**One-A-Day 55 Plus** tablets OTC *geriatric vitamin/mineral supplement* [multiple vitamins & minerals; folic acid; biotin] ±•400•30 μg

**One-A-Day Essential** tablets OTC *vitamin supplement* [multiple vitamins; folic acid] ±•400 μg

**One-A-Day Extras Antioxidant** softgel capsules OTC *vitamin/mineral supplement* [vitamins A, C, and E; multiple minerals] 5000 IU•250 mg•200 IU•±

**One-A-Day Kids** chewable tablets OTC *vitamin/mineral/iron supplement* [multiple vitamins & minerals; iron; folic acid; biotin] ±•18•0.4•0.03 mg

**One-A-Day Kids Scooby-Doo! Fizzy Vites** chewable tablets OTC *vitamin/ mineral/calcium/iron supplement* [multiple vitamins & minerals; calcium; iron (as ferrous fumarate); folic acid; biotin] •50•9•0.2•0.02 mg

**One-A-Day Maximum Formula** tablets OTC *vitamin/mineral/iron supplement* [multiple vitamins & minerals; iron; folic acid; biotin] ±•18• 0.4•0.03 mg

**One-A-Day Men's Vitamins** tablets OTC *vitamin supplement* [multiple vitamins; folic acid] ±•400 μg

**One-A-Day WeightSmart** tablets OTC *vitamin/mineral/calcium/iron supplement* [multiple vitamins & minerals; calcium; iron (as ferrous fumarate); folic acid] ±•300•18•0.4 mg

**One-A-Day Women's Formula** tablets OTC *vitamin/calcium/iron supplement* [multiple vitamins; calcium; iron; folic acid] ±•450•27•0.4 mg

**One-Alpha** ⒸⒶ⒩ capsules, oral solution, IV injection ℞ *vitamin D therapy; calcium regulator for hypocalcemia and osteodystrophy of chronic renal dialysis and hyperparathyroidism of chronic renal failure* [alfacalcidol] 0.25, 0.5, 1 μg; 0.2 μg/mL; 2 μg/mL

**1-alpha-D2** *investigational (Phase III) for secondary hyperparathyroidism in hemodialysis patients*

**1DMTX/6-MP (methotrexate [with leucovorin rescue], mercaptopurine)** *chemotherapy protocol for acute lymphocytic leukemia (ALL); the first-day initiation protocol* [also: MTX/6-MP (the ongoing continuation protocol)]

**One-Tablet-Daily** OTC *vitamin supplement* [multiple vitamins; folic acid] ±•400 μg

**One-Tablet-Daily with Iron** OTC *vitamin/iron supplement* [multiple vitamins; iron; folic acid] ±•18•0.4 mg

**One-Tablet-Daily with Minerals** OTC *vitamin/mineral/iron supplement* [multiple vitamins & minerals; iron; folic acid; biotin] ±•18•0.4•0.03 mg

**onion (***Allium cepa***)** bulb *medicinal herb used as an anthelmintic, antiseptic, antispasmodic, carminative, diuretic, expectorant, and stomachic*

**Onkolox** ℞ *investigational (orphan) agent for renal cell carcinoma* [coumarin]

**Ontak** frozen solution for IV injection ℞ *antineoplastic for recurrent or persistent cutaneous T-cell lymphoma (orphan)* [denileukin diftitox] 150 μg/mL

**ontazolast** USAN *antiasthmatic; leukotriene biosynthesis inhibitor*

**ontianil** INN

**Onxol** IV infusion ℞ *antineoplastic for ovarian and breast cancers, and non–small cell lung cancer (NSCLC), and AIDS-related Kaposi sarcoma (orphan)* [paclitaxel] 6 mg/mL

**Ony-Clear** topical solution OTC *antifungal* [benzalkonium chloride] 1%

**ONYX-015** *investigational (Phase III) adenovirus E1B, in combination with cisplatin and 5-FU, for recurrent head and neck cancer; investigational (Phase I) for Barrett esophageal metaplasia; investigational for primary liver tumors*

**OP-1 (osteogenic protein-1)** [q.v.]

**OPA (Oncovin, prednisone, Adriamycin)** *chemotherapy protocol for pediatric Hodgkin lymphoma*

**OPAL (Oncovin, prednisone, L-asparaginase)** *chemotherapy protocol*

**Opcon-A** eye drops OTC *topical ophthalmic decongestant, antihistamine, and lubricant* [naphazoline HCl; pheniramine maleate; hydroxypropyl methylcellulose] 0.027%•0.315%•0.5%

**OPEN (Oncovin, prednisone, etoposide, Novantrone)** *chemotherapy protocol*

**Operand** solution, prep pads, swab sticks, surgical scrub, perineal wash concentrate, aerosol, Iofoam skin cleanser, ointment OTC *broad-spectrum antimicrobial* [povidone-iodine] 1%; 1%; 1%; 7.5%; 1%; 0.5%; 1%; 1%

**Operand Douche** concentrate OTC *antiseptic/germicidal; vaginal cleanser and deodorizer* [povidone-iodine]

**Ophthalgan** eye drops (discontinued 2003) ℞ *corneal edema-reducing and clearing agent* [glycerin]

**Ophthetic** eye drops ℞ *topical ophthalmic anesthetic* [proparacaine HCl] 0.5%

**Ophthifluor** antecubital venous injection ℞ *ophthalmic diagnostic agent* [fluorescein sodium] 10%

**opiniazide** INN

**opipramol** INN *antidepressant; antipsychotic* [also: opipramol HCl]

**opipramol HCl** USAN *antidepressant; antipsychotic* [also: opipramol]

**opium** USP *narcotic analgesic; antiperistaltic; used in neonatal opioid withdrawal programs; widely abused as a street drug, which is highly addictive* 10% oral

**opium, powdered** USP *narcotic analgesic*

**Oplopanax horridus** *medicinal herb* [see: devil's club]

**OPP (Oncovin, procarbazine, prednisone)** *chemotherapy protocol*

**OPPA (Oncovin, prednisone, procarbazine, Adriamycin)** *chemotherapy protocol for pediatric Hodgkin lymphoma*

**oprelvekin** USAN *platelet growth factor for prevention of thrombocytopenia following chemotherapy or radiation*

*(orphan)* [also: interleukin 11, recombinant human]

**Opteform** moldable bone paste ℞ *human allograft material for orthopedic surgery* [demineralized bone powder; cortical bone chips]

**Opticare PMS** tablets OTC *vitamin/mineral supplement; digestive enzymes* [multiple vitamins & minerals; iron; folic acid; biotin; amylase; protease; lipase] ±•2.5 mg•0.033 mg•10.4 μg•2500 U•2500 U•200 U

**Opti-Clean** solution OTC *cleaning solution for hard, soft, or rigid gas permeable contact lenses*

**Opti-Clean II** solution OTC *cleaning solution for hard or soft contact lenses*

**Opti-Clean II Especially for Sensitive Eyes** solution OTC *cleaning solution for rigid gas permeable contact lenses*

**OptiClik** (trademarked insulin delivery device) *refillable subcu injector*

**Opticrom 4%** eye drops ℞ *ophthalmic mast cell stabilizer for vernal keratoconjunctivitis (orphan)* [cromolyn sodium]

**Opticyl** eye drops ℞ *cycloplegic; mydriatic* [tropicamide] 0.5%, 1%

**Opti-Free** solution OTC *chemical disinfecting solution for soft contact lenses* [note: one of four different products with the same name]

**Opti-Free** solution OTC *rewetting solution for soft contact lenses* [note: one of four different products with the same name]

**Opti-Free** solution OTC *surfactant cleaning solution for soft contact lenses* [note: one of four different products with the same name]

**Opti-Free** tablets OTC *enzymatic cleaner for soft contact lenses* [pork pancreatin] [note: one of four different products with the same name]

**Optigene** ophthalmic solution OTC *extraocular irrigating solution* [sterile isotonic solution]

**Optigene 3** eye drops OTC *topical ophthalmic decongestant and vasoconstrictor* [tetrahydrozoline HCl] 0.05%

**Optilets-500** Filmtabs (film-coated tablets) OTC *vitamin supplement* [multiple vitamins]

**Optilets-M-500** Filmtabs (film-coated tablets) OTC *vitamin/mineral/iron supplement* [multiple vitamins & minerals; iron] $\pm \bullet$ 20 mg

**OptiMARK** IV injection R *MRI contrast medium for imaging of the brain, head, and spine and liver structure and vascularity* [gadoversetamide] 330.9 mg

**Optimental** oral liquid OTC *enteral nutritional therapy* 237 mL

**Optimine** tablets (discontinued 2002) R *piperidine antihistamine for allergic rhinitis and chronic urticaria* [azatadine maleate] 1 mg

**Optimmune** R *investigational (orphan) tear stimulant for severe keratoconjunctivitis sicca in Sjögren syndrome* [cyclosporine]

**Optimoist** oral spray (discontinued 2003) OTC *saliva substitute*

**Optimox Prenatal** tablets OTC *vitamin/mineral/calcium/iron supplement* [multiple vitamins & minerals; calcium; iron; folic acid] $\pm \bullet$ 100 $\bullet$ 5 $\bullet$ 0.133 mg

**Opti-One** solution OTC *rewetting solution for soft contact lenses*

**Opti-One Multi-Purpose** solution OTC *chemical disinfecting solution for soft contact lenses*

**OptiPen One** (trademarked insulin delivery device) *cartridge-type subcu injector*

**OptiPranolol** eye drops R *topical antiglaucoma agent (β-blocker)* [metipranolol HCl] 0.3%

**Optiray 160; Optiray 240; Optiray 300; Optiray 320; Optiray 350** injection R *radiopaque contrast medium* [ioversol (47.3% iodine)] 339 mg/mL (160 mg/mL); 509 mg/mL (240 mg/mL); 636 mg/mL (300 mg/mL); 678 mg/mL (320 mg/mL); 741 mg/mL (350 mg/mL)

**Opti-Soft Especially for Sensitive Eyes** solution OTC *rinsing/storage solution for soft contact lenses* [sodium chloride (preserved saline solution)]

**Optison** injectable suspension *ultrasound contrast medium for cardiac imaging; investigational (Phase III) diagnostic aid for infertility due to obstructed fallopian tubes* [perflutren] 3 mL

**Opti-Tears** solution OTC *rewetting solution for hard or soft contact lenses*

**Optivar** eye drops R *selective $H_1$ antagonist; antihistamine; mast cell stabilizer* [azelastine HCl] 0.05%

**Optivite P.M.T.** tablets OTC *geriatric vitamin/mineral supplement* [multiple vitamins & minerals; folic acid; biotin] $\pm \bullet$ 30 $\bullet$ $\frac{?}{=}$ μg

**OptiZen** eye drops OTC *ophthalmic moisturizer/lubricant* [polysorbate 80] 0.5%

**Opti-Zyme Enzymatic Cleaner Especially for Sensitive Eyes** tablets OTC *enzymatic cleaner for soft or rigid gas permeable contact lenses* [pork pancreatin]

**Optrin** R *investigational (Phase I/II) photodynamic therapy for age-related macular degeneration* [motexafin lutetium]

**Optro** R *investigational agent for chronic anemia* [human hemoglobin, recombinant]

**OPV (oral poliovirus vaccine)** [see: poliovirus vaccine, live oral]

**ORA5** topical liquid OTC *oral anti-infective* [copper sulfate; iodine; potassium iodide]

**Orabase** gel OTC *mucous membrane anesthetic* [benzocaine] 15%

**Orabase Baby** gel OTC *topical oral anesthetic* [benzocaine] 7.5%

**Orabase HCA** oral paste R *topical corticosteroidal anti-inflammatory* [hydrocortisone acetate] 0.5%

**Orabase Lip Healer** cream OTC *topical oral anesthetic; antipruritic/counterirritant; vulnerary* [benzocaine; menthol; allantoin] 5% $\bullet$ 0.5% $\bullet$ 1.5%

**Orabase Soothe-N-Seal** topical liquid OTC *mucous membrane sealant and protectant for canker and mouth sores* [cyanoacrylate]

**Orabase-B** oral paste OTC *topical oral anesthetic* [benzocaine] 20% ⍰ Orinase

**Orabase-Plain** oral paste OTC *relief from minor oral irritations* [plasticized hydrocarbon gel]

**Oracit** solution ℞ *urinary alkalinizing agent* [sodium citrate; citric acid] 490•640 mg/5 mL

**OraDisc** ℞ *investigational (Phase III) agent for canker sores* [amlexanox]

**Oragrafin Sodium** capsules (discontinued 2001) ℞ *radiopaque contrast medium for cholecystography* [ipodate sodium (61.4% iodine)] 500 mg (307 mg)

**Orajel** topical liquid OTC *mucous membrane anesthetic* [benzocaine; alcohol 44.2%] 20%

**Orajel; Orajel Brace-aid; Orajel/d; Denture Orajel; Baby Orajel; Baby Orajel Nighttime Formula** gel OTC *mucous membrane anesthetic* [benzocaine] 20%; 20%; 10%; 10%; 7.5%; 10%

**Orajel Mouth-Aid** topical liquid, gel OTC *mucous membrane anesthetic* [benzocaine] 20%

**Orajel Perioseptic** oral liquid OTC *topical anti-inflammatory and anti-infective for braces* [carbamide peroxide] 15%

**Orajel P.M. Nighttime Formula Toothache Pain Relief** cream OTC *mucous membrane anesthetic* [benzocaine] 20%

**Orajel Tooth & Gum Cleanser, Baby** gel OTC *removes plaque-like film* [poloxamer 407; simethicone] 2%•0.12%

**Oralease** ℞ *investigational (Phase III) analgesic for pain due to oral ulcers*

**Oralet** (trademarked dosage form) *oral lozenge/lollipop*

**Oralgen; Oralin** Ⓒᴬᴺ ℞ *investigational (Phase II/III) oral insulin formulation*

**Oralone Dental** paste ℞ *topical corticosteroidal anti-inflammatory* [triamcinolone acetonide] 0.1%

**Oramorph SR** sustained-release tablets ℞ *narcotic analgesic* [morphine sulfate] 15, 30, 60, 100 mg

**orange flower oil** NF *flavoring agent; perfume*

**orange flower water** NF

**orange oil** NF

**orange peel tincture, sweet** NF

**orange root** *medicinal herb* [see: goldenseal]

**orange spirit, compound** NF

**orange swallow wort** *medicinal herb* [see: pleurisy root]

**orange syrup** NF

**Orap** tablets ℞ *antidyskinetic for Tourette syndrome* [pimozide] 1, 2 mg (4 mg available in Canada)

**Oraphen-PD** elixir OTC *analgesic; antipyretic* [acetaminophen] 120 mg/5 mL

**Orapred** oral solution ℞ *corticosteroid; anti-inflammatory* [prednisolone sodium phosphate; alcohol 2%] 15 mg/5 mL

**OraQuick Rapid HIV-1 Antibody Test** reagent kit for home use *in vitro diagnostic aid for HIV-1 and HIV-2 antibodies in a fingerstick blood sample and HIV-1 antibodies in oral fluid*

**Orarinse** ℞ *investigational (Phase II) mucositis treatment*

**orarsan** [see: acetarsone] ⍰ Oracin; Orasone

**Orasept** throat spray OTC *topical oral anesthetic; antiseptic* [benzocaine; methylbenzethonium chloride] 0.996%•1.037%

**Orasept** topical liquid OTC *oral astringent; antiseptic* [tannic acid; methylbenzethonium chloride; alcohol 53.31%] 12.16%•1.53%

**Orasol** topical liquid OTC *oral anesthetic; antipruritic/counterirritant; antiseptic* [benzocaine; phenol; alcohol 70%] 6.3%•0.5%

**OraSolv** (trademarked delivery system) *investigational (NDA filed)*

**Orasone** tablets ℞ *corticosteroid; anti-inflammatory; immunosuppressant* [prednisone] 1, 5, 10, 20, 50 mg ⍰ Oracin; orarsan

**OraSure** reagent kit for home use *in vitro diagnostic aid for HIV antibodies*

**OraSure HIV-1** reagent kit for professional use *in vitro diagnostic aid for HIV antibodies using oral mucosal transudate* [single-sample, three-test kit: two ELISA assays + Western Blot assay]

**Orathecin** capsules R *investigational (Phase III) antineoplastic for pancreatic cancer* [rubitecan]

**orazamide** INN

**Orazinc** capsules, tablets OTC *zinc supplement* [zinc sulfate] 220 mg; 110 mg

**orbofiban acetate** USAN *platelet aggregation inhibitor; fibrinogen receptor antagonist*

**orbutopril** INN

**OrCel** R *investigational bilayered cellular matrix for acute and chronic diabetic foot ulcers* [collagen sponge seeded with allogenic dermal and epidermal cells]

**orchanet** *medicinal herb* [see: henna (Alkanna)]

**orciprenaline** INN, BAN *bronchodilator* [also: metaproterenol polistirex]

**orciprenaline polistirex** [see: metaproterenol polistirex]

**orciprenaline sulfate** [see: metaproterenol sulfate]

**orconazole** INN *antifungal* [also: orconazole nitrate]

**orconazole nitrate** USAN *antifungal* [also: orconazole]

**Ordrine AT** extended-release capsules (discontinued 2002) R *antitussive; decongestant* [caramiphen edisylate; phenylpropanolamine HCl] 40•75 mg

**oregano** *medicinal herb* [see: marjoram]

**Oregon grape** *(Mahonia aquifolium)* rhizome and root *medicinal herb for acne, blood disorders, eczema, jaundice, liver disorders, promoting digestion, psoriasis, and staphylococcal infections*

**orestrate** INN

**orestrol** [see: diethylstilbestrol dipropionate]

**Oretic** tablets R *antihypertensive; diuretic* [hydrochlorothiazide] 25, 50 mg ⍰ Oreton

**Oreton Methyl** tablets, buccal tablets (discontinued 2001) R *androgen for hypogonadism or testosterone deficiency in men, delayed puberty in boys, and metastatic breast cancer in women; also abused as a street drug* [methyltestosterone] 10 mg ⍰ Oretic

**Orexin** chewable tablets OTC *vitamin supplement* [vitamins $B_1$, $B_6$, and $B_{12}$] 8.1 mg•4.1 mg•25 µg

**Orfadin** capsules R *adjunctive treatment for hereditary tyrosinemia type 1 (HT-1), a pediatric liver disease (orphan)* [nitisinone] 2, 5, 10 mg

**ORG 33062** *investigational (Phase III) antidepressant*

**Organidin NR** tablets, oral liquid R *expectorant* [guaifenesin] 200 mg; 100 mg/5 mL

**organoclay** [see: bentoquatam]

**Organan** deep subcu injection R *anticoagulant/antithrombotic for prevention of deep vein thrombosis (DVT) following hip replacement surgery* [danaparoid sodium] 750 anti-Xa U/0.6 mL

**orgotein** USAN, INN, BAN *anti-inflammatory; antirheumatic; investigational (orphan) for amyotrophic lateral sclerosis and to prevent donor organ reperfusion injury* [previously known as superoxide dismutase (SOD)]

**orgotein, recombinant human** *investigational (orphan) for bronchopulmonary dysplasia of premature neonates*

**orienticine A; orienticine D** [see: orientiparcin]

**orientiparcin** INN [a mixture of orienticine A and orienticine D]

**Origanum vulgare** *medicinal herb* [see: marjoram]

**Orimune** oral suspension (discontinued 2004) R *poliomyelitis vaccine* [poliovirus vaccine, live oral trivalent] 0.5 mL

**Orinase** tablets R *sulfonylurea antidiabetic* [tolbutamide] 500 mg ⍰ Orabase; Ornade; Ornex; Tolinase

**Orinase Diagnostic** powder for IV injection R *in vivo diagnostic aid for*

*pancreas function and diabetes* [tolbutamide sodium] 1 g

**Orlaam** IV injection (discontinued 2004) ℞ *narcotic analgesic for management of opiate addiction (orphan)* [levomethadyl acetate HCl] 10 mg/mL

**orlipastat** [see: orlistat]

**orlistat** USAN, INN *lipase inhibitor to suppress the absorption of dietary fats, leading to weight loss; investigational (Phase III) preventative for type 2 diabetes*

**ormaplatin** USAN *antineoplastic*

**ormetoprim** USAN, INN *antibacterial*

**Ornade** Spansules (sustained-release capsules) (discontinued 2001) ℞ *decongestant; antihistamine* [phenylpropanolamine HCl; chlorpheniramine maleate] 75•12 mg ② Orinase; Ornex

**Ornex No Drowsiness** caplets OTC *decongestant; analgesic; antipyretic* [pseudoephedrine HCl; acetaminophen] 30•325, 30•500 mg ② Orex; Orinase; Ornade

**ornidazole** USAN, INN *anti-infective*

**Ornidyl** IV injection concentrate ℞ *antiprotozoal for* Trypanosoma brucei gambiense *(sleeping sickness) infection (orphan); investigational (orphan) for* AIDS-related Pneumocystis carinii *pneumonia* [eflornithine HCl] 200 mg/mL

**ornipressin** INN

**ornithine (L-ornithine)** INN

**ornithine vasopressin** [see: ornipressin]

**ornoprostil** INN

**Oros** (trademarked delivery system) *patterned-release tablets*

**orotic acid** INN

**orotirelin** INN

**orpanoxin** USAN, INN *anti-inflammatory*

**orphenadine citrate** [see: orphenadrine citrate]

**orphenadrine** INN, BAN *skeletal muscle relaxant; antihistamine* [also: orphenadrine citrate]

**orphenadrine citrate** USP *skeletal muscle relaxant; antihistamine* [also: orphenadrine] 100 mg oral; 30 mg/mL injection

**orphenadrine HCl** *anticholinergic; antiparkinsonian*

**Orphengesic; Orphengesic Forte** tablets ℞ *skeletal muscle relaxant; analgesic* [orphenadrine citrate; aspirin; caffeine] 25•385•30 mg; 50•770•60 mg

**orpressin** [see: ornipressin]

**orris root (Iris florentina)** *medicinal herb used as a diuretic and stomachic*

**ortetamine** INN

**orthesin** [see: benzocaine]

**Ortho 0.5/35; Ortho 1/35** ⑭ tablets (in 21 or 28 packs) ℞ *monophasic oral contraceptive* [norethindrone; ethinyl estradiol] 0.5 mg•35 µg; 1 mg•35 µg

**Ortho 7/7/7** ⑭ tablets (in 21 or 28 packs) ℞ *triphasic oral contraceptive* [norethindrone; ethinyl estradiol] Phase 1 (7 days): 0.5 mg•35 µg; Phase 2 (7 days): 0.75 mg•35 µg; Phase 3 (7 days): 1 mg•35 µg

**Ortho Dienestrol** vaginal cream (discontinued 2003) ℞ *estrogen replacement for postmenopausal atrophic vaginitis* [dienestrol] 0.01%

**Ortho Evra** transdermal patch ℞ *once-weekly contraceptive* [norelgestromin; ethinyl estradiol] 150•20 µg/day

**Ortho Micronor** tablets (in Dialpaks of 28) ℞ *oral contraceptive (progestin only)* [norethindrone] 0.35 mg

**Ortho Tri-Cyclen** tablets (in Dialpaks and Veridates of 28) ℞ *triphasic oral contraceptive; treatment for acne vulgaris in females* [norgestimate; ethinyl estradiol] Phase 1 (7 days): 180•35 µg; Phase 2 (7 days): 215•35 µg; Phase 3 (7 days): 250•35 µg

**Ortho Tri-Cyclen Lo** tablets (in Dialpaks and Veridates of 28) ℞ *triphasic oral contraceptive* [norgestimate; ethinyl estradiol] Phase 1 (7 days): 180•25 µg; Phase 2 (7 days): 215•25 µg; Phase 3 (7 days): 250•25 µg

**Ortho-Cept** tablets (in Dialpaks and Veridates of 28) ℞ *monophasic oral*

*contraceptive* [desogestrel; ethinyl estradiol] 0.15 mg•30 μg

**Orthoclone OKT3** IV injection ℞ *immunosuppressant for renal, cardiac, and hepatic transplants* [muromonab-CD3] 5 mg/5 mL ⑨ Ortho-Creme

**orthocresol** NF

**Ortho-Cyclen** tablets (in Dialpaks and Veridates of 28) ℞ *monophasic oral contraceptive* [norgestimate; ethinyl estradiol] 0.25 mg•35 μg

**Ortho-Est** tablets ℞ *natural estrogen replacement therapy for the treatment of postmenopausal symptoms and prevention of postmenopausal osteoporosis* [estrone (from estropipate)] 0.625 (0.75), 1.25 (1.5) mg

**Ortho-Gynol** vaginal gel OTC *spermicidal contraceptive (for use with a diaphragm)* [octoxynol 9] 1%

**Ortho-Novum 1/35** tablets (in Dialpaks and Veridates of 28) ℞ *monophasic oral contraceptive* [norethindrone; ethinyl estradiol] 1 mg•35 μg

**Ortho-Novum 1/50** tablets (in Dialpaks of 28) ℞ *monophasic oral contraceptive* [norethindrone; mestranol] 1 mg•50 μg

**Ortho-Novum 7/7/7** tablets (in Dialpaks and Veridates of 28) ℞ *triphasic oral contraceptive* [norethindrone; ethinyl estradiol]
Phase 1 (7 days): 500•35 μg;
Phase 2 (7 days): 750•35 μg;
Phase 3 (7 days): 1000•35 μg

**Ortho-Novum 10/11** tablets (in Dialpaks of 28) ℞ *biphasic oral contraceptive* [norethindrone; ethinyl estradiol]
Phase 1 (10 days): 500•35 μg;
Phase 2 (11 days): 1000•35 μg

**Ortho-Prefest** tablets (in packs of 30) ℞ *hormone replacement therapy for postmenopausal symptoms* [estradiol-17β; norgestimate] 1•0 mg × 3 days; 1•0.09 mg × 3 days; repeat without interruption

**orthotolidine**

**Orthovisc** intra-articular injection in single-use vials ℞ *viscoelastic lubri-*

*cant and "shock absorber" for osteoarthritis of the knee* [hyaluronan] 30 mg

**OrthoWash** oral rinse ℞ *dental caries preventative* [sodium fluoride (as acidulated phosphate solution)] 0.044%

**Orthoxicol Cough** syrup (discontinued 2002) OTC *antitussive; decongestant; antihistamine* [dextromethorphan hydrobromide; phenylpropanolamine HCl; chlorpheniramine maleate; alcohol 8%] 6.7•8.3•1.3 mg/5 mL

**Orudis** capsules (discontinued 2004) ℞ *analgesic; antiarthritic; nonsteroidal anti-inflammatory drug (NSAID)* [ketoprofen] 25, 50, 75 mg

**Orudis KT** tablets OTC *analgesic; antiarthritic; antipyretic; nonsteroidal anti-inflammatory drug (NSAID)* [ketoprofen] 12.5 mg

**Oruvail** sustained-release pellets in capsules ℞ *once-daily antiarthritic; nonsteroidal anti-inflammatory drug (NSAID)* [ketoprofen] 100, 150, 200 mg

**oryzanol A, B, and C** *medicinal herb* [see: rice bran oil]

**Orzel** tablets ℞ *investigational (NDA filed) oral agent for colorectal cancer* [uracil; tegafur; leucovorin calcium]

**osalmid** INN

**osarsal** [see: acetarsone]

**Os-Cal 250+D; Os-Cal 500+D** film-coated tablets OTC *dietary supplement* [calcium carbonate; vitamin D] 250 mg Ca•125 IU; 500 mg Ca•200 IU

**Os-Cal 500** tablets, chewable tablets OTC *calcium supplement* [calcium carbonate] 1250 mg (500 mg Ca)

**Os-Cal Fortified** tablets OTC *vitamin/calcium/iron supplement* [multiple vitamins; calcium carbonate; iron] ±•250•5 mg

**Os-Cal Fortified Multivitamin & Minerals** tablets OTC *vitamin/mineral/calcium/iron supplement* [multiple vitamins & minerals; calcium carbonate; iron] ±•250•5 mg

**oseltamivir phosphate** USAN *antiviral neuraminidase inhibitor for influenza A and B*

**osmadizone** INN

**Osmitrol** IV infusion ℞ *antihypertensive; osmotic diuretic* [mannitol] 5%, 10%, 15%, 20%

**osmium** *element (Os)*

**Osmoglyn** solution ℞ *osmotic diuretic* [glycerin] 50%

**Osmolite; Osmolite HN** oral liquid OTC *enteral nutritional therapy* [lactose-free formula]

*Osmorhiza longistylis medicinal herb* [see: sweet cicely]

**osmotic diuretics** *a class of diuretics that increase excretion of sodium and chloride and decrease tubular absorption of water*

*Osmunda cinnamomea; O. regalis medicinal herb* [see: buckhorn brake]

**OspA** [see: lipoprotein OspA, recombinant]

**Ostac** ⒸⒶ⒩ capsules, IV infusion ℞ *bisphosphonate bone resorption inhibitor for hypercalcemia of malignancy and osteolysis due to bone metastasis of malignant tumors* [clodronate disodium] 400 mg; 30 mg/mL

**Osteocalcin** subcu or IM injection ℞ *calcium regulator for hypercalcemia, Paget disease, and postmenopausal osteoporosis* [calcitonin (salmon)] 200 IU/mL

**Osteo-D** ℞ *calcium regulator; investigational (orphan) for familial hypophosphatemic rickets* [secalciferol]

**Osteofil** injectable bone paste ℞ *human allograft material for orthopedic surgery* [demineralized bone powder]

**osteogenic protein-1 (OP-1)** *investigational (NDA filed) morphogenic protein that enhances motor function following stroke*

**OsteoMax** effervescent powder for oral solution OTC *dietary supplement* [calcium citrate; vitamin D; magnesium] 500 mg•200 IU•200 mg

**Osteo-Mins** powder OTC *dietary supplement* [multiple minerals; vitamins C and D] ≟•500 mg•100 IU

**Ostiderm** lotion OTC *for hyperhidrosis and bromhidrosis* [aluminum sulfate; zinc oxide] 14.5•≟ mg/g

**Ostiderm** roll-on OTC *for hyperhidrosis and bromhidrosis* [aluminum chlorohydrate; camphor; alcohol] ≟•≟•≟

**ostreogrycin** INN, BAN

**osvarsan** [see: acetarsone]

**Oswego tea** *(Monarda didyma)* leaves and flowers *medicinal herb used as a calmative, rubefacient, and stimulant*

**OT (old tuberculin)** [see: tuberculin]

**Otic Domeboro** ear drops ℞ *antibacterial; antifungal* [acetic acid; aluminum acetate] 2%•≟

**Otic-Care** ear drops, otic suspension ℞ *topical corticosteroidal anti-inflammatory; antibiotic* [hydrocortisone; neomycin sulfate; polymyxin B sulfate] 1%•5 mg•10 000 U per mL

**otilonium bromide** INN, BAN

**Oti-Med** ear drops ℞ *topical corticosteroidal anti-inflammatory; antibacterial; topical local anesthetic* [hydrocortisone; chloroxylenol; pramoxine HCl] 10•1•10 mg/mL

**otimerate sodium** INN

**OtiTricin** otic suspension ℞ *topical corticosteroidal anti-inflammatory; antibiotic* [hydrocortisone; neomycin sulfate; polymyxin B sulfate] 1%•5 mg•10 000 U per mL

**Otobiotic Otic** ear drops ℞ *topical corticosteroidal anti-inflammatory; antibiotic* [hydrocortisone; polymyxin B sulfate] 0.5%•10 000 U per mL ⊡ Urobiotic

**Otocain** ear drops ℞ *topical local anesthetic* [benzocaine] 20%

**Otocalm** ear drops ℞ *topical local anesthetic; analgesic* [benzocaine; antipyrine] 1.4%•5.4%

**Otocort** ear drops, otic suspension ℞ *topical corticosteroidal anti-inflammatory; antibiotic* [hydrocortisone; neomycin sulfate; polymyxin B sulfate] 1%•5 mg•10 000 U per mL

**Otomar-HC** ear drops ℞ *topical corticosteroidal anti-inflammatory; local anesthetic; antibacterial* [hydrocortisone; pramoxine HCl; chloroxylenol] 10•10•1 mg/mL

**Otomycet-HC** ear drops ℞ *topical corticosteroidal anti-inflammatory; antibacterial; antifungal* [hydrocortisone; acetic acid] 1%•2%

**Otomycin-HPN Otic** ear drops ℞ *topical corticosteroidal anti-inflammatory; antibiotic* [hydrocortisone; neomycin sulfate; polymyxin B sulfate] 1%•5 mg•10 000 U per mL

**Otosporin** ear drops ℞ *topical corticosteroidal anti-inflammatory; antibiotic* [hydrocortisone; neomycin sulfate; polymyxin B sulfate] 1%•5 mg• 10 000 U per mL

**Otrivin** nasal spray, nose drops, pediatric nose drops OTC *nasal decongestant* [xylometazoline HCl] 0.1%; 0.1%; 0.05% ℞ Lotrimin

**ouabain** USP

**Our Lady's mint** *medicinal herb* [see: spearmint]

**Outgro** solution OTC *pain relief for ingrown toenails* [tannic acid; chlorobutanol; isopropyl alcohol 83%] 25%•5%

**Ovace** foam ℞ *antibiotic for acute and chronic seborrheic dermatitis and secondary bacterial infections of the scalp and skin* [sulfacetamide sodium] 10%

**ovandrotone albumin** INN, BAN

**OvaRex** ℞ *investigational (Phase II, orphan) therapeutic vaccine for epithelial ovarian cancer* [monoclonal antibody B43.13] ℞ O-Vax

**Ovastat** ℞ *investigational (orphan) for ovarian cancer* [treosulfan] ℞ Novastan

**O-Vax** ℞ *investigational (Phase III, orphan) therapeutic vaccine for adjuvant treatment of ovarian cancer* [autologous cell (AC) vaccine] ℞ Ovarex

**Ovcon-35** caplets, chewable tablets (in packs of 21 or 28) ℞ *monophasic oral contraceptive* [norethindrone; ethinyl estradiol] 0.4 mg•35 μg

**Ovcon-50** caplets (in packs of 28) ℞ *monophasic oral contraceptive* [norethindrone; ethinyl estradiol] 1 mg•50 μg

**Ovide** lotion ℞ *pediculicide for lice* [malathion; isopropyl alcohol 78%] 0.5%

**Ovidrel** prefilled syringes for subcu injection ℞ *fertility stimulant for anovulatory women; adjuvant therapy for cryptorchidism* [choriogonadotropin alfa] 250 μg/0.5 mL

**ovine corticotropin-releasing hormone** [see: corticorelin ovine triflutate]

**Ovoid** (trademarked dosage form) *sugar-coated tablet*

**Ovral** tablets (in Pilpaks of 21 and 28) ℞ *monophasic oral contraceptive; emergency postcoital contraceptive* [norgestrel; ethinyl estradiol] 0.5 mg•50 μg

**Ovrette** tablets (in Pilpaks of 28) ℞ *oral contraceptive (progestin only)* [norgestrel] 0.075 mg

**OvuGen** test kit *in vitro diagnostic aid to predict ovulation time*

**OvuKIT Self-Test** kit for home use *in vitro diagnostic aid to predict ovulation time*

**Ovulation Scope** kit for home use *in vitro diagnostic aid to predict ovulation time from a saliva sample*

**OvuLite** kit for home use *in vitro diagnostic aid to predict ovulation time from a saliva sample*

**OvuQuick Self-Test** kit for home use *in vitro diagnostic aid to predict ovulation time*

**[$^{15}$O]water** [see: water O 15]

**ox bile extract** [see: bile salts]

**oxabolone cipionate** INN

**oxabrexine** INN

**22-oxacalcitriol (OCT)** [see: maxacalcitol]

**oxaceprol** INN

**oxacillin** INN *penicillinase-resistant penicillin antibiotic* [also: oxacillin sodium]

**oxacillin sodium** USAN, USP *penicillinase-resistant penicillin antibiotic* [also: oxacillin] 250 mg/5 mL oral; 0.5, 1, 2, 10 g IV injection

**oxadimedine** INN

**oxadimedine HCl** [see: oxadimedine]

**oxadoddy** *medicinal herb* [see: Culver root]

**oxaflozane** INN

**oxaflumazine** INN

**oxafuradene** [see: nifuradene]

**oxagrelate** USAN, INN *platelet antiaggregatory agent*

**oxalinast** INN

**oxaliplatin** USAN, INN *alkylating antineoplastic for metastatic ovarian and colorectal cancers (orphan); investigational (Phase III) for pancreatic cancer*

**Oxalis acetosella** *medicinal herb* [see: wood sorrel]

**oxamarin** INN *hemostatic* [also: oxamarin HCl]

**oxamarin HCl** USAN *hemostatic* [also: oxamarin]

**oxametacin** INN

**oxamisole** INN *immunoregulator* [also: oxamisole HCl]

**oxamisole HCl** USAN *immunoregulator* [also: oxamisole]

**oxamniquine** USAN, USP, INN *antischistosomal; anthelmintic for schistosomiasis (flukes)*

**oxamphetamine hydrobromide** [see: hydroxyamphetamine hydrobromide]

**oxamycin** [see: cycloserine]

**oxanamide** INN

**Oxandrin** gel ℞ *investigational (Phase II) steroid for AIDS-wasting syndrome* [oxandrolone]

**Oxandrin** tablets ℞ *anabolic steroid; investigational (orphan) for muscular dystrophy, AIDS-wasting syndrome, and alcoholic hepatitis; also abused as a street drug to increase muscle mass* [oxandrolone] 2.5, 10 mg

**oxandrolone** USAN, USP, INN, BAN, JAN *anabolic steroid; investigational (Phase III, orphan) for AIDS-wasting syndrome; investigational (orphan) for muscular dystrophy and alcoholic hepatitis; also abused as a street drug to increase muscle mass*

**oxantel** INN *anthelmintic* [also: oxantel pamoate]

**oxantel pamoate** USAN *anthelmintic* [also: oxantel]

**oxantrazole HCl** [see: piroxantrone HCl]

**oxapadol** INN

**oxapium iodide** INN

**oxaprazine**

**oxapropanium iodide** INN

**oxaprotiline** INN *antidepressant* [also: oxaprotiline HCl]

**oxaprotiline HCl** USAN *antidepressant* [also: oxaprotiline]

**oxaprozin** USAN, INN, BAN *antiarthritic; nonsteroidal anti-inflammatory drug (NSAID)* 600 mg oral

**oxaprozin potassium** *antiarthritic; nonsteroidal anti-inflammatory drug (NSAID)* (base=88.5%)

**oxarbazole** USAN, INN *antiasthmatic*

**oxarutine** [see: ethoxazorutoside]

**oxatomide** USAN, INN *antiallergic; antiasthmatic*

**oxazafone** INN

**oxazepam** USAN, USP, INN *benzodiazepine anxiolytic; sedative; alcohol withdrawal aid* 10, 15, 30 mg oral

**oxazidione** INN

**oxazolam** INN

**oxazolidin** [see: oxyphenbutazone]

**oxazolidinediones** *a class of anticonvulsants (no longer used)*

**oxazorone** INN

**oxcarbazepine** INN *anticonvulsant for partial seizures in adults or children*

**oxdralazine** INN

**oxeladin** INN, BAN

**oxendolone** USAN, INN *antiandrogen for benign prostatic hypertrophy*

**oxepinac** INN

**oxerutins** BAN

**oxetacaine** INN *topical anesthetic* [also: oxethazaine]

**oxetacillin** INN

**2-oxetanone** [see: propiolactone]

**oxethazaine** USAN, BAN *topical anesthetic* [also: oxetacaine]

**oxetorone** INN *migraine-specific analgesic* [also: oxetorone fumarate]

**oxetorone fumarate** USAN *migraine-specific analgesic* [also: oxetorone]

**Oxeze** ㊀ Turbuhaler (dry powder in a metered-dose inhaler) ℞ *twice-daily bronchodilator for asthma* [formoterol fumarate] 6, 12 μg/dose

**oxfenamide** [see: oxiramide]

**oxfendazole** USAN, INN *anthelmintic*

**oxfenicine** USAN, INN, BAN *vasodilator*

**oxibendazole** USAN, INN *anthelmintic*

**oxibetaine** INN

**oxibuprocaine chloride** [see: benoxinate HCl]

**oxichlorochine sulfate** [see: hydroxychloroquine sulfate]

**oxicinchophen** [see: oxycinchophen]

**oxiconazole** INN, BAN *broad-spectrum topical antifungal* [also: oxiconazole nitrate]

**oxiconazole nitrate** USAN *broad-spectrum topical antifungal* [also: oxiconazole]

**oxicone** [see: oxycodone]

**oxidized cellulose** [see: cellulose, oxidized]

**oxidized cholic acid** [see: dehydrocholic acid]

**oxidized regenerated cellulose** [see: cellulose, oxidized regenerated]

**oxidopamine** USAN, INN *ophthalmic adrenergic*

**oxidronate sodium** *parenteral radiopaque contrast medium*

**oxidronic acid** USAN, INN, BAN *calcium regulator*

**oxifenamate** [see: hydroxyphenamate]

**oxifentorex** INN

**Oxi-Freeda** tablets OTC *dietary supplement* [multiple vitamins & minerals; multiple amino acids]

**oxifungin** INN *antifungal* [also: oxifungin HCl]

**oxifungin HCl** USAN *antifungal* [also: oxifungin]

**oxilorphan** USAN, INN *narcotic antagonist*

**oximetazoline HCl** [see: oxymetazoline HCl]

**oximetholone** [see: oxymetholone]

**oximonam** USAN, INN *antibacterial*

**oximonam sodium** USAN *antibacterial*

**oxindanac** INN

**oxiniacic acid** INN

**oxiperomide** USAN, INN *antipsychotic*

**oxipertine** [see: oxypertine]

**oxipethidine** [see: hydroxypethidine]

**oxiphenbutazone** [see: oxyphenbutazone]

**oxiphencyclimine chloride** [see: oxyphencyclimine HCl]

**Oxipor VHC** lotion OTC *antipsoriatic; antiseborrheic; keratolytic* [coal tar; alcohol 79%] 5%

**oxiprocaine** [see: hydroxyprocaine]

**oxiprogesterone caproate** [see: hydroxyprogesterone caproate]

**oxipurinol** INN *xanthine oxidase inhibitor* [also: oxypurinol]

**oxiracetam** INN, BAN *investigational treatment for Alzheimer disease*

**oxiramide** USAN, INN *antiarrhythmic*

**Oxistat** cream, lotion ℞ *broad-spectrum topical antifungal* [oxiconazole nitrate] 1%

**oxistilbamidine isethionate** [see: hydroxystilbamidine isethionate]

**oxisuran** USAN, INN *antineoplastic*

**oxitefonium bromide** INN

**oxitetracaine** [see: hydroxytetracaine]

**oxitetracycline** [see: oxytetracycline]

**oxitriptan** INN

**oxitriptyline** INN

**oxitropium bromide** INN, BAN

**Oxizole** ⓒ cream, lotion ℞ *broad-spectrum topical antifungal* [oxiconazole nitrate] 1%

**oxmetidine** INN, BAN *antagonist to histamine $H_2$ receptors* [also: oxmetidine HCl]

**oxmetidine HCl** USAN *antagonist to histamine $H_2$ receptors* [also: oxmetidine]

**oxmetidine mesylate** USAN *antagonist to histamine $H_2$ receptors*

**oxodipine** INN

**oxogestone** INN *progestin* [also: oxogestone phenpropionate]

**oxogestone phenpropionate** USAN *progestin* [also: oxogestone]

**oxoglurate** INN *combining name for radicals or groups*

**oxolamine** INN

**oxolinic acid** USAN, INN *antibacterial*

**oxomemazine** INN

**oxonazine** INN

**4-oxopentanoic acid, calcium salt** [see: calcium levulinate]

**oxophenarsine** INN [also: oxophenarsine HCl]

**oxophenarsine HCl** USP [also: oxophenarsine]

**5-oxoproline** [see: pidolic acid]

**oxoprostol** INN, BAN

**oxozepam** [see: oxazepam]

**oxpentifylline** BAN *peripheral vasodilator; hemorheologic agent* [also: pentoxifylline]

**oxpheneridine** INN

**oxprenoate potassium** INN

**oxprenolol** INN *coronary vasodilator* [also: oxprenolol HCl]

**oxprenolol HCl** USAN, USP *coronary vasodilator* [also: oxprenolol]

**OxSODrol** ℞ *investigational (Phase III) anti-inflammatory and antirheumatic; investigational (Phase III) for the prevention of bronchopulmonary dysplasia* [orgotein (previously known as superoxide dismutase, or SOD)]

**Oxsoralen** lotion ℞ *psoralens for repigmentation of idiopathic vitiligo* [methoxsalen] 1%

**Oxsoralen-Ultra** gelcaps ℞ *systemic psoralens for the treatment of severe recalcitrant psoriasis* [methoxsalen] 10 mg

**oxtriphylline** USP *bronchodilator* [also: choline theophyllinate] 100, 200 mg oral; 50, 100 mg/5 mL oral

**Oxy 5 for Sensitive Skin, Advanced Formula; Advanced Formula Oxy for Sensitive Skin** gel (discontinued 2003) OTC *keratolytic for acne* [benzoyl peroxide] 5%; 2.5%

**Oxy 5 Tinted** lotion (discontinued 2003) OTC *keratolytic for acne* [benzoyl peroxide] 5%

**Oxy 10 Advanced Formula** gel (discontinued 2003) OTC *keratolytic for acne* [benzoyl peroxide] 10%

**Oxy Medicated Cleanser & Pads** OTC *keratolytic cleanser for acne* [salicylic acid; alcohol] 0.5%•22%, 0.5%•40%, 2%•50%

**Oxy Medicated Soap** bar OTC *medicated cleanser for acne* [triclosan] 1%

**Oxy Night Watch; Oxy Night Watch for Sensitive Skin** lotion OTC *keratolytic for acne* [salicylic acid] 2%; 1%

**Oxy Oil-Free Acne Wash** topical liquid OTC *keratolytic for acne* [benzoyl peroxide] 10%

**oxybenzone** USAN, USP, INN *ultraviolet screen*

**oxybuprocaine** INN, BAN *topical anesthetic* [also: benoxinate HCl; oxybuprocaine HCl]

**oxybuprocaine HCl** JAN *topical anesthetic* [also: benoxinate HCl; oxybuprocaine]

**oxybutynin** USAN, INN, BAN *anticholinergic; smooth muscle relaxant; urinary antispasmodic* [also: oxybutynin chloride]

**oxybutynin chloride** USAN, USP *anticholinergic; smooth muscle relaxant; urinary antispasmodic for urge urinary incontinence and frequency* [also: oxybutynin] 5 mg oral; 5 mg/5 mL oral

**Oxycel** pads, pledgets, strips ℞ *local hemostat for surgery* [cellulose, oxidized]

**oxychlorosene** USAN *topical anti-infective*

**oxychlorosene sodium** USAN *topical anti-infective*

**oxycinchophen** INN, BAN

**oxyclipine** INN *anticholinergic* [also: propenzolate HCl]

**oxyclipine HCl** [see: propenzolate HCl]

**oxyclozanide** INN, BAN

**Oxycocet** ⓒ tablets ℞ *narcotic analgesic* [oxycodone HCl; acetaminophen] 5•325 mg

**oxycodone** USAN, INN, BAN *narcotic analgesic; also abused as a street drug* ⊉ Roxicodone

**oxycodone HCl** USAN, USP *narcotic analgesic; also abused as a street drug* 10, 20, 40, 80 mg oral ⊉ Roxicodone

**oxycodone terephthalate** USP *narcotic analgesic; also abused as a street drug* ⊉ Roxicodone

**OxyContin** controlled-release tablets ℞ *narcotic analgesic* [oxycodone HCl] 10, 20, 40, 80, 160 mg

**Oxydess II** tablets ℞ *CNS stimulant; amphetamine* [dextroamphetamine sulfate] 10 mg

**oxydimethylquinazine** [see: antipyrine]

**oxydipentonium chloride** INN

**Oxydose** oral drops ℞ *narcotic analgesic* [oxycodone HCl] 20 mg/mL

**oxyethyltheophylline** [see: etofylline]

**OxyFast** oral drops ℞ *narcotic analgesic* [oxycodone HCl] 20 mg/mL

**oxyfedrine** INN, BAN

**oxyfenamate** INN *minor tranquilizer* [also: hydroxyphenamate]

**oxyfilcon A** USAN *hydrophilic contact lens material*

**oxygen (O₂)** USP *medicinal gas; element* (O)

**oxygen, polymeric** *investigational (orphan) for sickle cell anemia*

**oxygen 93 percent** USP *medicinal gas*

**Oxygent** emulsion ℞ *investigational (Phase III) intravascular oxygen carrier to reduce need for blood transfusions in surgical patients* [perflubron]

**OxyIR** immediate-release capsules ℞ *narcotic analgesic* [oxycodone HCl] 5 mg

**oxymesterone** INN, BAN

**oxymetazoline** INN, BAN *topical ocular vasoconstrictor; nasal decongestant* [also: oxymetazoline HCl] ⊘ oxymetholone

**oxymetazoline HCl** USAN, USP *topical ocular vasoconstrictor; nasal decongestant* [also: oxymetazoline] 0.05% nasal

**oxymetholone** USAN, USP, INN, BAN *androgen; anabolic steroid; also abused as a street drug* ⊘ oxymetazoline; oxymorphone

**oxymethylene urea** [see: polynoxylin]

**oxymorphone** INN, BAN *narcotic analgesic* [also: oxymorphone HCl] ⊘ oxymetholone

**oxymorphone HCl** USP *narcotic analgesic; investigational (orphan) for intractable pain in narcotic-tolerant patients* [also: oxymorphone]

**oxypendyl** INN

**oxypertine** USAN, INN *antidepressant*

**oxyphenbutazone** USP, INN *antiinflammatory; antirheumatic; antipyretic; analgesic*

**oxyphencyclimine** INN *anticholinergic* [also: oxyphencyclimine HCl]

**oxyphencyclimine HCl** USP *peptic ulcer adjunct* [also: oxyphencyclimine]

**oxyphenhydrazine** [see: carsalam]

**oxyphenisatin** BAN *laxative* [also: oxyphenisatin acetate; oxyphenisatine]

**oxyphenisatin acetate** USAN *laxative* [also: oxyphenisatine; oxyphenisatin]

**oxyphenisatine** INN *laxative* [also: oxyphenisatin acetate; oxyphenisatin]

**oxyphenonium bromide**

**oxyphylline** [see: etofylline]

**oxypurinol** USAN *xanthine oxidase inhibitor* [also: oxipurinol]

**oxypyrronium bromide** INN

**oxyquinoline** USAN *disinfectant/antiseptic*

**oxyquinoline benzoate** [see: benzoxiquine]

**oxyquinoline sulfate** USAN, NF *complexing agent*

**oxyridazine** INN

**Oxysept** solution + tablets OTC *two-step chemical disinfecting system for soft contact lenses* [hydrogen peroxide-based] 3%

**Oxysept 2** solution OTC *rinsing/storage solution for soft contact lenses* [sodium chloride (saline solution)]

**oxysonium iodide** INN

**oxytetracycline** USP, INN *tetracycline antibiotic; antirickettsial*

**oxytetracycline calcium** USP *tetracycline antibiotic; antirickettsial*

**oxytetracycline HCl** USP *tetracycline antibiotic; antirickettsial*

**oxytocics** *a class of posterior pituitary hormones that stimulate contraction of the myometrium (uterine muscle)*

**oxytocin** USP, INN *posterior pituitary hormone; oxytocic for induction of labor* 10 U/mL injection

**Oxytrol** transdermal patch ℞ *urinary antispasmodic for urge urinary incontinence and frequency* [oxybutynin chloride] 36 mg (3.9 mg/day)

**Oxyzal Wet Dressing** topical liquid OTC *antiseptic dressing for minor infections* [oxyquinoline sulfate; benzalkonium chloride]

**Oysco 500** chewable tablets OTC *calcium supplement* [calcium carbonate] 1250 mg (500 mg Ca)

**Oyst-Cal 500** film-coated tablets OTC *calcium supplement* [calcium carbonate] 1250 mg (500 mg Ca)

**Oyst-Cal-D** film-coated tablets OTC *dietary supplement* [calcium carbonate; vitamin D] 250 mg•125 IU

**Oyster Calcium** tablets OTC *dietary supplement* [calcium carbonate; vitamins A and D] 375 mg•800 IU•200 IU

**Oyster Calcium 500 + D** tablets OTC *dietary supplement* [calcium carbonate; vitamin D] 500 mg•125 IU

**Oyster Calcium with Vitamin D** tablets OTC *dietary supplement* [calcium carbonate; vitamin D] 250 mg• 125 IU

**Oyster Shell Calcium** tablets OTC *calcium supplement* [calcium carbonate] 1250 mg (500 mg Ca)

**Oyster Shell Calcium with Vitamin D** tablets OTC *dietary supplement* [calcium carbonate; vitamin D] 250 mg•125 IU

**Oystercal 500** tablets (discontinued 2002) OTC *calcium supplement* [calcium carbonate] 1250 mg (500 mg Ca)

**Oystercal-D 250** tablets OTC *dietary supplement* [calcium carbonate; vitamin D] 250 mg•125 IU

**oz; gamma-oz** *medicinal herb* [see: rice bran oil]

**ozagrel** INN *investigational antiasthmatic* [also: ozagrel sodium]

**ozagrel sodium** JAN *investigational antiasthmatic* [also: ozagrel]

**ozolinone** USAN, INN *diuretic*

**P & S** shampoo OTC *antiseborrheic; keratolytic* [salicylic acid] 2%

**P & S** topical liquid OTC *antimicrobial hair dressing* [phenol]

**P & S Plus** gel (discontinued 2003) OTC *antipsoriatic; antiseborrheic; keratolytic* [coal tar solution; salicylic acid] 8%•2%

**p30 protein** [see: ranpirnase]

**$^{32}$P** [see: chromic phosphate P 32]

**$^{32}$P** [see: polymetaphosphate P 32]

**$^{32}$P** [see: sodium phosphate P 32]

**p53 adenoviral gene** *investigational (Phase III) gene therapy for head and neck cancer* [also: adenoviral p53 gene]

**P-081** *investigational isoflavone that increases HDL cholesterol in menopausal women*

**$P_1E_1$; $P_2E_1$; $P_4E_1$; $P_6E_1$** Drop-Tainers (eye drops) (discontinued 2004) R *antiglaucoma agent* [pilocarpine HCl;

epinephrine bitartrate] 1%•1%; 2%•1%; 4%•1%; 6%•1%

**PAB (para-aminobenzoate)** [see: aminobenzoic acid]

**PABA (para-aminobenzoic acid)** [now: aminobenzoic acid]

**PABA sodium** [see: aminobenzoate sodium]

**Pabalate** enteric-coated tablets (discontinued 2000) OTC *analgesic; antipyretic; anti-inflammatory* [sodium salicylate; aminobenzoate sodium] 300•300 mg

**PAB-Esc-C (Platinol, Adriamycin, bleomycin, escalating doses of cyclophosphamide)** *chemotherapy protocol*

**pabestrol D** [see: diethylstilbestrol dipropionate]

**PAC; PAC-I (Platinol, Adriamycin, cyclophosphamide)** *chemotherapy protocol for ovarian and endometrial* cancer; "I" stands for "Indiana protocol," used for ovarian cancer only

**P-A-C Analgesic** tablets OTC *analgesic; antipyretic; anti-inflammatory* [aspirin; caffeine] 400•32 mg

**PACE (Platinol, Adriamycin, cyclophosphamide, etoposide)** *chemotherapy protocol*

**Pacerone** tablets ℞ *antiarrhythmic for acute ventricular tachycardia and fibrillation (orphan)* [amiodarone HCl] 100, 200 mg

**PA-CI (Adriamycin, cisplatin)** *chemotherapy protocol for pediatric hepatoblastoma*

**Pacis** powder for intravesical instillation (discontinued 2004) ℞ *antineoplastic for urinary bladder cancer* [BCG vaccine, Montreal strain] 120 mg (2.4–12 × 10⁸ CFU)

**Packer's Pine Tar** shampoo (discontinued 2003) OTC *antiseborrheic; antipsoriatic; antipruritic; antibacterial* [pine tar]

**Packer's Pine Tar** soap OTC *antiseborrheic; antipsoriatic; antipruritic; antibacterial* [pine tar]

**paclitaxel** USAN, INN, BAN *antineoplastic for AIDS-related Kaposi sarcoma (orphan), breast and ovarian cancers, and non–small cell lung cancer*

**paclitaxel & carboplatin & etoposide** *chemotherapy protocol for primary adenocarcinoma and small cell lung cancer (SCLC)*

**paclitaxel & trastuzumab** *chemotherapy protocol for breast cancer*

**paclitaxel & vinorelbine tartrate** *chemotherapy protocol for breast cancer*

**pacrinolol** INN

**padimate** INN *ultraviolet screen* [also: padimate A]

**padimate A** USAN *ultraviolet screen* [also: padimate]

**padimate O** USAN *ultraviolet screen*

*Paeonia officinalis* medicinal herb [see: peony]

**Pafase** ℞ *investigational (Phase II/III) platelet-activating factor for acute respiratory distress syndrome* [acetylhydrolase]

**pafenolol** INN

**paflufocon A** USAN *hydrophobic contact lens material*

**paflufocon B** USAN *hydrophobic contact lens material*

**paflufocon C** USAN *hydrophobic contact lens material*

**paflufocon D** USAN *hydrophobic contact lens material*

**paflufocon E** USAN *hydrophobic contact lens material*

**pagoclone** USAN *nonsedating anxiolytic; investigational (Phase III) for panic disorder; investigational (Phase II) for generalized anxiety disorder*

**PAH (para-aminohippurate)** [see: aminohippuric acid]

**PAHA (para-aminohippuric acid)** [see: aminohippuric acid]

**Pain Bust-R II** cream OTC *analgesic; counterirritant* [methyl salicylate; menthol] 17%•12%

**Pain Doctor** cream OTC *analgesic; topical anesthetic; antipruritic* [capsaicin; methyl salicylate; menthol] 0.025%•25%•10%

**Pain Gel Plus** OTC *topical analgesic; counterirritant* [menthol] 4%

**Pain Reliever** tablets (discontinued 2000) OTC *analgesic; antipyretic; anti-inflammatory* [acetaminophen; aspirin; caffeine] 250•250•65 mg

**Painaid** tablets OTC *analgesic; antipyretic; anti-inflammatory* [acetaminophen; aspirin; salicylamide; caffeine] 110•162•152•32.4 mg

**Painaid BRF** (Back Relief Formula) tablets OTC *analgesic; antipyretic; anti-inflammatory* [magnesium salicylate tetrahydrate; acetaminophen] 250•250 mg

**Painaid ESF** (Extra Strength Formula) tablets OTC *analgesic; antipyretic; anti-inflammatory* [acetaminophen; aspirin; caffeine] 250•250•65 mg

**Painaid PMF** (Premenstrual Formula) tablets OTC *analgesic; antipyretic; diuretic* [acetaminophen; pamabrom] 500•25 mg

**paint, Indian** *medicinal herb* [see: blood-root]

**paint, yellow Indian** *medicinal herb* [see: goldenseal]

**paint root, red** *medicinal herb* [see: bloodroot]

**Pain-X** gel OTC *topical analgesic; counterirritant* [capsaicin; menthol; camphor] 0.05%•5%•4%

**PALA disodium** [see: sparfosate sodium]

**palatrigine** INN, BAN

**paldimycin** USAN, INN *antibacterial*

**paldimycin A** [see: paldimycin]

**paldimycin B** [see: paldimycin]

**pale gentian** *medicinal herb* [see: gentian]

**palestrol** [see: diethylstilbestrol]

**Palgic** tablets, oral solution ℞ *antihistamine* [carbinoxamine maleate] 4 mg; 4 mg/5 mL

**Palgic-D** extended-release caplets ℞ *decongestant; antihistamine* [pseudoephedrine HCl; carbinoxamine maleate] 80•8 mg

**Palgic-DS** pediatric syrup ℞ *decongestant; antihistamine* [pseudoephedrine HCl; carbinoxamine maleate] 30•2 mg/5 mL

**palifermin** *keratinocyte growth factor; investigational (Phase III) for radiation- and chemotherapy-induced mucositis*

**palinavir** USAN *antiviral; HIV-1 protease inhibitor*

**palinum** [see: cyclobarbitone]

**palivizumab** *monoclonal antibody for prophylaxis of respiratory syncytial virus (RSV) in infants*

**palladium** *element (Pd)*

**palladium Pd 103** *investigational radioactive "seeds" for ultrasound-guided brachytherapy for adenocarcinoma of the prostate*

**palm, dwarf; dwarf palmetto; pan palm** *medicinal herb* [see: saw palmetto]

**palmidrol** INN

**Palmitate-A 5000** tablets OTC *vitamin supplement* [vitamin A palmitate] 5000 IU

**palmitic acid** USAN *ultrasound contrast medium for echocardiography*

**palmoxirate sodium** USAN *antidiabetic* [also: palmoxiric acid]

**palmoxiric acid** INN *antidiabetic* [also: palmoxirate sodium]

**palonosetron HCl** USAN *selective serotonin 5-HT$_3$ antagonist; antiemetic for chemotherapy-induced nausea and vomiting (CINV)*

**PALS** coated tablets OTC *systemic deodorant for ostomy, breath, and body odors* [chlorophyllin copper complex] 100 mg

**PAM; L-PAM (phenylalanine mustard)** [see: melphalan]

**2-PAM (2-pyridine aldoxime methylchloride)** [see: pralidoxime chloride]

**pamabrom** USAN *nonprescription diuretic*

**pamaqueside** USAN *hypocholesterolemic; cholesterol absorption inhibitor; antiatherosclerotic*

**pamaquine naphthoate** NF

**pamatolol** INN *antiadrenergic (β-receptor)* [also: pamatolol sulfate]

**pamatolol sulfate** USAN *antiadrenergic (β-receptor)* [also: pamatolol]

**Pamelor** capsules, oral solution ℞ *tricyclic antidepressant* [nortriptyline HCl] 10, 25, 50, 75 mg; 10 mg/5 mL ⓘ Dymelor; Panlor

**pamidronate disodium** USAN *bisphosphonate bone resorption inhibitor for Paget disease, hypercalcemia of malignancy, and bone metastases of breast cancer and multiple myeloma* 3, 6, 9 mg/mL injection

**pamidronic acid** INN, BAN

**Pamine; Pamine Forte** tablets ℞ *GI antispasmodic; anticholinergic; peptic ulcer treatment* [methscopolamine bromide] 2.5 mg; 5 mg

**Pamisyl** ℞ *investigational (orphan) for ulcerative colitis* [aminosalicylic acid]

**pamoate** USAN, USP *combining name for radicals or groups* [also: embonate]

**Pamprin, Nighttime** powder OTC *antihistaminic sleep aid; analgesic* [diphenhydramine HCl; acetaminophen] 50•650 mg

**Pamprin Maximum Pain Relief** caplets OTC *analgesic; antipyretic; diuretic* [acetaminophen; magnesium salicylate; pamabrom] 250•250•25 mg

**Pamprin Multi-Symptom** caplets, tablets OTC *analgesic; antipyretic; diuretic; antihistaminic sleep aid* [acetaminophen; pamabrom; pyrilamine maleate] 500•25•15 mg

**Pan C Ascorbate; Pan C-500** tablets OTC *vitamin C supplement with multiple bioflavonoids* [vitamin C; citrus bioflavonoids; hesperidin] 200•100•100 mg; 500•100•100 mg

**PAN-2400** capsules OTC *digestive enzymes* [lipase; protease; amylase] 9816•60 214•75 900 U

**Panacet 5/500** tablets ℞ *narcotic analgesic* [hydrocodone bitartrate; acetaminophen] 5•500 mg

**panadiplon** USAN, INN *anxiolytic*

**Panadol** tablets, caplets OTC *analgesic; antipyretic* [acetaminophen] 500 mg

**Panadol, Children's** chewable tablets, oral liquid OTC *analgesic; antipyretic* [acetaminophen] 80 mg; 160 mg/5 mL

**Panadol, Infants'** drops OTC *analgesic; antipyretic* [acetaminophen] 100 mg/mL

**Panadol, Junior** caplets OTC *analgesic; antipyretic* [acetaminophen] 160 mg

**Panafil** ointment ℞ *enzyme for wound debridement; vulnerary; wound deodorant* [papain; urea; chlorophyllin copper complex] 10%•10%•0.5%

**Panafil White** ointment ℞ *topical enzyme for wound debridement; vulnerary* [papain; urea] 10%•10%

**Panalgesic** cream OTC *analgesic; counterirritant* [methyl salicylate; menthol] 35%•4%

**Panalgesic Gold** liniment OTC *analgesic; counterirritant; antiseptic* [methyl salicylate; camphor; menthol; alcohol 22%] 55%•3.1%•1.25%

**Panasal 5/500** tablets ℞ *narcotic analgesic* [hydrocodone bitartrate; aspirin] 5•500 mg

**Panasol-S** tablets ℞ *corticosteroid; anti-inflammatory; immunosuppressant* [prednisone] 1 mg ② Panscol

**Panavir** ℞ *investigational (Phase II) antiviral for HIV and AIDS* [probucol]

*Panax ginseng; P. shin-seng* **(Korean ginseng)** *medicinal herb* [see: ginseng]

*Panax horridum* *medicinal herb* [see: devil's club]

*Panax pseudoginseng* **(Chikusetsu ginseng; Himalayan ginseng; Sanchi ginseng; Zhuzishen)** *medicinal herb* [see: ginseng]

*Panax quinquefolia* **(American ginseng)** *medicinal herb* [see: ginseng]

*Panax spp.* *medicinal herb* [see: ginseng]

*Panax trifolius* **(dwarf ginseng)** *medicinal herb* [see: ginseng]

**Pancof** syrup ℞ *narcotic antitussive; decongestant; antihistamine* [dihydrocodeine bitartrate; pseudoephedrine HCl; chlorpheniramine maleate] 7.5•15•2 mg/5 mL

**Pancof-EXP** syrup ℞ *narcotic antitussive; decongestant; expectorant* [dihydrocodeine bitartrate; pseudoephedrine HCl; guaifenesin] 7.5•15•100 mg/5 mL

**Pancof-HC** oral liquid (discontinued 2002) ℞ *narcotic antitussive; decongestant; antihistamine* [hydrocodone bitartrate; pseudoephedrine HCl; chlorpheniramine maleate] 3•15•2 mg/5 mL

**Pancof-PD** syrup ℞ *narcotic antitussive; decongestant; antihistamine* [dihydrocodeine bitartrate; phenylephrine HCl; chlorpheniramine maleate] 3•7.5•2 mg/5 mL

**Pancof-XP** oral liquid ℞ *narcotic antitussive; decongestant; expectorant* [hydrocodone bitartrate; pseudoephedrine HCl; guaifenesin] 2.5•15•100 mg/5 mL

**pancopride** USAN, INN *antiemetic; anxiolytic; peristaltic stimulant*

**Pancrease; Pancrease MT 4; Pancrease MT 10; Pancrease MT 16; Pancrease MT 20** capsules containing enteric-coated microtablets

℞ *porcine-derived digestive enzymes* [lipase; protease; amylase] 4.5•25• 25; 4•12•12; 10•30•30; 16•48•48; 20•44•56 thousand USP units

**pancreatin** USP *porcine-derived digestive enzymes; a combination of lipase, protease, and amylase*

**Pancreatin, 4X; Pancreatin, 8X** tablets (discontinued 2002) OTC *porcine-derived digestive enzymes* [pancreatin (lipase; protease; amylase)] 2400 mg (12 000•60 000•60 000 USP units); 7200 mg (22 500• 180 000•180 000 USP units)

**Pancrecarb MS-4; Pancrecarb MS-8** delayed-release capsules containing enteric-coated microspheres ℞ *porcine-derived digestive enzymes* [lipase; protease; amylase] 4000• 25 000•25 000 USP units; 8000• 45 000•40 000 USP units

**pancrelipase** USAN, USP *porcine-derived digestive enzymes; a combination of lipase, protease, and amylase* 4.5•25• 20, 8•30•30, 16•48•48, 16•60•60 thousand USP units

**Pancrezyme 4X** tablets (discontinued 2002) OTC *porcine-derived digestive enzymes* [pancreatin (lipase; protease; amylase)] 2400 mg (12 000• 60 000•60 000 USP units)

**pancuronium bromide** USAN, INN *nondepolarizing neuromuscular blocking agent; muscle relaxant; adjunct to tracheal intubation for general anesthesia or mechanical ventilation* 1, 2 mg/ mL injection

**Pandel** cream ℞ *corticosteroidal antiinflammatory* [hydrocortisone probutate] 0.1%

**Panfil G** capsules, syrup ℞ *antiasthmatic; bronchodilator; expectorant* [dyphylline; guaifenesin] 200•100 mg; 100•50 mg/5 mL

**Panglobulin NF** powder for IV infusion ℞ *passive immunizing agent for HIV and idiopathic thrombocytopenic purpura (ITP)* [immune globulin] 1, 3, 6, 12 g

**Panhematin** powder for IV injection ℞ *enzyme inhibitor for recurrent attacks of acute intermittent porphyria* [hemin] 301 mg/vial

**panidazole** INN, BAN

**Panitone-500** tablets OTC *analgesic; antipyretic* [acetaminophen] 500 mg

**Panixine DisperDose** tablets for oral suspension ℞ *cephalosporin antibiotic* [cephalexin] 125, 250 mg

**Panlor DC** capsules ℞ *narcotic antitussive; analgesic* [dihydrocodeine bitartrate; acetaminophen; caffeine] 16• 356.4•30 mg ② Pamelor

**Panlor SS** tablets ℞ *narcotic analgesic* [dihydrocodeine bitartrate; acetaminophen; caffeine] 32•712.8•60 mg

**PanMist-DM** extended-release caplets, syrup ℞ *antitussive; decongestant; expectorant* [dextromethorphan hydrobromide; pseudoephedrine HCl; guaifenesin] 32•48•595 mg; 15•40•100 mg/5 mL

**PanMist-JR** extended-release caplets ℞ *decongestant; expectorant* [pseudoephedrine HCl; guaifenesin] 48•595 mg

**PanMist-LA** extended-release caplets ℞ *decongestant; expectorant* [pseudoephedrine HCl; guaifenesin] 85•795 mg

**PanMist-S** syrup ℞ *decongestant; expectorant* [pseudoephedrine HCl; guaifenesin] 40•200 mg/5 mL

**Panmycin** capsules (discontinued 2003) ℞ *broad-spectrum antibiotic* [tetracycline HCl] 250 mg

**Pannaz** sustained-release tablets ℞ *decongestant; antihistamine; anticholinergic to dry mucosal secretions* [pseudoephedrine HCl; carbinoxamine maleate; methscopolamine bromide] 90•8•2.5 mg

**Pannaz S** syrup ℞ *decongestant; antihistamine; anticholinergic to dry mucosal secretions* [pseudoephedrine HCl; carbinoxamine maleate; methscopolamine nitrate] 15•2•1.25 mg/5 mL

**Panokase** tablets ℞ *porcine-derived digestive enzymes* [lipase; protease; amylase] 8000•30 000•30 000 USP units

**panomifene** INN

**Panoxyl** cleansing bar OTC *keratolytic for acne* [benzoyl peroxide] 5%, 10% ⧉ Benoxyl

**Panoxyl 5; Panoxyl 10** gel ℞ *keratolytic and antiseptic for acne* [benzoyl peroxide; alcohol] 5%•12%; 10%•20%

**Panoxyl AQ 2½; Panoxyl AQ 5; Panoxyl AQ 10** gel ℞ *keratolytic for acne* [benzoyl peroxide] 2.5%; 5%; 10%

**Panretin** capsules ℞ *investigational (Phase III, orphan) treatment for Kaposi sarcoma and acute promyelocytic leukemia (APL)* [alitretinoin]

**Panretin** gel ℞ *treatment for cutaneous lesions of AIDS-related Kaposi sarcoma (orphan)* [alitretinoin] 0.1%

**Panscol** lotion, ointment OTC *keratolytic* [salicylic acid] 3% ⧉ Panasol

**pansy (Viola tricolor)** plant *medicinal herb used as an anodyne, demulcent, diaphoretic, diuretic, expectorant, laxative, and vulnerary*

**pantenicate** INN

**panthenol** USAN, USP, INN *B complex vitamin*

**DL-panthenol** [see: dexpanthenol]

**Panthoderm** cream OTC *antipruritic; vulnerary; emollient* [dexpanthenol] 2%

**Panto IV** ⓒ powder for injection ℞ *proton pump inhibitor for erosive esophagitis associated with gastroesophageal reflux disease (GERD)* [pantoprazole sodium] 40 mg/vial

**Panto IV** ⓒ powder for IV injection ℞ *proton pump inhibitor for gastroesophageal reflux disease (GERD) and eradication of H. pylori infection* [pantoprazole sodium]

**Pantoloc** ⓒ enteric-coated tablets ℞ *proton pump inhibitor for erosive esophagitis associated with gastroesophageal reflux disease (GERD)* [pantoprazole sodium] 40 mg

**pantoprazole** USAN, INN, BAN *proton pump inhibitor for erosive esophagitis*

associated with gastroesophageal reflux disease (GERD)

**pantoprazole sodium** USAN *proton pump inhibitor for erosive esophagitis associated with gastroesophageal reflux disease (GERD) and Zollinger-Ellison syndrome*

**pantothenic acid (vitamin B₅)** BAN *water-soluble vitamin; enzyme cofactor* [also: calcium pantothenate]

**DL-pantothenic acid** [see: calcium pantothenate, racemic]

**pantothenol** [see: dexpanthenol]

**pantothenyl alcohol** [see: panthenol]

**D-pantothenyl alcohol** [see: dexpanthenol]

**Pantozol** ℞ *investigational proton pump inhibitor for gastroesophageal reflux disease (GERD)* [pantoprazole]

**panuramine** INN, BAN

**Panvac-VF** ℞ *investigational (Phase III) antineoplastic vaccine for metastatic pancreatic cancer*

**Panzem** ℞ *investigational (orphan) for multiple myeloma* [2-methoxyestradiol]

**papain** USP *topical proteolytic enzyme for necrotic tissue debridement*

**papaverine** BAN *peripheral vasodilator; smooth muscle relaxant; orphan status withdrawn 1996* [also: papaverine HCl]

**papaverine HCl** USP *peripheral vasodilator; smooth muscle relaxant for cerebral, myocardial, and peripheral ischemias* [also: papaverine] 150 mg oral; 30 mg/mL

**papaveroline** INN, BAN

**papaya (Carica papaya)** leaves, fruit, juice, and seeds *medicinal herb for aiding digestion, gas, insect bites, and intestinal worms*

**Papaya Enzyme** chewable tablets (discontinued 2002) OTC *digestive enzymes* [papain; amylase] 60•60 mg

**Papirine** ℞ *investigational antiviral*

**Paplex Ultra** topical solution ℞ *keratolytic* [salicylic acid in flexible collodion] 26%

**papoose root** *medicinal herb* [see: blue cohosh]

**Par Glycerol** elixir ℞ *expectorant* [iodinated glycerol] 60 mg/5 mL

**Para Special Lice and Nits** ⓒⒶⓃ spray, shampoo OTC *pediculicide* [piperonyl butoxide; bioallethrin] 2.64%•0.66%; 4.4%•1.1%

**para-aminobenzoate (PAB)** [see: aminobenzoic acid]

**Para-Aminobenzoic Acid** tablets, powder OTC *"possibly effective" for scleroderma and other skin diseases and Peyronie disease* [aminobenzoic acid] 100, 500 mg; 120 g

**para-aminobenzoic acid (PABA)** [now: aminobenzoic acid]

**para-aminohippurate (PAH)** [see: aminohippuric acid]

**para-aminohippurate sodium** [see: aminohippurate sodium]

**para-aminohippuric acid (PAHA)** [see: aminohippuric acid]

**para-aminosalicylate (PAS)** [see: aminosalicylic acid]

**para-aminosalicylic acid (PASA)** [see: aminosalicylic acid]

**Parabolan** *brand name for trenbolone hexahydrobenzylcarbonate, a European veterinary anabolic steroid abused as a street drug*

**parabromdylamine maleate** [see: brompheniramine maleate]

**paracetaldehyde** [see: paraldehyde]

**paracetamol** INN, BAN *analgesic; antipyretic* [also: acetaminophen]

**parachlorometaxylenol (PCMX)** *topical antiseptic; broad-spectrum antibacterial*

**parachlorophenol (PCP)** USP *topical antibacterial*

**parachlorophenol, camphorated** USP *topical dental anti-infective*

**paracodin** [see: dihydrocodeine]

**paraffin** NF *stiffening agent*

**paraffin, liquid** [see: mineral oil]

**paraffin, synthetic** NF *stiffening agent*

**Paraflex** caplets ℞ *skeletal muscle relaxant* [chlorzoxazone] 250 mg

**paraflutizide** INN

**Parafon Forte DSC** caplets ℞ *skeletal muscle relaxant* [chlorzoxazone] 500 mg ⑨ Pantopon

**paraformaldehyde** USP

**Paraguay tea** *medicinal herb* [see: yerba maté]

**Para-Hist HD** oral liquid (discontinued 2002) ℞ *narcotic antitussive; decongestant; antihistamine* [hydrocodone bitartrate; phenylephrine HCl; chlorpheniramine maleate] 1.67•5•2 mg/5 mL

**parahydrecin** [now: isomerol]

**Paral** oral liquid, rectal liquid ℞ *sedative; hypnotic* [paraldehyde]

**paraldehyde** USP *hypnotic; sedative; anticonvulsant* 1 g/mL oral or rectal

**paramethadione** USP, INN, BAN *anticonvulsant* ⑨ paramethasone

**paramethasone** INN *corticosteroid; anti-inflammatory* [also: paramethasone acetate] ⑨ paramethadione

**paramethasone acetate** USAN, USP *corticosteroid; anti-inflammatory* [also: paramethasone]

**para-nitrosulfathiazole** NF [also: nitrosulfathiazole]

**paranyline HCl** USAN *anti-inflammatory* [also: renytoline]

**parapenzolate bromide** USAN, INN *anticholinergic*

**Paraplatin** powder for IV injection ℞ *alkylating antineoplastic for ovarian and other cancers* [carboplatin] 50, 150, 450 mg

**parapropamol** INN

**pararosaniline embonate** INN *antischistosomal* [also: pararosaniline pamoate]

**pararosaniline pamoate** USAN *antischistosomal* [also: pararosaniline embonate]

**parasympathomimetics** *a class of agents that produce effects similar to those of the parasympathetic nervous system* [also called: cholinergic agonists]

**Parathar** powder for IV injection (discontinued 2004) ℞ *in vivo diagnostic aid for parathyroid-induced hypocalcemia (orphan)* [teriparatide acetate] 200 U

**parathesin** [see: benzocaine]

**parathiazine** INN

**parathyroid** USP *hormone*

**parathyroid hormone (1-34), biosynthetic human** [see: teriparatide]

**parathyroid hormone (1-84), recombinant human** *investigational (Phase III) agent to increase bone mineral content and density in postmenopausal osteoporosis*

**paraxazone** INN

**parbendazole** USAN, INN *anthelmintic*

**parconazole** INN *antifungal* [also: parconazole HCl]

**parconazole HCl** USAN *antifungal* [also: parconazole]

**Parcopa** RapiTab (orally disintegrating tablets) ℞ *antiparkinsonian; dopamine precursor; decarboxylase inhibitor* [carbidopa; levodopa] 10•100, 25•100, 25•250 mg

**parecoxib** USAN *COX-2 inhibitor; anti-inflammatory; analgesic*

**parecoxib sodium** USAN *COX-2 inhibitor; anti-inflammatory; analgesic*

**Paredrine** eye drops ℞ *mydriatic* [hydroxyamphetamine hydrobromide] 1%

**paregoric (PG)** (a preparation of opium, anise oil, benzoic acid, camphor, alcohol, and glycerin) USP *antiperistaltic; narcotic analgesic; used in neonatal opioid withdrawal programs; sometimes abused as a street drug* 2 mg/5 mL oral

**Paremyd** eye drops ℞ *mydriatic; weak cycloplegic* [hydroxyamphetamine hydrobromide; tropicamide] 1%•0.25%

**parenabol** [see: boldenone undecylenate]

**Parepectolin** concentrated oral liquid OTC *GI adsorbent; antidiarrheal* [attapulgite] 600 mg/15 mL

**pareptide** INN *antiparkinsonian* [also: pareptide sulfate]

**pareptide sulfate** USAN *antiparkinsonian* [also: pareptide]

**parethoxycaine** INN

**parethoxycaine HCl** [see: parethoxycaine]

**Par-F** tablets ℞ *vitamin/mineral/calcium/iron supplement* [multiple vitamins & minerals; calcium; iron; folic acid] ±•250•60•1 mg

**pargeverine** INN

**pargolol** INN

**pargyline** INN *antihypertensive* [also: pargyline HCl]

**pargyline HCl** USAN, USP *antihypertensive* [also: pargyline]

**paricalcitol** USAN *synthetic vitamin D analogue for osteodystrophy and hyperparathyroidism secondary to chronic renal failure*

**paridocaine** INN

**Parlodel** SnapTabs (scored tablets), capsules ℞ *dopamine agonist; antiparkinsonian; lactation preventative; treats acromegaly, infertility, and hypogonadism* [bromocriptine mesylate] 2.5 mg; 5 mg

**Par-Natal Plus 1 Improved** tablets ℞ *vitamin/calcium/iron supplement* [multiple vitamins; calcium; iron; folic acid] ±•200•65•1 mg

**Parnate** film-coated tablets ℞ *monoamine oxidase inhibitor (MAOI) for reactive depression (a major depressive episode without melancholia)* [tranylcypromine sulfate] 10 mg

**parodilol** INN

**parodyne** [see: antipyrine]

**paroleine** [see: mineral oil]

**paromomycin** INN, BAN *aminoglycoside antibiotic; amebicide* [also: paromomycin sulfate]

**Paromomycin** ℞ *investigational (orphan) agent for visceral leishmaniasis* [aminosidine]

**paromomycin sulfate** USP *aminoglycoside antibiotic; amebicide; investigational (Phase III) for visceral leishmaniasis* [also: paromomycin]

**paroxetine** USAN, INN, BAN *selective serotonin reuptake inhibitor (SSRI) for depression, obsessive-compulsive disorder, and panic disorder*

**paroxetine HCl** *selective serotonin reuptake inhibitor (SSRI) for depression,* obsessive-compulsive disorder, panic disorder, social anxiety disorder, generalized anxiety disorder, post-traumatic stress disorder, and premenstrual dysphoric disorder 10, 20, 30, 40 mg oral

**paroxetine mesylate** selective serotonin reuptake inhibitor (SSRI) for depression, obsessive-compulsive disorder, and panic disorder 10, 20, 30, 40 mg

**paroxyl** [see: acetarsone]

**paroxypropione** INN

**parpanit HCl** [see: caramiphen HCl]

**parsalmide** INN

**parsley (Petroselinum sativum)** leaves and root medicinal herb for amenorrhea, bladder infections, blood building and cleansing, body lice, colic, dysmenorrhea, flatulence, gallstones, inducing abortion, jaundice, nephritis, prostate disorders, and urinary retention

**parsley fern** medicinal herb [see: tansy]

**parsnip, cow; wooly parsnip** medicinal herb [see: masterwort]

**Partaject** R̶ investigational (Phase II/III) intravenous delivery device

**Parthenocissus quinquefolia** medicinal herb [see: American ivy]

**partricin** USAN, INN antifungal; antiprotozoal

**partridge berry** medicinal herb [see: squaw vine; wintergreen]

**Partuss LA** long-acting tablets (discontinued 2002) R̶ decongestant; expectorant [phenylpropanolamine HCl; guaifenesin] 75•400 mg

**parvaquone** INN, BAN ge

**Parvlex** tablets OTC hematinic [ferrous fumarate; multiple B vitamins & minerals; vitamin C; folic acid] 100• ± •50•0.1 mg

**PAS (para-aminosalicylate)** [see: aminosalicylic acid]

**PASA (para-aminosalicylic acid)** [see: aminosalicylic acid]

**Paser** delayed-release granules for oral solution R̶ treatment for multidrug-resistant tuberculosis (MDR-TB) (orphan) [aminosalicylic acid] 4 g/pkt.

**pasiniazid** INN

**pasque flower (Anemone patens)** plant medicinal herb used as a diaphoretic, diuretic, and rubefacient; not generally regarded as safe and effective due to toxicity

**passion flower (Passiflora incarnata)** plant medicinal herb for asthma, bronchitis, eye infections, fever, inflamed hemorrhoids, insomnia, menopause, nervousness, pain related to neurasthenia, and attention-deficit disorder, nervousness, and excitability in children

**Pastilles** (dosage form) troches

**Patanol** Drop-Tainers (eye drops) R̶ topical ophthalmic antihistamine and mast cell stabilizer for allergic conjunctivitis [olopatadine HCl] 0.1%

**PATCO (prednisone, ara-C, thioguanine, cyclophosphamide, Oncovin)** chemotherapy protocol

**Pathilon** film-coated tablets (discontinued 2001) R̶ peptic ulcer treatment adjunct [tridihexethyl chloride] 25 mg ⊘ Pathocil

**Pathocil** capsules, powder for oral suspension (discontinued 2002) R̶ penicillinase-resistant penicillin antibiotic [dicloxacillin sodium] 250, 500 mg; 62.5 mg/5 mL ⊘ Bactocill; Pathilon; Placidyl

**patience, garden** medicinal herb [see: yellow dock]

**patience dock** medicinal herb [see: bistort]

**pau d'arco (Lapacho colorado; L. morado)** inner bark medicinal herb for boils, blood cleansing, cancer, Candida albicans infections, chlorosis, diabetes, leukemia, skin wounds, syphilis, and pain

**Paullinia cupana; P. sorbilis** medicinal herb [see: guarana]

**paulomycin** USAN, INN antibacterial

**Pausinystalia johimbe** medicinal herb [see: yohimbe]

**pauson** medicinal herb [see: bloodroot]

**Pavabid** Plateau Caps (controlled-release capsules) R̶ peripheral vasodilator; smooth muscle relaxant for cerebral, myocardial, and peripheral

ischemias [papaverine HCl] 150 mg
⑦ Pavased

**Pavagen TD** timed-release capsules ℞ *peripheral vasodilator; smooth muscle relaxant for cerebral, myocardial, and peripheral ischemias* [papaverine HCl] 150 mg

**PAVe (procarbazine, Alkeran, Velban)** *chemotherapy protocol*

**Pavulon** IM injection (discontinued 2004) ℞ *nondepolarizing neuromuscular blocking agent; muscle relaxant; adjunct to tracheal intubation for general anesthesia or mechanical ventilation* [pancuronium bromide] 1, 2 mg/mL ⑦ Paverolan

**pawpaw (*Asimina triloba*)** fruit *medicinal herb used as an antimicrobial and antineoplastic*

**paxamate** INN

**Paxarel** tablets ℞ *anxiolytic; sedative* [acecarbromal] 250 mg

**Paxene** ℞ *investigational (Phase III) antineoplastic for AIDS-related Kaposi sarcoma* [paclitaxel]

**Paxil** film-coated tablets, oral suspension ℞ *selective serotonin reuptake inhibitor (SSRI) for depression, obsessive-compulsive disorder, panic disorder, social anxiety disorder, generalized anxiety disorder, and post-traumatic stress disorder* [paroxetine HCl] 10, 20, 30, 40 mg; 10 mg/5 mL

**Paxil CR** enteric-coated controlled-release tablets ℞ *selective serotonin reuptake inhibitor (SSRI) for depression, panic disorder, premenstrual dysphoric disorder (PMDD), and social anxiety disorder* [paroxetine HCl] 12.5, 25, 37.5 mg

**pazelliptine** INN

**pazinaclone** USAN *anxiolytic*

**Pazo Hemorrhoid** ointment OTC *temporary relief of hemorrhoidal symptoms; topical vasoconstrictor; counterirritant; astringent* [ephedrine sulfate; camphor; zinc oxide] 0.2%•2%•5%

**Pazo Hemorrhoid** suppositories OTC *temporary relief of hemorrhoidal symptoms; topical vasoconstrictor; astringent* [ephedrine sulfate; zinc oxide] 3.8•96.5 mg

**pazoxide** USAN, INN *antihypertensive*

**PBV (Platinol, bleomycin, vinblastine)** *chemotherapy protocol*

**PBZ** tablets (discontinued 2002) ℞ *antihistamine* [tripelennamine HCl] 25, 50 mg

**PBZ (pyribenzamine)** [see: tripelennamine]

**PBZ-SR** extended-release tablets (discontinued 2002) ℞ *antihistamine* [tripelennamine HCl] 100 mg

**PC (paclitaxel, carboplatin)** *chemotherapy protocol for bladder cancer and non–small cell lung cancer (NSCLC)*

**PC (paclitaxel, cisplatin)** *chemotherapy protocol for non–small cell lung cancer (NSCLC)*

**PC (phosphatidylcholine)** [see: lecithin]

**PCE** Dispertabs (delayed-release tablets) ℞ *macrolide antibiotic* [erythromycin] 333, 500 mg

**PCE (Platinol, cyclophosphamide, etoposide)** *chemotherapy protocol*

**PCE (polymer-coated erythromycin)** [see: erythromycin]

**PCMX (parachlorometaxylenol)** [q.v.]

**PCOs (procyanidolic oligomers)** [q.v.]

**PCP (parachlorophenol)** [q.v.]

**PCP (phenylcyclohexyl piperidine)** *a powerful veterinary analgesic/anesthetic widely abused as a hallucinogenic street drug* [medically known as phencyclidine HCl]

**PCV (procarbazine, CCNU, vincristine)** *chemotherapy protocol for brain tumors*

**PDE III (phosphodiesterase III) inhibitors** *a class of platelet aggregation inhibitors*

**PDGA (pteroyldiglutamic acid)**

**PDLA (phosphinicodilactic acid)** [see: foscolic acid]

**PDP Liquid Protein** (discontinued 2001) OTC *dietary supplement* [hydrolyzed protein; L-tryptophan] 15•⸛ g/30 mL

**PE (paclitaxel, estramustine)** *chemotherapy protocol for prostate cancer*

**PE (phenylephrine)** [q.v.]

**PE (polyethylene)** [q.v.]

**pea, ground squirrel** *medicinal herb* [see: twin leaf]

**pea, turkey; wild turkey pea** *medicinal herb* [see: turkey corn]

**peach** *(Prunus persica)* bark and leaves *medicinal herb for bladder disorders, chest congestion, chronic bronchitis, nausea, and water retention*

**peanut oil** NF *solvent*

**PEB (Platinol, etoposide, bleomycin)** *chemotherapy protocol*

**pecazine** INN, BAN

**pecazine acetate** [see: pecazine]

**pecilocin** INN, BAN

**pecocycline** INN

**pectin** USP *suspending agent; protectant; GI adsorbent*

**pectorals** *a class of agents that relieve disorders of the respiratory tract, such as expectorants*

**Pedameth** capsules, oral liquid ℞ *urinary acidifier to control ammonia production* [racemethionine] 200 mg; 75 mg/5 mL

**Pedia Relief Decongestant Plus Cough** infants' oral drops OTC *antitussive; decongestant* [dextromethorphan hydrobromide; pseudoephedrine HCl] 5•15 mg/1.6 mL

**PediaCare Allergy Formula** oral liquid OTC *antihistamine* [chlorpheniramine maleate] 1 mg/5 mL

**PediaCare Children's Cold & Allergy** oral liquid OTC *decongestant; antihistamine* [pseudoephedrine HCl; chlorpheniramine maleate] 30•2 mg/10 mL

**PediaCare Children's Long-Lasting Cough Plus Cold** oral liquid OTC *antitussive; decongestant* [dextromethorphan hydrobromide; pseudoephedrine HCl] 7.5•15 mg/5 mL

**PediaCare Children's Multi-Symptom Cold** chewable tablets OTC *pediatric antitussive, decongestant, and antihistamine* [dextromethorphan

hydrobromide; pseudoephedrine HCl; chlorpheniramine maleate] 5•15•1 mg

**PediaCare Cold-Allergy** chewable tablets (discontinued 2002) OTC *pediatric decongestant and antihistamine* [pseudoephedrine HCl; chlorpheniramine maleate] 15•1 mg

**PediaCare Cough-Cold** pediatric chewable tablets (discontinued 2002) OTC *antitussive; decongestant; antihistamine* [dextromethorphan hydrobromide; pseudoephedrine HCl; chlorpheniramine maleate] 5•15•1 mg

**PediaCare Cough-Cold; PediaCare Multi-Symptom Cold** pediatric oral liquid OTC *antitussive; decongestant; antihistamine* [dextromethorphan hydrobromide; pseudoephedrine HCl; chlorpheniramine maleate] 10•30•2 mg/10 mL

**PediaCare Fever** oral suspension, oral drops OTC *analgesic; antiarthritic; antipyretic; nonsteroidal anti-inflammatory drug (NSAID)* [ibuprofen] 100 mg/5 mL; 40 mg/mL

**PediaCare Infant's Decongestant** oral drops OTC *nasal decongestant* [pseudoephedrine HCl] 7.5 mg/0.8 mL

**PediaCare Infant's Decongestant & Cough** oral drops OTC *antitussive; decongestant* [dextromethorphan hydrobromide; pseudoephedrine HCl] 5•15 mg/1.6 mL

**PediaCare NightRest Cough & Cold** pediatric oral liquid OTC *antitussive; decongestant; antihistamine* [dextromethorphan hydrobromide; pseudoephedrine HCl; chlorpheniramine maleate] 15•30•2 mg/10 mL

**Pediacof** pediatric syrup (discontinued 2002) ℞ *narcotic antitussive; decongestant; antihistamine; expectorant* [codeine phosphate; phenylephrine HCl; chlorpheniramine maleate; potassium iodide; alcohol 5%] 5•2.5•0.75•75 mg/5 mL

**Pediacon DX** children's syrup, pediatric drops (discontinued 2002) OTC *pediatric antitussive, decongestant, and expectorant* [dextromethorphan hydrobromide; phenylpropanolamine HCl; guaifenesin] 5•6.25•100 mg/5 mL; 5•6.25•50 mg/mL

**Pediacon EX** pediatric drops (discontinued 2002) OTC *decongestant; expectorant* [phenylpropanolamine HCl; guaifenesin] 6.25•50 mg/mL

**Pediaflor** drops ℞ *dental caries preventative* [sodium fluoride] 1.1 mg/mL

**Pedialyte** oral solution, freezer pops OTC *electrolyte replacement* [sodium, potassium, and chloride electrolytes]

**Pediamist** low-pressure nasal spray OTC *nasal moisturizer for children* [sodium chloride (saline solution)]

**Pediapred** oral solution ℞ *corticosteroid; anti-inflammatory* [prednisolone sodium phosphate] 5 mg/5 mL

**Pediarix** IM injection ℞ *active immunizing agent for diphtheria, tetanus, pertussis, hepatitis B and D, and three types of poliovirus* [diphtheria & tetanus toxoids & acellular pertussis (DTaP) vaccine; hepatitis B virus vaccine; inactivated poliovirus vaccine Types 1, 2, and 3] 25 Lf•10 Lf•25 μg•10 μg•40 DU•8 DU•32 DU per 0.5 mL dose

**PediaSure; PediaSure with Fiber** ready-to-use oral liquid OTC *total or supplementary infant feeding*

**Pediatex** oral liquid ℞ *antihistamine* [carbinoxamine maleate] 1.75 mg/5 mL

**Pediatex-D** pediatric oral liquid ℞ *decongestant; antihistamine* [pseudoephedrine HCl; carbinoxamine maleate] 20•2 mg/5 mL

**Pediatex-DM** pediatric oral liquid ℞ *antitussive; decongestant; antihistamine* [dextromethorphan hydrobromide; pseudoephedrine HCl; carbinoxamine maleate] 15•15•2 mg/5 mL

**Pediatric Electrolyte** oral solution OTC *electrolyte replacement* [dextrose; multiple electrolytes] 1 L

**pediatric VAC** *chemotherapy protocol for pediatric sarcomas* [see: VAC pediatric]

**Pediazole** oral suspension ℞ *antibiotic* [erythromycin ethylsuccinate; sulfisoxazole acetyl] 200•600 mg/5 mL

**Pedi-Bath Salts** (discontinued 2000) OTC *bath emollient*

**Pedi-Boro Soak Paks** powder packets OTC *astringent wet dressing (modified Burow solution)* [aluminum sulfate; calcium acetate]

**Pedi-Cort V Creme** (discontinued 2000) ℞ *topical corticosteroidal anti-inflammatory; antifungal; antibacterial* [hydrocortisone; clioquinol] 1%•3%

**pediculicides** *a class of agents effective against head and pubic lice*

**Pedi-Dri** powder ℞ *topical antifungal* [nystatin] 100 000 U/g

**Pediotic** ear drop suspension ℞ *topical corticosteroidal anti-inflammatory; antibiotic* [hydrocortisone; neomycin sulfate; polymyxin B sulfate] 1%•5 mg•10 000 U per mL

**Pediox** pediatric chewable tablets ℞ *decongestant; antihistamine* [pseudoephedrine HCl; chlorpheniramine maleate] 15•2 mg

**Pedi-Pro** foot powder OTC *topical antifungal; anhidrotic* [zinc undecylenate; aluminum chlorohydrate; menthol; chloroxylenol]

**Pedituss Cough** pediatric syrup (discontinued 2002) ℞ *narcotic antitussive; decongestant; antihistamine; expectorant* [codeine phosphate; phenylephrine HCl; chlorpheniramine maleate; potassium iodide] 5•2.5•0.75•75 mg/5 mL

**Pedi-Vit-A Creme** OTC *moisturizer; emollient* [vitamin A] 100 000 U/30 g

**Pedotic** otic suspension ℞ *topical corticosteroidal anti-inflammatory; antibiotic* [hydrocortisone; neomycin sulfate; polymyxin B sulfate] 1%•5 mg•10 000 U per mL

**PedTE-Pak-4** IV injection ℞ *intravenous nutritional therapy* [multiple trace elements (metals)]

**Pedtrace-4** IV injection ℞ *intravenous nutritional therapy* [multiple trace elements (metals)]

**PedvaxHIB** IM injection ℞ *pediatric (2–71 months) vaccine for* Haemophilus influenzae *type b (HIB)* [Hemophilus b conjugate vaccine; *Neisseria meningitidis* OMPC] 7.5•125 μg/dose

**pefloxacin** USAN, INN, BAN *antibacterial*

**pefloxacin mesylate** USAN *antibacterial*

**PEG (polyethylene glycol)** [q.v.]

**pegacaristim** USAN *megakaryocyte stimulating factor for thrombocytopenia*

**PEG-ADA (polyethylene glycol-adenosine deaminase)** [see: pegademase bovine]

**pegademase** INN *adenosine deaminase (ADA) replacement* [also: pegademase bovine]

**pegademase bovine** USAN *adenosine deaminase (ADA) replacement for severe combined immunodeficiency disease (orphan)* [also: pegademase]

**PEG-adenosine deaminase (PEG-ADA)** [see: pegademase bovine]

**Peganone** tablets ℞ *hydantoin anticonvulsant* [ethotoin] 250, 500 mg

**pegaptanib sodium** *investigational (NDA filed) pegylated anti-VEGF (vascular endothelial growth factor) agent for wet age-related macular degeneration*

**PEG-L-asparaginase** [see: pegaspargase]

**pegaspargase (PEG-L-asparaginase)** USAN, INN *antineoplastic for acute lymphocytic leukemia (orphan) and acute lymphoblastic leukemia*

**Pegasys** subcu injection, prefilled syringes ℞ *immunomodulator for chronic hepatitis C; investigational (Phase III) for chronic hepatitis B; investigational (orphan) for renal cell carcinoma* [peginterferon alfa-2a] 180 μg/mL

**PEG-ES (polyethylene glycol–electrolyte solution)** [q.v.]

**pegfilgrastim** *recombinant human granulocyte colony-stimulating factor (G-CSF) in polyethylene glycol (PEG); hematopoietic stimulant for severe chronic neutropenia following cancer chemotherapy*

**PEG-glucocerebrosidase** *investigational (orphan) chronic enzyme replacement therapy for Gaucher disease*

**peginterferon alfa-2a** *immunomodulator for chronic hepatitis C; investigational (orphan) for renal cell carcinoma*

**peginterferon alfa-2b** *immunomodulator for chronic hepatitis C; investigational (Phase III) for malignant melanoma and chronic myelogenous leukemia*

**PEG-interleukin-2** *investigational (Phase II) cytokine for AIDS; investigational (orphan) for primary immunodeficiencies associated with T-cell defects*

**PEG-Intron** powder for subcu injection *antiviral; long-acting formulation of Intron A for chronic hepatitis C; investigational (Phase III) for malignant melanoma and chronic myelogenous leukemia* [peginterferon alfa-2b] 100, 160, 240, 300 μg/mL

**peglicol 5 oleate** USAN *emulsifying agent*

**pegnartograstim** USAN *immunostimulant adjunct to cancer chemotherapy*

**pegorgotein** USAN, INN *free-radical scavenger; investigational to prevent irreversible brain damage after head trauma*

**pegoterate** USAN, INN *suspending agent*

**pegoxol 7 stearate** USAN *emulsifying agent*

**PEG-SOD (polyethylene glycol-superoxide dismutase)** [see: pegorgotein]

**pegvisomant** USAN *growth hormone receptor antagonist for acromegaly (orphan)*

**pegylated megakaryocyte growth factor** [see: megakaryocyte growth and development factor, pegylated, recombinant human]

**pelanserin** INN *antihypertensive; vasodilator; serotonin adrenergic blocker* [also: pelanserin HCl]

**pelanserin HCl** USAN *antihypertensive; vasodilator; serotonin adrenergic blocker* [also: pelanserin]

**peldesine** USAN *purine nucleoside phosphorylase inhibitor for psoriasis; investigational (orphan) for cutaneous T-cell* lymphoma; investigational (Phase III) for HIV

**peliomycin** USAN, INN antineoplastic

**pellants** a class of agents that purify or cleanse the system, particularly the blood [also called: depurants; depuratives]

**pelretin** USAN, INN antikeratinizing agent

**pelrinone** INN cardiotonic [also: pelrinone HCl]

**pelrinone HCl** USAN cardiotonic [also: pelrinone]

**PemADD** tablets (discontinued 2003) ℞ CNS stimulant for attention-deficit hyperactivity disorder (ADHD) [pemoline] 18.75, 37.5, 75 mg

**PemADD CT** chewable tablets ℞ CNS stimulant for attention-deficit hyperactivity disorder (ADHD) [pemoline] 37.5 mg

**pemedolac** USAN, INN analgesic

**pemerid** INN antitussive [also: pemerid nitrate]

**pemerid nitrate** USAN antitussive [also: pemerid]

**pemetrexed disodium** USAN folic acid antagonist; thymidylate synthase inhibitor; dihydrofolate reductase inhibitor; glycinamide ribonucleotide formyl transferase inhibitor; antineoplastic for malignant pleural mesothelioma (MPM)

**pemirolast** INN ophthalmic antiallergic; mast cell stabilizer [also: pemirolast potassium]

**pemirolast potassium** USAN ophthalmic antiallergic; mast cell stabilizer [also: pemirolast]

**pemoline** USAN, INN, BAN, JAN CNS stimulant for attention-deficit hyperactivity disorder (ADHD) and narcolepsy 18.75, 37.5, 75 mg oral

**pempidine** INN, BAN

**penamecillin** USAN, INN, BAN antibacterial

**penbutolol** INN, BAN antiadrenergic (β-receptor) [also: penbutolol sulfate]

**penbutolol sulfate** USAN antiadrenergic (β-receptor) [also: penbutolol]

**penciclovir** USAN, INN, BAN topical antiviral for recurrent herpes labialis

**penciclovir sodium** USAN antiviral for herpes infections

**pendecamaine** INN, BAN

**pendiomide** [see: azamethonium bromide]

**Penecare** cream, lotion OTC moisturizer; emollient [lactic acid]

**Penecort** cream, solution ℞ topical corticosteroidal anti-inflammatory [hydrocortisone] 1%

**penems** a class of broad-spectrum antibiotics

**Penetrex** film-coated tablets (discontinued 2002) ℞ broad-spectrum fluoroquinolone antibiotic [enoxacin] 200, 400 mg

**PenFill** (trademarked form) insulin injector refill cartridge

**penfluridol** USAN, INN antipsychotic

**penflutizide** INN

**pengitoxin** INN

**penicillamine** USAN, USP, INN metal chelating agent; antirheumatic ⁊ penicillin

**penicillin aluminum**

**penicillin benzathine phenoxymethyl** [now: penicillin V benzathine]

**penicillin calcium** USP

**penicillin G benzathine** USP natural penicillin antibiotic [also: benzathine benzylpenicillin; benzathine penicillin; benzylpenicillin benzathine]

**penicillin G hydrabamine** natural penicillin antibiotic

**penicillin G potassium** USP natural penicillin antibiotic [also: benzylpenicillin potassium] 1, 2, 3, 5, 10, 20 million U injection

**penicillin G procaine** USP natural penicillin antibiotic [also: procaine penicillin] 600 000, 1 200 000 U injection

**penicillin G redox** [see: redox-penicillin G]

**penicillin G sodium** USP natural penicillin antibiotic [also: benzylpenicillin sodium] 5 million U injection

**penicillin hydrabamine phenoxy-
methyl** [now: penicillin V hydraba-
mine]

**penicillin N** [see: adicillin]

**penicillin O** [see: almecillin]

**penicillin O chloroprocaine**

**penicillin O potassium**

**penicillin O sodium**

**penicillin phenoxymethyl** [now:
penicillin V]

**penicillin potassium G** [see: penicillin G potassium]

**penicillin potassium phenoxymethyl**
[now: penicillin V potassium]

**penicillin V** USAN, USP *natural penicillin antibiotic* [also: phenoxymethyl-
penicillin]

**penicillin V benzathine** USAN, USP
*natural penicillin antibiotic*

**penicillin V hydrabamine** USAN, USP
*natural penicillin antibiotic*

**penicillin V potassium** USAN, USP
*natural penicillin antibiotic*

**Penicillin VK** tablets, powder for oral
solution ℞ *natural penicillin antibiotic*
[penicillin V potassium] 250, 500
mg; 125, 250 mg/5 mL

**penicillin-152 potassium** [see: phenethicillin potassium] 🄌 penicillamine; Polycillin

**penicillinase** INN, BAN

**penicillinase-resistant penicillins** *a
subclass of penicillins (q.v.)*

**penicillinphenyrazine** [see: phenyra-
cillin]

**penicillins** *a class of bactericidal antibiotics, divided into natural, penicillinase-
resistant, aminopenicillin, and extended-
spectrum penicillins, and effective against
both gram-positive and gram-negative
bacteria* [also called: "cillins"]

**penidural** [see: benzathine penicillin]

**penimepicycline** INN

**penimocycline** INN

**PenInject** (trademarked delivery
device) *prefilled self-injection syringe*

**penirolol** INN

**Pen-Kera** cream OTC *moisturizer; emollient*

**Penlac Nail Lacquer** topical solution
℞ *antifungal for onychomycosis*
[ciclopirox] 8%

**penmesterol** INN

**pennyroyal (*Hedeoma pulegeoides;
Mentha pulegium*)** plant *medicinal
herb for childbirth pain, colds, colic,
fever, gas, inducing abortion and menstruation, mouth sores, respiratory illnesses, and venomous bites; also used
as an insect repellent; not generally
regarded as safe and effective for ingestion due to toxicity*

**penoctonium bromide** INN

**penprostene** INN

**penta tea** *medicinal herb* [see: jiaogulan]

**pentabamate** USAN, INN *minor tranquilizer*

**Pentacarinat** IV or IM injection ℞
*antiprotozoal; treatment and prophy-
laxis of* Pneumocystis carinii *pneumonia (orphan)* [pentamidine isethio-
nate] 300 mg

**Pentacea** ℞ *investigational (orphan)
antineoplastic for small cell lung cancer*

**Pentacel** ℞ *investigational (Phase III)
vaccine for diphtheria, pertussis, tetanus (DPT), polio, and hemophilus
influenza type B*

**pentacosactride** BAN [also: norleusac-
tide]

**pentacynium chloride** INN

**pentacyone chloride** [see: pentacynium chloride]

**pentaerithritol tetranicotinate** [see:
niceritrol]

**pentaerithrityl tetranitrate** INN *vasodilator* [also: pentaerythritol tetranitrate]

**pentaerythritol tetranitrate (PETN)**
USP *coronary vasodilator; antianginal*
[also: pentaerithrityl tetranitrate]

**pentaerythritol trinitrate** [see: pen-
trinitrol]

**pentafilcon A** USAN *hydrophilic contact
lens material*

**pentafluranol** INN, BAN

**pentafuside** *investigational (Phase II)
antiviral fusion inhibitor for HIV and
AIDS*

**pentagastrin** USAN, INN, JAN *gastric secretion indicator*

**pentagestrone** INN

**pentalamide** INN, BAN

**pentalyte** USAN, USP, NF *electrolyte combination*

**Pentam 300** IV or IM injection ℞ *antiprotozoal; treatment and prophylaxis of* Pneumocystis carinii *pneumonia (orphan)* [pentamidine isethionate] 300 mg

**pentamethazene** [see: azamethonium bromide]

**pentamethonium bromide** INN, BAN

**pentamethylenetetrazol** [see: pentylenetetrazol]

**pentamidine** INN, BAN

**pentamidine isethionate** *antiprotozoal; treatment and prophylaxis of* Pneumocystis carinii *pneumonia (orphan)* 300 mg injection

**pentamin** [see: azamethonium bromide]

**pentamorphone** USAN, INN *narcotic analgesic*

**pentamoxane** INN

**pentamoxane HCl** [see: pentamoxane]

**pentamustine** USAN *antineoplastic* [also: neptamustine]

**pentanedial** [see: glutaral]

**pentanitrol** [see: pentaerythritol tetranitrate]

**pentaphonate**

**pentapiperide** INN

**pentapiperium methylsulfate** USAN *anticholinergic* [also: pentapiperium metilsulfate]

**pentapiperium metilsulfate** INN *anticholinergic* [also: pentapiperium methylsulfate]

**pentaquine** INN [also: pentaquine phosphate]

**pentaquine phosphate** USP [also: pentaquine]

**Pentasa** controlled-release capsules ℞ *anti-inflammatory for active ulcerative colitis, proctosigmoiditis, and proctitis* [mesalamine (5-aminosalicylic acid)] 250 mg

**pentasodium colistinmethanesulfonate** [see: colistimethate sodium]

**Pentaspan** ℞ *leukapheresis adjunct to improve leukocyte yield (orphan)* [pentastarch]

**pentastarch** USAN, BAN *leukapheresis adjunct; red cell sedimenting agent; centrifugal leukocyte harvesting aid (orphan)*

**pentavalent gas gangrene antitoxin**

**Pentazine VC with Codeine** oral liquid (discontinued 2002) ℞ *narcotic antitussive; antihistamine* [codeine phosphate; promethazine HCl] 10•6.25 mg/5 mL

**pentazocine** USAN, USP, INN, BAN *narcotic agonist-antagonist analgesic; also abused as a street drug*

**pentazocine HCl** USAN, USP *narcotic agonist-antagonist analgesic; also abused as a street drug*

**pentazocine HCl & acetaminophen** *narcotic analgesic* 25•650 mg oral

**pentazocine lactate** USAN, USP *analgesic*

**pentazocine & naloxone HCl** *narcotic agonist-antagonist analgesic; also abused as a street drug* 50•0.5 mg oral

**pentetate calcium trisodium (Ca-DTPA)** USAN *chelating agent for plutonium, americium, and curium; approved to treat contamination from radioactive materials (radiation sickness from "dirty bombs")* [also: calcium trisodium pentetate]

**pentetate calcium trisodium Yb 169** USAN *radioactive agent*

**pentetate disodium** [see: pentetic acid, sodium salts]

**pentetate indium disodium In 111** USAN *diagnostic aid; radioactive agent*

**pentetate monosodium** [see: pentetic acid, sodium salts]

**pentetate pentasodium** [see: pentetic acid, sodium salts]

**pentetate tetrasodium** [see: pentetic acid, sodium salts]

**pentetate trisodium** [see: pentetic acid, sodium salts]

**pentetate trisodium calcium** [see: pentetate calcium trisodium]

**pentetate zinc trisodium (Zn-DTPA)** *chelating agent for plutonium, ameri-*

*cium, and curium; approved to treat contamination from radioactive materials (radiation sickness from "dirty bombs")*

**pentethylcyclanone** [see: cyclexanone]

**pentetic acid** USAN, BAN *diagnostic aid*

**pentetic acid, sodium salts** *diagnostic aid*

**pentetrazol** INN [also: pentylenetetrazol]

**penthanil diethylenetriamine penta-acetic acid (DTPA)** [see: pentetic acid]

**penthienate bromide** NF

**Penthrane** liquid for vaporization ℞ *inhalation general anesthetic* [methoxyflurane]

**penthrichloral** INN, BAN

**pentiapine** INN *antipsychotic* [also: pentiapine maleate]

**pentiapine maleate** USAN *antipsychotic* [also: pentiapine]

**penticide** [see: chlorophenothane]

**pentifylline** INN, BAN

**pentigetide** USAN, INN *antiallergic*

**pentisomicin** USAN, INN *anti-infective*

**pentisomide** INN

**pentizidone** INN *antibacterial* [also: pentizidone sodium]

**pentizidone sodium** USAN *antibacterial* [also: pentizidone]

**pentobarbital** USP, INN *sedative; hypnotic; also abused as a street drug* [also: pentobarbitone; pentobarbital calcium] ⊘ phenobarbital

**pentobarbital calcium** JAN *sedative; hypnotic; also abused as a street drug* [also: pentobarbital; pentobarbitone]

**pentobarbital sodium** USP, JAN *sedative; hypnotic; also abused as a street drug* [also: pentobarbitone sodium] 100 mg oral; 50 mg/mL injection

**pentobarbitone** BAN *sedative; hypnotic; also abused as a street drug* [also: pentobarbital]

**pentobarbitone sodium** BAN *sedative; hypnotic; also abused as a street drug* [also: pentobarbital sodium]

**Pentolair** eye drops ℞ *mydriatic; cycloplegic* [cyclopentolate HCl] 1%

**pentolinium tartrate** NF [also: pentolonium tartrate]

**pentolonium tartrate** INN [also: pentolinium tartrate]

**pentolonum bitartrate** [see: pentolinium tartrate]

**pentomone** USAN, INN *prostate growth inhibitor*

**pentopril** USAN, INN *angiotensin-converting enzyme (ACE) inhibitor*

**pentorex** INN

**pentosalen** BAN

**pentosan polysulfate sodium** USAN, INN *urinary tract anti-inflammatory and analgesic for interstitial cystitis (orphan)* [also: pentosan polysulphate sodium]

**pentosan polysulphate sodium** BAN *urinary tract anti-inflammatory and analgesic* [also: pentosan polysulfate sodium]

**Pentostam** (available only from the Centers for Disease Control) ℞ *investigational anti-infective for leishmaniasis* [sodium stibogluconate]

**pentostatin** USAN, INN *potentiator; antibiotic antineoplastic for hairy cell leukemia (orphan); investigational (orphan) for chronic lymphocytic leukemia and cutaneous T-cell lymphoma; investigational (Phase III) for AIDS-related non-Hodgkin lymphoma*

**Pentothal** powder for IV injection ℞ *barbiturate general anesthetic* [thiopental sodium] 2%, 2.5% (20, 25 mg/mL) ⊘ pentrinitrol

**pentoxifylline** USAN, INN *peripheral vasodilator; hemorheologic agent* [also: oxpentifylline] 400 mg oral

**pentoxiverine citrate** [see: carbetapentane citrate]

**pentoxyverine** INN [also: carbetapentane citrate]

**pentoxyverine citrate** [see: carbetapentane citrate]

**Pentrax** shampoo OTC *antiseborrheic; antipsoriatic; antipruritic; antibacterial* [coal tar] 5%

**Pentrax Gold** shampoo (discontinued 2003) OTC *antiseborrheic; antipsoriatic; antipruritic; antibacterial* [coal tar] 4%

**pentrinitrol** USAN, INN *coronary vasodilator* ⊘ Pentothal *tert*-**pentyl alcohol** [see: amylene hydrate]

**6-pentyl-*m*-cresol** [see: amylmetacresol]

**pentylenetetrazol** NF [also: pentetrazol]

**pentymal** [see: amobarbital]

**Pen-Vee K** tablets, powder for oral solution (discontinued 2002) ℞ *natural penicillin antibiotic* [penicillin V potassium] 250, 500 mg; 125, 250 mg/5 mL

**peony (*Paeonia officinalis*) root** (other parts are poisonous) *medicinal herb used as an antispasmodic, diuretic, and sedative*

**Pepcid** film-coated tablets, powder for oral suspension, IV injection, preloaded syringes for IV ℞ *histamine H₂ antagonist for gastric and duodenal ulcers* [famotidine] 20, 40 mg; 40 mg/5 mL; 10 mg/mL; 20 mg

**Pepcid AC** ("acid controller") tablets, chewable tablets, gelcaps OTC *histamine H₂ antagonist for heartburn and acid indigestion* [famotidine] 10, 20 mg

**Pepcid Complete** chewable tablets OTC *combination antacid and histamine H₂ antagonist for heartburn and acid indigestion* [calcium carbonate; magnesium hydroxide; famotidine] 800•165•10 mg

**Pepcid RPD** rapidly disintegrating tablets ℞ *histamine H₂ antagonist for gastric and duodenal ulcers* [famotidine] 20, 40 mg

**pepleomycin** [see: peplomycin sulfate]

**peplomycin** INN *antineoplastic* [also: peplomycin sulfate]

**peplomycin sulfate** USAN *antineoplastic* [also: peplomycin]

**pepper, African red; American red pepper; bird pepper; cayenne pepper; chili pepper; cockspur pepper; garden pepper; red pepper; Spanish pepper** *medicinal herb* [see: cayenne]

**pepper, Jamaica** *medicinal herb* [see: allspice]

**pepper, java; tailed pepper** *medicinal herb* [see: cubeb]

**pepper, water** *medicinal herb* [see: knotweed]

**pepper, wild** *medicinal herb* [see: mezereon]

**pepperidge bush** *medicinal herb* [see: barberry]

**peppermint** NF *flavoring agent; perfume*

**peppermint (*Mentha piperita*) leaves** *medicinal herb for appetite stimulation, colds, colic, indigestion, fever, gas and heartburn, headache, shock, sore throat, and toothache*

**peppermint oil** NF *flavoring agent*

**peppermint spirit** USP *flavoring agent; perfume*

**peppermint water** NF *flavored vehicle*

**pepsin** *digestive aid*

**pepstatin** USAN, INN *pepsin enzyme inhibitor*

**Peptamen** ready-to-use oral liquid OTC *enteral nutritional therapy for GI impairment*

**Peptavlon** subcu injection (discontinued 2002) ℞ *in vivo diagnostic aid for gastrointestinal function* [pentagastrin] 250 μg/mL

**Peptic Relief** chewable tablets, oral liquid OTC *antidiarrheal; antinauseant* [bismuth subsalicylate] 262 mg; 262 mg/15 mL

**peptide YY (PYY)** *endogenous peptides manufactured in the GI tract postprandially in proportion to the caloric content of a meal; subdivided into PYY 1-36 (PYY-I) and PYY 3-36 (PYY-II); exogenous administration of PYY 3-36 is investigational for weight loss*

**Peptinex; Peptinex DT** oral liquid OTC *enteral nutritional treatment for patients with GI impairment* [whey protein–based] 8 oz./pkt.

**Pepto Diarrhea Control** oral solution OTC *antidiarrheal* [loperamide HCl] 1 mg/5 mL

**Pepto-Bismol** chewable tablets, caplets, oral liquid OTC *antidiarrheal; antinauseant* [bismuth subsalicylate] 262 mg; 262 mg; 262, 524 mg/15 mL

**peraclopone** INN

**peradoxime** INN

**perafensine** INN

**peralopride** INN

**peramivir** USAN *neuraminidase inhibitor for influenza A and B virus infections*

**peraquinsin** INN

**perastine** INN

**peratizole** INN, BAN

**perbufylline** INN

**Perchloracap** capsules ℞ *radioimaging adjunct* [potassium perchlorate] 200 mg

**Percocet** tablets ℞ *narcotic analgesic* [oxycodone HCl; acetaminophen] 2.5•325, 5•325, 7.5•325, 7.5•500, 10•325, 10•650 mg

**Percodan; Percodan-Demi** tablets ℞ *narcotic analgesic; also abused as a street drug* [oxycodone HCl; oxycodone terephthalate; aspirin] 4.5•0.38•325 mg; 2.25•0.19•325 mg ② Decadron

**Percogesic** tablets OTC *antihistamine; analgesic* [phenyltoloxamine citrate; acetaminophen] 30•325 mg

**Percogesic Extra Strength** caplets OTC *antihistamine; analgesic* [diphenhydramine HCl; acetaminophen] 12.5•500 mg

**Percolone** tablets ℞ *narcotic analgesic* [oxycodone HCl] 5 mg

**Perdiem** granules OTC *bulk laxative* [psyllium] 4.03 g/tsp. ② Pyridium

**Perdiem Overnight Relief** granules OTC *bulk laxative; stimulant laxative* [psyllium; senna] 3.25•0.74 g/tsp.

**Perfect Image** (CAM) capsules OTC *chromium supplement* [chromium chloride] 200 µg

**Perfectoderm** gel (discontinued 2003) OTC *keratolytic for acne* [benzoyl peroxide] 5%

**perfilcon A** USAN *hydrophilic contact lens material*

**perflenapent** USAN *ultrasound contrast medium*

**perflexane** USAN *investigational (NDA filed) ultrasound contrast medium for cardiac imaging*

**perflisopent** USAN *ultrasound contrast medium*

**perfluamine** INN, BAN

**perflubron** USAN, INN *blood substitute; oral MRI contrast medium; investigational (Phase III) agent for pediatric acute respiratory distress syndrome (ARDS); investigational (Phase III) intravascular oxygen carrier to reduce need for blood transfusions in surgery patients*

**perflunafene** INN, BAN

**perflutren** USAN *ultrasound contrast medium for cardiac imaging; investigational (Phase III) for gynecologic imaging*

**perfomedil** INN

**perfosfamide** USAN *antineoplastic*

**pergolide** INN, BAN *dopamine agonist; antiparkinsonian* [also: pergolide mesylate]

**pergolide mesylate** USAN *dopamine agonist; antiparkinsonian; investigational (orphan) for Tourette syndrome* [also: pergolide] 0.05, 0.25, 1 mg oral

**Pergonal** powder for IM injection ℞ *ovulation stimulant for women; spermatogenesis stimulant for men* [menotropins] 75, 150 IU

**perhexiline** INN *coronary vasodilator* [also: perhexiline maleate]

**perhexiline maleate** USAN *coronary vasodilator* [also: perhexiline]

**Periactin** syrup (discontinued 2001) ℞ *piperidine antihistamine* [cyproheptadine HCl] 2 mg/5 mL ② Taractan

**Periactin** tablets (discontinued 2002) ℞ *piperidine antihistamine* [cyproheptadine HCl] 4 mg ② Taractan

**periciazine** INN *phenothiazine antipsychotic* [also: pericyazine]

**Peri-Colace** capsules, syrup (discontinued 2003) OTC *stimulant laxative; stool softener* [casanthranol; docusate sodium] 30•100 mg; 30•60 mg/15 mL

**PeriColace** tablets OTC *stimulant laxative; stool softener* [sennosides; docusate sodium] 8.6•50 mg

**pericyazine** BAN *phenothiazine antipsychotic* [also: periciazine]

**Peridex** mouth rinse ℞ *antimicrobial; gingivitis treatment; investigational (orphan) for oral mucositis in bone mar-*

row transplant patients [chlorhexidine gluconate; alcohol 11.6%] 0.12%

**Peridin-C** tablets OTC *vitamin C supplement with bioflavonoids* [ascorbic acid; hesperidin] 200•200 mg

**Peri-Dose** softgels (discontinued 2003) OTC *stimulant laxative; stool softener* [casanthranol; docusate sodium] 30• 100 mg

**perilla (Perilla frutescens)** plant *medicinal herb for asthma, inducing sweating, nausea, gastrointestinal spasms, and sunstroke*

**perillyl alcohol (POH)** *investigational (Phase II) monoterpene antineoplastic for advanced colorectal carcinoma and pancreatic cancer*

**perimetazine** INN

**perindopril** USAN, INN, BAN *antihypertensive; angiotensin-converting enzyme (ACE) inhibitor*

**perindopril erbumine** USAN *antihypertensive; angiotensin-converting enzyme (ACE) inhibitor*

**perindoprilat** INN, BAN

**PerioChip** biodegradable polymer implant ℞ *antimicrobial adjunct to scaling and root planing procedures in periodontitis* [chlorhexidine gluconate] 2.5 mg

**PerioGard** mouth rinse ℞ *antimicrobial; gingivitis treatment* [chlorhexidine gluconate; alcohol 11.6%] 0.12%

**PerioMed** oral rinse ℞ *dental caries preventative* [stannous fluoride] 0.64%

**Periostat** capsules (discontinued 2001) ℞ *antibiotic for periodontal disease* [doxycycline hyclate] 20 mg

**Periostat** tablets ℞ *antibiotic for periodontal disease* [doxycycline hyclate] 20 mg

**peripheral vasodilators** *a class of cardiovascular drugs that cause dilation of the blood vessels*

*Periploca sylvestris* medicinal herb [see: gymnema]

**perisoxal** INN

**periwinkle (Catharanthus roseus)** plant *medicinal herb for cancer, diabetes, diarrhea, insect stings, nervous-*

ness, ocular inflammation, and ulcers; not generally regarded as safe and effective for ingestion because of toxicity

**perlapine** USAN, INN *hypnotic*

**Perles** (dosage form) *soft gelatin capsule*

**permanganic acid, potassium salt** [see: potassium permanganate]

**Permapen** Isoject (unit dose syringe) for deep IM injection ℞ *natural penicillin antibiotic* [penicillin G benzathine] 1 200 000 U

**Permax** tablets ℞ *dopamine agonist; antiparkinsonian; investigational (orphan) for Tourette syndrome* [pergolide mesylate] 0.05, 0.25, 1 mg

**permethrin** USAN, INN, BAN *ectoparasiticide for scabies and lice* 1%, 5% topical

**Permitil** tablets, oral concentrate (discontinued 2002) ℞ *conventional (typical) antipsychotic* [fluphenazine HCl] 2.5, 5, 10 mg; 5 mg/mL

*Perna canaliculus* natural remedy [see: New Zealand green-lipped mussel]

**Pernox Scrub; Pernox Lathering Lotion** OTC *abrasive cleanser for acne* [sulfur; salicylic acid]

**peroxide, dibenzoyl** [see: benzoyl peroxide]

**Peroxin A 5; Peroxin A 10** gel (discontinued 2003) ℞ *keratolytic for acne* [benzoyl peroxide] 5%; 10%

**peroxisome proliferator-activated receptor (PPAR) agonists** *a class of investigational agents that increase insulin receptor sensitivity in type 2 diabetes*

**Peroxyl** mouth rinse, oral gel OTC *cleansing of oral wounds* [hydrogen peroxide] 1.5%

**perphenazine** USP, INN *phenothiazine antipsychotic; antiemetic; intractable hiccough relief* 2, 4, 8, 16 mg oral; 16 mg/5 mL oral

**Persa-Gel; Persa-Gel W 5%; Persa-Gel W 10%** gel (discontinued 2003) ℞ *keratolytic for acne* [benzoyl peroxide] 5%, 10%; 5%; 10%

**Persantine** sugar-coated tablets ℞ *platelet aggregation inhibitor* [dipyridamole] 25, 50, 75 mg ⏣ Pertofrane

**Persantine IV** injection ℞ *diagnostic aid for coronary artery function* [dipyridamole] 10 mg

*Persea americana; P. gratissima* medicinal herb [see: avocado]

**Persian bark; Persian berries** medicinal herb [see: buckthorn]

**Persian walnut** medicinal herb [see: English walnut]

**persic oil** NF *vehicle*

**persilic acid** INN

**Pertropin** capsules (discontinued 2003) OTC *dietary lipotropic agent* [linolenic acid; multiple essential fatty acids] 7 mins.

**Pertussin CS; Pertussin ES** syrup (discontinued 2002) OTC *antitussive* [dextromethorphan hydrobromide] 3.5 mg/5 mL; 15 mg/5 mL

**pertussis immune globulin** USP *passive immunizing agent*

**pertussis immune human globulin** [now: pertussis immune globulin]

**pertussis vaccine** USP *active immunizing agent*

**pertussis vaccine, acellular** [see: diphtheria & tetanus toxoids & acellular pertussis (DTaP) vaccine, adsorbed]

**pertussis vaccine, component** (alternate name for acellular pertussis vaccine) [see: diphtheria & tetanus toxoids & acellular pertussis (DTaP) vaccine, adsorbed]

**pertussis vaccine, whole-cell** [see: diphtheria & tetanus toxoids & whole-cell pertussis (DTwP) vaccine, adsorbed]

**pertussis vaccine adsorbed** USP *active immunizing agent*

**Peruvian balsam** NF *topical local protectant; rubefacient*

**Peruvian balsam** *(Myroxylon balsamum; M. pereirae)* oil medicinal herb for edema, expelling worms, hemostasis, topical infections, and wound healing

**Peruvian bark; yellow Peruvian bark** medicinal herb [see: quinine]

**Peruvian ginseng** medicinal herb [see: maca]

*Petasites hybridus* medicinal herb [see: butterbur]

**pethidine** INN, BAN *narcotic analgesic; also abused as a street drug* [also: meperidine HCl]

**pethidine HCl** [see: meperidine HCl]

**PETN (pentaerythritol tetranitrate)** [q.v.]

**petrichloral** INN

**petrolatum** USP *ointment base; emollient/protectant* [also: yellow petrolatum]

**petrolatum, hydrophilic** USP *absorbent ointment base; topical protectant*

**petrolatum, liquid** [see: mineral oil]

**petrolatum, liquid emulsion** [see: mineral oil emulsion]

**petrolatum, white** USP, JAN *oleaginous ointment base; topical protectant*

**petrolatum gauze** [see: gauze, petrolatum]

**petroleum benzin** [see: benzin, petroleum]

**petroleum distillate inhalants** *vapors from butane, toluene, acetone, benzene, gasoline, etc. which produce psychoactive effects, abused as street drugs* [see also: nitrous oxide; volatile nitrites]

**petroleum jelly** [see: petrolatum]

*Petroselinum sativum* medicinal herb [see: parsley]

*Peumus boldus* medicinal herb [see: boldo]

**pexantel** INN

**Pexeva** tablets ℞ *selective serotonin reuptake inhibitor (SSRI) for depression, obsessive-compulsive disorder, panic disorder, social anxiety disorder, generalized anxiety disorder, and posttraumatic stress disorder* [paroxetine HCl] 10, 20, 30, 40 mg

**pexiganan acetate** USAN *investigational (NDA filed) broad-spectrum topical antibiotic for impetigo and diabetic foot ulcers*

**PFA (phosphonoformic acid)** [see: foscarnet sodium]

*Pfaffia paniculata* medicinal herb [see: suma]

**Pfeiffer's Cold Sore** lotion OTC *topical oral anesthetic; analgesic; counterirritant* [gum benzoin; camphor; menthol; eucalyptol; alcohol 85%] 7%• <u>?</u> • <u>?</u> • <u>?</u>

**Pfizerpen** powder for injection ℞ *natural penicillin antibiotic* [penicillin G potassium] 1, 5, 20 million U

**PFL (Platinol, fluorouracil, leucovorin [rescue])** *chemotherapy protocol for head, neck, and gastric cancer*

**PFT (L-phenylalanine mustard, fluorouracil, tamoxifen)** *chemotherapy protocol*

**PG (paregoric)** [q.v.]

**PG (prostaglandin)** [q.v.]

**PGA (pteroylglutamic acid)** [see: folic acid]

**PGE₁ (prostaglandin E₁)** [now: alprostadil]

**PGE₂ (prostaglandin E₂)** [now: dinoprostone]

**PGF₂α (prostaglandin F₂α)** [see: dinoprost]

**PGF₂α (prostaglandin F₂α) THAM** [see: dinoprost tromethamine]

**PGI₂ (prostaglandin I₂)** [now: epoprostenol]

**PGX (prostaglandin X)** [now: epoprostenol]

*Phaenicia sericata* natural treatment [see: maggots]

**Phanadex Cough** syrup (discontinued 2002) OTC *antitussive; decongestant; antihistamine; expectorant* [dextromethorphan hydrobromide; phenylpropanolamine HCl; pyrilamine maleate; guaifenesin] 15•25•40•100 mg/5 mL

**Phanatuss DM Cough** syrup OTC *antitussive; expectorant* [dextromethorphan hydrobromide; guaifenesin] 20•200 mg/10 mL

**phanchinone** [see: phanquinone; phanquone]

**phanquinone** INN [also: phanquone]

**phanquone** BAN [also: phanquinone]

**pharmaceutical glaze** [see: glaze, pharmaceutical]

**Pharmaflur; Pharmaflur df; Pharmaflur 1.1** chewable tablets ℞ *dental caries preventative* [sodium fluoride] 2.2 mg; 2.2 mg; 1.1 mg

**Pharmalgen** subcu or IM injection ℞ *venom sensitivity testing (subcu); venom desensitization therapy (IM)* [extracts of honeybee, yellow jacket, yellow hornet, white-faced hornet, mixed vespid, and wasp venom]

*Pharmia regina* natural treatment [see: maggots]

**Pharmorubicin PFS; Pharmorubicin RDF** ⓒⓐⓝ injection ℞ *antibiotic antineoplastic* [epirubicin HCl] 2 mg/mL; 10, 20, 50, 150 mg

**Phazyme** tablets, drops OTC *antiflatulent* [simethicone] 60 mg; 40 mg/0.6 mL ⑦ Pherazine

**Phazyme** ⓒⓐⓝ oral liquid OTC *antiflatulent* [simethicone] 125 mg/5 mL

**Phazyme 95** tablets OTC *antiflatulent* [simethicone] 95 mg

**Phazyme 125** softgels OTC *antiflatulent* [simethicone] 125 mg

**phebutazine** [see: febuverine]

**phebutyrazine** [see: febuverine]

**phemfilcon A** USAN *hydrophilic contact lens material*

**phenacaine** INN [also: phenacaine HCl]

**phenacaine HCl** USP [also: phenacaine]

**phenacemide** USP, INN, BAN *anticonvulsant*

**phenacetin** USP, INN *(withdrawn from market)* ⑦ phenazocine

**phenacon** [see: fenaclon]

**phenactropinium chloride** INN, BAN

**phenacyl 4-morpholineacetate** [see: mobecarb]

**N-phenacylhomatropinium chloride** [see: phenactropinium chloride]

**phenacylpivalate** [see: pibecarb]

**phenadoxone** INN, BAN

**Phenadoz** suppositories ℞ *antihistamine; sedative; antiemetic; motion sickness relief* [promethazine HCl] 12.5, 25 mg

**phenaglycodol** INN

**Phenahist-TR** sustained-release tablets (discontinued 2001) ℞ *deconges-*

*tant; antihistamine; anticholinergic* [phenylpropanolamine HCl; phenylephrine HCl; chlorpheniramine maleate; hyoscyamine sulfate; atropine sulfate; scopolamine hydrobromide] 50•25•8•0.19•0.04•0.01 mg

**phenamazoline** INN

**phenamazoline HCl** [see: phenamazoline]

**Phenameth DM** syrup (discontinued 2002) ℞ *antitussive; antihistamine* [dextromethorphan hydrobromide; promethazine HCl; alcohol] 15•6.25 mg/5 mL

**phenampromide** INN

**Phenapap** tablets OTC *decongestant; analgesic* [pseudoephedrine HCl; acetaminophen] 30•325 mg

**Phenapap Sinus Headache & Congestion** tablets (discontinued 2002) OTC *decongestant; antihistamine; analgesic* [pseudoephedrine HCl; chlorpheniramine maleate; acetaminophen] 30•2•325 mg

**Phenaphen with Codeine No. 3 & No. 4** capsules (discontinued 2004) ℞ *narcotic antitussive; analgesic* [codeine phosphate; acetaminophen] 30•325 mg; 60•325 mg

**phenaphthazine**

**phenarbutal** [see: phetharbital]

**phenarsone sulfoxylate** INN

**Phenaseptic** throat spray OTC *antipruritic/counterirritant; mild local anesthetic* [phenol] 1.4%

**Phenate** timed-release tablets (discontinued 2001) ℞ *decongestant; antihistamine; analgesic* [phenylpropanolamine HCl; chlorpheniramine maleate; acetaminophen] 40•4•325 mg

**PhenaVent LA; PhenaVent D** film-coated caplets ℞ *decongestant; expectorant* [phenylephrine HCl; guaifenesin] 30•600 mg; 40•1200 mg

**Phenazo** ⒸⒶ⒩ tablets ℞ *urinary analgesic* [phenazopyridine HCl] 100, 200 mg

**phenazocine** INN ⊡ phenacetin

**phenazocine hydrobromide** [see: phenazocine]

**phenazone** INN, BAN *analgesic* [also: antipyrine]

**phenazopyridine** INN, BAN *urinary tract analgesic* [also: phenazopyridine HCl]

**phenazopyridine HCl** USAN, USP *urinary tract analgesic* [also: phenazopyridine] 100, 200 mg oral

**phenbenicillin** BAN [also: fenbenicillin]

**phenbutazone sodium glycerate** USAN *anti-inflammatory*

**phenbutrazate** BAN [also: fenbutrazate]

**phencarbamide** USAN *anticholinergic* [also: fencarbamide]

**Phenchlor S.H.A.** sustained-release tablets (discontinued 2001) ℞ *decongestant; antihistamine; anticholinergic* [phenylpropanolamine HCl; phenylephrine HCl; chlorpheniramine maleate; hyoscyamine sulfate; atropine sulfate; scopolamine hydrobromide] 50•25•8•0.19•0.04•0.01 mg

**phencyclidine** INN *anesthetic* [also: phencyclidine HCl]

**phencyclidine HCl** USAN *anesthetic* [also: phencyclidine]

**phendimetrazine** INN *anorexiant* [also: phendimetrazine tartrate]

**phendimetrazine tartrate** USP *anorexiant; CNS stimulant* [also: phendimetrazine] 35 mg oral

**phenelzine** INN, BAN *antidepressant; MAO inhibitor* [also: phenelzine sulfate] ⊡ Phenazine; Phenylzin

**phenelzine sulfate** USP *antidepressant; MAO inhibitor* [also: phenelzine]

**phenemal** [see: phenobarbital]

**Phenerbel-S** tablets ℞ *GI anticholinergic; sedative; analgesic* [belladonna alkaloids; phenobarbital; ergotamine tartrate] 0.2•40•0.6 mg

**Phenergan** tablets, suppositories, injection ℞ *antihistamine; sedative; antiemetic; motion sickness relief* [promethazine HCl] 12.5, 25, 50 mg; 12.5, 25, 50 mg; 25, 50 mg/mL ⊡ Phenaphen; Theragran

**Phenergan Fortis** syrup (discontinued 2002) ℞ *antihistamine; sedative; antiemetic; motion sickness relief* [promethazine HCl; alcohol 1.5%] 25 mg/5 mL

**Phenergan Plain** syrup (discontinued 2002) ℞ *antihistamine; sedative; antiemetic; motion sickness relief* [promethazine HCl] 6.25 mg/5 mL

**Phenergan VC** syrup (discontinued 2004) ℞ *decongestant; antihistamine* [phenylephrine HCl; promethazine HCl; alcohol 7%] 5•6.25 mg/5 mL

**Phenergan VC with Codeine** syrup (discontinued 2002) ℞ *narcotic antitussive; decongestant; antihistamine* [codeine phosphate; phenylephrine HCl; promethazine HCl; alcohol 7%] 10•5•6.25 mg/5 mL

**Phenergan with Codeine** syrup (discontinued 2002) ℞ *narcotic antitussive; antihistamine* [codeine phosphate; promethazine HCl; alcohol 7%] 10•6.25 mg/5 mL

**Phenergan with Dextromethorphan** syrup (discontinued 2002) ℞ *antitussive; antihistamine* [dextromethorphan hydrobromide; promethazine HCl; alcohol 7%] 15•6.25 mg/5 mL

**pheneridine** INN

**phenethanol** [see: phenylethyl alcohol]

**phenethazine** [see: fenethazine]

**phenethicillin potassium** USP [also: pheneticillin]

**phenethyl alcohol** BAN *antimicrobial agent* [also: phenylethyl alcohol]

**N-phenethylanthranilic acid** [see: enfenamic acid]

**phenethylazocine bromide** [see: phenazocine hydrobromide]

**phenethylhydrazine sulfate** [see: phenelzine sulfate]

**pheneticillin** INN [also: phenethicillin potassium]

**pheneticillin potassium** [see: phenethicillin potassium]

**phenetsal** [see: acetaminosalol]

**pheneturide** INN, BAN [also: acetylpheneturide]

**Phenex-1** powder OTC *formula for infants with phenylketonuria*

**Phenex-2** powder OTC *enteral nutritional therapy for phenylketonuria (PKU)*

**phenformin** INN, BAN *biguanide hypoglycemic agent* [also: phenformin HCl]

**phenformin HCl** USP *hypoglycemic agent (removed from market by FDA in 1977, now available as an investigational drug)* [also: phenformin]

**phenglutarimide** INN, BAN

**Phenhist DH with Codeine** oral liquid (discontinued 2002) ℞ *narcotic antitussive; decongestant; antihistamine* [codeine phosphate; pseudoephedrine HCl; chlorpheniramine maleate; alcohol 5%] 10•30•2 mg/5 mL

**Phenhist Expectorant** oral liquid (discontinued 2002) ℞ *narcotic antitussive; decongestant; expectorant* [codeine phosphate; pseudoephedrine HCl; guaifenesin; alcohol 7.5%] 10•30•100 mg/5 mL

**phenicarbazide** INN

**phenidiemal** [see: phetharbital]

**phenindamine** INN *nonselective piperidine antihistamine* [also: phenindamine tartrate]

**phenindamine tartrate** USAN *nonselective piperidine antihistamine for allergic rhinitis* [also: phenindamine]

**phenindione** USP, INN *anticoagulant*

**pheniodol sodium** INN [also: iodoalphionic acid]

**peniprazine** INN, BAN

**peniprazine HCl** [see: peniprazine]

**pheniramine** INN [also: pheniramine maleate]

**pheniramine maleate** USAN *antihistamine* [also: pheniramine]

**pheniramine maleate & naphazoline HCl** *topical ocular antihistamine and decongestant* 0.3%•0.025% eye drops

**phenisonone hydrobromide**

**phenmetraline HCl** [see: phenmetrazine HCl]

**phenmetrazine** INN, BAN *anorexiant; CNS stimulant; also abused as a street drug* [also: phenmetrazine HCl]

**phenmetrazine HCl** USP *anorexiant; CNS stimulant; also abused as a street drug* [also: phenmetrazine]

**phenobamate** [see: febarbamate]

**phenobarbital** USP, INN, JAN *anticonvulsant; hypnotic; sedative; also abused as a street drug* [also: phenobarbitone] 15, 30, 60, 100 mg oral; 15, 20 mg/5 mL oral ☒ pentobarbital

**phenobarbital sodium** USP, INN, JAN *anticonvulsant; hypnotic; sedative; also abused as a street drug* 30, 60, 65, 130 mg/mL injection

**phenobarbitone** BAN *anticonvulsant; hypnotic; sedative; also abused as a street drug* [also: phenobarbital]

**phenobutiodil** INN

**phenododecinium bromide** [see: domiphen bromide]

**phenol** USP *topical antiseptic/antipruritic; local anesthetic; preservative*

**phenol, liquefied** USP *topical antipruritic*

**phenol, sodium salt** [see: phenolate sodium]

**phenol red** [see: phenolsulfonphthalein]

**phenolate sodium** USAN *disinfectant*

**Phenolated Calamine** lotion OTC *poison ivy treatment* [calamine; zinc oxide; phenol] 8%•8%•1%

**phenolphthalein** USP, INN *stimulant laxative* [banned in all OTC laxatives in 1998]

**phenolphthalein, white** [see: phenolphthalein]

**phenolphthalein, yellow** USP *stimulant laxative* [banned in all OTC laxatives in 1998]

**phenolsulfonphthalein** USP

**phenolsulphonate sodium** USP

**phenomorphan** INN, BAN

**phenomycilline** [see: penicillin V]

**phenoperidine** INN, BAN

**phenopryldiasulfone sodium** [see: solasulfone]

**Phenoptic** eye drops ℞ *topical ophthalmic decongestant and vasoconstrictor; mydriatic* [phenylephrine HCl] 2.5%

**phenosulfophthalein** [see: phenolsulfonphthalein]

**phenothiazine** NF, INN *antipsychotic*

**phenothiazines** *a class of dopamine receptor antagonists with antipsychotic, hypotensive, antiemetic, antispasmodic, and antihistaminic activity*

**phenothrin** INN, BAN

**phenoxazoline HCl** [see: fenoxazoline HCl]

**Phenoxine** tablets (discontinued 2001) OTC *diet aid* [phenylpropanolamine HCl] 25 mg ☒ Phenazine

**phenoxybenzamine** INN *antihypertensive* [also: phenoxybenzamine HCl]

**phenoxybenzamine HCl** USP *antihypertensive; pheochromocytomic agent* [also: phenoxybenzamine]

**phenoxymethylpenicillin** INN *natural penicillin antibiotic* [also: penicillin V]

**phenoxypropazine** BAN [also: fenoxypropazine]

**phenoxypropylpenicillin** [see: propicillin]

**phenozolone** [see: fenozolone]

**phenprobamate** INN, BAN

**phenprocoumon** USAN, USP, INN *anticoagulant*

**phenprocumone** [see: phenprocoumon]

**phenpromethadrine** [see: phenpromethamine]

**phenpromethamine** INN

**phenpropamine citrate** [see: alverine citrate]

**Phenserine** ℞ *investigational (Phase II) acetylcholinesterase (AChE) inhibitor to suppress the formation of beta-amyloid precursor protein (beta-APP) and beta-amyloid plaque to delay the progression of Alzheimer disease*

**phensuximide** USP, INN, BAN *succinimide anticonvulsant*

**phentermine** USAN, INN *anorexiant; CNS stimulant; an adrenergic isomer of amphetamine* ☒ phentolamine

**phentermine HCl** USP *anorexiant; CNS stimulant; the water-soluble form of phentermine for oral administration* 8, 15, 18.75, 30, 37.5 mg oral

**phenthiazine** [see: phenothiazine]

**phentolamine** INN, BAN *antihypertensive; pheochromocytomic agent* [also: phentolamine HCl] ☒ phentermine; Ventolin

**phentolamine HCl** USP *antihypertensive; pheochromocytomic agent* [also: phentolamine]

**phentolamine mesilate** INN, JAN *antiadrenergic; antihypertensive; pheochro-*

*mocytomic agent* [also: phentolamine mesylate]

**phentolamine mesylate** USP *antihypertensive; α-adrenergic blocker; pheochromocytomic agent; investigational (Phase III) oral treatment for erectile dysfunction* [also: phentolamine mesilate] 5 mg injection

**phentolamine methanesulfonate** [now: phentolamine mesylate]

**Phentrol 2; Phentrol 4; Phentrol 5** capsules ℞ *anorexiant; CNS stimulant* [phentermine HCl] 30 mg

**phentydrone**

**phenyl aminosalicylate** USAN, BAN *antibacterial; tuberculostatic* [also: fenamisal]

**phenyl salicylate** NF *analgesic; not generally regarded as safe and effective as an antidiarrheal*

**phenylalanine (L-phenylalanine)** USAN, USP, INN *essential amino acid; symbols: Phe, F*

**phenylalanine ammonia-lyase** *investigational (orphan) for hyperphenylalaninemia*

**phenylalanine mustard (PAM)** [see: melphalan]

**L-phenylalanine mustard (L-PAM)** [see: melphalan]

**Phenylase** *investigational (orphan) for hyperphenylalaninemia* [phenylalanine ammonia-lyase]

**phenylazo diamino pyridine HCl** [see: phenazopyridine HCl]

**phenylbenzyl atropine** [see: xenytropium bromide]

**phenylbutazone** USP, INN *antirheumatic; anti-inflammatory; antipyretic; analgesic*

**phenylbutylpiperadines** *a class of dopamine receptor antagonists with conventional (typical) antipsychotic activity* [also called: butyrophenones]

**phenylbutyrate sodium** [see: sodium phenylbutyrate]

**2-phenylbutyrylurea** [see: pheneturide; acetylpheneturide]

**phenylcarbinol** [see: benzyl alcohol]

**phenylcinchoninic acid** [now: cinchophen]

**α-phenyl-p-cresol carbamate** [see: diphenan]

**phenylcyclohexyl piperidine (PCP)** [see: PCP; phencyclidine HCl]

**2-phenylcyclopentylamine HCl** [see: cypenamine HCl]

**phenyldimazone** [see: normethadone]

**Phenyldrine** *timed-release tablets (discontinued 2001)* OTC *diet aid* [phenylpropanolamine HCl] 75 mg

**phenylephrine (PE)** INN, BAN *nasal decongestant; ocular vasoconstrictor; vasopressor for hypotensive or cardiac shock* [also: phenylephrine HCl]

**phenylephrine bitartrate** *bronchodilator; vasoconstrictor*

**phenylephrine HCl** USP *nasal decongestant; ocular vasoconstrictor; vasopressor for hypotensive or cardiac shock* [also: phenylephrine] 0.25%, 0.5%, 1% nose drops or spray; 2.5%, 10% eye drops; 1% injection

**phenylephrine HCl & phenylpropanolamine HCl & guaifenesin** *nasal decongestant; expectorant* PPA banned in all OTC products in 2001

**phenylephrine HCl & promethazine HCl** *decongestant; antihistamine* 5•6.25 mg/5 mL oral

**phenylephrine tannate** *nasal decongestant*

**phenylephrine tannate & chlorpheniramine tannate & pyrilamine tannate** *decongestant; antihistamine* 5•2•12.5 mg/5 mL oral

**phenylethanol** [see: phenylethyl alcohol]

**phenylethyl alcohol** USP *antimicrobial agent; preservative* [also: phenethyl alcohol]

**phenylethylmalonylurea** [see: phenobarbital]

**Phenylfenesin L.A.** *extended-action tablets (discontinued 2002)* ℞ *decongestant; expectorant* [phenylpropanolamine HCl; guaifenesin] 75•400 mg

**Phenylfenesin L.A.** *long-acting tablets (discontinued 2002)* ℞ *desconges-*

*tant; expectorant* [phenylpropanol-
amine HCl; guaifenesin] 75•400 mg

**Phenyl-Free** oral liquid, powder for
oral solution OTC *special diet for
infants with phenylketonuria (PKU)*

**Phenylgesic** tablets OTC *antihistamine;
analgesic* [phenyltoloxamine citrate;
acetaminophen] 30•325 mg

**phenylhydrazone** *investigational
(Phase I) antiviral for AIDS-related
Kaposi sarcoma*

**phenylindanedione** [see: phenindione]

**phenylmercuric acetate** NF *antimicrobial agent; preservative*

**phenylmercuric borate** INN

**phenylmercuric chloride** NF

**phenylmercuric nitrate** NF *antimicrobial agent; preservative; topical antiseptic*

**phenylone** [see: antipyrine]

**phenylpropanolamine (PPA)** INN,
BAN *vasoconstrictor; nasal decongestant; nonprescription diet aid* [also:
phenylpropanolamine HCl] banned
in all OTC products in 2001

**phenylpropanolamine HCl** USP
*vasoconstrictor; nasal decongestant;
nonprescription diet aid* [also: phenyl-
propanolamine] banned in all OTC
products in 2001

**phenylpropanolamine HCl &
chlorpheniramine maleate** *decongestant; antihistamine* [PPA banned in
all OTC products in 2001]

**phenylpropanolamine HCl & phen-
ylephrine HCl & guaifenesin**
*nasal decongestant; expectorant* [PPA
banned in all OTC products in 2001]

**phenylpropanolamine polistirex**
USAN *adrenergic; vasoconstrictor*
banned in all OTC products in 2001

**1-phenylsemicarbazide** [see: pheni-
carbazide]

**phenylthilone** [see: phenythilone]

**phenyltoloxamine** INN *antihistamine;
sleep aid*

**phenyltoloxamine citrate** *antihistamine; sleep aid*

**phenyltriazines** *a class of anticonvulsants*

**phenyracillin** INN

**phenyramidol HCl** USAN *analgesic;
skeletal muscle relaxant* [also: feny-
ramidol]

**Phenytek** extended-release capsules
R *once-daily hydantoin anticonvulsant*
[phenytoin sodium] 200, 300 mg

**phenythilone** INN

**phenytoin** USAN, USP, INN, BAN *hydantoin anticonvulsant* 125 mg/5 mL oral

**phenytoin redox** [see: redox-pheny-
toin]

**phenytoin sodium** USP *hydantoin anticonvulsant* 100 mg oral; 50 mg/mL
injection

**Pherazine DM** syrup (discontinued
2002) R *antitussive; antihistamine*
[dextromethorphan hydrobromide;
promethazine HCl; alcohol 7%] 15•
6.25 mg/5 mL

**Pherazine VC with Codeine** syrup
(discontinued 2002) R *narcotic antitussive; decongestant; antihistamine*
[codeine phosphate; phenylephrine
HCl; promethazine HCl; alcohol
7%] 10•5•6.25 mg/5 mL

**Pherazine with Codeine** syrup (discontinued 2002) R *narcotic antitussi-
sive; antihistamine* [codeine phosphate; promethazine HCl; alcohol
7%] 10•6.25 mg/5 mL

**phetharbital** INN

**phezathion** [see: fezatone]

**Phicon** cream OTC *topical anesthetic;
emollient* [pramoxine HCl; vitamins
A and E] 0.5%•7500 IU•2000 IU

**Phicon F** cream OTC *topical anesthetic;
antifungal* [pramoxine HCl; undecylenic acid] 0.05%•8%

**Phillips' Chewable** tablets OTC *antacid* [magnesium hydroxide] 311 mg

**Phillips' Liqui-Gels** OTC *laxative; stool
softener* [docusate sodium] 100 mg

**Phillips' Milk of Magnesia; Con-
centrated Phillips' Milk of Magnesia** oral liquid OTC *antacid; saline
laxative* [magnesium hydroxide] 400
mg/5 mL; 800 mg/5 mL

**pHisoDerm; pHisoDerm for Baby**
topical liquid OTC *soap-free therapeutic skin cleanser*

**pHisoDerm Cleansing Bar** (discontinued 2004) OTC *therapeutic skin cleanser*

**pHisoHex** topical liquid R *bacteriostatic skin cleanser* [hexachlorophene] 3% ⑦ Fostex

**phloropropiophenone** [see: flopropione]

**pholcodine** INN

**pholedrine** INN, BAN

**pholescutol** [see: folescutol]

*Phoradendron flavescens; P. serotinum; P. tomentosum medicinal herb* [see: mistletoe]

**PhosChol** softgels, oral liquid concentrate OTC *lipotropic* [phosphatidylcholine] 565, 900 mg; 3 g/5 mL

**phoscolic acid** [see: foscolic acid]

**Phos-Flur** oral rinse R *topical dental caries preventative* [acidulated phosphate fluoride] 0.44 mg/mL

**PhosLo** tablets, capsules, gelcaps R *buffering agent for hyperphosphatemia in end-stage renal disease* (orphan) [calcium acetate] 667 mg; 333.3, 667 mg; 667 mg

**Phos-NaK** powder for oral solution R *phosphorus/electrolyte supplement* [phosphorus; potassium; sodium] 250•280•160 mg/pkt.

**phosphate salt of tricyclic nucleoside** [now: triciribine phosphate]

**phosphatidylcholine (PC)** [see: lecithin]

**phosphatidylserine (PS)** *natural agent to improve neural function, maintain brain cell membrane integrity, and protect the brain against age-related functional deterioration*

**phosphinic acid** [see: hypophosphorous acid]

**2,2′-phosphinicodilactic acid (PDLA)** [see: foscolic acid]

**Phosphocol P 32** suspension for intracavitary instillation, interstitial injection R *radiopharmaceutical antineoplastic* [chromic phosphate P 32] 10, 15 mCi

**phosphocysteamine** *investigational (orphan) for cystinosis*

**phosphodiesterase III (PDE III) inhibitors** *a class of platelet aggregation inhibitors*

**Phospholine Iodide** powder for eye drops R *antiglaucoma agent; irreversible cholinesterase inhibitor miotic* [echothiophate iodide] 0.03%, 0.125%

**phosphonoformic acid (PFA)** [see: foscarnet sodium]

**phosphonomethoxypropyladenine (PMPA)** [see: tenofovir]

**phosphorated carbohydrate solution (hyperosmolar solution with phosphoric acid)** *antiemetic for nausea associated with influenza, morning sickness, motion sickness, inhalation anesthesia, or food and drink indiscretions*

**phosphoric acid** NF *solvent; acidifying agent*

**phosphoric acid, aluminum salt** [see: aluminum phosphate gel]

**phosphoric acid, calcium salt** [see: calcium phosphate, dibasic]

**phosphoric acid, chromium salt** [see: chromic phosphate Cr 51 & P 32]

**phosphoric acid, diammonium salt** [see: ammonium phosphate]

**phosphoric acid, dipotassium salt** [see: potassium phosphate, dibasic]

**phosphoric acid, disodium salt heptahydrate** [see: sodium phosphate, dibasic]

**phosphoric acid, disodium salt hydrate** [see: sodium phosphate, dibasic]

**phosphoric acid, magnesium salt** [see: magnesium phosphate]

**phosphoric acid, monopotassium salt** [see: potassium phosphate, monobasic]

**phosphoric acid, monosodium salt dihydrate** [see: sodium phosphate, monobasic]

**phosphoric acid, monosodium salt monohydrate** [see: sodium phosphate, monobasic]

**phosphorofluoridic acid, disodium salt** [see: sodium monofluorophosphate]

**phosphorothiolate deoxyribose** *investigational (orphan) agent for advanced malignant melanoma*

**phosphorus** *element (P)*

**Phospho-Soda** [see: Fleet Phospho-Soda]

**phosphothiamine** [see: monophosphothiamine]

**Photofrin PDT** powder for IV injection ℞ *laser light–activated antineoplastic for photodynamic therapy (PDT) of esophageal (orphan) and non–small cell lung cancers (NSCLC); used for ablation of high-grade dysplasia in Barrett esophagus (BE) patients; investigational (orphan) for bladder cancer* [porfimer sodium] 75 mg

**PhotoPoint** ℞ *investigational (Phase III) photosensitizer for wet age-related macular degeneration (AMD)* [tin ethyl etiopurpurin]

**phoxim** INN, BAN

**Phrenilin** tablets ℞ *analgesic; barbiturate sedative* [acetaminophen; butalbital] 325•50 mg

**Phrenilin Forte** capsules ℞ *analgesic; barbiturate sedative* [acetaminophen; butalbital] 650•50 mg

**PHRT (procarbazine, hydroxyurea, radiotherapy)** *chemotherapy protocol*

**phthalofyne** USAN *veterinary anthelmintic* [also: ftalofyne]

**phthalylsulfacetamide** NF

**phthalylsulfamethizole** INN

**phthalylsulfathiazole** USP, INN

**phylcardin** [see: aminophylline]

**phyllindon** [see: aminophylline]

**Phyllocontin** controlled-release tablets (discontinued 2004) ℞ *antiasthmatic; bronchodilator* [aminophylline] 225 mg

**phylloquinone** [see: phytonadione]

**Phylorinol** mouthwash/gargle OTC *topical antipruritic/counterirritant; mild local anesthetic* [phenol] 0.6%

**Phylorinol** topical liquid OTC *antipruritic/counterirritant; mild local anesthetic; antiseptic; astringent; oral deodorant* [phenol; boric acid; strong iodine solution; chlorophyllin copper complex] 0.6%• 2̱ • 2̱ • 2̱

**physic root** *medicinal herb* [see: Culver root]

**physiological irrigating solution** *for general irrigating, washing and rinsing; not for injection*

**Physiolyte** topical liquid ℞ *sterile irrigant* [physiological irrigating solution]

**PhysioSol** topical liquid ℞ *sterile irrigant* [physiological irrigating solution]

**Physiotens** ℞ *investigational centrally acting sympatholytic for hypertension, congestive heart failure, and type 2 diabetes* [moxonidine]

**physostigmine** USP, BAN *reversible cholinesterase inhibitor miotic for glaucoma* ⑨ pyridostigmine; Prostigmin

**physostigmine salicylate** USP *cholinergic to reverse anticholinergic overdose; investigational (orphan) for Friedreich and other inherited ataxias* 1 mg/mL injection

**physostigmine sulfate** USP *ophthalmic cholinergic for glaucoma; miotic*

**phytate persodium** USAN *pharmaceutic aid*

**phytate sodium** USAN *calcium-chelating agent*

**phytic acid** [see: fytic acid]

*Phytolacca americana; P. decandra; P. rigida medicinal herb* [see: pokeweed]

**phytomenadione (vitamin K₁)** INN, BAN *fat-soluble vitamin; prothrombogenic* [also: phytonadione]

**phytonadiol sodium diphosphate** INN

**phytonadione (vitamin K₁)** USP, JAN *fat-soluble vitamin; prothrombogenic* [also: phytomenadione] 2 mg/mL injection

**PIA (Platinol, ifosfamide, Adriamycin)** *chemotherapy protocol*

**pibecarb** INN

**piberaline** INN

**piboserod HCl** USAN *selective serotonin 5-HT₄ receptor antagonist for irritable bowel syndrome*

**pibrozelesin hydrobromide** USAN *antineoplastic*

**picafibrate** INN

**picartamide** INN

*Picea excelsa; P. mariana* medicinal herb [see: spruce tree]

**picenadol** INN *analgesic* [also: picenadol HCl]

**picenadol HCl** USAN *analgesic* [also: picenadol]

**picilorex** INN

**pick purse; pickpocket** *medicinal herb* [see: shepherd's purse]

**piclamilast** USAN *phosphodiesterase type IV inhibitor for asthma*

**piclonidine** INN

**piclopastine** INN

**picloxydine** INN, BAN

**picobenzide** INN

**picodralazine** INN

**picolamine** INN

**piconol** INN

**picoperine** INN

**picoprazole** INN

**picotrin** INN *keratolytic* [also: picotrin diolamine]

**picotrin diolamine** USAN *keratolytic* [also: picotrin]

**Picovir** ℞ *investigational (NDA filed) viral replication inhibitor for viral respiratory infections, including the common cold* [pleconaril]

*Picrasma excelsa* medicinal herb [see: quassia]

**picric acid** [see: trinitrophenol]

**picrotoxin** NF

**picumast** INN, BAN

**picumeterol** INN, BAN *bronchodilator* [also: picumeterol fumarate]

**picumeterol fumarate** USAN *bronchodilator* [also: picumeterol]

**pidolacetamol** INN

**pidolic acid** INN

**pifarnine** USAN, INN *gastric antiulcerative*

**pifenate** INN, BAN

**pifexole** INN

**piflutixol** INN

**pifoxime** INN

**pigeonberry** *medicinal herb* [see: pokeweed]

**piketoprofen** INN

**Pilagan** eye drops (discontinued 2004) ℞ *antiglaucoma agent; direct-acting miotic* [pilocarpine nitrate] 1%, 2%, 4%

**pildralazine** INN

**pilewort** (*Erechtites hieracifolia*) plant *medicinal herb used as an astringent and emetic*

**Pilocar** eye drops ℞ *antiglaucoma agent; direct-acting miotic* [pilocarpine HCl] 0.5%, 1%, 2%, 3%, 4%, 6%

**pilocarpine** USP, BAN *antiglaucoma agent; ophthalmic cholinergic*

**pilocarpine HCl** USP *ophthalmic cholinergic; antiglaucoma; miotic; treatment of xerostomia and keratoconjunctivitis sicca due to radiotherapy or Sjögren syndrome (orphan); also for dry mouth* 0.5%, 1%, 2%, 4%, 6%, 8% eye drops

**pilocarpine nitrate** USP *ophthalmic cholinergic; antiglaucoma; miotic*

**Pilopine HS** ophthalmic gel ℞ *topical antiglaucoma agent; direct-acting miotic* [pilocarpine HCl] 4%

**Piloptic-½; Piloptic-1; Piloptic-2; Piloptic-3; Piloptic-4; Piloptic-6** eye drops ℞ *topical antiglaucoma agent; direct-acting miotic* [pilocarpine HCl] 0.5%; 1%; 2%; 3%; 4%; 6%

**Pilopto-Carpine** eye drops ℞ *topical antiglaucoma agent; direct-acting miotic* [pilocarpine HCl] 4%

**Pilostat** eye drops ℞ *topical antiglaucoma agent; direct-acting miotic* [pilocarpine HCl] 0.5%, 1%, 2%, 3%, 4%, 6%

**Pilpak** (trademarked packaging form) *patient compliance package*

**Pima** syrup ℞ *expectorant* [potassium iodide] 325 mg/5 mL

**pimagedine HCl** USAN *advanced glycosylation inhibitor for type 1 diabetes; investigational (Phase III) for diabetics in end-stage renal disease*

**pimaricin** JAN *ophthalmic antibacterial/antifungal antibiotic* [also: natamycin]

**pimeclone** INN

**pimecrolimus** USAN *immunosuppressant for atopic dermatitis*

**pimefylline** INN

**pimelautide** INN

**Pimenta dioica; P. officinalis** *medicinal herb* [see: allspice]

**pimetacin** INN

**pimethixene** INN

**pimetine** INN *antihyperlipoproteinemic* [also: pimetine HCl]

**pimetine HCl** USAN *antihyperlipoproteinemic* [also: pimetine]

**pimetixene** [see: pimethixene]

**pimetremide** INN

**pimeverine** [see: pimetremide]

**piminodine** INN [also: piminodine esylate]

**piminodine esylate** NF [also: piminodine]

**piminodine ethanesulfonate** [see: piminodine esylate]

**pimobendan** USAN, INN *cardiotonic*

**pimonidazole** INN, BAN

**pimozide** USAN, USP, INN, BAN, JAN *antidyskinetic for Tourette syndrome; diphenylbutylpiperidine antipsychotic; neuroleptic*

**pimpernel; small pimpernel** *medicinal herb* [see: burnet]

**pimpernel, blue** *medicinal herb* [see: skullcap]

**pimpernel, water** *medicinal herb* [see: brooklime]

**Pimpinella anisum** *medicinal herb* [see: anise]

**Pimpinella magna; P. saxifrage** *medicinal herb* [see: burnet]

**pinacidil** USAN, INN *antihypertensive (approved in 1989, but not marketed by the manufacturer)*

**pinadoline** USAN, INN *analgesic*

**pinafide** INN

**pinaverium bromide** INN *GI antispasmodic*

**pinazepam** INN

**pincainide** INN

**pindolol** USAN, USP, INN, BAN *antianginal; antihypertensive; vasodilator; antiadrenergic (β-receptor)* 5, 10 mg oral

**pine, Norway** *medicinal herb* [see: spruce]

**pine, prince's** *medicinal herb* [see: pipsissewa]

**pine bark extract** *natural free radical scavenger for inflammatory collagen disease and peripheral vascular disease; contains 80%–85% procyanidolic oligomers (PCOs)*

**pine needle oil** NF

**pine tar** USP

**pineapple (Ananas comosus)** *fruit medicinal herb for constipation, jaundice, soft tissue inflammation, and topical wound debridement*

**Pink Bismuth** oral liquid OTC *antidiarrheal; antinauseant* [bismuth subsalicylate] 130, 262 mg/15 mL

**pinolcaine** INN

**pinoxepin** INN *antipsychotic* [also: pinoxepin HCl]

**pinoxepin HCl** USAN *antipsychotic* [also: pinoxepin]

**Pin-Rid** soft gel capsules, oral liquid OTC *anthelmintic for ascariasis (roundworm) and enterobiasis (pinworm)* [pyrantel pamoate] 180 mg; 50 mg/mL

**Pinus palustris** *natural remedy* [see: turpentine]

**Pinus strobus** *medicinal herb* [see: white pine]

**Pin-X** oral liquid OTC *anthelmintic for ascariasis (roundworm) and enterobiasis (pinworm)* [pyrantel pamoate] 50 mg/mL

**pioglitazone** INN *thiazolidinedione antidiabetic; increases cellular response to insulin without increasing insulin secretion* [also: pioglitazone HCl]

**pioglitazone HCl** USAN *thiazolidinedione antidiabetic; increases cellular response to insulin without increasing insulin secretion* [also: pioglitazone]

**pipacycline** INN

**pipamazine** INN

**pipamperone** USAN, INN *antipsychotic*

**pipaneperone** [see: pipamperone]

**pipazetate** INN *antitussive* [also: pipazethate]

**pipazethate** USAN *antitussive* [also: pipazetate]

**pipe plant; Dutchman's pipe; Indian pipe** *medicinal herb* [see: fit root]

**pipebuzone** INN

**pipecuronium bromide** USAN, INN, BAN *nondepolarizing neuromuscular blocking agent; muscle relaxant; adjunct to general anesthesia*

**pipemidic acid** INN

**pipenzolate bromide** INN

**pipenzolate methylbromide** [see: pipenzolate bromide]

**pipenzolone bromide** [see: pipenzolate bromide]

**pipequaline** INN

*Piper cubeba* medicinal herb [see: cubeb]

*Piper methysticum* medicinal herb [see: kava kava]

**piperacetazine** USAN, USP, INN *antipsychotic* ⊡ piperazine

**piperacillin** INN, BAN *extended-spectrum penicillin antibiotic* [also: piperacillin sodium]

**piperacillin sodium** USAN, USP, JAN *extended-spectrum penicillin antibiotic* [also: piperacillin] 2, 3, 4 g injection

**piperamide** INN *anthelmintic* [also: piperamide maleate]

**piperamide maleate** USAN *anthelmintic* [also: piperamide]

**piperamine** [see: bamipine]

**piperazine** USP *anthelmintic for enterobiasis (pinworm) and ascariasis (roundworm)* ⊡ piperacetazine

**piperazine calcium edetate** INN *anthelmintic* [also: piperazine edetate calcium]

**piperazine citrate** USP *anthelmintic* 250 mg oral; 500 mg/mL oral

**piperazine citrate hydrate** [see: piperazine citrate]

**piperazine edetate calcium** USAN *anthelmintic* [also: piperazine calcium edetate]

**piperazine estrone sulfate** [now: estropipate]

**piperazine hexahydrate** [see: piperazine citrate]

**piperazine phosphate**

**piperazine phosphate monohydrate** [see: piperazine phosphate]

**piperazine theophylline ethanoate** [see: acefylline piperazine]

**piperidine phosphate**

**piperidines** *a class of antihistamines*

**piperidolate** INN [also: piperidolate HCl]

**piperidolate HCl** USP [also: piperidolate]

**piperilate** [see: pipethanate]

**piperine** USP *natural pepper extract that increases the absorption of chrysin*

**piperocaine** INN [also: piperocaine HCl]

**piperocaine HCl** USP [also: piperocaine]

**piperonyl butoxide** *pediculicide for lice*

**piperoxan** INN

**piperphenidol HCl**

**piperylone** INN

**pipethanate** INN

**pipobroman** USAN, USP, INN *alkylating antineoplastic*

**pipoctanone** INN

**pipofezine** INN

**piposulfan** USAN, INN *antineoplastic*

**pipotiazine** INN *phenothiazine antipsychotic* [also: pipotiazine palmitate]

**pipotiazine palmitate** USAN *phenothiazine antipsychotic* [also: pipotiazine]

**pipoxizine** INN

**pipoxolan** INN *muscle relaxant* [also: pipoxolan HCl]

**pipoxolan HCl** USAN *muscle relaxant* [also: pipoxolan]

**Pipracil** *powder for IV or IM injection (discontinued 2004)* ℞ *extended-spectrum penicillin antibiotic* [piperacillin sodium] 2, 3, 4, 40 g/vial

**pipradimadol** INN

**pipradrol** INN [also: pipradrol HCl]

**pipradrol HCl** NF [also: pipradrol]

**pipramadol** INN

**pipratecol** INN

**piprinhydrinate** INN, BAN

**piprocurarium iodide** INN

**piprofurol** INN

**piprozolin** USAN, INN *choleretic*

**pipsissewa (Chimaphila umbellata)** plant *medicinal herb used as an astringent, diaphoretic, and diuretic*

**piquindone** INN *antipsychotic* [also: piquindone HCl]

**piquindone HCl** USAN *antipsychotic* [also: piquindone]

**piquizil** INN *bronchodilator* [also: piquizil HCl]

**piquizil HCl** USAN *bronchodilator* [also: piquizil]

**piracetam** USAN, INN, BAN *cognition adjuvant; investigational (orphan) for myoclonus* ② piroxicam

**pirandamine** INN *antidepressant* [also: pirandamine HCl]

**pirandamine HCl** USAN *antidepressant* [also: pirandamine]

**pirarubicin** INN

**piraxelate** INN

**pirazmonam** INN *antimicrobial* [also: pirazmonam sodium]

**pirazmonam sodium** USAN *antimicrobial* [also: pirazmonam]

**pirazofurin** INN *antineoplastic* [also: pyrazofurin]

**pirazolac** USAN, INN, BAN *antirheumatic*

**pirbenicillin** INN *antibacterial* [also: pirbenicillin sodium]

**pirbenicillin sodium** USAN *antibacterial* [also: pirbenicillin]

**pirbuterol** INN *sympathomimetic bronchodilator* [also: pirbuterol acetate]

**pirbuterol acetate** USAN *sympathomimetic bronchodilator* [also: pirbuterol]

**pirbuterol HCl** USAN *bronchodilator*

**pirdonium bromide** INN

**pirenoxine** INN

**pirenperone** USAN, INN, BAN *tranquilizer*

**pirenzepine** INN, BAN *tricyclic benzodiazepine for peptic ulcers* [also: pirenzepine HCl]

**pirenzepine HCl** USAN, JAN *investigational (NDA filed) tricyclic benzodiazepine for peptic ulcers* [also: pirenzepine]

**pirepolol** INN

**piretanide** USAN, INN *diuretic*

**pirfenidone** USAN, INN *analgesic; antiinflammatory; antipyretic*

**piribedil** INN

**piribenzyl methylsulfate** [see: bevonium metilsulfate]

**piridicillin** INN *antibacterial* [also: piridicillin sodium]

**piridicillin sodium** USAN *antibacterial* [also: piridicillin]

**piridocaine**

**piridocaine HCl** [see: piridocaine]

**piridoxilate** INN, BAN

**piridronate sodium** USAN *calcium regulator*

**piridronic acid** INN

**pirifibrate** INN

**pirinidazole** INN

**pirinitramide** [see: piritramide]

**pirinixic acid** INN

**pirinixil** INN

**piriprost** USAN *antiasthmatic*

**piriprost potassium** USAN *antiasthmatic*

**piriqualone** INN

**pirisudanol** INN

**piritramide** INN, BAN

**piritrexim** INN *antiproliferative agent* [also: piritrexim isethionate]

**piritrexim isethionate** USAN *antiproliferative; orphan status withdrawn 1996* [also: piritrexim]

**pirlimycin HCl** USAN *antibacterial*

**pirlindole** INN

**pirmagrel** USAN, INN *thromboxane synthetase inhibitor*

**pirmenol** INN *antiarrhythmic* [also: pirmenol HCl]

**pirmenol HCl** USAN *antiarrhythmic* [also: pirmenol]

**pirnabin** INN *antiglaucoma agent* [also: pirnabine]

**pirnabine** USAN *antiglaucoma agent* [also: pirnabin]

**piroctone** USAN, INN *antiseborrheic*

**piroctone olamine** USAN *antiseborrheic*

**pirodavir** USAN, INN, BAN *antiviral*

**pirogliride** INN *antidiabetic* [also: pirogliride tartrate]

**pirogliride tartrate** USAN *antidiabetic* [also: pirogliride]

**piroheptine** INN

**pirolate** USAN, INN *antiasthmatic*

**pirolazamide** USAN, INN *antiarrhythmic*

**piromidic acid** INN

**piroxantrone** INN *antineoplastic* [also: piroxantrone HCl]

**piroxantrone HCl** USAN *antineoplastic* [also: piroxantrone]

**piroxicam** USAN, USP, INN, BAN, JAN *antiarthritic; nonsteroidal anti-inflam-*

*matory drug (NSAID)* 10, 20 mg oral ⍰ piracetam

**piroxicam β-cyclodextrin** [see: piroxicam betadex]

**piroxicam betadex** USAN *analgesic; antirheumatic; nonsteroidal anti-inflammatory drug (NSAID)*

**piroxicam cinnamate** USAN *anti-inflammatory*

**piroxicam olamine** USAN *analgesic; anti-inflammatory*

**piroxicillin** INN

**piroximone** USAN, INN, BAN *cardiotonic*

**pirozadil** INN

**pirprofen** USAN, INN, BAN *anti-inflammatory*

**pirquinozol** USAN, INN *antiallergic*

**pirralkonium bromide** INN

**pirroksan** [now: proroxan HCl]

**pirsidomine** USAN, INN *vasodilator*

**pirtenidine** INN

**pistachio** *medicinal herb* [see: witch hazel]

**pitch tree, Canada; hemlock pitch tree** *medicinal herb* [see: hemlock]

**pitcher plant (Sarracenia purpurea)** root *medicinal herb used as an astringent, diuretic, and stimulant*

**pitenodil** INN

**Pitocin** IV, IM injection ℞ *oxytocic for induction of labor, postpartum bleeding, and incomplete abortion* [oxytocin] 10 U/mL ⍰ Pitressin

**pitofenone** INN

**Pitressin Synthetic** IM or subcu injection ℞ *pituitary antidiuretic hormone for diabetes insipidus or prevention of abdominal distention* [vasopressin] 20 U/mL ⍰ Pitocin

**Pitrex** Ⓒᴬᴺ cream OTC *topical antifungal* [tolnaftate] 1%

**pituitary, anterior**

**pituitary, posterior** USP *antidiuretic hormone*

**pituxate** INN

**pivalate** USAN, INN, BAN *combining name for radicals or groups*

**pivampicillin** INN *aminopenicillin antibiotic* [also: pivampicillin HCl]

**pivampicillin HCl** USAN *aminopenicillin antibiotic* [also: pivampicillin]

**pivampicillin pamoate** USAN *antibacterial*

**pivampicillin probenate** USAN *antibacterial*

**pivenfrine** INN

**pivmecillinam** INN, BAN *aminopenicillin antibiotic* [also: amdinocillin pivoxil; pivmecillinam HCl]

**pivmecillinam HCl** JAN *aminopenicillin antibiotic* [also: amdinocillin pivoxil; pivmecillinam]

**pivopril** USAN *antihypertensive*

**pivoxazepam** INN

**pivoxetil** USAN, INN *combining name for radicals or groups*

**pivoxil** USAN, INN *combining name for radicals or groups*

**pivsulbactam** BAN *β-lactamase inhibitor; penicillin/cephalosporin synergist* [also: sulbactam pivoxil]

**pix pini** [see: pine tar]

**Pixykine** ℞ *investigational second-generation colony stimulating factor for neutropenia and thrombocytopenia* [milodistim]

**pizotifen** INN, BAN *anabolic; antidepressant; serotonin inhibitor (migraine specific)* [also: pizotyline]

**pizotyline** USAN *anabolic; antidepressant; serotonin inhibitor (migraine specific)* [also: pizotifen]

**placebo** *an inert substance with no therapeutic value* [also: obecalp]

**placebo effect** [L. I will please] *a perceived therapeutic effect from an inert substance* [compare to: nocebo effect]

**Placidyl** capsules (discontinued 2004) ℞ *hypnotic* [ethchlorvynol] 200, 500, 750 mg ⍰ Pathocil

**plafibride** INN

**plague vaccine** USP *active bacterin for plague (Yersinia pestis)* $1.8–2.2 \times 10^8$ bacilli/mL IM injection

**Plan B** tablets (in packs of 2) ℞ (available from pharmacists without a prescription in some states) *emergency postcoital contraceptive (progestin only)* [levonorgestrel] 0.75 mg

**planadalin** [see: carbromal]

*Plantago lanceolata; P. major* **and other species** *medicinal herb* [see: plantain]

*Plantago ovata* **(psyllium)** *medicinal herb* [see: plantain]

**plantago seed** USP *laxative*

**plantain** (*Plantago lanceolata; P. major* **and other species**) leaves and seeds *medicinal herb for bed-wetting, bladder infections, blood poisoning, constipation, diarrhea, diverticulitis, edema, hyperlipidemia, kidney disorders, neuralgia, snake bites, sores, and topical inflammation*

**Plaquase** powder for injection R̥ *investigational (orphan) agent for Peyronie disease* [collagenase]

**Plaquenil** film-coated tablets R̥ *antimalarial; antirheumatic; lupus erythematosus suppressant* [hydroxychloroquine sulfate] 200 mg

**Plaretase 8000** tablets R̥ *porcine-derived digestive enzymes* [lipase; protease; amylase] 8000•30 000•30 000 USP units

**Plasbumin-5; Plasbumin-25** IV infusion R̥ *blood volume expander for shock, burns, and hypoproteinemia* [human albumin] 5%; 25%

**plasma, antihemophilic human** USP

**plasma concentrate factor IX** [see: factor IX complex]

**plasma expanders** *a class of therapeutic blood modifiers used to increase the volume of circulating blood* [also called: blood volume expanders]

**plasma protein fraction** USP *blood volume supporter*

**plasma protein fraction, human** [now: plasma protein fraction]

**plasma protein fractions** *a class of therapeutic blood modifiers used to regulate the volume of circulating blood*

**plasma thromboplastin component (PTC)** [see: factor IX]

**Plasma-Lyte 56** IV infusion (discontinued 2001) R̥ *intravenous electrolyte therapy* [combined electrolyte solution]

**Plasma-Lyte A pH 7.4; Plasma-Lyte R; Plasma-Lyte 148** IV infusion R̥ *intravenous electrolyte therapy* [combined electrolyte solution]

**Plasma-Lyte M (R; 56; 148) and 5% Dextrose** IV infusion R̥ *intravenous nutritional/electrolyte therapy* [combined electrolyte solution; dextrose]

**Plasmanate** IV infusion R̥ *blood volume expander for shock due to burns, trauma and surgery* [plasma protein fraction] 5%

**Plasma-Plex** IV infusion R̥ *blood volume expander for shock due to burns, trauma and surgery* [plasma protein fraction] 5%

**Plasmatein** IV infusion R̥ *blood volume expander for shock due to burns, trauma and surgery* [plasma protein fraction] 5%

**plasmin** BAN [also: fibrinolysin, human]

**Plateau Cap** (trademarked dosage form) *controlled-release capsule*

**platelet cofactor II** [see: factor IX]

**platelet concentrate** USP *platelet replenisher*

**Platinol-AQ** IV injection R̥ *alkylating antineoplastic for metastatic testicular tumors, metastatic ovarian tumors, and advanced bladder cancer* [cisplatin] 1 mg/mL

**platinum** *element (Pt)*

*cis*-**platinum** [now: cisplatin]

*cis*-**platinum II** [now: cisplatin]

**platinum diamminodichloride** [see: cisplatin]

**plaunotol** INN

**plauracin** USAN, INN *veterinary growth stimulant*

**Plavix** coated tablets R̥ *platelet aggregation inhibitor for stroke, myocardial infarction, peripheral artery disease, and acute coronary syndrome* [clopidogrel bisulfate] 75 mg

**Plax, Advanced Formula** mouthwash/gargle OTC [sodium pyrophosphate]

**pleconaril** USAN *investigational (NDA filed) viral replication inhibitor for treatment of viral respiratory infection and viral meningitis*

**Plegisol** solution ℞ *cardioplegic solution* [calcium chloride; magnesium chloride; potassium chloride; sodium chloride] 17.6•325.3•119.3•643 mg/100 mL

**Plenaxis** powder for IM injection *GnRH antagonist to suppress LH and FSH, leading to the cessation of testosterone production (medical castration, androgen ablation); treatment for prostate cancer; investigational for uterine fibroids, endometriosis, and precocious puberty* [abarelix] 100 mg/vial

**Plendil** extended-release tablets ℞ *antihypertensive; calcium channel blocker* [felodipine] 2.5, 5, 10 mg

**Pletal** tablets ℞ *vasodilator and platelet aggregation inhibitor for intermittent claudication* [cilostazol] 50, 100 mg

**pleurisy root (Asclepias tuberosa)** *medicinal herb for asthma, bronchitis, dysentery, emphysema, fever, pleurisy, and pneumonia*

**pleuromulin** INN

**Plexion** topical liquid ℞ *acne treatment* [sulfacetamide sodium; sulfur] 10%•5%

**Plexion SCT** cream ℞ *acne treatment* [sulfacetamide sodium; sulfur] 10%•5%

**Pliagel** solution OTC *surfactant cleaning solution for soft contact lenses*

**plicamycin** USAN, USP, INN *antibiotic antineoplastic*

**plomestane** USAN *antineoplastic; aromatase inhibitor*

**plum (Prunus americana; P. domestica; P. spinosa)** fruit and bark *medicinal herb used as an anthelmintic, astringent, and laxative*

**Plus Sinus** ⒸⒶⓃ extended-release caplets (discontinued 2001) OTC *nasal decongestant* [pseudoephedrine HCl] 120 mg

**plutonium** *element (Pu)*

**PM Caps** ⒸⒶⓃ OTC *vitamin supplement* [multiple vitamins; folic acid] ≐•0.2 mg

**pMDI** (dosage form) *pressurized metered-dose inhaler*

**PMMA (polymethylmethacrylate)** [q.v.]

**PMPA (phosphonomethoxypropyladenine)** [see: tenofovir]

**PMPA prodrug** [see: tenofovir disoproxil fumarate]

**PMS-Bezafibrate** ⒸⒶⓃ tablets ℞ *antihyperlipidemic* [bezafibrate] 200 mg

**PMS-Bromocriptine** ⒸⒶⓃ tablets, capsules ℞ *dopamine agonist for Parkinson disease; lactation inhibitor; growth hormone suppressant for acromegaly* [bromocriptine mesylate] 2.5 mg; 5 mg

**PMS-Captopril** ⒸⒶⓃ tablets ℞ *antihypertensive; angiotensin-converting enzyme (ACE) inhibitor* [captopril] 12.5, 25, 50, 100 mg

**PMS-Carbamazepine CR** ⒸⒶⓃ controlled-release tablets ℞ *anticonvulsant; analgesic for trigeminal neuralgia; antimanic* [carbamazepine] 200, 400 mg

**PMS-Conjugated Estrogens** ⒸⒶⓃ tablets ℞ *estrogen replacement therapy for postmenopausal symptoms* [conjugated estrogens] 0.3, 0.625, 0.9, 1.25 mg

**PMS-Desferoxamine** ⒸⒶⓃ powder for IM, IV, or subcu injection ℞ *adjunct treatment for iron intoxication or overload* [deferoxamine mesylate] 500 mg

**PMS-Dexamethasone** ⒸⒶⓃ injection ℞ *corticosteroidal anti-inflammatory* [dexamethasone sodium phosphate] 4, 10 mg/mL

**PMS-Dexamethasone** ⒸⒶⓃ tablets, elixir, eye drops, ear drops ℞ *corticosteroidal anti-inflammatory* [dexamethasone] 0.5, 0.75, 4 mg; 0.5 mg/5 mL; 0.1%; 0.1%

**PMS-Dicitrate** ⒸⒶⓃ oral solution ℞ *urinary alkalinizing agent* [sodium citrate; citric acid] 500•334 mg/5 mL

**PMS-Diclofenac** ⒸⒶⓃ tablets, suppositories ℞ *analgesic; antiarthritic; nonsteroidal anti-inflammatory drug (NSAID)* [diclofenac sodium] 25, 50 mg; 25, 50 mg

**PMS-Diclofenac SR** ⒸⒶⓃ slow-release tablets ℞ *analgesic; antiarthritic; nonste-*

*roidal anti-inflammatory drug (NSAID)* [diclofenac sodium] 75, 100 mg

**PMS-Dipivefrin** Ⓒ eye drops ℞ *topical antiglaucoma agent* [dipivefrin HCl] 0.1%

**PMS-Fenofibrate Micro** Ⓒ capsules ℞ *antihyperlipidemic* [fenofibrate, micronized] 200 mg

**PMS-Fluorometholone** Ⓒ eye drops ℞ *topical ophthalmic corticosteroidal anti-inflammatory* [fluorometholone] 0.1%

**PMS-Fluphenazine Decanoate** Ⓒ subcu or IM injection ℞ *conventional (typical) antipsychotic* [fluphenazine decanoate] 25, 100 mg/mL

**PMS-Fluvoxamine** Ⓒ film-coated tablets ℞ *selective serotonin reuptake inhibitor (SSRI) for depression and obsessive-compulsive disorder (OCD)* [fluvoxamine maleate] 50, 100 mg

**PMS-Gabapentin** Ⓒ capsules ℞ *anticonvulsant for partial-onset seizures* [gabapentin] 100, 300, 400 mg

**PMS-Haloperidol LA** Ⓒ IM injection ℞ *conventional (typical) antipsychotic; antidyskinetic for Tourette syndrome* [haloperidol decanoate] 50, 100 mg/mL

**PMS-Indapamide** Ⓒ tablets ℞ *antihypertensive; diuretic* [indapamide] 1.25, 2.5 mg

**PMS-Levobunolol** Ⓒ eye drops ℞ *topical antiglaucoma agent* [levobunolol HCl] 5 mg/mL

**PMS-Lithium Carbonate** Ⓒ capsules ℞ *antipsychotic for manic episodes* [lithium carbonate] 150, 300, 600 mg

**PMS-Lithium Citrate** Ⓒ syrup ℞ *antipsychotic for manic episodes* [lithium citrate] 300 mg/5 mL

**PMS-Minocycline** Ⓒ capsules ℞ *tetracycline antibiotic* [minocycline HCl] 50, 100 mg

**PMS-Moclobemide** Ⓒ tablets ℞ *antidepressant* [moclobemide] 100, 150 mg

**PMS-Nizatidine** Ⓒ capsules ℞ *histamine $H_2$ antagonist for treatment of gastric and duodenal ulcers* [nizatidine] 150, 300 mg

**PMS-Oxybutynin** Ⓒ tablets, syrup ℞ *urinary antispasmodic* [oxybutynin chloride] 2.5, 5 mg; 5 mg/5 mL

**PMS-Pindolol** Ⓒ tablets ℞ *antihypertensive; antianginal* [pindolol] 5, 10, 15, 80, 160 mg

**PMS-Polytrimethoprim** Ⓒ eye drops ℞ *topical ophthalmic antibiotic* [polymyxin B sulfate; trimethoprim sulfate] 10 000 U•1 mg per mL

**PMS-Ranitidine** Ⓒ film-coated tablets ℞ *histamine $H_2$ antagonist for gastric and duodenal ulcers* [ranitidine HCl] 150, 300 mg

**PMS-Sotalol** Ⓒ tablets ℞ *antiarrhythmic* [sotalol HCl] 80, 160 mg

**PMS-Sucralfate** Ⓒ tablets ℞ *cytoprotective agent for gastric ulcers* [sucralfate]

**PMS-Tamoxifen** Ⓒ tablets ℞ *antiestrogen antineoplastic for breast cancer* [tamoxifen citrate] 10, 20 mg

**PMS-Terazosin** Ⓒ tablets ℞ *antihypertensive (α-blocker); treatment for benign prostatic hyperplasia (BPH)* [terazosin HCl] 1, 2, 5, 10 mg

**PMS-Terbinafine** Ⓒ tablets ℞ *systemic allylamine antifungal* [terbinafine HCl] 250 mg

**PMS-Ticlopidine** Ⓒ film-coated tablets ℞ *platelet aggregation inhibitor for stroke* [ticlopidine HCl] 250 mg

**PMS-Tobramycin** Ⓒ eye drops ℞ *topical antibiotic* [tobramycin] 0.3%

**P-MVAC (Platinol, methotrexate, vinblastine, Adriamycin, carboplatin)** *chemotherapy protocol*

**PNCRM7** *investigational pneumococcal conjugate vaccine for otitis media*

**Pneumo 23** Ⓒ subcu or IM injection ℞ *active immunization against 23 strains of Streptococcus pneumoniae* [pneumococcal vaccine, polyvalent] 0.5 mL

**pneumococcal vaccine, 7-valent** *active bacterin for pneumococcal pneumonia (polysaccharide isolates of seven strains of Streptococcus pneumoniae: 4, 6B, 9V, 14, 18C, 19F, and 23F)*

**pneumococcal vaccine, polyvalent** *active bacterin for pneumococcal pneu-*

*monia (polysaccharide isolates of 23 strains of* Streptococcus pneumoniae)

**Pneumomist** sustained-release tablets (discontinued 2002) ℞ *expectorant* [guaifenesin] 600 mg

**Pneumopent** for inhalation ℞ *investigational (orphan) prophylaxis of* Pneumocystis carinii *pneumonia* [pentamidine isethionate]

**Pneumotussin** caplets ℞ *narcotic antitussive; expectorant* [hydrocodone bitartrate; guaifenesin] 2.5•300 mg

**Pneumotussin 2.5 Cough** syrup ℞ *narcotic antitussive; expectorant* [hydrocodone bitartrate; guaifenesin] 5•400 mg/10 mL

**Pneumotussin HC** syrup (discontinued 2002) ℞ *narcotic antitussive; expectorant* [hydrocodone bitartrate; guaifenesin] 5•100 mg/5 mL

**Pneumovax 23** subcu or IM injection ℞ *active immunization against 23 strains of* Streptococcus pneumoniae [pneumococcal vaccine, polyvalent] 25 μg of each strain per 0.5 mL dose

**Pnu-Imune 23** subcu or IM injection (discontinued 2002) ℞ *active immunization against 23 strains of* Streptococcus pneumoniae [pneumococcal vaccine, polyvalent] 25 μg of each strain per 0.5 mL dose

**pobilukast edamine** USAN *antiasthmatic*

**POC (procarbazine, Oncovin, CCNU)** *chemotherapy protocol for pediatric brain tumors*

**POCA (prednisone, Oncovin, cytarabine, Adriamycin)** *chemotherapy protocol*

**POCC (procarbazine, Oncovin, cyclophosphamide, CCNU)** *chemotherapy protocol*

**Pockethaler** (trademarked delivery device) *nasal inhalation aerosol*

**pod pepper** *medicinal herb* [see: cayenne]

**podilfen** INN

**Podocon-25** topical liquid ℞ *keratolytic for genital warts* [podophyllum resin] 25%

**podofilox** USAN *topical antimitotic for genital warts* [also: podophyllotoxin] 0.5% topical

**Podofin** topical liquid ℞ *keratolytic for genital warts* [podophyllum resin] 25% ⓓ podophyllin

**podophyllin** [see: podophyllum resin] ⓓ Podofin

**podophyllotoxin** BAN *topical antimitotic* [also: podofilox]

**podophyllotoxins** *a class of mitotic-inhibiting antineoplastics derived from podophyllotoxin*

**podophyllum** USP *caustic; cytotoxic agent for genital warts*

*Podophyllum peltatum medicinal herb* [see: mandrake]

**podophyllum resin** USP *caustic; cytotoxic agent for genital warts*

**poinsettia (Euphorbia pulcherrima; E. poinsettia; Poinsettia pulcherrima)** *plant and sap medicinal herb for fever, pain relief, stimulating lactation, toothache, and warts; also used as an antibacterial and depilatory*

**Point-Two** oral rinse ℞ *topical dental caries preventative* [sodium fluoride; alcohol 6%] 0.2%

**poison, dog** *medicinal herb* [see: dog poison]

**Poison Antidote Kit** (discontinued 2002) OTC *emergency treatment for various poisons* [syrup of ipecac; charcoal suspension] 30•60 mL

**poison ash** *medicinal herb* [see: fringe tree]

**poison flag** *medicinal herb* [see: blue flag]

**poison hemlock (Conium maculatum)** *plant medicinal herb that has been used for analgesia and sedation and as a method of execution; it is extremely poisonous*

**poison ivy extract, alum precipitated** USAN *ivy poisoning counteractant*

**poison oak (Tocicodendron diversilobum)** *extract medicinal herb used in homeopathic remedies for osteoarthritis*

**poison oak extract** USAN *antiallergic*

**Poison Oak-N-Ivy Armor** lotion (discontinued 2003) OTC *poison ivy protectant*

**poke root** *(Phytolacca decandra)* *medicinal herb* [see: pokeweed]

**pokeweed** *(Phytolacca americana; P. decandra; P. rigida)* root and young shoots *medicinal herb for arthritis, blood cleansing, bowel evacuation, dysmenorrhea, mucous membrane inflammation and discharge, mumps, pain, rheumatism, ringworm, scabies, syphilis, and tonsillitis; not generally regarded as safe and effective*

**polacrilex** [see: nicotine polacrilex]

**polacrilin** USAN, INN *pharmaceutic aid*

**polacrilin potassium** USAN, NF *tablet disintegrant*

**Polaramine** tablets, Repetabs (repeat-action tablets), syrup (discontinued 2002) ℞ *antihistamine* [dexchlorpheniramine maleate] 2 mg; 4, 6 mg; 2 mg/5 mL

**Polaramine Expectorant** oral liquid ℞ *decongestant; antihistamine; expectorant* [pseudoephedrine sulfate; dexchlorpheniramine maleate; guaifenesin; alcohol 7.2%] 20•2•100 mg/5 mL

**poldine methylsulfate** USAN, USP *anticholinergic* [also: poldine metilsulfate]

**poldine metilsulfate** INN *anticholinergic* [also: poldine methylsulfate]

**polecat weed** *medicinal herb* [see: skunk cabbage]

**policapram** USAN, INN *tablet binder*

**policosanol** *natural supplement from sugar cane plants; enhanced extract of octacosanol (q.v.) used for hypercholesterolemia; therapeutic effects are similar to statin drugs but without side effects such as liver dysfunction and muscle atrophy*

**policresulen** INN

**polidexide sulfate** INN

**polidocanol** INN, JAN, DCF *polyethylene glycol monododecyl ether*

**polifeprosan** INN *pharmaceutic aid; implantable, biodegradable drug carrier* [also: polifeprosan 20]

**polifeprosan 20** USAN *pharmaceutic aid; implantable, biodegradable drug carrier* [also: polifeprosan]

**poligeenan** USAN, INN *dispersing agent*

**poliglecaprone 25** USAN *absorbable surgical suture material*

**poliglecaprone 90** USAN *absorbable surgical suture coating*

**poliglusam** USAN *antihemorrhagic*

**polignate sodium** USAN *pepsin enzyme inhibitor*

**polihexanide** INN [also: polyhexanide]

**poliomyelitis vaccine** [now: poliovirus vaccine, inactivated]

**poliovirus vaccine, enhanced inactivated (eIPV)** *active immunizing agent for poliomyelitis*

**poliovirus vaccine, inactivated (IPV)** USP *active immunizing agent for poliomyelitis*

**poliovirus vaccine, live oral (OPV)** USP *active immunizing agent for poliomyelitis*

**polipropene 25** USAN *tablet excipient*

**polisaponin** INN

**politef** INN *prosthetic aid* [also: polytef]

**polixetonium chloride** USAN, INN *preservative*

**Polocaine** injection ℞ *injectable local anesthetic* [mepivacaine HCl] 1%, 2%, 3%

**Polocaine MPF** injection ℞ *injectable local anesthetic* [mepivacaine HCl] 1%, 1.5%, 2%

**Polocaine with levonordefrin** injection ℞ *injectable local anesthetic* [mepivacaine HCl; levonordefrin] 2%•1:20 000

**polonium** *element (Po)*

**poloxalene** USAN, INN, BAN *surfactant*

**poloxamer** USAN, NF, INN, BAN *ointment and suppository base; tablet binder*

**poloxamer 124** USAN *surfactant; emulsifier; solubilizer; stabilizer*

**poloxamer 188** USAN *surfactant; emulsifier; solubilizer; investigational (Phase III, orphan) for sickle cell crisis; investigational (orphan) for severe burns and vasospasm following cerebral aneurysm repair*

**poloxamer 237** USAN *surfactant; emulsifier; solubilizer; stabilizer*

**poloxamer 331** *investigational (orphan) for toxoplasmosis of AIDS*

**poloxamer 338** USAN *surfactant; emulsifier; solubilizer; stabilizer*

**poloxamer 407** USAN *surfactant; emulsifier; solubilizer; stabilizer*

**poly I: poly C12U** *investigational (Phase III, orphan) antiviral/immunomodulator for HIV, renal cell carcinoma, metastatic melanoma, and chronic fatigue syndrome*

**polyamine-methylene resin**

**polyanhydroglucose** [see: dextran]

**polyanhydroglucuronic acid** [see: dextran]

**polybenzarsol** INN

**polybutester** USAN *surgical suture material*

**polybutilate** USAN *surgical suture coating*

**polycarbokane** [see: polycarbophil]

**polycarbophil** USP, INN, BAN *bulk laxative; antidiarrheal*

**Polycitra** syrup ℞ *urinary alkalinizing agent* [potassium citrate; sodium citrate; citric acid] 550•500•334 mg/5 mL

**Polycitra-K** oral solution, crystals for oral solution ℞ *urinary alkalizing agent* [potassium citrate; citric acid] 1100•334 mg/5 mL; 3300•1002 mg/pkt.

**Polycitra-LC** solution ℞ *urinary alkalizing agent* [potassium citrate; sodium citrate; citric acid] 550•500•334 mg/5 mL

**Polycose** oral liquid, powder for oral liquid OTC *carbohydrate caloric supplement* [glucose polymers]

**polydextrose** USAN *food additive*

**polydimethylsiloxane** *surgical aid (retinal tamponade) for retinal detachment*

**Polydine** ointment, scrub, solution OTC *broad-spectrum antimicrobial* [povidone-iodine]

**polydioxanone** USAN *absorbable surgical suture material*

**polyelectrolyte 211** [see: sodium alginate]

**polyenes** *a class of antifungals produced by a species of* Streptomyces *that damage fungal cell membranes*

**polyestradiol phosphate** INN, BAN *antineoplastic; estrogen*

**polyetadene** INN *antacid* [also: polyethadene]

**polyethadene** USAN *antacid* [also: polyetadene]

**polyethylene excipient** NF *stiffening agent*

**polyethylene glycol (PEG)** NF *ophthalmic moisturizer; ointment and suppository base; solvent*

**polyethylene glycol** *n* (*n* refers to the molecular weight: 300, 1000, etc.)

**polyethylene glycol** *n* **dioleate** (*n* refers to the molecular weight: 300, 400, 1000, etc.)

**polyethylene glycol 8 monostearate** [see: polyoxyl 8 stearate]

**polyethylene glycol 1000 monocetyl ether** [see: cetomacrogol 1000]

**polyethylene glycol 1540** NF

**polyethylene glycol 4000** USP [also: macrogol 4000]

**polyethylene glycol 6000** USP

**polyethylene glycol–electrolyte solution (PEG-ES)** *pre-procedure bowel evacuant* [contains PEG 3350]

**polyethylene glycol monoleyl ether** [see: polyoxyl 10 oleyl ether]

**polyethylene glycol monomethyl ether** NF *excipient*

**polyethylene glycol monostearate** [see: polyoxyl 40 & 50 stearate]

**polyethylene glycol-superoxide dismutase (PEG-SOD)** [see: pegorgotein]

**polyethylene oxide** NF *suspending and viscosity agent; tablet binder*

**polyferose** USAN *hematinic*

*Polygala senega* *medicinal herb* [see: senega]

**Polygam** powder for IV infusion (discontinued 2001; replaced by Polygam S/D) ℞ *passive immunizing agent for HIV* [immune globulin] 50 mg/mL

**Polygam S/D** freeze-dried powder for IV infusion ℞ *passive immunizing*

*agent for HIV, idiopathic thrombocytopenic purpura, and B-cell chronic lymphocytic leukemia* [immune globulin, solvent/detergent treated] 50 mg/mL

**polygeline** INN, BAN

**polyglactin 370** USAN *absorbable surgical suture coating*

**polyglactin 910** USAN *absorbable surgical suture material*

**polyglycolic acid** USAN, INN *surgical suture material*

**polyglyconate** USAN, BAN *absorbable surgical suture material*

*Polygonatum multiflorum; P. odoratum medicinal herb* [see: Solomon's seal]

*Polygonum aviculare; P. hydropiper; P. persicaria; P. punctatum medicinal herb* [see: knotweed]

*Polygonum bistorta medicinal herb* [see: bistort]

*Polygonum multiflorum medicinal herb* [see: fo-ti; ho-shou-wu]

**PolyHeme** R *investigational (Phase III) blood substitute* [human hemoglobin cross-linked with glutaral]

**polyhexanide** BAN [also: polihexanide]

**Poly-Histine** elixir R *antihistamine for allergic and vasomotor rhinitis, allergic conjunctivitis, and mild urticaria* [pheniramine maleate; pyrilamine maleate; phenyltoloxamine citrate] 4•4•4 mg/5 mL

**Poly-Histine CS** syrup (discontinued 2002) R *narcotic antitussive; decongestant; antihistamine* [codeine phosphate; phenylpropanolamine HCl; brompheniramine maleate] 10•12.5•2 mg/5 mL

**Poly-Histine DM** syrup (discontinued 2002) R *antitussive; decongestant; antihistamine* [dextromethorphan hydrobromide; phenylpropanolamine HCl; brompheniramine maleate] 10•12.5•2 mg/5 mL

**Poly-Histine-D** sustained-release capsules, elixir (discontinued 2001) R *decongestant; antihistamine* [phenylpropanolamine HCl; phenyltoloxamine citrate; pyrilamine maleate;

pheniramine maleate] 50•16•16•16 mg; 12.5•4•4•4 mg/5 mL

**Poly-Histine-D Ped Caps** sustained-release capsules (discontinued 2001) R *pediatric decongestant and antihistamine* [phenylpropanolamine HCl; phenyltoloxamine citrate; pyrilamine maleate; pheniramine maleate] 25•8•8•8 mg

**poly-ICLC** *investigational (orphan) for primary brain tumors*

**polyloxyl 8 stearate** USAN *surfactant*

**polymacon** USAN *hydrophilic contact lens material*

**polymanoacetate** [now: acemannan]

**polymeric oxygen** [see: oxygen, polymeric]

**polymetaphosphate P 32** USAN *radioactive agent*

**polymethyl methacrylate (PMMA)** *rigid hydrophobic polymer used for hard contact lenses*

**polymixin E** [see: colistin sulfate]

**polymonine**

**polymyxin** BAN *bactericidal antibiotic* [also: polymyxin B sulfate; polymyxin B]

**polymyxin B** INN *bactericidal antibiotic* [also: polymyxin B sulfate; polymyxin]

**polymyxin B sulfate** USP *bactericidal antibiotic* [also: polymyxin B; polymyxin] 500 000 U/vial eye drops or injection

**polymyxin B sulfate & bacitracin zinc** *topical antibiotic* 10 000•500 U/g ophthalmic

**polymyxin B sulfate & bacitracin zinc & neomycin sulfate** *topical antibiotic* 10 000 U•400 U•5 mg per g ophthalmic

**polymyxin B sulfate & gramicidin & neomycin sulfate** *topical antibiotic* 10 000 U•0.025 mg•1.75 mg per mL eye drops

**polymyxin B sulfate & neomycin sulfate & dexamethasone** *topical ophthalmic antibiotic and corticosteroidal anti-inflammatory* 10 000 U/mL• 0.35%•0.1% eye drops

**polymyxin B sulfate & neomycin sulfate & hydrocortisone** *topical ophthalmic antibiotic and corticosteroidal anti-inflammatory* 10 000 U/mL • 0.35% • 1% eye drops

**polymyxin B sulfate & trimethoprim sulfate** *topical ophthalmic antibiotic* 10 000 U • 1 mg per mL eye drops

**polymyxin B₁** [see: polymyxin B]

**polymyxin B₂** [see: polymyxin B]

**polymyxin B₃** [see: polymyxin B]

**polymyxin E** [see: colistin sulfate]

**polynoxylin** INN, BAN

**polyolprepolymer** *topical base for gels and creams*

**polyoxyethylene 20 sorbitan monolaurate** [see: polysorbate 20]

**polyoxyethylene 20 sorbitan monooleate** [see: polysorbate 80]

**polyoxyethylene 20 sorbitan monopalmitate** [see: polysorbate 40]

**polyoxyethylene 20 sorbitan monostearate** [see: polysorbate 60]

**polyoxyethylene 20 sorbitan trioleate** [see: polysorbate 85]

**polyoxyethylene 20 sorbitan tristearate** [see: polysorbate 65]

**polyoxyethylene 50 stearate** [now: polyoxyl 50 stearate]

**polyoxyethylene glycol 1000 monocetyl ether** [see: cetomacrogol 1000]

**polyoxyethylene nonyl phenol** *surfactant/wetting agent*

**polyoxyl 10 oleyl ether** NF *surfactant*

**polyoxyl 20 cetostearyl ether** NF *surfactant*

**polyoxyl 35 castor oil** NF *emulsifying agent; surfactant*

**polyoxyl 40 hydrogenated castor oil** NF *emulsifying agent; surfactant*

**polyoxyl 40 stearate** USAN, NF *surfactant*

**polyoxyl 50 stearate** NF *surfactant; emulsifying agent*

**polyoxypropylene 15 stearyl ether** USAN *solvent*

**polyphosphoric acid, sodium salt** [see: sodium polyphosphate]

*Polypodium vulgare* *medicinal herb* [see: female fern]

**Poly-Pred** eye drop suspension ℞ *corticosteroidal anti-inflammatory; antibiotic* [prednisolone acetate; neomycin sulfate; polymyxin B sulfate] 0.5% • 0.35% • 10 000 U per mL

**polypropylene glycol** NF

**polyribonucleotide** [see: poly I: poly C12U]

**polysaccharide-iron complex** *hematinic; dietary iron supplement* 150 mg oral

**Polysorb Hydrate** cream OTC *moisturizer; emollient*

**polysorbate 20** USAN, NF, INN *surfactant/wetting agent*

**polysorbate 40** USAN, NF, INN *surfactant*

**polysorbate 60** USAN, NF, INN *surfactant*

**polysorbate 65** USAN, INN *surfactant*

**polysorbate 80** USAN, NF, INN *surfactant/wetting agent; viscosity-increasing agent*

**polysorbate 85** USAN, INN *surfactant*

**Polysporin** ointment, topical powder OTC *antibiotic* [polymyxin B sulfate; bacitracin zinc] 10 000 • 500 U/g

**Polysporin** ophthalmic ointment OTC *topical ophthalmic antibiotic* [polymyxin B sulfate; bacitracin zinc] 10 000 • 500 U/g

**Polytabs-F** chewable tablets ℞ *pediatric vitamin supplement and dental caries preventative* [multiple vitamins; fluoride; folic acid] ± • 1 • 0.3 mg

**Polytar** shampoo, soap OTC *antiseborrheic; antipsoriatic; antipruritic; antibacterial* [coal tar (solution includes pine tar and juniper tar)] 0.5% (4.5%); 0.5% ( 2.5%)

**Polytar Bath** oil (discontinued 2003) OTC *antipsoriatic; antiseborrheic; antipruritic; antibacterial* [coal tar (solution includes pine tar and juniper tar)] 0.5% (25%)

**polytef** USAN *prosthetic aid* [also: politef]

**polytetrafluoroethylene (PTFE)** [see: polytef]

**polythiazide** USAN, USP, INN *diuretic; antihypertensive*

**Polytrim** eye drops (discontinued 2003) ℞ *antibiotic* [polymyxin B sulfate; trimethoprim] 10 000 U•1 mg per mL

**Poly-Tussin** syrup ℞ *narcotic antitussive; decongestant; antihistamine* [hydrocodone bitartrate; phenylephrine HCl; chlorpheniramine maleate] 5•5•2 mg/5 mL

**polyurethane foam** USAN *internal bone splint*

**polyvalent Crotaline antivenin** [see: antivenin (Crotalidae) polyvalent]

**polyvalent gas gangrene antitoxin** [see: gas gangrene antitoxin, pentavalent]

**polyvidone** INN *dispersing, suspending and viscosity-increasing agent* [also: povidone]

**Poly-Vi-Flor** chewable tablets ℞ *pediatric vitamin supplement and dental caries preventative* [multiple vitamins; sodium fluoride; folic acid] ±•0.25•0.3, ±•0.5•0.3, ±•1•0.3 mg

**Poly-Vi-Flor** drops ℞ *pediatric vitamin supplement and dental caries preventative* [multiple vitamins; sodium fluoride] ±•0.25, ±•0.5 mg/mL

**Poly-Vi-Flor with Iron** chewable tablets ℞ *pediatric vitamin/iron supplement and dental caries preventative* [multiple vitamins & minerals; sodium fluoride; iron; folic acid] ±•0.25•12•0.3, ±•0.5•12•0.3, ±•1•12•0.3 mg

**Poly-Vi-Flor with Iron** drops ℞ *pediatric vitamin/iron supplement and dental caries preventative* [multiple vitamins & minerals; sodium fluoride; iron] ±•0.25•10, ±•0.5•10 mg/mL

**polyvinyl acetate phthalate** NF *coating agent*

**polyvinyl alcohol (PVA)** USP *ophthalmic moisturizer; viscosity-increasing agent*

**polyvinyl chloride, radiopaque** *oral radiopaque contrast medium for severe constipation*

**polyvinylpyrrolidone** [now: povidone]

**Poly-Vi-Sol** chewable tablets OTC *vitamin supplement* [multiple vitamins; folic acid] ±•0.3 mg

**Poly-** drops OTC *vitamin supplement* [multiple vitamins]

**Poly-Vi-Sol with Iron** chewable tablets OTC *vitamin/iron supplement* [multiple vitamins; iron; folic acid] ±•12•0.3 mg

**Poly-Vi-Sol with Iron** drops OTC *vitamin/iron supplement* [multiple vitamins; iron] ±•10 mg/mL

**Poly-Vitamin** drops OTC *vitamin supplement* [multiple vitamins]

**Polyvitamin Fluoride** chewable tablets ℞ *pediatric vitamin supplement and dental caries preventative* [multiple vitamins; fluoride; folic acid] ±•0.5•0.3, ±•1•0.3 mg

**Polyvitamin Fluoride** drops ℞ *pediatric vitamin supplement and dental caries preventative* [multiple vitamins; fluoride] ±•0.25, ±•0.5 mg/mL

**Polyvitamin Fluoride with Iron** chewable tablets ℞ *pediatric vitamin/iron supplement and dental caries preventative* [multiple vitamins & minerals; fluoride; iron; folic acid] ±•1•12•0.3 mg

**Poly-Vitamin with Iron** drops OTC *vitamin/iron supplement* [multiple vitamins; iron] ±•10 mg/mL

**Polyvitamin with Iron and Fluoride** drops ℞ *pediatric vitamin/iron supplement and dental caries preventative* [multiple vitamins; iron; fluoride] ±•10•0.25 mg/mL

**Polyvitamins with Fluoride and Iron** chewable tablets ℞ *pediatric vitamin/iron supplement and dental caries preventative* [multiple vitamins; fluoride; iron; folic acid] ±•0.5•12•0.3 mg

**pomegranate (Punica granatum)** seeds and fruit rind *medicinal herb used as an anthelmintic and astringent*

**POMP (prednisone, Oncovin, methotrexate, Purinethol)** *chemotherapy protocol*

**ponalrestat** USAN, INN, BAN *aldose reductase inhibitor*

**ponfibrate** INN

**Ponstel** capsules ℞ *analgesic; nonsteroidal anti-inflammatory drug*

*(NSAID)* [mefenamic acid] 250 mg ℞ Pronestyl

**Pontocaine** cream OTC *topical local anesthetic* [tetracaine HCl] 1%

**Pontocaine** ointment OTC *topical local anesthetic* [tetracaine; menthol] 0.5%•0.5%

**Pontocaine HCl** Mono-Drop (eye drops) ℞ *topical ophthalmic anesthetic* [tetracaine HCl] 0.5%

**Pontocaine HCl** solution ℞ *nose/throat anesthetic to abolish laryngeal and esophageal reflex* [tetracaine HCl; chlorobutanol] 2%•0.4%

**Pontocaine HCl** spinal injection, powder for reconstitution ℞ *injectable local anesthetic* [tetracaine HCl] 0.2%, 0.3%, 1%

**poplar *(Populus tremuloides)*** bark and buds *medicinal herb used as an antiperiodic, balsamic, febrifuge, and stomachic*

**poplar, balsam** *medicinal herb* [see: balm of Gilead]

**poplar, black** *medicinal herb* [see: black poplar]

**Po-Pon-S** sugar-coated tablets OTC *vitamin/mineral supplement* [multiple vitamins & minerals]

*Populus balsamifera; P. candicans medicinal herb* [see: balm of Gilead]

*Populus nigra; P. tremula medicinal herb* [see: black poplar]

*Populus tremuloides medicinal herb* [see: poplar]

**poractant alfa** BAN *porcine lung extract containing 90% phospholipids for emergency rescue and treatment of respiratory distress syndrome (RDS) in premature infants (orphan)*

**Porcelana** cream (discontinued 2003) OTC *hyperpigmentation bleaching agent* [hydroquinone] 2%

**Porcelana with Sunscreen** cream (discontinued 2003) OTC *hyperpigmentation bleaching agent* [hydroquinone (in a sunscreen base)] 2%

**porcine islet preparation, encapsulated** *investigational (orphan) antidiabetic for type 1 patients on immunosuppression*

**porfimer sodium** USAN, INN *laser light–activated antineoplastic for photodynamic therapy (PDT) of esophageal (orphan) and non–small cell lung cancers; used for ablation of high-grade dysplasia in Barrett esophagus (BE) patients; investigational (orphan) for bladder cancer*

**porfiromycin** USAN, INN, BAN *antibacterial; investigational (Phase III, orphan) antineoplastic for head, neck, and cervical cancers*

*Porites spp. natural material* [see: coral]

**porofocon A** USAN *hydrophobic contact lens material*

**porofocon B** USAN *hydrophobic contact lens material*

**Portagen** powder OTC *enteral nutritional therapy* [lactose-free formula]

**Portia** film-coated tablets (in packs of 21 or 28) ℞ *monophasic oral contraceptive; emergency postcoital contraceptive* [levonorgestrel; ethinyl estradiol] 0.15 mg•30 μg

**porton asparaginase** [see: Erwinia L-asparaginase]

**posaconazole** USAN *antifungal; investigational (Phase III) treatment for AIDS-related fungal infections*

**posatirelin** INN

**posedrine** [see: benzchlorpropamid]

**poskine** INN, BAN

**posterior pituitary** [see: pituitary, posterior]

**Posture** tablets OTC *calcium supplement* [calcium phosphate, tribasic] 600 mg Ca

**Posture-D** film-coated tablets OTC *dietary supplement* [calcium phosphate, tribasic; vitamin D] 600 mg•125 IU

**Potaba** tablets, capsules, Envules (powder for oral solution) ℞ *water-soluble vitamin; "possibly effective" for scleroderma and other skin diseases and Peyronie disease* [aminobenzoate potassium] 500 mg; 500 mg; 2 g

**Potable Aqua** tablets (discontinued 2002) OTC *emergency disinfectant for*

*drinking water* [tetraglycine hydroperiodide (source of iodine)] 16.7% (6.68%)

**Potasalan** oral liquid ℞ *potassium supplement* [potassium chloride; alcohol 4%] 20 mEq K/15 mL

**potash, sulfurated** USP *source of sulfides*

**potassic saline, lactated** NF

**potassium** *element (K)*

**potassium acetate** USP *electrolyte replenisher* 2, 4 mEq/mL injection

**potassium acid phosphate** *urinary acidifier*

**potassium alpha-phenoxyethyl penicillin** [see: phenethicillin potassium]

**potassium alum** [see: alum, potassium]

**potassium aminobenzoate** [see: aminobenzoate potassium]

**potassium aspartate** [see: L-aspartate potassium]

**potassium aspartate & magnesium aspartate** USAN *nutrient*

**potassium benzoate** NF *preservative*

**potassium benzyl penicillin** [see: penicillin G potassium]

**potassium bicarbonate** USP *pH buffer; electrolyte replacement*

**potassium bitartrate** USAN

**potassium borate** *pH buffer*

**potassium canrenoate** JAN *aldosterone antagonist* [also: canrenoate potassium; canrenoic acid]

**potassium carbonate** USP *alkalizing agent*

**potassium chloride (KCl)** USP *electrolyte replenisher* 600, 750, 1500 mg oral; 20, 40 mEq/15 mL oral; 20 mEq/pkt oral; 2, 10, 20, 30, 40, 60, 90 mEq/mL injection

**potassium chloride K 42** USAN *radioactive agent*

**potassium citrate** USP *electrolyte replacement; urinary alkalizer for nephrolithiasis and hypocitruria prevention (orphan)*

**potassium clavulanate & amoxicillin** [see: amoxicillin]

**potassium clavulanate & ticarcillin** [see: ticarcillin disodium]

**potassium dichloroisocyanurate** [see: troclosene potassium]

**potassium gamma hydroxybutyrate (KGHB)** [see: gamma hydroxybutyrate (GHB)]

**potassium glucaldrate** USAN, INN *antacid*

**potassium gluconate** USP *electrolyte replenisher* 500, 595 mg oral; 20 mEq/15 mL oral

**potassium guaiacolsulfonate** USP *expectorant* [also: sulfogaiacol]

**potassium hydroxide (KOH)** NF *alkalizing agent*

**potassium hydroxymethoxybenzenesulfonate hemihydrate** [see: potassium guaiacolsulfonate]

**potassium iodate** *prevents the uptake of radioactive iodine by the thyroid gland after a nuclear accident or attack*

**potassium iodide** USP *antifungal; expectorant; dietary iodine supplement; thyroid agent; prevents the uptake of radioactive iodine by the thyroid gland after a nuclear accident or attack* 1 g/mL oral

**potassium mercuric iodide** NF

**potassium metabisulfite** NF *antioxidant*

**potassium metaphosphate** NF *buffering agent*

**potassium nitrate** *tooth desensitizer*

**potassium nitrazepate** INN

**potassium para-aminobenzoate (PAB)** [see: aminobenzoate potassium]

**potassium penicillin G** [see: penicillin G potassium]

**potassium perchlorate** *radioimaging adjunct*

**potassium permanganate** USP *topical anti-infective*

**potassium phosphate, dibasic** USP *calcium regulator; phosphorus replacement; pH buffer*

**potassium phosphate, monobasic** NF *pH buffer; phosphorus replacement*

**potassium sodium tartrate** USP *laxative*

**potassium sorbate** NF *antimicrobial agent*

**potassium tetraborate** *pH buffer*

**potassium thiocyanate** NF

**potassium-sparing diuretics** *a class of diuretic agents that interfere with sodium reabsorption, thus decreasing potassium secretion*

**potato, wild; wild sweet potato vine** *medicinal herb* [see: wild jalap]

*Potentilla anserina; P. canadensis; P. reptans medicinal herb* [see: cinquefoil]

*Potentilla tormentilla medicinal herb* [see: tormentil]

**Povidine** ointment, scrub, solution OTC *broad-spectrum antimicrobial* [povidone-iodine] 10%, 5%, 10%

**povidone** USAN, USP *dispersing, suspending and viscosity-increasing agent* [also: polyvidone]

**povidone I 125** USAN *radioactive agent*

**povidone I 131** USAN *radioactive agent*

**povidone-iodine** USP, BAN *broad-spectrum antimicrobial* 10% topical

**powdered cellulose** [see: cellulose, powdered]

**powdered ipecac** [see: ipecac, powdered]

**powdered opium** [see: opium, powdered]

**PowerMate** tablets OTC *vitamin/mineral supplement* [multiple vitamins & minerals]

**PowerSleep** tablets OTC *vitamin/mineral supplement; nonprescription sleep aid* [multiple vitamins & minerals; 5-hydroxytryptophan; L-glutamine; melatonin; valerian] ±•250•25• 0.25•75 mg

**PowerVites** tablets OTC *vitamin/mineral supplement* [multiple vitamins & minerals; folic acid; biotin] ±•150•25 µg

**PPA (phenylpropanolamine)** [q.v.]

**PPAR (peroxisome proliferator-activated receptor) agonists** *a class of investigational agents that increase insulin receptor sensitivity in type 2 diabetes*

**PPD (purified protein derivative [of tuberculin])** [see: tuberculin]

**PPG-15 stearyl ether** [now: polyoxypropylene 15 stearyl ether]

**PPIs (proton pump inhibitors)** [q.v.]

**practolol** USAN, INN *antiadrenergic (β-receptor)*

**prajmalium bitartrate** INN, BAN

**pralidoxime chloride** USAN, USP *cholinesterase reactivator for organophosphate poisoning and anticholinesterase overdose* ⊡ pyridoxine; pramoxine

**pralidoxime iodide** USAN, INN *cholinesterase reactivator* ⊡ pyridoxine; pramoxine

**pralidoxime mesylate** USAN *cholinesterase reactivator* ⊡ pyridoxine; pramoxine

**pralmorelin dihydrochloride** USAN *growth hormone secretagogue*

**PrameGel** gel OTC *local anesthetic* [pramoxine HCl; menthol] 1%•0.5%

**Pramilet FA** Filmtabs (film-coated tablets) ℞ *prenatal vitamin/mineral/calcium/iron supplement* [multiple vitamins & minerals; calcium; iron; folic acid] ±•250•40•1 mg

**pramipexole** USAN, INN *dopamine agonist; antiparkinsonian; investigational for depression and schizophrenia*

**pramipexole dihydrochloride** USAN *dopamine agonist; antiparkinsonian; investigational for depression and schizophrenia*

**pramiracetam** INN *cognition adjuvant* [also: pramiracetam HCl]

**pramiracetam HCl** USAN *cognition adjuvant* [also: pramiracetam]

**pramiracetam sulfate** USAN *cognition adjuvant*

**pramiverine** INN, BAN

**pramlintide** USAN *synthetic amylin analogue to slow gastric emptying*

**pramlintide acetate** USAN *synthetic amylin analogue to slow gastric emptying; investigational (NDA filed) antidiabetic for type 1 and type 2 diabetes*

**pramocaine** INN *topical anesthetic* [also: pramoxine HCl; pramoxine]

**pramocaine HCl** [see: pramoxine HCl]

**Pramosone** cream, lotion, ointment ℞ *corticosteroidal anti-inflammatory; local anesthetic* [hydrocortisone acetate; pramoxine] 1%•1%, 2.5%•1%; 2.5%•1%; 2.5%•1% ⊡ pramoxine

**pramoxine** BAN *topical local anesthetic* [also: pramoxine HCl; pramocaine] ⌷ pralidoxime; Pramosone

**Pramoxine HC** anorectal aerosol foam ℞ *topical corticosteroidal anti-inflammatory; local anesthetic* [hydrocortisone acetate; pramoxine HCl] 1%•1%

**pramoxine HCl** USP *topical local anesthetic* [also: pramocaine; pramoxine]

**prampine** INN, BAN

**Prandase** ⓖⓐⓝ tablets ℞ *alpha-glucosidase inhibitor for type 2 diabetes* [acarbose] 50, 100 mg

**Prandin** tablets ℞ *oral antidiabetic agent that stimulates the release of insulin from the pancreas for type 2 diabetes* [repaglinide] 0.5, 1, 2 mg

**pranidipine** INN

**pranlukast** INN, BAN *investigational treatment for asthma*

**pranolium chloride** USAN, INN *antiarrhythmic*

**pranoprofen** INN

**pranosal** INN

**praseodymium** *element* (Pr)

**prasterone** INN *synthetic dehydroepiandrosterone (DHEA); investigational (NDA filed) agent to increase bone density in patients with systemic lupus erythematosus (SLE) on corticosteroid therapy*

**Pravachol** tablets ℞ *HMG-CoA reductase inhibitor for hyperlipidemia, hypertriglyceridemia, atherosclerosis, coronary procedures, and recurrent myocardial infarctions* [pravastatin sodium] 10, 20, 40, 80 mg ⌷ Primacor

**pravadoline** INN *analgesic* [also: pravadoline maleate]

**pravadoline maleate** USAN *analgesic* [also: pravadoline]

**pravastatin** INN, BAN *HMG-CoA reductase inhibitor for hyperlipidemia, atherosclerosis, coronary procedures, and recurrent myocardial infarctions* [also: pravastatin sodium]

**pravastatin sodium** USAN, JAN *HMG-CoA reductase inhibitor for hyperlipidemia, atherosclerosis, coronary proce-* dures, and recurrent myocardial infarctions [also: pravastatin]

**Pravigard PAC** combo pack (1 tablet of each per dose) ℞ *antihyperlipidemic; HMG-CoA reductase inhibitor; antiplatelet nonsteroidal anti-inflammatory drug (NSAID)* [pravastatin sodium; bufered aspirin] 20•81, 20•325, 40•81, 40•325, 80•81, 80•325 mg

**Prax** lotion, cream OTC *local anesthetic* [pramoxine HCl] 1%

**praxadine** INN

**prazarelix acetate** USAN *gonadotropin-releasing hormone (GnRH) antagonist for uterine fibroids, endometriosis, and prostate cancer*

**prazepam** USAN, USP, INN *sedative; anxiolytic* 5 mg oral ⌷ prazepine; prazosin

**prazepine** INN ⌷ prazepam

**praziquantel** USAN, USP, INN, BAN *anthelmintic for schistosomiasis (flukes)*

**prazitone** INN, BAN

**prazocillin** INN

**prazosin** INN, BAN *alpha₁-adrenergic blocker for hypertension* [also: prazosin HCl] ⌷ prazepam

**prazosin HCl** USAN, USP, JAN *alpha₁-adrenergic blocker for hypertension* [also: prazosin] 1, 2, 5 mg oral

**Pre-Attain** oral liquid OTC *enteral nutritional therapy* [lactose-free formula]

**PreCare Conceive** film-coated tablets ℞ *pre-conception vitamin/mineral/calcium/iron supplement* [multiple vitamins & minerals; calcium; iron; folic acid] ≛•200•30•1 mg

**PreCare Prenatal** film-coated caplet ℞ *vitamin/mineral/calcium/iron supplement for pregnancy and lactation* [multiple vitamins & minerals; calcium; iron; folic acid] ≛•250•40•1 mg

**precatory bean (Abrus precatorius)** plant *medicinal herb for eye inflammation, hastening labor, and stimulating abortion; not generally regarded as safe and effective as it is highly toxic and ingestion may be fatal*

**Precedex** IV infusion ℞ *sedative for intubated and ventilated patients in an intensive care setting; premedication to* anesthesia [dexmedetomidine HCl] 100 μg/mL

**precipitated calcium carbonate** JAN *antacid; dietary calcium supplement* [also: calcium carbonate]

**precipitated chalk** [see: calcium carbonate]

**precipitated sulfur** [see: sulfur, precipitated]

**Precision High Nitrogen Diet** powder OTC *enteral nutritional therapy* [lactose-free formula]

**Precision LR Diet** powder OTC *enteral nutritional therapy* [lactose-free formula]

**preclamol** INN

**Precose** tablets ℞ *antidiabetic agent for type 2 diabetes; alpha-glucosidase inhibitor that delays the digestion of dietary carbohydrates* [acarbose] 25, 50, 100 mg

**Pred Mild; Pred Forte** eye drop suspension ℞ *corticosteroidal anti-inflammatory* [prednisolone acetate] 0.12%; 1%

**Predalone 50** IM injection ℞ *corticosteroid; anti-inflammatory* [prednisolone acetate] 50 mg/mL

**Predcor-50** IM injection ℞ *corticosteroid; anti-inflammatory* [prednisolone acetate] 50 mg/mL

**Pred-G** eye drop suspension ℞ *topical ophthalmic corticosteroidal anti-inflammatory; antibiotic* [prednisolone acetate; gentamicin sulfate] 1%•0.3%

**Pred-G S.O.P.** ophthalmic ointment ℞ *ophthalmic topical corticosteroidal anti-inflammatory; antibiotic* [prednisolone acetate; gentamicin sulfate; chlorobutanol] 0.6%•0.3%•0.5%

**prednazate** USAN, INN *anti-inflammatory*

**prednazoline** INN

**prednicarbate** USAN, INN *corticosteroid; anti-inflammatory*

**Prednicen-M** tablets ℞ *corticosteroid; anti-inflammatory; immunosuppressant* [prednisone] 5 mg

**prednimustine** USAN, INN *antineoplastic; investigational for malignant non-Hodgkin lymphomas; orphan status withdrawn 1998*

**Prednisol TBA** intra-articular, intralesional, or soft tissue injection ℞ *corticosteroid; anti-inflammatory* [prednisolone tebutate] 20 mg/mL

**prednisolamate** INN, BAN

**prednisolone** USP, INN *corticosteroidal anti-inflammatory* 5 mg oral; 15 mg/5 mL oral ⍰ prednisone

**prednisolone acetate** USP, BAN *corticosteroidal anti-inflammatory* 1% eye drops; 25, 50 mg/mL injection

**prednisolone hemisuccinate** USP *corticosteroidal anti-inflammatory*

**prednisolone sodium phosphate** USP *corticosteroidal anti-inflammatory* 15 mg/5 mL oral; 0.125%, 1% eye drops

**prednisolone sodium succinate** USP *corticosteroidal anti-inflammatory*

**prednisolone steaglate** INN, BAN *corticosteroidal anti-inflammatory*

**prednisolone tebutate** USP *corticosteroidal anti-inflammatory* 20 mg/mL injection

**prednisone** USP, INN *corticosteroid; anti-inflammatory; immunosuppressant* 1, 5, 20 mg oral ⍰ prednisolone

**prednival** USAN *corticosteroid; anti-inflammatory*

**prednylidene** INN, BAN

**prefenamate** INN

**Prefest** [see: Ortho-Prefest]

**Prefill** (dosage form) *prefilled applicator*

**Preflex Daily Cleaner Especially for Sensitive Eyes** solution OTC *surfactant cleaning solution for soft contact lenses*

**Prefrin Liquifilm** eye drops OTC *topical ophthalmic decongestant* [phenylephrine HCl] 0.12%

**pregabalin** USAN *gabamimetic anticonvulsant; investigational (NDA filed) agent for neuropathic pain from diabetic neuropathy, peripheral neuropathy, and postherpetic neuropathy; investigational (Phase III) for generalized anxiety disorder (GAD)*

**pregelatinized starch** [see: starch, pregelatinized]

**Pregestimil** powder OTC *hypoallergenic infant food for severe malabsorption* disorders [enzymatically hydrolyzed protein formula]

**pregnandiol** JAN

**pregneninolone** [see: ethisterone]

**pregnenolone** INN *natural hormone precursor* [also: pregnenolone succinate]

**pregnenolone succinate** USAN *hormone precursor* [also: pregnenolone]

**Pregnosis** slide test for home use *in vitro diagnostic aid; urine pregnancy test* [latex agglutination test]

**Pregnyl** powder for IM injection ℞ *hormone for prepubertal cryptorchidism and hypogonadism; ovulation stimulant* [chorionic gonadotropin] 1000 U/mL

**Prehist** sustained-release capsules ℞ *decongestant; antihistamine* [phenylephrine HCl; chlorpheniramine maleate] 20•8 mg

**Prehist D** sustained-release capsules (discontinued 2002) ℞ *decongestant; antihistamine; anticholinergic to dry mucosal secretions* [phenylephrine HCl; chlorpheniramine maleate; methscopolamine nitrate] 20•8•2.5 mg

**Pre-Hist-D** sustained-release tablets ℞ *decongestant; antihistamine; anticholinergic to dry mucosal secretions* [phenylephrine HCl; chlorpheniramine maleate; methscopolamine nitrate] 20•8•2.5 mg

**Prelone** syrup ℞ *corticosteroid; antiinflammatory* [prednisolone; alcohol 5%] 5, 15 mg/5 mL

**Prelu-2** timed-release capsules ℞ *anorexiant; CNS stimulant* [phendimetrazine tartrate] 105 mg

**premafloxacin** USAN, INN *veterinary antibacterial*

**Premarin** tablets ℞ *a mixture of equine estrogens; hormone replacement therapy for the treatment of postmenopausal symptoms and prevention of postmenopausal osteoporosis; palliative therapy for prostate and breast cancer; investigational (Phase III) for Alzheimer disease* [conjugated estrogens] 0.3, 0.45, 0.625, 0.9, 1.25 mg

**Premarin Intravenous** IV or IM injection ℞ *a mixture of equine estrogens for the treatment of abnormal uterine bleeding due to hormonal imbalance* [conjugated estrogens] 25 mg

**Premarin Vaginal** cream ℞ *a mixture of equine estrogens; hormone replacement for postmenopausal atrophic vaginitis* [conjugated estrogens] 0.625 mg/g

**premazepam** INN, BAN

**PremesisRx** tablets ℞ *prenatal vitamin/mineral supplement* [vitamin $B_6$; vitamin $B_{12}$; folic acid; calcium carbonate] 75 mg•12 µg•1 mg•200 mg

**Premphase** tablets (28 per package, 14 of each phase) ℞ *hormone replacement therapy for postmenopausal symptoms* [Phase 1: conjugated estrogens; Phase 2: conjugated estrogens; medroxyprogesterone acetate] 0.625 mg; 0.625•5 mg

**Prempro** tablets ℞ *hormone replacement therapy for postmenopausal symptoms* [conjugated estrogens; medroxyprogesterone acetate] 0.3•1.5, 0.45•1.5, 0.625•2.5, 0.625•5 mg

**Prēmsyn PMS** caplets OTC *analgesic; antipyretic; diuretic; antihistaminic sleep aid* [acetaminophen; pamabrom; pyrilamine maleate] 500•25•15 mg

**prenalterol** INN, BAN *adrenergic* [also: prenalterol HCl]

**prenalterol HCl** USAN *adrenergic* [also: prenalterol]

**Prenatabs RX** film-coated tablets ℞ *vitamin/mineral/calcium/iron supplement* [multiple vitamins & minerals; calcium; iron; folic acid; biotin] ≚•200•29•1•0.03 mg

**Prenatal 19** tablets, chewable tablets ℞ *vitamin/mineral/calcium/iron supplement* [multiple vitamins & minerals; calcium; iron; folic acid] ≚•200•29•1 mg

**Prenatal AD** tablets ℞ *vitamin/mineral/calcium/iron supplement* [multiple vitamins & minerals; calcium; iron; folic acid] ≚•200•90•1 mg

**Prenatal H.P.** tablets ℞ *vitamin/calcium/iron supplement* [multiple vitamins; calcium; iron; folic acid] ≚•50•30•0.8 mg

**Prenatal Maternal** tablets ℞ *vitamin/ mineral/calcium/iron supplement* [multiple vitamins & minerals; calcium; iron; folic acid; biotin] ± •250•60• 1•0.03 mg

**Prenatal MR 90** delayed-release film-coated tablets ℞ *vitamin/calcium/iron supplement* [multiple vitamins; calcium; iron; folic acid] ± •250•90•1 mg

**Prenatal PC 40** film-coated caplets ℞ *vitamin/mineral/calcium/iron supplement* [multiple vitamins and minerals; calcium; iron; folic acid] ± • 250•40•1 mg

**Prenatal Plus; Prenatal Plus Improved** tablets ℞ *vitamin/calcium/ iron supplement* [multiple vitamins; calcium; iron; folic acid] ± •200• 65•1 mg

**Prenatal Plus Iron** tablets ℞ *vitamin/ calcium/iron supplement* [multiple vitamins; calcium; iron; folic acid] ± •200•27•1 mg

**Prenatal Plus with Betacarotene** tablets ℞ *vitamin/calcium/iron supplement* [multiple vitamins; calcium; iron; folic acid] ± •200•65•1 mg

**Prenatal Rx** tablets ℞ *vitamin/calcium/ iron supplement* [multiple vitamins; calcium; iron; folic acid] ± •175• 29.5•1 mg

**Prenatal Rx with Betacarotene** tablets ℞ *vitamin/calcium/iron supplement* [multiple vitamins; calcium; iron; folic acid; biotin] ± •200•60• 1•0.03 mg

**Prenatal with Folic Acid** tablets OTC *vitamin/calcium/iron supplement* [multiple vitamins; calciun; iron; folic acid] ± •200•60•0.8 mg

**Prenatal Z** delayed-release film-coated tablets ℞ *vitamin/calcium/iron supplement* [multiple vitamins; calcium; iron; folic acid] ± •300•65•1 mg

**Prenatal-1 + Iron** tablets ℞ *vitamin/ calcium/iron supplement* [multiple vitamins; calcium; iron; folic acid] ± •200•65•1 mg

**Prenatal-H** capsules ℞ *vitamin/mineral/iron supplement* [multiple vitamins & minerals; iron; folic acid] ± •106.5•1 mg

**Prenatal-S** tablets OTC *vitamin/calcium/ iron supplement* [multiple vitamins; calcium; iron; folic acid] ± •200• 60•0.8 mg

**Prenate Advance; Prenate 90** delayed-release film-coated tablets ℞ *prenatal vitamin/calcium/iron supplement* [multiple vitamins; calcium; iron; folic acid] ± •200•90•1 mg; ± •250•90•1 mg

**Prenate GT** delayed-release gel-coated tablets (discontinued 2004) ℞ *prenatal vitamin/calcium/iron supplement* [multiple vitamins; calcium; iron; folic acid] ± •200•90•1 mg

**Prenate Ultra** delayed-release film-coated tablets (discontinued 2000) ℞ *prenatal vitamin/calcium/iron supplement* [multiple vitamins; calcium; iron; folic acid] ± •200•90•1 mg

**Prenavite** tablets OTC *vitamin/calcium/ iron supplement* [multiple vitamins; calcium; iron; folic acid] ± •200• 60•0.8 mg

**prenisteine** INN

**prenoverine** INN

**prenoxdiazine** INN

**prenylamine** USAN, INN *coronary vasodilator*

**Preos** subcu injection ℞ *investigational (Phase III) recombinant human parathyroid hormone for postmenopausal osteoporosis in women*

**Preparation H** anorectal cream, anorectal ointment OTC *temporary relief of hemorrhoidal symptoms* [shark liver oil; phenylephrine HCl] 3%•0.25%

**Preparation H** cleansing tissues OTC *moisturizer and cleanser for external rectal/vaginal areas* [propylene glycol]

**Preparation H** rectal suppositories OTC *temporary relief of hemorrhoidal symptoms* [shark liver oil] 3%

**Preparation H Cooling Gel** OTC *temporary relief of hemorrhoidal symptoms* [phenylephrine HCl; hamamelis water; alcohol 7.5%] 0.25%•50%

**prepared chalk** [see: calcium carbonate]

**Prepcat** oral suspension ℞ *radiopaque contrast medium for gastrointestinal imaging* [barium sulfate] 1.5%

**Pre-Pen** solution for dermal scratch test ℞ *diagnostic aid for penicillin hypersensitivity* [benzylpenicilloyl polylysine] 0.25 mL

**Pre-Pen/MDM** solution for dermal scratch test ℞ *investigational (orphan) agent for penicillin hypersensitivity assessment* [benzylpenicillin]

**Prepidil** gel ℞ *prostaglandin for cervical ripening at term* [dinoprostone] 0.5 mg

**Prepulsid** ⒸⒶⓃ tablets, oral suspension (discontinued 2001) ℞ *treatment for nocturnal heartburn due to gastroesophageal reflux disease (GERD)* [cisapride] 5, 10, 20 mg; 1 mg/mL

**Prestara** ℞ *investigational (NDA filed) agent to increase bone density in patients with systemic lupus erythematosus (SLE) on corticosteroid therapy* [prasterone]

**pretamazium iodide** INN, BAN

**prethcamide**

**prethrombin** [see: prothrombin complex, activated]

**pretiadil** INN

**Pretts Diet-Aid** chewable tablets OTC *diet aid* [sodium carboxymethylcellulose; alginic acid; sodium bicarbonate] 100•200•70 mg

**Pretty Feet & Hands** cream OTC *moisturizer; emollient*

**Pretz** solution OTC *nasal moisturizer* [sodium chloride (saline solution)] 0.6%

**Pretz Irrigating** solution OTC *for postoperative irrigation* [sodium chloride (saline solution); glycerin; eriodictyon] 0.75%

**Pretz Moisturizing** nose drops OTC *nasal moisturizer* [sodium chloride (saline solution); glycerin; eriodictyon] 0.75%

**Pretz-D** nasal spray OTC *nasal decongestant* [ephedrine sulfate] 0.25%

**PretzPak** ointment (discontinued 2004) OTC *antimicrobial postoperative nasal pack* [benzyl alcohol; polyethylene glycol; carboxymethylcellulose; urea; allantoin]

**Prevacid** delayed-release capsules containing enteric-coated granules ℞ *proton pump inhibitor for gastric and duodenal ulcers, erosive esophagitis, gastroesophageal reflux disease (GERD), and other gastroesophageal disorders* [lansoprazole] 15, 30 mg

**Prevacid** enteric-coated granules for delayed-release oral suspension ℞ *proton pump inhibitor for gastric and duodenal ulcers, erosive esophagitis, gastroesophageal reflux disease (GERD), and other gastroesophageal disorders* [lansoprazole] 15, 30 mg

**Prevacid I.V.** infusion ℞ *proton pump inhibitor for erosive esophagitis in hospitalized patients* [lansoprazole] 30 mg/5 mL vial

**Prevacid NapraPAC** capsules + tablets in 7-day dose packs ℞ *proton pump inhibitor; nonsteroidal antiinflammatory; treatment for gastric and duodenal ulcers* [lansoprazole (capsules); naproxen (tablets)] 15•375, 15•500 mg

**Prevacid SoluTab** (delayed-release orally disintegrating tablets) ℞ *proton pump inhibitor for gastric and duodenal ulcers, erosive esophagitis, gastroesophageal reflux disease (GERD), and other gastroesophageal disorders* [lansoprazole] 15, 30 mg

**Prevalite** powder for oral suspension ℞ *cholesterol-lowering antihyperlipidemic; also used for biliary obstruction* [cholestyramine resin] 4 g/dose

**Preven** kit (4 film-coated tablets + pregnancy test) ℞ (available from pharmacists without a prescription in some states) *emergency postcoital contraceptive* [levonorgestrel; ethinyl estradiol] 0.25•0.05 mg ② Preveon

**Prevent-X** powder for oral solution OTC *dietary supplement* [multiple vitamins & minerals; multiple amino acids]

**PreviDent** dental gel (for self-application) ℞ *topical caries preventative* [sodium fluoride] 1.1%

**PreviDent 5000 Plus** dental cream (for self-application) ℞ *topical caries preventative* [sodium fluoride] 1.1%

**PreviDent Rinse** oral solution ("swish and spit") ℞ *dental caries preventative* [sodium fluoride] 0.2%

**Prevnar** IM injection ℞ *active immunization against seven strains of* Streptococcus pneumoniae *in infants and toddlers; investigational (Phase III) for adults over 50 years* [pneumococcal vaccine, 7-valent] 2–4 μg of each strain per 0.5 mL dose

**Prevpac** three-drug daily pack ℞ *triple therapy for* H. pylori: *an antisecretory and two antibiotics* [lansoprazole; clarithromycin; amoxicillin] 2 × 30 mg; 2 × 500 mg; 4 × 500 mg

**PreVue B. burgdorferi Antibody Detection Assay** reagent kit for professional use *in vitro diagnostic aid for Lyme disease*

**Prexige** ℞ *investigational (Phase III) antiarthritic for osteoarthritis; analgesic for acute pain; COX-2 inhibitor; nonsteroidal anti-inflammatory drug (NSAID)* [lumiracoxib] 100 mg

**prezatide copper acetate** USAN, INN *immunomodulator; investigational (Phase II) wound-healing gel for venous leg ulcers*

**Prezios** ℞ *investigational vitamin D₃ analogue for the topical treatment of psoriasis* [maxacalcitol]

**pribecaine** INN

**prickly ash (Xanthoxylum americanum; X. fraxineum)** bark *medicinal herb for fever, mouth sores, poor circulation, ulcers, and wounds*

**prickly juniper (Juniperus oxycedrus)** *medicinal herb* [see: juniper]

**prickly pear** *medicinal herb* [see: nopal]

**pride of China (Melia azedarach)** root bark and fruit *medicinal herb* used as an anthelmintic, astringent, bitter tonic, emetic, emmenagogue, and purgative

**pride weed** *medicinal herb* [see: fleabane; horseweed]

**pridefine** INN *antidepressant* [also: pridefine HCl]

**pridefine HCl** USAN *antidepressant* [also: pridefine]

**prideperone** INN

**pridinol** INN

**priest's crown** *medicinal herb* [see: dandelion]

**prifelone** USAN, INN *dermatologic anti-inflammatory*

**prifinium bromide** INN

**Priftin** film-coated tablets ℞ *antibacterial for tuberculosis (orphan); investigational (orphan) for AIDS-related* Mycobacterium avium *complex* [rifapentine] 150 mg

**prifuroline** INN

**priliximab** USAN, INN *monoclonal antibody to treat autoimmune lymphoproliferative diseases and in organ transplants; investigational (orphan) for multiple sclerosis*

**prilocaine** USAN, INN, BAN *topical local anesthetic*

**prilocaine HCl** USAN, USP *topical local anesthetic* [also: propitocaine HCl]

**Prilosec** delayed-release capsules ℞ *proton pump inhibitor for gastric and duodenal ulcers, erosive esophagitis, GERD, and other gastroesophageal disorders* [omeprazole] 10, 20, 40 mg ⊘ Prozac

**Prilosec OTC** delayed-release tablets OTC *proton pump inhibitor for frequent heartburn* [omeprazole magnesium] 20.6 mg (=20 mg base)

**primachine phosphate** [see: primaquine phosphate]

**Primacor** IV infusion ℞ *vasodilator for congestive heart failure* [milrinone lactate] 0.2, 1 mg/mL ⊘ Pravachol

**Primacor in 5% Dextrose** IV infusion ℞ *vasodilator for congestive heart failure* [milrinone lactate; dextrose] 200 μg/mL; 5% ⊘ Pravachol

**primaperone** INN

**primaquine** INN *antimalarial* [also: primaquine phosphate]

**primaquine phosphate** USP *antimalarial; prevention of malarial relapse* [also: primaquine] 26.3 mg oral

**primaquine phosphate & clindamycin HCl** *investigational (orphan) for AIDS-associated* Pneumocystis carinii *pneumonia*

**Primatene** tablets OTC *bronchodilator; decongestant; expectorant* [ephedrine HCl; guaifenesin] 12.5•200 mg

**Primatene Dual Action** tablets (discontinued 2000) OTC *antiasthmatic; bronchodilator; decongestant; expectorant* [theophylline; ephedrine HCl; guaifenesin] 60•12.5•100 mg

**Primatene Mist** inhalation aerosol OTC *sympathomimetic bronchodilator* [epinephrine] 0.2 mg/dose

**Primatuss Cough Mixture 4** oral liquid (discontinued 2002) OTC *antitussive; antihistamine* [dextromethorphan hydrobromide; chlorpheniramine maleate; alcohol 10%] 15•2 mg/5 mL

**Primatuss Cough Mixture 4D** oral liquid (discontinued 2002) OTC *antitussive; decongestant; expectorant* [dextromethorphan hydrobromide; pseudoephedrine HCl; guaifenesin; alcohol 10%] 10•20•67 mg/5 mL

**Primaxin I.M.** powder for injection ℞ *carbapenem antibiotic* [imipenem; cilastatin sodium] 500•500, 750•750 mg

**Primaxin I.V.** powder for injection ℞ *carbapenem antibiotic* [imipenem; cilastatin sodium] 250•250, 500•500 mg

**primidolol** USAN, INN *antihypertensive; antianginal; antiarrhythmic*

**primidone** USP, INN, BAN *anticonvulsant for grand mal, psychomotor, or focal epileptic seizures* 50, 250 mg oral

**Primobolan** *brand name for methenolone acetate, a European anabolic steroid abused as a street drug*

**Primobolan Depot** *brand name for methenolone enanthate, a European anabolic steroid abused as a street drug*

**Primsol** oral solution ℞ *antibiotic for otitis media in children and urinary tract infections in adults* [trimethoprim HCl] 50 mg/5 mL

**primycin** INN

**prince's pine** *medicinal herb* [see: pipsissewa]

**Principen** capsules, powder for oral suspension ℞ *aminopenicillin antibiotic* [ampicillin] 250, 500 mg; 125, 250 mg/5 mL

**Prinivil** tablets ℞ *antihypertensive; angiotensin-converting enzyme (ACE) inhibitor; adjunctive treatment for CHF* [lisinopril] 2.5, 5, 10, 20, 40 mg

**prinodolol** [see: pindolol]

**prinomastat** USAN *investigational (Phase III) matrix metalloprotease inhibitor for advanced non–small cell lung cancer (NSCLC) and prostate cancer (clinical trials discontinued 2000); investigational (Phase II) for age-related macular degeneration*

**prinomide** INN *antirheumatic* [also: prinomide tromethamine]

**prinomide tromethamine** USAN *antirheumatic* [also: prinomide]

**prinoxodan** USAN, INN *cardiotonic*

**Prinzide** tablets ℞ *antihypertensive; angiotensin-converting enzyme (ACE) inhibitor; diuretic* [hydrochlorothiazide; lisinopril] 12.5•10 mg

**Prinzide 12.5; Prinzide 25** tablets ℞ *antihypertensive; angiotensin-converting enzyme (ACE) inhibitor; diuretic* [hydrochlorothiazide; lisinopril] 12.5•20 mg; 25•20 mg

**Priorix** Ⓒ injection ℞ *active immunizing agent* [measles, mumps, and rubella virus vaccine, live attenuated] 0.5 mL

**Priscoline HCl** IV injection (discontinued 2002) ℞ *antiadrenergic; peripheral vasodilator for neonatal persistent pulmonary hypertension* [tolazoline HCl] 25 mg/mL ② Apresoline

**pristinamycin** INN, BAN

**privet, Egyptian** *medicinal herb* [see: henna (*Lawsonia*)]

**Privine** nasal spray, nose drops OTC *nasal decongestant* [naphazoline HCl] 0.05%

**prizidilol** INN, BAN *antihypertensive* [also: prizidilol HCl]

**prizidilol HCl** USAN *antihypertensive* [also: prizidilol]

**PRO 367** *investigational (Phase I/II) radiolabeled antigen-binding agent for HIV infection*

**PRO 542** *investigational (Phase I/II) recombinant fusion protein, antigen-binding agent, and HIV attachment inhibitor for HIV infection*

**PRO 2000** *investigational (Phase I) antiviral and microbicide gel for HIV infection*

**Pro Fem** cream OTC *natural progesterone from soy; hormone replacement therapy; postmenopausal osteoporosis preventative* [progesterone USP (in a liposomal base)] 2.5%

**Pro Skin** capsules OTC *vitamin/zinc supplement* [vitamins A, B₅, C, and E; zinc] 6250 IU•10 mg•100 mg•100 IU•10 mg

**Proact** ℞ *investigational (Phase III) immunomodulator for sarcoma*

**proadifen** INN *non-specific synergist* [also: proadifen HCl]

**proadifen HCl** USAN *non-specific synergist* [also: proadifen]

**ProAmatine** tablets ℞ *vasopressor for orthostatic hypotension (orphan)* [midodrine HCl] 2.5, 5, 10 mg

**proanthocyanidins** *natural free radical scavenger found in grape seed extract and pine bark extract* [also: procyanidolic oligomers (PCOs); procyanidins]

**Pro-Banthīne** tablets ℞ *GI antispasmodic; peptic ulcer treatment adjunct; antisecretory* [propantheline bromide] 7.5, 15 mg

**probarbital sodium** NF, INN

**Probax** gel OTC *relief from minor oral irritations* [propolis] 2%

**Probec-T** tablets OTC *vitamin supplement* [multiple B vitamins; vitamin C] ≛•600 mg

**probenecid** USP, INN, BAN *uricosuric for gout* 500 mg oral

**Probeta** ℞ *investigational investigational antihypertensive (β-blocker)* [bisoprolol]

**probicromil calcium** USAN *prophylactic antiallergic* [also: ambicromil]

**Pro-Bionate** capsules, powder OTC *dietary supplement; fever blister treatment; not generally regarded as safe and effective as an antidiarrheal* [Lactobacillus acidophilus] 2 billion U; 2 billion U/g

**probucol** USAN, USP, INN *antihyperlipidemic; investigational (Phase II) antiviral for HIV and AIDS*

**probutate** USAN *combining name for radicals or groups* [also: buteprate]

**procainamide** INN *antiarrhythmic* [also: procainamide HCl]

**procainamide HCl** USP *antiarrhythmic* [also: procainamide] 250, 375, 500, 750, 1000 mg oral; 500 mg/mL injection

**procaine** INN *local anesthetic* [also: procaine borate] ⌺ Procan

**procaine borate** NF *local anesthetic* [also: procaine] ⌺ Procan

**procaine HCl** USP *injectable local anesthetic; investigational (Phase II) for HIV infection; sometimes used as a treatment for the overall effects of aging such as alopecia, arthritis, cerebral atherosclerosis, hypertension, progressive dementia, and sexual dysfunction* 1%, 2% ⌺ Procan

**procaine penicillin** BAN *bactericidal antibiotic* [also: penicillin G procaine] ⌺ Procan

**ProcalAmine** IV infusion ℞ *peripheral parenteral nutrition* [multiple essential and nonessential amino acids; electrolytes]

**Procanbid** film-coated extended-release tablets ℞ *twice-daily antiarrhythmic* [procainamide HCl] 500, 1000 mg

**procarbazine** INN *antineoplastic* [also: procarbazine HCl] ⌺ dacarbazine

**procarbazine HCl** USAN, USP *antineoplastic for Hodgkin disease* [also: procarbazine]

**Procardia** capsules ℞ *antianginal; antihypertensive; calcium channel blocker* [nifedipine] 10, 20 mg

**Procardia XL** film-coated sustained-release tablets ℞ *antianginal; antihypertensive; calcium channel blocker* [nifedipine] 30, 60, 90 mg

**procaterol** INN, BAN *bronchodilator* [also: procaterol HCl]

**procaterol HCl** USAN *bronchodilator* [also: procaterol]

**Prochieve** vaginal gel ℞ *natural progestin; hormone replacement for secondary amenorrhea; hormone supplementation for assisted reproductive technology treatments* [progesterone] 4%, 8%

**prochlorperazine** USP, INN *phenothiazine antipsychotic; antiemetic* 25 mg suppositories

**prochlorperazine bimaleate** *phenothiazine antipsychotic; antiemetic*

**prochlorperazine edisylate** USP *phenothiazine antipsychotic; antiemetic* 5 mg/mL injection

**prochlorperazine ethanedisulfonate** [see: prochlorperazine edisylate]

**prochlorperazine maleate** USP *phenothiazine antipsychotic; antiemetic* 5, 10 mg oral

**prochlorperazine mesylate** *phenothiazine antipsychotic; antiemetic*

**procinolol** INN

**procinonide** USAN, INN *adrenocortical steroid*

**Proclim** ⓒ tablets (discontinued 2001) ℞ *progestin* [medroxyprogesterone acetate] 2.5, 5, 10 mg

**proclonol** USAN, INN *anthelmintic; antifungal*

**procodazole** INN

**proconvertin** [see: factor VII]

**Procort** cream, spray OTC *topical corticosteroidal anti-inflammatory* [hydrocortisone] 1%

**Procrit** IV or subcu injection ℞ *hematopoietic to stimulate RBC production for anemia of chronic renal failure, HIV, or chemotherapy (orphan)* [epoetin alfa] 2000, 3000, 4000, 10 000, 20 000, 40 000 U/mL

**Proctocort** anorectal cream, suppositories ℞ *topical corticosteroidal anti-inflammatory* [hydrocortisone] 1%; 30 mg

**ProctoCream-HC** anorectal cream (discontinued 2000) ℞ *corticosteroidal anti-inflammatory; local anesthetic* [hydrocortisone acetate; pramoxine HCl] 1%•1%

**ProctoCream-HC 2.5%** anorectal cream ℞ *corticosteroidal anti-inflammatory* [hydrocortisone acetate] 2.5%

**Proctodan-HC** ⓒ anorectal ointment, suppositories ℞ *topical corticosteroidal anti-inflammatory, local anesthetic, and astringent* [hydrocortisone acetate; pramoxine HCl; zinc sulfate] 0.5%•1%•0.5%; 10•20•10 mg

**ProctoFoam NS** anorectal aerosol foam OTC *topical local anesthetic* [pramoxine HCl] 1%

**Proctofoam-HC** anorectal aerosol foam ℞ *topical corticosteroidal anti-inflammatory; local anesthetic* [hydrocortisone acetate; pramoxine HCl] 1%•1%

**Pro-Cute** lotion OTC *moisturizer; emollient*

**procyanidolic oligomers (PCOs)** *natural free radical scavenger found in grape seed extract and pine bark extract* [also: proanthocyanidins; procyanidins]

**ProCycle Gold** tablets OTC *vitamin/mineral/iron supplement* [multiple vitamins & minerals; iron; folic acid; biotin] ±•3•0.067•± mg

**procyclidine HCl** USP *anticholinergic; antiparkinsonian; skeletal muscle relaxant* [also: procyclidine]

**procymate** INN

**Procysteine** ℞ *investigational (Phase II) immunomodulator for AIDS; investigational (orphan) for amyotrophic lateral sclerosis; investigational (Phase III, orphan) for adult respiratory distress syndrome (ARDS trials discontinued 1998)* [oxothiazolidine carboxylate]

**prodeconium bromide** INN

**Proderm** aerosol OTC *topical wound spray for decubitus ulcers* [castor oil; peruvian balsam] 650•72.5 mg/0.82 mL

**prodilidine** INN *analgesic* [also: prodilidine HCl]

**prodilidine HCl** USAN *analgesic* [also: prodilidine]

**prodipine** INN

**Prodium** tablets OTC *urinary analgesic* [phenazopyridine HCl] 95 mg

**prodolic acid** USAN, INN *anti-inflammatory*

**pro-drugs** *a class of agents which metabolize into a therapeutic or more potent form in the body*

**profadol** INN *analgesic* [also: profadol HCl]

**profadol HCl** USAN *analgesic* [also: profadol]

**Profasi** powder for IM injection R̟ *hormone for prepubertal cryptorchidism and hypogonadism; ovulation stimulant* [chorionic gonadotropin] 500, 1000 U/mL

**Pro-Fast HS; Pro-Fast SR** capsules R̟ *anorexiant; CNS stimulant* [phentermine HCl] 18.75 mg; 37.5 mg

**Pro-Fast SA** tablets R̟ *anorexiant; CNS stimulant* [phentermine HCl] 8 mg

**Profen II; Profen Forte** extended-release tablets R̟ *decongestant; expectorant* [pseudoephedrine HCl; guaifenesin] 45•800 mg; 90•800 mg

**Profen II DM** extended-release caplets R̟ *antitussive; decongestant; expectorant* [dextromethorphan hydrobromide; pseudoephedrine HCl; guaifenesin] 30•45•800 mg

**Profen II DM** oral liquid (discontinued 2004) R̟ *antitussive; decongestant; expectorant* [dextromethorphan hydrobromide; pseudoephedrine HCl; guaifenesin] 10•15•200 mg/5 mL

**Profen Forte DM** sustained-release caplets R̟ *antitussive; decongestant; expectorant* [dextromethorphan hydrobromide; pseudoephedrine HCl; guaifenesin] 60•90•800 mg

**Profen LA** timed-release tablets (discontinued 2002) R̟ *decongestant; expectorant* [phenylpropanolamine HCl; guaifenesin] 75•600 mg

**Profenal** Drop-Tainers (eye drops) R̟ *ocular nonsteroidal anti-inflammatory drug (NSAID); intraoperative miosis inhibitor* [suprofen] 1%

**profenamine** INN *antiparkinsonian* [also: ethopropazine HCl; ethopropazine]

**profenamine HCl** [see: ethopropazine HCl]

**profexalone** INN

**Profiber** oral liquid OTC *enteral nutritional therapy* [lactose-free formula]

**Profilnine SD** powder for IV injection R̟ *anticoagulant to correct factor IX deficiency (hemophilia B; Christmas disease)* [coagulation factor IX concentrate, solvent/detergent treated]

**Proflavanol C** Ⓒ tablets OTC *vitamin C supplement* [vitamin C as mixed ascorbates] 100 mg

**proflavine** INN [also: proflavine dihydrochloride]

**proflavine dihydrochloride** NF [also: proflavine]

**proflavine sulfate** NF

**proflazepam** INN

**ProFree/GP Weekly Enzymatic Cleaner** tablets OTC *enzymatic cleaner for rigid gas permeable contact lenses* [papain]

**progabide** USAN, INN *anticonvulsant; muscle relaxant*

**Progestasert** IUD R̟ *intrauterine contraceptive* [progesterone] 38 mg

**progesterone** USP, INN *natural progestin; intrauterine contraceptive; hormone replacement for secondary amenorrhea; hormone supplementation for assisted reproductive technology (ART) treatments; investigational (orphan) for in vitro fertilization and embryo transfer* 50 mg/mL injection

**progestins** *a class of sex hormones that cause a sloughing of the endometrial lining, also used as a hormonal antineoplastic*

**proglumetacin** INN

**proglumide** USAN, INN, BAN, JAN *anticholinergic*

**Proglycem** capsules, oral suspension R̟ *emergency antihypertensive; vasodilator; glucose-elevating agent* [diazoxide] 50 mg; 50 mg/mL

**Prograf** capsules, IV infusion ℞ *immunosuppressant for liver and kidney transplants; investigational for other transplants* [tacrolimus] 0.5, 1, 5 mg; 5 mg/mL

**proguanil** INN, BAN, DCF *antimalarial; dihydrofolate reductase inhibitor* [also: chloroguanide HCl]

**proguanil HCl** [see: chloroguanide HCl]

**ProHance** injection ℞ *MRI contrast media for brain and spine imaging* [gadoteridol] 279.3 mg/mL

**proheptazine** INN

**ProHIBiT** IM injection (discontinued 2000) ℞ *pediatric (1½–5 years) vaccine for Haemophilus influenzae type b (HIB)* [Hemophilus b conjugate vaccine (with a diphtheria conjugate carrier)] 25•(18) μg/0.5 mL

**proinsulin human** USAN *antidiabetic*

**Prolastin** powder for IV infusion ℞ *enzyme replacement therapy for hereditary alpha₁-proteinase inhibitor deficiency, which leads to progressive panacinar emphysema (orphan)* [alpha₁-proteinase inhibitor] ≥ 20 mg/mL (500, 1000 mg/vial)

**Proleukin** powder for IV infusion ℞ *antineoplastic for metastatic melanoma and renal cell carcinoma (orphan); investigational (Phase III, orphan) for immunodeficiency diseases and acute myelogenous leukemia (AML); investigational (Phase II) for non-Hodgkin lymphoma* [aldesleukin] 18 million IU/mL

**Prolex DH** oral liquid ℞ *narcotic antitussive; expectorant* [hydrocodone bitartrate; potassium guaiacolsulfonate] 4.5•300 mg/5 mL

**proligestone** INN

**proline (L-proline)** USAN, USP, INN *nonessential amino acid; symbols: Pro, P* ⑨ Prolene

**prolintane** INN *antidepressant* [also: prolintane HCl]

**prolintane HCl** USAN *antidepressant* [also: prolintane]

**Prolixin** tablets, elixir, oral concentrate, IM injection (discontinued 2002) ℞ *conventional (typical) antipsychotic* [fluphenazine HCl] 1, 2.5, 5, 10 mg; 2.5 mg/5 mL; 5 mg/mL; 2.5 mg/mL

**Prolixin Decanoate** subcu or IM injection ℞ *conventional (typical) antipsychotic* [fluphenazine decanoate] 25 mg/mL

**Prolixin Decanoate** Unimatic (pre-filled) syringe (discontinued 2003) ℞ *conventional (typical) antipsychotic* [fluphenazine decanoate] 25 mg/mL

**Prolixin Enanthate** subcu or IM injection (discontinued 2002) ℞ *conventional (typical) antipsychotic* [fluphenazine enanthate] 25 mg/mL

**prolonium iodide** INN

**Proloprim** tablets ℞ *anti-infective; antibacterial* [trimethoprim] 100, 200 mg

**ProMACE (prednisone, methotrexate [with leucovorin rescue], Adriamycin, cyclophosphamide, etoposide)** *chemotherapy protocol for non-Hodgkin lymphoma*

**ProMACE/cytaBOM (ProMACE [above], cytarabine, bleomycin, Oncovin, mitoxantrone)** *chemotherapy protocol for non-Hodgkin lymphoma*

**ProMACE/MOPP (full course of ProMACE, followed by MOPP)** *chemotherapy protocol for non-Hodgkin lymphoma*

**Promacet** tablets ℞ *sedative; barbiturate analgesic* [butalbital; acetaminophen] 50•650 mg

**promazine** INN *phenothiazine antipsychotic* [also: promazine HCl] ⑨ Promethazine

**promazine HCl** USP *phenothiazine antipsychotic* [also: promazine]

**Promega** Pearls (softgels) OTC *dietary supplement* [omega-3 fatty acids; multiple vitamins & minerals] 600• ≛, 1000• ≛ mg

**promegestone** INN

**promelase** INN

**ProMem** ℞ *investigational (NDA filed) acetylcholinesterase (AChE) inhibitor for Alzheimer dementia* [metrifonate]

**promestriene** INN

**Prometh VC Plain** syrup ℞ *decongestant; antihistamine* [phenylephrine HCl; promethazine HCl; alcohol 7%] 5•6.25 mg/5 mL

**Prometh VC with Codeine** syrup ℞ *narcotic antitussive; decongestant; antihistamine* [codeine phosphate; phenylephrine HCl; promethazine HCl; alcohol 7%] 10•5•6.25 mg/5 mL

**Prometh with Codeine** syrup ℞ *narcotic antitussive; antihistamine* [codeine phosphate; promethazine HCl; alcohol 7%] 10•6.25 mg/5 mL

**Prometh with Dextromethorphan** syrup ℞ *antitussive; antihistamine* [dextromethorphan hydrobromide; promethazine HCl; alcohol 7%] 15•6.25 mg/5 mL

**promethazine** INN *phenothiazine antihistamine; antiemetic; antidopaminergic; motion sickness relief* [also: promethazine HCl]

**Promethazine DM** syrup (discontinued 2002) ℞ *antitussive; antihistamine* [dextromethorphan hydrobromide; promethazine HCl; alcohol] 15•6.25 mg/5 mL

**promethazine HCl** USP *phenothiazine antihistamine; antiemetic; antidopaminergic; motion sickness relief* [also: promethazine] 25, 50 mg oral; 6.25 mg/5 mL oral; 25, 50 mg suppositories; 25, 50 mg/mL injection

**promethazine HCl & codeine phosphate** *antihistamine; narcotic antitussive* 6.25•10 mg/5 mL oral

**promethazine HCl & phenylephrine HCl** *antihistamine; decongestant* 6.25•5 mg/5 mL oral

**promethazine teoclate** INN *phenothiazine antihistamine*

**Promethazine VC** syrup (discontinued 2002) ℞ *decongestant; antihistamine* [phenylephrine HCl; promethazine HCl] 5•6.25 mg/5 mL

**Promethazine VC Plain** syrup (discontinued 2002) ℞ *decongestant; antihistamine* [phenylephrine HCl; promethazine HCl; alcohol 7%] 5•6.25 mg/5 mL

**Promethazine VC with Codeine** syrup ℞ *narcotic antitussive; decongestant; antihistamine* [codeine phosphate; phenylephrine HCl; promethazine HCl; alcohol 7.1%] 10•5•6.25 mg/5 mL

**Promethazine with Dextromethorphan Cough** syrup ℞ *antitussive; antihistamine* [dextromethorphan hydrobromide; promethazine HCl; alcohol 7%] 15•6.25 mg/5 mL

**promethestrol** [see: methestrol]

**Promethist with Codeine** syrup (discontinued 2002) ℞ *narcotic antitussive; decongestant; antihistamine* [codeine phosphate; phenylephrine HCl; promethazine HCl; alcohol] 10•5•6.25 mg/5 mL

**promethium** *element (Pm)*

**Prometrium** capsules ℞ *natural progestin for secondary amenorrhea and to prevent endometrial hyperplasia* [progesterone, micronized] 100, 200 mg

**Prominol** tablets ℞ *analgesic; antipyretic; sedative* [acetaminophen; butalbital] 650•50 mg

**Promit** IV injection ℞ *monovalent hapten for prevention of dextran-induced anaphylactic reactions; investigational (orphan) for cystic fibrosis* [dextran 1] 150 mg/mL

**ProMod** powder OTC *oral protein supplement* [D-whey protein concentrate; soy lecithin]

**promolate** INN

**promoxolane** INN

**prompt insulin zinc** [see: insulin zinc, prompt]

**Promycin** *investigational (Phase III, orphan) antineoplastic for head, neck, and cervical cancers* [porfiromycin]

**Pronemia Hematinic** capsules ℞ *hematinic* [ferrous fumarate; cyanocobalamin; ascorbic acid; intrinsic factor concentrate; folic acid] 115 mg•15 μg•150 mg•75 mg•1 mg

**Pronestyl** capsules, tablets, IV or IM injection (discontinued 2003) ℞ *antiarrhythmic* [procainamide HCl]

250, 375, 500 mg; 250, 375, 500 mg; 100, 500 mg/mL ⑨ Ponstel

**Pronestyl-SR** sustained-release tablets (discontinued 2003) ℞ *antiarrhythmic* [procainamide HCl] 500 mg

**pronetalol** INN [also: pronethalol]

**pronethalol** BAN [also: pronetalol]

**Pronto** shampoo OTC *pediculicide for lice* [pyrethrins; piperonyl butoxide] 0.33%•4%

**Propac** powder OTC *oral protein supplement* [whey protein; lactose]

**Propacet 100** film-coated tablets ℞ *narcotic analgesic* [propoxyphene napsylate; acetaminophen] 100•650 mg

**propacetamol** INN

**propafenone** INN, BAN *antiarrhythmic* [also: propafenone HCl]

**propafenone HCl** USAN *antiarrhythmic* [also: propafenone] 150, 225, 300 mg oral

**Propagest** tablets (discontinued 2001) OTC *nasal decongestant* [phenylpropanolamine HCl] 25 mg

**propamidine** INN, BAN, DCF

**propamidine isethionate** *investigational (orphan) eye drops for* Acanthamoeba keratitis

**propaminodiphen** [see: pramiverine]

**propane** NF *aerosol propellant*

**1,2-propanediol** [see: propylene glycol]

**propanidid** USAN, INN *intravenous anesthetic*

**propanocaine** INN

**propanoic acid, sodium salt hydrate** [see: sodium propionate]

**2-propanol** [see: isopropyl alcohol]

**2-propanone** [see: acetone]

**propantheline bromide** USP, INN *GI antispasmodic; peptic ulcer adjunct* 15 mg oral

**PROPApH Acne** cream OTC *keratolytic for acne* [salicylic acid] 2%

**PROPApH Astringent Cleanser** topical liquid OTC *keratolytic for acne* [salicylic acid; alcohol 55%] 2%

**PROPApH Cleansing; PROPApH Cleansing for Sensitive Skin; PROPApH Cleansing Maximum Strength** pads OTC *keratolytic for acne* [salicylic acid] 0.5%; 0.5%; 2%

**PROPApH Cleansing for Normal/ Combination Skin; PROPApH Cleansing for Oily Skin** lotion OTC *keratolytic for acne* [salicylic acid] 0.5%

**PROPApH Foaming Face Wash** topical liquid ℞ *keratolytic cleanser for acne* [salicylic acid] 2%

**PROPApH Peel-Off Acne Mask** OTC *keratolytic for acne* [salicylic acid] 2%

**proparacaine HCl** USP *topical ophthalmic anesthetic* [also: proxymetacaine] 0.5% eye drops

**proparacaine HCl & fluorescein sodium** *topical ophthalmic anesthetic; corneal disclosing agent* 0.5%•0.25%

**propatyl nitrate** USAN *coronary vasodilator* [also: propatylnitrate]

**propatylnitrate** INN *coronary vasodilator* [also: propatyl nitrate]

**propazolamide** INN

**Propecia** film-coated tablets ℞ *androgen hormone inhibitor for androgenic alopecia in men* [finasteride] 1 mg

**1-propene homopolymer** [see: polipropene 25]

**propenidazole** INN

**propentofylline** INN

*p*-**propenylanisole** [see: anethole]

**propenzolate HCl** USAN *anticholinergic* [also: oxyclipine]

**propericiazine** [see: periciazine]

**properidine** INN, BAN

**propetamide** INN

**propetandrol** INN

**prophenamine HCl** [see: ethopropazine HCl]

**Pro-Phree** powder OTC *supplement to breast milk* [protein-free formula with vitamins & minerals]

**Prophyllin** ointment OTC *topical antifungal; vulnerary; wound deodorant* [sodium propionate; chlorophyll derivatives] 5%•0.0125%

**propicillin** INN, BAN

**propikacin** USAN, INN *antibacterial*

**Propimex-1** powder OTC *formula for infants with propionic or methylmalon-icacidemia*

**Propimex-2** powder OTC *enteral nutritional therapy for propionic or methylmalonic acidemia*

**Propine** eye drops ℞ *topical antiglaucoma agent* [dipivefrin HCl] 0.1%

**propinetidine** INN

**propiodal** [see: prolonium iodide]

**propiolactone (β-propiolactone)** USAN, INN *disinfectant*

**propiomazine** USAN, INN *preanesthetic sedative*

**propiomazine HCl** USP *sedative; analgesic adjunct*

**propionic acid** NF *antimicrobial; acidifying agent*

**propionyl erythromycin lauryl sulfate** [see: erythromycin estolate]

**propipocaine** INN

**propiram** INN, BAN *narcotic agonist-antagonist analgesic* [also: propiram fumarate]

**propiram fumarate** USAN *investigational (Phase III) narcotic agonist-antagonist analgesic* [also: propiram]

**propisergide** INN

**propitocaine HCl** JAN *topical local anesthetic* [also: prilocaine HCl]

**propiverine** INN

**propizepine** INN

**Proplex T** IV infusion ℞ *antihemophilic to correct factor VII, VIII (hemophilia A), and IX (hemophilia B; Christmas disease) deficiencies* [coagulation factors II, VII, IX, and X, heat treated] 30 mL

**propofol** USAN, INN, BAN *rapid-acting general anesthetic* 1% injection

**propolis** *natural resin collected from the buds of certain trees by bees and used as an antibiotic, anti-inflammatory, antioxidant, antineoplastic, fungicide, immune system stimulant, and vulnerary*

**propoxate** INN

**propoxycaine** INN *local anesthetic* [also: propoxycaine HCl]

**propoxycaine HCl** USP *local anesthetic* [also: propoxycaine]

**propoxyphene HCl** USAN, USP *narcotic analgesic* [also: dextropropoxyphene HCl] 65 mg oral

**propoxyphene napsylate** USAN, USP *narcotic analgesic*

**propranolol** INN, BAN *antianginal; antiarrhythmic; antihypertensive; antiadrenergic (β-receptor); migraine preventative* [also: propranolol HCl]

**propranolol HCl** USAN, USP *antianginal; antiarrhythmic; antihypertensive; antiadrenergic (β-receptor); migraine preventative* [also: propranolol] 10, 20, 40, 60, 80, 90, 120, 160 mg oral; 4, 8, 80 mg/mL oral; 1 mg/mL injection

**Propulsid** tablets, oral suspension (discontinued 2000) ℞ *treatment for nocturnal heartburn due to gastroesophageal reflux disease (GERD)* [cisapride] 10, 20 mg; 1 mg/mL

**propyl p-aminobenzoate** [see: risocaine]

**propyl docetrizoate** INN, BAN

**propyl gallate** NF *antioxidant*

**propyl p-hydroxybenzoate** [see: propylparaben]

**propyl p-hydroxybenzoate, sodium salt** [see: propylparaben sodium]

**N-propylajmalinium tartrate** [see: prajmalinum bitartrate]

**propylene carbonate** NF *gelling agent*

**propylene glycol** USP *humectant; solvent; suspending and viscosity-increasing agent*

**propylene glycol alginate** NF *suspending agent; viscosity-increasing agent*

**propylene glycol diacetate** NF *solvent*

**propylene glycol ether of methylcellulose** [see: hydroxypropyl methylcellulose]

**propylene glycol monostearate** NF *emulsifying agent*

**propylhexedrine** USP, INN, BAN *vasoconstrictor; nasal decongestant*

**propyliodone** USP, INN *radiopaque contrast medium (56.7% iodine)*

**propylorvinol** [see: etorphine]

**propylparaben** USAN, NF *antifungal agent; preservative*

**propylparaben sodium** USAN, NF *antimicrobial preservative*

**2-propylpentanoic acid** [see: valproic acid]

**propylthiouracil (PTU)** USP, INN *thyroid inhibitor*

**2-propylvaleramide** [see: valpromide]

**propylvaleric acid** [see: valproic acid]

**propyperone** INN

**propyphenazone** INN, BAN

**propyromazine bromide** INN

**Pro-Q** foam OTC *skin protectant* [dimethicone; glycerin; parabens]

**proquamezine** BAN [also: aminopromazine]

**proquazone** USAN, INN *anti-inflammatory*

**proquinolate** USAN, INN *coccidiostat for poultry*

**prorenoate potassium** USAN, INN *aldosterone antagonist*

**proroxan** INN *antiadrenergic (α-receptor)* [also: proroxan HCl]

**proroxan HCl** USAN *antiadrenergic (α-receptor)* [also: proroxan]

**Proscar** film-coated tablets ℞ *androgen hormone inhibitor for benign prostatic hyperplasia (BPH)* [finasteride] 5 mg ⏺ Posicor

**proscillaridin** USAN, INN *cardiotonic*

**proscillaridin A** [see: proscillaridin]

**Prosed/DS** sugar-coated tablets ℞ *urinary antibiotic; antiseptic; analgesic; antispasmodic* [methenamine; phenyl salicylate; methylene blue; benzoic acid; atropine sulfate; hyoscyamine sulfate] 81.6•36.2•10.8•9•0.06•0.06 mg

**ProSight Lutein** capsules OTC *dietary supplement* [calcium; vitamins C and E; zinc; copper (but no lutein)] 22 mg•60 mg•30 IU•15 mg•2 mg

**ProSobee** oral liquid, powder for oral liquid OTC *hypoallergenic infant food* [soy protein formula]

**ProSobee LIPIL** oral liquid, powder for oral liquid OTC *hypoallergenic infant food fortified with omega-3 fatty acids* [soy protein formula]

**ProSol 20%** IV infusion ℞ *total parenteral nutrition* [multiple essential and nonessential amino acids] 20 g

**ProSom** tablets ℞ *sedative; hypnotic* [estazolam] 1, 2 mg

**Prosorba Column** for dialysis ℞ *treatment for rheumatoid arthritis* [protein A]

**prospidium chloride** INN

**prostacyclin** [now: epoprostenol]

**prostaglandin agonists** *a class of antiglaucoma agents that reduce intraocular pressure (IOP) by increasing the outflow of aqueous humor*

**prostaglandin $E_1$ (PGE$_1$)** [now: alprostadil]

**prostaglandin $E_1$ enol ester** *investigational (orphan) for advanced chronic critical limb ischemia*

**prostaglandin $E_2$ (PGE$_2$)** [see: dinoprostone]

**prostaglandin $F_{2\alpha}$ (PGF$_{2\alpha}$)** [see: dinoprost]

**prostaglandin $I_2$ (PGI$_2$)** [now: epoprostenol]

**prostaglandin X (PGX)** [now: epoprostenol]

**prostaglandins** *a class of agents that stimulate uterine contractions, used for abortions, cervical ripening, and postpartum hemorrhage*

**prostalene** USAN, INN *prostaglandin*

**ProstaScint** *imaging agent for prostate cancer and its metastases* [capromab pendetide]

**Pro-Stat 64; Pro-Stat 101** oral liquid OTC *enteral nutritional therapy* [collagen hydrolysate formula] 500 g protein per 946 mL

**ProStep** transdermal patch (discontinued 2001) ℞ *smoking deterrent; nicotine withdrawal aid* [nicotine] 11, 22 mg/day

**Prostigmin** subcu or IM injection ℞ *cholinergic urinary stimulant for postsurgical urinary retention; treatment for myasthenia gravis; antidote to neuromuscular blockers* [neostigmine methylsulfate] 1:1000 (1 mg/mL), 1:2000 (0.5 mg/mL), 1:4000 (0.25 mg/mL) (1:400 [2.5 mg/mL] available in Canada) ⏺ physostigmine

**Prostigmin** tablets ℞ *myasthenia gravis treatment; antidote for neuromuscular blockers* [neostigmine bromide] 15 mg

**Prostin E2** vaginal suppository ℞ *prostaglandin-type abortifacient* [dinoprostone] 20 mg

**Prostin VR Pediatric** IV injection ℞ *vasodilator; platelet aggregation inhibitor* [alprostadil] 500 μg/mL

**prosulpride** INN

**prosultiamine** INN

**ProSure** oral liquid OTC *enteral nutritional therapy for cancer patients* 8 oz.

**protactinium** *element* (Pa)

**protamine sulfate** USP, INN *antidote to heparin overdose* [also: protamine sulphate] 10 mg/mL IV infusion

**protamine sulphate** BAN *antidote to heparin overdose* [also: protamine sulfate]

**protamine zinc insulin (PZI)** INN *antidiabetic* [also: insulin, protamine zinc; insulin zinc protamine]

**protargin, mild** [see: silver protein, mild]

**protease** *digestive enzyme* [100 IU/mg in pancrelipase; 25 IU/mg in pancreatin]

**protease inhibitors** *a class of antivirals that block HIV replication*

**proteasome inhibitors** *a class of antineoplastics*

**ProTech First Aid Stick** topical liquid OTC *antiseptic; analgesic* [lidocaine; povidone-iodine] 2.5%•10%

**Protectol Medicated** powder OTC *topical antifungal* [calcium undecylenate] 15%

**Protegra** softgels OTC *vitamin/mineral supplement* [multiple vitamins & minerals]

**Protegrin** mouthwash ℞ *investigational (Phase III) rinse for oral mucositis* [IB-367 (code name—generic name not yet assigned)]

**protein A** *treatment for rheumatoid arthritis*

**protein C concentrate** *investigational (orphan) anticoagulant for protein C deficiency*

**protein hydrolysate** USP *fluid and nutrient replenisher*

**protein kinase C-beta inhibitor** *investigational (Phase II/III) treatment for diabetic neuropathy, retinopathy, and macular edema*

**α₁-proteinase inhibitor** [see: alpha₁-proteinase inhibitor]

**Protenate** IV infusion ℞ *blood volume expander for shock due to burns, trauma and surgery* [plasma protein fraction] 5%

**proterguride** INN

**protheobromine** INN

**Prothiaden** ℞ *investigational (NDA filed) tricyclic antidepressant* [dothiepin HCl]

**prothionamide** BAN [also: protionamide]

**prothipendyl** INN

**prothipendyl HCl** [see: prothipendyl]

**prothixene** INN

**prothrombin complex, activated** BAN

**Protilase** capsules containing enteric-coated spheres (discontinued 2002) ℞ *digestive enzymes* [lipase; protease; amylase] 4000•25 000•20 000 USP units

**ProTime** test kit for home use *in vitro diagnostic aid for the management of anticoagulation therapy*

**protiofate** INN

**protionamide** INN [also: prothionamide]

**protirelin** USAN, INN, BAN *prothyrotropin; diagnostic aid for thyroid function; investigational (orphan) for infant respiratory distress syndrome of prematurity*

**protizinic acid** INN

**protokylol HCl**

**proton pump inhibitors (PPIs)** *a class of gastric antisecretory agents that inhibit the ATPase "proton pump" within the gastric parietal cell* [also called: ATPase inhibitors; substituted benzimidazoles]

**Protonix** enteric-coated delayed-release tablets ℞ *proton pump inhibitor for erosive esophagitis associated with gastroesophageal reflux disease (GERD) and Zollinger-Ellison syndrome* [pantoprazole sodium] 20, 40 mg

**Protonix I.V.** powder for infusion ℞ *proton pump inhibitor for erosive esophagitis associated with gastroesophageal reflux disease (GERD) and Zollinger-Ellison syndrome* [pantoprazole sodium] 40 mg/vial

**Protopam Chloride** IV injection ℞ *antidote for organophosphate poisoning and anticholinesterase overdose* [pralidoxime chloride] 1 g ⧈ Protamine

**Protopic** ointment ℞ *topical treatment of eczema* [tacrolimus] 0.03%, 0.1%

**Protostat** tablets ℞ *antibiotic; antiprotozoal; amebicide* [metronidazole] 250, 500 mg

**protoveratrine A**

**Protovir** ℞ *investigational (Phase I) antiviral for AIDS-related cytomegalovirus* [sevirumab]

**Protox** ℞ *investigational (orphan) for toxoplasmosis of AIDS; investigational (Phase II) for treatment of bacterial and viral infections* [poloxamer 331]

**protriptyline** INN *tricyclic antidepressant* [also: protriptyline HCl]

**protriptyline HCl** USAN, USP *tricyclic antidepressant* [also: protriptyline] 5, 10 mg oral

**Protropin** powder for IM or subcu injection ℞ *growth hormone for congenital growth failure due to lack of endogenous growth hormone (orphan)* [somatrem] 5, 10 mg (15, 30 IU) per vial

**Protuss** oral liquid ℞ *narcotic antitussive; expectorant* [hydrocodone bitartrate; potassium guaiacolsulfonate] 5•300 mg/5 mL

**Protuss DM** sustained-release tablets (discontinued 2004) ℞ *antitussive; decongestant; expectorant* [dextromethorphan hydrobromide; pseudoephedrine HCl; guaifenesin] 30•60•600 mg

**Protuss-D** oral liquid ℞ *narcotic antitussive; decongestant; expectorant* [hydrocodone bitartrate; pseudoephedrine HCl; potassium guaiacolsulfonate] 5•30•300 mg/5 mL

**prourokinase** [see: saruplase]

**Provenge** ℞ *investigational (Phase III) theraccine for prostate cancer*

**Proventil** inhalation aerosol ℞ *sympathomimetic bronchodilator* [albuterol] 90 μg/dose

**Proventil** Repetabs (extended-release tablets) (discontinued 2004) ℞ *sympathomimetic bronchodilator* [albuterol sulfate] 4 mg

**Proventil** tablets, syrup, solution for inhalation ℞ *sympathomimetic bronchodilator* [albuterol sulfate] 2, 4 mg; 4 mg; 2 mg/5 mL; 0.083%, 0.5%

**Proventil HFA** CFC-free inhalation aerosol ℞ *sympathomimetic bronchodilator* [albuterol sulfate] 90 μg/dose

**Provera** tablets ℞ *synthetic progestin for secondary amenorrhea, abnormal uterine bleeding, and endometrial hyperplasia* [medroxyprogesterone acetate] 2.5, 5, 10 mg ⧈ Covera; Provir; Trovert

**Provigil** tablets ℞ *analeptic for excessive daytime sleepiness (orphan); investigational for fatigue associated with multiple sclerosis* [modafinil] 100, 200 mg

**Provir** ℞ *investigational (Phase III) treatment for AIDS-related diarrhea* [crofelemer] ⧈ Provera; Trovert

**Proviron** *brand name for mesterolone, an androgen abused with anabolic steroid street drugs*

**ProVisc** prefilled syringes ℞ *cohesive viscoelastic agent for ophthalmic surgery* [hyaluronate sodium] 0.55, 0.85 mL

**provitamin A** [see: beta carotene]

**Provocholine** powder for inhalation solution ℞ *bronchoconstrictor for in vivo pulmonary function challenge test* [methacholine chloride] 100 mg/5 mL

**proxazole** USAN, INN *smooth muscle relaxant; analgesic; anti-inflammatory*

**proxazole citrate** USAN *smooth muscle relaxant; analgesic; anti-inflammatory*

**proxetil** INN *combining name for radicals or groups*

**proxibarbal** INN

**proxibutene** INN

**proxicromil** USAN, INN *antiallergic*

**proxifezone** INN

**Proxigel** (discontinued 2002) OTC *topical oral anti-inflammatory and anti-*

infective for braces [carbamide peroxide] 10%

**proxorphan** INN *analgesic; antitussive* [also: proxorphan tartrate]

**proxorphan tartrate** USAN *analgesic; antitussive* [also: proxorphan]

**proxymetacaine** INN, BAN *topical ophthalmic anesthetic* [also: proparacaine HCl]

**proxymetacaine HCl** [see: proparacaine HCl]

**proxyphylline** INN, BAN

**Prozac** tablets, Pulvules (capsules), oral solution ℞ *selective serotonin reuptake inhibitor (SSRI) for major depression, obsessive-compulsive disorder, bulimia nervosa, and panic disorder; investigational (orphan) for autism* [fluoxetine HCl] 10 mg; 10, 20, 40 mg; 20 mg/5 mL ☒ Prilosec

**Prozac Weekly** enteric-coated delayed-release pellets in capsules ℞ *selective serotonin reuptake inhibitor (SSRI) for major depression, obsessive-compulsive disorder, and bulimia nervosa; once-weekly dosing for maintenance* [fluoxetine HCl] 90 mg

**prozapine** INN

**Prozine-50** IM injection ℞ *conventional (typical) antipsychotic* [promazine HCl] 50 mg/mL

**prucalopride HCl** USAN *investigational (Phase III) prokinetic agent for post-ileus and opioid-induced constipation*

**prucalopride succinate** USAN *investigational (Phase III) prokinetic agent for post-ileus and opioid-induced constipation*

*Prunella vulgaris* medicinal herb [see: woundwort]

*Prunus africana* medicinal herb [see: pygeum]

*Prunus americana; P. domestica; P. spinosa* medicinal herb [see: plum]

*Prunus amygdalus* medicinal herb [see: almond]

*Prunus armeniaca* medicinal herb [see: apricot]

*Prunus persica* medicinal herb [see: peach]

*Prunus serotina* medicinal herb [see: wild black cherry]

*Prunus virginiana* medicinal herb [see: wild cherry]

**Prussian blue** [see: ferric hexacyanoferrate]

**PSE (pseudoephedrine HCl)** [q.v.]

**PSE 120/MSC 2.5** sustained-release tablets ℞ *decongestant; anticholinergic to dry mucosal secretions* [pseudoephedrine HCl; methscopolamine nitrate] 120•2.5 mg

**PSE CPM** chewable tablets ℞ *pediatric decongestant and antihistamine* [pseudoephedrine HCl; chlorpheniramine maleate] 15•2 mg

**Pseudo** oral liquid (discontinued 2002) OTC *nasal decongestant* [pseudoephedrine HCl] 30 mg/5 mL

**Pseudo-Car DM** syrup (discontinued 2002) ℞ *antitussive; decongestant; antihistamine* [dextromethorphan hydrobromide; pseudoephedrine HCl; carbinoxamine maleate] 15•60•4 mg/5 mL

**Pseudo-Chlor** sustained-release capsules (discontinued 2002) ℞ *decongestant; antihistamine* [pseudoephedrine HCl; chlorpheniramine maleate] 120•8 mg

**pseudoephedrine** INN, BAN *vasoconstrictor; nasal decongestant* [also: pseudoephedrine HCl]

**pseudoephedrine HCl** USAN, USP *vasoconstrictor; nasal decongestant* [also: pseudoephedrine] 30, 60 mg oral; 30 mg/5 mL oral

**pseudoephedrine HCl & brompheniramine maleate** *decongestant; antihistamine* 60•4 mg/5 mL oral

**pseudoephedrine HCl & carbinoxamine maleate** *nasal decongestant; antihistamine* 60•4 mg/5 mL oral; 25•2 mg/mL oral

**pseudoephedrine HCl & carbinoxamine maleate & hydrocodone bitartrate** *nasal decongestant; antihistamine; antitussive* 30•2•50 mg/5 mL oral

**pseudoephedrine HCl & chlorpheniramine maleate** *decongestant; antihistamine* 120•8 mg oral

**pseudoephedrine HCl & guaifenesin** *decongestant; expectorant* 48•595, 60•600, 85•795 mg oral

**pseudoephedrine HCl & triprolidine HCl** *decongestant; antihistamine* 60•2.5 mg oral

**pseudoephedrine polistirex** USAN *nasal decongestant*

**pseudoephedrine sulfate** USAN, USP *bronchodilator; nasal decongestant*

**pseudoephedrine tannate** *bronchodilator; nasal decongestant*

**pseudoephedrine tannate & chlorpheniramine tannate** *decongestant; antihistamine* 4.5•75 mg/5 mL oral

**Pseudofrin** ⓒᴬᴺ tablets OTC *decongestant* [pseudoephedrine HCl] 60 mg

**Pseudo-Gest** tablets (discontinued 2002) OTC *nasal decongestant* [pseudoephedrine HCl] 30, 60 mg

**Pseudo-Gest Plus** tablets (discontinued 2002) OTC *decongestant; antihistamine* [pseudoephedrine HCl; chlorpheniramine maleate] 60•4 mg

*Pseudomonas aeruginosa* **purified extract** *investigational (orphan) agent to increase platelet count in immune thrombocytopenic purpura*

*Pseudomonas* **immune globulin** [see: mucoid exopolysaccharide *Pseudomonas* hyperimmune globulin]

**pseudomonic acid A** [see: mupirocin]

**Pseudostat** ℞ *investigational (Phase II) theraccine for chronic bronchitis*

**Pseudovent** sustained-release capsules ℞ *decongestant; expectorant* [pseudoephedrine HCl; guaifenesin] 120•250 mg

**Pseudovent-PED** sustained-release pediatric capsules ℞ *decongestant; expectorant* [pseudoephedrine HCl; guaifenesin] 60•300 mg

**psilocin** *a hallucinogenic street drug closely related to psilocybin*

**psilocybin** BAN *a hallucinogenic street drug derived from the* Psilocybe mexicana *mushroom* [also: psilocybine]

**psilocybine** INN, DCF *a hallucinogenic street drug derived from the* Psilocybe mexicana *mushroom* [also: psilocybin]

**psoralens** *a class of oral or topical skin photosensitizing agents used with ultraviolet A light (320–400 nm wavelength) for the treatment of severe recalcitrant psoriasis*

**Psor-a-set** bar OTC *keratolytic skin cleanser* [salicylic acid] 2%

**Psorcon** cream, ointment (name changed to Psorcon E in 2000)

**Psorcon E** cream, ointment ℞ *topical corticosteroidal anti-inflammatory* [diflorasone diacetate] 0.05%

**Psoriatec** cream ℞ *antipsoriatic* [anthralin] 1%

**PsoriGel** OTC *antipsoriatic; antiseborrheic; antiseptic* [coal tar solution; alcohol 28.3%] 7.5%

**psyllium** *(Plantago ovata) medicinal herb* [see: plantain]

**psyllium husk** USP *bulk laxative*

**psyllium hydrocolloid** *bulk laxative*

**psyllium hydrophilic mucilloid** *bulk laxative*

**psyllium seed** [see: plantago seed]

**P-Tanna 12** pediatric oral suspension ℞ *decongestant; antihistamine* [phenylephrine tannate; pyrilamine tannate] 5•30 mg/5 mL

**PTC (plasma thromboplastin component)** [see: factor IX]

**P.T.E.-4; P.T.E.-5** IV injection ℞ *intravenous nutritional therapy* [multiple trace elements (metals)]

**pterins** *a class of investigational antineoplastics*

**pteroyldiglutamic acid (PDGA)**

**pteroylglutamic acid (PGA)** [see: folic acid]

**PTFE (polytetrafluoroethylene)** [see: polytef]

**PTU (propylthiouracil)** [q.v.]

**Pt/VM (Platinol, VM-26)** *chemotherapy protocol for pediatric neuroblastoma*

**ptyalagogues** *a class of agents that stimulate the secretion of saliva* [also called: sialagogues]

**puccoon, yellow** *medicinal herb* [see: goldenseal]

*Pueraria lobata; P. thunbergiana* *medicinal herb* [see: kudzu]

**puffball** *medicinal herb* [see: dandelion]

**Pulmicort** Respules (single-dose ampule for inhalation) ℞ *corticosteroidal anti-inflammatory for chronic asthma in children* [budesonide] 0.25, 0.5 mg

**Pulmicort** Turbuhaler (dry powder in a metered-dose inhaler) ℞ *corticosteroidal anti-inflammatory for chronic asthma* [budesonide] 160 μg/dose

**Pulmocare** ready-to-use oral liquid OTC *enteral nutritional therapy for pulmonary problems*

*Pulmonaria officinalis* *medicinal herb* [see: lungwort]

**pulmonary surfactant replacement, porcine** [now: poractant alfa]

**Pulmozyme** solution for nebulization ℞ *reduces respiratory viscoelasticity of sputum in cystic fibrosis (orphan)* [dornase alfa] 1 mg/mL

**pulse VAC** *chemotherapy protocol for sarcomas* [see: VAC pulse]

**pulse VAC (vincristine, Adriamycin, cyclophosphamide)** *chemotherapy protocol* [also: VAC]

**PulsePak** (trademarked dosage form) *one-week dosage pack*

**Pulvule** (trademarked dosage form) *bullet-shaped capsule*

**pumice** USP *dental abrasive*

**pumitepa** INN

**Punctum Plug** ℞ *blocks the puncta and canaliculus to eliminate tear loss in keratitis sicca* [silicone plug]

*Punica granatum* *medicinal herb* [see: pomegranate]

**Puralube** ophthalmic ointment OTC *ocular moisturizer/lubricant* [white petrolatum; mineral oil]

**Puralube Tears** eye drops OTC *ophthalmic moisturizer/lubricant* [polyvinyl alcohol; polyethylene glycol 400] 1%•1%

**Puregon** (CAN) subcu or IM injection ℞ *recombinant follicle-stimulating hormone (FSH) for the induction of ovulation and development of multiple follicles for assisted reproductive technology (ART)* [follitropin beta] 50, 100 IU

**purgatives** *a class of agents that cause vigorous evacuation of the bowels by increasing bulk, stimulating peristaltic action, etc.* [also called: cathartics]

**Purge** oral liquid OTC *stimulant laxative* [castor oil] 95%

**purified cotton** [see: cotton, purified]

**purified protein derivative (PPD) of tuberculin** [see: tuberculin]

**purified rayon** [see: rayon, purified]

**purified siliceous earth** [see: siliceous earth, purified]

**purified water** [see: water, purified]

*H-purin-6-amine* [see: adenine]

**Purinethol** tablets ℞ *antimetabolite antineoplastic for multiple leukemias* [mercaptopurine] 50 mg

**puromycin** USAN, INN *antineoplastic; antiprotozoal (Trypanosoma)*

**puromycin HCl** USAN *antineoplastic; antiprotozoal (Trypanosoma)*

**purple angelica** *medicinal herb* [see: angelica]

**purple boneset** *medicinal herb* [see: boneset]

**purple cone flower** *medicinal herb* [see: echinacea]

**purple leptandra** *medicinal herb* [see: Culver root]

**Purpose Alpha Hydroxy Moisture** lotion, cream OTC *moisturizer; emollient; exfoliant* [glycolic acid] 8%

**Purpose Dry Skin** cream OTC *moisturizer; emollient*

**Purpose Soap** bar OTC *therapeutic skin cleanser*

**purshiana bark** *medicinal herb* [see: cascara sagrada]

**purslain, water** *medicinal herb* [see: brooklime]

**purvain** *medicinal herb* [see: blue vervain]

**pussywillow** *medicinal herb* [see: willow]

**PUVA** *an acronym for psoralens (P) and ultraviolet A (UVA) light, used as a treatment for severe recalcitrant psoriasis* [see: psoralens; methoxsalen]

**PVA (polyvinyl alcohol)** [q.v.]

**PVA (prednisone, vincristine, asparaginase)** *chemotherapy protocol for acute lymphocytic leukemia (ALL)*

**PVB (Platinol, vinblastine, bleomycin)** *chemotherapy protocol for testicular cancer and adenocarcinoma*

**PVC (polyvinyl chloride)** [see: polyvinyl chloride, radiopaque]

**PVDA (prednisone, vincristine, daunorubicin, asparaginase)** *chemotherapy protocol for acute lymphocytic leukemia (ALL)*

**PVP; PVP-16 (Platinol, VP-16)** *chemotherapy protocol*

**PVS Basics** ℞ *hydrophobic contact lens material* [paflufocon E]

**P-V-Tussin** caplets ℞ *narcotic antitussive; antihistamine* [hydrocodone bitartrate; pseudoephedrine HCl] 5•60 mg

**P-V-Tussin** syrup ℞ *narcotic antitussive; decongestant; antihistamine* [hydrocodone bitartrate; pseudoephedrine HCl; chlorpheniramine maleate; alcohol 5%] 5•60•4 mg/10 mL

*Pycnanthemum virginianum* medicinal herb [see: wild hyssop]

**Pycnogenol** *natural free radical scavenger; a registered trade name for pine bark extract* [see: pine bark extract]

**pygeum (*Prunus africana; Pygeum africanum*)** bark *medicinal herb for prostate gland enlargement and urinary disorders*

**Pylori-Check** test kit for professional use *in vivo diagnostic aid for H. pylori in the breath*

**Pylorid** Ⓐ film-coated tablets (discontinued 2001) ℞ *histamine H₂ antagonist for duodenal ulcers with H. pylori infection* [ranitidine bismuth citrate] 400 mg

**Pyloriset** reagent kit for professional use *in vitro diagnostic aid for GI disorders*

**pyrabrom** USAN *antihistamine*

**pyradone** [see: aminopyrine]

**pyrantel** INN *anthelmintic for ascariasis (roundworm) and enterobiasis (pinworm)* [also: pyrantel pamoate]

**pyrantel pamoate** USAN, USP *anthelmintic for ascariasis (roundworm) and enterobiasis (pinworm)* [also: pyrantel]

**pyrantel tartrate** USAN *anthelmintic*

**pyrathiazine HCl** [see: parathiazine]

**pyrazinamide (PZA)** USP, INN, BAN *bactericidal; primary tuberculostatic* 500 mg oral

**pyrazinecarboxamide** [see: pyrazinamide]

**pyrazofurin** USAN *antineoplastic* [also: pirazofurin]

**pyrazoline** [see: antipyrine]

**pyrazolopyrimidines** *a class of sedative/hypnotics with rapid onset and short duration of action, used in the short-term treatment of insomnia*

**pyrbenzindole** [see: benzindopyrine HCl]

**pyrbuterol HCl** [see: pirbuterol HCl]

**pyrethrins** *a class of natural pesticides derived from pyrethrum flowers, especially* Chrysanthemum cinerariaefolium *and* C. coccineum

***Pyrethrum parthenium*** medicinal herb [see: feverfew]

**pyribenzamine (PBZ)** [see: tripelennamine]

**pyricarbate** INN

**pyridarone** INN

**Pyridiate; Pyridate No. 2** tablets ℞ *urinary analgesic* [phenazopyridine HCl] 100 mg; 200 mg

**4-pyridinamine** [see: fampridine]

**2-pyridine aldoxime methylchloride (2-PAM)** [see: pralidoxime chloride]

**3-pyridinecarboxamide** [see: niacinamide]

**3-pyridinecarboxylic acid** [see: niacin]

**4-pyridinecarboxylic acid hydrazide** [see: isoniazid]

**3-pyridinecarboxylic acid methyl ester** [see: methyl nicotinate]

**3-pyridinemethanol** [see: nicotinyl alcohol]

**2-pyridinemethanol** [see: piconol]

**3-pyridinemethanol tartrate** [see: nicotinyl tartrate]

**Pyridium** tablets ℞ *urinary analgesic* [phenazopyridine HCl] 100, 200 mg 🄳 Dyrenium; pyridoxine; pyrithione; pyritidium

**Pyridium Plus** tablets ℞ *urinary analgesic; antispasmodic; sedative* [phenazopyridine HCl; hyoscyamine hydrobromide; butabarbital] 150•0.3•15 mg

**pyridofylline** INN

**pyridostigmine bromide** USP, INN *cholinergic/anticholinesterase muscle stimulant* 60 mg oral 🄳 physostigmine

**pyridoxal-5′-phosphate** [see: pyridoxine HCl]

**pyridoxamine** [see: pyridoxine HCl]

**pyridoxine (vitamin B$_6$)** INN *water-soluble vitamin; enzyme cofactor* [also: pyridoxine HCl] 🄳 pralidoxime; Pyridium

**pyridoxine HCl (vitamin B$_6$)** USP *water-soluble vitamin; enzyme cofactor* [also: pyridoxine] 50, 100, 250, 500 mg oral; 100 mg/mL injection 🄳 pralidoxime; Pyridium

**β-pyridylcarbinol** [see: nicotinyl alcohol]

**pyridylmethanol** *me+* [see: nicotinyl alcohol]

**pyrilamine maleate** USP *anticholinergic; antihistamine; sleep aid* [also: mepyramine]

**pyrilamine tannate & phenylephrine tannate & chlorpheniramine tannate** *antihistamine; decongestant* 12.5•5•2 mg/5 mL oral

**pyrimethamine** USP, INN *folic acid antagonist for malaria suppression and transmission control; toxoplasmosis treatment adjunct*

**pyrimethamine & sulfadiazine** *treatment for* Toxoplasma gondii *encephalitis (orphan)*

**pyrimidinedione** [see: uracil]

**pyrimitate** INN, BAN

**Pyrinex Pediculicide** shampoo (discontinued 2003) OTC *pediculicide for lice* [pyrethrins; piperonyl butoxide; deodorized kerosene] 0.2%•2%•0.8%

**pyrinoline** USAN, INN *antiarrhythmic*

**Pyrinyl** topical liquid (discontinued 2003) OTC *pediculicide for lice* [pyrethrins; piperonyl butoxide; deodorized kerosene] 0.2%•2%•0.8%

**Pyrinyl II** topical liquid (discontinued 2003) OTC *pediculicide for lice* [pyrethrins; piperonyl butoxide] 0.3%•3%

**Pyrinyl Plus** shampoo OTC *pediculicide for lice* [pyrethrins; piperonyl butoxide] 0.3%•4%

**pyrithen** [see: chlorothen citrate]

**pyrithione sodium** USAN *topical antimicrobial* 🄳 Pyridium

**pyrithione zinc** USAN, INN, BAN *antibacterial; antifungal; antiseborrheic*

**pyrithyldione** INN

**pyritidium bromide** INN 🄳 Pyridium

**pyritinol** INN, BAN

**pyrodifenium bromide** [see: prifinium bromide]

**pyrogallic acid** [see: pyrogallol]

**pyrogallol** NF

**pyrophendane** INN

**pyrophenindane** [see: pyrophendane]

**pyrovalerone** INN *CNS stimulant* [also: pyrovalerone HCl]

**pyrovalerone HCl** USAN *CNS stimulant* [also: pyrovalerone]

**pyroxamine** INN *antihistamine* [also: pyroxamine maleate]

**pyroxamine maleate** USAN *antihistamine* [also: pyroxamine]

**pyroxylin** USP, INN *pharmaceutic necessity for collodion*

**pyrrobutamine phosphate** USP

**pyrrocaine** USAN, INN *local anesthetic*

**pyrrocaine HCl** NF

**pyrrolifene** INN *analgesic* [also: pyrroliphene HCl]

**pyrrolifene HCl** [see: pyrroliphene HCl]

**pyrroliphene HCl** USAN *analgesic* [also: pyrrolifene]

**pyrrolnitrin** USAN, INN *antifungal*

**pyrroxane** [now: proroxan HCl]

**Pyrroxate** capsules (discontinued 2001) OTC *decongestant; antihistamine; analgesic* [phenylpropanolamine HCl; chlorpheniramine maleate; acetaminophen] 25•4•650 mg

*Pyrus malus* medicinal herb [see: apple]
**pyrvinium chloride** INN
**pyrvinium embonate** [see: pyrvinium pamoate]
**pyrvinium pamoate** USP *anthelmintic* [also: viprynium embonate]
**pytamine** INN

*diagnostic aid, while preg...*
**QTest Ovulation** test kit for professional use *in vitro diagnostic aid to predict ovulation time*
**Quad Tann** caplets ℞ *antitussive; decongestant; antihistamine* [carbetapentane tannate; phenylephrine tannate; ephedrine tannate; chlorpheniramine tannate] 60•10•10•5 mg
**quadazocine** INN, BAN *opioid antagonist* [also: quadazocine mesylate]
**quadazocine mesylate** USAN *opioid antagonist* [also: quadazocine]
**Quadra-Hist D; Quadra-Hist D Ped** extended-release capsules ℞ *decongestant; antihistamine* [pseudoephedrine HCl; phenyltoloxamine citrate; pyrilamine maleate; pheniramine maleate] 80•16•16•16 mg; 40•8•8•8 mg
**Quadramet** IV injection ℞ *radiopharmaceutical for treatment of bone pain from osteoblastic metastatic tumors* [samarium Sm 153 lexidronam] 1850 MBq/mL (50 mCi/mL)
**quadrosilan** INN
**quaking aspen** medicinal herb [see: poplar]
**Quantaffirm** reagent kit for professional use *in vitro diagnostic aid for mononucleosis*
**Quarzan** capsules (discontinued 2001) ℞ *anticholinergic; peptic ulcer treat-*

**PYY (peptide YY)** [q.v.]
**PZA (pyrazinamide)** [q.v.]
**PZI (protamine zinc insulin)** [q.v.]

ment [clidinium bromide] 2.5, 5 mg
⑨ Questran
**quassia (*Picrasma excelsa; Quassia amara*)** bark *medicinal herb used as an anthelmintic, antimalarial, appetizer, digestive aid, febrifuge, insecticide, pediculicide, and tonic*
**quatacaine** INN
**quaternium-18 bentonite** [see: bentoquatam]
**quazepam** USAN, INN *sedative; hypnotic*
**quazinone** USAN, INN *cardiotonic*
**quazodine** USAN, INN *cardiotonic; bronchodilator*
**quazolast** USAN, INN *antiasthmatic; mediator release inhibitor*
**Queen Anne's lace** medicinal herb [see: carrot]
**queen of the meadow** medicinal herb [see: boneset; meadowsweet]
**queen of the meadow (*Eupatorium purpureum*)** leaves *medicinal herb for bursitis, gallstones, kidney infections and stones, neuralgias, rheumatism, ringworm, urinary disorders, and water retention*
**Quelicin** IV or IM injection ℞ *neuromuscular blocker* [succinylcholine chloride] 20, 50, 100 mg/mL
**Quelidrine Cough** syrup (discontinued 2002) OTC *antitussive; decongestant; antihistamine; expectorant* [dextromethorphan hydrobromide; ephedrine HCl; phenylephrine HCl; chlorpheniramine maleate; ammonium chloride; ipecac; alcohol 2%]

10 mg•5 mg•5 mg•2 mg•40 mg• 0.005 mL per 5 mL

**quercetin** *natural flavonoid used to protect capillary walls; antioxidant; active flavonol of rutin*

**Quercetin** tablets OTC *dietary supplement* [eucalyptus bioflavonoids] 50, 250 mg

*Quercus alba medicinal herb* [see: white oak]

**Questran; Questran Light** powder for oral suspension ℞ *cholesterol-lowering antihyperlipidemic; also used for biliary obstruction* [cholestyramine resin] 4 g/dose

**quetiapine fumarate** USAN *dibenzothiazepine antipsychotic*

**Quibron; Quibron-300** capsules ℞ *antiasthmatic; bronchodilator; expectorant* [theophylline; guaifenesin] 150•90 mg; 300•180 mg

**Quibron-T** Dividose (multiple-scored tablets) ℞ *antiasthmatic; bronchodilator* [theophylline] 300 mg

**Quibron-T/SR** sustained-release Dividose (multiple-scored tablets) ℞ *antiasthmatic; bronchodilator* [theophylline] 300 mg

**Quick AC Enema Kit** concentrated rectal suspension (discontinued 2001) ℞ *radiopaque contrast medium for gastrointestinal imaging* [barium sulfate] 150%

**Quick Care** solutions OTC *two-step chemical disinfecting system for soft contact lenses* [hydrogen peroxide-based]

**Quick Pep** tablets (discontinued 2001) OTC *CNS stimulant; analeptic* [caffeine] 150 mg

**Quicklets** (trademarked dosage form) *quickly dissolving tablets*

**Quickscreen** test kit for home use *in vitro diagnostic aid for detection of multiple illicit drugs in the urine*

**quick-set** *medicinal herb* [see: hawthorn]

**QuickVue** *H. pylori* **gII** test kit for professional use *in vitro diagnostic aid for* H. pylori *in serum or plasma*

**QuickVue Influenza Test** for professional use *in vitro diagnostic aid for detection of influenza A and B from nasal excretions*

**QuickVue Pregnancy Test** cassettes for professional use *in vitro diagnostic aid; urine pregnancy test*

**quifenadine** INN

**quiflapon sodium** USAN *leukotriene biosynthesis inhibitor for asthma and inflammatory bowel disease*

**Quilimmune-M** ℞ *investigational (Phase II) vaccine against malaria*

**quillaia** *(Quillaja saponaria)* bark *medicinal herb for bronchitis and cough; also used topically for dandruff and scalp itchiness*

**quillifoline** INN

**quilostigmine** USAN *cholinesterase inhibitor for Alzheimer disease*

**quinacainol** INN

**quinacillin** INN, BAN

**quinacrine HCl** USP *antimalarial; anthelmintic for giardiasis and cestodiasis (tapeworm)* [also: mepacrine] ⊘ quinidine

**Quinaglute** Dura-Tabs (sustained-release tablets) (discontinued 2003) ℞ *antiarrhythmic* [quinidine gluconate] 324 mg

**Quinalan** sustained-release tablets (discontinued 2000) ℞ *antiarrhythmic* [quinidine gluconate] 324 mg

**quinalbarbitone sodium** BAN *hypnotic; sedative* [also: secobarbital sodium]

**quinaldine blue** USAN *obstetric diagnostic aid*

**quinambicide** [see: clioquinol]

**quinapril** INN, BAN *angiotensin-converting enzyme (ACE) inhibitor; antihypertensive; adjunct to CHF therapy* [also: quinapril HCl]

**quinapril HCl** USAN *antihypertensive; angiotensin-converting enzyme (ACE) inhibitor; adjunctive treatment for CHF* [also: quinapril]

**quinaprilat** USAN, INN *antihypertensive; angiotensin-converting enzyme (ACE) inhibitor*

**quinazosin** INN *antihypertensive* [also: quinazosin HCl]

**quinazosin HCl** USAN *antihypertensive* [also: quinazosin]

**quinbolone** USAN, INN *anabolic*

**quincarbate** INN

**quindecamine** INN *antibacterial* [also: quindecamine acetate]

**quindecamine acetate** USAN *antibacterial* [also: quindecamine]

**quindonium bromide** USAN, INN *antiarrhythmic*

**quindoxin** INN, BAN

**quinelorane** INN *antihypertensive; antiparkinsonian* [also: quinelorane HCl]

**quinelorane HCl** USAN *antihypertensive; antiparkinsonian* [also: quinelorane]

**quinestradol** INN, BAN

**quinestrol** USAN, USP, INN, BAN *estrogen replacement therapy for postmenopausal disorders*

**quinetalate** INN *smooth muscle relaxant* [also: quinetolate]

**quinethazone** USP, INN *diuretic; antihypertensive*

**quinetolate** USAN *smooth muscle relaxant* [also: quinetalate]

**quinezamide** INN

**quinfamide** USAN, INN *antiamebic*

**quingestanol** INN *progestin* [also: quingestanol acetate]

**quingestanol acetate** USAN *progestin* [also: quingestanol]

**quingestrone** USAN, INN *progestin*

**Quinidex** Extentabs (extended-release tablets) (discontinued 2004) ℞ *antiarrhythmic* [quinidine sulfate] 300 mg

**quinidine** NF, BAN *antiarrhythmic* ⬚ clonidine; quinacrine; Quinatime; quinine

**quinidine gluconate** USP *antiarrhythmic; antimalarial* (base=62%) 324 mg oral; 80 mg/mL injection

**quinidine polygalacturonate** *antiarrhythmic* (base=80%)

**quinidine sulfate** USP *antiarrhythmic* (base=83%) 200, 300 mg oral

**quinine** (*Cinchona calisaya; C. ledgeriana; C. succirubra*) NF, BAN bark *medicinal herb for cancer, fever, hemorrhoids, indigestion, inducing abortion, jaundice, malaria, mouth and throat diseases, parasites, stimulation of hair growth, and varicose veins* ⬚ quinidine

**quinine ascorbate** USAN *smoking deterrent*

**quinine biascorbate** [now: quinine ascorbate]

**quinine bisulfate** NF

**quinine dihydrochloride** NF *investigational anti-infective for pernicious malaria*

**quinine ethylcarbonate** NF

**quinine glycerophosphate** NF

**quinine HCl** NF

**quinine hydrobromide** NF

**quinine hypophosphite** NF

**quinine monohydrobromide** [see: quinine hydrobromide]

**quinine monohydrochloride** [see: quinine HCl]

**quinine monosalicylate** [see: quinine salicylate]

**quinine phosphate** NF

**quinine phosphinate** [see: quinine hypophosphite]

**quinine salicylate** NF

**quinine sulfate** USP *antimalarial cinchona alkaloid; treatment of nocturnal leg cramps* 200, 260, 325 mg oral

**quinine sulfate dihydrate** [see: quinine sulfate]

**quinine tannate** USP

**Quinine-Odan** ⒸⒶⓃ capsules OTC *antimalarial* [quinine sulfate] 200, 300 mg

**quinisocaine** INN [also: dimethisoquin HCl; dimethisoquin]

**quinocide** INN

**8-quinolinol** [see: oxyquinoline]

**8-quinolinol benzoate** [see: benzoxiquine]

**quinolizidines** *a class of antibiotics based on the quinolizidine (norlupinane) structure* [also called: norlupinanes]

**quinolones** [see: fluoroquinolones]

**Quinora** tablets (discontinued 2003) ℞ *antiarrhythmic* [quinidine sulfate] 300 mg

**quinoxyl** [see: chiniofon]

**quinpirole** INN *antihypertensive* [also: quinpirole HCl]

**quinpirole HCl** USAN *antihypertensive* [also: quinpirole]

**quinprenaline** INN *bronchodilator* [also: quinterenol sulfate]

**quinprenaline sulfate** [see: quinterenol sulfate]

**Quinsana Plus** powder OTC *topical antifungal* [tolnaftate] 1%

**quinsy berry** *medicinal herb* [see: currant]

**Quintabs** tablets OTC *vitamin supplement* [multiple vitamins; folic acid] ± ● 0.1 mg

**Quintabs-M** tablets OTC *vitamin/mineral/iron supplement* [multiple vitamins & minerals; iron; folic acid] ± ● 18●0.4 mg

**quinterenol sulfate** USAN *bronchodilator* [also: quinprenaline]

**quintiofos** INN, BAN

**3-quinuclidinol benzoate** [see: benzoclidine]

**quinuclium bromide** USAN, INN *antihypertensive*

**quinupramine** INN

**quinupristin** USAN, INN *streptogramin antibiotic; bacteriostatic to gram-positive infections*

**quipazine** INN *antidepressant; oxytocic* [also: quipazine maleate]

**quipazine maleate** USAN *antidepressant; oxytocic* [also: quipazine]

**quisultazine** INN

**quisultidine** [see: quisultazine]

**Quixin** eye drops ℞ *fluoroquinolone antibiotic for bacterial conjunctivitis* [levofloxacin] 0.5%

**Qvar** CFC-free pMDI (pressurized metered-dose inhaler) ℞ *antiasthmatic* [beclomethasone dipropionate] 40, 80 μg/puff

**R & C** shampoo (discontinued 2003) OTC *pediculicide for lice* [pyrethrins; piperonyl butoxide] 0.3%●3%

**R & D Calcium Carbonate/600** ℞ *investigational (orphan) agent for hyperphosphatemia of end-stage renal disease* [calcium carbonate]

**RA Lotion** OTC *topical acne treatment* [resorcinol; alcohol 43%] 3%

**RabAvert** IM injection ℞ *rabies vaccine for pre-exposure vaccination or post-exposure prophylaxis* [rabies vaccine, chick embryo cell] 2.5 IU

**rabeprazole** INN *proton pump inhibitor for duodenal ulcers, erosive or ulcerative gastroesophageal reflux disease (GERD), and other gastroesophageal disorders* [also: rabeprazole sodium]

**rabeprazole sodium** USAN *proton pump inhibitor for duodenal ulcers, erosive or ulcerative gastroesophageal reflux disease (GERD), and other gastroesophageal disorders* [also: rabeprazole]

**rabies immune globulin (RIG)** USP *passive immunizing agent*

**rabies vaccine** USP *active immunizing agent* Challenge Virus Standard (CVS)

**rabies vaccine, adsorbed (RVA)** [see: rabies vaccine]

**rabies vaccine, DCO (diploid cell origin)** [see: rabies vaccine]

**rabies vaccine, HDCV (human diploid cell vaccine)** [see: rabies vaccine]

**race ginger** *medicinal herb* [see: ginger]

**racecadotril** [see: acetorphan]

**racefemine** INN

**racefenicol** INN *antibacterial* [also: racephenicol]

**racemethadol** [see: dimepheptanol]

**racemethionine** USAN, USP *urinary acidifier* [also: methionine (the DL- form)]

**racemethorphan** INN, BAN

**racemetirosine** INN

**racemic** [def.] *A chemical compound with equal parts of* (+) *(formerly d- or dextro-) and* (−) *(formerly l- or levo-) enantiomers. Designated by the prefix* (±) *(formerly dl-).* [see also: isomer; enantiomer]

**racemic amphetamine phosphate**

**racemic amphetamine sulfate** [see: amphetamine sulfate]

**racemic calcium pantothenate** [see: calcium pantothenate, racemic]

**racemoramide** INN, BAN

**racemorphan** INN

**racephedrine HCl** USAN

**racephenicol** USAN *antibacterial* [also: racefenicol]

**racepinefrine** INN *sympathomimetic bronchodilator* [also: racepinephrine]

**racepinephrine** USP *sympathomimetic bronchodilator* [also: racepinefrine]

**racepinephrine HCl** USP *sympathomimetic bronchodilator*

**raclopride** INN, BAN

**raclopride C 11** USAN *radiopharmaceutical*

**racoonberry** *medicinal herb* [see: mandrake]

**ractopamine** INN *veterinary growth stimulant* [also: ractopamine HCl]

**ractopamine HCl** USAN *veterinary growth stimulant* [also: ractopamine]

**radio-chromated serum albumin** [see: albumin, chromated]

**radio-iodinated I 125 serum albumin** [see: albumin, iodinated]

**radio-iodinated I 131 serum albumin** [see: albumin, iodinated]

**radiomerisoprol** $^{197}$**Hg** [see: merisoprol Hg 197]

**radioselenomethionine** $^{75}$**Se** [see: selenomethionine Se 75]

**radiotolpovidone I 131** INN *hypoalbuminemia test; radioactive agent* [also: tolpovidone I 131]

**radish** (*Raphanus sativus*) *root medicinal herb used as an antispasmodic, astringent, cholagogue, and diuretic*

**radium** *element* (*Ra*)

**radon** *element* (*Rn*)

**rAd/p53 gene therapy** *investigational (Phase I) therapy for cancer*

**rafoxanide** USAN, INN *anthelmintic*

**ragged cup** (*Silphium perfoliatum*) *root and gum medicinal herb used as an antispasmodic, diaphoretic, and stimulant*

**ragwort** *medicinal herb* [see: life root]

**ralitoline** USAN, INN *anticonvulsant*

**raloxifene** INN *antiestrogen; selective estrogen receptor modulator (SERM) for the prevention for postmenopausal osteoporosis; investigational (Phase III) for breast cancer* [also: raloxifene HCl]

**raloxifene HCl** USAN *antiestrogen; selective estrogen receptor modulator (SERM) for the prevention and treatment of postmenopausal osteoporosis* [also: raloxifene]

**raltitrexed** USAN *antimetabolite antineoplastic; investigational (Phase III) thymidylate synthase inhibitor for advanced colorectal cancer*

**raluridine** USAN *antiviral*

**rambufaside** [see: meproscillarin]

**ramciclane** INN

**ramifenazone** INN

**ramipril** USAN, INN, BAN *angiotensin-converting enzyme (ACE) inhibitor for hypertension, myocardial infarction, CHF, and stroke*

**ramiprilat** INN

**ramixotidine** INN

**ramnodigin** INN

**ramoplanin** USAN, INN *investigational (Phase III) broad-spectrum glycolipodepsipeptide antibiotic for vancomycin-resistant* Enterococcus faecium *(VREF) and other vancomycin-resistant enterococci (VRE)*

**Ramses** *vaginal jelly (discontinued 2002)* OTC *spermicidal contraceptive* [nonoxynol 9] 5%

**Ramses Extra** *premedicated condom (discontinued 2002)* OTC *spermicidal/barrier contraceptive* [nonoxynol 9] 15%

**Ranexa** ℞ *investigational (NDA filed) antianginal for chronic unstable angina* [ranolazine HCl]

**Raniclor** chewable tablets ℞ *cephalosporin antibiotic* [cefaclor] 125, 187, 250, 375 mg

**ranimustine** INN

**ranimycin** USAN, INN *antibacterial*

**ranitidine** USAN, INN, BAN *histamine $H_2$ antagonist for gastric ulcers* 150, 300 mg oral

**ranitidine bismuth citrate** USAN *histamine $H_2$ antagonist for gastric ulcers with H. pylori infection* [also: ranitidine bismutrex]

**ranitidine bismutrex** BAN *histamine $H_2$ antagonist for gastric ulcers with H. pylori infection* [also: ranitidine bismuth citrate]

**ranitidine HCl** USP, JAN *histamine $H_2$ antagonist for gastric ulcers* 75 mg oral; 15 mg/mL oral

**ranolazine** INN *antianginal* [also: ranolazine HCl]

**ranolazine HCl** USAN *investigational (NDA filed) antianginal for chronic stable angina* [also: ranolazine]

**ranpirnase** USAN *investigational (Phase III) adjunct to chemotherapy for pancreatic, breast, colorectal, prostate, and small cell lung cancers*

**Ranunculus acris; R. bulbosus; R. sceleratus** *medicinal herb* [see: buttercup]

**rapacuronium bromide** USAN *neuromuscular blocker; adjunct to general anesthesia*

**Rapamune** tablets, oral solution ℞ *immunosuppressant for renal transplantation* [sirolimus] 1, 2 mg; 1 mg/mL

**rapamycin** [now: sirolimus]

**Raphanus sativus** *medicinal herb* [see: radish]

**Rapid Anthrax Test** reagents for use with LightCycler assay device *diagnostic aid for anthrax DNA in human and environmental samples* [polymerase chain reaction (PCR) test]

**RapidVue** test kit for home use *in vitro diagnostic aid; urine pregnancy test*

**Rapimelt** (trademarked delivery system) *orally disintegrating tablets*

**Rapinex** powder for oral suspension ℞ *investigational (NDA filed) to prevent upper GI bleeding* [omeprazole] 20 mg

**RapiTab** (trademarked delivery system) *orally disintegrating tablets*

**Raplon** IV injection (discontinued 2001) ℞ *rapid-onset, short-acting neuromuscular blocker for skeletal muscle relaxation as an adjunct to general anesthesia* [rapacuronium bromide] 100, 200 mg

**Raptiva** powder for subcu injection ℞ *immunosuppressant for plaque psoriasis* [efalizumab] 125 mg/dose

**rasagiline** INN

**rasagiline mesylate** USAN *investigational (NDA filed) monoamine oxidase B (MAO-B) inhibitor for Parkinson disease*

**rasburicase** USAN *antimetabolite antineoplastic for leukemia, lymphoma, and solid tumor malignancies*

**raspberry, ground** *medicinal herb* [see: goldenseal]

**raspberry, red; wild red raspberry** *medicinal herb* [see: red raspberry]

**raspberry [syrup]** USP

**rathyronine** INN

**rattleroot** *medicinal herb* [see: black cohosh]

**rattlesnake antivenin** [see: antivenin (Crotalidae) polyvalent]

**rattlesnake root** *medicinal herb* [see: birthroot; black cohosh; senega]

**rattleweed** *medicinal herb* [see: black cohosh]

**rauwolfia serpentina** USP *antihypertensive; peripheral antiadrenergic; antipsychotic*

**Rauzide** tablets ℞ *antihypertensive; diuretic* [bendroflumethiazide; rauwolfia serpentina] 4•50 mg

**Ravocaine & Novocaine with Levophed** injection (discontinued 2002) ℞ *injectable local anesthetic for dental procedures* [propoxycaine HCl; procaine; norepinephrine bitartrate] 7.2•36•0.12 mg/1.8 mL

**rayon, purified** USAN, USP *surgical aid*

**razinodil** INN

**razobazam** INN

**razoxane** INN, BAN

**86Rb** [see: rubidium chloride Rb 86]

**rBPI (bactericidal and permeability-increasing protein, recombinant)** [q.v.]

**rCD4 (recombinant soluble human CD4)** [see: CD4, recombinant soluble human]

**RCF** oral liquid OTC *hypoallergenic infant formula* [soy protein formula, carbohydrate free]

**Reabilan; Reabilan HN** ready-to-use oral liquid OTC *enteral nutritional therapy* [lactose-free formula]

**Reactine** ⓒ film-coated tablets, syrup ℞ *once-daily antihistamine* [cetirizine HCl] 5, 10, 20 mg; 5 mg/5 mL

**reactrol** [see: clemizole HCl]

**rebamipide** INN

**Rebetol** capsules ℞ *nucleoside antiviral; combination therapy for chronic hepatitis C infection* [ribavirin] 200 mg

**Rebetron** capsules + subcu or IM injection ℞ *combination treatment for chronic hepatitis C* [Rebetol (ribavirin capsules); Intron A (interferon alfa-2b injection)] 200 mg•3 million IU

**Rebif** ⓒ powder for subcu injection ℞ *immunomodulator for relapsing remitting multiple sclerosis and condyloma acuminata* [interferon beta-1a] 3, 12 MIU/vial

**Rebif** prefilled syringes for subcu injection ℞ *immunomodulator for relapsing remitting multiple sclerosis (orphan); investigational (orphan) for malignant melanoma, metastatic renal cell carcinoma, T-cell lymphoma, and Kaposi sarcoma* [interferon beta-1a] 22, 44 μg (6, 12 MIU)/0.5 mL syringe

**reboxetine** INN *investigational (NDA filed) fast-acting selective norepinephrine reuptake inhibitor for depression*

**reboxetine mesylate** USAN *investigational (NDA filed) fast-acting selective norepinephrine reuptake inhibitor for depression*

**recainam** INN, BAN *antiarrhythmic* [also: recainam HCl]

**recainam HCl** USAN *antiarrhythmic* [also: recainam]

**recainam tosylate** USAN *antiarrhythmic*

**recanescin** [see: deserpidine]

**Receptin** ℞ *investigational (Phase II) antiviral for AIDS; orphan status withdrawn 1997* [CD4, recombinant soluble human]

**reclazepam** USAN, INN *sedative*

**Reclomide** tablets ℞ *antidopaminergic; antiemetic for chemotherapy; peristaltic* [metoclopramide HCl] 10 mg

**Recombigen HIV-1 LA Test** reagent kit for professional use *in vitro diagnostic aid for HIV-1 antibodies in blood, serum, or plasma* [latex agglutination test]

**recombinant alpha₁ antitrypsin** [see: alpha₁ antitrypsin, recombinant]

**recombinant antihemophilic factor** [see: antihemophilic factor, recombinant]

**recombinant factor VIIa** [see: factor VIIa, recombinant]

**recombinant factor VIII** [see: antihemophilic factor, recombinant]

**recombinant human activated protein C (rhAPC)** [see: drotrecogan alfa]

**recombinant human CD4 immunoglobulin G** [CD4 immunoglobulin G, recombinant human]

**recombinant human deoxyribonuclease (rhDNase)** [see: dornase alfa]

**recombinant human erythropoietin** [see: erythropoietin, recombinant human]

**recombinant human growth hormone (rhGH)** [see: somatropin]

**recombinant human interferon beta** [see: interferon beta, recombinant human]

**recombinant human interleukin-1 receptor (rhIL-1R; rhu IL-1R)** [see: interleukin-1 receptor]

**recombinant human monoclonal antibodies to vascular endothelial growth factor (rhuMAb-VEGF)** [now: bevacizumab]

**recombinant human superoxide dismutase (SOD)** [see: superoxide dismutase, recombinant human]

**recombinant interferon alfa-2a** [see: interferon alfa-2a, recombinant]

**recombinant interferon alfa-2b** [see: interferon alfa-2b, recombinant]

**recombinant interferon beta** [see: interferon beta, recombinant]

**recombinant interleukin-2** [see: interleukin-2, recombinant]

**recombinant methionyl granulocyte CSF** [see: methionyl granulocyte CSF, recombinant]

**recombinant methionyl human granulocyte CSF** [see: methionyl human granulocyte CSF, recombinant]

**recombinant soluble human CD4 (rCD4)** [see: CD4, recombinant soluble human]

**recombinant tissue plasminogen activator (rtPA; rt-PA)** [see: alteplase]

**Recombinate** powder for IV injection ℞ *antihemophilic to correct coagulation deficiency* [antihemophilic factor concentrate, recombinant] 250, 500, 1000 IU

**Recombivax HB** adult IM injection, pediatric/adolescent IM injection, dialysis formulation ℞ *active immunizing agent for hepatitis B and D* [hepatitis B virus vaccine, recombinant] 10 μg/mL; 5 μg/0.5 mL; 40 μg/mL

**Rectacort** rectal suppositories ℞ *corticosteroidal anti-inflammatory* [hydrocortisone acetate] 10%

**Rectagene** rectal suppositories OTC *temporary relief of hemorrhoidal symptoms* [live yeast cell derivative; shark liver oil] 2000 SRF U/oz.

**Rectagene Medicated Rectal Balm** ointment OTC *temporary relief of hemorrhoidal symptoms* [shark liver oil; phenyl mercuric nitrate; live yeast cell derivative] 3%•1:10 000•66.67 U/g

**Rectolax** suppositories OTC *stimulant laxative* [bisacodyl] 10 mg

**red bay; red laurel** *medicinal herb* [see: magnolia]

**red bearberry** *medicinal herb* [see: uva ursi]

**red blood cells** [see: blood cells, red]

**red bush tea (*Aspalathus contaminata; A. linearis; Borbonia pinifolia*)** leaves and stems *medicinal herb used as a free radical scavenger; investigational antineoplastic; investigational for preventing brain damage caused by aging*

**red clover (*Trifolium pratense*)** flower *medicinal herb for blood cleansing, bronchitis, cancer, clearing toxins, nervous disorders, and spasms*

**Red Cross Toothache** topical liquid OTC *oral analgesic* [eugenol] 85%

**red currant (*Ribes rubrum*)** *medicinal herb* [see: currant]

**red elm** *medicinal herb* [see: slippery elm]

**red ferric oxide** [see: ferric oxide, red]

**red ink berries; red ink plant** *medicinal herb* [see: pokeweed]

**red laurel; red bay** *medicinal herb* [see: magnolia]

**red legs** *medicinal herb* [see: bistort]

**red mulberry (*Morus rubra*)** *medicinal herb* [see: mulberry]

**red oak (*Quercus rubra*)** *medicinal herb* [see: white oak]

**red paint root** *medicinal herb* [see: bloodroot]

**red pepper; African red pepper; American red pepper** *medicinal herb* [see: cayenne]

**red pimpernel (*Anagallis arvensis*)** plant *medicinal herb used as a cholagogue, diaphoretic, diuretic, expectorant, nervine, purgative, and stimulant*

**red puccoon** *medicinal herb* [see: bloodroot]

**red raspberry (*Rubus idaeus; R. strigosus*)** leaves *medicinal herb for childbirth afterpains, diarrhea and other bowel disorders, fever, flu, morning sickness, menstrual disorders, mouth sores, nausea, and vomiting*

**red root** *medicinal herb* [see: bloodroot; danshen; New Jersey tea]

**red sarsaparilla** *medicinal herb* [see: sarsaparilla]

**Red Throat Spray; Green Throat Spray** OTC *topical antipruritic/counterirritant; mild local anesthetic* [phenol] 1.4%

**red veterinarian petrolatum (RVP)** [see: petrolatum]

**red weed** *medicinal herb* [see: pokeweed]

**redberry** *medicinal herb* [see: ginseng]

**Redi Vial** (trademarked packaging form) *dual-compartment vial*

**Rediject** (trademarked delivery system) *prefilled disposable syringe*

**Redipak** (trademarked packaging form) *unit dose or unit-of-issue package*

**RediTabs** (trademarked dosage form) *rapidly disintegrating tablets*

**redmond clay (montmorillonite)** *natural remedy for bug bites and stings and other skin problems*

**Redutemp** tablets OTC *analgesic; antipyretic* [acetaminophen] 500 mg

**Reese's Pinworm** soft gel capsules, oral liquid OTC *anthelmintic for ascariasis (roundworm) and enterobiasis (pinworm)* [pyrantel pamoate] 180 mg; 50 mg/mL

**ReFacto** powder for injection *anticoagulant for long-term treatment of hemophilia A and for surgical procedures (orphan)* [antihemophilic factor, recombinant]

**Refensen Plus Severe Strength Cough & Cold Medicine** caplets OTC *decongestant; expectorant* [pseudoephedrine HCl; guaifenesin] 60•400 mg

**Refludan** powder for IV injection *anticoagulant for heparin-associated thrombocytopenia (HAT) (orphan)* [lepirudin] 50 mg

**Refresh** eye drops OTC *ophthalmic moisturizer/lubricant* [polyvinyl alcohol] 1.4%

**Refresh Plus; Refresh Tears** eye drops OTC *ophthalmic moisturizer/lubricant* [carboxymethylcellulose] 0.5%

**Refresh P.M.** ophthalmic ointment OTC *ocular moisturizer/lubricant* [white petrolatum; mineral oil; lanolin]

**refrigerants** *a class of agents that lower abnormal body heat (a term used in folk medicine)*

**Rēgain** snack bar OTC *enteral nutritional therapy for impaired renal function* [multiple essential amino acids] ⊡ Rogaine

**Regitine** IV or IM injection (discontinued 2004) ℞ *antihypertensive for pheochromocytoma; α-blocker* [phentolamine mesylate] 5 mg/mL

**Reglan** syrup (discontinued 2004) ℞ *antidopaminergic; antiemetic for chemotherapy; peristaltic* [metoclopramide HCl] 5 mg/5 mL ⊡ Regonol

**Reglan** tablets, IV infusion ℞ *antidopaminergic; antiemetic for chemotherapy; peristaltic* [metoclopramide HCl] 5, 10 mg; 5 mg/mL ⊡ Regonol

**Regonol** IM or IV injection (discontinued 2003) ℞ *cholinergic/anticholinesterase muscle stimulant; muscle relaxant reversal* [pyridostigmine bromide] 5 mg/mL ⊡ Reglan

**regramostim** USAN, INN *antineutropenic; hematopoietic stimulant; biologic response modifier; bone marrow stimulant*

**Regranex** gel ℞ *recombinant plateletderived growth factor B for chronic diabetic foot ulcers* [becaplermin] 0.01%

**Regroton** tablets ℞ *antihypertensive; diuretic* [chlorthalidone; reserpine] 50•0.25 mg ⊡ Hygroton

**Regular Iletin II** subcu injection OTC *antidiabetic* [insulin (pork)] 100 U/mL

**Regular Iletin II U-500 (concentrated)** subcu or IM injection (discontinued 2000) ℞ *antidiabetic* [insulin (pork)] 500 U/mL

**Regular Purified Pork Insulin** subcu injection (discontinued 2000) OTC *antidiabetic* [insulin] 100 U/mL

**regulator, female** *medicinal herb* [see: life root]

**Regulax SS** capsules OTC *laxative; stool softener* [docusate sodium] 100 mg

**Reguloid** powder OTC *bulk laxative* [psyllium hydrophilic mucilloid] 3.4 g/tsp.

**Rehydralyte** oral solution OTC *electrolyte replacement* [sodium, potassium, and chloride electrolytes]

**reishi mushrooms** *body and stem medicinal herb for AIDS, allergies, fatigue, heart problems, and insomnia*

**Rejuva-A** ⓒⒶⓃ cream ℞ *treatment for photodamaged skin* [tretinoin] 0.025%

**Rejuvenex** cream OTC *antioxidant, moisturizer, and sunscreen for the face*

**Relafen** film-coated tablets ℞ *antiarthritic; nonsteroidal anti-inflammatory drug (NSAID)* [nabumetone] 500, 750 mg

**relaxin** *investigational (orphan) for progressive systemic sclerosis; investigational (Phase II/III) for scleroderma*

**Release+** ⓒⒶⓃ capsules OTC *vitamin C/ manganese supplement* [calcium ascorbate; manganese citrate] 30•1.25 mg

**Release-Tabs** (dosage form) *timed-release tablets*

**Relenza** Rotadisks (powder for oral inhalation, for use with Diskhaler device) *influenza neuraminidase inhibitor for the treatment of acute influenza types A and B* [zanamivir] 5 mg

**Reliable Gentle Laxative** delayed-release enteric-coated tablets, suppositories OTC *stimulant laxative* [bisacodyl] 5 mg; 10 mg

**Relief** eye drops OTC *topical ophthalmic decongestant* [phenylephrine HCl] 0.12%

**relomycin** USAN, INN *antibacterial*

**Relora** tablets, capsules OTC *dietary supplement to relieve stress and anxiety by reducing cortisol levels and increasing DHEA levels; adjunct to weight reduction* [Magnolia officinalis extract; Phellodendron amurense extract] 250 mg

**Relpax** film-coated tablets ℞ *vascular serotonin 5-HT$_{1B/1D/1F}$ receptor agonist for the acute treatment of migraine* [eletriptan hydrobromide] 24.2, 48.5 mg (=20, 40 mg base)

**remacemide** INN *neuroprotective anticonvulsant* [also: remacemide HCl]

**remacemide HCl** USAN *neuroprotective anticonvulsant* [also: remacemide]

**Remeron** coated tablets ℞ *tetracyclic antidepressant* [mirtazapine] 15, 30, 45 mg ② Femiron

**Remeron** SolTabs (orally disintegrating tablets) ℞ *tetracyclic antidepressant* [mirtazapine] 15, 30, 45 mg

**Remicade** powder for IV infusion ℞ *anti-inflammatory; anti-TNFα (tumor necrosis factor alpha) monoclonal antibody for severe and fistulizing Crohn disease (orphan) and rheumatoid arthritis (with methotrexate)* [infliximab] 100 mg

**Remifemin Menopause** tablets OTC *natural remedy for postmenopausal symptoms* [black cohosh (standardized extract)] 20 mg (1 mg triterpene glycosides)

**remifentanil** INN, BAN *short-acting narcotic analgesic for general anesthesia* [also: remifentanil HCl]

**remifentanil HCl** USAN *short-acting narcotic analgesic for general anesthesia* [also: remifentanil]

**remikiren** INN

**Reminyl** film-coated tablets, oral drops ℞ *acetylcholinesterase inhibitor to increase cognition in Alzheimer disease* [galantamine hydrobromide] 4, 8, 12 mg; 4 mg/mL

**remiprostol** USAN, INN *antiulcerative*

**Remodulin** continuous subcu infusion ℞ *prostacyclin analogue for pulmonary arterial hypertension (orphan) and peripheral vascular disease (PVD); investigational (Phase II) for critical limb ischemia (CLI)* [treprostinil sodium] 1, 2.5, 5, 10 mg/mL

**remoxipride** USAN, INN, BAN *antipsychotic*

**remoxipride HCl** USAN *antipsychotic*

**Remular-S** tablets ℞ *skeletal muscle relaxant* [chlorzoxazone] 250 mg

**Remune** ℞ *investigational (Phase III) immunostimulant theraccine adjunct for HIV* [HIV-1 immunogen, gp120-depleted, inactivated]

**Renacidin** powder for solution ℞ *bladder and catheter irrigant for apatite or*

*struvite calculi (orphan)* [citric acid; D-gluconic acid lactone; magnesium hydroxycarbonate] 6.602•0.198•3.177 g/100 mL

**Renacidin Irrigation** solution ℞ *bladder and catheter irrigant for apatite or struvite calculi (orphan)* [citric acid; glucono-delta-lactone; magnesium carbonate]

**Renagel** capsules (discontinued 2004) ℞ *phosphate-binding polymer for hyperphosphatemia of end-stage renal disease (ESRD)* [sevelamer HCl] 403 mg

**RenAmin** IV infusion ℞ *nutritional therapy for renal failure* [multiple essential and nonessential amino acids; electrolytes]

**renanolone** INN

**Renax** film-coated caplets ℞ *nutritional therapy for azotemia (uremia)* [multiple vitamins & minerals; folic acid; biotin] ±•2.5•0.3 mg

**Renese** tablets (discontinued 2003) ℞ *diuretic; antihypertensive* [polythiazide] 1, 2, 4 mg

**Renese-R** tablets ℞ *antihypertensive; diuretic* [polythiazide; reserpine] 2•0.25 mg

**rennet, cheese** *medicinal herb* [see: bedstraw]

**Reno-30** intracavitary instillation ℞ *radiopaque contrast medium for urological imaging* [diatrizoate meglumine (46.67% iodine)] 300 mg/mL (141 mg/mL)

**RenoCal-76** injection ℞ *radiopaque contrast medium* [diatrizoate meglumine; diatrizoate sodium (48.7% total iodine)] 660•100 mg/mL (370 mg/mL)

**Reno-Dip; Reno-60** injection ℞ *radiopaque contrast medium* [diatrizoate meglumine (46.67% iodine)] 300 mg/mL (141 mg/mL); 600 mg/mL (282 mg/mL)

**Renografin-60** injection ℞ *radiopaque contrast medium* [diatrizoate meglumine; diatrizoate sodium (48.75% total iodine)] 520•80 mg/mL (292.5 mg/mL)

**Renoquid** tablets ℞ *broad-spectrum bacteriostatic* [sulfacytine] 250 mg

**Renova** cream ℞ *retinoid for photodamage, fine wrinkles, mottled hyperpigmentation, and roughness of facial skin* [tretinoin] 0.02%, 0.05%

**Rentamine Pediatric** oral suspension (discontinued 2002) ℞ *antitussive; decongestant; antihistamine* [carbetapentane tannate; phenylephrine tannate; ephedrine tannate; chlorpheniramine tannate] 30•5•5•4 mg/5 mL

**rentiapril** INN

**ReNu** solution OTC *rinsing/storage solution for soft contact lenses* [sodium chloride (preserved saline solution)]

**ReNu Effervescent Enzymatic Cleaner; ReNu Thermal Enzymatic Cleaner** tablets OTC *enzymatic cleaner for soft contact lenses* [subtilisin]

**ReNu Multi-Purpose** solution OTC *chemical disinfecting solution for soft contact lenses*

**renytoline** INN *anti-inflammatory* [also: paranyline HCl]

**renytoline HCl** [see: paranyline HCl]

**renzapride** INN, BAN

**ReoPro** IV injection ℞ *platelet aggregation inhibitor for PTCA and acute arterial occlusive disorders* [abciximab] 2 mg/mL

**Reosyn** ℞ *investigational antineoplastic* [reovirus]

**reovirus** *investigational antineoplastic*

**repaglinide** USAN *oral antidiabetic agent that stimulates the release of insulin from the pancreas for type 2 diabetes*

**Repan** capsules (discontinued 2000) ℞ *analgesic; barbiturate sedative* [acetaminophen; caffeine; butalbital] 325•40•50 mg ⃞ Riopan

**Repan** tablets ℞ *analgesic; barbiturate sedative* [acetaminophen; caffeine; butalbital] 325•40•50 mg ⃞ Riopan

**Repan CF** caplets ℞ *analgesic; barbiturate sedative* [acetaminophen; butalbital] 650•50 mg

**Repetab** (trademarked dosage form) *extended-release tablet*

**repirinast** USAN, INN *antiallergic; anti-asthmatic*

**Replagal** ℞ *investigational (NDA filed, orphan) enzyme replacement therapy for Fabry disease* [agalsidase alfa]

**Replens** vaginal gel OTC *lubricant* [glycerin; mineral oil]

**Replete** ready-to-use oral liquid OTC *enteral nutritional therapy* [lactose-free formula]

**rEPO (recombinant erythropoietin)** [see: epoetin alfa; epoetin beta]

**Reposans-10** capsules (discontinued 2003) ℞ *benzodiazepine anxiolytic; sedative* [chlordiazepoxide HCl] 10 mg

**repository corticotropin** [see: corticotropin, repository]

**Reprexain** tablets ℞ *narcotic analgesic* [hydrocodone bitartrate; ibuprofen] 5•200 mg

**repromicin** USAN, INN *antibacterial*

**Repronex** powder for IM or subcu injection ℞ *ovulation stimulant for women; spermatogenesis stimulant for men* [menotropins] 75, 150 IU

**reproterol** INN, BAN *bronchodilator* [also: reproterol HCl]

**reproterol HCl** USAN *bronchodilator* [also: reproterol]

**Requip** film-coated tablets ℞ *dopamine agonist; antiparkinsonian; investigational for restless leg syndrome (RLS)* [ropinirole HCl] 0.25, 0.5, 1, 2, 4, 5 mg

**Resaid** sustained-release capsules (discontinued 2001) ℞ *decongestant; antihistamine* [phenylpropanolamine HCl; chlorpheniramine maleate] 75•12 mg

**Rescaps-D S.R.** sustained-release capsules (discontinued 2002) ℞ *antitussive; decongestant* [caramiphen edisylate; phenylpropanolamine HCl] 40•75 mg

**rescimetol** INN

**rescinnamine** NF, INN, BAN *antihypertensive; rauwolfia derivative*

**Rescon** oral liquid (discontinued 2001) OTC *decongestant; antihistamine* [phenylpropanolamine HCl; chlorpheniramine maleate] 12.5•2 mg/5 mL

**Rescon 12-Hour** sustained-release capsules (discontinued 2003) ℞ *decongestant; antihistamine* [pseudoephedrine HCl; chlorpheniramine maleate] 120•12 mg

**Rescon-DM** oral liquid OTC *antitussive; decongestant; antihistamine* [dextromethorphan hydrobromide; pseudoephedrine HCl; chlorpheniramine maleate] 30•60•4 mg/10 mL

**Rescon-ED** controlled-release capsules (discontinued 2002) ℞ *decongestant; antihistamine* [pseudoephedrine HCl; chlorpheniramine maleate] 120•8 mg

**Rescon-GG** oral liquid OTC *decongestant; expectorant* [phenylephrine HCl; guaifenesin] 10•200 mg/10 mL

**Rescon-Jr.** sustained-release pediatric caplets ℞ *decongestant; antihistamine* [phenylephrine HCl; chlorpheniramine maleate] 20•4 mg

**Rescon-MX** sustained-release tablets ℞ *decongestant; antihistamine; anticholinergic to dry mucosal secretions* [phenylephrine HCl; chlorpheniramine maleate; methscopolamine nitrate] 40•8•2.5 mg

**Rescriptor** tablets ℞ *antiretroviral; non-nucleoside reverse transcriptase inhibitor (NNRTI) for HIV-1* [delavirdine mesylate] 100, 200 mg

**Rescue Pak** (trademarked dosage form) *unit dose package*

**Rescula** eye drops ℞ *prostaglandin $F_{2\alpha}$ analogue for glaucoma and ocular hypertension* [unoprostone isopropyl] 0.15%

**Resectisol** solution ℞ *genitourinary irrigant* [mannitol] 5 g/100 mL

**reserpine** USP, INN *antihypertensive; peripheral antiadrenergic; rauwolfia derivative* 0.1, 0.25 mg oral

**resibufogenin** [see: bufogenin]

**Resinol** ointment (discontinued 2003) OTC *poison ivy treatment* [calamine; zinc oxide; resorcinol] 6%•12%•2%

**resocortol butyrate** USAN *topical anti-inflammatory*

**Resol** oral solution OTC *electrolyte replacement* [sodium, potassium, chloride, calcium, magnesium, and phosphate electrolytes]

**Resolve/GP** solution OTC *cleaning solution for hard or rigid gas permeable contact lenses*

**resorantel** INN

**resorcin** [see: resorcinol]

**resorcin acetate** [see: resorcinol monoacetate]

**resorcin brown** NF

**resorcinol** USP *keratolytic; antifungal*

**resorcinol monoacetate** USP *antiseborrheic; keratolytic*

**Resource; Resource Plus; Resource Diabetic; Resource Just for Kids** ready-to-use oral liquid OTC *enteral nutritional therapy* [lactose-free formula]

**ReSource Arginaid** powder for oral liquid OTC *argine-rich enteral nutritional therapy to speed recovery of pressure ulcers, burns, or surgery*

**Resource Fruit Beverage** ready-to-use oral liquid OTC *enteral nutritional therapy* [whey protein–based] 237 mL/pkt.

**Respa A.R.** tablets ℞ *decongestant; antihistamine; anticholinergic to dry mucosal secretions* [pseudoephedrine HCl; chlorpheniramine maleate; belladonna alkaloids] 90•8•0.024 mg

**Respa-1st** sustained-release tablets ℞ *decongestant; expectorant* [pseudoephedrine HCl; guaifenesin] 58•600 mg

**Respa-DM** sustained-release tablets ℞ *antitussive; expectorant* [dextromethorphan hydrobromide; guaifenesin] 28•600 mg

**Respa-GF** sustained-release tablets (discontinued 2004) ℞ *expectorant* [guaifenesin] 600 mg

**Respahist** sustained-release capsules ℞ *decongestant; antihistamine* [pseudoephedrine HCl; brompheniramine maleate] 60•6 mg

**Respaire-60 SR; Respaire-120 SR** extended-release capsules ℞ *decongestant; expectorant* [pseudoephedrine HCl; guaifenesin] 60•200 mg; 120•250 mg

**Respalor** ready-to-use oral liquid OTC *enteral nutritional therapy for pulmonary problems*

**Respbid** sustained-release tablets (discontinued 2004) ℞ *antiasthmatic; bronchodilator* [theophylline] 250, 500 mg

**RespiGam** IV infusion ℞ *preventative for respiratory syncytial virus (RSV) infections in high-risk infants (orphan); investigational (orphan) treatment for RSV* [respiratory syncytial virus immune globulin (RSV-IG)] 2500 mg/dose (50 mg/mL)

**Respihaler** (trademarked delivery system) *oral inhalation aerosol*

**RespiPak** (trademarked packaging form) *tablets in daily compliance packaging*

**Respiracult-Strep** culture paddles for professional use *in vitro diagnostic test for Group A streptococci from throat and nasopharyngeal sources*

**respiratory syncytial virus immune globulin (RSV-IG)** *preventative for respiratory syncytial virus (RSV) infections in high-risk infants (orphan); investigational (orphan) treatment for RSV*

**Respirgard II** (trademarked delivery system) *nebulizer*

**Respules** (trademarked delivery system) *single-dose ampule for inhalation*

**Restasis** eye drop emulsion ℞ *immunomodulator and anti-inflammatory to increase tear production in patients with Sjögren keratoconjunctivitis sicca (orphan)* [cyclosporine] 0.05%

**restoratives** *a class of agents that promote a restoration of strength and vigor (a term used in folk medicine)*

**Restoril** capsules ℞ *benzodiazepine sedative; hypnotic* [temazepam] 7.5, 15, 30 mg ② Risperdal; Vistaril; Zestril

**Restylane** subcu injection in prefilled syringes ℞ *dermal filler for deep wrinkles and facial folds* [hyaluronic acid] 20 mg/mL

**Retavase** powder for IV infusion ℞ *thrombolytic; tissue plasminogen activa-*

tor *(tPA) for acute myocardial infarction* [reteplase] 18.8 mg (10.8 IU)

**retelliptine** INN

**reteplase** USAN, INN *thrombolytic; tissue plasminogen activator (tPA) for acute myocardial infarction*

**Retin-A** cream, gel, topical liquid ℞ *keratolytic for acne* [tretinoin] 0.025%, 0.05%, 0.1% (0.01% available in Canada); 0.01%, 0.025%, 0.1%; 0.05%

**Retin-A Micro** gel ℞ *keratolytic for acne* [tretinoin] 0.04%, 0.1%

**retinamide R-II** *investigational (orphan) for myelodysplastic syndrome*

**retinoic acid (all-*trans*-retinoic acid)** [see: tretinoin]

**9-*cis*-retinoic acid** [see: alitretinoin]

**13-*cis*-retinoic acid** [see: isotretinoin]

**retinoids** *a class of antineoplastics chemically related to vitamin A*

**Retinol** cream OTC *moisturizer; emollient* [vitamin A] 100 000 IU

**retinol** INN, BAN *vitamin A$_1$*

**Retinol-A** cream OTC *moisturizer; emollient* [vitamin A palmitate] 10 000 IU/g

**Retrovir** film-coated tablets, capsules, syrup, IV injection ℞ *nucleoside antiviral for AIDS and AIDS-related complex (orphan), HIV infection, and to prevent maternal-fetal HIV transfer* [zidovudine] 300 mg; 100 mg; 50 mg/5 mL; 10 mg/mL

**Revaproxyn** (European name for U.S. product Efaproxyn)

**Reveal Rapid HIV-1 Antibody Test** kit for professional use *in vitro diagnostic aid for HIV-1 in blood*

**revenast** INN

**Reversa UV with Cosmederm-7** CAN cream, lip balm OTC *moisturizer; emollient; exfoliant; anti-irritant* [glycolic acid; strontium chloride] 4% • ?, 8% • ?; 2% • ?

**reverse transcriptase (RT) inhibitors** *a class of antiretroviral drugs that inhibit the activity of reverse transcriptase in viral cells, preventing cell replication; subdivided into nucleoside*

*(purine- or pyrimidine-based) and non-nucleoside types* [reverse transcriptase is also known as DNA polymerase]

**reversible proton pump inhibitors** [see: proton pump inhibitors]

**Reversol** IV or IM injection ℞ *myasthenia gravis treatment; antidote to curare overdose* [edrophonium chloride] 10 mg/mL

**Revex** IV, IM, or subcu injection ℞ *narcotic antagonist; postanesthesia "stir-up"; antidote to opioid overdose* [nalmefene] 0.1, 1 mg/mL

**Rēv-Eyes** powder for eye drops ℞ *miotic to reverse iatrogenic mydriasis* [dapiprazole HCl] 0.5%

**ReVia** tablets ℞ *narcotic antagonist for opiate dependence or overdose (orphan) and alcoholism* [naltrexone HCl] 50 mg

**Revimid** ℞ *investigational (orphan) for multiple myeloma; investigational (Phase III) for malignant melanoma* [3-(4'-aminoisoindoline-1'-one)-1-piperidine-2,6-dione]

**revospirone** INN, BAN

**Rexigen Forte** sustained-release capsules (discontinued 2001) ℞ *anorexiant; CNS stimulant* [phendimetrazine tartrate] 105 mg

**Rexin-G** IV injection ℞ *investigational (NDA filed, orphan) tumor-targeted gene therapy for pancreatic cancer*

**Rexolate** IM injection ℞ *analgesic; antipyretic; anti-inflammatory; antirheumatic* [sodium thiosalicylate] 50 mg/mL

**Reyataz** capsules ℞ *antiviral; protease inhibitor for HIV-1 infection* [atazanavir sulfate] 100, 150, 200 mg

**Rezamid** lotion OTC *topical acne treatment* [sulfur; resorcinol; alcohol] 5% • 2% • 28%

**Rezipas** ℞ *investigational (orphan) for ulcerative colitis* [aminosalicylic acid]

**Rezulin** film-coated tablets (discontinued 2000) ℞ *thiazolidinedione antidiabetic; increases cellular response to insulin without increasing insulin secretion* [troglitazone] 200, 300, 400 mg

**rGCR (recombinant glucocerebrosidase)** [see: glucocerebrosidase, recombinant retroviral vector]

**rG-CSF (recombinant granulocyte colony-stimulating factor)** [see: lenograstim]

**R-Gel** OTC *topical analgesic* [capsaicin] 0.025%

**R-Gen** elixir ℞ *expectorant* [iodinated glycerol] 60 mg/5 mL

**R-gene 10** IV injection ℞ *diagnostic aid for pituitary (growth hormone) function* [arginine HCl] 10% (950 mOsm/L)

**RGG0853, E1A lipid complex** *investigational (orphan) for advanced ovarian cancer*

**rGM-CSF; rhGM-CSF; rhuGM-CSF (granulocyte-macrophage colony-stimulating factor)** [q.v.]

**rgp160; rgp160 IIIB; rgp160 MN (recombinant glycoprotein)** *investigational (Phase I–III) antiviral (treatment) and vaccine (preventative) for HIV* [also: AIDS vaccine]

*Rhamnus cathartica; R. frangula medicinal herb* [see: buckthorn]

*Rhamnus purshiana medicinal herb* [see: cascara sagrada]

**rhAPC (recombinant human activated protein C)** [see: drotrecogan alfa]

**(rhATIII) recombinant human antithrombin III** [see: antithrombin III]

**rHb1.1 (recombinant human hemoglobin)** [see: hemoglobin, recombinant human]

**rhDNase (recombinant human deoxyribonuclease)** [see: dornase alfa]

**Rheaban** caplets (discontinued 2004) OTC *antidiarrheal; GI adsorbent* [activated attapulgite] 750 mg

**rhenium** *element (Re)*

**Rheomacrodex** IV infusion ℞ *plasma volume expander for shock due to hemorrhage, burns, or surgery* [dextran 40] 10%

**rheotran (45)** [see: dextran 45]

**rhetinic acid** [see: enoxolone]

*Rheum palmatum medicinal herb* [see: rhubarb]

**Rheumatex** slide tests for professional use *in vitro diagnostic aid for rheumatoid factor in the blood* ☒ Rheumatrex

**rheumatism root** *medicinal herb* [see: twin leaf; wild yam]

**rheumatism weed** *medicinal herb* [see: pipsissewa]

**Rheumaton** slide tests for professional use *in vitro diagnostic aid for rheumatoid factor in serum or synovial fluid*

**Rheumatrex** Dose Pack (tablets) ℞ *antimetabolite antineoplastic for leukemia; systemic antipsoriatic; antirheumatic; investigational (orphan) for juvenile rheumatoid arthritis* [methotrexate] 2.5 mg ☒ Rheumatex

**rhFSH (recombinant human follicle-stimulating hormone)** [see: menotropins]

**rhGH (recombinant human growth hormone)** [see: somatropin]

**rhIGF-1 (recombinant human insulin-like growth factor-1)** [now: mecasermin]

**rhIL-1R; rhu IL-1R (recombinant human interleukin-1 receptor)** [see: interleukin-1 receptor]

**rhIL-11 (recombinant human interleukin-11)** [see: interleukin-11, recombinant human]

**rhIL-12 (recombinant human interleukin-12)** [see: interleukin-12]

**Rhinall** nasal spray, nose drops OTC *nasal decongestant* [phenylephrine HCl] 0.25%

**Rhinaris Lubricating Mist** nasal spray, nasal gel OTC *nasal moisturizer* [polyethylene glycol; propylene glycol] 15%•5%; 15%•20%

**Rhinatate** tablets (discontinued 2002) ℞ *decongestant; antihistamine* [phenylephrine tannate; chlorpheniramine tannate; pyrilamine tannate] 25•8•25 mg

**Rhinatate Pediatric** oral suspension ℞ *decongestant; antihistamine* [phenylephrine tannate; chlorpheniramine tannate; pyrilamine tannate] 5•2•12.5 mg/5 mL

**Rhinatate-NF Pediatric** oral suspension ℞ *decongestant; antihistamine* [phenylephrine tannate; chlorpheniramine tannate] 5•4.5 mg/5 mL

**Rhinocaps** capsules (discontinued 2001) OTC *decongestant; analgesic; antipyretic* [phenylpropanolamine HCl; acetaminophen; aspirin] 20•162•162 mg

**Rhinocort** nasal inhalation aerosol (discontinued 2004) ℞ *corticosteroidal anti-inflammatory for seasonal or perennial rhinitis* [budesonide] 32 μg/dose

**Rhinocort Aqua** nasal spray ℞ *corticosteroidal anti-inflammatory for seasonal or perennial rhinitis* [budesonide] 32 μg/dose

**Rhinolar-EX; Rhinolar-EX 12** sustained-release capsules (discontinued 2001) ℞ *decongestant; antihistamine* [phenylpropanolamine HCl; chlorpheniramine maleate] 75•8 mg; 75•12 mg

**Rhinosyn; Rhinosyn-PD** oral liquid (discontinued 2002) OTC *decongestant; antihistamine* [pseudoephedrine HCl; chlorpheniramine maleate; alcohol] 60•4 mg/5 mL; 30•2 mg/5 mL

**Rhinosyn-DM** oral liquid (discontinued 2002) OTC *antitussive; decongestant; antihistamine* [dextromethorphan hydrobromide; pseudoephedrine HCl; chlorpheniramine maleate; alcohol 1.4%] 15•30•2 mg/5 mL

**Rhinosyn-DMX** syrup (discontinued 2002) OTC *antitussive; expectorant* [dextromethorphan hydrobromide; guaifenesin] 15•100 mg/5 mL

**Rhinosyn-X** oral liquid (discontinued 2002) OTC *antitussive; decongestant; expectorant* [dextromethorphan hydrobromide; pseudoephedrine HCl; guaifenesin; alcohol 7.5%] 10•30•100 mg/5 mL

**Rh₀(D) immune globulin** USP *passive immunizing agent; treatment for immune thrombocytopenic purpura (orphan)*

**Rh₀(D) immune human globulin** [now: Rh₀(D) immune globulin]

**rhodine** [see: aspirin]

**rhodium** *element (Rh)*

**Rho-Fluphenazine** ⒸⒶⓃ subcu or IM injection ℞ *conventional (typical) antipsychotic* [fluphenazine decanoate] 25, 100 mg/mL

**RhoGAM** IM injection, prefilled syringes ℞ *obstetric Rh factor immunity suppressant* [Rh₀(D) immune globulin (gamma globulin)] 300 μg (5%)

**Rhophylac** IM injection in prefilled syringes ℞ *obstetric Rh factor immunity suppressant* [Rh₀(D) immune globulin (gamma globulin)] 1500 IU (300 μg)

**Rhoxal-amiodarone** ⒸⒶⓃ tablets ℞ *antiarrhythmic for acute ventricular tachycardia and fibrillation (orphan)* [amiodarone HCl] 200 mg

**Rhoxal-diltiazem CD** ⒸⒶⓃ (once daily) sustained-release capsules ℞ *antihypertensive; antianginal; antiarrhythmic; calcium channel blocker* [diltiazem HCl] 120, 180, 240, 300 mg

**Rhoxal-famotidine** ⒸⒶⓃ film-coated tablets ℞ *histamine H₂ antagonist for gastric and duodenal ulcers* [famotidine] 20, 40 mg

**Rhoxal-fluoxetine** ⒸⒶⓃ capsules ℞ *selective serotonin reuptake inhibitor (SSRI) for depression, obsessive-compulsive disorder (OCD), and bulimia nervosa* [fluoxetine HCl] 10, 20 mg

**Rhoxal-minocycline** ⒸⒶⓃ capsules ℞ *tetracycline antibiotic* [minocycline HCl] 50, 100 mg

**Rhoxal-orphenadrine** ⒸⒶⓃ sustained-release tablets ℞ *skeletal muscle relaxant* [orphenadrine citrate] 100 mg

**Rhoxal-oxaprozin** ⒸⒶⓃ film-coated caplets ℞ *antiarthritic; nonsteroidal anti-inflammatory drug (NSAID)* [oxaprozin] 600 mg

**Rhoxal-ranitidine** ⒸⒶⓃ film-coated tablets ℞ *histamine H₂ antagonist for gastric and duodenal ulcers* [ranitidine HCl] 150, 300 mg

**Rhoxal·ticlopidine** ⓒᴬᴺ film-coated tablets ℞ *platelet aggregation inhibitor for stroke* [ticlopidine HCl] 250 mg

**Rhoxal·timolol** ⓒᴬᴺ eye drops ℞ *topical antiglaucoma agent (β-blocker)* [timolol maleate] 0.25%, 0.5%

**Rhoxal·valproic** ⓒᴬᴺ capsules, enteric-coated capsules ℞ *anticonvulsant* [valproic acid] 250 mg; 500 mg

**rhubarb (*Rheum palmatum*)** root *medicinal herb for colon and liver disorders*

**Rhuli** gel (discontinued 2003) OTc *poison ivy treatment* [benzyl alcohol; menthol; camphor] 2%•0.3%•0.3%

**Rhuli** spray (discontinued 2003) OTc *poison ivy treatment* [benzocaine; calamine; camphor] 5%•13.8%•0.7%

**rhuMAb-E25 (recombinant human monoclonal antibodies E25)** [now: omalizumab]

**rhuMAb·VEGF (recombinant human monoclonal antibodies to vascular endothelial growth factor)** [now: bevacizumab]

*Rhus glabra medicinal herb* [see: sumach]

**Riba 3.0 SIA** reagent kit for professional use *in vitro diagnostic aid for hepatitis C* [strip immunoblot assay (SIA)]

**ribaminol** USAN, INN *memory adjuvant*

**Ribasphere** capsules ℞ *nucleoside antiviral; combination therapy for chronic hepatitis C infection* [ribavirin] 200 mg

**ribavirin** USP, INN *nucleoside antiviral for severe lower respiratory tract infections; combination therapy for chronic hepatitis C infection; investigational (orphan) for hemorrhagic fever with renal syndrome* [also: tribavirin] 200 mg oral

*Ribes nigrum; R. rubrum medicinal herb* [see: currant]

**ribgrass; ribwort** *medicinal herb* [see: plantain]

**riboflavin (vitamin B₂)** USP, INN *water-soluble vitamin; enzyme cofactor* 50, 100 mg oral

**riboflavin 5′-phosphate sodium** USP *vitamin*

**riboflavine** [see: riboflavin]

**riboprine** USAN, INN *antineoplastic*

**ribostamycin** INN, BAN

**riboxamide** [see: tiazofurin]

**ricainide** [see: indecainide HCl]

**rice bran oil (gamma oryzanol)** extract *medicinal herb used as a hypolipidemic and to treat gastrointestinal and menopausal symptoms*

**richweed** *medicinal herb* [see: black cohosh; stone root]

**ricin (blocked) conjugated murine monoclonal antibodies (MAb) (anti-MY9 MAb)** *investigational (orphan) for myeloid leukemia (including AML), ex vivo treatment of autologous bone marrow in AML, and blast crisis in CML*

**ricin (blocked) conjugated murine monoclonal antibodies (MAb) (CD6 MAb)** *investigational (orphan) for T-cell leukemias, lymphomas, and other mature T-cell malignancies*

**ricin (blocked) conjugated murine monoclonal antibodies (MAb) (N901 MAb)** *investigational (orphan) for small cell lung cancer*

**RID** shampoo, mousse (aerosol foam) OTc *pediculicide for lice* [pyrethrins; piperonyl butoxide] 0.33%•4%

**RID** topical liquid (discontinued 2003) OTc *pediculicide for lice* [pyrethrins; piperonyl butoxide; petroleum distillate] 0.3%•3•1.2%

**RID Pure Alternative** gel OTc *pediculicide for lice* [dimethicone] 100%

**Rid·A·Pain** gel OTc *topical oral anesthetic* [benzocaine] 10%

**Rid·A·Pain·HP** cream OTc *analgesic; counterirritant* [capsaicin] 0.075%

**Ridaura** capsules ℞ *antirheumatic* [auranofin] 3 mg

**ridazolol** INN

**RIDD (recombinant interleukin-2, dacarbazine, DDP)** *chemotherapy protocol*

**Ridenol** elixir OTc *analgesic; antipyretic* [acetaminophen] 80 mg/5 mL

**ridogrel** USAN, INN, BAN *thromboxane synthetase inhibitor*

**rifabutin** USAN, INN *antiviral; antibacterial; for prevention of* Mycobacterium avium *complex (MAC) in advanced HIV patients (orphan)*

**Rifadin** capsules, powder for IV injection ℞ *tuberculostatic (orphan)* [rifampin] 150, 300 mg; 600 mg ⧉ Ritalin

**rifalazil** USAN *investigational (Phase II) rifampin derivative for* Mycobacterium avium *complex (MAC) and* Mycobacterium *tuberculosis*

**Rifamate** capsules ℞ *tuberculostatic* [rifampin; isoniazid] 300•150 mg

**rifametane** USAN, INN *antibacterial*

**rifamexil** USAN *antibacterial*

**rifamide** USAN, INN *antibacterial*

**rifampicin** INN, BAN, JAN *antibacterial* [also: rifampin]

**rifampin** USAN, USP *antibacterial; antituberculosis agent (orphan)* [also: rifampicin] 150, 300 mg oral; 600 mg injection

**rifampin & isoniazid & pyrazinamide** *short-course treatment of tuberculosis (orphan)*

**rifamycin** INN, BAN

**rifamycin diethylamide** [see: rifamide]

**rifamycin M·14** [see: rifamide]

**rifapentine** USAN, INN, BAN *antibacterial for tuberculosis (orphan); investigational (orphan) for AIDS-related* Mycobacterium avium *complex (MAC)*

**Rifater** tablets ℞ *short-course treatment for tuberculosis (orphan)* [rifampin; isoniazid; pyrazinamide] 120•50•300 mg

**rifaxidin** [see: rifaximin]

**rifaximin** USAN, INN *broad-spectrum rifamycin antibiotic for traveler's diarrhea; investigational (orphan) for hepatic encephalopathy*

**rIFN-A (recombinant interferon alfa)** [see: interferon alfa-2a, recombinant]

**rIFN-α2 (recombinant interferon alfa-2)** [see: interferon alfa-2b, recombinant]

**rIFN-B (recombinant interferon beta)** [see: interferon beta-1b, recombinant]

**rIFN-beta** *investigational (orphan) for malignant melanoma, metastatic renal cell carcinoma, T-cell lymphoma, and Kaposi sarcoma*

**rifomycin** [see: rifamycin]

**RIG (rabies immune globulin)** [q.v.]

**RIGScan** *investigational imaging agent*

**rilapine** INN

**rilmazafone** INN

**rilmenidine** INN

**rilopirox** INN

**rilozarone** INN

**Rilutek** film-coated tablets ℞ *amyotrophic lateral sclerosis (ALS) treatment (orphan); investigational (orphan) for Huntington disease; investigational (Phase III) for Parkinson disease* [riluzole] 50 mg

**riluzole** USAN, INN *amyotrophic lateral sclerosis (ALS) treatment (orphan); investigational (orphan) for Huntington disease; investigational (Phase III) for Parkinson disease*

**Rimactane** capsules ℞ *tuberculostatic* [rifampin] 300 mg

**rimantadine** INN *antiviral* [also: rimantadine HCl]

**rimantadine HCl** USAN *antiviral* [also: rimantadine]

**rimazolium metilsulfate** INN

**rimcazole** INN *antipsychotic* [also: rimcazole HCl]

**rimcazole HCl** USAN *antipsychotic* [also: rimcazole]

**rimexolone** USAN, INN, BAN *ophthalmic corticosteroidal anti-inflammatory*

**rimiterol** INN *bronchodilator* [also: rimiterol hydrobromide]

**rimiterol hydrobromide** USAN *bronchodilator* [also: rimiterol]

**rimonabant** *investigational (Phase III) selective cannabinoid CB-1 blocker for smoking cessation, weight loss, increasing HDL, increasing insulin sensitivity, and decreasing C-reactive protein (CRP) levels*

**rimoprogin** INN

**Rimso-50** solution for bladder instillation ℞ *anti-inflammatory for symptomatic relief of interstitial cystitis* [dimethyl sulfoxide (DMSO)] 50%

**Rinade B.I.D.** sustained-release capsules ℞ *decongestant; antihistamine* [pseudoephedrine HCl; chlorpheniramine maleate] 120•8 mg

**Ringer injection** USP *fluid and electrolyte replenisher* [also: compound solution of sodium chloride]

**Ringer injection, lactated** USP *fluid and electrolyte replenisher; systemic alkalizer* [also: compound solution of sodium lactate]

**Ringer irrigation** USP *irrigation solution*

**Ringer solution** [now: Ringer irrigation]

**riodipine** INN

**Riomet** oral liquid ℞ *biguanide antidiabetic* [metformin HCl] 500 mg/5 mL

**Riopan** oral suspension OTC *antacid* [magaldrate] 540 mg/5 mL

**Riopan Plus** chewable tablets, oral suspension OTC *antacid; antiflatulent* [magaldrate; simethicone] 480•20, 1080•20 mg; 540•40, 1080•40 mg/5 mL

**rioprostil** USAN, INN *gastric antisecretory*

**ripazepam** USAN, INN *minor tranquilizer*

**ripple grass** *medicinal herb* [see: plantain]

**Riquent** ℞ *investigational (NDA filed, orphan) immunosuppressant for lupus-associated nephritis* [abetimus sodium]

**risedronate sodium** USAN *bisphosphonate bone resorption inhibitor for osteoporosis and Paget disease*

**rismorelin porcine** USAN *growth stimulant for growth hormone deficiencies*

**risocaine** USAN, INN *local anesthetic*

**risotilide HCl** USAN *antiarrhythmic*

**Risperdal** tablets, M-Tabs (orally disintegrating tablets), oral drops ℞ *novel (atypical) antipsychotic; treatment for manic episodes of a bipolar disorder* [risperidone] 0.25, 0.5, 1, 2, 3, 4 mg; 0.5, 1, 2 mg; 1 mg/mL ② Restoril

**Risperdal Consta** long-acting injection ℞ *novel (atypical) antipsychotic* [risperidone (encapsulated in polymer microspheres)] 25, 37.5, 50 mg ② Restoril

**risperidone** USAN, INN, BAN *benzisoxazole antipsychotic; neuroleptic; treat-*

*ment for manic episodes of a bipolar disorder*

**ristianol** INN, BAN *immunoregulator* [also: ristianol phosphate]

**ristianol phosphate** USAN *immunoregulator* [also: ristianol]

**ristocetin** USP, INN, BAN

**Ritadex** (name changed to Focalin upon marketing release in 2001)

**Ritalin** tablets ℞ *CNS stimulant for attention-deficit hyperactivity disorder (ADHD) and narcolepsy; also abused as a street drug* [methylphenidate HCl] 5, 10, 20 mg ② Ismelin; Rifadin

**Ritalin LA** dual-release capsules ℞ *CNS stimulant for attention-deficit hyperactivity disorder (ADHD)* [methylphenidate HCl] 20, 30, 40 mg (50% immediate release, 50% delayed release)

**Ritalin SR** sustained-release tablets ℞ *CNS stimulant for attention-deficit hyperactivity disorder (ADHD) and narcolepsy* [methylphenidate HCl] 20 mg

**ritamycin** *investigational (Phase III) antibiotic for bacterial infectious diarrhea (BID)*

**ritanserin** USAN, INN, BAN *investigational serotonin $S_2$ antagonist for various psychiatric illnesses and substance abuse*

**ritiometan** INN

**ritodrine** USAN, INN *smooth muscle relaxant*

**ritodrine HCl** USAN, USP *smooth muscle relaxant; uterine relaxant to arrest preterm labor* 10, 15 mg/mL injection

**Ritodrine HCl in 5% Dextrose** IV infusion in 500 mL LifeCare bags ℞ *uterine relaxant to arrest preterm labor* [ritodrine HCl; dextrose] 0.03%•5%

**ritolukast** USAN, INN *antiasthmatic; leukotriene antagonist*

**ritonavir** USAN, INN *antiviral protease inhibitor for HIV infection*

**ritonavir & lamivudine & saquinavir mesylate** *investigational (Phase II) protease inhibitor and nucleoside reverse transcriptase inhibitor combination for HIV infection*

**ritonavir & zidovudine & saquina-vir mesylate** *investigational (Phase II) protease inhibitor combination for HIV infection*

**ritropirronium bromide** INN

**ritrosulfan** INN

**Rituxan** IV infusion ℞ *monoclonal antibody for non-Hodgkin B-cell lymphoma (orphan); investigational (Phase III) for rheumatoid arthritis and chronic lymphocytic leukemia* [rituximab] 10 mg/mL

**rituximab** USAN *monoclonal antibody for non-Hodgkin B-cell lymphoma (orphan); investigational (Phase III) for rheumatoid arthritis and chronic lymphocytic leukemia*

**Riva-Diclofenac** ⒸⒶⓃ enteric-coated tablets ℞ *analgesic; antiarthritic; nonsteroidal anti-inflammatory drug (NSAID)* [diclofenac sodium] 50 mg

**Riva-Diclofenac-K** ⒸⒶⓃ film-coated slow-release tablets ℞ *analgesic; antiarthritic; nonsteroidal anti-inflammatory drug (NSAID)* [diclofenac potassium] 75 mg

**Riva-Loperamide** ⒸⒶⓃ caplets OTC *antidiarrheal* [loperamide HCl] 2 mg

**Riva-Lorazepam** ⒸⒶⓃ tablets ℞ *benzodiazepine anxiolytic* [lorazepam] 0.5, 1, 2 mg

**Riva-Naproxen** ⒸⒶⓃ tablets ℞ *analgesic; antiarthritic; nonsteroidal anti-inflammatory drug (NSAID)* [naproxen] 250, 375, 500 mg

**Riva-Norfloxacin** ⒸⒶⓃ film-coated tablets ℞ *broad-spectrum fluoroquinolone antibiotic* [norfloxacin] 400 mg

**rivastigmine** USAN *acetylcholinesterase inhibitor to increase cognition in Alzheimer disease*

**rivastigmine tartrate** *acetylcholinesterase inhibitor to increase cognition in Alzheimer disease*

**rivoglitazone** USAN *antidiabetic for type 2 diabetes*

**rizatriptan benzoate** USAN *vascular serotonin 5-HT$_{1B/1D}$ receptor agonist for the acute treatment of migraine*

**rizatriptan sulfate** USAN *vascular serotonin 5-HT$_{1B/1D}$ receptor agonist for the acute treatment of migraine*

**rizolipase** INN

**r-metHuLeptin** [see: metreleptin]

**RMP-7 (receptor-mediated permeabilizer)** [see: lobradimil]

**RMS** suppositories ℞ *narcotic analgesic* [morphine sulfate] 5, 10, 20, 30 mg

**rNPA (recombinant novel plasminogen activator)** [see: novel plasminogen activator]

**rob elder** *medicinal herb* [see: elderberry]

**Robafen AC Cough** syrup (discontinued 2002) ℞ *narcotic antitussive; expectorant* [codeine phosphate; guaifenesin; alcohol 3.5%] 10•100 mg/5 mL

**Robafen CF** oral liquid (discontinued 2002) OTC *antitussive; decongestant; expectorant* [dextromethorphan hydrobromide; phenylpropanolamine HCl; guaifenesin] 10•12.5•100 mg/5 mL

**Robafen DAC** syrup (discontinued 2002) ℞ *narcotic antitussive; decongestant; expectorant* [codeine phosphate; pseudoephedrine HCl; guaifenesin; alcohol 1.4%] 10•30•100 mg/5 mL

**Robafen DM** syrup (discontinued 2002) OTC *antitussive; expectorant* [dextromethorphan hydrobromide; guaifenesin; alcohol 1.4%] 10•100 mg/5 mL

**Robafen PE** oral liquid OTC *decongestant; expectorant* [pseudoephedrine HCl; guaifenesin] 60•200 mg/10 mL

**RoBathol Bath Oil** OTC *bath emollient*

**Robaxin** tablets, IV or IM injection ℞ *skeletal muscle relaxant* [methocarbamol] 500, 750 mg; 100 mg/mL

**Robaxisal** tablets (discontinued 2004) ℞ *skeletal muscle relaxant; analgesic* [methocarbamol; aspirin] 400•325 mg ② Robaxacet

**robenidine** INN *coccidiostat for poultry* [also: robenidine HCl]

**robenidine HCl** USAN *coccidiostat for poultry* [also: robenidine]

**Robicap** (trademarked dosage form) *capsule*

**Robinul** tablets, IV or IM injection ℞ *GI antispasmodic; anticholinergic; peptic ulcer treatment adjunct; antisecretory* [glycopyrrolate] 1 mg; 0.2 mg/5 mL

**Robinul Forte** tablets ℞ *GI antispasmodic; anticholinergic; peptic ulcer treatment adjunct; antisecretory* [glycopyrrolate] 2 mg

**Robitab** (trademarked dosage form) *tablet*

**Robitussin** oral liquid OTC *expectorant* [guaifenesin] 100 mg/5 mL

**Robitussin A-C** syrup (discontinued 2002) ℞ *narcotic antitussive; expectorant* [codeine phosphate; guaifenesin; alcohol 3.5%] 10•100 mg/5 mL

**Robitussin Allergy & Cough** oral liquid OTC *antitussive; decongestant; antihistamine* [dextromethorphan hydrobromide; pseudoephedrine HCl; brompheniramine maleate] 20•60•4 mg/10 mL

**Robitussin Cold, Cold & Congestion** caplets, softgels OTC *antitussive; decongestant; expectorant* [dextromethorphan hydrobromide; pseudoephedrine HCl; guaifenesin] 10•30•200 mg

**Robitussin Cold, Cold & Cough** softgels OTC *antitussive; decongestant; expectorant* [dextromethorphan hydrobromide; pseudoephedrine HCl; guaifenesin] 10•30•200 mg

**Robitussin Cold, Multi-Symptom Cold & Flu** caplets, softgels OTC *antitussive; decongestant; expectorant; analgesic* [dextromethorphan hydrobromide; pseudoephedrine HCl; guaifenesin; acetaminophen] 10•30•200•325 mg; 10•30•100•250 mg

**Robitussin Cold, Sinus & Congestion** caplets OTC *decongestant; expectorant; analgesic* [pseudoephedrine HCl; guaifenesin; acetaminophen] 30•200•325 mg

**Robitussin Cough** oral liquid OTC *antitussive* [dextromethorphan hydrobromide; alcohol 1.4%] 15 mg/5 mL

**Robitussin Cough Calmers** lozenges (discontinued 2002) OTC *antitussive* [dextromethorphan hydrobromide] 5 mg

**Robitussin Cough & Cold** infant oral drops OTC *antitussive; decongestant; expectorant* [dextromethorphan hydrobromide; pseudoephedrine HCl; guaifenesin] 5•15•100 mg/2.5 mL

**Robitussin Cough & Cold; Robitussin Honey Cough & Cold; Robitussin Pediatric Cough & Cold Formula** oral liquid OTC *antitussive; decongestant* [dextromethorphan hydrobromide; pseudoephedrine HCl] 30•60 mg/10 mL; 30•60 mg/15 mL; 7.5•15 mg/5 mL

**Robitussin Cough & Congestion Formula** oral liquid OTC *antitussive; expectorant* [dextromethorphan hydrobromide; guaifenesin] 20•400 mg/10 mL

**Robitussin Cough Drops** lozenge OTC *analgesic; mild local anesthetic* [menthol] 7.4, 10 mg

**Robitussin CoughGels** liquid-filled gelcaps OTC *antitussive* [dextromethorphan hydrobromide] 15 mg

**Robitussin Flu** oral liquid OTC *antitussive; decongestant; antihistamine; analgesic* [dextromethorphan hydrobromide; pseudoephedrine HCl; chlorpheniramine maleate; acetaminophen] 20•60•4•640 mg/20 mL

**Robitussin Honey Cough DM** ⓒⒶⓃ honey-based syrup OTC *antitussive* [dextromethorphan hydrobromide] 10 mg/5 mL

**Robitussin Honey Flu Multi-Symptom Relief** oral liquid OTC *antitussive; decongestant; analgesic* [dextromethorphan hydrobromide; pseudoephedrine HCl; acetaminophen] 20•60•500 mg/15 mL

**Robitussin Honey Flu Nighttime** syrup OTC *antitussive; decongestant; antihistamine; analgesic* [dextromethorphan hydrobromide; pseudoephedrine HCl; chlorpheniramine maleate; acetaminophen] 20•60•4•500 mg/pouch

**Robitussin Honey Flu Non-Drowsy** syrup for oral solution OTC *antitussive; decongestant; analgesic* [dextromethorphan hydrobromide; pseudoephedrine HCl; acetaminophen] 20•60•500 mg/pouch

**Robitussin Liquid Center Cough Drops** lozenges OTC *topical analgesic; counterirritant; mild local anesthetic* [menthol] 10 mg

**Robitussin Night Relief** oral liquid OTC *antitussive; decongestant; antihistamine; analgesic* [dextromethorphan hydrobromide; pseudoephedrine HCl; pyrilamine maleate; acetaminophen] 30•60•50•650 mg/30 mL

**Robitussin Pediatric Cough** oral liquid OTC *antitussive* [dextromethorphan hydrobromide] 7.5 mg/5 mL

**Robitussin Pediatric Night Relief Cough & Cold; Robitussin PM Cough & Cold** oral liquid OTC *antitussive; decongestant; antihistamine* [dextromethorphan hydrobromide; pseudoephedrine HCl; chlorpheniramine maleate] 15•30•2 mg/10 mL

**Robitussin Severe Congestion** Liqui-Gels (liquid-filled softgels) OTC *decongestant; expectorant* [pseudoephedrine HCl; guaifenesin] 30•200 mg

**Robitussin Sugar Free Cough** oral liquid OTC *antitussive; expectorant* [dextromethorphan hydrobromide; guaifenesin] 20•200 mg/10 mL

**Robitussin-CF** oral liquid (discontinued 2002) OTC *antitussive; decongestant; expectorant* [dextromethorphan hydrobromide; phenylpropanolamine HCl; guaifenesin; alcohol 4.75%] 10•12.5•100 mg/5 mL

**Robitussin-DAC** syrup (discontinued 2002) ℞ *narcotic antitussive; decongestant; expectorant* [codeine phosphate; pseudoephedrine HCl; guaifenesin; alcohol 1.9%] 10•30•100 mg/5 mL

**Robitussin-DM** oral liquid, infants' oral drops OTC *antitussive; expectorant* [dextromethorphan hydrobromide; guaifenesin] 20•200 mg/10 mL; 5•100 mg/2.5 mL

**Robitussin-PE** oral liquid OTC *decongestant; expectorant* [pseudoephedrine HCl; guaifenesin; alcohol 1.4%] 60•200 mg/10 mL

**Rocaltrol** capsules, oral solution ℞ *vitamin D therapy for hypoparathyroidism and hypocalcemia of chronic renal dialysis; decreases severity of psoriatic lesions* [calcitriol] 0.25, 0.5 μg; 1 μg/mL

**rocastine** INN *antihistamine* [also: rocastine HCl]

**rocastine HCl** USAN *antihistamine* [also: rocastine]

**Rocephin** powder or frozen premix for IV or IM injection ℞ *cephalosporin antibiotic* [ceftriaxone sodium] 0.25, 0.5, 1, 2, 10 g

**rochelle salt** [see: potassium sodium tartrate]

**rociverine** INN

**rock brake; rock polypod** *medicinal herb* [see: female fern]

**rock elm** *medicinal herb* [see: slippery elm]

**rock parsley** *medicinal herb* [see: parsley]

**rock rose (Helianthemum canadense)** plant *medicinal herb used as an astringent and tonic*

**Rocky Mountain grape** *medicinal herb* [see: Oregon grape]

**Rocky Mountain spotted fever vaccine** USP

**rocuronium bromide** USAN, INN, BAN *nondepolarizing neuromuscular blocking agent; muscle relaxant; adjunct to general anesthesia*

**rodocaine** USAN, INN *local anesthetic*

**rodorubicin** INN

**rofecoxib** *analgesic; antiarthritic; antipyretic; COX-2 inhibitor; nonsteroidal anti-inflammatory drug (NSAID); treatment for acute migraine*

**rofelodine** INN

**Roferon-A** subcu or IM injection in prefilled syringes ℞ *antineoplastic/ antiviral for hairy cell leukemia, hepatitis C, Kaposi sarcoma (orphan), and chronic myelogenous leukemia (orphan); investigational (orphan) for renal cell* carcinoma [interferon alfa-2a] 3, 6, 9 million IU

**roflurane** USAN, INN *inhalation anesthetic*

**Rogaine for Men; Rogaine for Women** topical solution OTC *hair growth stimulant* [minoxidil] 2%, 5%; 2% ⑨ Rēgain

**rogletimide** USAN, INN, BAN *antineoplastic; aromatase inhibitor*

**Rohypnol** (banned in the U.S.) ℞ *sedative and hypnotic; smuggled into the U.S. as a street drug, commonly called "roofies" or "the date rape drug"* [flunitrazepam]

**rokitamycin** INN

**Rolaids; Calcium Rich Rolaids** chewable tablets OTC *antacid* [magnesium hydroxide; calcium carbonate] 110•550, 135•675 mg; 80•412 mg

**Rolaids Multi-Symptom** chewable tablets OTC *antacid* [magnesium hydroxide; calcium carbonate; simethicone] 135•675•60 mg

**Rolatuss Expectorant** oral liquid (discontinued 2002) ℞ *narcotic antitussive; decongestant; antihistamine; expectorant* [codeine phosphate; phenylephrine HCl; chlorpheniramine maleate; ammonium chloride; alcohol 5%] 9.85•5•2•33.3 mg/5 mL

**Rolatuss Plain** oral liquid (discontinued 2002) OTC *decongestant; antihistamine* [phenylephrine HCl; chlorpheniramine maleate; alcohol 5%] 5•2 mg/5 mL

**Rolatuss with Hydrocodone** oral liquid (discontinued 2002) ℞ *narcotic antitussive; decongestant; antihistamine* [hydrocodone bitartrate; phenylpropanolamine HCl; phenylephrine HCl; pyrilamine maleate; pheniramine maleate] 1.7•3.3•5•3.3•3.3 mg/5 mL

**Rolazar** (name changed to Alimta upon marketing release in 2004)

**roletamide** USAN, INN *hypnotic*

**rolgamidine** USAN, INN, BAN *antidiarrheal*

**rolicton** [see: amisometradine]

**rolicyclidine** INN

**rolicypram** BAN *antidepressant* [also: rolicyprine]

**rolicyprine** USAN, INN *antidepressant* [also: rolicypram]

**rolipram** USAN, INN *tranquilizer*

**rolitetracycline** USAN, USP, INN *antibacterial*

**rolitetracycline nitrate** USAN *antibacterial*

**rolodine** USAN, INN *skeletal muscle relaxant*

**rolziracetam** INN, BAN

**Roman camomile** *medicinal herb* [see: chamomile]

**Roman laurel** *medicinal herb* [see: laurel]

**romazarit** USAN, INN, BAN *anti-inflammatory; antirheumatic*

**Romazicon** IV injection ℞ *benzodiazepine antagonist to reverse anesthesia or treat overdose* [flumazenil] 0.1 mg/mL

**rometin** [see: clioquinol]

**romifenone** INN

**romifidine** INN

**Romilar AC** oral liquid ℞ *narcotic antitussive; expectorant* [codeine phosphate; guaifenesin] 20•200 mg/10 mL

**romurtide** INN

**ronactolol** INN

**Rondamine-DM** pediatric oral drops (discontinued 2002) ℞ *antitussive; decongestant; antihistamine* [dextromethorphan hydrobromide; pseudoephedrine HCl; carbinoxamine maleate] 4•25•2 mg/5 mL

**Rondamine-DM** syrup ℞ *pediatric antitussive, decongestant, and antihistamine* [dextromethorphan hydrobromide; pseudoephedrine HCl; brompheniramine maleate] 15•60•4 mg/5 mL

**Rondec** chewable tablets (discontinued 2002) ℞ *decongestant; antihistamine* [pseudoephedrine HCl; brompheniramine maleate] 60•4 mg

**Rondec** syrup ℞ *decongestant; antihistamine* [pseudoephedrine HCl; brompheniramine maleate] 45•4 mg/5 mL

**Rondec** tablets, pediatric oral drops ℞ *decongestant; antihistamine* [pseudoephedrine HCl; carbinoxamine maleate] 60•4 mg; 15•1 mg/mL

**Rondec-DM** pediatric oral drops ℞ *antitussive; decongestant; antihistamine* [dextromethorphan hydrobromide; pseudoephedrine HCl; carbinoxamine maleate] 4•15•1 mg/mL

**Rondec-DM** syrup ℞ *antitussive; decongestant; antihistamine* [dextromethorphan hydrobromide; pseudoephedrine HCl; brompheniramine maleate] 15•45•4 mg/5 mL

**Rondec-TR** timed-release tablets ℞ *decongestant; antihistamine* [pseudoephedrine HCl; carbinoxamine maleate] 120•8 mg

**ronidazole** USAN, INN *antiprotozoal*

**ronifibrate** INN

**ronipamil** INN

**ronnel** USAN *systemic insecticide* [also: fenclofos; fenchlorphos]

**ropinirole** INN, BAN *dopamine agonist; antiparkinsonian* [also: ropinirole HCl]

**ropinirole HCl** USAN *dopamine agonist; antiparkinsonian* [also: ropinirole]

**ropitoin** INN *antiarrhythmic* [also: ropitoin HCl]

**ropitoin HCl** USAN *antiarrhythmic* [also: ropitoin]

**ropivacaine** INN *long-acting local anesthetic*

**ropivacaine HCl** *long-acting local anesthetic*

**ropizine** USAN, INN *anticonvulsant*

**roquinimex** USAN, INN *investigational (Phase II) immunomodulator for HIV; investigational for bone marrow transplant for leukemia*

*Rosa acicularis; R. canina; R. rugosa* **and other species** *medicinal herb* [see: rose]

**Rosac** cream ℞ *acne treatment* [sulfacetamide sodium; sulfur] 10%•5%

**rosamicin** [now: rosaramicin]

**rosamicin butyrate** [now: rosaramicin butyrate]

**rosamicin propionate** [now: rosaramicin propionate]

**rosamicin sodium phosphate** [now: rosaramicin sodium phosphate]

**rosamicin stearate** [now: rosaramicin stearate]

**Rosanil** cleanser ℞ *acne treatment* [sulfacetamide sodium; sulfur] 10%•5%

**rosaprostol** INN

**rosaramicin** USAN, INN *antibacterial*

**rosaramicin butyrate** USAN *antibacterial*

**rosaramicin propionate** USAN *antibacterial*

**rosaramicin sodium phosphate** USAN *antibacterial*

**rosaramicin stearate** USAN *antibacterial*

**rosary pea** *medicinal herb* [see: precatory bean]

**rose (*Rosa acicularis; R. canina; R. rugosa* and other species)** flowers and hips *medicinal herb for blood cleansing, cancer, colds, flu, infections, and sore throat; also used as a diuretic, mild laxative, and source of vitamin C*

**rose, sun** *medicinal herb* [see: rock rose]

**rose bengal** *diagnostic aid for corneal injury and pathology* 1.3 mg/strip

**rose bengal sodium ($^{131}$I)** INN *hepatic function test; radioactive agent* [also: rose bengal sodium I 131]

**rose bengal sodium I 125** USAN *radioactive agent*

**rose bengal sodium I 131** USAN, USP *hepatic function test; radioactive agent* [also: rose bengal sodium ($^{131}$I)]

**rose laurel** *medicinal herb* [see: mountain laurel]

**rose oil** NF *perfume*

**rose petal aqueous infusion** *ocular emollient*

**rose water, stronger** NF *perfume*

**rose water ointment** USP *emollient; ointment base*

**rosemary (*Rosmarinus officinalis*)** leaves *medicinal herb for flatulence, gastrointestinal spasm, halitosis, heart tonic, inducing diaphoresis, migraine headache, promoting menstrual flow, stimulating abortion, and stomach disorders*

**Rosets** ophthalmic strips OTC *diagnostic aid for corneal injury and pathology* [rose bengal] 1.3 mg

**rosiglitazone maleate** USAN *thiazolidinedione antidiabetic; increases cellular response to insulin without increasing insulin secretion*

**rosin** USP

**rosoxacin** USAN, INN *antibacterial* [also: acrosoxacin]

**rosterolone** INN

**Rosula** gel ℞ *treatment for acne, rosacea, and seborrheic dermatitis* [sulfacetamide sodium; sulfur; urea] 10%•5%•10%

**Rosula Aqueous Cleanser** topical liquid ℞ *treatment for acne and rosacea* [sulfacetamide sodium; sulfur; urea] 10%•5%•10%

**rosuvastatin calcium** USAN *HMG-CoA reductase inhibitor for hypercholesterolemia, mixed dyslipidemia, and hypertriglyceridemia*

**Rotacaps** (trademarked form) *encapsulated powder for inhalation*

**Rotadisk** (trademarked dosage form) *powder for inhalation* [used in a Diskhaler]

**rotamicillin** INN

**Rotamune** ℞ *investigational oral rotavirus vaccine*

**rotigotine** *investigational (Phase III) transdermal dopamine agonist; antiparkinsonian*

**rotoxamine** USAN, INN *antihistamine*

**rotoxamine tartrate** NF

**rotraxate** INN

**round-leaved plantain** *medicinal herb* [see: plantain]

**rovelizumab** USAN *immunomodulator; investigational (Phase III) cell adhesion inhibitor for ischemic stroke, acute myocardial infarction, and trauma-induced hemorrhagic shock*

**Rowasa** suppositories, rectal suspension enema ℞ *anti-inflammatory for active ulcerative colitis, proctosigmoiditis, and proctitis* [mesalamine (5-aminosalicylic acid)] 500 mg; 4 g/60 mL

**roxadimate** USAN, INN *sunscreen*

**Roxanol; Roxanol 100; Roxanol T** oral solution ℞ *narcotic analgesic* [morphine sulfate] 20 mg/mL; 100 mg/5 mL; 20 mg/mL

**Roxanol Rescudose; Roxanol UD** oral solution (discontinued 2001) ℞ *narcotic analgesic* [morphine sulfate] 10 mg/2.5 mL; 10 mg/2.5 mL, 20 mg/5 mL, 30 mg/1.5 mL

**roxarsone** USAN, INN *antibacterial*

**roxatidine** INN, BAN *histamine $H_2$ antagonist for gastric and duodenal ulcers* [also: roxatidine acetate HCl]

**roxatidine acetate HCl** USAN *investigational (NDA filed) histamine $H_2$ antagonist for gastric and duodenal ulcers* [also: roxatidine]

**roxibolone** INN

**Roxicet** tablets, oral solution ℞ *narcotic analgesic* [oxycodone HCl; acetaminophen] 5•325 mg; 5•325 mg/5 mL

**Roxicet 5/500** caplets ℞ *narcotic analgesic* [oxycodone HCl; acetaminophen] 5•500 mg

**Roxicodone** tablets, oral solution, Intensol (concentrated oral solution) ℞ *narcotic analgesic* [oxycodone HCl] 5, 15, 30 mg; 5 mg/5 mL; 20 mg/mL ⑨ oxycodone

**roxifiban acetate** USAN *antithrombotic; fibrinogen receptor antagonist*

**Roxilox** capsules ℞ *narcotic analgesic* [oxycodone HCl; acetaminophen] 5•500 mg

**Roxin** ℞ *investigational (NDA filed) histamine $H_2$ antagonist for duodenal and gastric ulcers* [roxatidine acetate HCl]

**roxindole** INN

**Roxiprin** tablets ℞ *narcotic analgesic* [oxycodone HCl; oxycodone terephthalate; aspirin] 4.5•0.38•325 mg

**roxithromycin** USAN, INN *macrolide antibiotic*

**roxolonium metilsulfate** INN

**roxoperone** INN

**royal jelly** *natural remedy for improving fertility and increasing longevity*

**rp24** *investigational antiviral for AIDS* [also: AIDS vaccine]

**rPA; r-PA (recombinant plasminogen activator)** *more properly called "recombinant tissue plasminogen activator" (rtPA)* [see: alteplase; anistreplase; lanoteplase; monteplase; reteplase; saruplase; tenecteplase]

**R/S** lotion OTC *topical acne treatment* [sulfur; resorcinol; alcohol] 5%•2%•28%

**RSV-IG (respiratory syncytial virus immune globulin)** [q.v.]

**RT (reverse transcriptase) inhibitors** [q.v.]

**R-Tanna** caplets ℞ *decongestant; antihistamine* [phenylephrine tannate; chlorpheniramine tannate] 25•9 mg

**R-Tanna 12** pediatric oral suspension ℞ *decongestant; antihistamine* [phenylephrine tannate; pyrilamine tannate] 5•30 mg/5 mL

**R-Tanna S Pediatric** oral suspension ℞ *decongestant; antihistamine* [phenylephrine tannate; chlorpheniramine tannate] 5•4.5 mg/5 mL

**R-Tannamine** tablets, pediatric oral suspension (discontinued 2002) ℞ *decongestant; antihistamine* [phenylephrine tannate; chlorpheniramine tannate; pyrilamine tannate] 25•8•25 mg; 5•2•12.5 mg/5 mL

**R-Tannate** tablets, pediatric oral suspension (discontinued 2002) ℞ *decongestant; antihistamine* [phenylephrine tannate; chlorpheniramine tannate; pyrilamine tannate] 25•8•25 mg; 5•2•12.5 mg/5 mL

**R-Tannic-S A/D** pediatric oral suspension (discontinued 2004) ℞ *decongestant; antihistamine* [phenylephrine tannate; pyrilamine tannate] 5•30 mg/5 mL

**rtPA; rt-PA (recombinant tissue plasminogen activator)** [see: alteplase; anistreplase; lanoteplase; monteplase; reteplase; saruplase; tenecteplase]

**Rubazyme** reagent kit for professional use *in vitro diagnostic aid for rubella virus IgG antibodies in serum* [enzyme immunoassay (EIA)]

**rubbing alcohol** [see: alcohol, rubbing]

**rubbing isopropyl alcohol** [see: isopropyl alcohol, rubbing]

**rubefacients** *a class of gentle local irritants that redden the skin by producing active or passive hyperemia*

**rubella & mumps virus vaccine, live** *active immunizing agent for rubella and mumps*

**rubella virus vaccine, live** USP *active immunizing agent for rubella*

**rubeola vaccine** [see: measles virus vaccine, live]

**Rubex** powder for IV injection (discontinued 2004) ℞ *anthracycline antibiotic antineoplastic* [doxorubicin HCl] 100 mg

**rubidium** *element (Rb)*

**rubidium chloride Rb 82** USAN *radioactive diagnostic aid for cardiac disease*

**rubidium chloride Rb 86** USAN *radioactive agent*

**rubitecan** USAN *topoisomerase I inhibitor; investigational (Phase III, orphan) for pancreatic cancer and pediatric HIV/AIDS infections*

**Rubramin PC** IM or subcu injection ℞ *hematinic; vitamin $B_{12}$ supplement* [cyanocobalamin] 100, 1000 μg/mL

*Rubus fructicosus; R. villosus medicinal herb* [see: blackberry]

*Rubus idaeus; R. strigosus medicinal herb* [see: red raspberry]

**rue (*Ruta bracteosa; R. graveolens; R. montana*)** plant *medicinal herb for cramps, hypertension, hysteria, muscle strains, neuralgia, nervous disorders, sciatica, stimulation of abortion and menstruation, tendon strains, and trauma*

**rufinamide** USAN *anticonvulsant*

**rufloxacin** INN

**rufocromomycin** INN, BAN *antineoplastic* [also: streptonigrin]

**Ru-lets M 500** film-coated tablets OTC *vitamin/mineral supplement* [multiple vitamins & minerals]

**Rulid** Ⓔⓤⓡ tablets ℞ *macrolide antibiotic* [roxithromycin] 150 mg

**RuLox** oral suspension OTC *antacid* [aluminum hydroxide; magnesium hydroxide] 225•200 mg/5 mL

**RuLox #1; RuLox #2** chewable tablets OTC *antacid* [aluminum hydroxide; magnesium hydroxide] 200•200 mg; 400•400 mg

**RuLox Plus** chewable tablets, oral suspension OTC *antacid; antiflatulent* [aluminum hydroxide; magnesium

hydroxide; simethicone] 200•200•
25 mg; 500•450•40 mg/5 mL

**rum cherry** *medicinal herb* [see: wild black cherry]

*Rumex acetosa* *medicinal herb* [see: sorrel]

*Rumex crispus* *medicinal herb* [see: yellow dock]

*Rumex hymenosepalus* *medicinal herb* [see: canaigre]

**Rum-K** oral liquid ℞ *potassium supplement* [potassium chloride] 30 mEq K/ 15 mL

**ruplizumab** USAN *treatment for immune thrombocytopenic purpura and systemic lupus erythematosus (SLE) (orphan)*

*Ruscus aculeatus* *medicinal herb* [see: butcher's broom]

**rush, sweet** *medicinal herb* [see: calamus]

*Ruta bracteosa; R. graveolens; R. montana* *medicinal herb* [see: rue]

**rutamycin** USAN, INN *antifungal*

**ruthenium** *element (Ru)*

**rutin** NF *a bioflavonoid (q.v.)* [also: rutoside]

**rutoside** INN [also: rutin]

**Ru-Tuss** oral liquid (discontinued 2000) OTC *decongestant; antihistamine* [phenylephrine HCl; chlorpheniramine maleate; alcohol 5%] 5•2 mg/5 mL

**Ru-Tuss DE** prolonged-action film-coated tablets (discontinued 2000) ℞ *decongestant; expectorant* [pseudoephedrine HCl; guaifenesin] 120• 600 mg

**Ru-Tuss Expectorant** oral liquid (discontinued 2000) OTC *antitussive; decongestant; expectorant* [dextromethorphan hydrobromide; pseudoephedrine HCl; guaifenesin; alcohol 10%] 10•30•100 mg/5 mL

**Ru-Tuss with Hydrocodone** oral liquid (discontinued 2000) ℞ *narcotic antitussive; decongestant; antihistamine* [hydrocodone bitartrate; phenylpropanolamine HCl; phenylephrine HCl; pyrilamine maleate; pheniramine maleate; alcohol 5%] 1.7• 3.3•5•3.3•3.3 mg/5 mL

**ruvazone** INN

**RVA (rabies vaccine, adsorbed)** [see: rabies vaccine]

**RVP (red veterinarian petrolatum)** [see: petrolatum]

**RxPak; ℞Pak** (trademarked form) *prescription package*

**Rymed** capsules (discontinued 2002) ℞ *decongestant; expectorant* [pseudoephedrine HCl; guaifenesin] 30• 250 mg

**Rymed** oral liquid (discontinued 2002) OTC *decongestant; expectorant* [pseudoephedrine HCl; guaifenesin; alcohol 1.4%] 30•100 mg/5 mL

**Rymed-TR** long-acting caplets (discontinued 2002) ℞ *decongestant; expectorant* [phenylpropanolamine HCl; guaifenesin] 75•400 mg

**Ryna** oral liquid OTC *decongestant; antihistamine* [pseudoephedrine HCl; chlorpheniramine maleate] 60•4 mg/10 mL

**Ryna-12** caplets ℞ *decongestant; antihistamine* [phenylephrine tannate; pyrilamine tannate] 25•60 mg

**Ryna-12 S** pediatric oral suspension ℞ *decongestant; antihistamine* [phenylephrine tannate; pyrilamine tannate] 5•30 mg/5 mL

**Ryna-12D S** oral suspension ℞ *pediatric antitussive, decongestant, and antihistamine* [carbetapentane tannate; phenylephrine tannate; pyrilamine tannate] 30•5•30 mg/5 mL

**Ryna-C** oral liquid ℞ *narcotic antitussive; decongestant; antihistamine* [codeine phosphate; pseudoephedrine HCl; chlorpheniramine maleate] 20•60•4 mg/10 mL

**Ryna-CX** oral liquid (discontinued 2002) ℞ *narcotic antitussive; decongestant; expectorant* [codeine phosphate; pseudoephedrine HCl; guaifenesin] 10•30•100 mg/5 mL

**Rynatan** pediatric oral suspension ℞ *decongestant; antihistamine* [phenylephrine tannate; chlorpheniramine tannate; pyrilamine tannate] 5•2• 12.5 mg/5 mL

**Rynatan** caplets ℞ *decongestant; antihistamine* [phenylephrine tannate; chlorpheniramine tannate] 25•9 mg

**Rynatan-12 S** oral suspension ℞ *pediatric decongestant and antihistamine* [phenylephrine tannate; pyrilamine tannate] 5•30 mg/5 mL

**Rynatan-S** oral suspension (discontinued 2002) ℞ *pediatric decongestant and antihistamine* [phenylephrine tannate; chlorpheniramine tannate; pyrilamine tannate] 5•2•12.5 mg/5 mL

**Rynatuss** tablets, pediatric oral suspension ℞ *antitussive; decongestant; antihistamine* [carbetapentane tannate; phenylephrine tannate; ephedrine tannate; chlorpheniramine tannate] 60•10•10•5 mg; 30•5•5•4 mg/5 mL

**Rythmol** film-coated tablets, extended-release capsules ℞ *antiarrhythmic* [propafenone HCl] 150, 225, 300 mg; 225, 325, 425 mg

**S-2** solution for inhalation OTC *sympathomimetic bronchodilator* [racepinephrine HCl] 2.25%

$^{35}$S [see: sodium sulfate S 35]

**SA (salicylic acid)** [q.v.]

**SA (serum albumin)** [see: albumin, human]

*Sabatia angularis* medicinal herb [see: American centaury]

**Sab-Betaxolol** ⓒ eye drops ℞ *topical antiglaucoma agent (β-blocker)* [betaxolol HCl] 0.5%

**sabcomeline HCl** USAN *muscarinic receptor agonist for Alzheimer disease*

**Sab-Cortimyxin** ⓒ ophthalmic ointment ℞ *topical ophthalmic corticosteroidal anti-inflammatory; antibiotic* [hydrocortisone; neomycin sulfate; polymyxin B sulfate] 1%•0.35%•10 000 U per mL

**sabeluzole** USAN, INN, BAN *anticonvulsant; antihypoxic*

**Sabin vaccine** [see: poliovirus vaccine, live oral]

**Sabril** (approved in 40 foreign countries) ℞ *investigational (NDA filed) anticonvulsant* [vigabatrin]

**saccharated ferric oxide** JAN *hematinic* [also: iron sucrose]

**saccharated iron; saccharated iron oxide** [see: iron sucrose; saccharated ferric oxide]

s...

s...

s...

s... ...rnal herb [see: cascara sagrada]

**sacrosidase** USAN *enzyme replacement therapy for congenital sucrase-isomaltase deficiency (orphan)*

**S-adenosyl-L-methionine (SAMe)** *natural amino acid derivative used to treat depression and protect the liver from toxic overload; regenerates liver function and restores hepatic glutathione levels when taken with vitamins $B_6$, $B_{12}$, and folic acid*

**Saf-Clens** spray OTC *wound cleanser*

**Safe Tussin** oral liquid OTC *antitussive; expectorant* [dextromethorphan hydrobromide; guaifenesin] 30•200 mg/10 mL

**safflower (Carthamus tinctorius)** flowers medicinal herb for delirium, digestive disorders, fever, gout, inducing sweating, jaundice, liver disorders, lowering cholesterol, promoting expectoration, uric acid build-up, and urinary disorders

**safflower oil** USP *oleaginous vehicle; essential fatty acid supplement*

**saffron (Crocus sativus)** flowers
*medicinal herb for fever, gout, inducing
sweating, measles, rheumatism, scarlet
fever, and sedation; also used as an
aphrodisiac and expectorant*

**saffron, American; bastard saffron**
*medicinal herb* [see: safflower]

**safingol** USAN *antipsoriatic; antineoplastic adjunct*

**safingol HCl** USAN *antipsoriatic; antineoplastic adjunct*

**safrole** USP

**sagackhomi** *medicinal herb* [see: uva ursi]

**sage (Salvia lavandulaefolia; S. lyrata;
S. officinalis)** leaves *medicinal herb
for cough, diarrhea, dysmenorrhea,
fever, gastritis, gum and mouth sores,
memory improvement, nausea, nervous
disorders, and sore throat*

**sailor's tobacco** *medicinal herb* [see:
mugwort]

**St. Benedict thistle** *medicinal herb*
[see: blessed thistle]

**St. James weed; St. James wort**
*medicinal herb* [see: shepherd's purse]

**St. John's wort (Hypericum perfora-
tum)** plant *medicinal herb for AIDS,
antiviral therapy, anxiety, bronchitis,
cancer, childbirth afterpains, depression,
gastritis, insomnia, and skin disorders*

**St. Joseph Adult Chewable Aspirin**
chewable tablets OTC *analgesic; antipyretic; anti-inflammatory* [aspirin] 81 mg

**St. Joseph Cold Tablets for Children**
chewable tablets (discontinued 2001)
OTC *pediatric decongestant and analgesic* [phenylpropanolamine HCl; acet-
aminophen] 3.125•80 mg

**St. Joseph Cough Suppressant** syrup
(discontinued 2002) OTC *antitussive*
[dextromethorphan hydrobromide]
7.5 mg/5 mL

**St. Josephwort** *medicinal herb* [see: basil]

**Saizen** powder for subcu or IM injection, cool.click (needle-free subcu
injector) ℞ *growth hormone for adults
or children with congenital or endogenous growth hormone deficiency, children with Turner syndrome or renal-
induced growth failure, or AIDS-*

*wasting syndrome (orphan)* [somatro-
pin] 5 mg (15 IU) per vial

**SalAc** topical liquid OTC *keratolytic
cleanser for acne* [salicylic acid] 2%

**salacetamide** INN

**salacetin** [see: aspirin]

**Sal-Acid** plaster OTC *keratolytic* [sali-
cylic acid in a collodion-like vehi-
cle] 40%

**Salactic Film** topical liquid OTC *keratolytic* [salicylic acid in a collodion-
like vehicle] 17%

**salafibrate** INN

**Salagen** film-coated tablets ℞ *treatment of xerostomia and keratoconjunctivitis sicca due to radiotherapy or Sjögren syndrome (orphan); also for dry
mouth* [pilocarpine HCl] 5, 7.5 mg

**salantel** USAN, INN *veterinary anthelmintic*

**salazodine** INN

**Salazopyrin** (European name for U.S.
product Azulfidine)

**salazosulfadimidine** INN [also: salazo-
sulphadimidine]

**salazosulfamide** INN

**salazosulfapyridine** JAN *broad-spectrum bacteriostatic; anti-inflammatory
for ulcerative colitis; antirheumatic*
[also: sulfasalazine; sulphasalazine]

**salazosulfathiazole** INN

**salazosulphadimidine** BAN [also: sala-
zosulfadimidine]

**salbutamol** INN, BAN *sympathomimetic
bronchodilator* [also: albuterol]

**Salbutamol Nebuamp** ⓒ solution
for nebulization ℞ *sympathomimetic
bronchodilator* [salbutamol sulfate]
2.5 mL/ampule

**salbutamol sulfate** JAN *sympathomimetic bronchodilator* [also: albuterol
sulfate]

**salcatonin** BAN *synthetic analogue of
calcitonin (salmon); calcium regulator;
investigational osteoporosis treatment*
[also: calcitonin salmon (synthesis)]

**salcetogen** [see: aspirin]

**Sal-Clens Acne Cleanser** gel OTC
*keratolytic for acne* [salicylic acid] 2%

**salcolex** USAN, INN *analgesic; anti-
inflammatory; antipyretic*

**SalEst** test kit for professional use *in vitro diagnostic aid for estriol levels in saliva, used to predict spontaneous preterm labor and delivery*

**saletamide** INN *analgesic* [also: salethamide maleate]

**saletamide maleate** [see: salethamide maleate]

**salethamide maleate** USAN *analgesic* [also: saletamide]

**saletin** [see: aspirin]

**Saleto** tablets OTC *analgesic; antipyretic; anti-inflammatory* [acetaminophen; aspirin; salicylamide; caffeine] 115•210•65•16 mg

**Saleto CF** tablets (discontinued 2002) OTC *antitussive; decongestant; analgesic* [dextromethorphan hydrobromide; phenylpropanolamine; acetaminophen] 10•12.5•325 mg

**Saleto-200** tablets (discontinued 2000) OTC *analgesic; antiarthritic; antipyretic; nonsteroidal anti-inflammatory drug (NSAID)* [ibuprofen] 200 mg

**Saleto-400; Saleto-600; Saleto-800** tablets (discontinued 2000) R *analgesic; antiarthritic; antipyretic; nonsteroidal anti-inflammatory drug (NSAID)* [ibuprofen] 400 mg; 600 mg; 800 mg

**Saleto-D** capsules (discontinued 2001) OTC *decongestant; analgesic; antipyretic* [phenylpropanolamine HCl; acetaminophen; salicylamide; caffeine] 18•240•120•16 mg

**Salex** cream R *keratolytic for acne* [salicylic acid] 6%

**Salflex** film-coated tablets OTC *analgesic; antipyretic; anti-inflammatory; antirheumatic* [salsalate] 500, 750 mg

**salfluverine** INN

**salicain** [now: salicyl alcohol]

**salicin** USP

**salicin willow** *medicinal herb* [see: willow]

**salicyl alcohol** USAN *local anesthetic*

**salicylamide** USP *analgesic*

**salicylanilide** NF

**salicylate meglumine** USAN *antirheumatic; analgesic*

**salicylates** *a class of drugs that have analgesic, antipyretic, and anti-inflammatory effects*

**salicylazosulfapyridine** [now: sulfasalazine]

**salicylic acid (SA)** USP *keratolytic; antiseborrheic; antipsoriatic*

**salicylic acid, bimolecular ester** [see: salsalate]

**salicylic acid acetate** [see: aspirin]

**Salicylic Acid and Sulfur Soap** bar OTC *medicated cleanser for acne* [salicylic acid; precipitated sulfur] 3%•10%

**Salicylic Acid Cleansing** bar OTC *medicated cleanser for acne* [salicylic acid] 2%

**salicylic acid dihydrogen phosphate** [see: fosfosal]

**salicylsalicylic acid** [see: salsalate]

**saligenin** [now: salicyl alcohol]

**saligenol** [now: salicyl alcohol]

**salinazid** INN, BAN

**saline, lactated potassic** [see: potassic saline, lactated]

**saline laxatives** *a subclass of laxatives that work by attracting and retaining water in the intestines to increase intraluminal pressure and cholecystokinin release* [see also: laxatives]

**saline solution (SS)** [also: normal saline]

**SalineX** nasal mist, nose drops OTC *nasal moisturizer* [sodium chloride (saline solution)] 0.4%

**saliniazid** [see: salinazid]

**salinomycin** INN, BAN

**Saliva Substitute** oral solution OTC *saliva substitute*

**Salivart** oral spray OTC *saliva substitute*

**Salix** lozenges (discontinued 2003) OTC *saliva substitute*

**Salix alba; S. caprea; S. nigra; S. purpurea** *medicinal herb* [see: willow]

**salmaterol** [see: salmeterol]

**salmefamol** INN, BAN

**salmeterol** USAN, INN, BAN *sympathomimetic bronchodilator*

**salmeterol xinafoate** USAN *adrenergic; sympathomimetic bronchodilator* (base=69%)

**salmisteine** INN

**salmon calcitonin** [see: salcatonin]

*Salmonella typhi* **vaccine** [see: typhoid vaccine]

**Salmonine** subcu or IM injection ℞ *calcium regulator for hypercalcemia, Paget disease, and postmenopausal osteoporosis* [calcitonin (salmon)] 200 IU/mL

**salmotin** [see: adicillin]

**salnacedin** USAN *topical anti-inflammatory*

**Salofalk** ⒸⒶⓃ enteric-coated tablets ℞ *anti-inflammatory for acute ulcerative colitis and the prevention of Crohn disease relapse following bowel resection* [mesalamine (5-aminosalicylic acid)] 250, 500 mg

**Salofalk** ⒸⒶⓃ suppositories, rectal suspension enema ℞ *anti-inflammatory for distal ulcerative colitis (DUC) and ulcerative proctitis* [mesalamine (5-aminosalicylic acid)] 250, 500 mg; 2, 4 g/58 mL

**Sal-Oil-T** hair dressing ℞ *antipsoriatic; antiseborrheic; keratolytic* [coal tar; salicylic acid] 10%●6%

**salol** [see: phenyl salicylate]

**Sal-Plant** gel OTC *keratolytic* [salicylic acid in a collodion-like vehicle] 17%

**Salprofen** IV injection ℞ *investigational (orphan) for patent ductus arteriosus* [ibuprofen]

**salprotoside** INN

**salsalate** USAN, USP, INN, BAN *analgesic; antipyretic; anti-inflammatory; antirheumatic* 500, 750 mg oral

**Salsitab** film-coated tablets ℞ *analgesic; antipyretic; anti-inflammatory; antirheumatic* [salsalate] 500, 750 mg

**salt** [def.] *The inactive part of a compound, made by combining an acid with an alkali. In naproxen sodium, for example, the base is* naproxen *(an acid) and the salt is* sodium *(from sodium hydroxide, an alkali).* [compare to: base]

**Sal-Tropine** tablets ℞ *GI/GU antispasmodic; antiparkinsonian; anticholinergic "drying agent" for the respiratory tract; antidote to insecticide poisoning* [atropine sulfate] 0.4 mg

**Saluron** tablets ℞ *diuretic; antihypertensive* [hydroflumethiazide] 50 mg

**Salutensin; Salutensin-Demi** tablets ℞ *antihypertensive* [hydroflumethiazide; reserpine] 50●0.125 mg; 25●0.125 mg Ⓓ Diutensen

**saluzide** [see: opiniazide]

**salvarsan** [see: arsphenamine]

**salverine** INN

*Salvia lavandulaefolia; S. lyrata; S. officinalis* medicinal herb [see: sage]

*Salvia miltiorrhiza* medicinal herb [see: danshen]

**samarium** *element (Sm)*

**samarium Sm 153 EDTMP (ethylenediaminetetramethylenephosphoric acid)** [see: samarium Sm 153 lexidronam]

**samarium Sm 153 lexidronam** USAN *radiopharmaceutical for treatment of bone pain from osteoblastic metastatic tumors*

*Sambucus canadensis; S. ebulus; S. nigra; S. racemosa* medicinal herb [see: elder flower; elderberry]

**SAMe (S-adenosyl-ʟ-methionine)** [q.v.]

**Sanchi ginseng (***Panax pseudoginseng***)** medicinal herb [see: ginseng]

**Sanctura** film-coated tablets ℞ *muscarinic receptor antagonist for urinary frequency, urgency, and incontinence* [trospium chloride] 20 mg

**sancycline** USAN, INN *antibacterial*

**sandalwood (***Santalum album***)** oil *medicinal herb for headache, stomach ache, and urogenital disorders; also used topically as an antiseptic and astringent*

**Sandimmune** gelcaps, oral solution, IV injection ℞ *immunosuppressant for allogenic kidney, liver, and heart transplants (orphan)* [cyclosporine] 25, 100 mg; 100 mg/mL; 50 mg/mL

**Sandimmune** ophthalmic ointment
Ŗ *investigational (orphan) for keratoconjunctivitis sicca, keratoplasty graft
rejection, and corneal melting syndrome*
[cyclosporine] 2%

**Sandimmune Neoral** Ⓐ soft gels,
oral solution [see: Neoral]

**Sandoglobulin** powder for IV infusion
(discontinued 2003) Ŗ *passive immunizing agent for HIV and idiopathic
thrombocytopenic purpura (ITP)*
[immune globulin] 1, 3, 6, 12 g

**SandoPak** (trademarked packaging
form) *unit dose blister package*

**Sandostatin** subcu or IV injection Ŗ
*gastric antisecretory for acromegaly and
severe diarrhea due to VIPomas and
other tumors (orphan)* [octreotide ace-
tate] 0.05, 0.1, 0.2, 0.5, 1 mg/mL ▣
simvastatin; zinostatin

**Sandostatin LAR Depot** suspension
for IM injection Ŗ *gastric antisecretory for acromegaly and severe diarrhea
due to VIPomas and other tumors
(orphan)* [octreotide acetate]

**sanfetrinem** INN, BAN *antibacterial*
[also: sanfetrinem sodium]

**sanfetrinem cilexetil** USAN *antibacterial*

**sanfetrinem sodium** USAN *antibacterial* [also: sanfetrinem]

**SangCya** oral solution (discontinued
2004) Ŗ *immunosuppressive to prevent solid organ transplant rejection
(orphan)* [cyclosporine; alcohol
10.5%] 100 mg/mL

*Sanguinaria canadensis* medicinal herb
[see: bloodroot]

**sanguinarine chloride** [now: sanguinarium chloride]

**sanguinarium chloride** USAN, INN *antifungal; antimicrobial; anti-inflammatory*

**sanicle** (*Sanicula europea; S. mari-
landica*) root *medicinal herb used as
an astringent, expectorant, discutient,
depurative, nervine, and vulnerary*

**Sani-Pak** (trademarked packaging
form) *sanitary dispensing box*

**Sani-Supp** suppositories OTC *hyperosmolar laxative* [glycerin]

**Sanorex** tablets (discontinued 2001)
Ŗ *anorexiant; CNS stimulant; investigational (orphan) treatment for
Duchenne muscular dystrophy* [mazin-
dol] 1, 2 mg

**Sansert** tablets (discontinued 2002) Ŗ
*agent for migraine and vascular head-
aches* [methysergide maleate] 2 mg

*Santalum album* medicinal herb [see:
sandalwood]

**santonin** NF

**Santyl** ointment Ŗ *topical enzyme for
biochemical debridement* [collagenase]
250 U/g

**saperconazole** USAN, INN, BAN *antifungal*

*Saponaria officinalis* medicinal herb
[see: soapwort]

**saprisartan** INN, BAN *antihypertensive;
angiotensin II antagonist* [also: saprisartan potassium]

**saprisartan potassium** USAN *antihypertensive; angiotensin II antagonist*
[also: saprisartan]

**sapropterin** INN

**saquinavir** USAN, INN, BAN *antiretroviral protease inhibitor for HIV infection*
[also: saquinavir mesylate]

**saquinavir & amprenavir** *investigational (Phase II) protease inhibitor
combination for AIDS*

**saquinavir mesylate** USAN *antiretroviral protease inhibitor for HIV infection*
[also: saquinavir]

**saquinavir mesylate & ritonavir &
lamivudine** *investigational (Phase II)
protease inhibitor and nucleoside
reverse transcriptase inhibitor combination for HIV infection*

**saquinavir mesylate & ritonavir &
zidovudine** *investigational (Phase II)
protease inhibitor combination for HIV
infection*

**Sarafem** capsules Ŗ *selective serotonin
reuptake inhibitor (SSRI) for premenstrual dysphoric disorder (PMDD)* [flu-
oxetine HCl] 10, 20 mg

**sarafloxacin** INN, BAN *anti-infective;
DNA gyrase inhibitor* [also: sarafloxacin HCl]

**sarafloxacin HCl** USAN *anti-infective; DNA gyrase inhibitor* [also: sarafloxacin]

**saralasin** INN *antihypertensive* [also: saralasin acetate]

**saralasin acetate** USAN *antihypertensive; investigational (Phase I/II) mouthwash for oral candidiasis* [also: saralasin]

**Sarasar** *investigational (Phase III) antineoplastic for lung cancer* [lonafarnib]

**Saratoga** ointment OTC *astringent; antiseptic; wound protectant* [zinc oxide; boric acid; eucalyptol]

**sarcolysin** INN

**L-sarcolysin** [see: melphalan]

**Sardo Bath & Shower** oil OTC *bath emollient*

**Sardoettes** towelettes OTC *moisturizer; emollient*

**sargramostim** USAN, INN, BAN *antineutropenic for bone marrow transplant and graft delay (orphan); investigational (Phase III) cytokine for HIV infection*

**sargramostim & HGP-30** *investigational (Phase I) combination for HIV infection*

**sarmazenil** INN

**sarmoxicillin** USAN, INN *antibacterial*

**Sarmustine** Ŗ *investigational (orphan) for malignant glioma* [2-chloroethyl-3-sarcosinamide-1-nitrosourea]

**Sarna Anti-Itch** foam, lotion OTC *topical analgesic; counterirritant* [camphor; menthol] 0.5%•0.5%

**saroten** [see: amitriptyline]

*Sarothamnus scoparius* *medicinal herb* [see: broom]

**sarpicillin** USAN, INN *antibacterial*

*Sarracenia purpurea* *medicinal herb* [see: pitcher plant]

**sarsaparilla (*Smilax* spp.)** root *medicinal herb for blood cleansing (binding and expulsion of endotoxins), joint aches including arthritis and rheumatism, hormonal disorders, skin diseases including leprosy and psoriasis, and syphilis*

**saruplase** INN *investigational (Phase III) prourokinase (pro-UK) clot-dissolving agent for stroke*

**sassafras (*Sassafras albidum*; *S. officinale*)** root and bark *medicinal herb for acne, blood cleansing, insect bites and stings, obesity, psoriasis, skin diseases, and water retention; not generally regarded as safe and effective and banned by the FDA as a carcinogen with other serious side effects*

**sassafras, swamp** *medicinal herb* [see: magnolia]

**SAStid Soap** bar OTC *medicated cleanser for acne* [precipitated sulfur] 10%

**saterinone** INN

**satinflower** *medicinal herb* [see: chickweed]

**satoribine** [now: isatoribine]

**satranidazole** INN

**Satraplatin** Ŗ *investigational (Phase III) platinum agent for prostate cancer*

**satraplatin** USAN *antineoplastic*

**satumomab** INN, BAN *radiodiagnostic monoclonal antibody for ovarian and colorectal carcinoma* [also: indium In 111 satumomab pendetide]

**satumomab pendetide** [see: indium In 111 satumomab pendetide]

*Satureja hortensis* *medicinal herb* [see: summer savory]

*Satureja montana*; *S. obovata* *medicinal herb* [see: winter savory]

**savory** *medicinal herb* [see: summer savory; winter savory]

**savoxepin** INN

**Savvy** vaginal gel Ŗ *investigational (Phase I/II) microbicide and spermicide for HIV infection*

**saw palmetto (*Serenoa repens*; *S. serrulata*)** berries *medicinal herb for benign prostatic hypertrophy (BPH) and genitourinary, glandular, and reproductive disorders; also used to enlarge breasts, increase sperm production, promote weight gain, and enhance sexual vigor*

**saxifrage, burnet; European burnet saxifrage; small burnet saxifrage;**

**small saxifrage** *medicinal herb* [see: burnet]

**saxifrax** *medicinal herb* [see: sassafras]

**SBR-Lipocream** OTC *emollient for dry skin* [oil-in-water emulsion] 70% oil•30• water

**SC (succinylcholine)** [see: succinyl-choline chlorine]

**SCA proteins (single-chain antigen-binding proteins)** *a class of investigational antineoplastics*

**scabicides** *a class of agents effective against scabies*

**scabwort** *medicinal herb* [see: elecampane]

**Scadan** scalp lotion OTC *antiseptic; anti-seborrheic* [myristyltrimethylammonium bromide; stearyl dimethyl benzyl ammonium chloride] 1%•0.1%

**Scalpicin** topical liquid OTC *antiseborrheic* [salicylic acid] 3%

**scaly dragon's claw** *medicinal herb* [see: coral root]

**scammony, wild** *medicinal herb* [see: wild jalap]

**scandium** *element (Sc)*

**Scar Cream** OTC *to reduce the appearance of surgical scars; sunscreens* [octinoxate; octisalate] 7.5%•5%

**scarlet bergamot** *medicinal herb* [see: Oswego tea]

**scarlet berry** *medicinal herb* [see: bittersweet nightshade]

**scarlet fever streptococcus toxin**

**scarlet red** NF *promotes wound healing*

**Scarlet Red Ointment Dressings** medication-impregnated gauze ℞ *wound dressing; vulnerary* [scarlet red] 5%

**scarlet sumach** *medicinal herb* [see: sumach]

**SCCS (simethicone-coated cellulose suspension)** [see: SonoRx]

**sCD4-PE40** [see: alvircept sudotox]

*Sceletium tortuosum medicinal herb* [see: kanna]

**SCF (stem cell factor)** [q.v.]

**SCH-58500** *investigational (Phase II) gene therapy for liver and colorectal tumors*

**Schamberg** lotion OTC *topical analgesic; antiseptic; astringent; antifungal; counterirritant* [zinc oxide; menthol; phenol] 8.25%•0.25%•1.5%

**Scheinpharm Tobramycin** ⓒᴬᴺ IV or IM injection (discontinued 2000) ℞ *aminoglycoside antibiotic* [tobramycin sulfate] 10, 40 mg/mL

**Schick test** [see: diphtheria toxin for Schick test]

**Schick test control** USP *dermal reactivity indicator*

**Schirmer Tear Test** ophthalmic strips *diagnostic tear flow test aid*

**schizandra (Schisandra arisanensis; S. chinensis; S. rubriflora; S. sphenanthera)** berries *medicinal herb for cough, gastrointestinal disorders, increasing energy and mental alertness, nervous disorders, respiratory illnesses, and stress; also used as a liver protectant*

**Scleromate** IV injection ℞ *sclerosing agent for varicose veins* [morrhuate sodium] 50 mg/mL

**Sclerosol** aerosol ℞ *treatment for malignant pleural effusion and pneumothorax via intrapleural thoracoscopy administration (orphan)* [talc, sterile]

**Sclerosol** ℞ *investigational (orphan) anti-inflammatory for the topical treatment for scleroderma* [dimethyl sulfoxide (DMSO)]

**scoke** *medicinal herb* [see: pokeweed]

**Scopace** tablets ℞ *GI antispasmodic; anticholinergic CNS depressant; motion sickness preventative* [scopolamine hydrobromine] 0.4 mg

**scopafungin** USAN *antibacterial; antifungal*

**Scope** mouthwash OTC *oral antiseptic* [cetylpyridinium chloride]

**scopolamine** *oral/transdermal motion sickness preventative*

**scopolamine hydrobromide** USP *GI antispasmodic; anticholinergic CNS depressant; motion sickness preventative; cycloplegic; mydriatic* [also: hyoscine hydrobromide] 0.3, 0.4, 0.86, 1 mg/mL injection

**scopolamine methyl nitrate** [see: methscopolamine nitrate]

**scopolamine methylbromide** [see: methscopolamine bromide]

**Scott's Emulsion** OTC *vitamin supplement* [vitamins A and D] 1250•100 IU/5 mL

**Scot-Tussin Allergy Relief Formula Clear** oral liquid OTC *antihistamine* [diphenhydramine HCl] 12.5 mg/5 mL

**Scot-Tussin DM** oral liquid OTC *antitussive; antihistamine* [dextromethorphan hydrobromide; chlorpheniramine maleate] 30•4 mg/10 mL

**Scot-Tussin DM Cough Chasers** lozenges OTC *antitussive* [dextromethorphan hydrobromide] 5 mg

**Scot-Tussin Expectorant** oral liquid OTC *expectorant* [guaifenesin] 100 mg/5 mL

**Scot-Tussin Original 5-Action Cold Formula** syrup, sugar-free oral liquid OTC *decongestant; antihistamine; analgesic* [phenylephrine HCl; pheniramine maleate; sodium citrate; sodium salicylate; caffeine citrate] 4.2•13.3•83.3•83.3•25 mg

**Scot-Tussin Senior Clear** oral liquid OTC *antitussive; expectorant* [dextromethorphan hydrobromide; guaifenesin] 15•200 mg/5 mL

**Scriptene** R̥ *investigational (Phase II) heterodimer antiviral for AIDS* [zidovudine; didanosine]

**scrofula plant** *medicinal herb* [see: figwort]

*Scrophularia nodosa* *medicinal herb* [see: figwort]

**scullcap** *medicinal herb* [see: skullcap]

**scuroforme** [see: butyl aminobenzoate]

*Scutellaria lateriflora* *medicinal herb* [see: skullcap]

**SD (streptodornase)** [q.v.]

**SDZ-ASM-981** *investigational (Phase III) nonsteroidal cream for atopic dermatitis*

**75Se** [see: selenomethionine Se 75]

**sea girdles** *medicinal herb* [see: kelp (*Laminaria*)]

**Sea Mist** nasal spray (discontinued 2002) OTC *nasal moisturizer* [sodium chloride (saline solution)] 0.65%

**Seale's Lotion Modified** OTC *topical acne treatment* [sulfur] 6.4%

**sealroot; sealwort** *medicinal herb* [see: Solomon's seal]

**Sea-Omega 30; Sea-Omega 50** softgels OTC *dietary supplement* [omega-3 fatty acids] 1200 mg; 1000 mg

**Seasonale** film-coated tablets (in packs of 91) R̥ *extended-cycle (3 months) monophasic oral contraceptive* [levonorgestrel; ethinyl estradiol] 0.15 mg•30 μg

**seawrack** *medicinal herb* [see: kelp (*Fucus*)]

**Seba-Nil Cleansing Mask** scrub OTC *abrasive cleanser for acne*

**Seba-Nil Oily Skin Cleanser** topical liquid OTC *cleanser for acne* [alcohol; acetone]

**Sebasorb** lotion OTC *keratolytic for acne* [salicylic acid; attapulgite] 2%•10%

**Sebazole** gel R̥ *investigational (Phase III) antifungal for seborrheic dermatitis* [ketoconazole]

**Sebex** shampoo OTC *antiseborrheic; keratolytic* [sulfur; salicylic acid] 2%•2%

**Sebex-T** shampoo OTC *antiseborrheic; antipsoriatic; keratolytic* [sulfur; salicylic acid; coal tar] 2%•2%•5%

**Sebizon** lotion (discontinued 2003) R̥ *antibiotic; antiseborrheic* [sulfacetamide sodium] 10%

**Sebucare** hair lotion OTC *antiseborrheic; keratolytic* [salicylic acid; alcohol 61%] 1.8%

**Sebulex with Conditioners** shampoo OTC *antiseborrheic; keratolytic* [sulfur; salicylic acid] 2%•2%

**secalciferol** USAN, INN, BAN *calcium regulator; investigational (orphan) for familial hypophosphatemic rickets*

**secbutabarbital sodium** INN *sedative; hypnotic* [also: butabarbital sodium]

**secbutobarbitone** BAN *sedative; hypnotic* [also: butabarbital]

**seclazone** USAN, INN *anti-inflammatory; uricosuric*

secnidazole INN, BAN

secobarbital USP, INN *hypnotic; sedative*

secobarbital sodium USP, JAN *hypnotic; sedative; also abused as a street drug* [also: quinalbarbitone sodium] 100 mg oral; 50 mg/mL injection

**Seconal Sodium** Pulvules (capsules) ℞ *sedative; hypnotic; also abused as a street drug* [secobarbital sodium] 100 mg

secoverine INN

**Secran** oral liquid OTC *vitamin supplement* [vitamins $B_1$, $B_3$, and $B_{12}$; alcohol 17%] 10 mg•10 mg•25 μg per 5 mL

**SecreFlo** powder for IV injection ℞ *diagnostic aid for pancreatic function* [secretin] 16 μg/vial

secretin INN, BAN *diagnostic aid for pancreatic function*

**Secretin Ferring** powder for IV injection (name changed to SecreFlo in 2002)

secretory leukocyte protease inhibitor *investigational (orphan) for congenital alpha$_1$-antitrypsin deficiency, cystic fibrosis, and bronchopulmonary dysplasia*

**Sectral** capsules ℞ *antianginal; antihypertensive; antiarrhythmic; β-blocker* [acebutolol HCl] 200, 400 mg

**Secule** (trademarked packaging form) *single-dose vial*

securinine INN

sedaform [see: chlorobutanol]

**Sedapap** caplets ℞ *analgesic; barbiturate sedative* [acetaminophen; butalbital] 650•50 mg

sedatine [see: antipyrine]

sedatives *a class of soothing agents that reduce excitement, nervousness, distress, or irritation* [also called: calmatives]

sedecamycin USAN, INN *veterinary antibacterial*

sedeval [see: barbital]

sedge, sweet *medicinal herb* [see: calamus]

sedoxantrone trihydrochloride [now: ledoxantrone trihydrochloride]

seganserin INN, BAN

seglitide INN *antidiabetic* [also: seglitide acetate]

seglitide acetate USAN *antidiabetic* [also: seglitide]

selamectin USAN *veterinary antiparasitic*

**Selecor** tablets ℞ *investigational (NDA filed) antihypertensive; antianginal; β-blocker* [celiprolol HCl]

**Select-A-Jet** (trademarked delivery system) *syringe system*

selective estrogen receptor modulators (SERMs) *a class of osteoporosis prevention agents that reduce bone resorption and decrease overall bone turnover in postmenopausal women*

selective serotonin 5-HT$_3$ (hydroxytryptamine) blockers *a class of antiemetic and antinauseant agents used primarily after emetogenic cancer chemotherapy* [also called: 5-HT$_3$ receptor antagonists]

selective serotonin and norepinephrine reuptake inhibitors (SSNRIs) *a class of oral antidepressants that inhibit neuronal uptake of serotonin (5-HT) and norepinephrine, CNS neurotransmitters*

selective serotonin reuptake inhibitors (SSRIs) *a class of oral antidepressants that inhibit neuronal uptake of serotonin (5-HT), a CNS neurotransmitter*

selegiline INN, BAN *dopaminergic antiparkinsonian; investigational (Phase III) transdermal treatment for depression* [also: selegiline HCl]

selegiline HCl USAN *dopaminergic antiparkinsonian (orphan)* [also: selegiline]

selenious acid USP *dietary selenium supplement (61% elemental selenium)* 65.4 μg/mL (40 μg Se/mL) injection

selenium *element (Se)*

selenium dioxide, monohydrated [see: selenious acid]

selenium sulfide USP *antiseborrheic; antipsoriatic; antifungal for tinea versicolor* 1%, 2.5% topical

selenomethionine ($^{75}$Se) INN *pancreas function test; radioactive agent* [also: selenomethionine Se 75]

**selenomethionine Se 75** USAN, USP *pancreas function test; radioactive agent* [also: selenomethionine ($^{75}$Se)]

**Sele-Pak** IV injection ℞ *selenium supplement* [selenious acid (61% elemental selenium)] 65.4 μg/mL (40 μg Se/mL)

**Selepen** IV injection ℞ *selenium supplement* [selenious acid (61% elemental selenium)] 65.4 μg/mL (40 μg Se/mL)

**selfotel** USAN *NMDA (N-methyl-D-aspartate) antagonist for treatment of stroke-induced impairment*

**Seloken** (foreign name for U.S. product Lopressor)

**Seloken ZOC** (foreign name for U.S. product Toprol XL)

**selprazine** INN

**Selsun** lotion/shampoo ℞ *antiseborrheic; antipsoriatic; antifungal for tinea versicolor* [selenium sulfide] 2.5%

**Selsun Blue** lotion/shampoo OTC *antiseborrheic; dandruff treatment* [selenium sulfide] 1%

**Selsun Gold for Women** lotion/shampoo (discontinued 2004) OTC *antiseborrheic; dandruff treatment* [selenium sulfide] 1%

**sematilide** INN *antiarrhythmic* [also: sematilide HCl]

**sematilide HCl** USAN *antiarrhythmic* [also: sematilide]

**semduramicin** USAN, INN *coccidiostat*

**semduramicin sodium** USAN *coccidiostat*

**Semicid** vaginal suppositories OTC *spermicidal contraceptive* [nonoxynol 9] 100 mg

**semisodium valproate** BAN *anticonvulsant; antipsychotic for manic episodes; migraine prophylaxis* [also: divalproex sodium; valproate semisodium]

**semparatide acetate** USAN *parathyroid hormone analogue to enhance fracture healing*

**Semprex-D** capsules ℞ *decongestant; antihistamine* [pseudoephedrine HCl; acrivastine] 60•8 mg

**semustine** USAN, INN *antineoplastic*

**senecio, golden** *medicinal herb* [see: life root]

***Senecio aureus; S. jacoboea; S. vulgaris*** *medicinal herb* [see: life root]

**senega (*Polygala senega*)** root *medicinal herb used as an antitussive for asthma, chronic bronchitis, croup, lung congestion, and pneumonia*

**Senexon** tablets OTC *stimulant laxative* [sennosides] 8.6 mg

**Senilezol** elixir ℞ *vitamin/iron supplement* [multiple B vitamins; ferric pyrophosphate] ≗•3.3 mg

**senna** USP *stimulant laxative*

**senna (*Cassia acutifolia; C. angustifolia; C. senna*)** leaves *medicinal herb for bowel evacuation before gastrointestinal procedures, constipation, edema, and expelling worms*

**Senna-Gen** tablets OTC *stimulant laxative* [sennosides] 8.6 mg

**SennaPrompt** capsules OTC *bulk/stimulant laxative* [psyllium; sennosides] 500•9 mg

**sennosides** USP *stimulant laxative*

**Senokot** tablets, granules, syrup OTC *stimulant laxative* [sennosides] 8.6 mg; 15 mg/5 mL; 8.8 mg/5 mL

**Senokot-S** tablets OTC *stimulant laxative; stool softener* [sennosides; docusate sodium] 8.6•50 mg

**SenokotXtra** tablets OTC *stimulant laxative* [sennosides] 17 mg

**Sensability** kit OTC *breast self-examination aid*

**Sensipar** film-coated tablets ℞ *calcimimetic agent for hypercalcemia due to parathyroid carcinoma (orphan) and secondary hyperparathyroidism (SHPT) due to chronic kidney disease* [cinacalcet HCl] 33, 66, 99 mg (=30, 60, 90 mg base)

**Sensitive Eyes; Sensitive Eyes Plus** solution OTC *rinsing/storage solution for soft contact lenses* [sodium chloride (preserved saline solution)]

**Sensitive Eyes Daily Cleaner; Sensitive Eyes Saline/Cleaning Solution** OTC *surfactant cleaning solution for soft contact lenses*

**Sensitive Eyes Drops** OTC *rewetting solution for soft contact lenses*

**Sensitivity Protection Crest** toothpaste OTC *tooth desensitizer; topical dental caries preventative* [potassium nitrate; sodium fluoride]

**Sensodyne Cool Gel** toothpaste OTC *tooth desensitizer; topical dental caries preventative* [potassium nitrate; sodium fluoride]

**Sensodyne Fresh Mint** toothpaste OTC *tooth desensitizer; dental caries preventative* [potassium nitrate; sodium monofluorophosphate]

**Sensodyne-SC** toothpaste OTC *tooth desensitizer* [strontium chloride hexahydrate] 10%

**SensoGARD** gel OTC *topical oral anesthetic* [benzocaine] 20%

**Sensorcaine** injection R̥ *injectable local anesthetic* [bupivacaine HCl] 0.25%, 0.5%

**Sensorcaine** injection R̥ *injectable local anesthetic* [bupivacaine HCl; epinephrine] 0.25%•1:200 000; 0.5%•1:200 000

**Sensorcaine MPF** injection R̥ *injectable local anesthetic* [bupivacaine HCl] 0.25%, 0.5%, 0.75%

**Sensorcaine MPF** injection R̥ *injectable local anesthetic* [bupivacaine HCl; epinephrine] 0.25%•1:200 000, 0.5%•1:200 000, 0.75%•1:200 000

**Sensorcaine MPF Spinal** injection R̥ *injectable local anesthetic* [bupivacaine HCl] 0.75%

**Sentinel** test kit for professional use *urine test for HIV-1 antibodies* ⚕ fentanyl

**sepazonium chloride** USAN, INN *topical anti-infective*

**seperidol HCl** USAN *antipsychotic* [also: clofluperol]

**Seprafilm** hydrated gel film *to reduce the incidence, extent, and severity of postoperative adhesions* [hyaluronate sodium; carboxymethylcellulose]

**seprilose** USAN *antirheumatic*

**seproxetine HCl** USAN *antidepressant*

**Septa** ointment (discontinued 2001) OTC *topical antibiotic* [polymyxin B sulfate; neomycin sulfate; bacitracin] 5000 U•3.5 mg•400 U per g ⚕ Cipro; Septra

**Septi-Soft** solution R̥ *antiseptic; disinfectant* [triclosan] 0.25%

**Septisol** foam R̥ *bacteriostatic skin cleanser* [hexachlorophene; alcohol 56%] 0.23%

**Septisol** solution R̥ *antiseptic; disinfectant* [triclosan] 0.25%

**Septocaine** intraoral injection R̥ *local anesthetic for dentistry* [articaine HCl; epinephrine] 4%•1:100 000

**septomonab** [see: nebacumab]

**Septopal** polymethyl methacrylate (PMMA) beads on surgical wire R̥ *investigational (orphan) agent for chronic osteomyelitis* [gentamicin sulfate]

**Septra** tablets, oral suspension R̥ *anti-infective; antibacterial* [trimethoprim; sulfamethoxazole] 80•400 mg; 40•200 mg/5 mL ⚕ Cipro; Septa

**Septra DS** tablets R̥ *anti-infective; antibacterial* [trimethoprim; sulfamethoxazole] 160•800 mg

**Septra IV** infusion R̥ *anti-infective; antibacterial* [trimethoprim; sulfamethoxazole] 80•400 mg/5 mL

**Sequels** (trademarked dosage form) *sustained-release capsule or tablet*

**sequential AC/paclitaxel (Adriamycin, cyclophosphamide; paclitaxel)** *chemotherapy protocol for breast cancer*

**sequential DOX→ CMF (doxorubicin; cyclophosphamide, methotrexate, fluorouracil)** *chemotherapy protocol for breast cancer*

**sequifenadine** INN

**seractide** INN *adrenocorticotropic hormone* [also: seractide acetate]

**seractide acetate** USAN *adrenocorticotropic hormone* [also: seractide]

**Ser-Ap-Es** tablets R̥ *antihypertensive; vasodilator; diuretic* [hydrochlorothiazide; reserpine; hydralazine HCl] 15•0.1•25 mg ⚕ Catapres

**seratrodast** USAN, INN *anti-inflammatory; antiasthmatic; thromboxane receptor antagonist*

**Serax** capsules, tablets ℞ *benzodiazepine anxiolytic; sedative; alcohol withdrawal aid* [oxazepam] 10, 15, 30 mg; 15 mg ⊡ Eurax; Urex; Xerac

**serazapine HCl** USAN *anxiolytic*

**Serdolect** ℞ *investigational (NDA filed) novel (atypical) antipsychotic; neuroleptic* [sertindole]

**Sereine** solution OTC *cleaning solution for hard contact lenses* [note: one of three different products with the same name]

**Sereine** solution OTC *wetting solution for hard contact lenses* [note: one of three different products with the same name]

**Sereine** solution OTC *wetting/soaking solution for hard contact lenses* [note: one of three different products with the same name]

*Serenoa repens; S. serrulata medicinal herb* [see: saw palmetto]

**Serentil** IM injection (discontinued 2003) ℞ *conventional (typical) antipsychotic* [mesoridazine besylate] 25 mg/mL ⊡ Surital

**Serentil** oral concentrate (discontinued 2004) ℞ *conventional (typical) antipsychotic* [mesoridazine besylate] 25 mg/mL ⊡ Surital

**Serentil** tablets (discontinued 2004) ℞ *conventional (typical) antipsychotic* [mesoridazine besylate] 10, 50 mg ⊡ Surital

**Serevent** oral metered dose inhaler (discontinued 2004) ℞ *twice-daily sympathomimetic bronchodilator for asthma and bronchospasm* [salmeterol xinafoate] 25 μg/dose

**Serevent Diskus** oral inhalation powder ℞ *twice-daily sympathomimetic bronchodilator for asthma and bronchospasm* [salmeterol xinafoate] 50 μg/dose

**serfibrate** INN

**sergolexole** INN *antimigraine* [also: sergolexole maleate]

**sergolexole maleate** USAN *antimigraine* [also: sergolexole]

**serine (L-serine)** USAN, USP, INN *nonessential amino acid; symbols: Ser, S*

**L-serine diazoacetate** [see: azaserine]

**84-L-serineplasminogen activator** [see: monteplase]

**sermetacin** USAN, INN *anti-inflammatory*

**sermorelin** INN, BAN *growth hormone deficiency diagnosis and treatment* [also: sermorelin acetate]

**sermorelin acetate** USAN *diagnostic aid for pituitary function; treatment for growth hormone deficiency (orphan), anovulation, and AIDS-related weight loss* [also: sermorelin]

**SERMs (selective estrogen receptor modulators)** [q.v.]

**SeroJet** (trademarked device) *needle-free subcutaneous injector for Serostim (somatropin)*

**Seromycin** Pulvules (capsules) ℞ *tuberculostatic* [cycloserine] 250 mg

**Serophene** tablets ℞ *ovulation stimulant* [clomiphene citrate] 50 mg

**Seroquel** film-coated tablets ℞ *novel (atypical) antipsychotic for schizophrenia and manic episodes of a bipolar disorder* [quetiapine fumarate] 25, 100, 200, 300 mg

**Serostim** powder for subcu injection ℞ *growth hormone for adults or children with congenital or endogenous growth hormone deficiency, children with Turner syndrome or renal-induced growth failure, or AIDS-wasting syndrome (orphan)* [somatropin] 5, 6 mg (15, 18 IU) per vial

**serotonin (5-hydroxytriptamine₁; 5-HT₁)** [see: selective serotonin reuptake inhibitors; vascular serotonin receptor antagonists]

**Seroxat** (European name for U.S. product Paxil)

**SERPACWA (Skin Exposure Reduction Paste Against Chemical Warfare Agents)** cream ℞ *to delay absorption of chemical warfare agents through the skin when applied before exposure; used in conjunction with MOPP (Mis-*

sion Oriented Protective Posture) gear
[polytef; perfluoroalkylpolyether]

**serrapeptase** INN

*Serratia marcescens* **extract (polyribosomes)** *investigational (orphan) for
primary brain malignancies*

**sertaconazole** INN *topical antifungal*

**sertaconazole nitrate** *topical antifungal*

**sertindole** USAN, INN *investigational
(NDA filed) novel (atypical) antipsychotic; neuroleptic*

**Sertoli cells, porcine** *investigational
(orphan) intracerebral implant for stage
4 and 5 Parkinson disease (for co-
implantation with fetal neural cells)*

**sertraline** INN, BAN *selective serotonin
reuptake inhibitor (SSRI) for depression, obsessive-compulsive disorder
(OCD), panic disorder, post-traumatic
stress disorder, premenstrual dysphoric
disorder (PMDD), and social anxiety
disorder* [also: sertraline HCl]

**sertraline HCl** USAN *selective serotonin
reuptake inhibitor (SSRI) for depression, obsessive-compulsive disorder
(OCD), panic disorder, post-traumatic
stress disorder, premenstrual dysphoric
disorder (PMDD), and social anxiety
disorder* [also: sertraline]

**serum albumin (SA)** [see: albumin,
human]

**serum albumin, iodinated ($^{125}$I)
human** [see: albumin, iodinated I
125 serum]

**serum albumin, iodinated ($^{131}$I)
human** [see: albumin, iodinated I
131 serum]

**serum fibrinogen (SF)** [see: fibrinogen, human]

**serum globulin (SG)** [see: globulin,
immune]

**serum gonadotrophin** [see: gonadotrophin, serum]

**serum gonadotropin** [see: gonadotrophin, serum]

**serum prothrombin conversion
accelerator (SPCA) factor** [see:
factor VII]

**Serutan** granules OTC *bulk laxative*
[psyllium] 2.5 g/tsp.

**Serzone** tablets (discontinued 2004
due to safety concerns) ℞ *antidepressant* [nefazodone HCl] 50, 100, 150,
200, 250 mg

**Serzone-5HT₂** Ⓐ tablets ℞ *antidepressant* [nefazodone HCl] 50, 100,
150, 200 mg

**sesame oil** NF *solvent; oleaginous vehicle*

**Sesame Street Complete** chewable
tablets OTC *vitamin/mineral/calcium/
iron supplement* [multiple vitamins &
minerals; calcium; iron; folic acid;
biotin] ±•80•10•0.2•0.015 mg

**Sesame Street Plus Extra C** chewable tablets (discontinued 2004) OTC
*vitamin supplement* [multiple vitamins; folic acid] ±•0.2 mg

**Sesame Street Plus Iron** chewable
tablets OTC *vitamin/iron supplement*
[multiple vitamins; iron; folic acid]
±•10•0.2 mg

**setastine** INN

**setazindol** INN

**setiptiline** INN

**setoperone** USAN, INN *antipsychotic*

**setwall** *medicinal herb* [see: valerian]

**Seudotabs** tablets (discontinued
2002) OTC *nasal decongestant* [pseu-
doephedrine HCl] 30 mg

**sevelamer HCl** USAN *phosphate-binding polymer for hyperphosphatemia of
end-stage renal disease (ESRD)*

**7 + 3 protocol (cytarabine, dauno-
rubicin)** *chemotherapy protocol for
acute myelocytic leukemia (AML)*

**7 + 3 protocol (cytarabine, idarubi-
cin)** *chemotherapy protocol for acute
myelocytic leukemia (AML)*

**7 + 3 protocol (cytarabine, mito-
xantrone)** *chemotherapy protocol for
acute myelocytic leukemia (AML)*

**7 + 3 + 7 protocol (cytarabine,
daunorubicin, etoposide)** *chemotherapy protocol for acute myelocytic
leukemia (AML)*

**seven barks** *medicinal herb* [see:
hydrangea]

**7E3 monoclonal antibodies (MAb)**
[see: abciximab]

**Severe Congestion Tussin** softgels OTC *decongestant; expectorant* [pseudoephedrine HCl; guaifenesin] 30•200 mg

**sevirumab** USAN, INN *investigational (Phase I) antiviral for AIDS; orphan status withdrawn 1996*

**sevitropium mesilate** INN

**sevoflurane** USAN, INN *inhalation general anesthetic*

**sevopramide** INN

**sezolamide HCl** USAN *carbonic anhydrase inhibitor*

**SF (serum fibrinogen)** [see: fibrinogen, human]

**SFC** lotion OTC *soap-free therapeutic skin cleanser*

**sfericase** INN

**SG (serum globulin)** [see: globulin, immune]

**SG (soluble gelatin)** [see: gelatin]

**shamrock, Indian** *medicinal herb* [see: birthroot]

**shamrock, water** *medicinal herb* [see: buckbean]

**shark cartilage (derived from Sphyrna lewini, Squalus acanthias, and other species)** *natural remedy for cancer* [also: squalamine]

**shark liver oil** *emollient/protectant*

**shavegrass** *medicinal herb* [see: horsetail]

**sheep laurel** *medicinal herb* [see: mountain laurel]

**Sheik Elite** premedicated condom OTC *spermicidal/barrier contraceptive* [nonoxynol 9] 8%

**shell flower** *medicinal herb* [see: turtlebloom]

**shellac** NF *tablet coating agent*

**Shellgel** intraocular injection R̸ *viscoelastic agent for ophthalmic surgery* [hyaluronate sodium] 12 mg/mL

**Shepard's Cream Lotion; Shepard's Skin Cream** OTC *moisturizer; emollient*

**shepherd's club** *medicinal herb* [see: mullein]

**shepherd's heart** *medicinal herb* [see: shepherd's purse]

**shepherd's purse (Capsella bursa-pastoris)** plant *medicinal herb for bleed-*

*ing, ear disease, hypertension, painful menstruation, and urinary bleeding*

**shigoka** *medicinal herb* [see: Siberian ginseng]

**shiitake mushrooms (Lentinula edodes; Tricholomopsis edodes)** stem and cap *medicinal herb for boosting the immune system, cancer, lowering cholesterol, and viral illnesses*

**Shohl solution, modified (sodium citrate & citric acid)** *urinary alkalizer; compounding agent*

**short chain fatty acids** *investigational (orphan) for left-sided ulcerative colitis and chronic radiation proctitis*

**short-leaved buchu** *medicinal herb* [see: buchu]

**Shur-Clens** solution OTC *wound cleanser* [poloxamer 188] 20%

**Shur-Seal** vaginal gel OTC *spermicidal contraceptive (for use with a diaphragm)* [nonoxynol 9] 2%

**siagoside** INN

**sialagogues** *a class of agents that stimulate the secretion of saliva* [also called: ptyalagogues]

**Sibelium** R̸ *investigational (orphan) vasodilator for alternating hemiplegia* [flunarizine HCl]

**sibenadet HCl** USAN *treatment for chronic obstructive pulmonary disease (COPD)*

**Siberian ginseng (Acanthopanax senticosus; Eleutherococcus senticosus)** root *medicinal herb for age spots, blood diseases, depression, hemorrhage, immune system stimulation, increasing endurance and longevity, normalizing blood pressure, platelet aggregation inhibition, sexual stimulation, and stress* [also see: ginseng]

**sibopirdine** USAN *cognition enhancer for Alzheimer disease; nootropic*

**sibrafiban** USAN *platelet inhibitor; fibrinogen receptor antagonist; investigational (Phase III) oral glycoprotein IIb/IIIa receptor antagonist for acute coronary syndrome*

**sibutramine** INN, BAN *anorexiant for the treatment of obesity; monoamine* reuptake inhibitor antidepressant [also: sibutramine HCl]

**sibutramine HCl** USAN *anorexiant for the treatment of obesity; monoamine reuptake inhibitor antidepressant* [also: sibutramine]

**siccanin** INN

**Sickledex** *test kit for professional use in vitro diagnostic aid for hemoglobin S (sickle cell)*

**sicklewort** *medicinal herb* [see: woundwort]

**side-flowering skullcap** *medicinal herb* [see: skullcap]

**SigPak** *(trademarked packaging form) unit-of-use package*

**Sigtab** *tablets* OTC *vitamin supplement* [multiple vitamins; folic acid] ± •0.4 mg

**Sigtab-M** *tablets* OTC *vitamin/mineral/calcium/iron supplement* [multiple vitamins & minerals; calcium; iron; folic acid; biotin] ± •200•18•0.4•0.045 mg

**siguazodan** INN, BAN

**Silace** *syrup* OTC *laxative; stool softener* [docusate sodium] 60 mg/15 mL

**Silace-C** *syrup (discontinued 2003)* OTC *stimulant laxative; stool softener* [casanthranol; docusate sodium; alcohol 10%] 30•60 mg/15 mL

**Siladryl** *elixir* OTC *antihistamine* [diphenhydramine HCl] 12.5 mg/5 mL

**Silafed** *syrup* OTC *decongestant; antihistamine* [pseudoephedrine HCl; triprolidine HCl] 60•2.5 mg/10 mL

**silafilcon A** USAN *hydrophilic contact lens material*

**silafocon A** USAN *hydrophobic contact lens material*

**Silaminic Cold** *syrup (discontinued 2002)* OTC *decongestant; antihistamine* [phenylpropanolamine HCl; chlorpheniramine maleate] 12.5•2 mg/5 mL

**Silaminic Expectorant** *syrup (discontinued 2002)* OTC *decongestant; expectorant* [phenylpropanolamine HCl; guaifenesin; alcohol 5%] 12.5•100 mg/5 mL

**silandrone** USAN, INN *androgen*

**Silapap, Children's** *oral liquid* OTC *analgesic; antipyretic* [acetaminophen] 80 mg/2.5 mL

**Silapap, Infant's** *drops* OTC *analgesic; antipyretic* [acetaminophen] 100 mg/mL

**Sildec-DM** *pediatric oral drops* R *antitussive; decongestant; antihistamine* [dextromethorphan hydrobromide; pseudoephedrine HCl; carbinoxamine maleate] 4•15•2 mg/mL

**Sildec-DM** *syrup* R *antitussive; decongestant; antihistamine* [dextromethorphan hydrobromide; pseudoephedrine HCl; brompheniramine maleate] 15•60•4 mg/5 mL

**sildenafil citrate** USAN *phosphodiesterase type 5 (PDE5) inhibitor; selective vasodilator for erectile dysfunction (ED)*

**Sildicon-E** *pediatric oral drops (discontinued 2002)* OTC *decongestant; expectorant* [phenylpropanolamine HCl; guaifenesin] 6.25•30 mg/mL

**Silfedrine, Children's** *oral liquid* OTC *nasal decongestant* [pseudoephedrine HCl] 30 mg/5 mL

**silibinin** INN

**silica, dental-type** NF *pharmaceutic aid*

**silica gel** [now: silicon dioxide]

**siliceous earth, purified** NF *filtering medium*

**silicic acid, magnesium salt** [see: magnesium trisilicate]

**silicon** *element (Si)*

**silicon dioxide** NF *dispersing and suspending agent*

**silicon dioxide, colloidal** NF *suspending agent; tablet and capsule diluent*

**silicone**

**Silicone No. 2** *ointment* OTC *skin protectant* [silicone; hydrophobic starch derivative] 10%• ±

**silicone oil** [see: polydimethylsiloxane]

**silicristin** INN

**silidianin** INN

**silkweed** *medicinal herb* [see: milkweed; pleurisy root]

**silky swallow wort; Virginia silk** *medicinal herb* [see: milkweed]

**silodrate** USAN *antacid* [also: simaldrate]

**Silphen Cough** syrup OTC *antihistamine; antitussive* [diphenhydramine HCl; alcohol 5%] 12.5 mg/5 mL

**Silphen DM** syrup OTC *antitussive* [dextromethorphan hydrobromide; alcohol 5%] 10 mg/5 mL

*Silphium perfoliatum* medicinal herb [see: ragged cup]

**Siltapp with Dextromethorphan Cold & Cough** elixir (discontinued 2002) ℞ *antitussive; decongestant; antihistamine* [dextromethorphan hydrobromide; phenylpropanolamine HCl; brompheniramine maleate] 10•12.5•2 mg/5 mL

**Sil-Tex** oral liquid (discontinued 2002) ℞ *decongestant; expectorant* [phenylpropanolamine HCl; phenylephrine HCl; guaifenesin; alcohol 5%] 20• 5•100 mg/5 mL

**Siltussin CF** oral liquid (discontinued 2002) OTC *antitussive; decongestant; expectorant* [dextromethorphan hydrobromide; phenylpropanolamine HCl; guaifenesin; alcohol 4.75%] 10•12.5•100 mg/5 mL

**Siltussin DAS** oral liquid OTC *expectorant* [guaifenesin] 100 mg/5 mL

**Siltussin DM Cough** syrup OTC *antitussive; expectorant* [dextromethorphan hydrobromide; guaifenesin] 20•200 mg/10 mL

**Siltussin SA** oral liquid OTC *expectorant* [guaifenesin] 100 mg/5 mL

**Silvadene** cream ℞ *broad-spectrum bactericidal for adjunctive burn treatment* [silver sulfadiazine] 10 mg/g ☒ Azulfidine

**silver** *element* (Ag)

**silver nitrate** USP *ophthalmic neonatal anti-infective; strong caustic* 1% eye drops; 10%, 25%, 50%, 75% topical

**silver nitrate, toughened** USP *caustic*

**silver protein, mild** NF *ophthalmic antiseptic; ophthalmic surgical aid*

**silver sulfadiazine (SSD)** USAN, USP *broad-spectrum bactericidal; adjunct to burn therapy* [also: sulfadiazine silver]

**silverweed; silver cinquefoil** *medicinal herb* [see: cinquefoil]

*Silybum marianum* medicinal herb [see: milk thistle]

**Simaal Gel** oral liquid (discontinued 2000) OTC *antacid; antiflatulent* [aluminum hydroxide; magnesium hydroxide; simethicone] 200•200• 20 mg/5 mL

**Simaal Gel 2** oral liquid OTC *antacid; antiflatulent* [aluminum hydroxide; magnesium hydroxide; simethicone] 500•400•40 mg/5 mL

**simaldrate** INN *antacid* [also: silodrate]

**Simdax** (approved in several European countries) *investigational (Phase III) calcium sensitizer and vasodilator for decompensated heart failure* [levosimendan]

**simethicone** USAN, USP *antiflatulent; adjunct to gastrointestinal imaging* 80 mg oral; 40 mg/0.6 mL oral

**simethicone-coated cellulose suspension (SCCS)** [see: SonoRx]

**simetride** INN

**simfibrate** INN

**Similac Advance with Iron** ready-to-use oral liquid, powder for oral liquid OTC *infant formula fortified with omega-3 fatty acids*

**Similac Human Milk Fortifier** powder OTC *supplement to breast milk* 900 mg/pkt.

**Similac Low Iron** oral liquid, powder for oral liquid OTC *total or supplementary infant feeding*

**Similac PM 60/40 Low-Iron** oral liquid OTC *formula for infants predisposed to hypocalcemia* [whey formula with lowered mineral levels]

**Similac with Iron** oral liquid, powder for oral liquid OTC *total or supplementary infant feeding*

**simple syrup** [see: syrup]

**Simpler's joy** *medicinal herb* [see: blue vervain]

**Simplet** tablets OTC *decongestant; antihistamine; analgesic* [pseudoephedrine HCl; chlorpheniramine maleate; acetaminophen] 60•4•650 mg ☒ Singlet

**Simply Cough** oral liquid OTC *antitussive* [dextromethorphan hydrobromide] 5 mg/5 mL

**Simply Saline** nasal spray OTC *nasal moisturizer* [sodium chloride (saline solution)]

**Simply Sleep** tablets OTC *antihistaminic sleep aid* [diphenhydramine HCl] 25 mg

**Simply Stuffy** tablets, oral liquid OTC *nasal decongestant* [pseudoephedrine HCl] 30 mg; 15 mg/5 mL

**Simron Plus** capsules OTC *vitamin/iron supplement* [multiple vitamins; ferrous gluconate; folic acid] ±•10•0.1 mg

**simtrazene** USAN, INN *antineoplastic*

**Simulect** powder for IV infusion *immunosuppressant; IL-2 receptor antagonist for the prevention of acute rejection of renal transplants (orphan)* [basiliximab] 20 mg

**simvastatin** USAN, INN, BAN *HMG-CoA reductase inhibitor for hyperlipidemia, hypertriglyceridemia, and coronary heart disease* ▣ Sandostatin; zinostatin

**Sinapils** tablets (discontinued 2001) OTC *decongestant; antihistamine; analgesic* [phenylpropanolamine HCl; chlorpheniramine maleate; acetaminophen; caffeine] 12.5•2•325•32.5 mg

*Sinapis alba* medicinal herb [see: mustard]

**sinapultide** USAN *pulmonary surfactant for respiratory distress syndrome*

**Sinarest; Sinarest Sinus** tablets (discontinued 2002) OTC *decongestant; antihistamine; analgesic* [pseudoephedrine HCl; chlorpheniramine maleate; acetaminophen] 30•2•500 mg; 30•2•325 mg

**Sinarest, No Drowsiness** tablets (discontinued 2002) OTC *decongestant; analgesic; antipyretic* [pseudoephedrine HCl; acetaminophen] 30•500 mg

**Sinarest 12 Hour** nasal spray (discontinued 2002) OTC *nasal decongestant* [oxymetazoline HCl] 0.05%

**sincalide** USAN, INN *choleretic; diagnostic aid for gallbladder function*

**Sine-Aid** tablets, caplets, gelcaps (discontinued 2002) OTC *decongestant; analgesic; antipyretic* [pseudoephedrine HCl; acetaminophen] 30•500 mg

**Sine-Aid IB** caplets (discontinued 2002) OTC *decongestant; analgesic* [pseudoephedrine HCl; ibuprofen] 30•200 mg

**sinefungin** USAN, INN *antifungal*

**Sinemet 10-100; Sinemet 25-100; Sinemet 25-250** tablets ℞ *antiparkinsonian; dopamine precursor; decarboxylase inhibitor* [carbidopa; levodopa] 10•100 mg; 25•100 mg; 25•250 mg

**Sinemet CR** sustained-release tablets ℞ *antiparkinsonian; dopamine precursor; decarboxylase inhibitor* [carbidopa; levodopa] 25•100, 50•200 mg

**Sine-Off Night Time Formula Sinus, Cold, & Flu Medicine** gelcaps OTC *decongestant; antihistamine; analgesic* [pseudoephedrine HCl; diphenhydramine HCl; acetaminophen] 30•25•500 mg

**Sine-Off No Drowsiness Formula** caplets OTC *decongestant; analgesic; antipyretic* [pseudoephedrine HCl; acetaminophen] 30•500 mg

**Sine-Off Sinus Medicine** caplets OTC *decongestant; antihistamine; analgesic* [pseudoephedrine HCl; chlorpheniramine maleate; acetaminophen] 30•2•500 mg

**Sinequan** capsules, concentrate for oral solution ℞ *tricyclic antidepressant; anxiolytic* [doxepin HCl] 10, 25, 50, 75, 100, 150 mg; 10 mg/mL

**Sinex 12-Hour Long Acting; Sinex 12-Hour Ultra Fine Mist for Sinus Relief** nasal spray OTC *nasal decongestant* [oxymetazoline HCl] 0.05%

**Sinex Ultra Fine Mist** nasal spray OTC *nasal decongestant* [phenylephrine HCl] 0.5%

**single-chain antigen-binding proteins (SCA proteins)** *a class of investigational antineoplastics*

**SingleJect** (trademarked dosage form) *prefilled syringe*

**Singlet for Adults** tablets OTC *decongestant; antihistamine; analgesic* [pseudoephedrine HCl; chlorpheniramine maleate; acetaminophen] 60•4•650 mg ② Simplet

**Singulair** film-coated tablets, chewable tablets, granules for oral solution ℞ *leukotriene receptor inhibitor for allergic rhinitis and the prophylaxis and chronic treatment of asthma* [montelukast sodium] 10 mg; 4, 5 mg; 4 mg/pkt.

**Sinografin** intracavitary instillation ℞ *radiopaque contrast medium for gynecological imaging* [diatrizoate meglumine; iodipamide meglumine (47.8% total iodine)] 727•268 mg/mL (380 mg/mL)

**sinorphan** [now: ecadotril]

**sintropium bromide** INN

**Sinufed** Timecelles (sustained-release capsules) (discontinued 2002) ℞ *decongestant; expectorant* [pseudoephedrine HCl; guaifenesin] 60•300 mg

**Sinulin** tablets (discontinued 2001) OTC *decongestant; antihistamine; analgesic* [phenylpropanolamine HCl; chlorpheniramine maleate; acetaminophen] 25•4•650 mg

**Sinumist-SR** sustained-release Capsulets (capsule-shaped tablet) (discontinued 2002) ℞ *expectorant* [guaifenesin] 600 mg

**Sinupan** controlled-release capsules (discontinued 2002) ℞ *decongestant; expectorant* [phenylephrine HCl; guaifenesin] 40•200 mg

**Sinus Headache & Congestion** tablets (discontinued 2002) OTC *decongestant; antihistamine; analgesic* [pseudoephedrine HCl; chlorpheniramine maleate; acetaminophen] 30•2•500 mg

**Sinus Relief** caplets OTC *decongestant; analgesic* [pseudoephedrine HCl; acetaminophen] 30•500 mg

**Sinustop** capsules OTC *nasal decongestant* [pseudoephedrine HCl] 60 mg

**Sinutab Non-Drying** liquid-filled capsules OTC *decongestant; expectorant* [pseudoephedrine HCl; guaifenesin] 30•200 mg

**Sinutab Sinus Allergy** caplets OTC *decongestant; antihistamine; analgesic* [pseudoephedrine HCl; chlorpheniramine maleate; acetaminophen] 30•2•500 mg

**Sinutab Sinus Without Drowsiness** tablets, caplets OTC *decongestant; analgesic; antipyretic* [pseudoephedrine HCl; acetaminophen] 30•325 mg; 30•500 mg

**SINUtuss DM** caplets ℞ *antitussive; decongestant; expectorant* [dextromethorphan hydrobromide; phenylephrine HCl; guaifenesin] 30•15•60 mg

**SINUvent** long-acting tablets (discontinued 2002) ℞ *decongestant; expectorant* [phenylpropanolamine HCl; guaifenesin] 75•600 mg

**SINUvent PE** extended-release caplets ℞ *decongestant; expectorant* [phenylephrine HCl; guaifenesin] 15•600 mg

**Sirdalud** (foreign name for U.S. product Zanaflex)

**sirolimus** USAN *immunosuppressant for renal transplantation* ② temsirolimus

**sisomicin** USAN, INN *antibacterial* [also: sissomicin]

**sisomicin sulfate** USAN, USP *antibacterial*

**sissomicin** BAN *antibacterial* [also: sisomicin]

**sitafloxacin** USAN *antibacterial; DNA-gyrase inhibitor*

**sitalidone** INN

**sitofibrate** INN

**sitogluside** USAN, INN *antiprostatic hypertrophy*

**sitosterols** NF

**Sitzmarks** capsules ℞ *radiopaque contrast medium for severe constipation* [polyvinyl chloride, radiopaque] 24 rings/capsule

**666 Cold Preparation** oral liquid OTC *antitussive; decongestant; analgesic* [dextromethorphan hydrobromide;

pseudoephedrine HCl; acetamino-phen] 20•60•650 mg/30 mL

**sizofiran** INN

**SK (streptokinase)** [q.v.]

**Skeeter Stik** topical liquid OTC *local anesthetic; counterirritant* [lidocaine; menthol] 4%•1%

**Skelaxin** tablets ℞ *skeletal muscle relaxant* [metaxalone] 400, 800 mg

**Skelid** tablets ℞ *bisphosphonate bone resorption inhibitor for Paget disease* [tiludronate disodium] 240 mg

**skin respiratory factor (SRF)** *claimed to promote wound healing*

**Skin Shield** topical liquid OTC *skin protectant; local anesthetic* [dyclonine HCl; benzethonium chloride] 0.75%•0.2%

**Skinoren** (German name for U.S. product Azelex)

**skullcap** *(Scutellaria lateriflora)* plant *medicinal herb for convulsions, epilepsy, fever, hypertension, infertility, insomnia, nervous disorders, rabies, and restlessness*

**skunk cabbage** *(Symplocarpus foetidus)* root *medicinal herb used as an antispasmodic, diuretic, emetic, expectorant, pectoral, stimulant, and sudorific*

**skunk weed** *medicinal herb* [see: skunk cabbage]

**SL (sodium lactate)** [q.v.]

**Sleep-Eze 3** tablets (discontinued 2003) OTC *antihistaminic sleep aid* [diphenhydramine HCl] 25 mg

**Sleepinal** capsules, soft gels OTC *antihistaminic sleep aid* [diphenhydramine HCl] 50 mg

**Sleepwell 2-nite** tablets OTC *antihistaminic sleep aid* [diphenhydramine HCl] 25 mg

**Slidecase** (packaging form) *patient compliance package for oral contraceptives*

**Slim-Mint** gum (discontinued 2001) OTC *decrease taste perception of sweetness* [benzocaine] 6 mg

**slippery elm** *(Ulmus fulva; U. rubra)* inner bark *medicinal herb for asthma, blackened or bruised eyes, boils, bronchitis, burns, cold sores, colitis, cough,*

*diaper rash, diarrhea, indigestion, lung disorders, sore throat, and urinary tract inflammation*

**slippery root** *medicinal herb* [see: comfrey]

**Slo-bid** Gyrocaps (extended-release capsules) ℞ *antiasthmatic; bronchodilator* [theophylline] 50, 75, 100, 125, 200, 300 mg

**Slocaps** (trademarked form) *sustained-release capsules*

**Slo-Niacin** controlled-release tablets OTC *vitamin B₃ supplement; antihyperlipidemic* [niacin] 250, 500, 750 mg

**Slonnon** (Japanese name for U.S. product Acova)

**Slo-phyllin** tablets, syrup, Gyrocaps (extended-release capsules) ℞ *antiasthmatic; bronchodilator* [theophylline] 100, 200 mg; 80 mg/15 mL; 60, 125, 250 mg

**Slo-phyllin GG** capsules, syrup (discontinued 2004) ℞ *antiasthmatic; bronchodilator; expectorant* [theophylline; guaifenesin] 150•90 mg; 150•90 mg/15 mL

**Slo-Salt-K** slow-release tablets OTC *electrolyte replacement; dehydration preventative* [sodium chloride; potassium chloride] 410•150 mg

**slow channel blockers** *a class of coronary vasodilators that inhibit cardiac muscle contraction and slow cardiac electrical conduction velocity* [also called: calcium channel blockers; calcium antagonists]

**Slow Fe** slow-release tablets OTC *hematinic* [ferrous sulfate, dried (source of iron)] 160 mg (50 mg)

**Slow Fe with Folic Acid** slow-release tablets OTC *hematinic* [ferrous sulfate; folic acid] 50•0.4 mg

**Slow-K** controlled-release tablets (discontinued 2004) ℞ *potassium supplement* [potassium chloride] 600 mg (8 mEq K)

**Slow-Mag** delayed-release enteric-coated tablets OTC *magnesium supplement* [magnesium chloride] 535 mg
②  Flomax; Zomig

**Slow-Mag** enteric-coated tablets OTC *magnesium supplement* [magnesium chloride hexahydrate] 64 mg Mg

**Slow-Release Iron** extended-release tablets OTC *hematinic* [ferrous fumarate (source of iron)] 150 mg (50 mg)

**SLT** hair lotion OTC *antiseborrheic; antipsoriatic; keratolytic; antiseptic* [coal tar; salicylic acid; lactic acid; alcohol 65%] 2%•3%•5%

**small burnet saxifrage** *medicinal herb* [see: burnet]

**small pimpernel** *medicinal herb* [see: burnet]

**small saxifrage** *medicinal herb* [see: burnet]

**smallpox vaccine** USP *active immunizing agent*

**SMART anti-CD3 antibody** *investigational (Phase I) immunosuppressant*

**SMART anti-gpIIb/IIIa monoclonal antibody** *investigational cardiovascular antiplatelet agent*

**SMART anti-tac; humanized anti-tac** [now: dacliximab]

**SMART M195 antibody** *investigational (Phase III) agent for acute myelogenous leukemia*

**SmartMist** (trademarked form) *handheld inhalation device*

**smartweed; water smartweed** *medicinal herb* [see: knotweed]

**SMF (streptozocin, mitomycin, fluorouracil)** *chemotherapy protocol for pancreatic cancer*

*Smilax* **spp.** *medicinal herb* [see: sarsaparilla]

**smooth sumach** *medicinal herb* [see: sumach]

**SMX; SMZ (sulfamethoxazole)** [q.v.]

**SMZ-TMP (sulfamethoxazole & trimethoprim)** [q.v.]

**SN (streptonigrin)** [q.v.]

**snake bite** *medicinal herb* [see: birthroot]

**snake head** *medicinal herb* [see: turtlebloom]

**snake lily** *medicinal herb* [see: blue flag]

**snake weed** *medicinal herb* [see: bistort; plantain]

**snakebite antivenin** [see: antivenin, Crotalidae & Micrurus fulvius]

**snakeroot** *medicinal herb* [see: echinacea]

**snakeroot, black** *medicinal herb* [see: black cohosh; sanicle]

**Snaplets-DM** granules for pediatric oral solution (discontinued 2002) OTC *antitussive; decongestant* [dextromethorphan hydrobromide; phenylpropanolamine HCl] 5•6.25 mg/pkt.

**Snaplets-EX** granules for pediatric oral solution (discontinued 2002) OTC *decongestant; expectorant* [phenylpropanolamine HCl; guaifenesin] 6.25•50 mg/pkt.

**Snaplets-Multi** granules for pediatric oral solution (discontinued 2002) OTC *antitussive; decongestant; antihistamine* [dextromethorphan hydrobromide; phenylpropanolamine HCl; chlorpheniramine maleate] 5•6.25•1 mg/pkt.

**snapping hazel** *medicinal herb* [see: witch hazel]

**SnapTab** (trademarked dosage form) *scored tablet*

**Snooze Fast** tablets OTC *antihistaminic sleep aid* [diphenhydramine HCl] 50 mg

**Sno-Strips** ophthalmic strips *diagnostic tear flow test aid*

**snout, swine** *medicinal herb* [see: dandelion]

**snowball, wild** *medicinal herb* [see: New Jersey tea]

**snowdrop tree; snowflower** *medicinal herb* [see: fringe tree]

**Soac-Lens** solution OTC *wetting/soaking solution for hard contact lenses*

**soap, green** USP *detergent*

**soapwort (Saponaria officinalis)** plant and roots *medicinal herb for acne, boils, eczema, poison ivy rash and psoriasis; also used in skin disinfectants and soaps*

**SOD (superoxide dismutase)** [see: orgotein]

**soda lime** NF *carbon dioxide absorbent*

**sodium** *element (Na)*

**sodium acetate** USP *dialysis aid; electrolyte replenisher; pH buffer* 2, 4 mEq/mL (16.4%, 32.8%) injection

**sodium acetate trihydrate** [see: sodium acetate]

**sodium acetrizoate** INN, BAN [also: acetrizoate sodium]

**sodium acetylsalicylate** *analgesic*

**sodium acid phosphate** *urinary acidifier*

**sodium alginate** NF *suspending agent*

**sodium amidotrizoate** INN *oral/rectal/parenteral radiopaque contrast medium (59.87% iodine)* [also: diatrizoate sodium; sodium diatrizoate]

**sodium aminobenzoate** [see: aminobenzoate sodium]

**sodium amylopectin sulfate** [see: sodium amylosulfate]

**sodium amylosulfate** USAN *enzyme inhibitor*

**sodium anoxynaphthonate** BAN *blood volume and cardiac output test* [also: anazolene sodium]

**sodium antimony gluconate** [see: sodium stibogluconate]

**sodium antimonylgluconate** BAN

**sodium apolate** INN, BAN *anticoagulant* [also: lyapolate sodium]

**sodium arsenate, exsiccated** NF

**sodium arsenate As 74** USAN *radioactive agent*

**sodium ascorbate (vitamin C)** USP, INN *water-soluble vitamin; antiscorbutic*

**sodium aurothiomalate** INN *antirheumatic* [also: gold sodium thiomalate]

**sodium aurotiosulfate** INN [also: gold sodium thiosulfate]

**sodium azodisalicylate** [now: olsalazine sodium]

**sodium benzoate** USAN, NF, JAN *antihyperammonemic; antifungal agent; preservative*

**sodium benzoate & caffeine** *analeptic for respiratory depression due to an overdose of CNS depressants* 250 mg/mL injection

**sodium benzoate & sodium phenylacetate** *to prevent and treat hyperammonemia of urea cycle enzymopathy (orphan)*

**sodium benzyl penicillin** [see: penicillin G sodium]

**sodium bicarbonate** USP *electrolyte replenisher; systemic alkalizer; antacid* 325, 600, 650 mg oral; 0.5, 0.6, 0.9, 1 mEq/mL (4.2%, 5%, 7.5%, 8.4%) injection

**sodium biphosphate** *urinary acidifier; pH buffer*

**sodium bisulfite** NF *antioxidant*

**sodium bitionolate** INN *topical anti-infective* [also: bithionolate sodium]

**sodium borate** NF *alkalizing agent; antipruritic; bacteriostatic agent in cold creams, eye washes, and mouth rinses*

**sodium borocaptate ($^{10}$B)** INN *antineoplastic; radioactive agent* [also: borocaptate sodium B 10]

**sodium cacodylate** NF

**sodium calcium edetate** INN *heavy metal chelating agent* [also: edetate calcium disodium; sodium calciumedetate; calcium disodium edetate]

**sodium calciumedetate** BAN *heavy metal chelating agent* [also: edetate calcium disodium; sodium calcium edetate; calcium disodium edetate]

**sodium caprylate** *antifungal*

**sodium carbonate** NF *alkalizing agent*

**sodium chloride (NaCl)** USP *ophthalmic hypertonic; electrolyte replacement; abortifacient* [sterile isotonic solution] 650, 1000, 2250 mg oral; 0.45%, 0.9%, 3%, 5%, 14.6%, 23.4% injection/diluent

**0.45% sodium chloride (½ normal saline; ½ NS)** *electrolyte replacement*

**0.9% sodium chloride (normal saline; NS)** *electrolyte replacement* [also: saline solution]

**sodium chloride, compound solution of** INN *fluid and electrolyte replenisher* [also: Ringer's injection]

**sodium chloride Na 22** USAN *radioactive agent*

**sodium chondroitin sulfate** [see: chondroitin sulfate sodium]

**sodium chromate ($^{51}$Cr)** INN *blood volume test; radioactive agent* [also: sodium chromate Cr 51]

**sodium chromate Cr 51** USAN *blood volume test; radioactive agent* [also: sodium chromate ($^{51}$Cr)]

**sodium citrate** USP *systemic alkalizer; pH buffer; antacid; investigational (orphan) adjunct to leukapheresis procedures*

**sodium colistin methanesulfonate** [see: colistimethate sodium]

**sodium cromoglycate** [see: cromolyn sodium]

**sodium cyclamate** NF, INN

**sodium cyclohexanesulfamate** [see: sodium cyclamate]

**sodium dehydroacetate** NF *antimicrobial preservative*

**sodium dehydrocholate** INN [also: dehydrocholate sodium]

**sodium denyl** [see: phenytoin sodium]

**sodium diatrizoate** BAN *oral/rectal/parenteral radiopaque contrast medium (59.87% iodine)* [also: diatrizoate sodium; sodium amidotrizoate]

**sodium dibunate** INN, BAN

**sodium dicloroacetate (sodium DCA)** USAN *pyruvate dehydrogenase activator; investigational (orphan) for acute head trauma and neurologic injury; investigational (orphan) for lactic acidosis and homozygous familial hypercholesterolemia*

**sodium diethyldithiocarbamate** [see: ditiocarb sodium]

**sodium diiodomethanesulfonate** [see: dimethiodal sodium]

**sodium dioctyl sulfosuccinate** INN *stool softener; surfactant* [also: docusate sodium]

**sodium diphenylhydantoin** [see: phenytoin sodium]

**sodium diprotrizoate** INN, BAN [also: diprotrizoate sodium]

**Sodium Diuril** powder for IV injection ℞ *diuretic* [chlorothiazide] 500 mg

**sodium edetate** [see: edetate sodium]

**sodium estrone sulfate** *estrogen replacement therapy for postmenopausal disorders* 0.625, 1.25, 2.5, 5 mg oral

**sodium etasulfate** INN *detergent* [also: sodium ethasulfate]

**sodium ethasulfate** USAN *detergent* [also: sodium etasulfate]

**sodium feredetate** INN [also: sodium ironedetate]

**sodium ferric gluconate** *hematinic for iron deficiency of chronic hemodialysis with epoetin therapy*

**sodium fluoride** USP *fluoride replacement therapy; dental caries preventative; investigational agent for treatment of postmenopausal osteoporosis* 1.1, 2.2 mg oral; 0.125 mg/drop oral

**sodium fluoride F 18** USP

**sodium fluoride & phosphoric acid** USP *dental caries prophylactic*

**sodium formaldehyde sulfoxylate** NF *preservative*

**sodium gamma hydroxybutyrate (NaGHB)** [see: gamma hydroxybutyrate (GHB); sodium oxybate]

**sodium gammahydroxyburate** [see: sodium oxybate]

**sodium gentisate** INN

**sodium glucaspaldrate** INN, BAN

**sodium gluconate** USP *electrolyte replenisher*

**sodium glucosulfone** USP

**sodium glutamate**

**sodium glycerophosphate** NF

**sodium glycocholate** [see: bile salts]

**sodium gualenate** INN [also: azulene sulfonate sodium]

**sodium hyaluronate** [see: hyaluronate sodium]

**sodium hydroxide** NF *alkalizing agent*

**sodium hydroxybenzenesulfonate** [see: phenolsulphonate sodium]

**sodium 4-hydroxybutyrate** [see: sodium oxybate]

**sodium hypochlorite** USP, JAN *disinfectant; bleach; used for utensils and equipment*

**sodium hypochlorite, diluted** NF [also: antiformin, dental]

**sodium hypophosphite** NF

**sodium iodide** USP *dietary iodine supplement (85% elemental iodine)*

**sodium iodide ($^{123}$I)** JAN *thyroid function test; radioactive agent* [also: sodium iodide I 123]

**sodium iodide ($^{125}$I)** INN *thyroid function test; radioactive agent* [also: sodium iodide I 125]

**sodium iodide ($^{131}$I)** JAN *antineoplastic for thyroid carcinoma; radioactive agent for hyperthyroidism* [also: sodium iodide I 131]

**sodium iodide I 123** USP *diagnostic aid for thyroid function; radioactive agent* [also: sodium iodide ($^{123}$I)] 3.7, 7.4 MBq oral

**sodium iodide I 125** USAN, USP *thyroid function test; radioactive agent* [also: sodium iodide ($^{125}$I)]

**sodium iodide I 131** USAN, USP, INN *antineoplastic for thyroid carcinoma; radioactive agent for hyperthyroidism* [also: sodium iodide ($^{131}$I)] 0.75–100 mCi, 3.5–150 mCi oral

**sodium iodohippurate ($^{131}$I)** INN, JAN *renal function test; radioactive agent* [also: iodohippurate sodium I 131]

**sodium iodomethanesulfonate** [see: methiodal sodium]

**sodium iopodate** JAN *oral radiopaque contrast medium for cholecystography (61.4% iodine)* [also: ipodate sodium; sodium ipodate]

**sodium iotalamate ($^{125}$I)** INN *radioactive agent* [also: iothalamate sodium I 125]

**sodium iotalamate ($^{131}$I)** INN *radioactive agent* [also: iothalamate sodium I 131]

**sodium iothalamate** BAN *parenteral radiopaque contrast medium (59.9% iodine)* [also: iothalamate sodium]

**sodium ioxaglate** BAN *radiopaque contrast medium* [also: ioxaglate sodium]

**sodium ipodate** INN, BAN *oral radiopaque contrast medium for cholecystography (61.4% iodine)* [also: ipodate sodium; sodium iopodate]

**sodium ironedetate** BAN [also: sodium feredetate]

**sodium lactate (SL)** USP *electrolyte replenisher* 167 mEq/L (1/6 molar) injection

**sodium lactate, compound solution of** INN *electrolyte and fluid replenisher; systemic alkalizer* [also: Ringer's injection, lactated]

**sodium lauryl sulfate** NF *surfactant/wetting agent* [also: laurilsulfate]

**sodium lignosulfonate** [see: polignate sodium]

**sodium metabisulfite** NF *antioxidant*

**sodium metrizoate** INN *radiopaque contrast medium* [also: metrizoate sodium]

**sodium monododecyl sulfate** [see: sodium lauryl sulfate]

**sodium monofluorophosphate** USP *dental caries prophylactic*

**sodium monomercaptoundecahydro-closo-dodecaborate** *investigational (orphan) for boron neutron capture therapy (BNCT) for glioblastoma multiforme*

**sodium morrhuate** INN *sclerosing agent* [also: morrhuate sodium]

**sodium nitrite** USP *antidote to cyanide poisoning* 30 mg/mL injection

**sodium nitroferricyanide** [see: sodium nitroprusside]

**sodium nitroferricyanide dihydrate** [see: sodium nitroprusside]

**sodium nitroprusside** USP *emergency antihypertensive; vasodilator* 50 mg/dose injection

**sodium noramidopyrine methanesulfonate** [see: dipyrone]

**sodium oxybate** USAN *adjunct to anesthesia; CNS depressant for narcolepsy, cataplexy, sleep paralysis, and hypnagogic hallucinations* (orphan)

**sodium oxychlorosene** [see: oxychlorosene sodium]

**sodium paratoluenesulfan chloramide** [see: chloramine-T]

**sodium PCA; Na PCA (sodium pyrrolidone carboxylic acid)** [q.v.]

**sodium penicillin G** [see: penicillin G sodium]

**sodium pentosan polysulfate** [see: pentosan polysulfate sodium]

**sodium perborate** *topical antiseptic/germicidal*

**sodium perborate monohydrate** USAN

**sodium pertechnetate Tc 99m** USAN, USP *radioactive agent*

**sodium phenolate** [see: phenolate sodium]

**sodium phenylacetate** USAN *antihyperammonemic*

**sodium phenylacetate & sodium benzoate** *to prevent and treat hyperammonemia of urea cycle enzymopathy (orphan)*

**sodium phenylbutyrate** USAN *antihyperammonemic for urea cycle disorders (orphan); investigational (orphan) for various sickling disorders*

**sodium phosphate ($^{32}$P)** INN *antineoplastic; antipolycythemic; neoplasm test* [also: sodium phosphate P 32]

**sodium phosphate, dibasic** USP *saline laxative; phosphorus replacement; pH buffer*

**sodium phosphate, monobasic** USP *saline laxative; phosphorus replacement; pH buffer*

**sodium phosphate P 32** USAN, USP *antipolycythemic; radiopharmaceutical antineoplastic for various leukemias and skeletal metastases* [also: sodium phosphate ($^{32}$P)] 0.67 mCi/mL

**sodium picofosfate** INN

**sodium picosulfate** INN

**sodium polyphosphate** USAN *pharmaceutic aid*

**sodium polystyrene sulfonate** USP *potassium-removing ion-exchange resin for hyperkalemia 15 g/60 mL oral*

**sodium propionate** NF *preservative; antifungal*

**sodium propionate hydrate** [see: sodium propionate]

**sodium 2-propylvalerate** [see: valproate sodium]

**sodium psylliate** NF

**sodium pyrophosphate** USAN *pharmaceutic aid*

**sodium pyrrolidone carboxylic acid (sodium PCA; Na PCA)** *natural skin moisturizing factor; humectant*

**sodium radiochromate** [see: sodium chromate Cr 51]

**sodium rhodanate** [see: thiocyanate sodium]

**sodium salicylate (SS)** USP *analgesic; antipyretic; anti-inflammatory; antirheumatic* 325, 650 mg oral

**sodium starch glycolate** NF *tablet excipient*

**sodium stearate** NF *emulsifying and stiffening agent*

**sodium stearyl fumarate** NF *tablet and capsule lubricant*

**sodium stibocaptate** INN [also: stibocaptate]

**sodium stibogluconate** INN, BAN, DCF *investigational antiparasitic for leishmaniasis and trypanosomiasis*

**Sodium Sulamyd** eye drops, ophthalmic ointment ℞ *antibiotic* [sulfacetamide sodium] 10%, 30%; 10%

**sodium sulfacetamide** [see: sulfacetamide sodium]

**sodium sulfate** USP *calcium regulator*

**sodium sulfate S 35** USAN *radioactive agent*

**sodium sulfocyanate** [see: thiocyanate sodium]

**sodium taurocholate** [see: bile salts]

**sodium tetradecyl (STD) sulfate** INN *sclerosing agent; investigational (orphan) for bleeding esophageal varices*

**sodium thiomalate, gold** [see: gold sodium thiomalate]

**sodium thiosalicylate** *analgesic; antipyretic; anti-inflammatory; antirheumatic* 50 mg/mL injection

**sodium thiosulfate** USP *antidote to cyanide poisoning; antiseptic; antifungal* 10%, 25% (100, 250 mg/mL) injection

**sodium thiosulfate, gold** [see: gold sodium thiosulfate]

**sodium thiosulfate & hydroxocobalamin** *investigational (orphan) for severe acute cyanide poisoning*

**sodium thiosulfate pentahydrate** [see: sodium thiosulfate]

**sodium timerfonate** INN *topical anti-infective* [also: thimerfonate sodium]

**sodium trimetaphosphate** USAN *pharmaceutic aid*

**sodium tyropanoate** INN *oral radiopaque contrast medium for cholecystography (57.4% iodine)* [also: tyropanoate sodium]

**sodium valproate** [see: valproate sodium]

**Sodol Compound** tablets ℞ *skeletal muscle relaxant; analgesic* [carisoprodol; aspirin] 200•325 mg

**sofalcone** INN

**Sofenol 5** lotion OTC *moisturizer; emollient*

**Sof-lax** softgels OTC *laxative; stool softener* [docusate sodium] 100 mg

**Soft Mate Comfort Drops for Sensitive Eyes** OTC *rewetting solution for soft contact lenses*

**Soft Mate Consept** solution + aerosol spray OTC *two-step chemical disinfecting system for soft contact lenses* [hydrogen peroxide based] 3%

**Soft Mate Disinfecting for Sensitive Eyes** solution OTC *chemical disinfecting solution for soft contact lenses*

**Soft Mate Hands Off Daily Cleaner** solution OTC *surfactant cleaning solution for soft contact lenses*

**soft pine** *medicinal herb* [see: white pine]

**Soft Sense** lotion OTC *moisturizer; emollient*

**Softabs** (trademarked dosage form) *chewable tablets*

**softgels** (dosage form) *soft gelatin capsules*

**SoftWear** solution OTC *rinsing/storage solution for soft contact lenses* [sodium chloride (preserved saline solution)]

**Solagé** topical solution ℞ *depigmenting agent for solar lentigines* [mequinol; tretinoin; alcohol 77.8%] 2%•0.01%

**Solanum dulcamara** *medicinal herb* [see: bittersweet nightshade]

**solapsone** BAN [also: solasulfone]

**Solaquin** cream OTC *hyperpigmentation bleaching agent* [hydroquinone in a sunscreen base] 2%

**Solaquin Forte** cream, gel ℞ *hyperpigmentation bleaching agent* [hydroquinone (in a sunscreen base)] 4%

**Solaraze** gel ℞ *topical treatment for actinic keratosis* [diclofenac potassium] 3%

**Solarcaine** aerosol spray, lotion OTC *topical local anesthetic; antiseptic* [benzocaine; triclosan] 20%•0.13%

**Solarcaine Aloe Extra Burn Relief** spray, gel, cream OTC *topical local anesthetic* [lidocaine] 0.5%

**solasulfone** INN [also: solapsone]

**soldier's woundwort** *medicinal herb* [see: yarrow]

**Solfoton** tablets, capsules ℞ *long-acting barbiturate sedative, hypnotic and anticonvulsant* [phenobarbital] 16 mg

**Solganal** IM injection ℞ *antirheumatic* [aurothioglucose] 50 mg/mL

**Solia** tablets (in packs of 28) ℞ *monophasic oral contraceptive* [desogestrel; ethinyl estradiol] 0.15 mg•30 μg

**Solidago nemoralis; S. odora; S. virgaurea** *medicinal herb* [see: goldenrod]

**solifenacin succinate** *investigational (NDA filed) selective muscarinic M₃ receptor antagonist for overactive bladder with urinary incontinence, urgency, and frequency*

**Solomon's seal (Polygonatum multiflorum; P. odoratum)** root *medicinal herb used as an astringent, demulcent, emetic, and expectorant*

**solpecainol** INN

**SolTabs** (trademarked dosage form) *orally disintegrating tablets*

**Soltice Quick-Rub** OTC *analgesic; counterirritant* [methyl salicylate; camphor; menthol; eucalyptus oil]

**soluble complement receptor** [see: complement receptor type I, soluble recombinant human]

**soluble ferric pyrophosphate** [see: ferric pyrophosphate, soluble]

**soluble gelatin (SG)** [see: gelatin]

**Soluble T4** ℞ *investigational (orphan) treatment for AIDS* [CD4 human truncated 369 AA polypeptide]

**Solu-Cortef** powder for IV or IM injection ℞ *corticosteroid; anti-inflammatory* [hydrocortisone sodium succinate] 100, 250, 500, 1000 mg/vial

**Solu-Medrol** powder for IV or IM injection ℞ *corticosteroid; anti-inflammatory; immunosuppressant* [methylprednisolone sodium succinate] 40, 125, 500, 1000, 2000 mg/vial

**Solumol** OTC *ointment base*

**Solurex** intra-articular, intralesional, soft tissue, or IM injection ℞ *corticosteroid; anti-inflammatory* [dexamethasone sodium phosphate] 4 mg/mL

**Solurex LA** intralesional, intra-articular, soft tissue, or IM injection ℞ *corticosteroid; anti-inflammatory* [dexamethasone acetate] 8 mg/mL

**Soluspan** (trademarked form) *injectable suspension*

**Soluvite C.T.** chewable tablets ℞ *pediatric vitamin supplement and dental caries preventative* [multiple vitamins; fluoride; folic acid] ≟•1•0.3 mg

**Soluvite-f** drops ℞ *pediatric vitamin supplement and dental caries preventative* [vitamins A, C, and D; fluoride] 1500 IU•35 mg•400 IU•0.25 mg per 0.6 mL

**Solvent-G** OTC *liquid base*

**Solvet** (trademarked dosage form) *soluble tablet*

**solypertine** INN *antiadrenergic* [also: solypertine tartrate]

**solypertine tartrate** USAN *antiadrenergic* [also: solypertine]

**Soma** tablets ℞ *skeletal muscle relaxant* [carisoprodol] 350 mg

**Soma Compound** tablets ℞ *skeletal muscle relaxant; analgesic* [carisoprodol; aspirin] 200•325 mg

**Soma Compound with Codeine** tablets ℞ *skeletal muscle relaxant; narcotic antitussive; analgesic* [carisoprodol; aspirin; codeine phosphate] 200•325•16 mg

**Somagard** ℞ *investigational (orphan) LHRH agonist for central precocious puberty* [deslorelin]

**somagrebove** USAN *veterinary galactopoietic agent*

**somalapor** USAN, INN, BAN *porcine growth hormone*

**somantadine** INN *antiviral* [also: somantadine HCl]

**somantadine HCl** USAN *antiviral* [also: somantadine]

**SomatoKine** ℞ *investigational (Phase II, orphan) agent for treatment of muscle degradation following severe burns and hip fracture surgery; investigational (Phase II) for type 1 diabetes* [IGF-BP3 complex]

**somatomedin-C** [see: mecasermin]

**somatorelin** INN *growth hormone-releasing factor (GH-RF)*

**somatostatin (SS)** INN, BAN *growth hormone-release inhibiting factor; investigational (orphan) for cutaneous gastrointestinal fistulas and bleeding esophageal varices*

**SomatoTher** ℞ *investigational (orphan) radiotherapeutic agent for somatostatin receptor–positive neuroendocrine tumors* [indium In 111 pentetreotide]

**somatotropin, human** [see: somatropin]

**Somatrel** ℞ *investigational (orphan) diagnostic aid for pituitary release of growth hormone* [NG-29 (code name—generic name not yet assigned)]

**somatrem** USAN, INN, BAN *growth hormone for congenital growth failure due to lack of endogenous growth hormone (orphan)*

**somatropin** USAN, INN, BAN, JAN *growth hormone for adults or children with congenital or endogenous growth hormone deficiency, children with Turner syndrome or renal-induced growth failure, short bowel syndrome, or AIDS-wasting syndrome (orphan); investigational (orphan) for severe burns* [also: human growth hormone]

**somatropin & glutamine** *investigational (orphan) for GI malabsorption due to short bowel syndrome*

**Somavert** subcu injection ℞ *growth hormone receptor antagonist for acromegaly (orphan)* [pegvisomant] 10, 15, 20 mg/dose

**somavubove** USAN, INN *veterinary galactopoietic agent*

**somenopor** USAN *porcine growth hormone*

**sometribove** USAN, INN, BAN *veterinary growth stimulant*

**sometripor** USAN, INN, BAN *veterinary growth stimulant*

**somfasepor** USAN *veterinary growth stimulant*

**somidobove** USAN, INN *synthetic bovine growth hormone*

**Sominex** tablets, caplets OTC *antihistaminic sleep aid* [diphenhydramine HCl] 25 mg; 50 mg

**Sominex Pain Relief** tablets OTC *antihistaminic sleep aid; analgesic* [diphenhydramine HCl; acetaminophen] 25•500 mg

**Somnote** capsules ℞ *sedative; hypnotic* [chloral hydrate] 500 mg

**Sonata** capsules ℞ *rapid-onset, short-duration hypnotic for the short-term treatment of insomnia* [zaleplon] 5, 10 mg

**Sonazoid** ℞ *investigational (NDA filed) ultrasound imaging agent*

**sonepiprazole mesylate** USAN *dopamine $D_4$ antagonist; antipsychotic*

**SonoRx** oral suspension ℞ *ultrasound imaging agent to reduce gas shadowing* [simethicone-coated cellulose] 7.5 mg/mL

**SonoVue** ℞ *investigational ultrasound imaging agent* [sulfur hexafluoride]

**Soothaderm** lotion OTC *local anesthetic; antihistamine; emollient* [pyrilamine maleate; benzocaine; zinc oxide] 2.07•2.08•41.35 mg/mL

**sopecainol** [see: solpecainol]

**sopitazine** INN

**sopromidine** INN

**soproxil** USAN *combining name for radicals or groups* [also: disoproxil]

**soquinolol** INN

**sorb apple** *medicinal herb* [see: mountain ash]

**sorbic acid** NF *antimicrobial agent; preservative*

**sorbide nitrate** [see: isosorbide dinitrate]

**sorbimacrogol laurate 300** [see: polysorbate 20]

**sorbimacrogol oleate 300** [see: polysorbate 80]

**sorbimacrogol palmitate 300** [see: polysorbate 40]

**sorbimacrogol stearate** [see: polysorbate 60]

**sorbimacrogol tristearate 300** [see: polysorbate 65]

**sorbinicate** INN

**sorbinil** USAN, INN, BAN *aldose reductase enzyme inhibitor*

**sorbitan laurate** INN *surfactant* [also: sorbitan monolaurate]

**sorbitan monolaurate** USAN, NF *surfactant* [also: sorbitan laurate]

**sorbitan monooleate** USAN, NF *surfactant* [also: sorbitan oleate]

**sorbitan monopalmitate** USAN, NF *surfactant* [also: sorbitan palmitate]

**sorbitan monostearate** USAN, NF *surfactant* [also: sorbitan stearate]

**sorbitan oleate** INN *surfactant* [also: sorbitan monooleate]

**sorbitan palmitate** INN *surfactant* [also: sorbitan monopalmitate]

**sorbitan sesquioleate** USAN, INN *surfactant*

**sorbitan stearate** INN *surfactant* [also: sorbitan monostearate]

**sorbitan trioleate** USAN, INN *surfactant*

**sorbitan tristearate** USAN, INN *surfactant*

**sorbitol** NF *flavoring agent; tablet excipient; urologic irrigant* 3%, 3.3%

**sorbitol (solution)** USP *flavoring agent; tablet excipient*

**Sorbitrate** sublingual tablets (discontinued 2004) ℞ *antianginal; vasodilator* [isosorbide dinitrate] 2.5, 5 mg

**Sorbitrate** tablets, chewable tablets ℞ *antianginal; vasodilator* [isosorbide dinitrate] 5, 10, 20, 30, 40 mg; 5, 10 mg

**Sorbsan** pads *absorbent dressing for wet wounds* [calcium alginate fiber]

***Sorbus americana; S. aucuparia*** *medicinal herb* [see: mountain ash]

**Soriatane** capsules ℞ *systemic antipsoriatic* [acitretin] 10, 25 mg

**sorivudine** USAN, INN, BAN *antiviral for varicella zoster and herpes zoster in* *immunocompromised patients; orphan status withdrawn 1997*

**sornidipine** INN

**sorrel (Rumex acetosa)** *plant medicinal herb used as an antiscorbutic, astringent, diuretic, laxative, refrigerant, and vermifuge*

**sorrel, common; mountain sorrel; white sorrel** *medicinal herb* [see: wood sorrel]

**sorrel, Jamaica** *medicinal herb* [see: hibiscus]

**sotalol** INN, BAN *antiarrhythmic; antiadrenergic (β-receptor)* [also: sotalol HCl]

**sotalol HCl** USAN *antiarrhythmic (β-blocker) for ventricular arrhythmias (orphan)* [also: sotalol] 80, 120, 160, 240 mg oral

**Sotalol HCl AF** *tablets* ℞ *antiarrhythmic (β-blocker) for atrial fibrillation or atrial flutter* [sotalol HCl] 80, 120, 160 mg

**soterenol** INN *adrenergic; bronchodilator* [also: soterenol HCl]

**soterenol HCl** USAN *adrenergic; bronchodilator* [also: soterenol]

**Sotradecol** IV injection, Dosette (unit-of-use injection) ℞ *sclerosing agent; investigational (orphan) for bleeding esophageal varices* [sodium tetradecyl sulfate] 1%, 3%

**Sotret** *softgels* ℞ *keratolytic for severe recalcitrant cystic acne* [isotretinoin] 10, 20, 30, 40 mg

**sour dock** *medicinal herb* [see: yellow dock]

**sourberry; sowberry** *medicinal herb* [see: barberry]

**sourgrass** *medicinal herb* [see: sorrel]

**Southern ginseng** *medicinal herb* [see: jiaogulan]

**Soviet gramicidin** [see: gramicidin S]

**sowberry; sourberry** *medicinal herb* [see: barberry]

**soy; soya; soybean (Glycine max)** *medicinal herb and food crop; isoflavone compounds provide phytoestrogens to alleviate menopausal symptoms, including osteoporosis, and provide antineoplastic, cardiovascular, and gastrointestinal benefits*

**Soyalac; I-Soyalac** *oral liquid, powder for oral liquid* OTC *hypoallergenic infant food* [soy protein formula]

**soybean oil** USP *pharmaceutic necessity*

**spaglumic acid** INN

**Span C** *tablets* OTC *vitamin C supplement with bioflavonoids* [ascorbic acid and rose hips; citrus bioflavonoids] 200•300 mg

**Spancap No. 1** *sustained-release capsules* ℞ *CNS stimulant* [dextroamphetamine sulfate] 15 mg

**Spancaps** (dosage form) *timed-release capsules*

**Spanidin** *investigational (orphan) immunosuppressant for acute renal graft rejection* [gusperimus]

**Spanish chestnut** *medicinal herb* [see: horse chestnut]

**Spanish pepper** *medicinal herb* [see: cayenne]

**Spansule** (trademarked dosage form) *sustained-release capsule*

**sparfloxacin (SPFX)** USAN, INN, BAN *broad-spectrum fluoroquinolone antibiotic*

**sparfosate sodium** USAN *antineoplastic* [also: sparfosic acid]

**sparfosic acid** INN *antineoplastic* [also: sparfosate sodium]

**Sparine** *tablets* (discontinued 2001) ℞ *conventional (typical) antipsychotic* [promazine HCl] 25, 50 mg

**Sparkles** *effervescent granules* OTC *antacid; aid in endoscopic examination* [sodium bicarbonate; citric acid; simethicone] 2000•1500• ≟ mg/dose

**sparsomycin** USAN, INN *antineoplastic*

**Spartaject** ℞ *investigational (Phase II/III) intravenous delivery device*

**Spartaject Busulfan** ℞ *investigational (orphan) alkylating antineoplastic for neoplastic meningitis and primary brain malignancies* [busulfan]

**sparteine** INN *oxytocic* [also: sparteine sulfate]

**sparteine sulfate** USAN *oxytocic* [also: sparteine]

**Spasmolin** *tablets* ℞ *GI antispasmodic; anticholinergic; sedative* [atropine sulfate; scopolamine hydrobromide; hyo-

scyamine hydrobromide; phenobarbi-
tal] 0.0194•0.0065•0.1037•16.2 mg

**SPCA (serum prothrombin conver-
sion accelerator) factor** [see: factor VII]

**spearmint** NF

**spearmint (Mentha spicata)** leaves
*medicinal herb for colds, colic, flu, gas,
nausea, and vomiting*

**spearmint oil** NF

**Spec-T** lozenges OTC *topical oral anesthetic* [benzocaine] 10 mg

**Spec-T Sore Throat/Cough Sup-
pressant** lozenges (discontinued
2002) OTC *topical oral anesthetic; antitussive* [benzocaine; dextromethorphan hydrobromide] 10•10 mg

**Spec-T Sore Throat/Decongestant**
lozenges (discontinued 2001) OTC
*decongestant; topical oral anesthetic*
[phenylpropanolamine HCl; phenylephrine HCl; benzocaine] 10.5•5•
10 mg

**Spectazole** cream ℞ *antifungal* [econa-
zole nitrate] 1%

**spectinomycin** INN *antibiotic* [also:
spectinomycin HCl]

**spectinomycin HCl** USAN, USP *antibiotic for gonorrhea* [also: spectinomycin]

**Spectracef** capsules ℞ *broad-spectrum
cephalosporin antibiotic* [cefditoren
pivoxil] 200, 400 mg

**Spectrobid** film-coated tablets (discontinued 2002) ℞ *aminopenicillin
antibiotic* [bacampicillin HCl] 400 mg

**Spectrocin Plus** ointment OTC *antibiotic; local anesthetic* [polymyxin B
sulfate; neomycin sulfate; bacitracin
zinc; pramoxine HCl] 10 000 U•3.5
mg•500 U•10 mg per g

**Spectro-Jel** topical liquid OTC *soap-
free therapeutic skin cleanser*

**speedwell (Veronica officinalis)** flowering plant *medicinal herb used as a
diuretic, expectorant, and stomachic*

**speedwell, tall** *medicinal herb* [see:
Culver root]

**spenbolic** [see: methandriol]

**spermaceti, synthetic** [see: cetyl
esters wax]

**spermicides** *a class of topical contraceptive agents that kill the male sperm*

**Spexil** ℞ *investigational (Phase III)
broad-spectrum aminocyclitol antibiotic
for respiratory, gynecologic, and
abdominal infections* [trospectomycin]

**SPFX (sparfloxacin)** [q.v.]

**Spheramine** ℞ *investigational (Phase
II, orphan) dopamine-producing brain
implants for stage 3 and 4 Parkinson
disease* [human retinal pigment
epithelial (RPE) cells on spherical
cell-coated microcarriers (CCM)]

**Spherulin** intradermal injection ℞
*diagnostic aid for coccidioidomycosis*
[coccidioidin] 1:100, 1:10

**spiceberry** *medicinal herb* [see: winter-
green]

**spiclamine** INN

**spiclomazine** INN

**spicy wintergreen** *medicinal herb* [see:
wintergreen]

**spider bite antivenin** [see: antivenin
(Latrodectus mactans)]

**spignet** *medicinal herb* [see: spikenard]

**spikenard (Aralia racemosa)** root
*medicinal herb for asthma, childbirth,
cough, and rheumatism*

**spindle tree** *medicinal herb* [see: wahoo]

**spiperone** USAN, INN *antipsychotic*

**spiradoline** INN *analgesic* [also: spiradoline mesylate]

**spiradoline mesylate** USAN *analgesic*
[also: spiradoline]

**spiramide** INN

**spiramycin** USAN, INN, BAN *macrolide
antibiotic* [also: acetylspiramycin]

**spirapril** INN, BAN *angiotensin-converting enzyme (ACE) inhibitor* [also: spirapril HCl]

**spirapril HCl** USAN *angiotensin-converting enzyme (ACE) inhibitor* [also:
spirapril]

**spiraprilat** USAN, INN *angiotensin-converting enzyme (ACE) inhibitor*

**spirazine** INN

**spirazine HCl** [see: spirazine]

**spirendolol** INN

**spirgetine** INN

**spirilene** INN, BAN

**spirit of nitrous ether** [see: ethyl nitrite]

**Spiriva** powder in capsules for inhalation (used with HandiHaler device) ℞ *once-daily bronchodilator for chronic obstructive pulmonary disease (COPD)* [tiotropium bromide] 18 µg/dose

**spirobarbital sodium**

**spirofylline** INN

**spirogermanium** INN, BAN *antineoplastic* [also: spirogermanium HCl]

**spirogermanium HCl** USAN *antineoplastic* [also: spirogermanium]

**spirohydantoin mustard** [now: spiromustine]

**spiromustine** USAN, INN *antineoplastic*

**spironolactone** USP, INN, BAN, JAN *antihypertensive; potassium-sparing diuretic; aldosterone antagonist* 25, 50, 100 mg oral

**spiroplatin** USAN, INN, BAN *antineoplastic*

**spirorenone** INN

**Spiros** (trademarked delivery system) ℞ *investigational inhaler*

**spirotriazine HCl** [see: spirazine]

**spiroxamide** [see: spiroxatrine]

**spiroxasone** USAN, INN *diuretic*

**spiroxatrine** INN

**spiroxepin** INN

**spirulina** (*Spirulina pratensis*) plant *medicinal herb for chronic disease, enhancing antibody production, lowering serum lipids and triglycerides, and reducing gastric secretory activity; also used as a blood builder and food supplement*

**spizofurone** INN

**SPL (staphage lysate)** [q.v.]

**SPL-Serologic types I and III** solution for subcu injection, nasal aerosol, nasal drop, oral, or topical irrigation (discontinued 2000) ℞ *staphylococcal or polymicrobial vaccine* [staphage lysate (*Staphylococcus aureus* vaccine; *Staphylococcus* bacteriophage plaque-forming units)]

**spoonwood** *medicinal herb* [see: linden tree]

**Sporanox** capsules, PulsePak (one-week dose package), IV infusion ℞ *systemic*

*triazole antifungal* [itraconazole] 100 mg; 28 × 100 mg; 10 mg/mL

**Sporanox** oral solution ("swish and swallow") ℞ *antifungal for esophageal and oropharyngeal candidiasis* [itraconazole] 10 mg/mL

**Sporidin-G** ℞ *investigational (orphan) treatment of cryptosporidiosis-induced diarrhea in immunocompromised patients* [*Cryptosporidium parvum* bovine colostrum IgG concentrate]

**Sports Spray** OTC *analgesic; counterirritant; antiseptic* [methyl salicylate; menthol; camphor; alcohol 58%] 3.5% • 10% • 5%

**Sportscreme** OTC *topical analgesic* [trolamine salicylate] 10%

**Sportscreme Ice** gel OTC *topical analgesic; counterirritant* [trolamine; menthol] ≟ • 2%

**spotted alder** *medicinal herb* [see: witch hazel]

**spotted comfrey** *medicinal herb* [see: lungwort]

**spotted cranesbill** *medicinal herb* [see: alum root]

**spotted geranium** *medicinal herb* [see: alum root]

**spotted hemlock; spotted cowbane; spotted parsley** *medicinal herb* [see: poison hemlock]

**spotted lungwort** *medicinal herb* [see: lungwort]

**spotted thistle** *medicinal herb* [see: blessed thistle]

**spp.** plural of *species*

**SPPG (sulfated polysaccharide peptidoglycan)** [see: tecogalan sodium]

**Spray-U-Thin** oral spray (discontinued 2001) OTC *diet aid* [phenylpropanolamine HCl] 6.58 mg

**spring wintergreen** *medicinal herb* [see: wintergreen]

**Sprinkle Caps** (trademarked form) *powder*

**Sprintec** tablets (in packs of 28) ℞ *monophasic oral contraceptive* [norgestimate; ethinyl estradiol] 0.25 mg • 35 µg

**sprodiamide** USAN *heart and CNS imaging aid for MRI*

**spruce (Picea excelsa; P. mariana)** young shoots *medicinal herb used as a calmative, diaphoretic, expectorant, and pectoral*

**spruce, Norway** *medicinal herb* [see: spruce]

**spruce, weeping** *medicinal herb* [see: hemlock]

**SPS** oral suspension R *potassium-removing agent for hyperkalemia* [sodium polystyrene sulfonate] 15 g/60 mL

**S·P·T** liquid-filled capsules (discontinued 2000) R *thyroid replacement therapy for hypothyroidism or thyroid cancer* [thyroid, desiccated (porcine)] 60, 120, 180, 300 mg

**spurge laurel; spurge olive** *medicinal herb* [see: mezereon]

**squalamine** *natural remedy; investigational (Phase III) angiogenesis inhibitor for the treatment of solid tumors; investigational (Phase II) for advanced non–small cell lung cancer (NSCLC)* [also: shark cartilage]

**squalane** NF *oleaginous vehicle*

**square, carpenter's** *medicinal herb* [see: figwort]

**squaw balm; squaw mint** *medicinal herb* [see: pennyroyal]

**squaw root** *medicinal herb* [see: black cohosh; blue cohosh]

**squaw tea** *medicinal herb* [see: ephedra]

**squaw vine (Mitchella repens)** plant *medicinal herb for easing childbirth, lactation, and menstruation and for uterine disorders*

**squaw weed** *medicinal herb* [see: life root]

**squawberry** *medicinal herb* [see: squaw vine]

**squill (Urginea indica; U. maritima; U. scilla)** bulb *medicinal herb for edema and inducing emesis and expectoration; also used as a rat poison*

**squirrel pea, ground** *medicinal herb* [see: twin leaf]

**SR-57746** *investigational (Phase III) agent for Alzheimer disease*

**$^{85}$Sr** [see: strontium chloride Sr 85]

**$^{85}$Sr** [see: strontium nitrate Sr 85]

**$^{85}$Sr** [see: strontium Sr 85]

**SRC Expectorant** oral liquid (discontinued 2002) R *narcotic antitussive; decongestant; expectorant* [hydrocodone bitartrate; pseudoephedrine HCl; guaifenesin; alcohol 12.5%] 5•60•200 mg/5 mL

**SRF (skin respiratory factor)** [q.v.]

**SS (saline solution)**

**SS (sodium salicylate)** [q.v.]

**SS (somatostatin)** [q.v.]

**SSD (silver sulfadiazine)** [q.v.]

**SSD; SSD AF** cream R *broad-spectrum bactericidal for adjunctive burn treatment* [silver sulfadiazine] 10 mg/g

**SSKI** oral solution R *expectorant* [potassium iodide] 1 g/mL

**SSNRIs (selective serotonin and norepinephrine reuptake inhibitors)** [q.v.]

**SSRIs (selective serotonin reuptake inhibitors)** [q.v.]

**S.S.S. High Potency Vitamin Tablets** OTC *vitamin/mineral/iron supplement* [multiple vitamins & minerals; iron; biotin] ≛•27•0.0225 mg

**S.S.S. Vitamin and Mineral Complex** oral liquid OTC *vitamin/mineral/iron supplement* [multiple vitamins & minerals; iron; biotin; alcohol 6.6%] ≛•3•0.1 mg

**S.T. 37** solution OTC *topical antiseptic* [hexylresorcinol] 0.1%

**S·T Cort** lotion R *topical corticosteroidal anti-inflammatory* [hydrocortisone] 0.5%

**S·T Forte** syrup, oral liquid (discontinued 2002) R *narcotic antitussive; decongestant; antihistamine; expectorant* [hydrocodone bitartrate; phenylephrine HCl; phenylpropanolamine HCl; pheniramine maleate; guaifenesin; alcohol 5%] 2.5•5•5•13.33•80 mg/5 mL

**S·T Forte 2** oral liquid R *narcotic antitussive; antihistamine* [hydrocodone bitartrate; chlorpheniramine maleate] 2.5•2 mg/5 mL

**Staarvisc** intraocular injection ℞ *viscoelastic agent for ophthalmic surgery* [hyaluronate sodium]

**stable factor** [see: factor VII]

*Stachys officinalis medicinal herb* [see: betony]

**Stadol** IV or IM injection ℞ *narcotic agonist-antagonist analgesic* [butorphanol tartrate] 1, 2 mg/mL

**Stadol NS** nasal spray ℞ *narcotic agonist-antagonist analgesic; antimigraine agent* [butorphanol tartrate] 10 mg/mL

**staff vine** *medicinal herb* [see: bittersweet nightshade]

**Stagesic** capsules ℞ *narcotic analgesic* [hydrocodone bitartrate; acetaminophen] 5•500 mg

**staggerweed** *medicinal herb* [see: turkey corn]

**staghorn** *medicinal herb* [see: club moss]

**Stahist** sustained-release tablets ℞ *decongestant; antihistamine; anticholinergic to dry mucosal secretions* [phenylephrine HCl; pseudoephedrine HCl; chlorpheniramine maleate; hyoscyamine sulfate; atropine sulfate; scopolamine hydrobromide] 25•40•8•0.19•0.04•0.01 mg

**Stalevo 50; Stalevo 100; Stalevo 150** tablets ℞ *multi-modal antiparkinsonian: dopamine precursor + dopadecarboxylase inhibitor + catechol-O-methyltransferase (COMT) inhibitor* [levodopa; carbidopa; entacapone] 50•12.5•200 mg; 100•25•200 mg; 150•37.5•200 mg

**stallimycin** INN *antibacterial* [also: stallimycin HCl]

**stallimycin HCl** USAN *antibacterial* [also: stallimycin]

**Stamoist E** sustained-release film-coated caplets ℞ *decongestant; expectorant* [pseudoephedrine HCl; guaifenesin] 120•500 mg

**Stamoist LA** sustained-release tablets (discontinued 2002) ℞ *decongestant; expectorant* [phenylpropanolamine HCl; guaifenesin] 75•400 mg

**Stanate** ℞ *investigational bilirubin inhibitor for neonatal hyperbilirubinemia*

**standard VAC** *chemotherapy protocol for sarcomas* [see: VAC standard]

**Stanford V (mechlorethamine, doxorubicin, vinblastine, vincristine, bleomycin, etoposide, prednisone)** *chemotherapy protocol for Hodgkin lymphoma*

**stannous chloride** USAN *pharmaceutic aid*

**stannous fluoride** USP *dental caries prophylactic* 0.4%, 0.63% topical oral

**stannous pyrophosphate** USAN *skeletal imaging aid*

**stannous sulfur colloid** USAN *bone, liver and spleen imaging aid*

**stannsoporfin** USAN *investigational bilirubin inhibitor for neonatal hyperbilirubinemia*

**stanolone** BAN *investigational (orphan) for AIDS-wasting syndrome* [also: androstanolone]

**stanozolol** USAN, USP, INN, BAN *androgen; anabolic steroid*

**staphage lysate (SPL)** *active bacterin for staphylococcal infections*

**StaphVAX** ℞ *investigational (Phase III) vaccine against Staphylococcus aureus infection of end-stage renal disease*

*Staphylococcus aureus vaccine* [see: staphage lysate]

**star anise (Illicium anisatum; I. verum)** seeds *medicinal herb used as a carminative, stimulant, and stomachic; also added to other herbal medications to improve digestibility and taste*

**star chickweed; starweed** *medicinal herb* [see: chickweed]

**star grass (Aletris farinosa)** root and rhizome *medicinal herb for diarrhea, dysmenorrhea and menstrual discomfort, gas and colonic cramps, and rheumatism*

**star root** *medicinal herb* [see: star grass]

**starch** NF *dusting powder; pharmaceutic aid*

**starch, pregelatinized** NF *tablet excipient*

**starch, topical** USP *dusting powder*

**starch carboxymethyl ether, sodium salt** [see: sodium starch glycolate]

**starch glycerite** NF

**starch 2-hydroxyethyl ether** [see: hetastarch; pentastarch]

**Starlix** tablets ℞ *antidiabetic agent that stimulates the release of insulin from the pancreas for type 2 diabetes* [nateglinide] 60, 120 mg

**Starnoc** Ⓒᴬᴺ capsules ℞ *rapid-onset, short-duration hypnotic for the short-term treatment of insomnia* [zaleplon] 5, 10 mg

**Star-Otic** ear drops OTC *antibacterial; antifungal* [acetic acid; aluminum acetate; boric acid]

**Starsis** (Japanese name for U.S. product Starlix)

**Starvisc** [see: Staarvisc]

**starwort; mealy starwort** *medicinal herb* [see: chickweed; star grass]

**Stat-Crit** electrode device for professional use *in vitro diagnostic aid for hemoglobin/hematocrit measurement*

**STATdose** (trademarked device) *pre-filled syringes for self-administration*

**Staticin** topical solution ℞ *antibiotic for acne* [erythromycin; alcohol 55%] 1.5%

**"statins"** *brief term for a class of antihyperlipidemics that include atorvastatin, cerivastatin, fluvastatin, lovastatin, pravastatin, rosuvastatin, and simvastatin* [properly called: HMG-CoA reductase inhibitors]

**statolon** USAN *antiviral* [also: vistatolon]

**Stat-One** gel (discontinued 2004) OTC *antiseptic* [hydrogen peroxide] 3%

**Stat-One** gel (discontinued 2004) OTC *antiseptic* [isopropyl alcohol] 70%

**Stat-Pak** (trademarked packaging form) *unit-dose package*

**Statuss Expectorant** oral liquid (discontinued 2002) ℞ *narcotic antitussive; decongestant; expectorant* [codeine phosphate; phenylpropanolamine HCl; guaifenesin; alcohol 5%] 10•12.5•100 mg/5 mL

**Statuss Green** oral liquid ℞ *narcotic antitussive; decongestant; antihistamine* [hydrocodone bitartrate; phenylephrine HCl; pseudoephedrine HCl; chlorpheniramine maleate; pyril-

amine maleate] 5•10•6.6•4•6.6 mg/10 mL

**staunch, blood** *medicinal herb* [see: fleabane; horseweed]

**stavudine** USAN, INN *nucleoside reverse transcriptase inhibitor; antiviral for HIV-1 infection*

**Stay Alert** tablets (discontinued 2001) OTC *CNS stimulant; analeptic* [caffeine] 200 mg

**Stay Awake** tablets OTC *CNS stimulant; analeptic* [caffeine] 200 mg

**Stay-Wet 3; Stay-Wet 4** solution OTC *disinfecting/wetting/soaking solution for rigid gas permeable contact lenses*

**STD (sodium tetradecyl sulfate)** [q.v.]

**steaglate** INN *combining name for radicals or groups*

**STEAM (streptonigrin, thioguanine, cyclophosphamide, actinomycin, mitomycin)** *chemotherapy protocol*

**stearethate 40** [see: polyoxyl 40 stearate]

**stearic acid** NF *emulsion adjunct; tablet and capsule lubricant*

**stearyl alcohol** NF *emulsion adjunct*

**stearyl dimethyl benzyl ammonium chloride**

**stearylsulfamide** INN

**Stedicor** *investigational antiarrhythmic* [azimilide dihydrochloride]

**steffimycin** USAN, INN *antibacterial; antiviral*

**Stelazine** film-coated tablets (discontinued 2003) ℞ *conventional (typical) antipsychotic; anxiolytic* [trifluoperazine HCl] 5 mg

**Stelazine** IM injection (discontinued 2003) ℞ *conventional (typical) antipsychotic; anxiolytic* [trifluoperazine HCl] 2 mg/mL

**Stelazine** oral concentrate (discontinued 2002) ℞ *conventional (typical) antipsychotic; anxiolytic* [trifluoperazine HCl] 10 mg/mL

**Stellaria media** *medicinal herb* [see: chickweed]

**Stemetil** Ⓒᴬᴺ film-coated tablets ℞ *conventional (typical) antipsychotic; anti-*

*emetic* [prochlorperazine bimaleate] 5, 10 mg

**Stemetil** ⓒ oral liquid, IV or IM injection ℞ *conventional (typical) antipsychotic; antiemetic* [prochlorperazine mesylate] 5 mg/5 mL; 5 mg/mL

**Stemetil** ⓒ suppositories ℞ *conventional (typical) antipsychotic; antiemetic* [prochlorperazine] 10 mg

**Stemgen** ⓒ powder for subcu injection ℞ *recombinant human stem cell factor; hematopoietic growth factor; adjunct to myelosuppressive and myeloablative therapy (investigational (NDA filed, orphan) in the U.S.)* [ancestim] 187.5 mg/vial

**stenbolone** INN *anabolic steroid; also abused as a street drug* [also: stenbolone acetate]

**stenbolone acetate** USAN *anabolic steroid; also abused as a street drug* [also: stenbolone]

**Step 2** creme rinse (discontinued 2003) OTC *for use following a pediculicide shampoo to remove lice eggs from hair*

**stepronin** INN

**Sterapred; Sterapred DS** tablets, Unipak (dispensing pack) ℞ *corticosteroid; anti-inflammatory* [prednisone] 5 mg; 10 mg

*Sterculia tragacantha; S. urens; S. villosa medicinal herb* [see: karaya gum]

**stercuronium iodide** INN

**Steri-Dose** (trademarked delivery system) *prefilled disposable syringe*

**SteriNail** solution OTC *topical antifungal* [undecylenic acid; tolnaftate] ② • ②

**Steri-Vial** (trademarked packaging form) *ampule*

**Sterules** (trademarked dosage form) *solution for nebulization*

**stevaladil** INN

*stevia (Stevia rebaudiana)* leaves *medicinal herb used as a non-caloric sugar substitute; also used for diabetes, food cravings, hypertension, obesity, and tobacco cravings*

**stibamine glucoside** INN, BAN

**stibocaptate** BAN [also: sodium stibocaptate]

**stibophen** NF

**stibosamine** INN

**stickwort; sticklewort** *medicinal herb* [see: agrimony]

**stigmata maidis (corn silk)** *medicinal herb* [see: Indian corn]

**stilbamidine isethionate** [see: stilbamidine isetionate]

**stilbamidine isetionate** INN

**stilbazium iodide** USAN, INN *anthelmintic*

**stilbestroform** [see: diethylstilbestrol]

**stilbestrol** [see: diethylstilbestrol] ② Stilphostrol

**stilbestronate** [see: diethylstilbestrol dipropionate]

**stilboestroform** [see: diethylstilbestrol]

**stilboestrol** BAN *estrogen* [also: diethylstilbestrol]

**stilboestrol DP** [see: diethylstilbestrol dipropionate]

*stillingia (Stillingia ligustina)* root *medicinal herb for acne, eczema, and other skin disorders, blood cleansing, liver disorders, respiratory illnesses, and syphilis*

**Stilnoct; Stilnox** (European name for U.S. product Ambien)

**stilonium iodide** USAN, INN *antispasmodic*

**Stilphostrol** tablets, IV injection (discontinued 2001) ℞ *hormonal antineoplastic for palliative therapy of advanced prostatic carcinoma* [diethylstilbestrol diphosphate] 50 mg; 250 mg ② Disophrol; stilbestrol

**stilronate** [see: diethylstilbestrol dipropionate]

**Stimate** nasal spray ℞ *posterior pituitary hormone for hemophilia A and von Willebrand disease (orphan)* [desmopressin acetate] 150 μg (600 IU)/dose

**stimulant laxatives** *a subclass of laxatives that work by direct action on the intestinal mucosa and nerve plexus to increase peristaltic action* [see also: laxatives]

**stimulants** *a class of agents that excite the activity of physiological processes*

**Sting-Eze** concentrate OTC *topical antihistamine; antipruritic; anesthetic; bacteriostatic* [diphenhydramine HCl; camphor; phenol; benzocaine; eucalyptol]

**stinging nettle** *medicinal herb* [see: nettle]

**Sting-Kill** swabs OTC *topical local anesthetic* [benzocaine; menthol] 20%•1%

**stingless nettle** *medicinal herb* [see: blind nettle]

**stinking nightshade** *medicinal herb* [see: henbane]

**stirimazole** INN, BAN

**stiripentol** USAN, INN *anticonvulsant*

**stirocainide** INN

**stirofos** USAN *veterinary insecticide*

**stitchwort** *medicinal herb* [see: chickweed]

**Stoko Gard** cream (discontinued 2003) OTC *protection from the effects of poison ivy*

**stomachics** *a class of agents that promote the functional activity of the stomach*

**stone root (Collinsonia canadensis)** roots and leaves *medicinal herb used as a diuretic and vulnerary*

**Stool Softener** capsules OTC *laxative; stool softener* [docusate sodium] 100, 250 mg

**Stool Softener; Stool Softener DC** capsules OTC *laxative; stool softener* [docusate calcium] 240 mg

**stool-softening laxatives** *a subclass of laxatives that work by increasing the amount of fat and water in the stool to ease its movement through the intestines* [see also: laxatives]

**Stop** gel ℞ *topical dental caries preventative* [stannous fluoride] 0.4%

**storax** USP

**storax (Liquidambar orientalis; L. styraciflua)** leaves and gum *medicinal herb for diarrhea, inducing expectoration, parasitic infections, promoting sweating and diuresis, skin sores and wounds, and sore throat*

**Storzfen** eye drops ℞ *topical ophthalmic decongestant and vasoconstrictor; mydriatic* [phenylephrine HCl] 2.5%

**Storzine 2** eye drops ℞ *topical antiglaucoma agent; direct-acting miotic* [pilocarpine HCl] 2%

**Storz-N-D** eye drops ℞ *topical ophthalmic corticosteroidal anti-inflammatory; antibiotic* [dexamethasone sodium phosphate; neomycin sulfate] 0.1%•0.35%

**Storz-N-P-D** eye drop suspension ℞ *topical ophthalmic corticosteroidal anti-inflammatory; antibiotic* [dexamethasone; neomycin sulfate; polymyxin B sulfate] 0.1%•0.35%•10 000 U/mL

**Storz-Sulf** eye drops ℞ *antibiotic* [sulfacetamide sodium] 10%

**stramonium** [see: jimsonweed]

**Strattera** capsules ℞ *non-stimulant treatment for attention-deficit hyperactivity disorder (ADHD); investigational (orphan) for Tourette syndrome* [atomoxetine HCl] 10, 18, 25, 40, 60 mg

**strawberry (Fragaria vesca)** leaves *medicinal herb for blood cleansing, diarrhea, eczema, intestinal disorders, preventing miscarriage, and stomach cleansing*

**strawberry bush; strawberry tree** *medicinal herb* [see: wahoo]

**Strep Detect** slide tests for professional use *in vitro diagnostic aid for streptococcal antigens in throat swabs*

**Streptase** powder for IV or intracoronary infusion ℞ *thrombolytic enzyme for lysis of thrombi and catheter clearance* [streptokinase] 250 000, 750 000, 1 500 000 IU ⊡ Streptonase

**streptodornase (SD)** INN, BAN

**streptoduocin** USP

**streptogramins** *a class of antibiotics, isolated from Streptomyces pristinaespirales, used for gram-positive infections*

**streptokinase (SK)** INN *thrombolytic enzymes for myocardial infarction, thrombosis or embolism* ⊡ Streptonase

**streptomycin** INN, BAN *aminoglycoside antibiotic; primary tuberculostatic* [also: streptomycin sulfate]

**streptomycin sulfate** USP *aminoglycoside antibiotic; primary tuberculostatic* [also: streptomycin] 1 g injection

**Streptonase-B** test kit for professional use *in vitro diagnostic test for DNAse-B streptococcal antigens in serum* ② Streptase; streptokinase

**streptoniazid** INN *antibacterial* [also: streptonicozid]

**streptonicozid** USAN *antibacterial* [also: streptoniazid]

**streptonigrin (SN)** USAN *antineoplastic* [also: rufocromomycin]

**streptovarycin** INN

**streptozocin** USAN, INN *nitrosourea-type alkylating antineoplastic for metastatic islet cell carcinoma of the pancreas*

**streptozotocin** [see: streptozocin]

**Streptozyme** slide tests for professional use *in vitro diagnostic test for streptococcal extracellular antigens in blood, plasma, and serum*

**Stress 600 with Zinc** tablets OTC *vitamin/mineral supplement* [multiple vitamins & minerals; folic acid; biotin] ± •400•45 μg

**Stress B Complex** tablets OTC *vitamin/mineral supplement* [multiple vitamins & minerals; folic acid; biotin] ± •400•45 μg

**Stress B Complex with Vitamin C** timed-release tablets OTC *vitamin/mineral supplement* [multiple B vitamins; vitamin C; zinc] ± •300•15 mg

**Stress Formula 600** tablets OTC *vitamin supplement* [multiple vitamins; folic acid; biotin] ± •400•45 μg

**Stress Formula Vitamins** capsules, tablets OTC *vitamin supplement* [multiple vitamins; folic acid; biotin] ± •400•45 μg

**Stress Formula with Iron** film-coated tablets OTC *vitamin/iron supplement* [multiple B vitamins; vitamins C and E; ferrous fumarate; folic acid; biotin] ± •500 mg•30 IU•27 mg•0.4 mg•45 μg

**Stress Formula with Zinc** tablets OTC *vitamin/iron supplement* [multiple B vitamins; vitamins C and E; multiple minerals; folic acid; biotin] ± •500 mg•30 IU• ± •0.4 mg•45 μg

**StressForm "605" with Iron** tablets (discontinued 2003) OTC *vitamin/iron supplement* [multiple B vitamins; vitamins C and E; iron; folic acid; biotin] ± •605 mg•30 IU•27 mg•0.4 mg•45 μg

**Stresstabs** tablets OTC *vitamin supplement* [multiple vitamins; folic acid; biotin] ± •400•45 μg

**Stresstabs + Iron** film-coated tablets OTC *vitamin/iron supplement* [multiple B vitamins; vitamins C and E; ferrous fumarate; folic acid; biotin] ± •500 mg•30 IU•18 mg•0.4 mg•45 μg

**Stresstabs + Zinc** film-coated tablets OTC *vitamin/mineral supplement* [multiple vitamins & minerals; folic acid; biotin] ± •400•45 μg

**Stresstein** powder OTC *enteral nutritional therapy for moderate to severe stress or trauma* [multiple branched chain amino acids]

**Striant** mucoadhesive buccal tablets ℞ *hormone replacement therapy for male hypogonadism* [testosterone] 30 mg

**Stri-Dex** pads OTC *keratolytic cleanser* [salicylic acid; alcohol] 0.5%•28%, 2%•44%, 2%•54%

**Stri-Dex Cleansing** bar OTC *medicated cleanser for acne* [triclosan] 1%

**Stri-Dex Clear** gel OTC *keratolytic cleanser for acne* [salicylic acid; alcohol] 2%•9.3%

**Stri-Dex Face Wash** solution OTC *medicated cleanser for acne* [triclosan] 1%

**strinoline** INN

**striped alder** medicinal herb [see: winterberry; witch hazel]

**Stromectol** tablets ℞ *anthelmintic for strongyloidiasis and onchocerciasis* [ivermectin] 3, 6 mg

**strong ammonia solution** [see: ammonia solution, strong]

**Strong Iodine** solution, tincture ℞ *thyroid-blocking therapy; topical antimicrobial* [iodine; potassium iodide] 5%•10%; 7%•5%

**stronger rose water** [see: rose water, stronger]

**StrongStart** caplets ℞ *vitamin/mineral/ calcium/iron supplement; stool softener* [multiple vitamins & minerals; calcium; iron; folic acid; docusate sodium] ± • 200 • 29 • 1 • 25 mg

**StrongStart** chewable tablets ℞ *vitamin/ mineral/calcium/iron supplement* [multiple vitamins & minerals; calcium; iron; folic acid] ± • 200 • 29 • 1 mg

**strontium** *element (Sr)*

**strontium chloride** *topical anti-irritant*

**strontium chloride Sr 85** USAN *radioactive agent*

**strontium chloride Sr 89** USAN *radioactive agent; analgesic for metastatic bone pain*

**strontium nitrate Sr 85** USAN *radioactive agent*

**strontium salicylate** NF

**strontium Sr 85** USP

**Strovite** tablets ℞ *vitamin supplement* [multiple B vitamins; vitamin C; folic acid] ± • 500 • 0.5 mg

**Strovite Advance; Strovite Forte; Strovite Plus** caplets ℞ *geriatric vitamin/mineral therapy* [multiple vitamins & minerals; folic acid; biotin] ± • 1000 • 100 μg; ± • 1000 • 150 μg; ± • 800 • 150 μg

**structum** *natural remedy* [see: chondroitin sulfate]

**strychnine** NF *an extremely poisonous CNS stimulant; occasionally abused as a street drug in combination with LSD*

**strychnine glycerophosphate** NF

**strychnine nitrate** NF

**strychnine phosphate** NF

**strychnine sulfate** NF

**strychnine valerate** NF

**Stuart Formula** tablets OTC *vitamin/ mineral/iron supplement* [multiple vitamins & minerals; iron; folic acid] ± • 18 • 0.1 mg

**Stuart Prenatal** tablets OTC *vitamin/ calcium/iron supplement* [multiple vitamins; calcium; iron; folic acid] ± • 200 • 28 • 0.8 mg

**StuartNatal Plus** tablets (discontinued 2003) ℞ *vitamin/calcium/iron supplement* [multiple vitamins; calcium; iron; folic acid] ± • 200 • 65 • 1 mg

**StuartNatal Plus 3** tablets ℞ *vitamin/ calcium/iron supplement* [multiple vitamins; calcium; iron; folic acid] ± • 200 • 28 • 1 mg

**stugeron** [see: cinnarizine]

**stutgin** [see: cinnarizine]

**Stye** ophthalmic ointment OTC *emollient* [white petrolatum; mineral oil; boric acid]

**styptics** *a class of hemostatic agents that stop bleeding of the skin by astringent action* [see also: astringents; hemostatics]

**Stypto-Caine** solution OTC *to stop bleeding of minor cuts* [aluminum chloride; tetracaine HCl; oxyquinoline sulfate] 250 • 2.5 • 1 mg/g

**styramate** INN

**styronate resins**

**SU-5416** *investigational (Phase III) angiogenesis inhibitor for colorectal and non–small cell lung cancers (NSCLC); investigational (Phase II/III) for AIDS-related Kaposi sarcoma*

**subathizone** INN

**Subdue** ⓒ oral liquid OTC *enteral nutritional therapy for patients with inflammatory bowel disease*

**subendazole** INN

**Sublimaze** IV or IM injection ℞ *narcotic analgesic; anesthetic* [fentanyl citrate] 0.05 mg/mL

**sublimed sulfur** [see: sulfur, sublimed]

**Sublingual B Total** drops OTC *vitamin supplement* [multiple B vitamins; vitamin C] ± • 60 mg/mL

**Suboxone** sublingual tablets ℞ *narcotic agonist-antagonist analgesic for outpatient maintenance of opiate dependence (orphan)* [buprenorphine HCl; naloxone HCl] 2 • 0.5, 8 • 2 mg

**substance F** [see: demecolcine]

**substituted benzimidazoles** *a class of gastric antisecretory agents that inhibit the ATPase "proton pump" within the gastric parietal cell* [also called: proton pump inhibitors; ATPase inhibitors]

**Subutex** sublingual tablets ℞ *narcotic agonist-antagonist analgesic for inpatient treatment of opiate dependence (orphan)* [buprenorphine HCl] 2, 8 mg

**Suby G solution; Suby solution G (citric acid, magnesium oxide, sodium carbonate)** *urologic irrigant to dissolve phosphatic calculi*

**succimer** USAN, INN, BAN *heavy metal chelating agent for lead poisoning (orphan); investigational (orphan) for mercury poisoning and cysteine kidney stones*

**succinchlorimide** NF

**succinimides** *a class of anticonvulsants*

**succinylcholine chloride** USP *neuromuscular blocker; muscle relaxant; anesthesia adjunct* [also: suxamethonium chloride] 20 mg/mL injection

**succinyldapsone** [see: succisulfone]

**succinylsulfathiazole** USP

**succisulfone** INN

**succory** *medicinal herb* [see: chicory]

**Succus Cineraria Maritima** eye drops ℞ *treatment for optic opacity caused by cataract* [senecio compositae; hamamelis water; boric acid]

**suclofenide** INN, BAN

**Sucraid** oral solution ℞ *enzyme replacement therapy for congenital sucrase-isomaltase deficiency (orphan)* [sacrosidase] 8500 IU/mL

**sucralfate** USAN, INN, BAN *cytoprotective agent for gastric ulcers; investigational (orphan) for oral mucositis and stomatitis following cancer radiation or chemotherapy* 1 g oral; 1 g/10 mL oral

**sucralose** BAN

**sucralox** INN, BAN

**Sucrets** throat spray OTC *antipruritic/counterirritant; mild local anesthetic* [dyclonine HCl] 0.1%

**Sucrets Children's Sore Throat; Vapor Lemon Sucrets; Sucrets Maximum Strength** lozenges OTC *antipruritic/counterirritant; mild local anesthetic* [dyclonine HCl] 1.2 mg; 2 mg; 3 mg

**Sucrets Cough Control; Sucrets 4-Hour Cough** lozenges (discontinued 2002) OTC *antitussive* [dextromethorphan hydrobromide] 5 mg; 15 mg

**Sucrets Sore Throat** lozenges OTC *oral antiseptic* [hexylresorcinol] 2.4 mg

**sucrose** NF *flavoring agent; tablet excipient* ⁇ sucrase

**sucrose octaacetate** NF *alcohol denaturant*

**sucrosofate potassium** USAN *antiulcerative*

**Sudafed** tablets OTC *nasal decongestant* [pseudoephedrine HCl] 30, 60 mg

**Sudafed, Children's** chewable tablets OTC *nasal decongestant* [pseudoephedrine HCl] 15 mg

**Sudafed, Children's Non-Drowsy** oral liquid OTC *nasal decongestant* [pseudoephedrine HCl] 15 mg/5 mL

**Sudafed Children's Non-Drowsy Cold & Cough** oral liquid OTC *antitussive; decongestant* [dextromethorphan hydrobromide; pseudoephedrine HCl] 5•15 mg/5 mL

**Sudafed Cold & Allergy** tablets OTC *decongestant; antihistamine* [pseudoephedrine HCl; chlorpheniramine maleate] 60•4 mg

**Sudafed Cold & Sinus Non-Drowsy** Liqui-Caps (liquid-filled gelcaps) OTC *decongestant; analgesic; antipyretic* [pseudoephedrine HCl; acetaminophen] 30•325 mg

**Sudafed Multi-Symptom Cold & Cough** liquid caps OTC *antitussive; decongestant; expectorant; analgesic* [dextromethorphan hydrobromide; pseudoephedrine HCl; guaifenesin; acetaminophen] 10•30•100•250 mg

**Sudafed Non-Drowsy** tablets OTC *nasal decongestant* [pseudoephedrine HCl] 30 mg

**Sudafed Non-Drowsy 12 Hour Long Acting** extended-release caplets OTC *nasal decongestant* [pseudoephedrine HCl] 120 mg

**Sudafed Non-Drowsy 24 Hour Long Acting** dual-release tablets OTC *nasal decongestant* [pseudoephedrine HCl] 240 mg (60 mg immediate release, 180 mg extended release)

**Sudafed Non-Drowsy Non-Drying Sinus** liquid-filled capsules OTC *decongestant; expectorant* [pseudoephedrine HCl; guaifenesin] 30•120 mg

**Sudafed Non-Drowsy Severe Cold Formula** caplets OTC *antitussive; decongestant; analgesic* [dextromethorphan hydrobromide; pseudoephedrine HCl; acetaminophen] 15•30•500 mg

**Sudafed Plus** tablets (name changed to Sudafed Cold & Allergy in 2002)

**Sudafed Severe Cold** tablets (discontinued 2002) OTC *antitussive; decongestant; analgesic* [dextromethorphan hydrobromide; pseudoephedrine HCl; acetaminophen] 15•30•500 mg

**Sudafed Sinus Advance** ⒸⒶⓃ caplets OTC *decongestant; analgesic; antipyretic* [pseudoephedrine HCl; ibuprofen] 30•200 mg

**Sudafed Sinus Headache Non-Drowsy** tablets, caplets OTC *decongestant; analgesic; antipyretic* [pseudoephedrine HCl; acetaminophen] 30•500 mg

**Sudafed Sinus Nighttime** tablets OTC *decongestant; antihistamine* [pseudoephedrine HCl; triprolidine HCl] 60•2.5 mg

**Sudafed Sinus Nighttime Plus Pain Relief** caplets OTC *decongestant; antihistamine; analgesic* [pseudoephedrine HCl; diphenhydramine HCl; acetaminophen] 30•25•500 mg

**Sudal 60/500** sustained-release caplets ℞ *decongestant; expectorant* [pseudoephedrine HCl; guaifenesin] 60•500 mg

**Sudal-DM** sustained-release tablets ℞ *antitussive; expectorant* [dextromethorphan hydrobromide; guaifenesin] 30•500 mg

**sudexanox** INN

**sudismase** INN

**Sudodrin** tablets OTC *nasal decongestant* [pseudoephedrine HCl] 30 mg

**SudoGest** tablets OTC *decongestant* [pseudoephedrine HCl] 60 mg

**SudoGest Children's Syrup** OTC *antitussive; decongestant* [dextromethor-

phan hydrobromide; pseudoephedrine HCl] 5•15 mg/5 mL

**SudoGest Cold & Allergy** tablets OTC *decongestant; antihistamine* [pseudoephedrine HCl; chlorpheniramine maleate] 60•4 mg

**SudoGest Sinus** tablets OTC *decongestant; analgesic; antipyretic* [pseudoephedrine HCl; acetaminophen] 30•500 mg

**sudorifics** a class of agents that promote profuse perspiration [also called: diaphoretics]

**sudoxicam** USAN, INN *anti-inflammatory*

**Sufenta** IV injection ℞ *narcotic analgesic; anesthetic* [sufentanil citrate] 50 μg/mL

**sufentanil** USAN, INN, BAN *narcotic analgesic; investigational (Phase III) for cancer-related pain*

**sufentanil citrate** USAN *narcotic analgesic* 50 μg/mL injection

**sufosfamide** INN

**sufotidine** USAN, INN, BAN *antagonist to histamine $H_2$ receptors*

**sugar, compressible** NF *flavoring agent; tablet excipient*

**sugar, confectioner's** NF *flavoring agent; tablet excipient*

**sugar, invert (50% dextrose & 50% fructose)** USP *fluid and nutrient replenisher; caloric replacement*

**sugar spheres** NF *solid carrier vehicle*

**sulamserod HCl** USAN *selective 5-$HT_4$ receptor antagonist; antiarrhythmic; treatment for urge incontinence*

**Sulamyd** [see: Sodium Sulamyd]

**Sular** extended-release tablets ℞ *calcium channel blocker for hypertension* [nisoldipine] 10, 20, 30, 40 mg

**sulazepam** USAN, INN *minor tranquilizer*

**sulbactam** INN, BAN *β-lactamase inhibitor; penicillin/cephalosporin synergist*

**sulbactam benzathine** USAN *β-lactamase inhibitor; penicillin/cephalosporin synergist*

**sulbactam pivoxil** USAN *β-lactamase inhibitor; penicillin/cephalosporin synergist* [also: pivsulbactam]

**sulbactam sodium** USAN, USP *β-lactamase inhibitor; penicillin/cephalosporin synergist*

**sulbenicillin** INN

**sulbenox** USAN, INN *veterinary growth stimulant*

**sulbentine** INN

**sulbutiamine** INN [also: bisibutiamine]

**sulclamide** INN

**sulconazole** INN, BAN *antifungal* [also: sulconazole nitrate]

**sulconazole nitrate** USAN, USP *topical antifungal* [also: sulconazole]

**sulergine** [see: disulergine]

**sulesomab** USAN *monoclonal antibody; diagnostic aid for infectious lesions* [also: technetium Tc 99m sulesomab]

**Sulf-10** eye drops R *ophthalmic antibiotic* [sulfacetamide sodium] 10% ⑨ Sulten-10

**sulfabenz** USAN, INN *antibacterial; coccidiostat for poultry*

**sulfabenzamide** USAN, USP, INN *bacteriostatic antibiotic*

**sulfabromomethazine sodium** NF

**sulfacarbamide** INN [also: sulphaurea]

**sulfacecole** INN

**sulfacetamide** USP, INN *bacteriostatic antibiotic*

**sulfacetamide sodium** USP *bacteriostatic antibiotic* 10%, 30% eye drops

**Sulfacet-R** lotion R *acne treatment* [sulfacetamide sodium; sulfur] 10%•5%

**sulfachlorpyridazine** INN

**sulfachrysoidine** INN

**sulfacitine** INN *antibacterial* [also: sulfacytine]

**sulfaclomide** INN

**sulfaclorazole** INN

**sulfaclozine** INN

**sulfacombin** [see: sulfadiazine]

**sulfacytine** USAN *broad-spectrum bacteriostatic* [also: sulfacitine]

**sulfadiasulfone sodium** INN *antibacterial; leprostatic* [also: acetosulfone sodium]

**sulfadiazine** USP, INN, JAN *broad-spectrum sulfonamide bacteriostatic* [also: sulphadiazine] 500 mg oral

**sulfadiazine & pyrimethamine** *oral Toxoplasma gondii encephalitis treatment (orphan)*

**sulfadiazine silver** JAN *broad-spectrum bactericidal; adjunct to burn therapy* [also: silver sulfadiazine]

**sulfadiazine sodium** USP, INN *antibacterial* [also: sulphadiazine sodium]

**sulfadicramide** INN, DCF

**sulfadicrolamide** [see: sulfadicramide]

**sulfadimethoxine** NF [also: sulphadimethoxine]

**sulfadimidine** INN, BAN *antibacterial* [also: sulfamethazine]

**sulfadoxine** USAN, USP *bacteriostatic; antimalarial adjunct*

**sulfaethidole** NF, INN [also: sulphaethidole]

**sulfafurazole** INN *broad-spectrum sulfonamide bacteriostatic* [also: sulfisoxazole; sulphafurazole]

**sulfaguanidine** NF, INN

**sulfaguanole** INN

**sulfaisodimidine** [see: sulfisomidine]

**sulfalene** USAN, INN *antibacterial* [also: sulfametopyrazine]

**sulfaloxic acid** INN [also: sulphaloxic acid]

**sulfamates** *a class of broad-spectrum anticonvulsants*

**sulfamazone** INN

**sulfamerazine** USP, INN *broad-spectrum bacteriostatic*

**sulfamerazine sodium** NF, INN

**sulfameter** USAN *antibacterial* [also: sulfametoxydiazine; sulfamethoxydiazine]

**sulfamethazine** USP *broad-spectrum bacteriostatic* [also: sulfadimidine]

**sulfamethizole** USP, INN, JAN *broad-spectrum sulfonamide bacteriostatic* [also: sulphamethizole] ⑨ sulfamethoxazole

**sulfamethoxazole (SMX; SMZ)** USAN, USP, INN, JAN *broad-spectrum sulfonamide antibiotic* [also: sulphamethoxazole; acetylsulfamethoxazole; sulfamethoxazole sodium] ⑨ sulfamethizole

**sulfamethoxazole sodium** JAN *broad-spectrum sulfonamide antibiotic* [also:

sulfamethoxazole; sulphamethoxazole; acetylsulfamethoxazole]

**sulfamethoxydiazine** BAN *antibacterial*
[also: sulfameter; sulfametoxydiazine]

**sulfamethoxypyridazine** USP, INN
[also: sulphamethoxypyridazine]

**sulfamethoxypyridazine acetyl**

**sulfametin** [see: sulfameter]

**sulfametomidine** INN

**sulfametopyrazine** BAN *antibacterial*
[also: sulfalene]

**sulfametoxydiazine** INN *antibacterial*
[also: sulfameter; sulfamethoxydiazine]

**sulfametrole** INN, BAN

**sulfamidothiodiazol** [see: glybuzole]

**sulfamonomethoxine** USAN, INN,
BAN *antibacterial*

**sulfamoxole** USAN, INN *antibacterial*
[also: sulphamoxole]

**p-sulfamoylbenzoic acid** [see: carze-
nide]

**4′-sulfamoylsuccinanilic acid** [see:
sulfasuccinamide]

**Sulfamylon** cream ℞ *broad-spectrum
bacteriostatic for second- and third-degree
burns* [mafenide acetate] 85 mg/g

**Sulfamylon** powder for topical solution ℞ *broad-spectrum bacteriostatic
to prevent meshed autograft loss on sec-
ond- and third-degree burns (orphan)*
[mafenide acetate] 5%

**sulfanilamide** NF, INN *broad-spectrum
sulfonamide antibiotic* 15% topical

**sulfanilanilide** [see: sulfabenz]

**sulfanilate zinc** USAN *antibacterial*

**N-sulfanilylacetamide** [see: sulfaceta-
mide]

**N-sulfanilylacetamide monosodium
salt monohydrate** [see: sulfacetamide sodium]

**N-p-sulfanilylphenylglycine sodium**
[see: acediasulfone sodium]

**N-sulfanilylstearamide** [see: stearyl-
sulfamide]

**4′-sulfanilylsuccinanilic acid** [see:
succisulfone]

**sulfanilylurea** [see: sulfacarbamide]

**sulfanitran** USAN, INN, BAN *antibacterial; coccidiostat for poultry*

**sulfaperin** INN

**sulfaphenazole** INN [also: sulpha-
phenazole]

**sulfaphtalythiazol** [see: phthalysulfa-
thiazole]

**sulfaproxyline** INN [also: sulpha-
proxyline]

**sulfapyrazole** INN, BAN *antibacterial*
[also: sulfazamet]

**sulfapyridine** USP, INN *investigational
(orphan) dermatitis herpetiformis suppressant* [also: sulphapyridine]

**sulfapyridine sodium** NF

**sulfaquinoxaline** INN, BAN

**sulfarsphenamine** NF, INN

**sulfasalazine** USAN, USP, INN *broad-
spectrum bacteriostatic; antirheumatic;
anti-inflammatory for ulcerative colitis*
[also: sulphasalazine; salazosulfapyri-
dine] 500 mg oral

**sulfasomizole** USAN, INN *antibacterial*
[also: sulphasomizole]

**sulfastearyl** [see: stearylsulfamide]

**sulfasuccinamide** INN

**sulfasymazine** INN

**sulfated polysaccharide peptidogly-
can (SPPG)** [see: tecogalan sodium]

**sulfathiazole** USP, INN *bacteriostatic
antibiotic* [also: sulphathiazole] ② sulfisoxazole

**sulfathiazole sodium** NF

**sulfathiocarbamide** [see: sulfathiourea]

**sulfathiourea** INN

**sulfatolamide** INN

**Sulfatrim** oral suspension ℞ *anti-infective; antibacterial* [trimethoprim; sul-
famethoxazole] 40•200 mg/5 mL

**sulfatroxazole** INN

**sulfatrozole** INN

**sulfazamet** USAN *antibacterial* [also:
sulfapyrazole]

**sulfinalol** INN *antihypertensive* [also:
sulfinalol HCl]

**sulfinalol HCl** USAN *antihypertensive*
[also: sulfinalol]

**sulfinpyrazone** USP, INN *uricosuric for
gout* [also: sulphinpyrazone] 100, 200
mg oral

**sulfiram** INN [also: monosulfiram]

**sulfisomidine** [also: sulphasomidine]

**sulfisoxazole** USP, JAN *broad-spectrum sulfonamide antibiotic* [also: sulfafurazole; sulphafurazole] 500 mg oral ⑨ sulfathiazole

**sulfisoxazole acetyl** USP *broad-spectrum sulfonamide antibiotic*

**sulfisoxazole diolamine** USAN, USP *broad-spectrum sulfonamide antibiotic*

**Sulfoam** shampoo OTC *antiseborrheic; keratolytic* [sulfur] 2%

**sulfobenzylpenicillin** [see: sulbenicillin]

**sulfobromophthalein sodium** USP *hepatic function test*

**sulfobromphthalein sodium** [see: sulfobromophthalein sodium]

**sulfocon B** USAN *hydrophobic contact lens material*

**sulfogaiacol** INN *expectorant* [also: potassium guaiacolsulfonate]

**Sulfoil** topical liquid OTC *soap-free therapeutic skin cleanser* [sulfonated castor oil]

**sulfomyxin** USAN, INN *antibacterial* [also: sulphomyxin sodium]

**sulfonal** [see: sulfonmethane]

**sulfonamides** *a class of broad-spectrum bacteriostatic antibiotics effective against both gram-positive and gram-negative organisms*

**sulfonated hydrogenated castor oil** [see: hydroxystearin sulfate]

**sulfonethylmethane** NF

**sulfonmethane** NF

**sulfonterol** INN *bronchodilator* [also: sulfonterol HCl]

**sulfonterol HCl** USAN *bronchodilator* [also: sulfonterol]

**sulfonylureas** *a class of antidiabetic agents that stimulate insulin production in the pancreas*

**Sulforcin** lotion OTC *topical acne treatment* [sulfur; resorcinol; alcohol] 5%•2%•11.65%

**sulforidazine** INN

**sulfosalicylic acid**

**sulfoxone sodium** USP *antibacterial; leprostatic* [also: aldesulfone sodium]

**Sulfoxyl Regular; Sulfoxyl Strong** lotion ℞ *keratolytic for acne* [benzoyl peroxide; sulfur] 5%•2%; 10%•5%

**sulfur** *element (S)* [see: sulfur, precipitated; sulfur, sublimed]

**sulfur, precipitated** USP *scabicide; topical antibacterial; topical exfoliant*

**sulfur, sublimed** USP *scabicide; topical antibacterial; topical exfoliant*

**sulfur dioxide** NF *antioxidant*

**sulfur hexafluoride** USAN *ultrasound imaging agent*

**Sulfur Soap** bar OTC *medicated cleanser for acne* [precipitated sulfur] 10%

**sulfurated lime solution** [see: lime, sulfurated]

**sulfurated potash** [see: potash, sulfurated]

**sulfuric acid** NF *acidifying agent*

**sulfuric acid, aluminum ammonium salt, dodecahydrate** [see: alum, ammonium]

**sulfuric acid, aluminum potassium salt, dodecahydrate** [see: alum, potassium]

**sulfuric acid, aluminum salt, hydrate** [see: aluminum sulfate]

**sulfuric acid, barium salt** [see: barium sulfate]

**sulfuric acid, calcium salt** [see: calcium sulfate]

**sulfuric acid, copper salt pentahydrate** [see: cupric sulfate]

**sulfuric acid, disodium salt decahydrate** [see: sodium sulfate]

**sulfuric acid, magnesium salt** [see: magnesium sulfate]

**sulfuric acid, manganese salt** [see: manganese sulfate]

**sulfuric acid, zinc salt hydrate** [see: zinc sulfate]

**sulfurous acid, monosodium salt** [see: sodium bisulfite]

**sulglicotide** INN [also: sulglycotide]

**sulglycotide** BAN [also: sulglicotide]

**sulicrinat** INN

**sulindac** USAN, USP, INN, BAN *antiarthritic; nonsteroidal anti-inflammatory drug (NSAID) for ankylosing spondyli-*

*tis and acute bursitis/tendinitis* 150, 200 mg oral ⒹⒷ Zoladex

**sulisatin** INN

**sulisobenzone** USAN, INN *ultraviolet screen*

**sulmarin** USAN, INN *hemostatic*

**Sulmasque** mask OTC *antibacterial and exfoliant for acne* [sulfur] 6.4%

**sulmazole** INN

**sulmepride** INN

**sulnidazole** USAN, INN *antiprotozoal (Trichomonas)*

**sulocarbilate** INN

**suloctidil** USAN, INN, BAN *peripheral vasodilator*

**sulodexide** INN *investigational (Phase III) glycosaminoglycan for diabetic neuropathy*

**sulofenur** USAN, INN *antineoplastic*

**sulopenem** USAN, INN *antibacterial*

**sulosemide** INN

**sulotroban** USAN, INN, BAN *treatment for glomerulonephritis*

**suloxifen** INN *bronchodilator* [also: suloxifen oxalate]

**suloxifen oxalate** USAN *bronchodilator* [also: suloxifen]

**sulphabutin** [see: busulfan]

**sulphadiazine** BAN *broad-spectrum bacteriostatic* [also: sulfadiazine]

**sulphadiazine sodium** BAN *antibacterial* [also: sulfadiazine sodium]

**sulphadimethoxine** BAN [also: sulfadimethoxine]

**sulphaethidole** BAN [also: sulfaethidole]

**sulphafurazole** BAN *broad-spectrum sulfonamide bacteriostatic* [also: sulfisoxazole; sulfafurazole]

**sulphaloxic acid** BAN [also: sulfaloxic acid]

**sulphamethizole** BAN *broad-spectrum sulfonamide bacteriostatic* [also: sulfamethizole]

**sulphamethoxazole** BAN *broad-spectrum sulfonamide bacteriostatic* [also: sulfamethoxazole; acetylsulfamethoxazole; sulfamethoxazole sodium]

**sulphamethoxypyridazine** BAN [also: sulfamethoxypyridazine]

**sulphamoxole** BAN *antibacterial* [also: sulfamoxole]

**sulphan blue** BAN *lymphangiography aid* [also: isosulfan blue]

**sulphaphenazole** BAN [also: sulfaphenazole]

**sulphaproxyline** BAN [also: sulfaproxyline]

**sulphapyridine** BAN *dermatitis herpetiformis suppressant* [also: sulfapyridine]

**sulphasalazine** BAN *broad-spectrum bacteriostatic; antirheumatic; antiinflammatory for ulcerative colitis* [also: sulfasalazine; salazosulfapyridine]

**sulphasomidine** BAN [also: sulfisomidine]

**sulphasomizole** BAN *antibacterial* [also: sulfasomizole]

**sulphathiazole** BAN *antibacterial* [also: sulfathiazole]

**sulphaurea** BAN [also: sulfacarbamide]

**sulphinpyrazone** BAN *uricosuric for gout* [also: sulfinpyrazone]

**sulphocarbolate sodium** [see: phenolsulphonate sodium]

**Sulpho-Lac** cream, soap OTC *antibacterial and exfoliant for acne* [sulfur] 5%

**Sulpho-Lac Acne Medication** cream OTC *antibacterial; exfoliant* [sulfur; zinc sulfate] 5%•27%

**sulphomyxin sodium** BAN *antibacterial* [also: sulfomyxin]

**sulphonal** [see: sulfonmethane]

**sulpiride** USAN, INN *antidepressant*

**sulprosal** INN

**sulprostone** USAN, INN *prostaglandin*

**sultamicillin** USAN, INN, BAN *antibacterial*

**sulthiame** USAN *anticonvulsant* [also: sultiame]

**sultiame** INN *anticonvulsant* [also: sulthiame]

**sultopride** INN

**sultosilic acid** INN

**Sultrin Triple Sulfa** vaginal inserts, vaginal cream (discontinued 2001) ℞ *broad-spectrum antibiotic* [sulfathiazole; sulfacetamide; sulfabenzamide] 172.5•143.75•184 mg; 3.42%•2.86%•3.7%

**sultroponium** INN

**sulukast** USAN, INN *antiasthmatic; leukotriene antagonist*

**sulverapride** INN

**suma** *(Pfaffia paniculata)* bark and root *medicinal herb for circulatory disorders, chronic disease, fatigue, hormone regulation, immune system stimulation, lowering cholesterol levels, and stress; also used as a tonic*

**Sumacal** powder OTC *carbohydrate caloric supplement* [glucose polymers]

**sumacetamol** INN, BAN

**sumach** *(Rhus glabra)* bark, leaves, and berries *medicinal herb used as an antiseptic, astringent, diaphoretic, diuretic, emmenagogue, febrifuge, and refrigerant*

**sumarotene** USAN, INN *keratolytic*

**sumatriptan** INN, BAN *vascular serotonin 5-HT$_1$ receptor agonist for the acute treatment of migraine headaches* [also: sumatriptan succinate]

**sumatriptan succinate** USAN *vascular serotonin 5-HT$_1$ receptor agonist for the acute treatment of migraine and cluster headaches* [also: sumatriptan]

**sumetizide** INN

**summer savory** *(Calamintha hortensis; Satureja hortensis)* leaves and stems *medicinal herb for diarrhea, nausea, promoting expectoration, relieving gas and flatulence, and stimulation of menstruation; also used as an aphrodisiac*

**Summer's Eve Disposable Douche** solution OTC *antifungal; vaginal cleanser and deodorizer; acidity modifier* [sodium benzoate; citric acid]

**Summer's Eve Disposable Douche; Summer's Eve Disposable Douche Extra Cleansing** solution OTC *vaginal cleanser and deodorizer; acidity modifier* [vinegar (acetic acid)]

**Summer's Eve Feminine Bath** topical liquid OTC *for external perivaginal cleansing*

**Summer's Eve Feminine Powder** OTC *absorbs vaginal moisture* [cornstarch; benzethonium chloride]

**Summer's Eve Feminine Wash** topical liquid, wipes OTC *for external perivaginal cleansing*

**Summer's Eve Medicated Disposable Douche** solution OTC *antiseptic/germicidal; vaginal cleanser and deodorizer* [povidone-iodine] 0.3%

**Summer's Eve Post-Menstrual Disposable Douche** solution OTC *vaginal cleanser and deodorizer; acidity modifier* [monosodium phosphate; disodium phosphate]

**Summit Extra Strength** coated caplets OTC *analgesic; antipyretic; anti-inflammatory* [acetaminophen; aspirin; caffeine] 250•250•65 mg

**Sumycin** syrup ℞ *broad-spectrum antibiotic* [tetracycline HCl] 125 mg/5 mL

**Sumycin '250'; Sumycin '500'** capsules, tablets ℞ *broad-spectrum antibiotic* [tetracycline HCl] 250 mg; 500 mg

**sun rose** *medicinal herb* [see: rock rose]

**sunagrel** INN

**suncillin** INN *antibacterial* [also: suncillin sodium]

**suncillin sodium** USAN *antibacterial* [also: suncillin]

**sunepitron HCl** USAN *anxiolytic; antidepressant*

**SunKist Multivitamins Complete, Children's** chewable tablets OTC *vitamin/mineral/iron supplement* [multiple vitamins & minerals; iron; folic acid; biotin] ≐•18 mg•400 µg•40 µg

**SunKist Multivitamins + Extra C** chewable tablets OTC *vitamin supplement* [multiple vitamins; folic acid] ≐•0.3 mg

**SunKist Multivitamins + Iron, Children's** chewable tablets (discontinued 2004) OTC *vitamin/iron supplement* [multiple vitamins; iron; folic acid] ≐•15•0.3 mg

**SunKist Vitamin C** chewable tablets OTC *vitamin C supplement* [ascorbic acid and sodium ascorbate] 60, 250, 500 mg

**Supac** tablets (discontinued 2000) OTC *analgesic; antipyretic; anti-inflam-*

*matory* [acetaminophen; aspirin; caffeine] 160•230•32 mg

**Supartz** intra-articular injection in prefilled syringes ℞ *viscoelastic lubricant and "shock absorber" for osteoarthritis and TMJ syndrome* [hyaluronate sodium] 25 mg/2.5 mL ② *sports*

**Orthovisc** intra-articular injection in single-use vials ℞ *viscoelastic lubricant and "shock absorber" for osteoarthritis of the knee* [hyaluronan] 30 mg

**Super 2 Daily** softgels OTC *vitamin/mineral supplement* [multiple vitamins & minerals; fish oil concentrate; lecithin; phosphatidyl choline; bioflavonoids; lutein] ≛•385•30•25•12.5•0.025 mg

**Super CalciCaps** tablets OTC *dietary supplement* [dibasic calcium phosphate; calcium gluconate; calcium carbonate; vitamin D] 400 mg (Ca)•42 mg (P)•133 IU

**Super CalciCaps M-Z** tablets OTC *dietary supplement* [vitamins A and D; multiple minerals] 1667 mg•133 IU• ≛

**Super Calcium '1200'** softgels OTC *dietary supplement* [calcium; vitamin D] 600 mg•200 IU

**Super Carnosine** capsules OTC *anti-aging supplement* [carnosine] 500 mg

**Super D** Perles (capsules) OTC *vitamin supplement* [vitamins A and D] 10 000•400 IU

**Super Flavons; Super Flavons-300** tablets OTC *dietary supplement* [mixed bioflavonoids] 300 mg

**Super Hi Potency** tablets OTC *vitamin/mineral supplement* [multiple vitamins & minerals; folic acid; biotin] ≛•0.4 mg•0.075 mg

**Super Ivy-Dry** lotion OTC *poison ivy treatment* [zinc acetate; benzyl alcohol; isopropanol] 2%•10%•35%

**Super MiraForte with Chrysin** capsules OTC *natural supplement to increase free testosterone levels in men* [chrysin; muira puama; maca; nettle; ginger; piperine; zinc] 375•212.5•80•70.5•12.5•3.75•3.75 mg

**Super Quints-50** tablets OTC *vitamin supplement* [multiple B vitamins; folic acid; biotin] ≛•400•50 μg

**Superdophilus** powder OTC *dietary supplement; fever blister treatment; not generally regarded as safe and effective as an antidiarrheal* [Lactobacillus acidophilus] 2 billion U/g

**SuperEPA 1200; SuperEPA 2000** softgels OTC *dietary supplement* [omega-3 fatty acids] 1200 mg; 1000 mg

**superoxide dismutase (SOD)** [see: orgotein]

**Superplex-T** tablets OTC *vitamin supplement* [multiple B vitamins; vitamin C] ≛•500 mg

**supidimide** INN

**Suplena** ready-to-use oral liquid OTC *enteral nutritional therapy for renal failure* [multiple essential amino acids]

**Supprelin** subcu injection ℞ *gonadotropin-releasing hormone for central precocious puberty (orphan)* [histrelin acetate] 120, 300, 600 μg/0.6 mL

**Suppress** lozenges (discontinued 2002) OTC *antitussive* [dextromethorphan hydrobromide] 7.5 mg

**Supprette** (trademarked dosage form) *suppository*

**Suprane** liquid for vaporization ℞ *inhalation general anesthetic* [desflurane]

**Suprax** film-coated tablets, powder for oral suspension ℞ *cephalosporin antibiotic* [cefixime] 200, 400 mg; 100 mg/5 mL

**Suprefact** Ⓒᴬᴺ nasal solution ℞ *LHRH analogue; hormonal antineoplastic for prostatic cancer and endometriosis* [buserelin acetate] 1 mg/mL

**Suprefact; Suprefact Depot** Ⓒᴬᴺ subcu injection ℞ *LHRH analogue; hormonal antineoplastic for prostatic cancer and endometriosis* [buserelin acetate] 1 mg/mL; 6.6 mg/dose

**suproclone** USAN, INN *sedative*

**suprofen** USAN, INN, BAN *ocular non-steroidal anti-inflammatory drug (NSAID); antimiotic*

**Supule** (trademarked dosage form) *suppository*

**suramin hexasodium** USAN *investigational (NDA filed, orphan) growth factor antagonist for prostate cancer*

**suramin sodium** USP, BAN *antiparasitic for African trypanosomiasis and onchocerciasis*

**Surbex** Filmtabs (film-coated tablets) OTC *vitamin supplement* [multiple B vitamins]

**Surbex 750 with Iron** Filmtabs (film-coated tablets) OTC *vitamin/iron supplement* [multiple B vitamins; vitamins C and E; ferrous sulfate, dried; folic acid] ± • 750 mg • 30 IU • 27 mg • 0.4 mg

**Surbex 750 with Zinc** Filmtabs (film-coated tablets) OTC *vitamin/zinc supplement* [multiple vitamins; zinc sulfate; folic acid] ± • 22.5 • 0.4 mg

**Surbex-T; Surbex with C** Filmtabs (film-coated tablets) OTC *vitamin supplement* [multiple B vitamins; vitamin C] ± • 500 mg; ± • 250 mg

**Surbu-Gen-T** film-coated tablets OTC *vitamin supplement* [multiple B vitamins; vitamin C] ± • 500 mg

**Sure Cell Chlamydia Test** reagent kit for professional use *in vitro diagnostic aid for Chlamydia trachomatis* [monoclonal antibody-based enzyme-linked immunosorbent assay]

**Sure Cell Herpes (HSV) Test** reagent kit for professional use *in vitro diagnostic aid for herpes simplex virus in genital, rectal, oral, or dermal swabs* [monoclonal antibody-based enzyme-linked immunosorbent assay (ELISA)]

**Sure Cell Pregnancy** test kit for professional use *in vitro diagnostic aid; urine pregnancy test* [monoclonal/polyclonal antibody ELISA test]

**Sure Cell Streptococci** test kit for professional use *in vitro diagnostic aid for Group A streptococcal antigens in blood and throat swabs* [enzyme-linked immunosorbent assay (ELISA)]

**SureLac** chewable tablets OTC *digestive aid for lactose intolerance* [lactase enzyme] 3000 U

**surface active extract of saline lavage of bovine lungs** [see: beractant]

**surfactant laxatives** *a subclass of laxatives that work by increasing the amount of fat and water in the stool to ease its movement through the intestines* [more commonly called stool softeners]

**surfactant TA** [see: beractant]

**surfactant TA, modified bovine lung surfactant extract** [see: beractant]

**Surfak** Liquigels (capsules) OTC *laxative; stool softener* [docusate calcium] 240 mg

**Surfaxin** ℞ *investigational (Phase II/III, orphan) KL4 pulmonary surfactant for acute respiratory distress syndrome (ARDS) and meconium aspiration syndrome (MAS)* [lucinactant]

**surfilcon A** USAN *hydrophilic contact lens material*

**Surfol Post-Immersion Bath Oil** OTC *bath emollient*

**surfomer** USAN, INN *hypolipidemic*

**Surgel** vaginal gel OTC *lubricant* [propylene glycol; glycerin]

**surgibone** USAN *internal bone splint*

**surgical catgut** [see: suture, absorbable surgical]

**surgical gut** [see: suture, absorbable surgical]

**Surgicel** strips, Nu-knit pads ℞ *topical local hemostat for surgery* [cellulose, oxidized]

**suricainide** INN *antiarrhythmic* [also: suricainide maleate]

**suricainide maleate** USAN, INN *antiarrhythmic* [also: suricainide]

**suriclone** INN, BAN

**Surinam wood** *medicinal herb* [see: quassia]

**suritozole** USAN, INN *antidepressant*

**Surmontil** capsules ℞ *tricyclic antidepressant* [trimipramine maleate] 25, 50, 100 mg

**Surodex** intraocular injection ℞ *investigational (Phase II) corticosteroidal anti-inflammatory* [dexamethasone]

**suronacrine** INN *cholinesterase inhibitor* [also: suronacrine maleate]

**suronacrine maleate** USAN *cholinesterase inhibitor* [also: suronacrine]

**Surpass** chewing gum OTC *antacid; calcium supplement* [calcium carbonate] 300, 450 mg

**Survanta** suspension for intratracheal instillation ℞ *pulmonary surfactant for neonatal respiratory distress syndrome or respiratory failure (orphan)* [beractant] 25 mg/mL

**Susano** elixir ℞ *GI antispasmodic; anticholinergic; sedative* [atropine sulfate; scopolamine hydrobromide; hyoscyamine hydrobromide; phenobarbital] 0.0194•0.0065•0.1037•16.2 mg/5 mL

**Sus-Phrine** subcu injection (discontinued 2001) ℞ *sympathomimetic bronchodilator for bronchial asthma, bronchospasm, and COPD; vasopressor for shock* [epinephrine] 1:200 (5 mg/mL)

**Sustacal** powder OTC *enteral nutritional therapy* [milk-based formula]

**Sustacal** pudding OTC *enteral nutritional therapy* [milk-based formula]

**Sustacal** ready-to-use oral liquid OTC *enteral nutritional therapy* [lactose-free formula]

**Sustacal Basic; Sustacal Plus** ready-to-use oral liquid OTC *enteral nutritional therapy* [lactose-free formula]

**Sustagen** powder OTC *enteral nutritional therapy* [milk-based formula]

**Sustain** tablets ℞ *electrolyte replacement; dehydration preventative* [sodium chloride; potassium chloride; calcium carbonate] 220•15•18 mg

**Sustaire** timed-release tablets (discontinued 2004) ℞ *antiasthmatic; bronchodilator* [theophylline] 100, 300 mg

**Sustiva** capsules, film-coated caplets ℞ *antiviral non-nucleoside reverse transcriptase inhibitor (NNRTI) for HIV infection* [efavirenz] 50, 100, 200 mg; 600 mg

**sutilains** USAN, USP, INN, BAN *topical proteolytic enzymes for necrotic tissue debridement*

**sutoprofen** [see: suprofen]

**suture, absorbable surgical** USP *surgical aid*

**suture, nonabsorbable surgical** USP *surgical aid*

**Su-Tuss DM** oral liquid ℞ *antitussive; expectorant* [dextromethorphan hydrobromide; guaifenesin; alcohol 5%] 20•200 mg/5 mL

**Su-Tuss HD** elixir ℞ *narcotic antitussive; decongestant; expectorant* [hydrocodone bitartrate; pseudoephedrine HCl; guaifenesin] 5•60•200 mg/10 mL

**suxamethone** [see: succinylcholine chloride]

**suxamethonium chloride** INN, BAN *neuromuscular blocking agent* [also: succinylcholine chloride]

**suxemerid** INN *antitussive* [also: suxemerid sulfate]

**suxemerid sulfate** USAN *antitussive* [also: suxemerid]

**suxethonium chloride** INN

**suxibuzone** INN

**swallow wort, orange** *medicinal herb* [see: pleurisy root]

**swallow wort, silky** *medicinal herb* [see: milkweed]

**swamp cabbage** *medicinal herb* [see: skunk cabbage]

**swamp laurel; swamp sassafras** *medicinal herb* [see: magnolia]

**sweet, mountain** *medicinal herb* [see: New Jersey tea]

**sweet, winter** *medicinal herb* [see: marjoram]

**sweet anise; sweet chervil** *medicinal herb* [see: sweet cicely]

**sweet balm** *medicinal herb* [see: lemon balm]

**sweet basil** *medicinal herb* [see: basil]

**sweet bay** *medicinal herb* [see: laurel]

**sweet birch** *medicinal herb* [see: birch]

**sweet birch oil** [see: methyl salicylate]

**sweet cicely (Osmorhiza longistylis)** root *medicinal herb used as a carminative, expectorant, and stomachic*

**sweet clover** *medicinal herb* [see: melilot]

**sweet dock** *medicinal herb* [see: bistort]

**sweet elder** *medicinal herb* [see: elderberry]

**sweet elm** *medicinal herb* [see: slippery elm]

**sweet fennel** *medicinal herb* [see: fennel]

**sweet flag** *medicinal herb* [see: calamus]

**sweet grass** *medicinal herb* [see: calamus]

**sweet leaf** *medicinal herb* [see: stevia]

**sweet magnolia** *medicinal herb* [see: magnolia]

**sweet marjoram** *medicinal herb* [see: marjoram]

**sweet myrtle** *medicinal herb* [see: calamus]

**sweet orange peel tincture** [see: orange peel tincture, sweet]

**sweet potato vine, wild** *medicinal herb* [see: wild jalap]

**sweet root** *medicinal herb* [see: calamus]

**sweet rush** *medicinal herb* [see: calamus]

**sweet sedge** *medicinal herb* [see: calamus]

**sweet spirit of nitre** [see: ethyl nitrite]

**sweet vernal grass (Anthoxanthum odoratum)** *natural flavoring banned by the FDA as it is not generally regarded as safe and effective*

**sweet violet** *medicinal herb* [see: violet]

**sweet water lily; sweet-scented water lily** *medicinal herb* [see: white pond lily]

**sweet weed** *medicinal herb* [see: marsh mallow]

**sweet woodruff (Asperula odorata; Galium odoratum)** *plant medicinal herb for diuresis, inducing expectoration, liver disorders, promoting wound healing, relieving gastrointestinal spasms, and sedation*

**Sweet'n Fresh Clotrimazole-7** cream, vaginal suppositories (discontinued 2001) OTC *antifungal* [clotrimazole] 1%; 100 mg

**sweet-scented pond lily; sweet-scented water lily** *medicinal herb* [see: white pond lily]

**sweetwood** *medicinal herb* [see: licorice]

**Swim-Ear** ear drops OTC *antiseptic* [isopropyl alcohol] 95%

**swine snout** *medicinal herb* [see: dandelion]

**Syllact** powder OTC *bulk laxative* [psyllium husks] 3.3 g/tsp.

**Symax-SL** sublingual tablets ℞ *GI/GU antispasmodic; antiparkinsonian; anticholinergic "drying agent" for allergic rhinitis and hyperhidrosis* [hyoscyamine sulfate] 0.125 mg

**Symax-SR** sustained-release caplets ℞ *GI/GU antispasmodic; antiparkinsonian; anticholinergic "drying agent" for allergic rhinitis and hyperhidrosis* [hyoscyamine sulfate] 0.375 mg

**Symbicort 100; Symbicort 200** ⓒᴬᴺ Turbuhaler (dry powder in a metered-dose inhaler) ℞ *corticosteroidal anti-inflammatory and bronchodilator combination for chronic asthma* [budesonide; formoterol] 100•6 μg; 200•6 μg

**Symbyax** capsules ℞ *antipsychotic plus selective serotonin reuptake inhibitor (SSRI) for depressive episodes of a bipolar disorder* [olanzapine; fluoxetine HCl] 6•25, 6•50, 12•25, 12•50 mg

**symclosene** USAN, INN *topical anti-infective*

**symetine** INN *antiamebic* [also: symetine HCl]

**symetine HCl** USAN *antiamebic* [also: symetine]

**Symlin** subcu injection ℞ *synthetic amylin analogue to slow gastric emptying; investigational (NDA filed) antidiabetic for type 1 and type 2 diabetes* [pramlintide acetate]

**Symmetrel** tablets, syrup ℞ *antiviral for influenza A infections; dopaminergic antiparkinson agent* [amantadine HCl] 100 mg; 50 mg/5 mL

**sympatholytics** *a class of cardiovascular drugs that block the passage of impulses through the sympathetic nervous system* [also called: antiadrenergics]

**sympathomimetics** *a class of bronchodilators that relax the bronchial muscles, reducing bronchospasm; a class of cardiac agents that increase myocardial contractility, causing a vasopressor effect to counteract shock (inadequate tissue perfusion)* [also called: adrenergic agonists]

**Symphytum officinale; S. tuberosum** *medicinal herb* [see: comfrey]

**Symplocarpus foetidus** *medicinal herb* [see: skunk cabbage]

**Synacol CF** tablets (discontinued 2002) OTC *antitussive; expectorant* [dextromethorphan hydrobromide; guaifenesin] 15•200 mg

**Synacort** cream ℞ *topical corticosteroidal anti-inflammatory* [hydrocortisone] 1%, 2.5%

**Synagis** powder for IM injection ℞ *monoclonal antibody for prophylaxis of respiratory syncytial virus (RSV) in infants* [palivizumab] 50, 100 mg/vial

**Synalar** cream, ointment, topical solution ℞ *topical corticosteroidal anti-inflammatory* [fluocinolone acetonide] 0.01, 0.25%; 0.025%; 0.01%

**Synalar-HP** cream ℞ *topical corticosteroidal anti-inflammatory* [fluocinolone acetonide] 0.2%

**Synalgos-DC** capsules ℞ *narcotic analgesic* [dihydrocodeine bitartrate; aspirin; caffeine] 16•356.4•30 mg

**Synarel** nasal spray ℞ *gonadotropin-releasing hormone for central precocious puberty (orphan) and endometriosis* [nafarelin acetate] 2 mg/mL (200 μg/spray)

**SynBiotics-3** capsules OTC *dietary supplement; fever blister treatment; not generally regarded as safe and effective as an antidiarrheal* [Bifidobacterium longum; Lactobacillus rhamnosus A; L. plantarum; Saccharomyces boulardii] 4.5 billion CFU

**Synemol** cream ℞ *corticosteroidal anti-inflammatory* [fluocinolone acetonide] 0.025%

**Synercid** powder for IV infusion ℞ *semi-synthetic streptogramin antibiotic for life-threatening infections* [quinupristin; dalfopristin] 150•350 mg/10 mL

**synestrin** [see: diethylstilbestrol]

**synnematin B** [see: adicillin]

**Synophylate-GG** syrup ℞ *antiasthmatic; bronchodilator; expectorant* [theophylline; guaifenesin; alcohol 10%] 150•100 mg/15 mL

**Syn-Rx** controlled-release tablets (14-day, 56-tablet treatment regimen) (discontinued 2002) ℞ *decongestant; expectorant* [pseudoephedrine HCl; guaifenesin] 60•600 mg

**Synsorb Cd** ℞ *investigational (Phase III) antidiarrheal for AIDS-related diarrhea due to* Clostridium difficile *infection*

**Synsorb-Pk** ℞ *investigational (Phase III, orphan)* E. coli *neutralizer for traveler's diarrhea and hemolytic uremic syndrome (HUS)* [8-methoxycarbonyloctyl oligosaccharides]

**Syntest D.S.** sugar-coated tablets (discontinued 2004) ℞ *hormone replacement therapy for postmenopausal symptoms* [esterified estrogens; methyltestosterone] 1.25•2.5 mg

**Syntest H.S.** sugar-coated tablets (discontinued 2004) ℞ *hormone replacement therapy for postmenopausal symptoms* [esterified estrogens; methyltestosterone] 0.625•1.25 mg

**synthestrin** [see: diethylstilbestrol]

**synthetic conjugated estrogens** [see: estrogens, synthetic conjugated (A and B)]

**synthetic lung surfactant** [see: colfosceril palmitate]

**synthetic monosaccharides** *a class of investigational synthetic carbohydrates with immunomodulatory and anti-inflammatory effects being evaluated for the treatment of rheumatic arthritis*

**synthetic paraffin** [see: paraffin, synthetic]

**synthetic spermaceti** [now: cetyl esters wax]

**synthoestrin** [see: diethylstilbestrol]

**Synthroid** tablets, powder for injection ℞ *synthetic thyroid hormone ($T_4$ fraction only)* [levothyroxine sodium] 25, 50, 75, 88, 100, 112, 125, 137, 150, 175, 200, 300 μg; 200, 500 μg

**synvinolin** [now: simvastatin]

**Synvisc** intra-articular injection ℞ *viscoelastic lubricant and "shock absorber" for osteoarthritis and TMJ syndrome* [hylan G-F 20] 16 mg/2 mL

**Syprine** capsules ℞ *copper chelating agent for Wilson disease (orphan)* [trientine HCl] 250 mg

**Syracol CF** tablets (discontinued 2002) OTC *antitussive; expectorant* [dextromethorphan hydrobromide; guaifenesin] 15•200 mg

**syrosingopine** NF, INN, BAN

**syrup** NF *flavoring agent*

**T₄ (levothyroxine sodium)** [q.v.]

**T4 endonuclease V (T4N5), liposome encapsulated** *investigational (orphan) for prevent cutaneous neoplasms in xeroderma pigmentosum*

**T-10 protocol (methotrexate, doxorubicin, cisplatin, bleomycin, cyclophosphamide, dactinomycin)** *chemotherapy protocol*

**T-67** *investigational (Phase III) tubulin antagonist for liver cancer*

**T-1249** *investigational for HIV infection*

**Tab-A-Vite** tablets OTC *vitamin supplement* [multiple vitamins; folic acid] ≟•0.4 mg

**Tab-A-Vite + Iron** tablets OTC *vitamin/iron supplement* [multiple vitamins; iron; folic acid] ≟•18•0.4 mg

*Tabebuia avellanedae; T. impetiginosa medicinal herb* [see: pau d'arco]

*Tabernanthe iboga street drug* [see: iboga]

**tabilautide** INN

**Tabloid** (trademarked dosage form) *tablet with raised lettering*

**Tabules** (dosage form) *tablets*

**Tac-3** IM, intra-articular, intrabursal, intradermal injection ℞ *corticosteroid; anti-inflammatory* [triamcinolone acetonide] 3 mg/mL

**syrupus cerasi** [see: cherry juice]

**Syrvite** oral liquid OTC *vitamin supplement* [multiple vitamins]

**Systane** eye drops OTC *moisturizer; lubricant* [polyethylene glycol 400; polypropylene glycol] 0.4%•0.3%

*Syzygium aromaticum medicinal herb* [see: cloves]

**(S)-zopiclone** [see: esopiclone]

**Tac-40** suspension for injection ℞ *corticosteroid; anti-inflammatory* [triamcinolone acetonide] 40 mg/mL

**taclamine** INN *minor tranquilizer* [also: taclamine HCl]

**taclamine HCl** USAN *minor tranquilizer* [also: taclamine]

**tacmahac** *medicinal herb* [see: balm of Gilead]

**tacrine** INN, BAN *reversible cholinesterase inhibitor; cognition adjuvant for Alzheimer dementia* [also: tacrine HCl]

**tacrine HCl** USAN *reversible cholinesterase inhibitor; cognition adjuvant for Alzheimer dementia* [also: tacrine]

**tacrolimus** USAN, INN *immunosuppressant for liver and kidney transplants; topical treatment for eczema; investigational (Phase III) treatment for rheumatoid arthritis*

**TAD (thioguanine, ara-C, daunorubicin)** *chemotherapy protocol for acute myelocytic leukemia (AML)* [also: DAT; DCT]

**tadalafil** *phosphodiesterase type 5 (PDE5) inhibitor; selective vasodilator for erectile dysfunction (ED); investigational for female sexual dysfunction*

**taeniacides** *a class of agents that destroy tapeworms* [see also: anthelmintics; vermicides; vermifuges]

**Tagamet** film-coated tablets ℞ *histamine H₂ antagonist for gastric and duodenal ulcers and gastric hypersecretory* conditions [cimetidine] 300, 400, 800 mg ② Tegopen

**Tagamet** oral liquid, IV or IM injection, premixed injection ℞ *histamine H₂ antagonist for gastric and duodenal ulcers and gastric hypersecretory conditions* [cimetidine HCl] 300 mg/5 mL; 300 mg/2 mL; 300 mg/vial

**Tagamet 100** (British name for U.S. product Tagamet HB [100 mg tablets])

**Tagamet HB** film-coated tablets, oral suspension OTC *histamine H₂ antagonist for episodic heartburn and acid indigestion* [cimetidine] 100, 200 mg; 200 mg

**taglutimide** INN

**taheebo** *medicinal herb* [see: pau d'arco]

**TA-HPV** ℞ *investigational (orphan) for cervical cancer* [vaccinia virus vaccine for human papillomavirus (HPV), recombinant]

**tail, colt's; cow's tail; horse tail; mare's tail** *medicinal herb* [see: fleabane; horseweed]

**tail, lion's** *medicinal herb* [see: motherwort]

**tailed cubebs; tailed pepper** *medicinal herb* [see: cubeb]

**TAK-603** *investigational (orphan) for Crohn disease*

**Talacen** caplets ℞ *narcotic agonist-antagonist analgesic; antipyretic* [pentazocine HCl; acetaminophen] 25•650 mg

**talampicillin** INN *antibacterial* [also: talampicillin HCl]

**talampicillin HCl** USAN *antibacterial* [also: talampicillin]

**talastine** INN

**talbutal** USP, INN *sedative; hypnotic*

**talc** USP, JAN *dusting powder; tablet and capsule lubricant*

**talc, sterile aerosol** *treatment for malignant pleural effusion and pneumothorax via intrapleural thoracoscopy administration (orphan)*

**taleranol** USAN, INN *gonadotropin enzyme inhibitor*

**talinolol** INN

**talipexole** INN

**talisomycin** USAN, INN *antineoplastic*

**tall speedwell** *medicinal herb* [see: Culver root]

**tall veronica** *medicinal herb* [see: Culver root]

**tallimustine** INN *investigational antineoplastic for leukemia and solid tumors*

**tallow shrub** *medicinal herb* [see: bayberry]

**tallysomycin A** [now: talisomycin]

**talmetacin** USAN, INN *analgesic; anti-inflammatory; antipyretic*

**talmetoprim** INN

**talnetant HCl** USAN NK₃ *receptor antagonist for urinary frequency, urgency, and incontinence*

**talniflumate** USAN, INN *anti-inflammatory; analgesic*

**talopram** INN *catecholamine potentiator* [also: talopram HCl]

**talopram HCl** USAN *catecholamine potentiator* [also: talopram]

**talosalate** USAN, INN *analgesic; anti-inflammatory*

**Taloxa** (foreign name for U.S. product Felbatol)

**taloximine** INN, BAN

**talsaclidine** INN

**talsaclidine fumarate** USAN *muscarinic M₁ agonist for Alzheimer disease*

**talsupram** INN

**taltibride** [see: metibride]

**taltrimide** INN

**taludipine** [see: teludipine]

**taludipine HCl** [see: teludipine HCl]

**Talwin** IV, subcu or IM injection ℞ *narcotic agonist-antagonist analgesic; also abused as a street drug* [pentazocine lactate] 30 mg/mL

**Talwin Compound** caplets ℞ *narcotic agonist-antagonist analgesic; antipyretic; also abused as a street drug* [pentazocine HCl; aspirin] 12.5•325 mg

**Talwin NX** tablets ℞ *narcotic agonist-antagonist analgesic; also abused as a street drug* [pentazocine HCl; naloxone HCl] 50•0.5 mg

**tamarind** (*Tamarindus indica*) fruit and leaves *medicinal herb used as an anthelmintic, laxative, and refrigerant*

**Tambocor** tablets ℞ *antiarrhythmic* [flecainide acetate] 50, 100, 150 mg

**tameridone** USAN, INN, BAN *veterinary sedative*

**tameticillin** INN

**tametraline** INN *antidepressant* [also: tametraline HCl]

**tametraline HCl** USAN *antidepressant* [also: tametraline]

**Tamiflu** capsules, powder for oral suspension ℞ *antiviral for the prophylaxis and treatment of influenza A and B infections* [oseltamivir phosphate] 75 mg; 12 mg/mL

**Tamine S.R.** sustained-release tablets (discontinued 2001) ℞ *decongestant; antihistamine* [phenylpropanolamine HCl; phenylephrine HCl; brompheniramine maleate] 15•15•12 mg

**tamitinol** INN

**tamoxifen** INN, BAN *antiestrogen antineoplastic for breast cancer* [also: tamoxifen citrate]

**tamoxifen citrate** USAN, USP, JAN *antiestrogen antineoplastic for breast cancer; also for breast cancer prevention in high-risk patients* [also: tamoxifen] 10, 20 mg oral

**tamoxifen & DTIC** *chemotherapy protocol for malignant melanoma*

**tamoxifen & epirubicin** *chemotherapy protocol for breast cancer*

**tampramine** INN *antidepressant* [also: tampramine fumarate]

**tampramine fumarate** USAN *antidepressant* [also: tampramine]

**Tamp-R-Tel** (trademarked packaging form) *tamper-evident cartridge-needle unit*

**tamsulosin** INN *alpha₁-adrenergic blocker for benign prostatic hyperplasia (BPH)* [also: tamsulosin HCl]

**tamsulosin HCl** USAN, JAN *alpha₁-adrenergic blocker for benign prostatic hyperplasia (BPH)* [also: tamsulosin]

**Tanac** gel OTC *oral anesthetic; vulnerary* [dyclonine HCl; allantoin] 1%•0.5%

**Tanac** topical liquid OTC *oral anesthetic; antiseptic* [benzocaine; benzalkonium chloride] 10%•0.12%

**Tanac Dual Core** stick OTC *topical oral anesthetic; antiseptic; astringent* [benzocaine; benzalkonium chloride; tannic acid] 7.5%•0.12%•6%

**Tanacetum parthenium** *medicinal herb* [see: feverfew]

**Tanacetum vulgare** *medicinal herb* [see: tansy]

**Tanafed** oral suspension (discontinued 2003) ℞ *decongestant; antihistamine* [pseudoephedrine tannate; chlorpheniramine tannate] 150•9 mg/10 mL

**Tanafed DM** pediatric oral suspension (discontinued 2003) ℞ *decongestant; antihistamine; antitussive* [pseudoephedrine tannate; chlorpheniramine tannate; dextromethorphan tannate] 75•4.5•25 mg/5 mL

**Tanafed DMX** pediatric oral suspension ℞ *decongestant; antihistamine; antitussive* [pseudoephedrine tannate; dexchlorpheniramine tannate; dextromethorphan tannate] 75•2.5•25 mg/5 mL

**Tanafed DP** pediatric oral suspension ℞ *decongestant; antihistamine* [pseudoephedrine tannate; dexchlorpheniramine tannate] 75•2.5 mg/5 mL

**tanaproget** *investigational (Phase III) oral progesterone receptor antagonist contraceptive that inhibits ovulation*

**tandamine** INN *antidepressant* [also: tandamine HCl]

**tandamine HCl** USAN *antidepressant* [also: tandamine]

**tandospirone** INN, BAN *anxiolytic* [also: tandospirone citrate]

**tandospirone citrate** USAN *anxiolytic* [also: tandospirone]

**taniplon** INN

**tannic acid** USP, JAN *astringent; topical mucosal protectant*

**tannic acid acetate** [see: acetyltannic acid]

**Tannic-12** caplets ℞ *antitussive; antihistamine* [carbetapentane tannate; chlorpheniramine tannate] 60•5 mg

**Tannic-12** pediatric oral suspension ℞ *antitussive; decongestant; antihistamine* [carbetapentane tannate; phenylephrine tannate; chlorpheniramine tannate] 30•5•4 mg/5 mL

**tannin** [see: tannic acid]

**tannyl acetate** [see: acetyltannic acid]

**Tanoral** tablets (discontinued 2002) ℞ *decongestant; antihistamine* [phenylephrine tannate; chlorpheniramine tannate; pyrilamine tannate] 25•8•25 mg

**tansy (Chrysanthemum vulgare; Tanacetum vulgare)** leaves and seeds *medicinal herb for inducing diaphoresis, promoting wound healing, relieving spasms, stimulating menstruation, and treating worm infections*

**tantalum** *element (Ta)*

**Tantum** ℞ *investigational (orphan) radioprotectant for oral mucosa following radiation therapy for head and neck cancer* [benzydamine HCl]

**Tao** capsules (discontinued 2004) ℞ *macrolide antibiotic* [troleandomycin] 250 mg

**taoryi edisylate** [see: caramiphen edisylate]

**Tapanol** tablets, caplets, gelcaps OTC *analgesic; antipyretic* [acetaminophen] 325, 500 mg; 500 mg; 500 mg

**Tapazole** tablets ℞ *antithyroid agent* [methimazole] 5, 10 mg

**tape, adhesive** USP *surgical aid*

**taprostene** INN

**tar** [see: coal tar]

**tarweed** *medicinal herb* [see: yerba santa]

**Tarabine PFS** subcu, intrathecal, or IV injection ℞ *antimetabolite antineoplastic for various leukemias* [cytarabine] 20 mg/mL

**Taraphilic** ointment OTC *antipsoriatic; antiseborrheic* [coal tar] 1%

**Taraxacum officinale** *medicinal herb* [see: dandelion]

**Tarceva** ℞ *investigational (Phase III) antineoplastic for lung, breast, and pancreatic cancers; investigational (orphan) for non-Hodgkin lymphoma* [erlotinib HCl]

**Targocid** (approved in 13 foreign countries) ℞ *investigational (NDA filed) glycopeptide antibiotic* [teicoplanin]

**Targretin** capsules, gel ℞ *synthetic retinoid analogue antineoplastic for cutaneous T-cell lymphoma (orphan); investigational (Phase III) for lung cancer* [bexarotene] 75 mg; 1% ⊡

Tegopen; Tegrin

**tariquidar** *investigational (Phase III) p-glycoprotein pump inhibitor for lung cancer*

**Tarka** film-coated combination-release tablets ℞ *once-daily antihypertensive; angiotensin-converting enzyme (ACE) inhibitor; calcium channel blocker* [trandolapril (immediate release); verapamil HCl (extended release)] 2•180, 1•240, 2•240, 4•240 mg

**Tarlene** hair lotion OTC *antiseborrheic; antipsoriatic; keratolytic* [salicylic acid; coal tar] 2.5%•2%

**Taro-Desoximetasone** ⓒᴬᴺ cream, gel (name changed to Desoxi in 2001)

**Taro-Warfarin** ⓒᴬᴺ tablets ℞ *coumarin-derivative anticoagulant* [warfarin sodium] 1, 2, 2.5, 3, 4, 5, 6, 7.5, 10 mg

**tarragon (Artemisia dracunculus)** flowering plant *medicinal herb used as a diuretic, emmenagogue, hypnotic, and stomachic*

**Tarsum** shampoo OTC *antipsoriatic; antiseborrheic; keratolytic* [coal tar; salicylic acid] 10%•5%

**tartar emetic** [see: antimony potassium tartrate]

**tartaric acid** NF *buffering agent*

**Tasmar** film-coated tablets ℞ *COMT inhibitor; adjunct to carbidopa and levodopa for Parkinson disease* [tolcapone] 100, 200 mg

**tasosartan** USAN, INN *antihypertensive; angiotensin II antagonist*

**tasuldine** INN

**TAT antagonist** *investigational (Phase I/II) antiviral for HIV infection*

**taurine** INN [also: aminoethylsulfonic acid]

**taurocholate sodium** [see: sodium taurocholate]

**taurolidine** INN, BAN *investigational antitoxin for the treatment of sepsis*

**tauromustine** INN *investigational treatment for renal cancer and multiple sclerosis*

**tauroselcholic acid** INN, BAN

**taurultam** INN, BAN

**Tavist** tablets, syrup (discontinued 2002) ℞ *antihistamine* [clemastine fumarate] 2.68 mg; 0.67 mg/5 mL

**Tavist Allergy** tablets OTC *antihistamine* [clemastine fumarate] 1.34 mg

**Tavist Allergy/Sinus/Headache** caplets OTC *decongestant; antihistamine; analgesic* [pseudoephedrine HCl; clemastine fumarate; acetaminophen] 30•0.335•500 mg

**Tavist ND** tablets OTC *nonsedating antihistamine for allergic rhinitis and chronic idiopathic urticaria* [loratadine] 10 mg

**Tavist Sinus** caplets OTC *decongestant; analgesic; antipyretic* [pseudoephedrine HCl; acetaminophen] 30•500 mg

**Tavist-D** film-coated sustained-release tablets (discontinued 2001) OTC *decongestant; antihistamine* [phenylpropanolamine HCl; clemastine fumarate] 75•1.34 mg

**taxanes; taxoids** *a class of antineoplastics that inhibits cancer cell mitosis by disrupting the cells' microtubular network*

**Taxol** IV infusion ℞ *antineoplastic for AIDS-related Kaposi sarcoma (orphan), breast and ovarian cancers, and non–small cell lung cancer (NSCLC)* [paclitaxel] 30 mg/5 mL

**Taxoprexin** ℞ *investigational (orphan) taxane for hormone-refractory prostate cancer, pancreatic cancer, malignant melanoma, and adenocarcinoma of the GI tract; investigational (Phase III) for breast cancer* [docosahexaenoic acid (DHA); paclitaxel]

**Taxotere** IV infusion ℞ *antineoplastic for advanced or metastatic breast, prostate, and non–small cell lung cancer (NSCLC); investigational (Phase III) for head and neck cancers* [docetaxel] 20, 80 mg/vial

***Taxus bacatta* and other species** *medicinal herb* [see: yew]

**tazadolene** INN *analgesic* [also: tazadolene succinate]

**tazadolene succinate** USAN *analgesic* [also: tazadolene]

**tazanolast** INN

**tazarotene** USAN, INN *retinoid prodrug; topical keratolytic for acne and psoriasis; adjuvant treatment for facial wrinkles, hyper- and hypopigmentation, and benign lentigines*

**tazasubrate** INN, BAN

**tazeprofen** INN

**Tazicef** powder or frozen premix for IV or IM injection ℞ *cephalosporin antibiotic* [ceftazidime] 1, 2, 6 g

**Tazidime** powder for IV or IM injection ℞ *cephalosporin antibiotic* [ceftazidime] 0.5, 1, 2, 6 g

**tazifylline** INN *antihistamine* [also: tazifylline HCl]

**tazifylline HCl** USAN *antihistamine* [also: tazifylline]

**taziprinone** INN

**tazobactam** USAN, INN, BAN *β-lactamase inhibitor; penicillin synergist*

**tazobactam sodium** USAN *β-lactamase inhibitor; penicillin synergist*

**Tazocin** (European name for U.S. product Zosyn)

**tazofelone** USAN *investigational (Phase II) treatment for ulcerative colitis and Crohn disease*

**tazolol** INN *cardiotonic* [also: tazolol HCl]

**tazolol HCl** USAN *cardiotonic* [also: tazolol]

**tazomeline citrate** USAN *cholinergic agonist for Alzheimer disease*

**Tazorac** cream, gel ℞ *retinoid pro-drug; keratolytic for acne and psoriasis* [tazarotene] 0.05%, 0.1%

**Taztia XT** extended-release capsules ℞ *antihypertensive; calcium channel blocker* [diltiazem HCl] 120, 180, 240, 300, 360 mg

**TBC-3B** *investigational (Phase I) vaccine for AIDS*

**TBZ (thiabendazole)** [q.v.]

**TC (thioguanine, cytarabine)** *chemotherapy protocol*

**3TC** [now: lamivudine]

**99mTc** [see: macrosalb (99mTc)]

**99mTc** [see: sodium pertechnetate Tc 99m]

**99mTc** [see: technetium Tc 99m albumin]

**99mTc** [see: technetium Tc 99m albumin aggregated]

**99mTc** [see: technetium Tc 99m albumin colloid]

**99mTc** [see: technetium Tc 99m albumin microaggregated]

**99mTc** [see: technetium Tc 99m antimony trisulfide colloid]

**99mTc** [see: technetium Tc 99m biciromab]

**99mTc** [see: technetium Tc 99m bicisate]

**99mTc** [see: technetium Tc 99m disofenin]

**99mTc** [see: technetium Tc 99m etidronate]

**99mTc** [see: technetium Tc 99m exametazine]

**99mTc** [see: technetium Tc 99m ferpentetate]

**99mTc** [see: technetium Tc 99m furifosmin]

**99mTc** [see: technetium Tc 99m gluceptate]

**99mTc** [see: technetium Tc 99m lidofenin]

**99mTc** [see: technetium Tc 99m mebrofenin]

**99mTc** [see: technetium Tc 99m medronate]

**99mTc** [see: technetium Tc 99m medronate disodium]

**99mTc** [see: technetium Tc 99m mertiatide]

**99mTc** [see: technetium Tc 99m oxidronate]

**99mTc** [see: technetium Tc 99m pentetate]

**99mTc** [see: technetium Tc 99m pentetate calcium trisodium]

**99mTc** [see: technetium Tc 99m (pyro- & trimeta-) phosphates]

**99mTc** [see: technetium Tc 99m pyrophosphate]

**99mTc** [see: technetium Tc 99m red blood cells]

**99mTc** [see: technetium Tc 99m sestamibi]

**99mTc** [see: technetium Tc 99m siboroxime]

**99mTc** [see: technetium Tc 99m succimer]

**99mTc** [see: technetium Tc 99m sulfur colloid]

**99mTc** [see: technetium Tc 99m teboroxime]

**99mTc** [see: technetium Tc 99m tetrofosmin]

**99mTc** [see: technetium Tc 99m tiatide]

**TCC (trichlorocarbanilide)** [see: triclocarban]

**T-cell gene therapy** *investigational (Phase III) treatment for HIV infection*

**TCF (Taxol, cisplatin, fluorouracil)** *chemotherapy protocol for esophageal cancer*

**TCI Ovulation Tester** test kit for home use OTC *in vitro diagnostic aid to predict ovulation time from a saliva sample*

**TD; Td (tetanus & diphtheria [toxoids])** *the designation TD (or DT) denotes the pediatric vaccine; Td denotes the adult vaccine* [see: diphtheria & tetanus toxoids, adsorbed]

**tea, Canada; mountain tea; redberry tea** *medicinal herb* [see: wintergreen]

**tea tree oil (Melaleuca alternifolia)** *medicinal herb for acne, boils, burns, Candida infections, cold sores, joint pain, skin disorders, staphylococcal and streptococcal infections, and sunburn; also used as a douche for trichomonal cervicitis and vaginal candidiasis*

**TEAB (tetraethylammonium bromide)** [see: tetrylammonium bromide]

**teaberry oil** [see: methyl salicylate]

**TEAC (tetraethylammonium chloride)** [q.v.]

**teamster's tea** *medicinal herb* [see: ephedra]

**TearGard** eye drops OTC *ocular moisturizer/lubricant* [hydroxyethylcellulose]

**Teargen** eye drops OTC *ophthalmic moisturizer/lubricant* [polyvinyl alcohol]

**Tearisol** eye drops OTC *ophthalmic moisturizer/lubricant* [hydroxypropyl methylcellulose] 0.5%

**Tears Naturale; Tears Naturale II; Tears Naturale Free** eye drops OTC *ophthalmic moisturizer/lubricant* [hydroxypropyl methylcellulose] 0.3%

**Tears Naturale P.M.** ⊕ ophthalmic ointment OTC *ocular moisturizer/lubricant* [white petrolatum; mineral oil; lanolin]

**Tears Plus** eye drops OTC *ophthalmic moisturizer/lubricant* [polyvinyl alcohol] 1.4%

**Tears Renewed** eye drops OTC *ophthalmic moisturizer/lubricant* [hydroxypropyl methylcellulose] 0.3%

**Tears Renewed** ophthalmic ointment OTC *ocular moisturizer/lubricant* [white petrolatum; mineral oil]

**TearSaver Punctum Plugs** ℞ *blocks the puncta and canaliculus to eliminate tear loss in keratitis sicca* [silicone plug]

**Tebamide** suppositories, pediatric suppositories ℞ *antiemetic; anticholinergic* [trimethobenzamide HCl; benzocaine] 200 mg•2%; 100 mg•2%

**tebatizole** INN

**tebethion** [see: thioacetazone; thiacetazone]

**tebufelone** USAN, INN *analgesic; antiinflammatory*

**tebuquine** USAN, INN *antimalarial*

**tebutate** USAN, INN *combining name for radicals or groups*

**TEC (thiotepa, etoposide, carboplatin)** *chemotherapy protocol*

**teceleukin** USAN, INN, BAN *immunostimulant; investigational (orphan) for metastatic renal cell carcinoma and metastatic malignant melanoma*

**teceleukin & interferon alfa-2a** *investigational (orphan) for metastatic renal cell carcinoma and metastatic malignant melanoma*

**technetium** *element (Tc)*

**technetium ($^{99m}$Tc) dimercaptosuccinic acid** JAN *diagnostic aid for renal function testing* [also: technetium Tc 99m succimer]

**technetium ($^{99m}$Tc) human serum albumin** JAN *radioactive agent*

**technetium ($^{99m}$Tc) labeled macroaggregated human albumin** JAN [also: macrosalb ($^{99m}$Tc)]

**technetium ($^{99m}$Tc) methylenediphosphonate** JAN *radioactive diagnostic aid for skeletal imaging* [also: technetium Tc 99m medronate]

**technetium ($^{99m}$Tc) phytate** JAN *radioactive agent*

**technetium Tc 99m albumin** USP *radioactive agent*

**technetium Tc 99m albumin aggregated** USAN, USP *radioactive diagnostic aid for lung imaging*

**technetium Tc 99m albumin colloid** USAN, USP *radioactive agent*

**technetium Tc 99m albumin microaggregated** USAN *radioactive agent*

**technetium Tc 99m antimelanoma murine monoclonal antibodies (MAb)** *investigational (orphan) for diagnostic imaging agent for metastases of malignant melanoma*

**technetium Tc 99m antimony trisulfide colloid** USAN *radioactive agent*

**technetium Tc 99m apcitide** *radiopharmaceutical diagnostic aid for acute venous thrombosis*

**technetium Tc 99m arcitumomab** USAN *radiopharmaceutical diagnostic aid for recurrent or metastatic thyroid and colorectal cancers*

**technetium Tc 99m bectumomab** *monoclonal antibody; investigational (Phase III, orphan) diagnostic aid for non-Hodgkin B-cell lymphoma, AIDS-related lymphomas, and other acute and chronic B-cell leukemias* [also: bectumomab]

**technetium Tc 99m biciromab** *radioactive diagnostic aid for deep vein thrombosis*

**technetium Tc 99m bicisate** USAN, INN, BAN *radioactive diagnostic aid for brain imaging*

**technetium Tc 99m disofenin** USP *radioactive diagnostic aid for hepatobiliary function testing*

**technetium Tc 99m DMSA (dimer-captosuccinic acid)** [see: technetium Tc 99m succimer]

**technetium Tc 99m DTPA (diethylenetriaminepentaacetic acid)** [see: technetium Tc 99m pentetate]

**technetium Tc 99m etidronate** USP *radioactive agent*

**technetium Tc 99m exametazine** USAN *radioactive agent*

**technetium Tc 99m ferpentetate** USP *radioactive agent*

**technetium Tc 99m furifosmin** USAN, INN *radioactive agent; diagnostic aid for cardiac disease*

**technetium Tc 99m gluceptate** USP *radioactive agent*

**technetium Tc 99m HSA (human serum albumin)** [see: technetium Tc 99m albumin]

**technetium Tc 99m iron ascorbate pentetic acid complex** [now: technetium Tc 99m ferpentetate]

**technetium Tc 99m lidofenin** USAN, USP *radioactive agent*

**technetium Tc 99m MAA (microaggregated albumin)** [see: technetium Tc 99m albumin aggregated]

**technetium Tc 99m MDP (methylenediphosphonate)** [see: technetium Tc 99m medronate]

**technetium Tc 99m mebrofenin** USAN, USP *radioactive agent*

**technetium Tc 99m medronate** USP *radioactive diagnostic aid for skeletal imaging* [also: technetium ($^{99m}$Tc) methylenediphosphonate]

**technetium Tc 99m medronate disodium** USAN *radioactive agent*

**technetium Tc 99m mertiatide** USAN *radioactive diagnostic aid for renal function testing*

**technetium Tc 99m murine monoclonal antibodies (MAb) to human alpha-fetoprotein (AFP)** *investigational (orphan) diagnostic aid for AFP-producing tumors, hepatoblastoma, and hepatocellular carcinoma*

**technetium Tc 99m murine monoclonal antibodies (MAb) to human chorionic gonadotropin (hCG)** *investigational (orphan) diagnostic aid for hCG-producing tumors*

**technetium Tc 99m murine monoclonal antibodies (MAb) IgG$_2$a to B cell** [now: technetium Tc 99m bectumomab]

**technetium Tc 99m oxidronate** USP *radioactive diagnostic aid for skeletal imaging*

**technetium Tc 99m pentetate** USP *radioactive agent* [also: human serum albumin diethylenetriaminepentaacetic acid technetium ($^{99m}$Tc)]

**technetium Tc 99m pentetate calcium trisodium** USAN *radioactive agent*

**technetium Tc 99m pentetate sodium** [now: technetium Tc 99m pentetate]

**technetium Tc 99m (pyro- and trimeta-) phosphates** USP *radioactive agent*

**technetium Tc 99m pyrophosphate** USP, JAN *radioactive agent*

**technetium Tc 99m red blood cells** USAN *radioactive agent*

**technetium Tc 99m sestamibi** USAN, INN, BAN *radioactive/radiopaque diagnostic aid for cardiac perfusion imaging and mammography*

**technetium Tc 99m siboroxime** USAN, INN *radioactive diagnostic aid for brain imaging*

**technetium Tc 99m sodium gluceptate** [now: technetium Tc 99m gluceptate]

**technetium Tc 99m succimer** USP *diagnostic aid for renal function testing* [also: technetium ($^{99m}$Tc) dimercaptosuccinic acid]

**technetium Tc 99m sulesomab** *monoclonal antibody; diagnostic aid for infectious lesions* [also: sulesomab]

**technetium Tc 99m sulfur colloid (TSC)** USAN, USP *radioactive agent*

**technetium Tc 99m teboroxime** USAN, INN, BAN *radioactive/radiopaque diagnostic aid for cardiac perfusion imaging*

**technetium Tc 99m tetrofosmin**
*radioactive agent for cardiovascular imaging*

**technetium Tc 99m tiatide** BAN

**technetium Tc 99m TSC (technetium sulfur colloid)** [see: technetium Tc 99m sulfur colloid]

**technetium Tc 99m-labeled CEA scan** [see: arcitumomab]

**teclothiazide** INN, BAN

**teclozan** USAN, INN *antiamebic*

**Tecnu Outdoor Skin Cleanser** lotion OTC *for the removal of toxic oils from poison ivy, oak, or sumac; use before or as soon as rash appears; can also be used to clean clothing and equipment* [deodorized mineral spirits; propylene glycol; fatty acid soap]

**Tecnu Poison Oak-N-Ivy** topical liquid (name changed to Tecnu Outdoor Skin Cleanser in 2003) OTC *poison ivy preventative* [deodorized mineral spirits]

**tecogalan sodium** USAN *antiangiogenic antineoplastic*

**Teczem** film-coated extended-release tablets Ɽ *antihypertensive; angiotensin-converting enzyme (ACE) inhibitor; calcium channel blocker* [diltiazem maleate; enalapril maleate] 180•5 mg

**tedisamil** INN *investigational calcium channel blocker for ischemic heart disease and arrhythmias*

**Tedrigen** tablets OTC *antiasthmatic; bronchodilator; decongestant; sedative* [theophylline; ephedrine HCl; phenobarbital] 120•22.5•7.5 mg

**tefazoline** INN

**tefenperate** INN

**tefludazine** INN

**teflurane** USAN, INN *inhalation anesthetic*

**teflutixol** INN

**tegafur** USAN, INN, BAN *antineoplastic; prodrug of fluorouracil*

**tegaserod** USAN *selective serotonin 5-HT$_4$ receptor antagonist for irritable bowel syndrome (IBS)*

**tegaserod maleate** *selective serotonin 5-HT$_4$ receptor antagonist for irritable bowel syndrome (IBS) and chronic constipation in women*

**Tegison** capsules (discontinued 2002) Ɽ *systemic antipsoriatic* [etretinate] 10, 25 mg

**Tegretol** chewable tablets, tablets, oral suspension Ɽ *anticonvulsant; analgesic for trigeminal neuralgia; antipsychotic* [carbamazepine] 100 mg; 200 mg; 100 mg/5 mL ⊡ Tegrin

**Tegretol-XR** extended-release tablets Ɽ *twice-daily anticonvulsant; antipsychotic* [carbamazepine] 100, 200, 400 mg

**Tegrin for Psoriasis** cream, lotion, soap (discontinued 2003) OTC *antipsoriatic; antiseborrheic; antiseptic* [coal tar solution] 5% ⊡ Targretin; Tegopen; Tegretol

**Tegrin Medicated** gel shampoo, lotion shampoo (discontinued 2003) OTC *antiseborrheic; antipsoriatic; antipruritic; antibacterial* [coal tar] 5%

**Tegrin Medicated Extra Conditioning; Advanced Formula Tegrin** shampoo (discontinued 2003) OTC *antiseborrheic; antipsoriatic; antipruritic; antibacterial* [coal tar] 7%

**Tegrin-HC** ointment OTC *topical corticosteroidal anti-inflammatory* [hydrocortisone] 1%

**Tegrin-LT** shampoo/conditioner (discontinued 2003) OTC *pediculicide for lice* [pyrethrins; piperonyl butoxide technical] 0.33%•3.15%

**teholamine** [see: aminophylline]

**TEIB (triethyleneiminobenzoquinone)** [see: triaziquone]

**teicoplanin** USAN, INN, BAN *investigational (NDA filed) glycopeptide antibiotic*

**teicoplanin A$_{2-1}$, A$_{2-2}$, A$_{2-3}$, A$_{2-4}$, A$_{2-5}$, and A$_{3-1}$** *components of teicoplanin*

**Teladar** cream Ɽ *corticosteroidal anti-inflammatory* [betamethasone dipropionate] 0.05%

**telbermin** USAN *angiogenic growth factor; vascular endothelial growth factor, recombinant human (rhVEGF); investigational (Phase II, orphan) for peripheral vascular disease and coronary artery disease*

**Telcyta** ℞ *investigational (Phase III) antineoplastic for ovarian cancer*

**Teldrin 12-Hour Allergy Relief** sustained-release capsules (discontinued 2001) OTC *decongestant; antihistamine* [phenylpropanolamine HCl; chlorpheniramine maleate] 75•8 mg

**Tel-E-Amp** (trademarked packaging form) *unit dose ampule*

**Tel-E-Dose** (trademarked packaging form) *unit dose package*

**Tel-E-Ject** (trademarked delivery system) *prefilled disposable syringe*

**telenzepine** INN

**Tel-E-Pack** (trademarked packaging form) *packaging system*

**Telepaque** tablets ℞ *radiopaque contrast medium for cholecystography* [iopanoic acid (66.68% iodine)] 500 mg (333.4 mg)

**Tel-E-Vial** (trademarked packaging form) *unit dose vial*

**telinavir** USAN *antiviral; HIV protease inhibitor*

**telithromycin** *broad-spectrum ketolide antibiotic for respiratory tract infections*

**tellurium** *element (Te)*

**telmisartan** USAN *long-acting antihypertensive; angiotensin II receptor antagonist*

**teloxantrone** INN *antineoplastic* [also: teloxantrone HCl]

**teloxantrone HCl** USAN *antineoplastic* [also: teloxantrone]

**teludipine** INN, BAN *antihypertensive; calcium channel antagonist* [also: teludipine HCl]

**teludipine HCl** USAN *antihypertensive; calcium channel antagonist* [also: teludipine]

**Telzir** (European name for U.S. product Lexiva)

**temafloxacin** INN, BAN *antibacterial; microbial DNA topoisomerase inhibitor* [also: temafloxacin HCl]

**temafloxacin HCl** USAN *antibacterial; microbial DNA topoisomerase inhibitor* [also: temafloxacin]

**temarotene** INN

**tematropium methylsulfate** USAN *anticholinergic* [also: tematropium metilsulfate]

**tematropium metilsulfate** INN *anticholinergic* [also: tematropium methylsulfate]

**temazepam** USAN, INN *benzodiazepine hypnotic; minor tranquilizer* 7.5, 15, 30 mg oral

**Temazin Cold** syrup (discontinued 2001) OTC *decongestant; antihistamine* [phenylpropanolamine HCl; chlorpheniramine maleate] 12.5•2 mg/5 mL

**Tembid** (trademarked dosage form) *sustained-action capsule*

**temefos** USAN, INN *veterinary ectoparasiticide*

**temelastine** USAN, INN, BAN *antihistamine*

**temocapril HCl** USAN *antihypertensive*

**temocillin** USAN, INN, BAN *antibacterial*

**Temodal** ⒸⒶⓃ capsules ℞ *alkylating antineoplastic for refractory anaplastic astrocytoma and recurrent malignant glioma* [temozolomide] 5, 20, 100, 250 mg

**Temodar** capsules ℞ *alkylating antineoplastic for refractory anaplastic astrocytoma; investigational (NDA filed) for recurrent malignant glioma and metastatic malignant melanoma* [temozolomide] 5, 20, 100, 250 mg

**temodox** USAN, INN *veterinary growth stimulant*

**temoporfin** USAN, INN, BAN *photosensitizer for photodynamic cancer therapy; investigational (NDA filed) for head and neck cancer*

**Temovate** ointment, gel, cream, scalp application ℞ *corticosteroidal anti-inflammatory* [clobetasol propionate] 0.05%

**Temovate Emollient** cream ℞ *corticosteroidal anti-inflammatory* [clobetasol propionate in an emollient base] 0.05%

**temozolomide** INN, BAN *alkylating antineoplastic for refractory anaplastic astrocytoma; investigational (NDA* filed) for malignant glioma and metastatic malignant melanoma

**TEMP (tamoxifen, etoposide, mitoxantrone, Platinol)** chemotherapy protocol

**Temp Tab** tablets OTC electrolyte replacement [sodium, potassium, and chloride electrolytes] 180•15•287 mg

**Tempium** ℞ investigational treatment for Alzheimer disease [lazabemide HCl]

**Tempo** chewable tablets OTC antacid; antiflatulent [aluminum hydroxide; magnesium hydroxide; calcium carbonate; simethicone] 133•81•414•20 mg

**Tempra** ⒸⒶⓃ chewable tablets, syrup, oral drops OTC pediatric analgesic and antipyretic [acetaminophen] 80 mg; 80, 160 mg/5 mL; 80 mg/mL

**Tempra 1** drops OTC analgesic; antipyretic [acetaminophen] 100 mg/mL

**Tempra 2** syrup OTC analgesic; antipyretic [acetaminophen] 160 mg/5 mL

**Tempra 3** chewable tablets OTC analgesic; antipyretic [acetaminophen] 80, 160 mg

**Tempra FirsTabs** ⒸⒶⓃ (quick dissolving tablets) OTC pediatric analgesic and antipyretic [acetaminophen] 160 mg

**Tempra Quicklets** (quickly dissolving tablets) OTC analgesic; antipyretic [acetaminophen] 80, 160 mg

**Tempule** (trademarked dosage form) timed-release capsule or tablet

**temsirolimus** investigational (Phase III) antineoplastic for renal cell carcinoma, metastatic breast cancer, and mantle cell lymphoma; investigational (Phase II) immunosuppressant for rheumatoid arthritis and multiple sclerosis ⍰ sirolimus

**temurtide** USAN, INN, BAN vaccine adjuvant

**10 Benzagel; 5 Benzagel** gel ℞ topical keratolytic for acne [benzoyl peroxide] 10%; 5%

**10% LMD** IV injection ℞ plasma volume expander for shock due to hemorrhage, burns, or surgery [dextran 40] 10%

**tenamfetamine** INN

**Tencet** capsules ℞ analgesic; antipyretic; sedative [acetaminophen; caffeine; butalbital] 325•40•50 mg

**Tencon** capsules ℞ analgesic; barbiturate sedative [acetaminophen; butalbital] 650•50 mg

**tendamistat** INN

**Tenecteplase** ℞ investigational (NDA filed) thrombolytic

**tenecteplase** USAN thrombolytic for acute myocardial infarction; genetically engineered mutation of tissue plasminogen activator (tPA)

**Tenex** tablets ℞ antihypertensive; antiadrenergic [guanfacine HCl] 1, 2 mg ⍰ Xanax

**tenidap** USAN, INN investigational (NDA filed) anti-inflammatory for osteoarthritis and rheumatoid arthritis; cytokine inhibitor

**tenidap sodium** USAN anti-inflammatory for osteoarthritis and rheumatoid arthritis

**tenilapine** INN

**teniloxazine** INN

**tenilsetam** INN

**teniposide** USAN, INN, BAN antineoplastic for refractory childhood acute lymphocytic leukemia (orphan)

**Ten-K** controlled-release tablets ℞ potassium supplement [potassium chloride] 750 mg (10 mEq K)

**tenoate** INN combining name for radicals or groups

**tenocyclidine** INN

**tenofovir** USAN antiviral; nucleotide reverse transcriptase inhibitor (NRTI)

**tenofovir disoproxil fumarate (tenofovir DF)** oral antiviral; nucleotide reverse transcriptase inhibitor (NRTI) for HIV-1 infection (base=82%)

**tenonitrozole** INN

**Tenoretic 50; Tenoretic 100** tablets ℞ antihypertensive; β-blocker; diuretic [chlorthalidone; atenolol] 25•50 mg; 25•100 mg

**Tenormin** tablets, IV injection ℞ antianginal; antihypertensive; β-

*blocker* [atenolol] 25, 50, 100 mg; 5 mg/10 mL

**Tenovil** ℞ *investigational (Phase I) immunomodulator for HIV infection; investigational (Phase II) for psoriasis* [interleukin-10]

**tenoxicam** USAN, INN, BAN *anti-inflammatory*

**Tensilon** IV or IM injection ℞ *myasthenia gravis treatment; antidote to curare overdose* [edrophonium chloride] 10 mg/mL

**Ten-Tab** (trademarked dosage form) *controlled-release tablet*

**Tenuate** tablets, Dospan (controlled-release tablets) ℞ *anorexiant; CNS stimulant* [diethylpropion HCl] 25 mg; 75 mg

**tenylidone** INN

**teoclate** INN *combining name for radicals or groups* [also: theoclate]

**teopranitol** INN

**teoprolol** INN

**tepirindole** INN

**tepoxalin** USAN, INN *antipsoriatic*

**teprenone** INN

**teprosilate** INN *combining name for radicals or groups*

**teprotide** USAN, INN *angiotensin-converting enzyme (ACE) inhibitor*

**Tequin** film-coated tablets, IV infusion ℞ *broad-spectrum fluoroquinolone antibiotic* [gatifloxacin] 200, 400 mg; 200, 400 mg/vial

**Terak with Polymyxin B Sulfate** ophthalmic ointment ℞ *topical ophthalmic antibiotic* [oxytetracycline HCl; polymyxin B sulfate] 5 mg• 10 000 U per g

**Terazol 3** vaginal suppositories, vaginal cream ℞ *antifungal* [terconazole] 80 mg; 0.8%

**Terazol 7** vaginal cream ℞ *antifungal* [terconazole] 0.4%

**terazosin** INN, BAN *alpha$_1$-adrenergic blocker for hypertension and benign prostatic hyperplasia (BPH)* [also: terazosin HCl]

**terazosin HCl** USAN *alpha$_1$-adrenergic blocker for hypertension and benign*

*prostatic hyperplasia (BPH)* [also: terazosin] 1, 2, 5, 10 mg oral

**terbinafine** USAN, INN, BAN *systemic allylamine antifungal* [also: terbinafine HCl]

**terbinafine HCl** JAN *allylamine antifungal* [also: terbinafine]

**terbium** *element (Tb)*

**terbogrel** USAN *platelet aggregation inhibitor*

**terbucromil** INN

**terbufibrol** INN

**terbuficin** INN

**terbuprol** INN

**terbutaline** INN, BAN *sympathomimetic bronchodilator* [also: terbutaline sulfate]

**terbutaline sulfate** USAN, USP *sympathomimetic bronchodilator* [also: terbutaline] 2.5, 5 mg oral

**terciprazine** INN

**terconazole** USAN, INN, BAN *vaginal antifungal* 0.4%, 0.8% vaginal

**terfenadine** USAN, USP, INN, JAN *piperidine antihistamine*

**terflavoxate** INN

**terfluranol** INN

**terguride** INN *investigational dopamine agonist for central nervous system disorders*

**teriparatide** USAN, INN *human parathyroid hormone, recombinant; osteoporosis treatment that stimulates new bone formation; diagnostic aid for parathyroid-induced hypocalcemia*

**teriparatide acetate** USAN, JAN *diagnostic aid for parathyroid-induced hypocalcemia (orphan)*

**terizidone** INN

**terlakiren** USAN *antihypertensive; renin inhibitor*

**terlipressin** INN, BAN *investigational (orphan) for bleeding esophageal varices*

**ternidazole** INN

**terodiline** INN, BAN, JAN *coronary vasodilator* [also: terodiline HCl]

**terodiline HCl** USAN *coronary vasodilator; investigational agent for urinary incontinence* [also: terodiline]

**terofenamate** INN

**teroxalene** INN *antischistosomal* [also: teroxalene HCl]

**teroxalene HCl** USAN *antischistosomal* [also: teroxalene]

**teroxirone** USAN, INN *antineoplastic*

**terpin hydrate** USP (*disapproved for use as an expectorant in 1991*)

**terpinol** [see: terpin hydrate]

**Terra-Cortril** eye drop suspension (discontinued 2000) ℞ *topical ophthalmic corticosteroidal anti-inflammatory; antibiotic* [hydrocortisone acetate; oxytetracycline HCl] 1.5%•0.5%

**terrafungine** [see: oxytetracycline]

**Terramycin** capsules (discontinued 2003) ℞ *broad-spectrum tetracycline antibiotic* [oxytetracycline HCl] 250 mg ⊡ Garamycin; Theramycin

**Terramycin** IM or IV injection ℞ *broad-spectrum tetracycline antibiotic* [oxytetracycline; lidocaine] 100 mg•2%, 250 mg•2% per 2 mL dose

**Terramycin with Polymyxin B** ophthalmic ointment ℞ *ophthalmic antibiotic* [oxytetracycline HCl; polymyxin B sulfate] 5 mg•10 000 U per g

**Terrell** liquid for vaporization ℞ *inhalation general anesthetic* [isoflurane]

**Tersaseptic** shampoo/cleanser OTC *soap-free therapeutic cleanser*

**tertatolol** INN, BAN

**tertiary amyl alcohol** [see: amylene hydrate]

***tert*-pentyl alcohol** [see: amylene hydrate]

**Tesamone** IM injection (discontinued 2001) ℞ *androgen replacement for delayed puberty or breast cancer* [testosterone] 100 mg/mL

**tesicam** USAN, INN *anti-inflammatory*

**tesimide** USAN, INN *anti-inflammatory*

**Teslac** tablets ℞ *adjunctive hormonal chemotherapy for advanced postmenopausal breast carcinoma* [testolactone] 50 mg

**Teslascan** IV injection ℞ *MRI contrast medium for liver imaging* [mangofodipir trisodium] 37.9 mg/mL (50 μmol/mL)

**tesmilifene HCl** USAN *antihistamine; chemopotentiator for adjunctive treatment of malignant tumors*

**TESPA (triethylenethiophosphoramide)** [see: thiotepa]

**Tessalon** Perles (capsules) ℞ *antitussive* [benzonatate] 100, 200 mg

**Test Pack** kit for professional use *in vitro diagnostic aid for Group A streptococcal antigens in throat swabs* [enzyme immunoassay]

**Testandro** IM injection (discontinued 2001) ℞ *androgen replacement for delayed puberty or breast cancer* [testosterone] 100 mg/mL

**Testim** gel ℞ *hormone replacement therapy for male hypogonadism* [testosterone; alcohol 74%] 1% (50 mg/pkt.)

**Testoderm; Testoderm with Adhesive** transdermal patch (for scrotal area) ℞ *hormone replacement therapy for male hypogonadism* [testosterone] 4, 6 mg/day (10, 15 mg total)

**Testoderm TTS** transdermal patch (for nonscrotal skin) (discontinued 2003) ℞ *hormone replacement therapy for hypogonadism* [testosterone] 5 mg/day

**testolactone** USAN, USP, INN *antineoplastic; androgen hormone* ⊡ testosterone

**Testopel** pellets for subcu implantation ℞ *hormone replacement therapy for hypogonadism* [testosterone] 75 mg

**testosterone** USP, INN, BAN *androgen for hypogonadism and testosterone deficiency in men; investigational (Phase II, orphan) for AIDS-wasting syndrome and delay of growth and puberty in boys* ⊡ testolactone

**Testosterone Aqueous** IM injection ℞ *androgen for hypogonadism, delayed puberty, and androgen-responsive metastatic cancers* [testosterone] 25, 50, 100 mg/mL

**testosterone cyclopentanepropionate** [see: testosterone cypionate]

**testosterone cyclopentylpropionate** [see: testosterone cypionate]

**testosterone cypionate** USP *parenteral androgen; sometimes abused as a street drug* 100, 200 mg/mL injection

**testosterone enanthate** USP *parenteral androgen for testosterone deficiency in men, delayed puberty in boys, and metastatic breast cancer in women; sometimes abused as a street drug*

**testosterone heptanoate** [see: testosterone enanthate]

**testosterone ketolaurate** USAN, INN *androgen*

**testosterone 3-oxododecanoate** [see: testosterone ketolaurate]

**testosterone phenylacetate** USAN *androgen*

**testosterone propionate** USP *parenteral androgen; investigational (orphan) for vulvar dystrophies* 100 mg/mL injection

**TestPack** [see: Abbott TestPack]

**Testred** capsules ℞ *androgen for hypogonadism or testosterone deficiency in men, delayed puberty in boys, and metastatic breast cancer in women; also abused as a street drug* [methyltestosterone] 10 mg

**tetanus antitoxin** USP *passive immunizing agent*

**tetanus & gas gangrene antitoxins** NF

**tetanus & gas gangrene polyvalent antitoxin** [see: tetanus & gas gangrene antitoxins]

**tetanus immune globulin (TIG)** USP *passive immunizing agent*

**tetanus immune human globulin** [now: tetanus immune globulin]

**tetanus toxoid** USP *active immunizing agent*

**tetanus toxoid, adsorbed** USP *active immunizing agent*

**tetiothalein sodium** [see: iodophthalein sodium]

**tetnicoran** [see: nicofurate]

**tetrabarbital** INN

**tetrabenazine** INN, BAN *investigational (orphan) for Huntington disease and severe tardive dyskinesia*

**TetraBriks** (trademarked delivery form) *ready-to-use liquid containers*

**tetracaine** USP, INN *topical local anesthetic* [also: amethocaine]

**tetracaine HCl** USP, JAN *topical local anesthetic* [also: amethocaine HCl]

**Tetracap** capsules (discontinued 2003) ℞ *broad-spectrum antibiotic* [tetracycline HCl] 250 mg

**tetrachlorodecaoxide** *investigational (Phase III) immunomodulator and growth factor for HIV and AIDS*

**tetrachloroethylene** USP

**tetrachloromethane** [see: carbon tetrachloride]

**tetracosactide** INN *adrenocorticotropic hormone* [also: cosyntropin; tetracosactrin]

**tetracosactrin** BAN *adrenocorticotropic hormone* [also: cosyntropin; tetracosactide]

**tetracyclics** *a class of antidepressants which enhance noradrenergic and serotonergic activity by blocking norepinephrine or serotonin uptake*

**tetracycline** USP, INN, BAN *bacteriostatic antibiotic; antirickettsial*

**tetracycline HCl** USP *bacteriostatic antibiotic; antirickettsial* 250, 500 mg oral

**tetracycline phosphate complex** USP, BAN *antibacterial*

**tetracyclines** *a class of bacteriostatic, antimicrobial antibiotics*

**tetradecanoic acid, methylethyl ester** [see: isopropyl myristate]

**tetradonium bromide** INN

**tetraethylammonium bromide (TEAB)** [see: tetrylammonium bromide]

**tetraethylammonium chloride (TEAC)**

**tetraethylthiuram disulfide** [see: disulfiram]

**tetrafilcon A** USAN *hydrophilic contact lens material*

**Tetra-Formula** lozenges OTC *antitussive; topical oral anesthetic* [dextromethorphan hydrobromide; benzocaine] 10•15 mg

**tetraglycine hydroperiodide** *source of iodine for disinfecting water*

**tetrahydroacridinamine (THA)** [see: tacrine HCl]

**tetrahydroaminoacridine (THA)**
[see: tacrine HCl]

**tetrahydrocannabinol (THC)** [see:
dronabinol]

**tetrahydrolipstatin** [see: orlistat]

**tetrahydrozoline** BAN *vasoconstrictor;
nasal decongestant; topical ophthalmic
decongestant* [also: tetrhydrozoline
HCl; tetryzoline]

**tetrahydrozoline HCl** USP *vasoconstrictor; nasal decongestant; topical ophthalmic decongestant* [also: tetryzoline;
tetrahydrozoline] 0.05% eye drops

**tetraiodophenolphthalein sodium**
[see: iodophthalein sodium]

**tetrallobarbital** [see: butalbital]

**tetramal** [see: tetrabarbital]

**tetrameprozine** [see: aminopromazine]

**tetramethrin** INN

**tetramethylene dimethanesulfo-
nate** [see: busulfan]

**tetramisole** INN *anthelmintic* [also:
tetramisole HCl]

**tetramisole HCl** USAN *anthelmintic*
[also: tetramisole]

**Tetramune** IM injection (discontinued 2001) ℞ *pediatric vaccine for
diphtheria, pertussis, tetanus and* Haemophilus influenzae *type b* [diphthe-
ria & tetanus toxoids & whole-cell
pertussis (DTwP) vaccine; Hemophilus b conjugate vaccine] 0.5 mL

**tetranitrol** [see: erythrityl tetranitrate]

**tetrantoin**

**TetraPaks** (trademarked delivery form)
*ready-to-use open system containers*

**Tetrasine; Tetrasine Extra** eye drops
OTC *topical ophthalmic decongestant
and vasoconstrictor* [tetrahydrozoline
HCl] 0.05%

**tetrasodium ethylenediaminetetra-
acetate** [see: edetate sodium]

**tetrasodium pyrophosphate** [see:
sodium pyrophosphate]

**tetrazepam** INN

**tetrazolast** INN *antiallergic; antiasthmatic* [also: tetrazolast meglumine]

**tetrazolast meglumine** USAN *antiallergic; antiasthmatic* [also: tetrazolast]

**tetridamine** INN *analgesic; anti-inflammatory* [also: tetrydamine]

**tetriprofen** INN

**tetrofosmin** USAN, INN, BAN *diagnostic
aid*

**tetronasin** BAN [also: tetronasin 5930]

**tetronasin 5930** INN [also: tetronasin]

**tetroquinone** USAN, INN *systemic keratolytic*

**tetroxoprim** USAN, INN *antibacterial*

**tetrydamine** USAN *analgesic; anti-
inflammatory* [also: tetridamine]

**tetrylammonium bromide** INN

**tetryzoline** INN *vasoconstrictor; nasal
decongestant; topical ocular decongestant* [also: tetrahydrozoline HCl; tet-
rahydrozoline]

**tetryzoline HCl** [see: tetrahydrozoline
HCl]

**tetterwort** *medicinal herb* [see: bloodroot; celandine]

**Teveten** film-coated caplets *antihypertensive; angiotensin II receptor antagonist* [eprosartan mesylate] 400, 600 mg

**Teveten HCT** film-coated caplets ℞
*antihypertensive; angiotensin II recep-
tor antagonist; diuretic* [eprosartan
mesylate; hydrochlorothiazide] 600•
12.5, 600•25 mg

**Tev-Tropin** powder for subcu injection
℞ *growth hormone for adults or children with congenital or endogenous
growth hormone deficiency, children
with Turner syndrome or renal-induced
growth failure* [somatropin] 5 mg (15
IU) per vial

**Texacort** solution ℞ *topical corticosteroidal anti-inflammatory* [hydrocorti-
sone] 1%

**texacromil** INN

**tezacitabine** USAN *antineoplastic for
colon and rectal cancers*

**tezosentan** *investigational (Phase III)
parenteral vasoconstrictor and endothelin receptor antagonist for acute heart
failure, pulmonary edema, and hepatorenal syndrome*

**6-TG (6-thioguanine)** [see: thiogua-
nine]

**TG (thyroglobulin)** [q.v.]

**T-Gen** suppositories, pediatric suppositories ℞ *antiemetic; anticholinergic* [trimethobenzamide HCl; benzocaine] 200 mg•2%; 100 mg•2%

**T-Gesic** capsules ℞ *narcotic analgesic* [hydrocodone bitartrate; acetaminophen] 5•500 mg

**αTGI (α-triglycidyl isocyanurate)** [see: teroxirone]

**TH (theophylline)** [q.v.]

**TH (thyroid hormone)** [see: levothyroxine sodium]

**THA (tetrahydroaminoacridine or tetrahydroacridinamine)** [see: tacrine HCl]

**thalidomide** USAN, INN, BAN *immunomodulator for erythema nodosum leprosum (ENL) (orphan); investigational (Phase III, orphan) cytokine inhibitor for graft vs. host disease, AIDS-wasting syndrome, lupus, and mycobacterial infections; investigational (Phase II/III, orphan) for various cancers; investigational (Phase III) for aphthous ulcers*

**Thalitone** tablets ℞ *antihypertensive; diuretic* [chlorthalidone] 15, 25 mg

**thallium** *element (Tl)* ⊡ Valium

**thallous chloride Tl 201** USAN, USP *radiopaque contrast medium; radioactive agent*

**Thalomid** capsules ℞ *immunomodulator for erythema nodosum leprosum (ENL) (orphan); investigational (Phase III, orphan) for graft vs. host disease, AIDS-wasting syndrome, lupus, and mycobacterial infections; investigational (Phase II/III, orphan) for various cancers; investigational (Phase III) for aphthous ulcers* [thalidomide] 50, 100, 200 mg

**Tham** IV infusion ℞ *systemic alkalizer; corrects acidosis associated with cardiac bypass surgery or cardiac arrest* [tromethamine] 18 g/500 mL (150 mEq/500 mL)

**thaumatin** BAN

**THC (tetrahydrocannabinol)** [see: dronabinol]

**THC (thiocarbanidin)**

**theanine (L-theanine)** *natural extract of green tea that produces calming and relaxing effects without drowsiness; effective in controlling PMS symptoms; increases brain levels of the neurotransmitters GABA and dopamine, which increase alpha brain wave activity*

**thebacon** INN, BAN

**theine** [see: caffeine]

**thenalidine** INN

**thenium closilate** INN *veterinary anthelmintic* [also: thenium closylate]

**thenium closylate** USAN *veterinary anthelmintic* [also: thenium closilate]

**thenyldiamine** INN

**thenylpyramine HCl** [see: methapyrilene HCl]

**Theo-24** timed-release capsules ℞ *antiasthmatic; bronchodilator* [theophylline] 100, 200, 300 mg

**Theobid** Duracaps (sustained-release capsules) (discontinued 2004) ℞ *antiasthmatic; bronchodilator* [theophylline] 260 mg

**theobromine** NF

**theobromine calcium salicylate** NF

**theobromine sodium acetate** NF

**theobromine sodium salicylate** NF

*Theobromo cacao* medicinal herb [see: cocoa]

**Theochron** extended-release tablets ℞ *antiasthmatic; bronchodilator* [theophylline] 100, 200, 300, 450 mg

**theoclate** BAN *combining name for radicals or groups* [also: teoclate]

**Theoclear L.A.** extended-release capsules (discontinued 2004) ℞ *antiasthmatic; bronchodilator* [theophylline] 130, 260 mg

**Theoclear-80** oral solution (discontinued 2004) ℞ *antiasthmatic; bronchodilator* [theophylline] 80 mg/15 mL ⊡ Theolair

**theodrenaline** INN, BAN

**Theodrine** tablets OTC *antiasthmatic; bronchodilator; decongestant* [theophylline; ephedrine HCl] 120•22.5 mg

**Theo-Dur** extended-release tablets (discontinued 2003) ℞ *antiasthmatic;*

*bronchodilator* [theophylline] 100, 200, 300, 450 mg

**theofibrate** USAN *antihyperlipoprotein-emic* [also: etofylline clofibrate]

**Theolair** oral liquid (discontinued 2004) ℞ *antiasthmatic; bronchodilator* [theophylline] 80 mg/15 mL

**Theolair** tablets ℞ *antiasthmatic; bronchodilator* [theophylline] 125 mg ⑨ Theoclear; Thyrolar

**Theolair-SR** sustained-release tablets ℞ *antiasthmatic; bronchodilator* [theophylline] 200, 250, 300, 500 mg

**Theolate** oral liquid ℞ *antiasthmatic; bronchodilator; expectorant* [theophylline; guaifenesin] 150•90 mg/15 mL

**Theomax DF** pediatric syrup ℞ *antiasthmatic; bronchodilator; decongestant; antihistamine* [theophylline; ephedrine sulfate; hydroxyzine HCl; alcohol 5%] 97.5•18.75•7.5 mg/15 mL

**theophyldine** [see: aminophylline]

**theophyllamine** [see: aminophylline]

**Theophyllin KI** elixir ℞ *antiasthmatic; bronchodilator; expectorant* [theophylline; potassium iodide] 80•130 mg/15 mL

**theophylline (TH)** USP, BAN *bronchodilator* 100, 125, 200, 300, 400, 450, 600 mg oral

**theophylline aminoisobutanol** [see: ambuphylline]

**theophylline calcium salicylate** *bronchodilator*

**theophylline ethylenediamine** [now: aminophylline]

**theophylline monohydrate** [see: theophylline]

**theophylline olamine** USP

**theophylline sodium acetate** NF

**theophylline sodium glycinate** USP *smooth muscle relaxant*

**Theo-Sav** controlled-release tablets (discontinued 2004) ℞ *antiasthmatic; bronchodilator* [theophylline] 100, 200, 300 mg

**Theospan-SR** timed-release capsules (discontinued 2003) ℞ *antiasthmatic; bronchodilator* [theophylline] 130, 260 mg

**Theostat 80** syrup (discontinued 2003) ℞ *antiasthmatic; bronchodilator* [theophylline; alcohol 1%] 80 mg/15 mL

**Theovent** timed-release capsules (discontinued 2004) ℞ *antiasthmatic; bronchodilator* [theophylline] 125, 250 mg

**Theo-X** controlled-release tablets (discontinued 2004) ℞ *antiasthmatic; bronchodilator* [theophylline] 100, 200, 300 mg

**Thera Hematinic** tablets OTC *hematinic; vitamin supplement* [ferrous fumarate; multiple vitamins; folic acid] 66.7•±•0.33 mg

**Thera Multi-Vitamin** oral liquid OTC *vitamin supplement* [multiple vitamins]

**Therabid** tablets OTC *vitamin supplement* [multiple vitamins]

**Therac** lotion OTC *topical acne treatment* [colloidal sulfur] 10%

**theraccines** *a class of vaccines with therapeutic action, usually used to help prevent the spread of cancer*

**TheraCys** powder for intravesical instillation ℞ *antineoplastic for urinary bladder cancer* [BCG vaccine, live] 81 mg (1.8–19.2 × 10$^8$ CFU)

**TheraDerm** transdermal patch ℞ *investigational (orphan) for AIDS-wasting syndrome* [testosterone]

**Therafectin** ℞ *investigational (NDA filed) synthetic monosaccharide anti-inflammatory for rheumatoid arthritis* [amiprilose HCl]

**TheraFlu Cold & Cough Night Time; TheraFlu Flu, Cold & Cough** powder for oral solution OTC *antitussive; decongestant; antihistamine; analgesic* [dextromethorphan hydrobromide; pseudoephedrine HCl; chlorpheniramine maleate; acetaminophen] 20•60•4•650 mg/pkt. ⑨ Thera-Flur

**TheraFlu Flu, Cold & Cough; TheraFlu Flu & Congestion Non-Drowsy** powder for oral solution OTC *antitussive; decongestant; expectorant; analgesic* [dextromethorphan hydrobromide; pseudoephedrine

HCl; guaifenesin; acetaminophen] 30•60•400•1000 mg/pkt

**TheraFlu Flu, Cold & Cough Night Time; TheraFlu Flu, Cold & Cough, and Sore Throat; Thera-Flu Flu & Cough Night Time; TheraFlu Severe Cold & Congestion** powder for oral solution OTC *antitussive; decongestant; antihistamine; analgesic* [dextromethorphan hydrobromide; pseudoephedrine HCl; chlorpheniramine maleate; acetaminophen] 20•60•4•1000 mg/pkt. ⍰ Thera-Flur

**TheraFlu Flu & Cold Medicine for Sore Throat; TheraFlu Flu & Sore Throat; TheraFlu Flu & Sore Throat Night Time** powder for oral solution OTC *decongestant; antihistamine; analgesic* [pseudoephedrine HCl; chlorpheniramine maleate; acetaminophen] 60•4•1000 mg/pkt.

**TheraFlu Flu & Cold Medicine Original Formula** powder for oral solution OTC *decongestant; antihistamine; analgesic* [pseudoephedrine HCl; chlorpheniramine maleate; acetaminophen] 60•4•650 mg/pkt.

**TheraFlu NightTime Formula Flu, Cold, & Cough Medicine** caplets OTC *antitussive; decongestant; antihistamine; analgesic* [dextromethorphan hydrobromide; pseudoephedrine HCl; chlorpheniramine maleate; acetaminophen] 15•30•2•500 mg

**TheraFlu Non-Drowsy Flu, Cold & Cough; TheraFlu Severe Cold & Congestion Non-Drowsy** powder for oral solution OTC *antitussive; decongestant; analgesic* [dextromethorphan hydrobromide; pseudoephedrine HCl; acetaminophen] 30•60•100 mg/pkt.

**TheraFlu Non-Drowsy Formula** caplets OTC *antitussive; decongestant; analgesic* [dextromethorphan hydrobromide; pseudoephedrine HCl; acetaminophen] 15•30•500 mg

**TheraFlu Vapor Stick** OTC *topical counterirritant* [camphor; menthol] 4.8%•2.6%

**Thera-Flur; Thera-Flur-N** gel (for self-application) ℞ *topical dental caries preventative* [sodium fluoride] 1.1% ⍰ TheraFlu

**Thera-Gesic** cream OTC *analgesic; counterirritant* [methyl salicylate; menthol] 15%• ≛

**Theragran** caplets OTC *vitamin supplement* [multiple vitamins; folic acid; biotin] ≛•400•30 µg ⍰ Theragyn

**Theragran** oral liquid OTC *vitamin supplement* [multiple vitamins] ⍰ Phenergan

**Theragran AntiOxidant** softgels OTC *vitamin/mineral supplement* [vitamins A, C, and E; multiple minerals] 5000 IU•250 mg•200 IU• ≛

**Theragran Hematinic** tablets (discontinued 2003) ℞ *hematinic; vitamin/mineral supplement* [ferrous fumarate; multiple vitamins & minerals; folic acid] 66.7• ≛ •0.33 mg

**Theragran Stress Formula** tablets OTC *vitamin/iron supplement* [multiple B vitamins; vitamins C and E; ferrous fumarate; folic acid; biotin] ≛•600 mg•30 IU•27 mg•0.4 mg•45 µg

**Theragran-M** caplets OTC *vitamin/mineral/calcium/iron supplement* [multiple vitamins & minerals; calcium; iron; folic acid; biotin] ≛•40•27•0.4•0.03 mg

**Thera-Hist Cold & Allergy** pediatric syrup OTC *decongestant; antihistamine* [pseudoephedrine HCl; chlorpheniramine maleate] 30•2 mg/10 mL

**Thera-Hist Cold & Cough** pediatric syrup OTC *antitussive; decongestant; antihistamine* [dextromethorphan hydrobromide; pseudoephedrine HCl; chlorpheniramine maleate] 10•30•2 mg/10 mL

**Thera-Hist Expectorant Chest Congestion** pediatric oral liquid OTC *decongestant; expectorant* [pseudoephedrine HCl; guaifenesin] 15•50 mg/5 mL

**Thera-Ject** (trademarked delivery system) *prefilled disposable syringe*

**Thera-M** tablets OTC *vitamin/mineral/ iron supplement* [multiple vitamins & minerals; iron; folic acid; biotin] ± • 27 mg•0.4 mg•35 μg

**Theramycin Z** topical solution (discontinued 2003) ℞ *antibiotic for acne* [erythromycin] 2% ⊠ Garamycin; Terramycin

**TheraPatch** patch OTC *analgesic; counterirritant* [methyl salicylate; menthol; camphor]

**TheraPatch Cold Sore** patch OTC *topical local anesthetic and antipruritic* [lidocaine; camphor; aloe vera; eucalyptus oil] 4%•0.5%• ± • ±

**TheraPatch Vapor Patch for Kids** OTC *counterirritant; cough suppressant* [camphor; menthol] 4.7%•2.6%

**Therapeutic** tablets OTC *vitamin supplement* [multiple vitamins; folic acid; biotin] ± •400•30 μg

**Therapeutic B with C** capsules OTC *vitamin supplement* [multiple B vitamins; vitamin C] ± •300 mg

**Therapeutic Bath** lotion, oil OTC *moisturizer; emollient*

**Therapeutic Mineral Ice; Therapeutic Mineral Ice Exercise Formula** gel OTC *topical analgesic; counterirritant* [menthol] 2%; 4%

**Therapeutic-H** tablets OTC *hematinic; vitamin supplement* [ferrous fumarate; multiple vitamins; folic acid] 66.7• ± •0.33 mg

**Therapeutic-M** tablets OTC *vitamin/ mineral/iron supplement* [multiple vitamins & minerals; iron; folic acid; biotin] ± •27 mg•0.4 mg•30 μg

**Theraplex T** shampoo (discontinued 2003) OTC *antiseborrheic; antipsoriatic; antipruritic; antibacterial* [coal tar] 1%

**Theraplex Z** shampoo (discontinued 2003) OTC *antiseborrheic; antibacterial; antifungal* [pyrithione zinc] 2%

**Theraseed** ℞ *investigational radioactive "seeds" for ultrasound-guided brachytherapy for adenocarcinoma of the* prostate [palladium Pd 103] 0.665 Gy (66.5 rads)

**TheraTears** ophthalmic gel OTC *ocular moisturizer/lubricant* [carboxymethylcellulose sodium] 1%

**Theratope-STn** ℞ *investigational (Phase III) theraccine for recurrent or metastatic breast and colorectal cancer and adenocarcinoma*

**Theravee** tablets OTC *vitamin supplement* [multiple vitamins; folic acid; biotin] ± •400•15 μg

**Theravee Hematinic** tablets OTC *hematinic; vitamin supplement* [ferrous fumarate; multiple vitamins; folic acid] 66.7• ± •0.33 mg

**Theravee-M** tablets OTC *vitamin/mineral/iron supplement* [multiple vitamins & minerals; iron; folic acid; biotin] ± •27 mg•0.4 mg•15 μg

**Theravim** tablets OTC *vitamin supplement* [multiple vitamins; folic acid; biotin] ± •400•35 μg

**Theravim-M** tablets OTC *vitamin/mineral/iron supplement* [multiple vitamins & minerals; iron; folic acid; biotin] ± •27 mg•0.4 mg•30 μg

**Theravite** oral liquid OTC *vitamin supplement* [multiple vitamins] ⊠ Therevac

**Therems** tablets OTC *vitamin supplement* [multiple vitamins; folic acid; biotin] ± •400•15 μg

**Therems-M** tablets OTC *vitamin/mineral/iron supplement* [multiple vitamins & minerals; iron; folic acid; biotin] ± •27 mg•0.4 mg•30 μg

**Therevac-Plus** disposable enema OTC *hyperosmotic laxative; stool softener; local anesthetic* [glycerin; docusate sodium; benzocaine] 275•283•20 mg ⊠ Theravite

**Therevac-SB** disposable enema OTC *hyperosmotic laxative; stool softener* [glycerin; docusate sodium] 275• 283 mg

**Thermazene** cream ℞ *broad-spectrum bactericidal for adjunctive burn treatment* [silver sulfadiazine] 10 mg/g

**ThexForte** caplets OTC *vitamin supplement* [multiple B vitamins; vitamin C] ≛ •500 mg

**THF (thymic humoral factor)** [q.v.]

**thiabendazole (TBZ)** USAN, USP *anthelmintic for strongyloidiasis (threadworm), larva migrans, and trichinosis* [also: tiabendazole]

**thiabutazide** [see: buthiazide]

**thiacetarsamide sodium** INN

**thiacetazone** BAN [also: thioacetazone]

**thialbarbital** INN [also: thialbarbitone]

**thialbarbitone** BAN [also: thialbarbital]

**thialisobumal sodium** [see: buthalital sodium]

**thiamazole** INN *thyroid inhibitor* [also: methimazole]

**thiambutosine** INN, BAN

**Thiamilate** enteric-coated tablets OTC *vitamin B₁ supplement* [thiamine HCl] 20 mg

**thiamine (vitamin B₁)** INN *water-soluble vitamin; enzyme cofactor* [also: thiamine HCl]

**thiamine HCl (vitamin B₁)** USP *water-soluble vitamin; enzyme cofactor* [also: thiamine] 50, 100, 250 mg oral; 100 mg/mL injection

**thiamine mononitrate** USP *vitamin B₁; enzyme cofactor*

**thiamine propyl disulfide** [see: prosultiamine]

**thiaminogen** *medicinal herb* [see: rice bran oil]

**thiamiprine** USAN *antineoplastic* [also: tiamiprine]

**thiamphenicol** USAN, INN, BAN *antibacterial*

**thiamylal** USP *barbiturate general anesthetic*

**thiamylal sodium** USP, JAN *barbiturate general anesthetic*

**thiazesim HCl** USAN *antidepressant* [also: tiazesim]

**thiazides** *a class of diuretic agents that increase urinary excretion of sodium and chloride in approximately equal amounts*

**thiazinamium chloride** USAN *antiallergic*

**thiazinamium metilsulfate** INN

**4-thiazolidinecarboxylic acid** [see: timonacic]

**thiazolidinediones** *a class of antidiabetic agents that increase insulin sensitivity and reduce plasma insulin levels*

**thiazolsulfone** [see: thiazosulfone]

**thiazosulfone** INN

**thiazothielite** [see: antienite]

**thiazothienol** [see: antazonite]

**thienamycins** *a class of antibiotics*

**thienobenzodiazepines** *a class of novel (atypical) antipsychotic agents*

**thiethylperazine** USAN, INN *antiemetic; antidopaminergic*

**thiethylperazine malate** USP *antiemetic; antipsychotic*

**thiethylperazine maleate** USAN, USP *antiemetic*

**thihexinol methylbromide** NF, INN

**thimbleberry** *medicinal herb* [see: blackberry]

**thimerfonate sodium** USAN *topical anti-infective* [also: sodium timerfonate]

**thimerosal** USP *topical anti-infective; preservative (49% mercury)* [also: thiomersal] 1:1000 topical

**thioacetazone** INN, DCF [also: thiacetazone]

**thiocarbanidin (THC)**

**thiocarlide** BAN [also: tiocarlide]

**thiocolchicine glycoside** [see: thiocolchicoside]

**thiocolchicoside** INN

**thioctan; thioctacid; thioctic acid** *natural antioxidant* [see: alpha lipoic acid]

**thiocyanate sodium** NF

**thiodiglycol** INN

**thiodiphenylamine** [see: phenothiazine]

**thiofuradene** INN

**thioguanine (6-TG)** USAN, USP *antimetabolite antineoplastic* [also: tioguanine] 40 mg oral

**thiohexallymal** [see: thialbarbital]

**thiohexamide** INN

**Thiola** sugar-coated tablets ℞ *prevention of cystine nephrolithiasis in homozygous cystinuria (orphan)* [tiopronin] 100 mg

**thiomebumal sodium** [see: thiopental sodium]

**thiomersal** INN, BAN *topical anti-infective; preservative* [also: thimerosal]

**thiomesterone** BAN [also: tiomesterone]

**thiomicid** [see: thioacetazone; thiacetazone]

**thioparamizone** [see: thioacetazone; thiacetazone]

**thiopental sodium** USP, INN, JAN *barbiturate general anesthetic; anticonvulsant* [also: thiopentone sodium] 2%, 2.5% (20, 25 mg/mL) injection

**thiopentone sodium** BAN *general anesthetic; anticonvulsant* [also: thiopental sodium]

**thiophanate** BAN

**thiophosphoramide** [see: thiotepa]

**Thioplex** powder for IV, intracavitary, or intravesical injection ℞ *alkylating antineoplastic for lymphomas and carcinoma of the breast, ovary, or bladder* [thiotepa] 15 mg

**thiopropazate** INN [also: thiopropazate HCl]

**thiopropazate HCl** NF [also: thiopropazate]

**thioproperazine** INN, BAN *phenothiazine antipsychotic* [also: thioproperazine mesylate]

**thioproperazine mesylate** *phenothiazine antipsychotic* [also: thioproperazine]

**thioproperazine methanesulfonate** [see: thioproperazine mesylate]

**thioridazine** USAN, USP, INN *phenothiazine antipsychotic; sedative*

**thioridazine HCl** USP *phenothiazine antipsychotic; sedative* 10, 15, 25, 50, 100, 150, 200 mg oral

**thiosalan** USAN *disinfectant* [also: tiosalan]

**Thiosulfil Forte** tablets (discontinued 2001) ℞ *broad-spectrum sulfonamide bacteriostatic* [sulfamethizole] 500 mg

**thiosulfuric acid, disodium salt pentahydrate** [see: sodium thiosulfate]

**thiotepa** USP, INN, BAN, JAN *alkylating antineoplastic for lymphomas and carcinoma of the breast, ovary, or bladder* 15 mg/vial injection

**thiotetrabarbital** INN

**thiothixene** USAN, USP, BAN *thioxanthene antipsychotic* [also: tiotixene] 1, 2, 5, 10 mg oral

**thiothixene HCl** USAN, USP *thioxanthene antipsychotic*

**thiouracil**

**thiourea** *antioxidant*

**thioxanthenes** *a class of dopamine receptor antagonists with conventional (typical) antipsychotic activity*

**thioxolone** BAN [also: tioxolone]

**thiphenamil HCl** USAN *smooth muscle relaxant* [also: tifenamil]

**thiphencillin potassium** USAN *antibacterial* [also: tifencillin]

**thiram** USAN, INN *antifungal*

**thistle, bitter; holy thistle; Saint Benedict thistle; spotted thistle** *medicinal herb* [see: blessed thistle]

**thistle, carline; ground thistle** *medicinal herb* [see: carline thistle]

**thonzonium bromide** USAN, USP *detergent; surface-active agent* [also: tonzonium bromide]

**thonzylamine HCl** USAN, INN

**Thorazine** Spansules (capsules) (discontinued 2003) ℞ *conventional (typical) antipsychotic; antiemetic* [chlorpromazine] 30, 75, 150 mg

**Thorazine** syrup (discontinued 2003) ℞ *conventional (typical) antipsychotic; antiemetic* [chlorpromazine] 10 mg/5 mL

**Thorazine** tablets, IV or IM injection, suppositories, oral concentrate ℞ *conventional (typical) antipsychotic; antiemetic* [chlorpromazine] 25, 50, 100, 200 mg; 25 mg/mL; 100 mg; 100 mg/mL

**thorium** *element (Th)*

**thorn, Egyptian** *medicinal herb* [see: acacia]

**thorn-apple** *medicinal herb* [see: hawthorn; jimsonweed]

**thousand-leaf; thousand seal** *medicinal herb* [see: yarrow]

**thozalinone** USAN *antidepressant* [also: tozalinone]

**THQ (tetrahydroxybenzoquinone)** [see: tetroquinone]

**THR (trishydroxyethyl rutin)** [see: troxerutin]

**Threamine DM** syrup (discontinued 2002) OTC *antitussive; decongestant; antihistamine* [dextromethorphan hydrobromide; phenylpropanolamine HCl; chlorpheniramine maleate] 10•12.5•2 mg/5 mL

**Threamine Expectorant** oral liquid (discontinued 2002) OTC *decongestant; expectorant* [phenylpropanolamine HCl; guaifenesin; alcohol 5%] 12.5•100 mg/5 mL

**3 in 1 Toothache Relief** topical liquid, gum, lotion/gel OTC *oral anesthetic* [benzocaine]

**three-leaved nightshade** *medicinal herb* [see: birthroot]

**3TC** [now: lamivudine]

**threonine (L-threonine)** USAN, USP, INN *essential amino acid; symbols: Thr, T; investigational (orphan) for familial spastic paraparesis and amyotrophic lateral sclerosis* 500 mg oral

**Threostat** ℞ *investigational (orphan) for familial spastic paraparesis and amyotrophic lateral sclerosis* [L-threonine] ⑨ Triostat

**Throat Discs** lozenges OTC *analgesic; counterirritant* [capsicum; peppermint oil]

**throatwort** *medicinal herb* [see: figwort; foxglove]

**Thrombate III** powder for IV infusion ℞ *for thrombosis and pulmonary emboli of congenital AT-III deficiency (orphan)* [antithrombin III] 500, 1000 IU

**thrombin** USP, INN *topical local hemostatic*

**Thrombinar** powder ℞ *topical local hemostatic for surgery* [thrombin] 1000, 5000, 50 000 U

**Thrombin-JMI** powder ℞ *topical local hemostatic for surgery* [thrombin] 10 000, 20 000, 50 000 U

**thrombinogen (prothrombin)**

**Thrombogen** powder ℞ *topical local hemostatic for surgery* [thrombin] 1000, 5000, 10 000, 20 000 U

**thrombolytics** *a class of enzymes that dissolve blood clots, used emergently to treat stroke, pulmonary embolus, and myocardial infarct*

**thromboplastin** USP

**thrombopoietin, recombinant human** *investigational (orphan) adjunct to hematopoietic stem cell transplantation*

**Thrombostat** powder ℞ *topical local hemostatic for surgery* [thrombin] 5000, 10 000, 20 000 U

**throw-wort** *medicinal herb* [see: motherwort]

**thulium** *element (Tm)*

**thunder god vine (*Tripterygium wilfordii*)** plant *medicinal herb for abscesses, autoimmune diseases, boils, fever, inflammation, tumors, and viruses; also used as an insecticide to kill maggots or larvae and as a rat and bird poison* [also: triptolide]

**thymalfasin** USAN *vaccine enhancer for hepatitis C, cancer, and infectious diseases; investigational (Phase III, orphan) for chronic active hepatitis B; investigational (orphan) for DiGeorge syndrome with immune defects; investigational (orphan) for hepatocellular carcinoma*

**thyme (*Thymus serpyllum; T. vulgaris*)** plant *medicinal herb for acute bronchitis, colic, digestive disorders, gas, gout, headache, laryngitis, lung congestion, sciatica, and throat disorders*

**thymic tissue for transplantation, cultured, partially T-cell depleted** *investigational (orphan) agent for primary immune deficiency due to athymia associated with complete DiGeorge syndrome*

**thymidylate synthase (TS) inhibitors** *a class of folate-based antineoplastics*

**Thymitaq** ℞ *investigational (Phase III) thymidylate synthase inhibitor for liver cancer* [nolatrexed dihydrochloride]

**thymocartin** INN

**thymoctonan** INN *investigational antiviral for HIV infection, genital herpes, and chronic viral hepatitis*

**Thymoglobulin** powder for IV infusion ℞ *passive immunizing agent to prevent allograft rejection of renal transplants (orphan); investigational (orphan) for myelodysplastic syndrome (MDS)* [antithymocyte globulin, rabbit] 25 mg

**thymol** NF *stabilizer; topical antiseptic*

**thymol iodide** NF

**thymopentin** USAN, INN, BAN *immunoregulator; investigational (Phase III) for asymptomatic HIV infection*

**thymopoietin 32-36** [now: thymopentin]

**thymosin alpha-1** [now: thymalfasin]

**thymostimulin** INN *investigational (Phase III) immunomodulator for AIDS*

**thymotrinan** INN

**thymoxamine** BAN [also: moxisylyte]

***Thymus serpyllum; T. vulgaris*** *medicinal herb* [see: thyme]

**Thypinone** IV injection (discontinued 2003) ℞ *diagnostic aid for thyroid function* [protirelin] 500 μg/mL

**Thyrel TRH** IV injection (discontinued 2003) ℞ *diagnostic aid for thyroid function* [protirelin] 500 μg/mL

**Thyro-Block** tablets ℞ *thyroid-blocking therapy* [potassium iodide] 130 mg

**thyrocalcitonin** [see: calcitonin]

**Thyrogen** injection ℞ *recombinant human thyroid-stimulating hormone (rhTSH); diagnostic aid for thyroid cancer (orphan); investigational (NDA filed, orphan) treatment for thyroid cancer* [thyrotropin alfa] 1.1 mg

**thyroglobulin (TG)** USAN, USP, INN *thyroid hormone*

**thyroid** USP *natural thyroid hormone (a 4:1 mixture of $T_4$ and $T_3$)* 32.5, 65, 130, 195 mg oral

**thyroid hormone (TH)** [see: levothyroxine sodium]

**thyroid-stimulating hormone (TSH)** [see: thyrotropin]

**Thyrolar** tablets ℞ *synthetic thyroid hormone (a 4:1 mixture of $T_4$ and $T_3$)* [liotrix] 15, 30, 60, 120, 180 mg ② Theolair; Thyrar

**thyromedan HCl** USAN *thyromimetic* [also: tyromedan]

**thyropropic acid** INN

**Thyro-Tabs** tablets ℞ *synthetic thyroid hormone ($T_4$ fraction only)* [levothyroxine sodium] 25, 50, 75, 88, 100, 112, 125, 150, 175, 200, 300 μg

**thyrotrophic hormone** [see: thyrotrophin]

**thyrotrophin** INN *thyroid-stimulating hormone* [also: thyrotropin]

**thyrotropin** *thyroid-stimulating hormone; in vivo diagnostic aid for thyroid function* [also: thyrotrophin]

**thyrotropin alfa** USAN *recombinant human thyroid-stimulating hormone (rhTSH); diagnostic aid for thyroid cancer (orphan); investigational (NDA filed, orphan) treatment for thyroid cancer*

**thyrotropin-releasing hormone (TRH)** [see: protirelin]

**thyroxine** BAN *synthetic thyroid hormone ($T_4$ fraction only)* [also: levothyroxine sodium

**D-thyroxine** [see: dextrothyroxine sodium]

**L-thyroxine** [see: levothyroxine sodium]

**thyroxine I 125** USAN *radioactive agent*

**thyroxine I 131** USAN *radioactive agent*

**Thytropar** powder for IM or subcu injection (discontinued 2001) ℞ *thyroid-stimulating hormone (TSH); in vivo diagnostic aid for thyroid function* [thyrotropin] 10 IU

**tiabendazole** INN *anthelmintic* [also: thiabendazole]

**tiacrilast** USAN, INN *antiallergic*

**tiacrilast sodium** USAN *antiallergic*

**tiadenol** INN

**tiafibrate** INN

**tiagabine** INN *anticonvulsant adjunct for partial seizures*

**tiagabine HCl** USAN *anticonvulsant adjunct for partial seizures*

**Tiamate** extended-release film-coated tablets (discontinued 2002) ℞ *antihypertensive; antianginal; antiarrhythmic; calcium channel blocker* [diltiazem maleate] 120, 180, 240 mg

**tiamenidine** USAN, INN *antihypertensive*

**tiamenidine HCl** USAN *antihypertensive*

**tiametonium iodide** INN

**tiamiprine** INN *antineoplastic* [also: thiamiprine]

**tiamizide** INN *diuretic; antihypertensive* [also: diapamide]

**tiamulin** USAN, INN *veterinary antibacterial*

**tiamulin fumarate** USAN *veterinary antibacterial*

**tianafac** INN

**tianeptine** INN

**tiapamil** INN, BAN *antagonist to calcium* [also: tiapamil HCl]

**tiapamil HCl** USAN *antagonist to calcium* [also: tiapamil]

**tiapirinol** INN

**tiapride** INN

**tiaprofenic acid** INN *nonsteroidal anti-inflammatory drug (NSAID)*

**tiaprost** INN

**tiaramide** INN, BAN *antiasthmatic* [also: tiaramide HCl]

**tiaramide HCl** USAN *antiasthmatic* [also: tiaramide]

**Tiazac** extended-release capsules ℞ *antihypertensive; antianginal; antiarrhythmic; calcium channel blocker* [diltiazem HCl] 120, 180, 240, 300, 360, 420 mg ⊘ Dyazide; thiazides

**tiazesim** INN *antidepressant* [also: thiazesim HCl]

**tiazesim HCl** [see: thiazesim HCl]

**tiazofurin** USAN *investigational (Phase II/III, orphan) antineoplastic for chronic myelogenous leukemia* [also: tiazofurine]

**tiazofurine** INN *antineoplastic* [also: tiazofurin]

**tiazuril** USAN, INN *coccidiostat for poultry*

**tibalosin** INN

**tibenelast sodium** USAN *antiasthmatic; bronchodilator*

**tibenzate** INN

**tibezonium iodide** INN

**tibolone** USAN, INN, BAN *investigational (NDA filed) synthetic steroid for osteoporosis and other postmenopausal symptoms*

**tibric acid** USAN, INN *antihyperlipoproteinemic*

**tibrofan** USAN, INN *disinfectant*

**ticabesone** INN *corticosteroid; anti-inflammatory* [also: ticabesone propionate]

**ticabesone propionate** USAN *corticosteroid; anti-inflammatory* [also: ticabesone]

**Ticar** powder for IV or IM injection ℞ *extended-spectrum penicillin antibiotic* [ticarcillin disodium] 3 g/vial ⊘ Tigan

**ticarbodine** USAN, INN *anthelmintic*

**ticarcillin** INN *extended-spectrum penicillin antibiotic* [also: ticarcillin disodium]

**ticarcillin cresyl sodium** USAN *extended-spectrum penicillin antibiotic*

**ticarcillin disodium** USAN, USP *extended-spectrum penicillin antibiotic* [also: ticarcillin]

**Tice BCG** dermal puncture injection for TB, intravesical instillation for cancer ℞ *tuberculosis immunizing agent; antineoplastic for urinary bladder cancer* [BCG vaccine, Tice strain] 50 mg (1–8 × 10$^8$ CFU)

**tickweed** *medicinal herb* [see: pennyroyal]

**ticlatone** USAN, INN *antibacterial; antifungal*

**Ticlid** film-coated tablets ℞ *platelet aggregation inhibitor for stroke* [ticlopidine HCl] 250 mg

**ticlopidine** INN, BAN *platelet aggregation inhibitor* [also: ticlopidine HCl]

**ticlopidine HCl** USAN *platelet aggregation inhibitor for stroke* [also: ticlopidine] 250 mg oral

**ticolubant** USAN *leukotriene B$_4$ receptor antagonist for psoriasis*

**Ticon** IM injection ℞ *antiemetic; anticholinergic* [trimethobenzamide HCl] 100 mg/mL

**ticrynafen** USAN *diuretic; uricosuric; antihypertensive* [also: tienilic acid]

**tidembersat** USAN *antimigraine*

**tidiacic** INN

**tiemonium iodide** INN, BAN

**tienilic acid** INN *diuretic; uricosuric; antihypertensive* [also: ticrynafen]

**tienocarbine** INN

**tienopramine** INN

**tienoxolol** INN

**tifacogin** USAN *anticoagulant; lipoprotein-associated coagulation inhibitor (LACI); investigational (Phase III) recombinant tissue factor pathway inhibitor*

**tifemoxone** INN

**tifenamil** INN *smooth muscle relaxant* [also: thiphenamil HCl]

**tifenamil HCl** [see: thiphenamil HCl]

**tifencillin** INN *antibacterial* [also: thiphencillin potassium]

**tifencillin potassium** [see: thiphencillin potassium]

**tiflamizole** INN

**tiflorex** INN

**tifluadom** INN

**tiflucarbine** INN

**Tifolar** (name changed to Alimta upon marketing release in 2004)

**tiformin** INN [also: tyformin]

**tifurac** INN *analgesic* [also: tifurac sodium]

**tifurac sodium** USAN *analgesic* [also: tifurac]

**TIG (tetanus immune globulin)** [q.v.]

**Tigan** capsules, IM injection ℞ *antiemetic; anticholinergic* [trimethobenzamide HCl] 100, 250, 300 mg; 100 mg/mL ☑ Ticar; Triban

**Tigan** suppositories, pediatric suppositories ℞ *antiemetic; anticholinergic* [trimethobenzamide HCl; benzocaine] 200 mg•2%; 100 mg•2% ☑ Ticar; Triban

**tigecycline** *investigational (Phase III) broad-spectrum antibiotic*

**tigemonam** INN *antimicrobial* [also: tigemonam dicholine]

**tigemonam dicholine** USAN *antimicrobial* [also: tigemonam]

**tigestol** USAN, INN *progestin*

**tigloidine** INN, BAN

**tiglylpseudotropine** [see: tigloidine]

**tiglyltropeine** [see: tropigline]

**Tikosyn** capsules ℞ *antiarrhythmic; potassium channel blocker* [dofetilide] 125, 250, 500 μg

**tilactase** INN *digestive enzyme*

**Tilad** (Spanish name for U.S. product Tilade)

**Tilade** oral inhalation aerosol ℞ *respiratory anti-inflammatory; mast cell stabilizer; antiasthmatic; bronchodilator* [nedocromil sodium] 1.75 mg/dose

**tilbroquinol** INN

**tiletamine** INN *anesthetic; anticonvulsant* [also: tiletamine HCl]

**tiletamine HCl** USAN *anesthetic; anticonvulsant* [also: tiletamine]

**Tilia americana; T. cordata; T. europaea; T. platyphyllos** *medicinal herb* [see: linden tree]

**tilidate HCl** BAN *analgesic* [also: tilidine HCl; tilidine]

**tilidine** INN *analgesic* [also: tilidine HCl; tilidate HCl]

**tilidine HCl** USAN *analgesic* [also: tilidine; tilidate HCl]

**tiliquinol** INN

**tilisolol** INN

**tilmicosin** USAN, INN, BAN *veterinary antibacterial*

**tilmicosin phosphate** USAN *veterinary antibacterial*

**tilomisole** USAN, INN *immunoregulator*

**tilorone** INN *antiviral* [also: tilorone HCl]

**tilorone HCl** USAN *antiviral* [also: tilorone]

**tilozepine** INN

**tilsuprost** INN

**Tiltab** (trademarked dosage form) *film-coated tablets*

**tiludronate disodium** USAN *bisphosphonate bone resorption inhibitor for Paget disease*

**tiludronic acid** INN

**timcodar dimesylate** USAN *antineoplastic adjunct to prevent emergence of multidrug-resistant tumors*

**Timecap** (trademarked dosage form) *sustained-release capsule*

**Timecelle** (trademarked dosage form) *timed-release capsule*

**timefurone** USAN, INN *antiatherosclerotic*

**timegadine** INN

**Time-Hist** sustained-release capsules R *decongestant; antihistamine* [pseudoephedrine HCl; chlorpheniramine maleate] 120•8 mg

**timelotem** INN

**Timentin** powder or frozen premix for IV infusion R *extended-spectrum penicillin antibiotic plus synergist* [ticarcillin disodium; clavulanate potassium] 3• 0.1 g

**timepidium bromide** INN

**Timespan** (trademarked dosage form) *timed-release tablets*

**Timesules** (dosage form) *sustained-release capsules*

**timiperone** INN

**timobesone** INN *topical adrenocortical steroid* [also: timobesone acetate]

**timobesone acetate** USAN *topical adrenocortical steroid* [also: timobesone]

**timofibrate** INN

**Timolide 10·25** tablets R *antihypertensive; β-blocker; diuretic* [timolol maleate; hydrochlorothiazide] 10•25 mg

**timolol** USAN, INN, BAN *topical antiglaucoma agent (β-blocker)* ☑ atenolol

**timolol hemihydrate** *topical antiglaucoma agent (β-blocker)*

**timolol maleate** USAN, USP *antianginal; antihypertensive; antiadrenergic (β-receptor); topical antiglaucoma agent; migraine prophylaxis* 5, 10, 20 mg oral; 0.25%, 0.5% eye drops

**timonacic** INN

**timoprazole** INN

**Timoptic** Ocumeter (eye drops), Ocudose (single-use eye drop dispenser) R *topical antiglaucoma agent (β-blocker)* [timolol maleate] 0.25%, 0.5%

**Timoptic-XE** gel-forming Ocumeter (eye drops) R *topical once-daily antiglaucoma agent (β-blocker)* [timolol maleate] 0.25%, 0.5%

**Timunox** R *investigational (Phase III) immunomodulator for asymptomatic HIV infection* [thymopentin]

**tin** *element (Sn)*

**tin chloride dihydrate** [see: stannous chloride]

**tin ethyl etiopurpurin** *investigational (Phase III) treatment for various cancers by photodynamic therapy; investigational (Phase III) for wet age-related macular degeneration (AMD)*

**tin fluoride** [see: stannous fluoride]

**tinabinol** USAN, INN *antihypertensive*

**Tinactin** cream, powder, spray powder, spray liquid, topical solution OTC *antifungal* [tolnaftate] 1% ☑ Taractan

**Tinactin for Jock Itch** cream, spray powder OTC *topical antifungal* [tolnaftate] 1%

**Tinactin Plus** CAN powder, aerosol powder (discontinued 2000) OTC *antifungal* [tolnaftate] 1%

**tinazoline** INN

**TinBen** tincture OTC *skin protectant* [benzoin; alcohol 75−83%]

**Tincture of Green Soap** topical liquid OTC *antiseptic cleanser* [green soap; alcohol 28−32%]

**Tindamax** film-coated tablets R *antiprotozoal; amebicide; treatment for trichomoniasis* [tinidazole] 250, 500 mg

**Tine Test OT** [see: Tuberculin Tine Test, Old]

**Tine Test PPD** single-use intradermal puncture test device (discontinued 2002) *tuberculosis skin test* [tuberculin purified protein derivative] 5 U

**Ting** cream OTC *topical antifungal* [tolnaftate] 1%

**Ting** spray powder OTC *antifungal* [miconazole nitrate] 2%

**tinidazole** USAN, INN *antiprotozoal; amebicide; treatment for trichomoniasis*

**tinisulpride** INN

**tinofedrine** INN

**tinoridine** INN

**Tinver** lotion R *antifungal; keratolytic; antipruritic; anesthetic* [sodium thiosulfate; salicylic acid; alcohol 10%] 25%•1%

**tinzaparin sodium** USAN, INN, BAN *a low molecular weight heparin−type anticoagulant and antithrombotic for the prevention of deep vein thrombosis (DVT)*

**tiocarlide** INN [also: thiocarlide]

**tioclomarol** INN

**tioconazole** USAN, USP, INN, BAN, JAN *antifungal*

**tioctilate** INN

**tiodazosin** USAN, INN *antihypertensive*

**tiodonium chloride** USAN, INN *antibacterial*

**tiofacic** [see: stepronin]

**tioguanine** INN *antineoplastic* [also: thioguanine]

**tiomergine** INN

**tiomesterone** INN [also: thiomesterone]

**tioperidone** INN *antipsychotic* [also: tioperidone HCl]

**tioperidone HCl** USAN *antipsychotic* [also: tioperidone]

**tiopinac** USAN, INN *anti-inflammatory; analgesic; antipyretic*

**tiopronin** INN *prevention of cystine nephrolithiasis in homozygous cystinuria (orphan)*

**tiopropamine** INN

**tiosalan** INN *disinfectant* [also: thiosalan]

**tiosinamine** [see: allylthiourea]

**tiospirone** INN *antipsychotic* [also: tiospirone HCl]

**tiospirone HCl** USAN *antipsychotic* [also: tiospirone]

**tiotidine** USAN, INN *antagonist to histamine $H_2$ receptors*

**tiotixene** INN *thioxanthene antipsychotic* [also: thiothixene]

**tiotropium bromide** *long-acting anticholinergic bronchodilator for chronic obstructive pulmonary disease (COPD)*

**tioxacin** INN

**tioxamast** INN

**tioxaprofen** INN

**tioxidazole** USAN, INN *anthelmintic*

**tioxolone** INN [also: thioxolone]

**TIP (Taxol, isosfamide [with mesna rescue], Platinol)** *chemotherapy protocol for head, neck, and esophageal cancers*

**tipentosin** INN, BAN *antihypertensive* [also: tipentosin HCl]

**tipentosin HCl** USAN *antihypertensive* [also: tipentosin]

**tipepidine** INN

**tipetropium bromide** INN

**tipifarnib** USAN *antineoplastic for advanced pancreatic, colorectal, and non–small cell lung cancers*

**tipindole** INN

**tipranavir disodium** USAN *antiviral protease inhibitor; investigational (Phase III) for HIV infection*

**tipredane** USAN, INN, BAN *topical adrenocortical steroid*

**tiprenolol** INN *antiadrenergic (β-receptor)* [also: tiprenolol HCl]

**tiprenolol HCl** USAN *antiadrenergic (β-receptor)* [also: tiprenolol]

**tiprinast** INN *antiallergic* [also: tiprinast meglumine]

**tiprinast meglumine** USAN *antiallergic* [also: tiprinast]

**tipropidil** INN *vasodilator* [also: tipropidil HCl]

**tipropidil HCl** USAN *vasodilator* [also: tipropidil]

**tiprostanide** INN, BAN

**tiprotimod** INN

**tiqueside** USAN, INN *antihyperlipidemic*

**tiquinamide** INN *gastric anticholinergic* [also: tiquinamide HCl]

**tiquinamide HCl** USAN *gastric anticholinergic* [also: tiquinamide]

**tiquizium bromide** INN

**tirapazamine** USAN, INN *antineoplastic; investigational (Phase III) for head, neck, and lung cancers*

**tiratricol** INN

**tiratricol & levothyroxine sodium** *investigational (orphan) to suppress thyroid-stimulating hormone (TSH) in thyroid cancer*

**tirilazad** INN, BAN *antioxidant; lipid peroxidation inhibitor; 21-aminosteroid (lazaroid)* [also: tirilazad mesylate]

**tirilazad mesylate** USAN *antioxidant; lipid peroxidation inhibitor; investigational (NDA filed) 21-aminosteroid (lazaroid) for subarachnoid hemorrhage (SAH), ischemic stroke, spinal cord and head injuries; investigational (Phase I/II) protease inhibitor for HIV infection* [also: tirilazad]

**tirofiban HCl** USAN *glycoprotein (GP) IIb/IIIa receptor antagonist; platelet aggregation inhibitor for acute coronary syndrome, unstable angina, myocardial infarction, and cardiac surgery*

**tiropramide** INN

**tisilfocon A** USAN *hydrophobic contact lens material*

**Tisit** *topical liquid, gel, shampoo* OTC *pediculicide for lice* [pyrethrins; piperonyl butoxide] 0.3%•2%; 0.3%•3%; 0.3%•4%

**Tisit Blue** *gel (discontinued 2003)* OTC *pediculicide for lice* [pyrethrins; piperonyl butoxide; petroleum distillate] 0.3%•3%•1.2%

**tisocromide** INN

**TiSol** *solution* OTC *anesthetic and antimicrobial throat irrigation* [benzyl alcohol; menthol] 1%•0.04%

**tisopurine** INN

**tisoquone** INN

**tissue factor** [see: thromboplastin]

**tissue plasminogen activator (tPA; t-PA)** [see: alteplase]

**Tis-U-Sol** *solution* ℞ *sterile irrigant* [physiological irrigating solution]

**TIT (methotrexate, cytarabine, hydrocortisone)** *chemotherapy protocol for CNS prophylaxis of pediatric acute lymphocytic leukemia; intrathecal (IT) administration*

**Titan** *solution* OTC *cleaning solution for hard contact lenses*

**titanium** *element (Ti)*

**titanium dioxide** USP *topical protectant; astringent*

**titanium oxide** [see: titanium dioxide]

**Titradose** *(trademarked dosage form) scored tablet*

**Titralac** *chewable tablets* OTC *antacid* [calcium carbonate] 420, 750 mg

**Titralac Plus** *chewable tablets, oral liquid* OTC *antacid; antiflatulent* [calcium carbonate; simethicone] 420•21 mg; 500•20 mg/5 mL

**tivanidazole** INN

**tivazine** [see: piperazine citrate]

**tixadil** INN

**tixanox** USAN *antiallergic* [also: tixanoxum]

**tixanoxum** INN *antiallergic* [also: tixanox]

**tixocortol** INN *topical anti-inflammatory* [also: tixocortol pivalate]

**tixocortol pivalate** USAN *topical anti-inflammatory* [also: tixocortol]

**Tixogel VP** *investigational topical skin protectant for allergic contact dermatitis* [bentoquatam]

**tizabrin** INN

**tizanidine** INN, BAN *antispasmodic; central α₂ agonist* [also: tizanidine HCl]

**tizanidine HCl** USAN, JAN *antispasmodic for multiple sclerosis and spinal cord injury (orphan); central α₂ agonist* [also: tizanidine] 2, 4 mg oral

**tizolemide** INN

**tizoprolic acid** INN

**T-Koff** *oral liquid (discontinued 2002)* ℞ *narcotic antitussive; decongestant; antihistamine* [codeine phosphate; phenylpropanolamine HCl; phenylephrine HCl; chlorpheniramine maleate] 10•20•20•5 mg/5 mL

**²⁰¹Tl** [see: thallous chloride Tl 201]

**TLK286** *investigational (Phase III) antineoplastic for ovarian cancer*

**T-lymphotrophic virus antigens** [see: human T-lymphotropic virus type III (HTLV-III) gp-160 antigens]

**TMB (trimedoxime bromide)** [q.v.]

**TMG (trimethylglycine)** [q.v.]

**TMP (trimethoprim)** [q.v.]

**TMP-SMZ (trimethoprim & sulfamethoxazole)** [q.v.]

**TNF (tumor necrosis factor)** [q.v.]

**TNKase** *powder for IV injection* ℞ *thrombolytic/fibrinolytic for the treatment of acute myocardial infarction* [tenecteplase] 50 mg/vial

**TNK-tPA** *a genetically engineered mutation of tissue plasminogen activator (tPA); "TNK" refers to the three specific sites of genetic modification* [see: tenecteplase]

**TOAP (thioguanine, Oncovin, [cytosine] arabinoside, prednisone)** *chemotherapy protocol*

**tobacco** *dried leaves of the* Nicotiana tabacum *plant; sedative narcotic; emetic; diuretic; heart depressant; antispasmodic* [also see: nicotine]

**tobacco, British** *medicinal herb* [see: coltsfoot]

**tobacco, Indian; wild tobacco** *medicinal herb* [see: lobelia]

**tobacco, sailor's** *medicinal herb* [see: mugwort]

**tobacco wood** *medicinal herb* [see: witch hazel]

**TOBI** solution for inhalation ℞ *antibiotic for* Pseudomonas aeruginosa *lung infections in cystic fibrosis patients (orphan); investigational (Phase II) for bronchiectasis and pulmonary tuberculosis* [tobramycin] 300 mg/5 mL

**toborinone** USAN *cardiotonic*

**TobraDex** eye drop suspension ℞ *topical ophthalmic corticosteroidal anti-inflammatory; antibiotic* [dexamethasone; tobramycin] 0.1%•0.3% ⧉ Tobrex

**TobraDex** ophthalmic ointment ℞ *topical ophthalmic corticosteroidal anti-inflammatory; antibiotic* [dexamethasone; tobramycin; chlorobutanol] 0.1%•0.3%•0.5%

**tobramycin** USAN, USP, INN, BAN *aminoglycoside antibiotic; inhalant for* Pseudomonas aeruginosa *lung infections in cystic fibrosis patients (orphan)* 0.3% eye drops ⧉ Trobicin

**tobramycin sulfate** USP *aminoglycoside antibiotic* 10, 40 mg/mL injection

**Tobrex** Drop-Tainers (eye drops), ophthalmic ointment ℞ *topical ophthalmic antibiotic* [tobramycin] 0.3%; 3 mg/g ⧉ TobraDex

**tobuterol** INN

**tocainide** USAN, INN, BAN *antiarrhythmic*

**tocainide HCl** USP *antiarrhythmic*

**tocamphyl** USAN, INN *choleretic*

*Tocicodendron diversilobum medicinal herb* [see: poison oak]

**tocladesine** USAN *immunomodulator; antineoplastic*

**tocofenoxate** INN

**tocofersolan** INN *dietary vitamin E supplement* [also: tocophersolan]

**tocofibrate** INN

**tocolytics** *a class of drugs used to inhibit uterine contractions*

**tocopherol, d-alpha** [see: vitamin E]

**tocopherol, dl-alpha** [see: vitamin E]

**tocopherols, mixed** [see: vitamin E]

**tocopherols excipient** NF *antioxidant*

**tocophersolan** USAN *dietary vitamin E supplement* [also: tocofersolan]

**tocopheryl acetate, d-alpha** [see: vitamin E]

**tocopheryl acetate, dl-alpha** [see: vitamin E]

**tocopheryl acid succinate, d-alpha** [see: vitamin E]

**tocopheryl acid succinate, dl-alpha** [see: vitamin E]

**tocopheryl polyethylene glycol succinate (TPGS)** [see: tocophersolan]

**todralazine** INN, BAN

**tofenacin** INN *anticholinergic* [also: tofenacin HCl]

**tofenacin HCl** USAN *anticholinergic* [also: tofenacin]

**tofesilate** INN *combining name for radicals or groups*

**tofetridine** INN

**tofisoline**

**tofisopam** INN

**Tofranil** sugar-coated tablets ℞ *tricyclic antidepressant; treatment for childhood enuresis* [imipramine HCl] 10, 25, 50 mg ⧉ Tepanil

**Tofranil-PM** capsules ℞ *tricyclic antidepressant* [imipramine pamoate] 75, 100, 125, 150 mg

**tolamolol** USAN, INN *vasodilator; antiarrhythmic; antiadrenergic (β-receptor)*

**tolazamide** USAN, USP, INN, BAN *sulfonylurea antidiabetic* 100, 250, 500 mg oral

**tolazoline** INN *antiadrenergic; peripheral vasodilator for hypertension* [also: tolazoline HCl]

**tolazoline HCl** USP *antiadrenergic; peripheral vasodilator for neonatal persistent pulmonary hypertension* [also: tolazoline]

**tolboxane** INN

**tolbutamide** USP, INN, BAN *sulfonyl-urea antidiabetic* 500 mg oral

**tolbutamide sodium** USP *diagnostic aid for diabetes*

**tolcapone** USAN, INN *antiparkinsonian; catechol-O-methyltransferase (COMT) inhibitor*

**tolciclate** USAN, INN *antifungal*

**tolclotide** [see: disulfamide]

**toldimfos** INN, BAN

**Tolectin 200; Tolectin 600** tablets ℞ *antiarthritic; nonsteroidal anti-inflammatory drug (NSAID) for ankylosing spondylitis and acute bursitis/tendinitis* [tolmetin sodium] 200 mg; 600 mg

**Tolectin DS** capsules ℞ *antiarthritic; nonsteroidal anti-inflammatory drug (NSAID) for ankylosing spondylitis and acute bursitis/tendinitis* [tolmetin sodium] 400 mg

**Tolerex** powder OTC *enteral nutritional therapy* [lactose-free formula]

**tolfamide** USAN, INN *urease enzyme inhibitor*

**tolfenamic acid** INN, BAN

**Tolfrinic** film-coated tablets OTC *hematinic* [ferrous fumarate; cyanocobalamin; ascorbic acid] 200 mg•25 μg•100 mg

**tolgabide** USAN, INN, BAN *anticonvulsant*

**tolhexamide** [see: glycyclamide]

**tolimidone** USAN, INN *antiulcerative*

**Tolinase** tablets ℞ *sulfonylurea antidiabetic* [tolazamide] 100, 250, 500 mg ▣ Orinase

**tolindate** USAN, INN *antifungal*

**toliodium chloride** USAN, INN *veterinary food additive*

**toliprolol** INN

**tolmesoxide** INN

**tolmetin** USAN, INN *antiarthritic; nonsteroidal anti-inflammatory drug (NSAID) for ankylosing spondylitis and acute bursitis/tendinitis*

**tolmetin sodium** USAN, USP *antiarthritic; nonsteroidal anti-inflammatory drug (NSAID) for ankylosing spondylitis and acute bursitis/tendinitis* 200, 400, 600 mg oral

**tolnaftate** USAN, USP, INN, BAN *antifungal* 1% topical

**tolnapersine** INN

**tolnidamine** INN

**toloconium metilsulfate** INN

**tolofocon A** USAN *hydrophobic contact lens material*

**tolonidine** INN

**tolonium chloride** INN *blue dye used in histology; diagnostic aid for oral cancer*

**toloxatone** INN

**toloxichloral** [see: toloxychlorinol]

**toloxychlorinol** INN

**tolpadol** INN

**tolpentamide** INN, BAN

**tolperisone** INN, BAN

**tolpiprazole** INN, BAN

**tolpovidone I 131** USAN *hypoalbuminemia test; radioactive agent* [also: radiotolpovidone I 131]

**tolpronine** INN, BAN

**tolpropamine** INN, BAN

**tolpyrramide** USAN, INN *antidiabetic*

**tolquinzole** INN

**tolrestat** USAN, INN, BAN *investigational (NDA filed) aldose reductase inhibitor for diabetic neuropathy*

**tolterodine** USAN *anticholinergic; muscarinic receptor antagonist for urinary frequency, urgency, and incontinence*

**tolterodine tartrate** USAN *anticholinergic; muscarinic receptor antagonist for urinary frequency, urgency, and incontinence*

**toltrazuril** USAN, INN, BAN *veterinary coccidiostat*

**tolu balsam** USP *pharmaceutic aid*

***p*-toluenesulfone dichloramine** [see: dichloramine T]

**tolufazepam** INN

**toluidine blue O** [see: tolonium chloride]

**toluidine blue O chloride** [see: tolonium chloride]

**Tolu-Sed DM** oral liquid OTC *antitussive; expectorant* [dextromethorphan hydrobromide; guaifenesin; alcohol 10%] 10•100 mg/5 mL

**tolycaine** INN, BAN

**tomelukast** USAN, INN *antiasthmatic; leukotriene antagonist*

**Tomocat** concentrated oral suspension R̄ *radiopaque contrast medium for gastrointestinal imaging* [barium sulfate] 5%

**tomoglumide** INN

**tomoxetine** INN *antidepressant* [also: tomoxetine HCl]

**tomoxetine HCl** USAN *antidepressant* [also: tomoxetine]

**tomoxiprole** INN

**Tom's of Maine Natural Cough & Cold Rub** vaporizing ointment OTC *counterirritant; cough suppressant* [menthol; camphor] 4.8%•2.6%

**Tomudex** R̄ *antimetabolite antineoplastic; investigational (Phase III) thymidylate synthase inhibitor for colorectal cancer* [raltitrexed]

**Tomycine** ⓒᴬᴺ eye drops R̄ *topical antibiotic* [tobramycin] 0.3%

**tonazocine** INN *analgesic* [also: tonazocine mesylate]

**tonazocine mesylate** USAN *analgesic* [also: tonazocine]

**tongue grass** *medicinal herb* [see: chickweed]

**tonics** *a class of agents that restore normal tone to tissue and strengthen or invigorate organs (a term used in folk medicine)*

**tonka bean (*Dipteryx odorata; D. oppositifolia*)** fruit and seed *medicinal herb for cramps, nausea, and schistosomiasis*

**Tonocard** film-coated tablets (discontinued 2004) R̄ *antiarrhythmic* [tocainide HCl] 400, 600 mg

**Tonopaque** powder for oral suspension R̄ *radiopaque contrast medium for gastrointestinal imaging* [barium sulfate] 95%

**tonzonium bromide** INN *detergent; surface-active agent* [also: thonzonium bromide]

**tooth, lion's** *medicinal herb* [see: dandelion]

**Toothache** gel OTC *topical oral anesthetic* [benzocaine]

**toothache bush; toothache tree** *medicinal herb* [see: prickly ash]

**Top Care Flu, Cold, & Cough Medicine Night Time** powder for oral solution OTC *antitussive; decongestant; antihistamine; analgesic* [dextromethorphan hydrobromide; pseudoephedrine HCl; chlorpheniramine maleate; acetaminophen] 20•60•4•1000 mg/pkt.

**Top Care Multi-Symptom Pain Relief Cold** caplets OTC *antitussive; decongestant; analgesic* [dextromethorphan hydrobromide; pseudoephedrine HCl; acetaminophen] 15•30•325 mg

**Top Care Multi-Symptom Pain Relief Cold** caplets OTC *antitussive; decongestant; antihistamine; analgesic* [dextromethorphan hydrobromide; pseudoephedrine HCl; chlorpheniramine maleate; acetaminophen] 15•30•2•325 mg

**Top Care Nite Time Multi-Symptom Cold/Flu Relief** LiquiCaps (liquid-filled capsules) OTC *antitussive; decongestant; antihistamine; analgesic* [dextromethorphan hydrobromide; pseudoephedrine HCl; doxylamine succinate; acetaminophen] 10•30•6.25•250 mg

**Top Care Soothing Cough & Head Congestion Relief D** oral liquid OTC *antitussive; decongestant* [dextromethorphan hydrobromide; pseudoephedrine HCl; alcohol 5%] 30•60 mg/15 mL

**Topamax** coated tablets, sprinkle caps R̄ *broad-spectrum sulfamate anticonvulsant for partial-onset and generalized tonic-clonic seizures; also for the prophylaxis of migraine headaches; investigational (orphan) for Lennox-Gastaut syndrome* [topiramate] 25, 50, 100, 200 mg; 15, 25 mg

**Topic** gel OTC *topical analgesic; counterirritant* [benzyl alcohol; camphor; menthol; alcohol 30%] 5%• ²⁄ • ²⁄ ⑨ Topicort

**topical starch** [see: starch, topical]

**TopiCare** (trademarked ingredient) *topical polyolprepolymer base for creams and gels*

**Topicort** ointment, cream, gel ℞ *corticosteroidal anti-inflammatory* [desoximetasone] 0.25%; 0.25%; 0.05% ⊡ Topic

**Topicort LP** cream ℞ *topical corticosteroidal anti-inflammatory* [desoximetasone] 0.05%

**Topicycline** solution (discontinued 2003) ℞ *antibiotic for acne* [tetracycline HCl] 2.2 mg/mL

**Topiglan** gel ℞ *investigational (Phase III) topical therapy for erectile dysfunction* [alprostadil]

**topiramate** USAN, INN, BAN *broad-spectrum sulfamate anticonvulsant for partial-onset and generalized tonic-clonic seizures; also for the prophylaxis of migraine headaches; investigational (orphan) for Lennox-Gastaut syndrome*

**topo/CTX (topotecan, cyclophosphamide [with mesna rescue])** *chemotherapy protocol for pediatric bone and soft tissue sarcomas*

**topoisomerase I inhibitors** *a class of hormonal antineoplastics that prevent DNA replication of tumors by inhibiting the re-ligation of naturally occurring single-strand breaks*

**Toposar** IV injection ℞ *antineoplastic for testicular and small cell lung cancers* [etoposide; alcohol 30.5%] 20 mg/mL

**topotecan** INN, BAN *topoisomerase I inhibitor; antineoplastic for ovarian and small cell lung cancers* [also: topotecan HCl]

**topotecan HCl** USAN *topoisomerase I inhibitor; antineoplastic for ovarian and small cell lung cancers; investigational (Phase II) for AIDS-related progressive multifocal leukoencephalopathy (PML)* [also: topotecan]

**toprilidine** INN

**Toprol-XL** film-coated extended-release tablets ℞ *antihypertensive; long-term antianginal; antiadrenergic (β-blocker)* [metoprolol succinate] 25, 50, 100, 200 mg

**topterone** USAN, INN *antiandrogen*

**TOPV (trivalent oral poliovirus vaccine)** [see: poliovirus vaccine, live oral]

**toquizine** USAN, INN *anticholinergic*

**Toradol** film-coated tablets, Tubex (prefilled syringes) for IM or IV injection ℞ *nonsteroidal anti-inflammatory drug (NSAID); analgesic for acute, moderately severe, opioid-level pain* [ketorolac tromethamine] 10 mg; 15, 30 mg/mL

**torasemide** INN, BAN *antihypertensive; loop diuretic* [also: torsemide]

**torbafylline** INN

**torcetrapib** *investigational (Phase III) antihyperlipidemic; cholesterol ester transfer protein (CETP) inhibitor that raises HDL cholesterol*

**Torecan** IM injection ℞ *antiemetic* [thiethylperazine maleate] 5 mg/mL

**Torecan** tablets (discontinued 2004) ℞ *antiemetic* [thiethylperazine maleate] 10 mg

**toremifene** INN, BAN *antiestrogen; antineoplastic* [also: toremifene citrate]

**toremifene citrate** USAN *antiestrogen antineoplastic for metastatic breast cancer in postmenopausal women (orphan); investigational (orphan) for desmoid tumors* [also: toremifene]

**toripristone** INN

**tormentil (Potentilla tormentilla; Tormentilla erecta)** root *medicinal herb used as an antiphlogistic, antiseptic, astringent, and hemostatic*

**Tornalate** oral inhalation aerosol, solution for inhalation (discontinued 2001) ℞ *sympathomimetic bronchodilator* [bitolterol mesylate] 0.8%; 0.2%

**torsemide** USAN *antihypertensive; loop diuretic* [also: torasemide] 5, 10, 20, 100 mg oral

**tosactide** INN [also: octacosactrin]

**tosifen** USAN, INN *antianginal*

**tosilate** INN *combining name for radicals or groups* [also: tosylate]

**tositumomab** *cytotoxic monoclonal antibody to non-Hodgkin lymphoma (NHL)* [see also: iodine I 131 tositumomab]

**Tostrex** transdermal gel ℞ *investiga-tional (Phase III) hormone for male hypogonadism* [testosterone]

**tosufloxacin** USAN, INN *antibacterial*

**tosulur** INN

**tosylate** USAN, BAN *combining name for radicals or groups* [also: tosilate]

**tosylchloramide sodium** INN [also: chloramine-T]

**Totacillin** capsules, powder for oral suspension (discontinued 2002) ℞ *aminopenicillin antibiotic* [ampicillin] 250, 500 mg; 125, 250 mg/5 mL

**Total** solution OTC *cleaning/soaking/wet-ting solution for hard contact lenses*

**Total Formula; Total Formula-2** tablets OTC *vitamin/mineral/iron supplement* [multiple vitamins & miner-als; iron; folic acid; biotin] ± • 20 • 0.4 • 0.3 mg

**Total Formula-3 without Iron** tab-lets OTC *vitamin/mineral supplement* [multiple vitamins & minerals; folic acid; biotin] ± • 0.4 • 0.3 mg

**touch-me-not; pale touch-me-not** *medicinal herb* [see: celandine; jewel-weed; Siberian ginseng]

**toughened silver nitrate** [see: silver nitrate, toughened]

**Touro A & H** timed-release capsules (name changed to Touro Allergy in 2000)

**Touro Allergy** sustained-release cap-sules ℞ *decongestant; antihistamine* [pseudoephedrine HCl; brompheni-ramine maleate] 60 • 5.75 mg

**Touro CC** sustained-release caplets ℞ *antitussive; decongestant; expectorant* [dextromethorphan hydrobromide; pseudoephedrine HCl; guaifenesin] 30 • 60 • 575 mg

**Touro DM** sustained-release tablets ℞ *antitussive; expectorant* [dextrometh-orphan hydrobromide; guaifenesin] 30 • 575 mg

**Touro Ex** sustained-release caplets (discontinued 2004) ℞ *expectorant* [guaifenesin] 575 mg

**Touro LA** sustained-release caplets ℞ *decongestant; expectorant* [pseudo-ephedrine HCl; guaifenesin] 120 • 525 mg

**toxoids** *a class of drugs used for active immunization that produce endogenous antibodies to toxins*

**toywort** *medicinal herb* [see: shepherd's purse]

**tozalinone** INN *antidepressant* [also: thozalinone]

**TP-10** *investigational (Phase I/II) com-plement inhibitor for severe burns, adult respiratory distress syndrome; investiga-tional (Phase I/II, orphan) for reperfu-sion injury* [also: sCR1]

**tPA; t-PA (tissue plasminogen acti-vator)** [see: alteplase; anistreplase; lanoteplase; monteplase; reteplase; saruplase; tenecteplase]

**TPCH (thioguanine, procarbazine, CCNU, hydroxyurea)** *chemother-apy protocol*

**TPDCV (thioguanine, procarba-zine, DCD, CCNU, vincristine)** *chemotherapy protocol*

**TPGS (tocopheryl polyethylene gly-col succinate)** [see: tocophersolan]

**T-Phyl** timed-release tablets ℞ *anti-asthmatic; bronchodilator* [theophyl-line] 200 mg

**TPM Test** kit for professional use *in vitro diagnostic aid for* Toxoplasma gondii *antibodies in serum* [indirect hemagglutination test]

**TPN Electrolytes; TPN Electrolytes II; TPN Electrolytes III** IV admix-ture ℞ *intravenous electrolyte therapy* [combined electrolyte solution]

**traboxopine** INN

**Trac Tabs 2X** tablets ℞ *urinary antibi-otic; analgesic; antispasmodic; acidifier* [methenamine; phenyl salicylate; atropine sulfate; hyoscyamine sul-fate; benzoic acid; methylene blue] 120 • 30 • 0.06 • 0.03 • 7.5 • 6 mg

**tracazolate** USAN, INN, BAN *sedative*

**Trace Metals Additive in 0.9% NaCl** IV injection ℞ *intravenous nutritional therapy* [multiple trace elements (metals)]

**Tracelyte; Tracelyte II; Tracelyte with Double Electrolytes; Tracelyte II with Double Electrolytes** IV admixture (discontinued 2003) ℞ *intravenous nutritional therapy* [multiple trace elements (metals); electrolytes]

**Tracleer** film-coated tablets ℞ *endothelin receptor antagonist (ERA) for pulmonary arterial hypertension (orphan)* [bosentan] 62.5, 125 mg

**Tracrium** IV infusion ℞ *nondepolarizing neuromuscular blocker; adjunct to anesthesia* [atracurium besylate] 10 mg/mL

**trafermin** USAN *investigational (Phase II/III) fibroblast growth factor for stroke and coronary artery disease*

**tragacanth** NF *suspending agent*

**tralonide** USAN, INN *corticosteroid; anti-inflammatory*

**tramadol** INN *central analgesic* [also: tramadol HCl]

**tramadol HCl** USAN *central analgesic* [also: tramadol] 50 mg oral

**tramazoline** INN *adrenergic* [also: tramazoline HCl]

**tramazoline HCl** USAN *adrenergic* [also: tramazoline]

**Trandate** film-coated tablets, IV injection ℞ *antihypertensive; α- and β-blocker* [labetalol HCl] 100, 200, 300 mg; 5 mg/mL

**trandolapril** INN, BAN *antihypertensive; angiotensin converting enzyme (ACE) inhibitor; treatment for CHF*

**trandolaprilat** INN

**tranexamic acid** USAN, INN, BAN *systemic hemostatic; orphan status withdrawn 1996*

**tranilast** USAN, INN *antiasthmatic*

**trans AMCHA (*trans*-aminomethyl cyclohexanecarboxylic acid)** [see: tranexamic acid]

**transcainide** USAN, INN *antiarrhythmic*

**transclomiphene** [now: zuclomiphene]

**Transderm Scōp** transdermal patch ℞ *motion sickness preventative* [scopolamine hydrobromide] 1.5 mg (1 mg dose over 3 days)

**Transderm-Nitro** transdermal patch ℞ *antianginal; vasodilator* [nitroglycerin] 12.5, 25, 50, 75, 100 mg (0.1, 0.2, 0.4, 0.6, 0.8 mg/hr.)

**transforming growth factor beta 2** *investigational (orphan) growth stimulator for full-thickness macular holes*

**trans-π-oxocamphor** JAN *topical antipruritic; mild local anesthetic; counterirritant* [also: camphor]

**trans-retinoic acid** [see: tretinoin]

**Trans-Ver-Sal Adult-Patch; Trans-Ver-Sal Pedia-Patch; Trans-Ver-Sal Plantar-Patch** patch OTC *keratolytic* [salicylic acid] 15%

**trantelinium bromide** INN

**Tranxene** T-Tabs ("T"-imprinted tablets) ℞ *benzodiazepine anxiolytic; minor tranquilizer; alcohol withdrawal aid; anticonvulsant adjunct* [clorazepate dipotassium] 3.75, 7.5, 15 mg

**Tranxene-SD; Tranxene-SD Half Strength** single-dose tablets ℞ *benzodiazepine anxiolytic; minor tranquilizer; alcohol withdrawal aid; anticonvulsant adjunct* [clorazepate dipotassium] 22.5 mg; 11.25 mg

**tranylcypromine** INN, BAN *antidepressant; MAO inhibitor* [also: tranylcypromine sulfate]

**tranylcypromine sulfate** USP *antidepressant; MAO inhibitor* [also: tranylcypromine]

**trapencaine** INN

**trapidil** INN

**trapymin** [see: trapidil]

**trastuzumab** *antineoplastic monoclonal antibody to HER-2 (human epidermal growth factor receptor 2) protein for metastatic breast cancer*

**trastuzumab & paclitaxel** *chemotherapy protocol for breast cancer*

**Trasylol** IV infusion ℞ *systemic hemostatic for coronary artery bypass graft (CABG) surgery (orphan)* [aprotinin] 10 000 KIU/mL (Kallikrein inhibitor units) ⊠ Travasol

**TraumaCal** ready-to-use oral liquid OTC *enteral nutritional therapy for mod-*

*erate to severe stress or trauma* [multiple branched chain amino acids]

**Travasol 2.75% in 5% (10%, 25%) Dextrose; Travasol 4.25% in 5% (10%, 25%) Dextrose** IV infusion ℞ *total parenteral nutrition; peripheral parenteral nutrition* [multiple essential and nonessential amino acids; dextrose] ⊘ Trasylol

**Travasol 3.5% (5.5%, 8.5%) with Electrolytes** IV infusion ℞ *total parenteral nutrition (all except 3.5%); peripheral parenteral nutrition (all)* [multiple essential and nonessential amino acids; electrolytes]

**Travasol 5.5% (8.5%, 10%)** IV infusion ℞ *total parenteral nutrition; peripheral parenteral nutrition* [multiple essential and nonessential amino acids]

**Travasorb HN; Travasorb MCT; Travasorb STD** powder OTC *enteral nutritional therapy* [lactose-free formula]

**Travatan** Drop-Tainers (eye drops) ℞ *prostaglandin* $F_{2\alpha}$ *analogue for glaucoma and ocular hypertension* [travoprost] 0.004%

**traveler's joy** *medicinal herb* [see: blue vervain; woodbine]

**5% Travert and Electrolyte No. 2; 10% Travert and Electrolyte No. 2** IV infusion ℞ *intravenous nutritional/electrolyte therapy* [combined electrolyte solution; invert sugar (50% dextrose + 50% fructose)]

**travoprost** USAN *topical prostaglandin* $F_{2\alpha}$ *analogue for glaucoma and ocular hypertension*

**traxanox** INN

**traxoprodil mesylate** USAN *selective NMDA receptor antagonist for traumatic brain injury*

**Traypak** (trademarked packaging form) *multivial carton*

**trazitiline** INN

**trazium esilate** INN

**trazodone** INN *triazolopyridine antidepressant for panic disorder, aggressive behavior, alcoholism, and cocaine withdrawal; serotonin uptake inhibitor* [also: trazodone HCl]

**trazodone HCl** USAN *triazolopyridine antidepressant for panic disorder, aggressive behavior, alcoholism, and cocaine withdrawal; serotonin uptake inhibitor* [also: trazodone] 50, 100, 150, 300 mg oral

**trazolopride** INN

**trebenzomine** INN *antidepressant* [also: trebenzomine HCl]

**trebenzomine HCl** USAN *antidepressant* [also: trebenzomine]

**trecadrine** INN

**Trecator-SC** tablets ℞ *tuberculostatic* [ethionamide] 250 mg

**trecetilide fumarate** USAN *antiarrhythmic*

**trecovirsen sodium** USAN *antisense antiviral for HIV and AIDS*

**trefentanil HCl** USAN *analgesic*

**trefoil, bean; bitter trefoil; marsh trefoil** *medicinal herb* [see: buckbean]

**treloxinate** USAN, INN *antihyperlipoproteinemic*

**Trelstar Depot** IM injection (once monthly) ℞ *gonadotropin-releasing hormone (GnRH) antineoplastic for palliative treatment of advanced prostate cancer* [triptorelin pamoate] 3.75 mg

**Trelstar LA** IM injection (three-month depot) ℞ *gonadotropin-releasing hormone (GnRH) agonist; antineoplastic for palliative treatment of advanced prostate cancer* [triptorelin pamoate] 11.25 mg

**tremacamra** USAN *antiviral; inhibits viral attachment to host cells*

**trembling poplar; trembling tree** *medicinal herb* [see: poplar]

**trenbolone** INN, BAN *veterinary anabolic steroid, also abused as a street drug* [also: trenbolone acetate]

**trenbolone acetate** USAN *veterinary anabolic steroid, also abused as a street drug* [also: trenbolone]

**trenbolone hexahydrobenzylcarbonate** *veterinary anabolic steroid, also abused as a street drug*

**trengestone** INN

**trenizine** INN

**Trental** film-coated controlled-release tablets ℞ *peripheral vasodilator to improve blood microcirculation in intermittent claudication* [pentoxifylline] 400 mg

**treosulfan** INN, BAN *investigational (orphan) for ovarian cancer*

**trepibutone** INN

**trepipam** INN *sedative* [also: trepipam maleate]

**trepipam maleate** USAN *sedative* [also: trepipam]

**trepirium iodide** INN

**treprostinil sodium** *prostacyclin analogue for pulmonary arterial hypertension (orphan) and peripheral vascular disease (PVD); investigational (Phase II) for critical limb ischemia*

**treptilamine** INN

**trequinsin** INN

**trestolone** INN *antineoplastic; androgen* [also: trestolone acetate]

**trestolone acetate** USAN *antineoplastic; androgen* [also: trestolone]

**tretamine** INN, BAN [also: triethylenemelamine]

**trethinium tosilate** INN

**trethocanic acid** INN

**trethocanoic acid** [see: trethocanic acid]

**tretinoin** USAN, USP, INN, BAN *topical keratolytic for acne; treatment for acute promyelocytic leukemia (orphan); investigational (orphan) for other leukemias and ophthalmic squamous metaplasia; investigational (Phase II) for AIDS-related Kaposi sarcoma and non-Hodgkin lymphoma* 0.01%, 0.025%, 0.05%, 0.1% topical

**tretoquinol** INN

**Trexall** film-coated tablets ℞ *antimetabolite antineoplastic for leukemia; systemic antipsoriatic; antirheumatic* [methotrexate] 5, 7.5, 10, 15 mg

**Trexima** ℞ *investigational (Phase III) combination 5-HT$_{1B/1D}$ agonist and nonsteroidal anti-inflammatory drug (NSAID) for the acute treatment of migraine headaches* [sumatriptan; naproxen sodium]

**TRH (thyrotropin-releasing hormone)** [see: protirelin]

**Tri Vit with Fluoride** drops ℞ *pediatric vitamin supplement and dental caries preventative* [vitamins A, C, and D; fluoride] 1500 IU•35 mg•400 IU•0.25 mg, 1500 IU•35 mg•400 IU•0.5 mg per mL

**TRIAC (triiodothyroacetic acid)** [q.v.]

**Triacana** ℞ *investigational (orphan) for suppression of thyroid-stimulating hormone (TSH) in thyroid cancer* [tiratricol; levothyroxine sodium]

**Triacet** cream ℞ *topical corticosteroidal anti-inflammatory* [triamcinolone acetonide] 0.1%

**triacetin** USP, INN *antifungal*

**triacetyloleandomycin** BAN *macrolide antibiotic* [also: troleandomycin]

**Triacin-C Cough** syrup ℞ *narcotic antitussive; decongestant; antihistamine* [codeine phosphate; pseudoephedrine HCl; triprolidine HCl; alcohol 4.3%] 20•60•2.5 mg/10 mL

**triaconazole** [now: terconazole]

**Triactin** syrup (discontinued 2001) OTC *decongestant; antihistamine* [phenylpropanolamine HCl; chlorpheniramine maleate] 6.25•1 mg/5 mL

**Triacting** pediatric oral liquid OTC *decongestant; expectorant* [pseudoephedrine HCl; guaifenesin] 15•50 mg/5 mL

**Triacting Cold & Allergy** pediatric oral liquid OTC *decongestant; antihistamine* [pseudoephedrine HCl; chlorpheniramine maleate] 30•2 mg/10 mL

**Tri-Acting Cold & Allergy** pediatric syrup OTC *decongestant; antihistamine* [pseudoephedrine HCl; chlorpheniramine maleate] 30•2 mg/10 mL

**Tri-Acting Cold & Cough** pediatric syrup OTC *antitussive; decongestant; antihistamine* [dextromethorphan hydrobromide; pseudoephedrine HCl; chlorpheniramine maleate] 10•30•2 mg/10 mL

**Triad** capsules ℞ *sedative; barbiturate analgesic* [acetaminophen; caffeine; butalbital] 325•40•50 mg

**Triafed with Codeine** syrup (discontinued 2000) (discontinued 2002) ℞ *narcotic antitussive; decongestant; antihistamine* [codeine phosphate; pseudoephedrine HCl; triprolidine HCl] 10•30•1.25 mg/5 mL

**triafungin** USAN, INN *antifungal*

**Trial AG** (Anti-Gas) tablets OTC *antacid; antiflatulent* [aluminum hydroxide; magnesium hydroxide; simethicone] 200•200•25 mg

**Trial Antacid** tablets OTC *antacid; calcium supplement* [calcium carbonate] 420 mg

**Triam Forte** IM injection ℞ *corticosteroid; anti-inflammatory* [triamcinolone diacetate] 40 mg/mL

**Triam-A** IM, intra-articular, intrabursal, intradermal injection ℞ *corticosteroid; anti-inflammatory* [triamcinolone acetonide] 40 mg/mL

**triamcinolone** USP, INN, BAN, JAN *corticosteroid* 4 mg oral ⑨ Triaminicin

**triamcinolone acetonide** USP, JAN *corticosteroidal anti-inflammatory; treatment for chronic asthma and rhinitis* 0.025%, 0.1%, 0.5% topical; 40 mg/mL injection

**triamcinolone acetonide sodium phosphate** USAN *corticosteroid*

**triamcinolone benetonide** INN *corticosteroid*

**triamcinolone diacetate** USP, JAN *corticosteroid* 40 mg/mL injection

**triamcinolone furetonide** INN *corticosteroid*

**triamcinolone hexacetonide** USAN, USP, INN, BAN *corticosteroid*

**Triaminic** oral infant drops (discontinued 2000) ℞ *decongestant; antihistamine* [phenylpropanolamine HCl; pyrilamine maleate; pheniramine maleate] 20•10•10 mg/mL

**Triaminic** pediatric syrup (discontinued 2001) OTC *decongestant; antihistamine* [phenylpropanolamine HCl; chlorpheniramine maleate] 6.25•0.5 mg; 6.25•1 mg/5 mL ⑨ Triaminicin; TriHemic

**Triaminic Allergy; Triaminic Cold** tablets (discontinued 2001) OTC *decongestant; antihistamine* [phenylpropanolamine HCl; chlorpheniramine maleate] 25•4 mg; 12.5•2 mg

**Triaminic Allergy, Sinus, & Headache Softchews** (pediatric chewable tablets) OTC *decongestant; analgesic; antipyretic* [pseudoephedrine HCl; acetaminophen] 15•150 mg

**Triaminic Allergy Congestion** Softchews (chewable tablets), pediatric oral liquid OTC *nasal decongestant* [pseudoephedrine HCl] 15 mg; 15 mg/5 mL

**Triaminic AM Decongestant Formula** syrup (discontinued 2002) OTC *decongestant* [pseudoephedrine HCl] 15 mg/5 mL

**Triaminic AM Non-Drowsy Cough & Decongestant** pediatric oral liquid OTC *antitussive; decongestant* [dextromethorphan hydrobromide; pseudoephedrine HCl] 7.5•15 mg/5 mL

**Triaminic Chest Congestion** pediatric oral liquid OTC *decongestant; expectorant* [pseudoephedrine HCl; guaifenesin] 15•50 mg/5 mL

**Triaminic Cold, Cough, & Fever** pediatric oral liquid OTC *antitussive; decongestant; antihistamine; analgesic; antipyretic* [dextromethorphan hydrobromide; pseudoephedrine HCl; chlorpheniramine maleate; acetaminophen] 15•30•2•320 mg/10 mL

**Triaminic Cold & Allergy** pediatric oral liquid OTC *decongestant; antihistamine* [pseudoephedrine HCl; chlorpheniramine maleate] 6.25•1 mg/5 mL

**Triaminic Cold & Cough; Triaminic Cold & Night Time Cough** pediatric oral liquid OTC *antitussive; decongestant; antihistamine* [dextromethorphan hydrobromide; pseudoephedrine HCl; chlorpheniramine maleate] 10•30•2 mg/10 mL; 15•30•2 mg/10 mL

**Triaminic Cold & Cough; Triaminic Cough** pediatric soft chews OTC *antitussive; decongestant; antihistamine* [dextromethorphan hydrobromide; pseudoephedrine HCl; chlorpheniramine maleate] 5•15•1 mg

**Triaminic Cough & Congestion** pediatric oral liquid OTC *antitussive; decongestant* [dextromethorphan hydrobromide; pseudoephedrine HCl] 7.5•15 mg/5 mL

**Triaminic Cough & Sore Throat** pediatric oral liquid OTC *antitussive; decongestant; analgesic* [dextromethorphan hydrobromide; pseudoephedrine HCl; acetaminophen] 7.5•15•160 mg/5 mL

**Triaminic Decongestant** oral infant drops OTC *pediatric decongestant* [pseudoephedrine HCl] 7.5 mg/0.8 mL

**Triaminic DM** syrup (discontinued 2002) OTC *antitussive; decongestant* [dextromethorphan hydrobromide; phenylpropanolamine HCl] 5•6.25 mg/5 mL

**Triaminic Expectorant** oral liquid (discontinued 2002) OTC *decongestant; expectorant* [phenylpropanolamine HCl; guaifenesin] 6.25•50 mg/5 mL

**Triaminic Expectorant DH** oral liquid (discontinued 2002) ℞ *narcotic antitussive; decongestant; antihistamine; expectorant* [hydrocodone bitartrate; phenylpropanolamine HCl; pyrilamine maleate; pheniramine maleate; guaifenesin; alcohol 5%] 1.67•12.5•6.25•6.25•100 mg/5 mL

**Triaminic Expectorant with Codeine** oral liquid (discontinued 2002) ℞ *narcotic antitussive; decongestant; expectorant* [codeine phosphate; phenylpropanolamine HCl; guaifenesin; alcohol 5%] 10•12.5•100 mg/5 mL

**Triaminic Nite Light** pediatric oral liquid (name changed to Triaminic Cold & Night Time Cough in 2002)

**Triaminic Severe Cold & Fever** pediatric oral liquid (name changed to Triaminic Cold, Cough, & Fever in 2002)

**Triaminic Softchews** (pediatric chewable tablets) OTC *decongestant; antihistamine* [pseudoephedrine HCl; chlorpheniramine maleate] 15•1 mg ☒ Triaminicin; TriHemic

**Triaminic Throat Pain & Cough** pediatric soft chews OTC *antitussive; decongestant; analgesic* [dextromethorphan hydrobromide; pseudoephedrine HCl; acetaminophen] 5•15•160 mg

**Triaminic Vapor Patch** OTC *counterirritant; cough suppressant* [camphor; menthol] 4.7%•2.6%

**Triaminic-12** sustained-release tablets (discontinued 2001) OTC *decongestant; antihistamine* [phenylpropanolamine HCl; chlorpheniramine maleate] 75•12 mg

**Triaminicin Cold, Allergy, Sinus Medicine** tablets OTC *decongestant; antihistamine; analgesic* [pseudoephedrine HCl; chlorpheniramine maleate; acetaminophen] 60•4•650 mg ☒ triamcinolone; Triaminic

**Triaminicol Multi-Symptom Cough and Cold** tablets (discontinued 2002) OTC *antitussive; decongestant; antihistamine* [dextromethorphan hydrobromide; phenylpropanolamine HCl; chlorpheniramine maleate] 10•12.5•2 mg

**Triaminicol Multi-Symptom Relief** oral liquid (discontinued 2002) OTC *antitussive; decongestant; antihistamine* [dextromethorphan hydrobromide; phenylpropanolamine HCl; chlorpheniramine maleate] 10•12.5•2 mg/5 mL

**Triaminicol Multi-Symptom Relief Colds with Cough** pediatric oral liquid (discontinued 2002) OTC *antitussive; decongestant; antihistamine* [dextromethorphan hydrobromide; phenylpropanolamine HCl; chlorpheniramine maleate] 5•6.25•1 mg/5 mL

**Triamolone 40** IM injection ℞ *corticosteroid; anti-inflammatory* [triamcinolone diacetate] 40 mg/mL

**Triamonide 40** IM, intra-articular, intrabursal, intradermal injection ℞ *corticosteroid; anti-inflammatory* [triamcinolone acetonide] 40 mg/mL

**triampyzine** INN *anticholinergic* [also: triampyzine sulfate]

**triampyzine sulfate** USAN *anticholinergic* [also: triampyzine]

**triamterene** USAN, USP, INN, BAN, JAN *antihypertensive; potassium-sparing diuretic* 🔲 trimipramine

**triamterene & hydrochlorothiazide** *antihypertensive; potassium-sparing diuretic* 37.5•25 mg oral

**trianisestrol** [see: chlorotrianisene]

**Triapine** ℞ *investigational (Phase I) anticancer agent* 🔲 Triaprim

**Triavil** tablets ℞ *conventional (typical) antipsychotic; antidepressant* [perphenazine; amitriptyline HCl] 2•10 mg; 2•25 mg; 4•10 mg; 4•25 mg

**Triavil 4-50** tablets (discontinued 2000) ℞ *conventional (typical) antipsychotic; antidepressant* [perphenazine; amitriptyline HCl] 4•50 mg

**Tri-A-Vite F** drops ℞ *pediatric vitamin supplement and dental caries preventative* [vitamins A, C, and D; fluoride] 1500 IU•35 mg•400 IU•0.5 mg per mL

**Triaz** gel, topical liquid (discontinued 2003) ℞ *keratolytic for acne* [benzoyl peroxide] 3%, 6%, 9%, 10%

**Triaz** skin cleanser (discontinued 2003) ℞ *keratolytic for acne* [benzoyl peroxide] 9%, 10%

**triaziquone** INN, BAN

**triazolam** USAN, USP, INN *benzodiazepine sedative; hypnotic* 0.125, 0.25 mg oral

**Triban; Pediatric Triban** suppositories ℞ *antiemetic; anticholinergic* [trimethobenzamide HCl; benzocaine] 200 mg•2%; 100 mg•2% 🔲 Tigan

**tribasic calcium phosphate** [see: calcium phosphate, tribasic]

**tribavirin** BAN *antiviral for severe lower respiratory tract infections* [also: ribavirin]

**tribendilol** INN

**tribenoside** USAN, INN *sclerosing agent*

**Tribiotic Plus** ointment (discontinued 2001) OTC *topical antibiotic; anesthetic* [polymyxin B sulfate; bacitracin; neomycin sulfate; lidocaine] 5000 U•500 U•3.5 mg•40 mg per g

**Tri-Biozene** ointment OTC *antibiotic; local anesthetic* [polymyxin B sulfate; neomycin sulfate; bacitracin zinc; pramoxine HCl] 10 000 U•3.5 mg•500 U•10 mg per g

**tribromoethanol** NF

**tribromomethane** [see: bromoform]

**tribromsalan** USAN, INN *disinfectant*

**tribuzone** INN

**tricalcium phosphate** [see: calcium phosphate, tribasic]

**tricarbocyanine dye** [see: indocyanine green]

**tricetamide** USAN *sedative*

**Trichinella extract** USP

**Tri-Chlor** topical liquid ℞ *cauterant; keratolytic* [trichloroacetic acid] 80%

**trichlorethoxyphosphamide** [see: defosfamide]

**trichlorfon** USP *veterinary anthelmintic; investigational (NDA filed) acetylcholinesterase inhibitor for Alzheimer dementia* [also: metrifonate; metriphonate]

**trichlorisobutylalcohol** [see: chlorobutanol]

**trichlormethiazide** USP, INN *diuretic; antihypertensive* 4 mg oral

**trichlormethine** INN [also: trimustine]

**trichloroacetic acid** USP *strong keratolytic/cauterant*

**trichlorocarbanilide (TCC)** [see: triclocarban]

**trichloroethylene** NF, INN

**trichlorofluoromethane** [see: trichloromonofluoromethane]

**trichlorofon** [see: metrifonate]

**trichloromonofluoromethane** NF *aerosol propellant; topical anesthetic*

**trichlorphon** [see: metrifonate]

*Tricholomopsis edodes* medicinal herb [see: shiitake mushrooms]

**Trichophyton extract** *diagnosis and treatment of Trichophyton-induced skin infections*

**trichorad** [see: acinitrazole]

*Trichosanthes kirilowii medicinal herb* [see: Chinese cucumber]

**trichosanthin** *investigational (Phase II) antiviral for AIDS*

**Trichotine Douche** powder OTC *antiseptic/germicidal; vaginal cleanser and deodorizer; acidity modifier* [sodium perborate]

**Trichotine Douche** solution OTC *antiseptic/germicidal; vaginal cleanser and deodorizer; acidity modifier* [sodium borate]

**triciribine** INN *antineoplastic* [also: triciribine phosphate]

**triciribine phosphate** USAN *antineoplastic* [also: triciribine]

**tricitrates (sodium citrate, potassium citrate, and citric acid)** USP *systemic alkalizer; urinary alkalizer; antiurolithic*

**triclabendazole** INN

**triclacetamol** INN

**triclazate** INN

**triclobisonium chloride** NF, INN

**triclocarban** USAN, INN *disinfectant*

**triclodazol** INN

**triclofenate** INN *combining name for radicals or groups*

**triclofenol piperazine** USAN, INN *anthelmintic*

**triclofos** INN *hypnotic; sedative* [also: triclofos sodium]

**triclofos sodium** USAN *hypnotic; sedative* [also: triclofos]

**triclofylline** INN

**triclonide** USAN, INN *anti-inflammatory*

**triclosan** USAN, INN, BAN *disinfectant/ antiseptic*

**Tricodene Cough and Cold** oral liquid ℞ *narcotic antitussive; antihistamine* [codeine phosphate; pyrilamine maleate] 16.4•25 mg/10 mL

**Tricodene Forte; Tricodene NN** oral liquid (discontinued 2002) OTC *antitussive; decongestant; antihistamine* [dextromethorphan hydrobromide; phenylpropanolamine HCl;

chlorpheniramine maleate] 10•12.5• 2 mg/5 mL

**Tricodene Pediatric Cough & Cold** oral liquid (discontinued 2002) OTC *antitussive; decongestant* [dextromethorphan hydrobromide; phenylpropanolamine HCl] 10•12.5 mg/5 mL

**Tricodene Sugar Free** oral liquid OTC *antitussive; antihistamine* [dextromethorphan hydrobromide; chlorpheniramine maleate] 20•4 mg/10 mL

**TriCor** capsules (discontinued 2002) ℞ *antihyperlipidemic for primary hypercholesterolemia (types IIa and IIb hyperlipidemia), hypertriglyceridemia (types IV and V hyperlipidemia), and mixed dyslipidemia* [fenofibrate] 67, 134, 200 mg

**TriCor** tablets ℞ *antihyperlipidemic for primary hypercholesterolemia (types IIa and IIb hyperlipidemia), hypertriglyceridemia (types IV and V hyperlipidemia), and mixed dyslipidemia* [fenofibrate] 54, 160 mg

**tricosactide** INN

**Tricosal** film-coated tablets ℞ *analgesic; antipyretic; antirheumatic* [choline magnesium trisalicylate] 500, 750, 1000 mg

**tricyclamol chloride** INN

**Tri-Cyclen** [see: Ortho Tri-Cyclen]

**tricyclics** *a class of antidepressants that inhibit reuptake of amines, norepinephrine, and serotonin*

**Triderm** cream ℞ *topical corticosteroidal anti-inflammatory* [triamcinolone acetonide] 0.1%

**Tridesilon** cream, ointment ℞ *corticosteroidal anti-inflammatory* [desonide] 0.05%

**Tridesilon Otic** [see: Otic Tridesilon]

**tridihexethyl chloride** USP *peptic ulcer treatment adjunct*

**tridihexethyl iodide** INN

**Tridil** IV infusion (discontinued 2004) ℞ *antianginal; vasodilator; perioperative antihypertensive; for congestive heart failure with myocardial infarction* [nitroglycerin] 0.5, 5 mg/mL

**Tridione** capsules, Dulcets (chewable tablets) (discontinued 2004) ℞ *anticonvulsant for absence (petit mal) seizures* [trimethadione] 300 mg; 150 mg

**tridolgosir HCl** USAN *chemoprotectant for solid tumor chemotherapy*

**Tridrate Bowel Cleansing System** oral solution + 3 tablets + 1 suppository OTC *pre-procedure bowel evacuant* [magnesium citrate (solution); bisacodyl (tablets and suppository)] 300 mL; 5 mg; 10 mg

**trientine** INN *copper chelating agent* [also: trientine HCl; trientine dihydrochloride]

**trientine dihydrochloride** BAN *copper chelating agent* [also: trientine HCl; trientine]

**trientine HCl** USAN, USP *copper chelating agent for Wilson disease (orphan)* [also: trientine; trientine dihydrochloride]

**triest; triestrogen** [see: estriol]

**triethanolamine** [now: trolamine]

**triethyl citrate** NF *plasticizer*

**triethyleneiminobenzoquinone (TEIB)** [see: triaziquone]

**triethylenemelamine** NF [also: tretamine]

**triethylenethiophosphoramide (TSPA; TESPA)** [see: thiotepa]

**Trifed-C Cough** syrup (discontinued 2002) ℞ *narcotic antitussive; decongestant; antihistamine* [codeine phosphate; pseudoephedrine HCl; triprolidine HCl; alcohol 4.4%] 10•30• 1.25 mg/5 mL

**trifenagrel** USAN, INN *antithrombotic*

**trifezolac** INN

**triflocin** USAN, INN *diuretic*

**Tri-Flor-Vite with Fluoride** drops ℞ *pediatric vitamin supplement and dental caries preventative* [vitamins A, C, and D; fluoride] 1500 IU•35 mg• 400 IU•0.25 mg per mL

**triflubazam** USAN, INN *minor tranquilizer*

**triflumidate** USAN, INN *anti-inflammatory*

**trifluomeprazine** INN, BAN

**trifluoperazine** INN *phenothiazine antipsychotic; sedative* [also: trifluoperazine HCl]

**trifluoperazine HCl** USP *phenothiazine antipsychotic; sedative; anxiolytic* [also: trifluoperazine] 1, 2, 5, 10 mg oral

**trifluorothymidine** [see: trifluridine]

**trifluperidol** USAN, INN *antipsychotic*

**triflupromazine** USP, INN *phenothiazine antipsychotic; antiemetic*

**triflupromazine HCl** USP *phenothiazine antipsychotic; antiemetic*

**trifluridine** USAN, INN *ophthalmic antiviral* 1% eye drops

**triflusal** INN *investigational treatment for stroke and vascular dementia*

**triflutate** USAN, INN *combining name for radicals or groups*

*Trifolium pratense* medicinal herb [see: red clover]

**trigevolol** INN

**α-triglycidyl isocyanurate (αTGI)** [see: teroxirone]

*Trigonella foenum-graecum* medicinal herb [see: fenugreek]

**TriHemic 600** film-coated tablets ℞ *hematinic* [ferrous fumarate; cyanocobalamin; ascorbic acid; vitamin E; intrinsic factor concentrate; docusate sodium; folic acid] 115 mg•25 μg•600 mg•30 IU•75 mg•50 mg• 1 mg ⑦ Triaminic

**Trihexy-2; Trihexy-5** tablets ℞ *anticholinergic; antiparkinsonian* [trihexyphenidyl HCl] 2 mg; 5 mg

**trihexyphenidyl** INN *anticholinergic; antiparkinsonian* [also: trihexyphenidyl HCl; benzhexol]

**trihexyphenidyl HCl** USP *anticholinergic; antiparkinsonian* [also: trihexyphenidyl; benzhexol] 2, 5 mg oral

**TriHIBit** IM injection ℞ *active immunizing agent for diphtheria, tetanus, pertussis, and Haemophilus influenzae type B* [diphtheria & tetanus toxoids & acellular pertussis (DTaP) vaccine; Hemophilus B conjugate vaccine] supplied as separate 0.5 mL vials of Tripedia (q.v.) and ActHib (q.v.)

**Tri-Hydroserpine** tablets ℞ *antihypertensive; vasodilator; diuretic* [hydrochlorothiazide; reserpine; hydralazine HCl] 15•0.1•25 mg

**Tri-Immunol** IM injection (discontinued 2001) ℞ *active immunizing agent for diphtheria, tetanus and pertussis* [diphtheria & tetanus toxoids & whole-cell pertussis (DTwP) vaccine, adsorbed] 12.5 LfU•5 LfU•4 U/0.5 mL

**3,5,3′-triiodothyroacetate** *investigational (orphan) for thyroid carcinoma*

**triiodothyroacetic acid (TRIAC)** *thyroid hormone analogue*

**triiodothyronine sodium, levo** [see: liothyronine sodium]

**Tri-K** oral liquid ℞ *potassium supplement* [potassium acetate; potassium bicarbonate; potassium citrate] 45 mEq K/15 mL

**trikates** USP *electrolyte replenisher*

**Trikof-D** sustained-release tablets (discontinued 2002) OTC *antitussive; decongestant; expectorant* [dextromethorphan hydrobromide; phenylpropanolamine HCl; guaifenesin] 30•37.5•600 mg

**Tri-Kort** IM, intra-articular, intrabursal, or intradermal injection ℞ *corticosteroid; anti-inflammatory* [triamcinolone acetonide] 40 mg/mL

**Trilafon** coated tablets, IV or IM injection (discontinued 2003) ℞ *conventional (typical) antipsychotic; antiemetic* [perphenazine] 2, 4, 8, 16 mg; 5 mg/ml

**Trilafon** oral concentrate (discontinued 2002) ℞ *conventional (typical) antipsychotic; antiemetic* [perphenazine] 2, 4, 8, 16 mg; 16 mg/5 mL; 5 mg/mL

**Trileptal** film-coated tablets, oral suspension ℞ *anticonvulsant for partial seizures* [oxcarbazepine] 150, 300, 600 mg; 300 mg/5 mL

**triletide** INN

**Tri-Levlen** film-coated tablets (in Slidecases of 21 or 28) ℞ *triphasic oral contraceptive; emergency postcoital contraceptive* [levonorgestrel; ethinyl estradiol]

Phase 1 (6 days): 50•30 μg;
Phase 2 (5 days): 75•40 μg;
Phase 3 (10 days): 125•30 μg

**Trilisate** tablets, oral liquid (discontinued 2004) ℞ *analgesic; antipyretic; anti-inflammatory; antirheumatic* [choline salicylate; magnesium salicylate] 750, 1000 mg; 500 mg/5 mL

**trilithium citrate tetrahydrate** [see: lithium citrate]

***Trillium erectum; T. grandiflorum; T. pendulum*** *medicinal herb* [see: birthroot]

**Trilog** IM, intra-articular, intrabursal, intradermal injection ℞ *corticosteroid; anti-inflammatory* [triamcinolone acetonide] 40 mg/mL

**Trilone** IM injection ℞ *corticosteroid; anti-inflammatory* [triamcinolone diacetate] 40 mg/mL

**trilostane** USAN, INN, BAN *adrenocortical suppressant; antisteroidal antineoplastic*

**Tri-Luma** cream ℞ *short-term treatment for melasma of the face* [hydroquinone; fluocinolone acetonide; tretinoin] 4%•0.01%•0.05%

**TriLyte** powder for oral solution ℞ *pre-procedure bowel evacuant* [polyethylene glycol–electrolyte solution (PEG 3350)]

**Trimazide** capsules (discontinued 2000) ℞ *antiemetic; anticholinergic* [trimethobenzamide HCl] 100 mg

**Trimazide** suppositories, pediatric suppositories ℞ *antiemetic; anticholinergic* [trimethobenzamide HCl] 200 mg; 100 mg

**trimazosin** INN, BAN *antihypertensive* [also: trimazosin HCl]

**trimazosin HCl** USAN *antihypertensive* [also: trimazosin]

**trimebutine** INN GI *antispasmodic*

**trimecaine** INN

**trimedoxime bromide** INN

**trimegestone** USAN *progestin for postmenopausal hormone deficiency*

**trimeperidine** INN, BAN

**trimeprazine** BAN *phenothiazine antihistamine; antipruritic* [also: trimepra-

zine tartrate; alimemazine; alimemazine tartrate] ⑤ trimipramine

**trimeprazine tartrate** USP *phenothiazine antihistamine; antipruritic* [also:
alimemazine; trimeprazine; alimemazine tartrate]

**trimeproprimine** [see: trimipramine]

**trimetamide** INN

**trimetaphan camsilate** INN *antihypertensive* [also: trimethaphan camsylate; trimetaphan camsylate]

**trimetaphan camsylate** BAN *antihypertensive* [also: trimethaphan camsylate; trimetaphan camsilate]

**trimetazidine** INN, BAN

**trimethadione** USP, INN *oxazolidinedione anticonvulsant for absence (petit
mal) seizures* [also: troxidone]

**trimethamide** [see: trimetamide]

**trimethaphan camphorsulfonate**
[see: trimethaphan camsylate] ⑤ trimethoprim

**trimethaphan camsylate** USP *emergency antihypertensive* [also: trimetaphan camsilate; trimetaphan camsy-
late]

**trimethidinium methosulfate** NF, INN

**trimethobenzamide** INN *antiemetic;
anticholinergic* [also: trimethobenzamide HCl]

**trimethobenzamide HCl** USP *antiemetic; anticholinergic* [also: trimetho-
benzamide] 250, 300 mg oral; 100,
200 mg suppositories; 100 mg/mL
injection

**trimethoprim (TMP)** USAN, USP,
INN, BAN *antibacterial antibiotic* 100,
200 mg oral ⑤ trimethaphan

**trimethoprim sulfate** USAN *antibiotic*

**trimethoprim sulfate & polymyxin
B sulfate** *topical ophthalmic antibiotic*
1 mg•10 000 U per mL eye drops

**trimethoquinol** [see: tretoquinol]

**trimethylammonium chloride car-
bamate** [see: bethanechol chloride]

**3,3,5-trimethylcyclohexyl salicyl-
ate** [see: homosalate]

**trimethylene** [see: cyclopropane]

**trimethylglycine (TMG)** *natural
methylation agent used to prevent cardiovascular disease by lowering homo-
cysteine levels, to boost neurological
function by remyelinating nerve cells,
and to slow cellular aging by protecting
DNA; precursor to SAMe (q.v.)*

**trimethyltetradecylammonium bro-
mide** [see: tetradonium bromide]

**trimetozine** USAN, INN *sedative*

**trimetrexate** USAN, INN, BAN *antimetabolic antineoplastic; systemic antiprotozoal*

**trimetrexate glucuronate** USAN *antimetabolic antineoplastic; antiprotozoal
for* Pneumocystis carinii *pneumonia
of AIDS (orphan); investigational
(orphan) for multiple cancers*

**trimexiline** INN

**Triminol Cough** syrup (discontinued
2002) OTC *antitussive; decongestant;
antihistamine* [dextromethorphan
hydrobromide; phenylpropanolamine HCl; chlorpheniramine male-
ate] 10•12.5•2 mg/5 mL

**trimipramine** USAN, INN *tricyclic antidepressant* ⑤ imipramine; triamterene; trimeprazine

**trimipramine maleate** USAN *tricyclic
antidepressant*

**trimolide** [see: trimetozine]

**trimopam maleate** [now: trepipam
maleate]

**trimoprostil** USAN, INN *gastric antisecretory*

**Trimo-San** vaginal jelly OTC *antibacterial; astringent; antipruritic* [oxyquino-
line sulfate; boric acid; sodium
borate] 0.025%•1%•0.7%

**Trimox** chewable tablets, capsules, powder for oral suspension ℞ *aminopenicillin antibiotic* [amoxicillin] 125, 250
mg; 250, 500 mg; 125, 250 mg/5 mL

**Trimox** pediatric drops (discontinued
2002) ℞ *aminopenicillin antibiotic*
[amoxicillin] 50 mg/mL

**trimoxamine** INN *antihypertensive*
[also: trimoxamine HCl]

**trimoxamine HCl** USAN *antihypertensive* [also: trimoxamine]

**Trimpex** tablets ℞ *anti-infective; antibacterial* [trimethoprim] 100 mg

**trimustine** BAN [also: trichlormethine]

**Trinalin** Repetabs (sustained-release tablets) ℞ *decongestant; antihistamine* [pseudoephedrine sulfate; azatadine maleate] 120•1 mg

**Trinam** reservoir delivery device ℞ *investigational (Phase II, orphan) gene-based therapy for neointimal hyperplasia disease* [vascular endothelial growth factor (VEGF)]

**Tri-Nasal** nasal spray (discontinued 2002) ℞ *once-daily corticosteroidal anti-inflammatory for chronic allergic rhinitis* [triamcinolone acetonide] 50 μg/spray

**Trinate** tablets ℞ *vitamin/mineral/calcium/iron supplement* [multiple vitamins & minerals; calcium; iron; folic acid] ≛•200•28•1 mg

**trinecol (pullus)** USAN *collagen derivative for treatment of rheumatoid arthritis*

**Tri-Nefrin** tablets (discontinued 2001) OTC *decongestant; antihistamine* [phenylpropanolamine HCl; chlorpheniramine maleate] 25•4 mg

**TriNessa** tablets (in packs of 28) ℞ *triphasic oral contraceptive* [norgestimate; ethinyl estradiol]
Phase 1 (7 days): 180•35 μg;
Phase 2 (7 days): 215•35 μg;
Phase 3 (7 days): 250•35 μg

**Trinipatch** ⓒ transdermal patch ℞ *antianginal; vasodilator* [nitroglycerin] 22.4, 44.8, 67.2 mg (0.2, 0.4, 0.6 mg/hr.)

**trinitrin** [see: nitroglycerin]

**trinitrophenol** NF

**Tri-Norinyl** tablets (in Wallettes of 28) ℞ *triphasic oral contraceptive* [norethindrone; ethinyl estradiol]
Phase 1 (7 days): 500•35 μg;
Phase 2 (9 days): 1000•35 μg;
Phase 3 (5 days): 500•35 μg

**Trinsicon** capsules ℞ *hematinic* [ferrous fumarate; cyanocobalamin; ascorbic acid; intrinsic factor concentrate; folic acid] 110 mg•15 μg•75 mg•240 mg•0.5 mg

**2′,3′,5′-tri-o-acetyluridine** *investigational (orphan) treatment for mitochondrial disease*

**Triofed** syrup (discontinued 2002) OTC *decongestant; antihistamine* [pseudoephedrine HCl; triprolidine HCl] 30•1.25 mg/5 mL

**triolein I 125** USAN *radioactive agent*

**triolein I 131** USAN *radioactive agent*

**trional** [see: sulfonethylmethane]

**Trionate** caplets ℞ *antitussive; antihistamine* [carbetapentane tannate; chlorpheniramine tannate] 60•5 mg

**Triostat** IV injection ℞ *synthetic thyroid hormone ($T_3$ fraction only) for myxedema coma or precoma (orphan)* [liothyronine sodium] 10 μg/mL ⊘ Threostat

**Triotann** tablets (discontinued 2002) ℞ *decongestant; antihistamine* [phenylephrine tannate; chlorpheniramine tannate; pyrilamine tannate] 25•8•25 mg

**Triotann Pediatric; Triotann-S Pediatric** oral suspension ℞ *decongestant; antihistamine* [phenylephrine tannate; chlorpheniramine tannate; pyrilamine tannate] 5•2•12.5 mg/5 mL

**Tri-Otic** ear drops ℞ *topical corticosteroidal anti-inflammatory; topical local anesthetic; antiseptic* [hydrocortisone; pramoxine HCl; chloroxylenol] 10•10•1 mg/mL

**trioxifene** INN *antiestrogen* [also: trioxifene mesylate]

**trioxifene mesylate** USAN *antiestrogen* [also: trioxifene]

**trioxsalen** USAN, USP *systemic psoralens for repigmentation of idiopathic vitiligo; also used to enhance pigmentation and increase tolerance to sunlight* [also: trioxysalen]

**trioxyethylrutin** [see: troxerutin]

**trioxymethylene** [see: paraformaldehyde]

**trioxysalen** INN *systemic psoralens for repigmentation of idiopathic vitiligo; also used to enhance pigmentation and increase tolerance to sunlight* [also: trioxsalen]

**Tri-P** oral infant drops (discontinued 2001) ℞ *decongestant; antihistamine* [phenylpropanolamine HCl; pyrilamine maleate; pheniramine maleate] 20•10•10 mg/mL

**tripamide** USAN, INN *antihypertensive; diuretic*

**triparanol** INN *(withdrawn from market)*

**Tripedia** IM injection ℞ *immunization against diphtheria, tetanus and pertussis* [diphtheria & tetanus toxoids & acellular pertussis (DTaP) vaccine, adsorbed] 6.7 LfU•5 LfU•46.8 µg per 0.5 mL dose

**tripelennamine** INN *ethylenediamine antihistamine* [also: tripelennamine citrate]

**tripelennamine citrate** USP *ethylenediamine antihistamine* [also: tripelennamine]

**tripelennamine HCl** USP *ethylenediamine antihistamine*

**Triphasil** tablets (in packs of 21 or 28) ℞ *triphasic oral contraceptive; emergency postcoital contraceptive* [levonorgestrel; ethinyl estradiol]
Phase 1 (6 days): 50•30 µg;
Phase 2 (5 days): 75•40 µg;
Phase 3 (10 days): 125•30 µg

**Tri-Phen-Chlor** syrup, pediatric syrup, pediatric drops (discontinued 2001) ℞ *decongestant; antihistamine* [phenylpropanolamine HCl; phenylephrine HCl; chlorpheniramine maleate; phenyltoloxamine citrate] 20•5•2.5•7.5 mg/5 mL; 5•1.25•0.5•2 mg/5 mL; 5•1.25•0.5•2 mg/mL

**Tri-Phen-Chlor T.R.** timed-release tablets (discontinued 2002) ℞ *decongestant; antihistamine* [phenylpropanolamine HCl; phenylephrine HCl; chlorpheniramine maleate; phenyltoloxamine citrate] 40•10•5•15 mg

**Tri-Phen-Mine** syrup, oral drops (discontinued 2001) ℞ *pediatric decongestant and antihistamine* [phenylpropanolamine HCl; phenylephrine HCl; chlorpheniramine maleate; phenyltoloxamine citrate] 5•1.25•0.5•2 mg/5 mL; 5•1.25•0.5•2 mg/mL

**Tri-Phen-Mine S.R.** timed-release tablets (discontinued 2002) ℞ *decongestant; antihistamine* [phenyl-

propanolamine HCl; phenylephrine HCl; chlorpheniramine maleate; phenyltoloxamine citrate] 40•10•5•15 mg

**Triphenyl** syrup (discontinued 2001) OTC *decongestant; antihistamine* [phenylpropanolamine HCl; chlorpheniramine maleate] 6.25•1 mg/5 mL

**Triphenyl Expectorant** oral liquid (discontinued 2002) OTC *decongestant; expectorant* [phenylpropanolamine HCl; guaifenesin; alcohol 5%] 12.5•100 mg/5 mL

**Triple Antibiotic** ointment OTC *antibiotic* [polymyxin B sulfate; neomycin sulfate; bacitracin] 5000 U•3.5 mg•400 U per g

**Triple Antibiotic** ophthalmic ointment (discontinued 2000) ℞ *antibiotic* [polymyxin B sulfate; neomycin sulfate; bacitracin zinc] 5000 U•3.5 mg•400 U per g

**Triple Antibiotic Plus** ointment (discontinued 2003) OTC *antibiotic; local anesthetic* [polymyxin B sulfate; neomycin sulfate; bacitracin zinc; pramoxine HCl] 10 000 U•3.5 mg•500 U•10 mg per g

**Triple Sulfa** vaginal cream (discontinued 2001) ℞ *broad-spectrum antibiotic* [sulfathiazole; sulfacetamide; sulfabenzamide] 3.42%•2.86%•3.7%

**triple sulfa (sulfathiazole, sulfacetamide, and sulfabenzamide)** [q.v.]

**Triple Vitamin ADC with Fluoride** drops ℞ *pediatric vitamin supplement and dental caries preventative* [vitamins A, C, and D; fluoride] 1500 IU•35 mg•400 IU•0.5 mg per mL

**Triple X Kit** topical liquid + shampoo (discontinued 2003) OTC *pediculicide for lice* [pyrethrins; piperonyl butoxide; petroleum distillate] 0.3%•3%• ?

**Triposed** tablets, syrup (discontinued 2002) OTC *decongestant; antihistamine* [pseudoephedrine HCl; triprolidine HCl] 60•2.5 mg; 30•1.25 mg/5 mL

**tripotassium citrate monohydrate** [see: potassium citrate]

**Tri-Previfem** tablets (in packs of 28) ℞ *triphasic oral contraceptive* [norgestimate; ethinyl estradiol]
Phase 1 (7 days): 180•35 µg;
Phase 2 (7 days): 215•35 µg;
Phase 3 (7 days): 250•35 µg

**triproamylin** [see: pramlintide]

**triprolidine** INN *antihistamine* [also: triprolidine HCl]

**triprolidine HCl** USP *antihistamine* [also: triprolidine]

**triprolidine HCl & pseudoephedrine HCl** *antihistamine; decongestant* 2.5•60 mg oral

**Tripterygium wilfordii** *medicinal herb* [see: thunder god vine]

**triptolide** *investigational immunosuppressive and antineoplastic*

**Triptone** long-acting caplets OTC *antinauseant; antiemetic; antivertigo; motion sickness preventative* [dimenhydrinate] 50 mg

**triptorelin** USAN, INN *gonadotropin-releasing hormone (GnRH) antineoplastic*

**triptorelin pamoate** *gonadotropin-releasing hormone (GnRH) antineoplastic for palliative treatment of advanced prostate cancer*

**trisaccharides A & B** *investigational (orphan) for newborn hemolytic disease and ABO blood incompatibility of organ or bone marrow transplants*

**Trisan** ⒸⒶⓃ foaming gel OTC *medicated cleanser for acne* [triclosan] 0,25%

**Trisenox** injection ℞ *antineoplastic for acute promyelocytic leukemia (orphan); investigational (NDA filed) for renal cell carcinoma; investigational (orphan) for multiple myeloma and myelodysplastic syndromes* [arsenic trioxide] 10 mg/10 mL

**trisodium citrate** [see: sodium citrate]

**trisodium citrate dihydrate** [see: sodium citrate]

**trisodium hydrogen ethylenediaminetetraacetate** [see: edetate trisodium]

**Trisoralen** tablets (discontinued 2003) ℞ *systemic psoralens for repigmentation of idiopathic vitiligo; also used to enhance pigmentation and increase tolerance to sunlight* [trioxsalen] 5 mg

**Tri-Sprintec** tablets (in packs of 28) ℞ *triphasic oral contraceptive* [norgestimate; ethinyl estradiol]
Phase 1 (7 days): 180•35 µg;
Phase 2 (7 days): 215•35 µg;
Phase 3 (7 days): 250•35 µg

**Tri-Statin II** cream ℞ *topical corticosteroidal anti-inflammatory; antifungal* [triamcinolone acetonide; nystatin] 0.1%•100 000 U per g

**Tristoject** IM injection ℞ *corticosteroid; anti-inflammatory* [triamcinolone diacetate] 40 mg/mL

**trisulfapyrimidines** USP (a mixture of sulfadiazine, sulfamerazine, and sulfamethazine) *broad-spectrum bacteriostatic*

**Tri-Super Flavons 1000** tablets OTC *dietary supplement* [mixed bioflavonoids] 1000 mg

**Tritan** tablets (discontinued 2002) ℞ *decongestant; antihistamine* [phenylephrine tannate; chlorpheniramine tannate; pyrilamine tannate] 25•8•25 mg

**Tri-Tannate** tablets, pediatric oral suspension (discontinued 2002) ℞ *decongestant; antihistamine* [phenylephrine tannate; chlorpheniramine tannate; pyrilamine tannate] 25•8•25 mg; 5•2•12.5 mg/5 mL

**Tri-Tannate Plus Pediatric** oral suspension (discontinued 2002) ℞ *antitussive; decongestant; antihistamine* [carbetapentane tannate; phenylephrine tannate; ephedrine tannate; chlorpheniramine tannate] 30•5•5•4 mg/5 mL

**Tritec** film-coated tablets (discontinued 2004) ℞ *histamine $H_2$ antagonist for duodenal ulcers with H. pylori infection* [ranitidine bismuth citrate] 400 mg

**tritheon** [see: acinitrazole]

**tritiated water** USAN *radioactive agent*

**Triticum repens** *medicinal herb* [see: couch grass]

**tritiozine** INN

**tritoqualine** INN

**Triva Douche** powder (discontinued 2003) OTC *antiseptic/germicidal; vaginal cleanser and deodorizer* [oxyquinoline sulfate] 2%

**Trivagizole 3** vaginal cream OTC *topical antifungal for yeast infections* [clotrimazole] 2%

**trivalent oral poliovirus vaccine (TOPV)** [see: poliovirus vaccine, live oral]

**Tri-Vi-Flor** chewable tablets, drops ℞ *pediatric vitamin supplement and dental caries preventative* [vitamins A, C, and D; sodium fluoride] 2500 IU•60 mg•400 IU•1 mg; 1500 IU•35 mg•400 IU•0.25 mg, 1500 IU•35 mg•400 IU•0.5 mg per mL

**Tri-Vi-Flor with Iron** drops ℞ *pediatric vitamin/iron supplement and dental caries preventative* [vitamins A, C, and D; iron; sodium fluoride] 1500 IU•35 mg•400 IU•0.25 mg per mL

**Tri-Vi-Sol** drops OTC *pediatric vitamin supplement* [vitamins A, C, and D] 1500 IU•35 mg•400 IU per mL

**Tri-Vi-Sol with Iron** drops OTC *vitamin/iron supplement* [vitamins A, C, and D; ferrous sulfate] 1500 IU•35 mg•400 IU•10 mg per mL

**Trivitamin Fluoride** chewable tablets, drops ℞ *pediatric vitamin supplement and dental caries preventative* [vitamins A, C, and D; fluoride] 2500 IU•60 mg•400 IU•1 mg; 1500 IU•35 mg•400 IU•0.25 mg, 1500 IU•35 mg•400 IU•0.5 mg per mL

**Tri-Vitamin Infants' Drops** OTC *vitamin supplement* [vitamins A, C, and D] 1500 IU•35 mg•400 IU per mL

**Tri-Vitamin with Fluoride** drops ℞ *pediatric vitamin supplement and dental caries preventative* [vitamins A, C, and D; fluoride] 1500 IU•35 mg•400 IU•0.5 mg per mL

**Trivora** tablets (in packs of 28) ℞ *triphasic oral contraceptive* [levonorgestrel; ethinyl estradiol]
Phase 1 (6 days): 50•30 µg;
Phase 2 (5 days): 75•40 µg;
Phase 3 (10 days): 125•30 µg

**trixolane** INN

**Trizivir** film-coated caplets ℞ *antiretroviral nucleoside reverse transcriptase inhibitor (NRTI) for HIV infection* [abacavir sulfate; zidovudine; lamivudine] 300•300•150 mg

**trizoxime** INN

**Trizyme** (ingredient) OTC *digestive enzymes* [amylolytic, proteolytic and cellulolytic enzymes (amylase; protease; cellulase)]

**Trobicin** powder for IM injection ℞ *antibiotic for gonorrhea* [spectinomycin HCl] 400 mg/mL ☒ tobramycin

**Trocade** ℞ *matrix metalloproteinase inhibitor; investigational cartilage protective agent for rheumatoid arthritis* [cipemastat]

**Trocaine** lozenges OTC *topical oral anesthetic* [benzocaine] 10 mg

**Trocal** lozenges OTC *antitussive* [dextromethorphan hydrobromide] 7.5 mg

**trocimine** INN

**troclosene potassium** USAN, INN *topical anti-infective*

**trofosfamide** INN

**troglitazone** USAN, INN *thiazolidinedione antidiabetic; increases cellular response to insulin without increasing insulin secretion*

**trolamine** USAN, NF *alkalizing agent; analgesic*

**trolamine polypeptide oleate-condensate** *cerumenolytic to emulsify and disperse ear wax*

**trolamine salicylate** *topical analgesic*

**troleandomycin** USAN, USP *macrolide antibiotic; investigational (orphan) for severe asthma* [also: triacetyloleandomycin]

**trolnitrate** INN

**trolnitrate phosphate** [see: trolnitrate]

**tromantadine** INN

**trometamol** INN, BAN *alkalizer for cardiac bypass surgery* [also: tromethamine]

**tromethamine** USAN, USP *alkalizer for cardiac bypass surgery* [also: trometamol]

**Tronolane** anorectal cream OTC *topical local anesthetic* [pramoxine HCl] 1% ⊡ Tronothane

**Tronolane** rectal suppositories OTC *astringent; emollient* [zinc oxide] 11%

**Tronothane HCl** cream OTC *topical local anesthetic* [pramoxine HCl] 1% ⊡ Tronolane

**tropabazate** INN

*Tropaeolum majus* medicinal herb [see: Indian cress]

**tropanserin** INN, BAN *migraine-specific serotonin receptor antagonist* [also: tropanserin HCl]

**tropanserin HCl** USAN *migraine-specific serotonin receptor antagonist* [also: tropanserin]

**tropapride** INN

**tropatepine** INN

**tropenziline bromide** INN

**TrophAmine 6%; TrophAmine 10%** IV infusion ℞ *total parenteral nutrition; peripheral parenteral nutrition* [multiple essential and nonessential amino acids]

**Trophite + Iron** oral liquid OTC *hematinic* [ferric pyrophosphate; vitamins $B_1$ and $B_{12}$] 60 mg•30 mg•75 μg per 15 mL

**trophosphamide** [see: trofosfamide]

**Tropicacyl** eye drops ℞ *cycloplegic; mydriatic* [tropicamide] 0.5%, 1%

**tropicamide** USAN, USP, INN *ophthalmic anticholinergic; cycloplegic; short-acting mydriatic*

**tropigline** INN, BAN

**tropirine** INN

**tropisetron** INN, BAN *investigational treatment for nausea and vomiting related to chemotherapy*

**Tropi-Storz** eye drops ℞ *cycloplegic; mydriatic* [tropicamide] 0.5%, 1%

**tropodifene** INN

**troquidazole** INN

**trospectomycin** INN, BAN *investigational (Phase III) broad-spectrum aminocyclitol antibiotic* [also: trospectomycin sulfate]

**trospectomycin sulfate** USAN *broad-spectrum aminocyclitol antibiotic* [also: trospectomycin]

**trospium chloride** INN *muscarinic receptor antagonist for urinary frequency, urgency, and incontinence*

**trovafloxacin mesylate** USAN *broad-spectrum fluoroquinolone antibiotic*

**Trovan** film-coated tablets ℞ *broad-spectrum fluoroquinolone antibiotic* [trovafloxacin mesylate] 100, 200 mg

**Trovan** IV infusion ℞ *broad-spectrum fluoroquinolone antibiotic* [alatrofloxacin mesylate] 5 mg/mL ⊡ Atrovent

**Trovan/Zithromax Compliance Pak** ℞ *single-dose antibiotic treatment for sexually transmitted diseases* [Trovan (trovafloxacin mesylate); Zithromax (azithromycin)] 100 mg tablet; 1 g pkt. of powder for oral suspension

**Trovert** ℞ *investigational (Phase II, orphan) growth hormone antagonist for acromegaly* [B2036-PEG (code name —generic name not yet assigned)] ⊡ Provir; Provera

**troxacitabine** USAN *antineoplastic for various leukemias and solid tumors*

**troxerutin** INN, BAN *vitamin $P_4$*

**troxidone** BAN *anticonvulsant* [also: trimethadione]

**troxipide** INN

**troxolamide** INN

**troxonium tosilate** INN [also: troxonium tosylate]

**troxonium tosylate** BAN [also: troxonium tosilate]

**troxundate** INN *combining name for radicals or groups*

**troxypyrrolium tosilate** INN [also: troxypyrrolium tosylate]

**troxypyrrolium tosylate** BAN [also: troxypyrrolium tosilate]

**true ivy** medicinal herb [see: English ivy]

**T.R.U.E. Test** patch *diagnostic aid for contact dermatitis* [skin test antigens (23 different) plus 1 negative control]

**Trugene** genetic testing system for professional use *in vitro diagnostic aid* for HIV mutations that cause resistance to anti-AIDS drugs; used to determine which treatment regimen is most effective in individual patients

**Truphylline** suppositories ℞ *antiasthmatic; bronchodilator* [aminophylline] 250, 500 mg

**Trusopt** eye drops ℞ *topical carbonic anhydrase inhibitor for glaucoma* [dorzolamide HCl] 2%

**Truvada** caplets ℞ *once-daily nucleoside reverse transcriptase inhibitor (NRTI) antiviral combination for HIV infections* [emtricitabine; tenofovir disoproxil fumarate] 200•300 mg

**truxicurium iodide** INN

**truxipicurium iodide** INN

**trypaflavine** [see: acriflavine HCl]

**tryparsamide** USP, INN

**trypsin, crystallized** USP *topical proteolytic enzyme; necrotic tissue debridement*

**tryptizol** [see: amitriptyline]

**tryptizol HCl** [see: amitriptyline HCl]

**tryptophan (L-tryptophan)** USAN, USP, INN *essential amino acid; serotonin precursor* (The FDA has banned all OTC tryptophan supplements.)

**Trysul** vaginal cream (discontinued 2001) ℞ *broad-spectrum antibiotic* [sulfathiazole; sulfacetamide; sulfabenzamide] 3.42%•2.86%•3.7%

**TSC (technetium sulfur colloid)** [see: technetium Tc 99m sulfur colloid]

**T/Scalp** topical liquid OTC *corticosteroidal anti-inflammatory* [hydrocortisone] 1%

**TSH (thyroid-stimulating hormone)** [see: thyrotropin]

**TSPA (triethylenethiophosphoramide)** [see: thiotepa]

**TST (tuberculin skin test)** [see: tuberculin]

**T-Stat** topical solution, medicated pads ℞ *antibiotic for acne* [erythromycin; alcohol 71.2%] 2%

**Tsuga canadensis** medicinal herb [see: hemlock]

**T-Tabs** (trademarked form) *tablets with a "T" imprint*

**tuaminoheptane** USP, INN *adrenergic; vasoconstrictor*

**tuaminoheptane sulfate** USP

**tuberculin** USP *tuberculosis skin test*

**tuberculin, crude** [see: tuberculin]

**tuberculin, old (OT)** [see: tuberculin]

**tuberculin purified protein derivative (PPD)** [see: tuberculin]

**Tuberculin Tine Test, Old** single-use intradermal puncture test device (discontinued 2002) *tuberculosis skin test* [old tuberculin] 5 U

**tuberculosis vaccine** [see: BCG vaccine]

**Tubersol** intradermal injection ℞ *tuberculosis skin test* [tuberculin purified protein derivative] 5 U/0.1 mL

**Tubex** (trademarked delivery system) *cartridge-needle unit*

**tubocurarine chloride** USP, INN, BAN *neuromuscular blocker; muscle relaxant* 3 mg (20 U)/mL injection

**tubocurarine chloride HCl pentahydrate** [see: tubocurarine chloride]

**tubulozole** INN *antineoplastic; microtubule inhibitor* [also: tubulozole HCl]

**tubulozole HCl** USAN, INN *antineoplastic; microtubule inhibitor* [also: tubulozole]

**tucaresol** INN, BAN *investigational (Phase II) immunopotentiator for HIV infection*

**Tucks; Tucks Take-Alongs** cleansing pads OTC *moisturizer and cleanser for the perineal area; astringent* [witch hazel; glycerin] 50%•10%

**Tucks Clear** gel OTC *astringent* [hamamelis water; glycerin] 50%•10%

**tuclazepam** INN

**Tuinal** Pulvules (capsules) ℞ *sedative; hypnotic; also abused as a street drug* [amobarbital sodium; secobarbital sodium] 50•50, 100•100 mg ⯑ Luminal; Tylenol

**tulobuterol** INN, BAN, JAN [also: tulobuterol HCl]

**tulobuterol HCl** JAN [also: tulobuterol]

**tulopafant** INN

**tumeric root** medicinal herb [see: goldenseal]

**tumor necrosis factor (TNF)** *investigational (Phase I) antiviral for HIV infection* [also see: anti-TNF MAb]

**tumor necrosis factor-binding protein I and II** *investigational (orphan) for symptomatic AIDS patients*

**Tums; Tums E-X; Tums Ultra; Tums Calcium for Life PMS; Tums Calcium for Life Bone Health** chewable tablets OTC *antacid; calcium supplement* [calcium carbonate] 500 mg (200 mg Ca); 750 mg (300 mg Ca); 1 g (400 mg Ca); 750 mg (300 mg Ca); 1250 mg (500 mg Ca)

**Tums 500** chewable tablets (discontinued 2000) OTC *antacid; calcium supplement* [calcium carbonate] 1250 mg (500 mg Ca)

**Tums Smooth Dissolve** (orally disintegrating tablets) OTC *antacid; calcium supplement* [calcium carbonate] 750 mg (300 mg Ca)

**tung seed (*Aleurites cordata; A. moluccana*)** seed and oil *medicinal herb for asthma, bowel evacuation, and tumors; not generally regarded as safe and effective as it is highly toxic*

**tungsten** *element (W)*

**Turbinaire** (trademarked delivery system) *nasal inhalation aerosol*

**Turbuhaler** (trademarked delivery system) *dry powder in a metered-dose inhaler*

**turkey corn (*Corydalis formosa*)** root *medicinal herb used as an antisyphilitic, bitter tonic, and diuretic*

**turkey pea; wild turkey pea** *medicinal herb* [see: turkey corn]

**turmeric (*Curcuma domestica; C. longa*)** rhizomes *medicinal herb for flatulence, hemorrhage, hepatitis and jaundice, topical analgesia, and ringworm*

**Turnera aphrodisiaca; T. diffusa; T. microphylla** *medicinal herb* [see: damiana]

**turosteride** INN

**turpentine (*Pinus palustris*)** gum *natural treatment for colds, cough, and toothache; also used topically as a coun-*terirritant for muscle pain and rheumatic disorders*

**turtlebloom (*Chelone glabra*)** leaves *medicinal herb used as an anthelmintic, aperient, cholagogue, and detergent*

**Tusibron** syrup (discontinued 2002) OTC *expectorant* [guaifenesin; alcohol 3.5%] 100 mg/5 mL ⊡ Tussigon

**Tusibron-DM** syrup (discontinued 2002) OTC *antitussive; expectorant* [dextromethorphan hydrobromide; guaifenesin] 15•100 mg/5 mL

**Tusquelin** syrup (discontinued 2002) ℞ *antitussive; decongestant; antihistamine; analgesic* [dextromethorphan hydrobromide; phenylpropanolamine HCl; phenylephrine HCl; chlorpheniramine maleate; alcohol 5%] 15•5•5•2 mg/5 mL

**Tussafed** pediatric oral drops (discontinued 2002) ℞ *antitussive; decongestant; antihistamine* [dextromethorphan hydrobromide; pseudoephedrine HCl; carbinoxamine maleate; menthol] 4•25•2 mg/mL ⊡ Tussafin

**Tussafed** syrup ℞ *antitussive; decongestant; antihistamine* [dextromethorphan hydrobromide; pseudoephedrine HCl; carbinoxamine maleate; menthol] 15•60•4 mg/5 mL ⊡ Tussafin

**Tussafed HC** syrup ℞ *narcotic antitussive; decongestant; expectorant* [hydrocodone bitartrate; phenylephrine HCl; guaifenesin] 5•15•100 mg/10 mL

**Tussafed-LA** sustained-release caplets ℞ *antitussive; decongestant; expectorant* [dextromethorphan hydrobromide; pseudoephedrine HCl; guaifenesin] 30•60•600 mg

**Tussafin Expectorant** oral liquid (discontinued 2002) ℞ *narcotic antitussive; decongestant; expectorant* [hydrocodone bitartrate; pseudoephedrine HCl; guaifenesin; alcohol 12.5%] 5•60•200 mg/5 mL ⊡ Tussafed

**Tuss-Allergine Modified T.D.** capsules (discontinued 2002) ℞ *antitussive; decongestant* [caramiphen edisy-

late; phenylpropanolamine HCl]
40•75 mg

**Tussanil DH** syrup (discontinued 2002) ℞ *narcotic antitussive; decongestant; antihistamine* [hydrocodone bitartrate; phenylephrine HCl; chlorpheniramine maleate; alcohol 5%] 2.5•10•4 mg/5 mL

**Tussanil DH** tablets (discontinued 2002) ℞ *narcotic antitussive; decongestant; expectorant; analgesic* [hydrocodone bitartrate; phenylpropanolamine HCl; guaifenesin; salicylamide] 1.66•25•100•300 mg

**Tussar DM** syrup (discontinued 2002) OTC *antitussive; decongestant; antihistamine* [dextromethorphan hydrobromide; pseudoephedrine HCl; chlorpheniramine maleate] 15•30•2 mg/5 mL

**Tussar SF; Tussar-2** oral liquid (discontinued 2002) ℞ *narcotic antitussive; antihistamine; expectorant* [codeine phosphate; pseudoephedrine HCl; guaifenesin; alcohol 2.5%] 10•30•100 mg/5 mL

**Tuss-DM** tablets OTC *antitussive; expectorant* [dextromethorphan hydrobromide; guaifenesin] 10•200 mg

**Tussend** caplets ℞ *narcotic antitussive; decongestant; antihistamine* [hydrocodone bitartrate; pseudoephedrine HCl; chlorpheniramine maleate] 5•60•4 mg

**Tussend** syrup ℞ *narcotic antitussive; decongestant; antihistamine* [hydrocodone bitartrate; pseudoephedrine HCl; chlorpheniramine maleate; alcohol 5%] 5•60•4 mg/10 mL

**Tussex Cough** syrup (discontinued 2002) OTC *antitussive; decongestant; expectorant* [dextromethorphan hydrobromide; phenylephrine HCl; guaifenesin] 10•5•100 mg/5 mL ⊡ Tussionex; Tussirex

**Tussi-12** caplets, pediatric oral suspension ℞ *antitussive; antihistamine* [carbetapentane tannate; chlorpheniramine tannate] 60•5 mg; 30•4 mg/5 mL

**Tussi-12 D** caplets ℞ *decongestant; antihistamine; antitussive* [phenylephrine tannate; pyrilamine tannate; carbetapentane tannate] 10•40•60 mg

**Tussi-12D S** oral suspension ℞ *decongestant; antihistamine; antitussive* [phenylephrine tannate; pyrilamine tannate; carbetapentane tannate] 5•30•30 mg/5 mL

**Tussi-bid** sustained-release caplets ℞ *antitussive; expectorant* [dextromethorphan hydrobromide; guaifenesin] 60•1200 mg

**Tussigon** tablets ℞ *narcotic antitussive; anticholinergic* [hydrocodone bitartrate; homatropine methylbromide] 5•1.5 mg ⊡ Tusibron

**Tussilago farfara** *medicinal herb* [see: coltsfoot]

**Tussionex Pennkinetic** extended-release oral suspension ℞ *narcotic antitussive; antihistamine* [hydrocodone polistirex; chlorpheniramine polistirex] 10•8 mg/5 mL ⊡ Tussex; Tussirex

**Tussi-Organidin DM NR** oral liquid ℞ *antitussive; expectorant* [dextromethorphan hydrobromide; guaifenesin] 20•200 mg/10 mL

**Tussi-Organidin NR; Tussi-Organidin-S NR** oral liquid (S includes a 10 mL oral syringe) ℞ *narcotic antitussive; expectorant* [codeine phosphate; guaifenesin] 20•200 mg/10 mL

**Tussirex** syrup, sugar-free oral liquid (discontinued 2002) ℞ *narcotic antitussive; decongestant; antihistamine; expectorant; analgesic* [codeine phosphate; phenylephrine HCl; pheniramine maleate; sodium citrate; sodium salicylate; caffeine citrate] 10•4.17•13.33•83.3•83.33•25 mg/5 mL ⊡ Tussex; Tussionex

**Tussizone-12 RF** caplets, pediatric oral suspension ℞ *antitussive; antihistamine* [carbetapentane tannate; chlorpheniramine tannate] 60•5 mg; 30•4 mg/5 mL

**Tuss-LA** sustained-release tablets (discontinued 2002) ℞ *decongestant;*

*expectorant* [pseudoephedrine HCl; guaifenesin] 120•500 mg

**Tusso-DM** oral liquid (discontinued 2002) ℞ *antitussive; expectorant* [dextromethorphan hydrobromide; iodinated glycerol] 10•30 mg/5 mL

**Tussogest** extended-release capsules (discontinued 2002) ℞ *antitussive; decongestant* [caramiphen edisylate; phenylpropanolamine HCl] 40•75 mg

**Tuss-Tan** tablets, pediatric oral suspension ℞ *antitussive; decongestant; antihistamine* [carbetapentane tannate; phenylephrine tannate; ephedrine tannate; chlorpheniramine tannate] 60•10•10•5 mg; 30•5•5•4 mg/5 mL

**Tusstat** syrup ℞ *antihistamine* [diphenhydramine HCl; alcohol 5%] 12.5 mg/5 mL

**tuvatidine** INN

**tuvirumab** USAN, INN *investigational (Phase II) antiviral monoclonal antibody for hepatitis B*

**T-Vites** tablets OTC *vitamin/mineral supplement* [multiple vitamins & minerals; biotin] ≟•30 μg

**12 Hour** nasal spray OTC *nasal decongestant* [oxymetazoline HCl] 0.05%

**12 Hour Cold** sustained-release tablets (discontinued 2002) OTC *decongestant; antihistamine* [pseudoephedrine sulfate; dexbrompheniramine maleate] 120•6 mg

**Twelve Resin-K** tablets OTC *vitamin B$_{12}$ supplement* [cyanocobalamin on resin] 1000 μg

**Twice-A-Day 12-Hour** nasal spray OTC *nasal decongestant* [oxymetazoline HCl] 0.05%

**Twilite** caplets OTC *antihistaminic sleep aid* [diphenhydramine HCl] 50 mg

**twin leaf** (*Jeffersonia diphylla*) root *medicinal herb used as an antirheumatic, antispasmodic, antisyphilitic, diuretic, emetic, and expectorant*

**Twinject** injection ℞ *sympathomimetic bronchodilator for bronchial asthma, bronchospasm, and COPD; vasopressor for shock* [epinephrine HCl]

**Twin-K** oral liquid ℞ *potassium supplement* [potassium gluconate; potassium citrate] 20 mEq K/15 mL

**Twinrix** IM injection ℞ *immunizing agent for hepatitis A, B, and D in adults* [hepatitis A vaccine, inactivated; hepatitis B virus vaccine, recombinant] 720 EL.U.•20 μg per mL

**TwoCal HN** ready-to-use oral liquid OTC *enteral nutritional therapy* [lactose-free formula]

**tybamate** USAN, NF, INN, BAN *minor tranquilizer*

**tyformin** BAN [also: tiformin]

**Tygacil** injection ℞ *investigational (Phase III) broad-spectrum antibiotic* [tigecycline]

**tylcalsin** [see: calcium acetylsalicylate]

**tylemalum** [see: carbubarb]

**Tylenol** tablets, caplets, gelcaps, oral liquid OTC *analgesic; antipyretic* [acetaminophen] 325, 500 mg; 325, 650 mg; 500 mg; 500 mg/15 mL ⑫ Tuinal

**Tylenol, Children's** chewable tablets, oral liquid OTC *analgesic; antipyretic* [acetaminophen] 80 mg; 160 mg/5 mL

**Tylenol, Children's** ⑭ oral suspension OTC *analgesic; antipyretic* [acetaminophen] 32 mg/mL

**Tylenol 8 Hour** extended-release geltabs, extended-release caplets OTC *analgesic; antipyretic* [acetaminophen] 650 mg

**Tylenol Allergy Sinus** caplets, gelcaps, geltabs OTC *decongestant; antihistamine; analgesic* [pseudoephedrine HCl; chlorpheniramine maleate; acetaminophen] 30•2•500 mg

**Tylenol Allergy Sinus NightTime** caplets OTC *decongestant; antihistamine; analgesic* [pseudoephedrine HCl; diphenhydramine HCl; acetaminophen] 30•25•500 mg

**Tylenol Arthritis Extended Relief** extended-release caplets OTC *analgesic; antipyretic* [acetaminophen] 650 mg

**Tylenol Children's Cold** chewable tablets, oral liquid OTC *decongestant; antihistamine; analgesic* [pseudoephedrine HCl; chlorpheniramine

maleate; acetaminophen] 7.5•0.5•
80 mg; 15•1•160 mg/10 mL

**Tylenol Children's Cold Plus Cough**
chewable tablets, oral suspension
OTC *antitussive; decongestant; antihis-*
*tamine; analgesic* [dextromethorphan
hydrobromide; pseudoephedrine
HCl; chlorpheniramine maleate;
acetaminophen] 2.5•7.5•0.5•80
mg; 10•30•2•320 mg/10 mL

**Tylenol Children's Flu** oral suspension OTC *antitussive; decongestant;*
*antihistamine; analgesic* [dextromethe-
orphan hydrobromide; pseudoephedrine HCl; chlorpheniramine maleate; acetaminophen] 15•30•2•320
mg/10 mL

**Tylenol Children's Sinus** oral suspension OTC *decongestant; analgesic;*
*antipyretic* [pseudoephedrine HCl;
acetaminophen] 15•160 mg/5 mL

**Tylenol Cold, Children's** chewable
tablets, oral liquid OTC *pediatric decon-*
*gestant, antihistamine and analgesic*
[pseudoephedrine HCl; chlorpheniramine maleate; acetaminophen] 7.5•
0.5•80 mg; 15•1•160 mg/5 mL

**Tylenol Cold, Multi-Symptom** caplets, tablets (name changed to Tylenol
Cold Complete Formula in 2002)

**Tylenol Cold Day Non-Drowsy** caplets, gelcaps OTC *antitussive; deconges-*
*tant; analgesic* [dextromethorphan
hydrobromide; pseudoephedrine HCl;
acetaminophen] 15•30•325 mg

**Tylenol Cold Multi Symptom Plus
Cough, Children's** oral liquid
(name changed to Tylenol Children's Flu in 2002)

**Tylenol Cold Night Time Complete
Formula** caplets OTC *antitussive;*
*decongestant; antihistamine; analgesic*
[dextromethorphan hydrobromide;
pseudoephedrine HCl; chlorpheniramine maleate; acetaminophen] 15•
30•2•325 mg

**Tylenol Cold No Drowsiness** caplets,
gelcaps (name changed to Tylenol
Cold Non-Drowsy Formula in 2002)

**Tylenol Cough, Multi-Symptom**
oral liquid (discontinued 2002) OTC
*antitussive; analgesic* [dextromethor-
phan hydrobromide; acetaminophen;
alcohol 5%] 10•216.7 mg/5 mL

**Tylenol Cough with Decongestant,
Multi-Symptom** oral liquid (discontinued 2002) OTC *antitussive;*
*decongestant; analgesic* [dextrometh-
orphan hydrobromide; pseudoephedrine HCl; acetaminophen; alcohol
5%] 10•20•200 mg/5 mL

**Tylenol Extended Relief** (name
changed to Tylenol Arthritis
Extended Relief in 1998)

**Tylenol Flu, Tylenol Flu Night Time**
gelcaps OTC *decongestant; antihista-*
*mine; analgesic* [pseudoephedrine
HCl; diphenhydramine HCl; aceta-
minophen] 30•25•500 mg

**Tylenol Flu Night Time** oral liquid
OTC *antitussive; decongestant; antihista-*
*mine; analgesic* [dextromethorphan
hydrobromide; pseudoephedrine HCl;
doxylamine succinate; acetamino-
phen] 30•60•12.5•1000 mg/30 mL

**Tylenol Flu NightTime** powder for
oral solution (discontinued 2002)
OTC *decongestant; antihistamine; anal-*
*gesic* [pseudoephedrine HCl; diphenhydramine HCl; acetaminophen]
60•50•1000 mg/pkt.

**Tylenol Flu Non-Drowsy** gelcaps
OTC *antitussive; decongestant; analge-*
*sic* [dextromethorphan hydrobromide; pseudoephedrine HCl; aceta-
minophen] 15•30•500 mg

**Tylenol Fruit; Tylenol Junior Fruit**
CAN chewable tablets OTC *analgesic;*
*antipyretic* [acetaminophen] 80 mg;
160 mg

**Tylenol Headache Plus** caplets (discontinued 2000) OTC *analgesic; anti-*
*pyretic; antacid* [acetaminophen; calcium carbonate] 500•250 mg

**Tylenol Infant's Cold** concentrated
oral drops OTC *decongestant; analgesic;*
*antipyretic* [pseudoephedrine HCl;
acetaminophen] 15•160 mg/1.6 mL

**Tylenol Infants' Cold, Decongestant, & Fever Reducer Plus
Cough** concentrated oral drops OTC
*antitussive; decongestant; analgesic;
antipyretic* [dextromethorphan hydrobromide; pseudoephedrine HCl; acetaminophen] 5•15•160 mg/1.6 mL
**Tylenol Infants' Drops** ⓒ oral suspension OTC *analgesic; antipyretic*
[acetaminophen] 80 mg/mL
**Tylenol Infants' Drops** solution OTC
*analgesic; antipyretic* [acetaminophen]
100 mg/mL
**Tylenol Junior Strength** chewable
tablets OTC *analgesic; antipyretic*
[acetaminophen] 160 mg
**Tylenol Menstrual** ⓒ tablets OTC
*analgesic; diuretic; antihistamine* [acetaminophen; pamabrom; pyrilamine
maleate] 500•25•15 mg
**Tylenol Multi-Symptom Cold
Severe Congestion** caplets OTC
*antitussive; decongestant; expectorant;
analgesic* [dextromethorphan hydrobromide; pseudoephedrine HCl;
guaifenesin; acetaminophen] 15•
30•200•325 mg
**Tylenol Multi-Symptom Hot Medication** powder for oral solution (discontinued 2002) OTC *antitussive;
decongestant; antihistamine; analgesic*
[dextromethorphan hydrobromide;
pseudoephedrine HCl; chlorpheniramine maleate; acetaminophen] 30•
60•4•650 mg/pkt.
**Tylenol Multi-Symptom Menstrual
Relief, Women's** caplets OTC *analgesic; diuretic* [acetaminophen; pamabrom] 500•25 mg
**Tylenol No. 2, No. 3, and No. 4**
[see: Tylenol with Codeine]
**Tylenol PM** tablets, caplets, gelcaps
OTC *analgesic; antihistaminic sleep aid*
[acetaminophen; diphenhydramine
HCl] 500•25 mg
**Tylenol Severe Allergy** caplets OTC
*antihistamine; analgesic* [diphenhydramine HCl; acetaminophen] 12.5•
500 mg

**Tylenol Sinus Night Time** caplets
OTC *decongestant; antihistamine; analgesic* [pseudoephedrine HCl; doxylamine succinate; acetaminophen]
30•6.25•500 mg
**Tylenol Sinus Non-Drowsy** caplets,
geltabs, gelcaps OTC *decongestant;
analgesic; antipyretic* [pseudoephedrine
HCl; acetaminophen] 30•500 mg
**Tylenol Sinus Severe Congestion**
caplets OTC *decongestant; expectorant;
analgesic* [pseudoephedrine HCl;
guaifenesin; acetaminophen] 30•
200•325 mg
**Tylenol Sore Throat** oral liquid OTC
*analgesic; antipyretic* [acetaminophen]
1000 mg/30 mL
**Tylenol with Codeine** elixir ℞ *narcotic antitussive; analgesic* [codeine
phosphate; acetaminophen] 12•120
mg/5 mL
**Tylenol with Codeine No. 2, No. 3,
and No. 4** tablets ℞ *narcotic antitussive; analgesic; sometimes abused as a
street drug* [codeine phosphate; acetaminophen] 15•300 mg; 30•300
mg; 60•300 mg
**tylosin** INN, BAN
**Tylox** capsules ℞ *narcotic analgesic*
[oxycodone HCl; acetaminophen]
5•500 mg
**tyloxapol** USAN, USP, INN, BAN *detergent; wetting agent; cleaner/lubricant
for artificial eyes; investigational
(orphan) for cystic fibrosis*
**Tympagesic** ear drops ℞ *topical local
anesthetic; analgesic; decongestant*
[benzocaine; antipyrine; phenylephrine HCl] 5%•5%•0.25%
**Typherix** ⓒ IM injection in prefilled
syringe ℞ *typhoid vaccine for adults
and children over 2 years* [typhoid
vaccine (Ty-2), Vi polysaccharide]
25μg/0.5 mL
**Typhim Vi** IM injection ℞ *typhoid
vaccine for adults and children over 2
years* [typhoid vaccine (Ty-2), Vi
polysaccharide] 25μg/0.5 mL dose

**typhoid vaccine** USP *active bacterin for typhoid fever (Salmonella typhi Ty21a, attenuated)*

**Typhoid Vaccine (AKD)** subcu injection by jet injectors only ℞ *typhoid vaccine for military use only* [typhoid vaccine (Ty-2), acetone-killed and dried] 8 U/mL

**Typhoid Vaccine (H-P)** subcu injection (discontinued 2003) ℞ *typhoid vaccine for adults and children* [typhoid vaccine (Ty-2), heat- and phenol-inactivated] 8 U/mL

**typhoid Vi capsular polysaccharide vaccine** *active bacterin for typhoid fever (Salmonella typhi Ty-2, inactivated)*

**typhus vaccine** USP

**"typical" antipsychotics** [see: conventional antipsychotics]

**Tyrex-2** powder OTC *enteral nutritional therapy for tyrosinemia type II*

**Tyrodone** oral liquid (discontinued 2002) ℞ *antitussive; decongestant* [hydrodocone bitartrate; pseudoephedrine HCl; alcohol 5%] 5•60 mg/5 mL

**tyromedan** INN *thyromimetic* [also: thyromedan HCl]

**tyromedan HCl** [see: thyromedan HCl]

**Tyromex-1** powder OTC *formula for infants with tyrosinemia type I*

**tyropanoate sodium** USAN, USP *oral radiopaque contrast medium for cholecystography (57.4% iodine)* [also: sodium tyropanoate]

**tyrosine (L-tyrosine)** USAN, USP, INN *nonessential amino acid; symbols: Tyr, Y*

**Tyrosum Cleanser** topical liquid, packets OTC *cleanser for acne* [isopropanol; acetone] 50%•10%

**tyrothricin** USP, INN *antibacterial*

**Tyzine** nasal spray, nose drops, pediatric nose drops ℞ *nasal decongestant* [tetrahydrozoline HCl] 0.1%; 0.1%; 0.05%

**UAA** sugar-coated tablets ℞ *urinary antibiotic; analgesic; antispasmodic; acidifier* [methenamine; phenyl salicylate; atropine sulfate; methylene blue; hyoscyamine sulfate; benzoic acid] 40.8•18.1•0.03•5.4•0.03•4.5 mg

**UAD Otic** ear drop suspension ℞ *topical corticosteroidal anti-inflammatory; antibiotic* [hydrocortisone; neomycin sulfate; polymyxin B sulfate] 1%•5 mg•10 000 U per mL

**ubenimex** INN

**ubidecarenone** INN

**ubiquinone** [see: coenzyme Q10]

**ubisindine** INN

**UBT Breath Test for H. pylori** test for professional use *diagnostic aid for the detection of ulcers*

**Ucephan** oral solution ℞ *to prevent and treat hyperammonemia of urea cycle enzymopathy (orphan)* [sodium benzoate; sodium phenylacetate] 10•10 g/100 mL

**UCG Beta Slide Monoclonal II** slide tests for professional use *in vitro diagnostic aid; urine pregnancy test*

**UCG Slide** tests for professional use *in vitro diagnostic aid; urine pregnancy test* [latex agglutination test]

**U-Cort** cream ℞ *corticosteroidal anti-inflammatory* [hydrocortisone acetate] 1%

**UDIP** (trademarked packaging form) *unit-dose identification package*

**Udo's Choice Oil** oral liquid OTC *a blend of natural seed oils that supply a balance of essential fatty acids* [omega-3 oils; omega-6 oils; omega-9 oils; medium-chain triglycerides] 6.4•3.2•3•0.231 g/15 mL

**Uendex** ℞ *investigational (orphan) inhalant for cystic fibrosis* [dextran sulfate]

**ufenamate** INN

**ufiprazole** INN

**UFT** capsules ℞ *antimetabolite antineoplastic; investigational (NDA filed) adjunct to leucovorin calcium for advanced colorectal cancer* [uracil; tegafur] 1:4

**U-Ject** (trademarked delivery system) *prefilled disposable syringe*

**Ulcerease** mouth rinse OTC *topical antipruritic/counterirritant; mild local anesthetic* [phenol] 0.6%

**uldazepam** USAN, INN *sedative*

**ulinastatin** INN

*Ulmus fulva; U. rubra medicinal herb* [see: slippery elm]

**ulobetasol** INN *topical corticosteroidal anti-inflammatory* [also: halobetasol propionate]

**ULR-LA** long-acting tablets (discontinued 2002) ℞ *decongestant; expectorant* [phenylpropanolamine HCl; guaifenesin] 75•400 mg

**Ultane** liquid for vaporization ℞ *inhalation general anesthetic* [sevoflurane]

**Ultiva** powder for IV infusion ℞ *short-acting narcotic analgesic for general anesthesia* [remifentanil HCl] 1 mg/mL

**Ultra Derm** lotion, bath oil (discontinued 2004) OTC *moisturizer; emollient*

**Ultra KLB6** tablets OTC *dietary supplement* [vitamin $B_6$; multiple food supplements] 16.7• ± mg

**Ultra Mide 25** lotion OTC *moisturizer; emollient; keratolytic* [urea] 25%

**Ultra Tears** eye drops OTC *ophthalmic moisturizer/lubricant* [hydroxypropyl methylcellulose] 1%

**Ultra Vent** (trademarked delivery system) *jet nebulizer*

**Ultra Vita Time** tablets OTC *dietary supplement* [multiple vitamins & minerals; multiple food products; iron; folic acid; biotin] ± •6•0.4•1 mg

**UltraBrom** extended-release capsules ℞ *decongestant; antihistamine* [pseudoephedrine HCl; brompheniramine maleate] 120•12 mg

**UltraBrom PD** extended-release pediatric capsules ℞ *decongestant; antihistamine* [pseudoephedrine HCl; brompheniramine maleate] 60•6 mg

**Ultracal** oral liquid OTC *enteral nutritional therapy* [lactose-free formula]

**Ultra-Care** solution + tablets OTC *two-step chemical disinfecting system for soft contact lenses* [hydrogen peroxide-based] 3%

**Ultracet** film-coated caplets ℞ *central analgesic for acute pain* [tramadol HCl; acetaminophen] 37.5•325 mg

**Ultra-Freeda; Ultra Freeda, Iron Free** tablets OTC *geriatric vitamin/ mineral supplement* [multiple vitamins & minerals; folic acid; biotin] ± •270•100 μg

**UltraJect** prefilled syringe ℞ *narcotic analgesic* [morphine sulfate]

**Ultralan** oral liquid OTC *enteral nutritional therapy* [lactose-free formula]

**Ultram** film-coated caplets ℞ *central analgesic* [tramadol HCl] 50 mg

**Ultram XL** ℞ *investigational (Phase III) extended-release formulation* [tramadol HCl]

**UltraMide 25** ⓒⒶⓃ lotion OTC *moisturizer; emollient* [urea] 25%

**Ultra-NatalCare** tablets ℞ *vitamin/ mineral/iron supplement for pregnancy and lactation* [multiple vitamins & minerals; carbonyl iron; folic acid] ± •90 mg iron•1 mg

**Ultrase; Ultrase MT 12; Ultrase MT 18; Ultrase MT 20** capsules containing enteric-coated microspheres ℞ *porcine-derived digestive enzymes* [lipase; protease; amylase] 4500• 25 000•20 000; 12 000•39 000• 39 000; 18 000•58 500•58 500; 20 000•65 000•65 000 USP units

**Ultravate** ointment, cream ℞ *topical corticosteroidal anti-inflammatory* [halobetasol propionate] 0.05%

**Ultravist** IV injection ℞ *radiopaque contrast medium for imaging of the head, heart, peripheral vascular system, and genitourinary tract* [iopromide (39% iodine)] 311.7, 498.72, 623.4, 768.86 mg/mL (150, 240, 300, 370 mg/mL)

**Ultrazyme Enzymatic Cleaner** effervescent tablets OTC *enzymatic cleaner for soft contact lenses* [subtilisin A]

**Ultrex** gel in unit-dose packs OTC *hydrogel wound dressing* [acemannan]

**Umecta** emulsion ℞ *moisturizer; emollient; keratolytic* [urea] 40%

**umespirone** INN

**uña de gato** *medicinal herb* [see: cat's claw]

**UN-Aspirin** tablets OTC *analgesic; antipyretic* [acetaminophen] 500 mg

**Unasyn** powder for IV or IM injection ℞ *aminopenicillin antibiotic plus synergist* [ampicillin sodium; sulbactam sodium] 1•0.5, 2•1, 10•5 g ⑨ Anacin; Unisom

*Uncaria guianensis; U. tomentosa* medicinal herb [see: cat's claw]

**10-undecenoic acid** [see: undecylenic acid]

**10-undecenoic acid, calcium salt** [see: calcium undecylenate]

**undecoylium chloride-iodine**

**undecylenic acid** USP *antifungal*

**Unguentine** cream OTC *local anesthetic; antifungal* [benzocaine; resorcinol] 5%•2%

**Unguentine** ointment OTC *minor burn treatment* [phenol; zinc oxide; eucalyptus oil] 1%• ⑨ • ⑨

**Unguentine Plus** cream OTC *topical local anesthetic* [lidocaine HCl; phenol] 2%•0.5%

**Unguentum Bossi** cream (discontinued 2003) ℞ *topical antipsoriatic; anti-infective; bactericidal* [ammoniated mercury; methenamine sulfosalicylate; coal tar] 5%•2%•2%

**Uni-Ace** drops OTC *analgesic; antipyretic* [acetaminophen] 100 mg/mL

**Uni-Amp** (trademarked packaging form) *single-dose ampule*

**Unibase** OTC *ointment base*

**Uni-Bent Cough** syrup (discontinued 2002) OTC *antihistamine; antitussive* [diphenhydramine HCl; alcohol 5%] 12.5 mg/5 mL

**Unicap** capsules, tablets OTC *vitamin supplement* [multiple vitamins; folic acid] ⬚•0.4 mg

**Unicap Jr.** chewable tablets OTC *vitamin supplement* [multiple vitamins; folic acid] ⬚•0.4 mg

**Unicap M; Unicap T** tablets OTC *vitamin/mineral/iron supplement* [multiple vitamins & minerals; iron; folic acid] ⬚•18•0.4 mg

**Unicap Plus Iron** tablets OTC *vitamin/iron supplement* [multiple vitamins; iron; folic acid] ⬚•22.5•0.4 mg

**Unicap Sr.** tablets OTC *vitamin/mineral/iron supplement* [multiple vitamins & minerals; iron; folic acid] ⬚•10•0.4 mg

**Unicomplex T & M** tablets OTC *vitamin/mineral/iron supplement* [multiple vitamins & minerals; iron; folic acid] ⬚•18•0.4 mg

**Uni-Decon** sustained-release tablets (discontinued 2001) ℞ *decongestant; antihistamine* [phenylpropanolamine HCl; phenylephrine HCl; chlorpheniramine maleate; phenyltoloxamine citrate] 40•10•5•15 mg

**Unidet** ⓒ extended-release capsules ℞ *anticholinergic; muscarinic receptor antagonist for urinary frequency, urgency, and incontinence* [tolterodine tartrate] 2, 4 mg

**Uni-Dur** extended-release tablets (discontinued 2003) ℞ *once-daily antiasthmatic/bronchodilator* [theophylline] 400, 600 mg

**Unifiber** powder OTC *bulk laxative* [cellulose powder]

**unifocon A** USAN *hydrophobic contact lens material*

**Unimatic** (trademarked delivery system) *prefilled disposable syringe*

**Uni-nest** (trademarked packaging form) *ampule*

**Unipak** (packaging form) *dispensing pack*

**Unipen** capsules (discontinued 2002) ℞ *penicillinase-resistant penicillin antibiotic* [nafcillin sodium] 250 mg ⑨ Omnipen

**Uniphyl** timed-release tablets ℞ *anti-asthmatic; bronchodilator* [theophylline] 400, 600 mg

**Uniprost** (name changed to Remodulin for the NDA in 2001)

**Uniquin** (foreign name for U.S. product Maxaquin)

**Uniretic** tablets ℞ *antihypertensive; angiotensin-converting enzyme (ACE) inhibitor; diuretic* [moexipril HCl; hydrochlorothiazide] 7.5•12.5, 15•12.5, 15•25 mg

**Uni-Rx** (trademarked packaging form) *unit-dose containers and packages*

**Unisert** (trademarked dosage form) *suppository*

**Unisol; Unisol 4** solution OTC *rinsing/storage solution for soft contact lenses* [sodium chloride (saline solution)]

**Unisol Plus** aerosol solution OTC *rinsing/storage solution for soft contact lenses* [sodium chloride (saline solution)]

**Unisom Natural Source** Ⓒ gel capsules OTC *herbal sleep aid* [valerian extract (from valerian root)] 100 mg (400 mg)

**Unisom Nighttime Sleep-Aid** tablets OTC *antihistaminic sleep aid* [doxylamine succinate] 25 mg ☑ Anacin; Unasyn

**Unisom SleepGels** (capsules) OTC *antihistaminic sleep aid* [diphenhydramine HCl] 50 mg ☑ Anacin; Unasyn

**Unisom with Pain Relief** tablets OTC *antihistaminic sleep aid; analgesic* [diphenhydramine citrate; acetaminophen] 50•650 mg ☑ Anacin; Unasyn

**Unistep hCG** test kit for professional use *in vitro diagnostic aid; urine pregnancy test*

**Unithroid** tablets ℞ *synthetic thyroid hormone (T₄ fraction only)* [levothyroxine sodium] 25, 50, 75, 88, 100, 112, 125, 150, 175, 200, 300 μg

**Unitrol** timed-release capsules (discontinued 2001) OTC *diet aid* [phenylpropanolamine HCl] 75 mg

**Unituss HC** syrup (discontinued 2002) ℞ *narcotic antitussive; decongestant; antihistamine* [hydrocodone bitartrate; phenylephrine HCl; chlorpheniramine maleate] 2.5•5•2 mg/5 mL

**Uni-Tussin** syrup (discontinued 2002) OTC *expectorant* [guaifenesin; alcohol 3.5%] 100 mg/5 mL

**Uni-Tussin DM** syrup (discontinued 2002) OTC *antitussive; expectorant* [dextromethorphan hydrobromide; guaifenesin] 10•100 mg/5 mL

**Univasc** tablets ℞ *antihypertensive; angiotensin-converting enzyme (ACE) inhibitor* [moexipril HCl] 7.5, 15 mg

**Univial** (trademarked form) *single-dose vials*

**Unna's boot** [see: Dome-Paste bandage]

**unoprostone isopropyl** *topical prostaglandin F₂α analogue for glaucoma and ocular hypertension*

**Uprima** sublingual tablets ℞ *investigational (NDA filed) dopamine receptor agonist for erectile dysfunction* [apomorphine HCl] 2, 3, 4 mg

**Uracid** capsules ℞ *urinary acidifier to control ammonia production* [racemethionine] 200 mg ☑ uracil; Urised; Urocit

**uracil** USAN *antineoplastic potentiator for tegafur (not available separately; combined with tegafur in a 1:4 ratio)*

**uracil mustard** USAN, USP *nitrogen mustard-type alkylating antineoplastic* [also: uramustine] ☑ Uracel; Uracid

**Uracyst-S; Uracyst-S Concentrate** Ⓒ liquid for bladder instillation ℞ *glycosaminoglycan temporary replacement* [chondroitan sulfate sodium] 2 mg/mL; 20 mg/mL

**uradal** [see: carbromal]

**uralenic acid** [see: enoxolone]

**uramustine** INN, BAN *nitrogen mustard-type alkylating antineoplastic* [also: uracil mustard]

**uranin** [see: fluorescein sodium]

**uranium** *element (U)*

**urapidil** INN, BAN

**urea** USP *osmotic diuretic; keratolytic; emollient* 40% topical

**urea peroxide** [see: carbamide peroxide]

**Ureacin-10** lotion OTC *moisturizer; emollient; keratolytic* [urea] 10%

**Ureacin-20** cream OTC *moisturizer; emollient; keratolytic* [urea] 20%

**Ureaphil** IV infusion ℞ *osmotic diuretic* [urea] 40 g/150 mL

**Urecholine** subcu injection (discontinued 2001) ℞ *cholinergic urinary stimulant for postsurgical and postpartum urinary retention* [bethanechol chloride] 5 mg/mL

**Urecholine** tablets ℞ *cholinergic urinary stimulant for postsurgical and postpartum urinary retention* [bethanechol chloride] 25 mg

**uredepa** USAN, INN *antineoplastic*

**uredofos** USAN, INN *veterinary anthelmintic*

**urefibrate** INN

*p*-**ureidobenzenearsonic acid** [see: carbarsone]

**Urelle** sugar-coated tablets ℞ *urinary antibiotic; antiseptic; analgesic; antispasmodic* [methenamine; sodium phosphate; phenyl salicylate; methylene blue; hyoscyamine sulfate] 81•40.8•32.4•10.8•0.12 mg

**urethan** NF [also: urethane]

**urethane** INN, BAN [also: urethan]

**urethane polymers** [see: polyurethane foam]

**Uretron D/S** sugar-coated tablets ℞ *urinary antibiotic; antiseptic; analgesic; antispasmodic* [methenamine; sodium biphosphate; phenyl salicylate; methylene blue; hyoscyamine sulfate] 120•40.8•36.2•10.8•0.12 mg

**Urex** tablets ℞ *urinary antibiotic* [methenamine hippurate] 1 g ②
Eurax; Serax

*Urginea indica; U. maritima; U. scilla* medicinal herb [see: squill]

**Uricult** culture paddles for professional use *in vitro diagnostic aid for nitrate, uropathogens, or bacteria in the urine*

**uridine 5′-triphosphate** *investigational (Phase I/II, orphan) for cystic fibrosis and primary ciliary dyskinesia*

**Uridon Modified** sugar-coated tablets ℞ *urinary antibiotic; analgesic; antispasmodic; acidifier* [methenamine; phenyl salicylate; atropine sulfate;

methylene blue; hyoscyamine sulfate; benzoic acid] 40.8•18.1•0.03•5.4•0.03•4.5 mg

**Urimar-T** tablets ℞ *urinary antibiotic; antiseptic; analgesic; antispasmodic* [methenamine; sodium biphosphate; phenyl salicylate; methylene blue; hyoscyamine sulfate] 81.6•40.8•36.2•10.8•0.12 mg

**Urimax** film-coated tablets ℞ *urinary antibiotic; analgesic; antispasmodic; acidifier* [methenamine; phenyl salicylate; methylene blue; hyoscyamine sulfate; sodium biphosphate] 81.6•36.2•10.8•0.12•40.8 mg

**Urinary Antiseptic No. 2** tablets ℞ *urinary antibiotic; analgesic; antispasmodic; acidifier* [methenamine; phenyl salicylate; atropine sulfate; methylene blue; hyoscyamine sulfate; benzoic acid] 40.8•18.1•0.03•5.4•0.03•4.5 mg

**Urised** sugar-coated tablets ℞ *urinary antibiotic; analgesic; antispasmodic; acidifier* [methenamine; phenyl salicylate; atropine sulfate; methylene blue; hyoscyamine sulfate; benzoic acid] 40.8•18.1•0.03•5.4•0.03•4.5 mg ② Uracel; Uracid; Urispas

**Urisedamine** tablets ℞ *urinary antibiotic; antispasmodic* [methenamine mandelate; hyoscyamine] 500•0.15 mg

**Uriseptic** film-coated tablets ℞ *urinary antibiotic; antiseptic; analgesic; antispasmodic* [methenamine; phenyl salicylate; methylene blue; benzoic acid; atropine sulfate; hyoscyamine sulfate] 40.8•18.1•5.4•4.5•0.03•0.03 mg

**Urispas** film-coated tablets ℞ *urinary antispasmodic* [flavoxate HCl] 100 mg (200 mg available in Canada) ② Urised

**Uristat** tablets ℞ *urinary analgesic* [phenazopyridine HCl] 95 mg

**Uristix; Uristix 4** reagent strips *in vitro diagnostic aid for multiple urine products*

**Uritact DS** caplets ℞ *urinary antibiotic; analgesic; antispasmodic; acidifier* [methenamine; phenyl salicylate;

atropine sulfate; methylene blue; hyoscyamine sulfate; benzoic acid] 81.6•36.2•0.06•10.8•0.06•9 mg

**Uritin** tablets ℞ *urinary antibiotic; analgesic; antispasmodic; acidifier* [methenamine; phenyl salicylate; atropine sulfate; methylene blue; hyoscyamine sulfate; benzoic acid] 40.8•18.1•0.03•5.4•0.03•4.5 mg

**Uro Blue** sugar-coated tablets ℞ *urinary antibiotic; antiseptic; analgesic; antispasmodic* [methenamine; sodium biphosphate; phenyl salicylate; methylene blue; hyoscyamine sulfate] 81.6•40.8•36.2•10.8•0.12 mg

**Urobak** tablets (discontinued 2001) ℞ *broad-spectrum bacteriostatic* [sulfamethoxazole] 500 mg

**urocidin** *investigational (Phase III) mycobacterial cell wall complex (MCC) for bladder cancer*

**Urocit-K** tablets ℞ *urinary alkalizer for nephrolithiasis and hypocitruria prevention (orphan)* [potassium citrate] 5, 10 mEq K ⊡ Uracid

**urofollitrophin** BAN *follicle-stimulating hormone (FSH)* [also: urofollitropin]

**urofollitropin** USAN, INN *follicle-stimulating hormone (FSH); ovulation stimulant for polycystic ovarian disease (orphan) and assisted reproductive techniques (ARTs); investigational (orphan) for spermatogenesis in hormone-deficient males* [also: urofollitrophin]

**urogastrone** *investigational (orphan) for recovery from corneal transplant surgery*

**Urogesic** tablets ℞ *urinary analgesic* [phenazopyridine HCl] 100 mg

**Urogesic Blue** sugar-coated tablets ℞ *urinary antibiotic; antiseptic; analgesic; antispasmodic* [methenamine; sodium biphosphate; phenyl salicylate; methylene blue; hyoscyamine sulfate] 81.6•40.8•36.2•10.8•0.12 mg

**urokinase** USAN, INN, BAN, JAN *plasminogen activator; thrombolytic enzyme*

**urokinase alfa** USAN *plasminogen activator; thrombolytic enzyme*

**Uro-KP-Neutral** film-coated caplets ℞ *urinary acidifier; phosphorus supplement* [sodium phosphate; potassium phosphate; monobasic sodium phosphate] 250 mg P

**Urolene Blue** tablets ℞ *urinary anti-infective and antiseptic; antidote to cyanide poisoning* [methylene blue] 65 mg

**Uro-Mag** capsules OTC *antacid; magnesium supplement* [magnesium oxide] 140 mg (84.5 mg Mg)

**uronal** [see: barbital]

**Uro-Phosphate** film-coated tablets ℞ *urinary antibiotic; acidifier* [methenamine; sodium biphosphate] 300•434.78 mg

**Uroqid-Acid No. 2** film-coated tablets ℞ *urinary antibiotic; acidifier* [methenamine mandelate; sodium acid phosphate] 500•500 mg

**Uroxatral** extended-release tablets ℞ *α₁-adrenergic blocker for benign prostatic hyperplasia (BPH)* [alfuzosin HCl] 10 mg

**Ursinus** Inlay-Tabs (tablets) (discontinued 2002) OTC *decongestant; analgesic; antipyretic* [pseudoephedrine HCl; aspirin] 30•325 mg

**Urso** tablets ℞ *bile acid for primary biliary cirrhosis (orphan); investigational for hypercholesterolemia, type IIa and IIb* [ursodiol] 250 mg

**ursodeoxycholic acid** INN, BAN *naturally occurring bile acid; anticholelithogenic* [also: ursodiol]

**ursodiol** USAN *naturally occurring bile acid for primary biliary cirrhosis (orphan); gallstone dissolving agent; investigational for hypercholesterolemia, type IIa and IIb* [also: ursodeoxycholic acid] 300 mg oral

**ursulcholic acid** INN

**Urtica dioica; U. urens** *medicinal herb* [see: nettle]

**UT-15** *investigational (NDA filed) non-intravenous prostacyclin analogue for pulmonary hypertension*

**uva ursi (Arbutus uva ursi; Arctostaphylos uva ursi)** leaves *medicinal herb for bladder and kidney infections, Bright disease, constipation, diabetes,* gonorrhea, nephritis, spleen disorders, urethritis, and uterine ulcerations

**Uvadex** extracorporeal solution (leukocytes are collected, photoactivated with the UVAR Photopheresis System, then reinfused) ℞ palliative treatment for cutaneous T-cell lymphoma (CTCL); investigational (orphan) treatment of diffuse systemic sclerosis and to prevent rejection of cardiac allografts [methoxsalen] 20 μg/mL

VAD; VAB-I (vinblastine, actinomycin D, bleomycin) chemotherapy protocol

**VAB-II** (vinblastine, actinomycin D, bleomycin, cisplatin) chemotherapy protocol

**VAB-III** (vinblastine, actinomycin D, bleomycin, cisplatin, chlorambucil, cyclophosphamide) chemotherapy protocol

**VAB-V** (vinblastine, actinomycin D, bleomycin, cyclophosphamide, cisplatin) chemotherapy protocol

**VAB-6** (vinblastine, actinomycin D, bleomycin, cyclophosphamide, cisplatin) chemotherapy protocol for testicular cancer

**VABCD** (vinblastine, Adriamycin, bleomycin, CCNU, DTIC) chemotherapy protocol

**VAC** (vincristine, Adriamycin, cisplatin) chemotherapy protocol

**VAC** (vincristine, Adriamycin, cyclophosphamide) chemotherapy protocol for small cell lung cancer (SCLC) [also: CAV]

**VAC pediatric** (vincristine, actinomycin D, cyclophosphamide) chemotherapy protocol for pediatric sarcomas

**VAC pulse; VAC standard** (vincristine, actinomycin D, cyclophosphamide) chemotherapy protocol for sarcomas

**VACA** (vincristine, actinomycin D, cyclophosphamide, Adriamycin) chemotherapy protocol

**VACAD** (vincristine, actinomycin D, cyclophosphamide, Adriamycin, dacarbazine) chemotherapy protocol

**VACAdr** (vincristine, actinomycin D, cyclophosphamide, Adriamycin) chemotherapy protocol for pediatric bone and soft tissue sarcomas

**VACAdr-IfoVP** (vincristine, actinomycin D, cyclophosphamide, Adriamycin, ifosfamide, VePesid) chemotherapy protocol

**vaccines** a class of drugs used for active immunization that consist of antigens which induce endogenous production of antibodies

**vaccinia immune globulin (VIG)** USP passive immunizing agent

**vaccinia immune human globulin** [now: vaccinia immune globulin]

**vaccinia virus vaccine for human papillomavirus (HPV), recombinant** investigational (orphan) for cervical cancer

*Vaccinium edule; V. erythrocarpum; V. macrocarpon; V. oxycoccos; V. vitis* medicinal herb [see: cranberry]

*Vaccinium myrtillus* medicinal herb [see: bilberry]

**VACP** (VePesid, Adriamycin, cyclophosphamide, Platinol) chemotherapy protocol

**VAD** (vincristine, Adriamycin, dactinomycin) chemotherapy protocol for pediatric Wilms tumor

**VAD (vincristine, Adriamycin, dexamethasone)** *chemotherapy protocol for multiple myeloma and acute lymphocytic leukemia (ALL)*

**Vademin-Z** capsules OTC *vitamin/mineral supplement* [multiple vitamins & minerals]

**vadocaine** INN

**VAdrC (vincristine, Adriamycin, cyclophosphamide)** *chemotherapy protocol*

**VAD/V (vincristine, Adriamycin, dexamethasone, verapamil)** *chemotherapy protocol*

**VAFAC (vincristine, amethopterin, fluorouracil, Adriamycin, cyclophosphamide)** *chemotherapy protocol*

**Vagifem** film-coated vaginal tablets ℞ *synthetic estrogen; hormone replacement for postmenopausal atrophic vaginitis* [estradiol hemihydrate] 25.8 μg (=25 mg base)

**Vagi-Gard; Vagi-Gard Advanced Sensitive Formula** vaginal cream OTC *topical local anesthetic; keratolytic; antifungal* [benzocaine; resorcinol] 20%•3%; 5%•2%

**Vaginex** vaginal cream OTC *topical antihistamine* [tripelennamine HCl]

**Vagisec Douche** solution ℞ *vaginal cleanser and deodorizer*

**Vagisec Plus** vaginal suppositories ℞ *antibacterial* [aminacrine HCl] 6 mg

**Vagisil** cream OTC *topical local anesthetic; antipruritic; antifungal* [benzocaine; resorcinol] 5%•2%

**Vagisil** powder OTC *absorbs vaginal moisture* [cornstarch; aloe]

**Vagistat-1** vaginal ointment in pre-filled applicator OTC *antifungal* [tioconazole] 6.5%

**VAI (vincristine, actinomycin D, ifosfamide)** *chemotherapy protocol*

**valaciclovir** INN *oral antiviral for herpes simplex virus types 1 and 2 (HSV-1, cold sores; HSV-2, genital herpes) and herpes zoster (shingles) infections; suppressive therapy for recurrent outbreaks* [also: valacyclovir HCl]

**valacyclovir HCl** USAN *oral antiviral for herpes simplex virus types 1 and 2 (HSV-1, cold sores; HSV-2, genital herpes) and herpes zoster (shingles) infections; suppressive therapy for recurrent outbreaks* [also: valaciclovir]

**valconazole** INN

**Valcyte** tablets ℞ *nucleoside analogue antiviral for AIDS-related cytomegalovirus (CMV) retinitis; CMV prevention in organ transplants* [valganciclovir HCl] 450 mg

**valdecoxib** USAN *COX-2 inhibitor; nonsteroidal anti-inflammatory drug (NSAID) for osteoarthritis (OA), rheumatoid arthritis (RA), and menstrual pain*

**valdetamide** INN

**valdipromide** INN

**valepotriate** [see: valtrate]

**Valergen 20; Valergen 40** IM injection (discontinued 2003) ℞ *estrogen replacement therapy for the treatment of postmenopausal symptoms; hormonal antineoplastic for prostate cancer* [estradiol valerate in oil] 20 mg/mL; 40 mg/mL

**valerian (*Valeriana officinalis*)** root *medicinal herb for convulsions, hypertension, hysteria, hypochondria, nervousness, pain, and sedation*

**valerian, false** *medicinal herb* [see: life root]

**Valertest No. 1** IM injection (discontinued 2003) ℞ *hormone replacement therapy for postmenopausal symptoms* [estradiol valerate; testosterone enanthate] 4•90 mg/mL

**valethamate bromide** NF

**valganciclovir HCl** USAN *nucleoside analogue antiviral for AIDS-related cytomegalovirus (CMV) retinitis; CMV prevention in organ transplants; oral prodrug of ganciclovir*

**valine (L-valine)** USAN, USP, INN, JAN *essential amino acid; symbols: Val, V*

**valine & isoleucine & leucine** *investigational (orphan) for hyperphenylalaninemia*

**Valisone** ointment, cream, lotion ℞ *topical corticosteroidal anti-inflammatory* [betamethasone valerate] 0.1%

**Valisone Reduced Strength** cream ℞ *topical corticosteroidal anti-inflammatory* [betamethasone valerate] 0.01%

**Valium** IV or IM injection, Tel-E-Ject syringes (discontinued 2003) ℞ *benzodiazepine sedative; anxiolytic; skeletal muscle relaxant; anticonvulsant; alcohol withdrawal aid; also abused as a street drug* [diazepam] 5 mg/mL; 10 mg ⊠ thallium; Valpin

**Valium** tablets ℞ *benzodiazepine sedative; anxiolytic; skeletal muscle relaxant; anticonvulsant; alsohol withdrawal aid; also abused as a street drug* [diazepam] 2, 5, 10 mg ⊠ thallium; Valpin

**valnoctamide** USAN, INN *tranquilizer*

**valofane** INN

**valomaciclovir stearate** USAN *DNA polymerase inhibitor antiviral for herpes zoster infections*

**valperinol** INN

**valproate pivoxil** INN

**valproate semisodium** INN *anticonvulsant; antipsychotic for manic episodes; migraine prophylaxis* [also: divalproex sodium; semisodium valproate]

**valproate sodium** USAN *anticonvulsant; investigational for migraine relief* 250 mg/5 mL oral; 500 mg injection

**valproic acid** USAN, USP, INN, BAN *anticonvulsant* 250 mg oral

**valpromide** INN

**valrubicin** USAN *anthracycline antibiotic antineoplastic for bladder cancer (orphan)*

**valsartan** USAN, INN *angiotensin II receptor antagonist; antihypertensive; treatment for congestive heart failure (CHF)*

**valspodar** USAN *investigational (Phase III) cyclosporine-derived P-glycoprotein (P-gp) inhibitor for multi-drug–resistant (MDR) cancers, including acute myelogenous leukemia (AML), multiple myeloma, and ovarian cancer*

**Valstar** intravesical solution (discontinued 2004) ℞ *anthracycline antibiotic antineoplastic for bladder cancer (orphan)* [valrubicin] 40 mg/mL

**Valtaxin** ⓒᴬᴺ intravesical solution ℞ *anthracycline antibiotic antineoplastic for bladder cancer (orphan)* [valrubicin] 40 mg/mL

**valtrate** INN

**Valtrex** film-coated caplets ℞ *antiviral for herpes simplex virus types 1 and 2 (HSV-1, cold sores; HSV-2, genital herpes) and herpes zoster (shingles) infections; suppressive therapy for recurrent outbreaks* [valacyclovir HCl] 500, 1000 mg

**VAM (vinblastine, Adriamycin, mitomycin)** *chemotherapy protocol*

**VAM (VP-16-213, Adriamycin, methotrexate)** *chemotherapy protocol*

**VAMP (vincristine, actinomycin, methotrexate, prednisone)** *chemotherapy protocol*

**VAMP (vincristine, Adriamycin, methylprednisolone)** *chemotherapy protocol*

**VAMP (vincristine, amethopterin, mercaptopurine, prednisone)** *chemotherapy protocol*

**vanadium** *element (V)*

**Vanamide** cream ℞ *keratolytic for the removal of dystrophic nails* [urea] 40%

**Vancenase** Pockethaler (nasal inhalation aerosol) (discontinued 2004) ℞ *corticosteroidal anti-inflammatory for seasonal or perennial rhinitis* [beclomethasone dipropionate] 42 μg/dose

**Vancenase AQ** nasal spray (discontinued 2004) ℞ *corticosteroidal anti-inflammatory for seasonal or perennial rhinitis* [beclomethasone dipropionate] 0.084% (100 μg/dose)

**Vanceril; Vanceril Double Strength** oral inhalation aerosol (discontinued 2002) ℞ *corticosteroidal anti-inflammatory for chronic asthma* [beclomethasone dipropionate] 42 μg/dose; 84 μg/dose

**Vancocin** Pulvules (capsules), powder for oral solution, powder for IV or IM injection ℞ *tricyclic glycopeptide*

*antibiotic* [vancomycin HCl] 125, 250 mg; 1, 10 g; 0.5, 1, 10 g

**Vancoled** powder for IV or IM injection ℞ *tricyclic glycopeptide antibiotic* [vancomycin HCl] 0.5, 1, 5 g

**vancomycin** INN, BAN *tricyclic glycopeptide antibiotic* [also: vancomycin HCl]

**vancomycin HCl** USP *tricyclic glycopeptide antibiotic* [also: vancomycin] 1 g oral; 0.5, 1, 5, 10 g/vial injection

**vaneprim** INN

**Vanex Expectorant** oral liquid (discontinued 2002) ℞ *narcotic antitussive; decongestant; expectorant* [hydrocodone bitartrate; pseudoephedrine HCl; guaifenesin; alcohol 5%] 2.5•30•100 mg/5 mL

**Vanex Forte** sustained-release caplets (discontinued 2001) ℞ *decongestant; antihistamine* [phenylpropanolamine HCl; phenylephrine HCl; chlorpheniramine maleate; pyrilamine maleate] 50•10•4•25 mg

**Vanex Forte-R** sustained-release capsules (discontinued 2001) ℞ *decongestant; antihistamine* [phenylpropanolamine HCl; chlorpheniramine maleate] 75•12 mg

**Vanex HD** oral liquid ℞ *narcotic antitussive; decongestant; antihistamine* [hydrocodone bitartrate; phenylephrine HCl; chlorpheniramine maleate] 3.33•10•4 mg/10 mL

**Vanicream** OTC *cream base*

**vanilla** NF *flavoring agent*

**vanilla** (*Vanilla fragrans; V. planifolia; V. tahitensis*) bean *medicinal herb for CNS stimulation, fever, and flatulence; also used as an aphrodisiac*

**vanillin** NF *flavoring agent*

**N-vanillylnonamide** [see: nonivamide]

**N-vanillyloleamide** [see: olvanil]

**Vaniqa** cream ℞ *hair growth inhibitor for unwanted facial hair on women* [eflornithine HCl] 13.9%

**vanitiolide** INN

**Vanlev** ℞ *vasopeptidase inhibitor (VPI); investigational (NDA filed) endopeptidase and angiotensin-converting enzyme*

*(ACE) inhibitor for hypertension and congestive heart failure* [omapatrilat]

**Vanocin** lotion ℞ *acne treatment* [sulfacetamide sodium; sulfur] 10%•5%

**Vanoxide** lotion (discontinued 2003) OTC *keratolytic for acne* [benzoyl peroxide] 5%

**Vanoxide-HC** lotion ℞ *topical corticosteroidal anti-inflammatory and keratolytic for acne* [benzoyl peroxide; hydrocortisone] 5%•0.5%

**Vanquish** caplets OTC *analgesic; antipyretic; anti-inflammatory* [acetaminophen; aspirin (buffered with magnesium hydroxide and aluminum hydroxide); caffeine] 194•227•(50•25)•33 mg

**Vansil** capsules (discontinued 2001) ℞ *anthelmintic for schistosomiasis (flukes)* [oxamniquine] 250 mg

**Vanticon** (German name for U.S. product Accolate)

**Vantin** film-coated tablets, granules for suspension ℞ *broad-spectrum cephalosporin antibiotic* [cefpodoxime proxetil] 100, 200 mg; 50, 100 mg/5 mL ⃞ Banthine; Bantron

**vanyldisulfamide** INN

**VAP (vinblastine, actinomycin D, Platinol)** *chemotherapy protocol*

**VAP (vincristine, Adriamycin, prednisone)** *chemotherapy protocol*

**VAP (vincristine, Adriamycin, procarbazine)** *chemotherapy protocol*

**VAP (vincristine, asparaginase, prednisone)** *chemotherapy protocol*

**vapiprost** INN, BAN *antagonist to thromboxane $A_2$* [also: vapiprost HCl]

**vapiprost HCl** USAN *antagonist to thromboxane $A_2$* [also: vapiprost]

**Vaporole** (trademarked dosage form) *crushable ampule for inhalation*

**vapreotide** USAN *antineoplastic*

**Vaqta** adult IM injection, pediatric IM injection ℞ *immunization against hepatitis A virus (HAV)* [hepatitis A vaccine, inactivated] 50 U/mL; 25 U/0.5 mL

**vardenafil HCl** USAN *phosphodiesterase type 5 (PDE5) inhibitor; selective vasodilator for erectile dysfunction (ED)*

**varicella virus vaccine** *live, attenuated vaccine for chickenpox*

**varicella-zoster immune globulin (VZIG)** USP *passive immunizing agent* 10%–18% (125 U/2.5 mL)

**Varivax** powder for subcu injection ℞ *vaccine for chickenpox* [varicella virus vaccine, live attenuated] 1350 PFU/0.5 mL

*Varoniscastrum virgincum medicinal herb* [see: Culver root]

**VAS-972** *investigational immune modulation therapy for contact hypersensitivity*

**Vascor** film-coated tablets (discontinued 2003) ℞ *antianginal* [bepridil HCl] 200, 300 mg

**Vascoray** injection (discontinued 2001) ℞ *radiopaque contrast medium* [iothalamate meglumine; iothalamate sodium (51.3% total iodine)] 520●260 mg/mL (400 mg/mL)

**vascular endothelial growth factor (VEGF)** *investigational (Phase II, orphan) gene-based therapy for neointimal hyperplasia disease*

**vascular serotonin 5-HT₁ receptor agonists** *a class of antimigraine agents that constrict cranial blood vessels and inhibit the release of inflammatory neuropeptides*

**Vaseretic 5-12.5; Vaseretic 10-25** tablets ℞ *antihypertensive; angiotensin-converting enzyme (ACE) inhibitor; diuretic* [enalapril maleate; hydrochlorothiazide] 5●12.5 mg; 10●25 mg

**vasoactive intestinal polypeptide (VIP)** *investigational (NDA filed) treatment for male sexual dysfunction; investigational (orphan) for acute esophageal food impaction*

**Vasocidin** eye drops ℞ *corticosteroidal anti-inflammatory; antibiotic* [prednisolone sodium phosphate; sulfacetamide sodium] 0.25%●10% ⑨ Vasodilan

**Vasocidin** ophthalmic ointment (discontinued 2002) ℞ *corticosteroidal anti-inflammatory; antibiotic* [prednisolone acetate; sulfacetamide sodium] 0.5%●10%

**Vasocine** ophthalmic ointment (discontinued 2003) ℞ *corticosteroidal anti-inflammatory; antibiotic* [prednisolone acetate; sulfacetamide sodium] 0.5%●10% ⑨ Vaseline

**VasoClear** eye drops OTC *decongestant; lubricant* [naphazoline HCl; polyvinyl alcohol; polyethylene glycol 400] 0.02%●0.25%●1% ⑨ VasoCare

**VasoClear A** eye drops OTC *decongestant; astringent* [naphazoline HCl; zinc sulfate] 0.02%●0.25%

**Vasocon Regular** eye drops ℞ *topical ophthalmic decongestant and vasoconstrictor* [naphazoline HCl] 0.1%

**Vasocon-A** eye drops ℞ *ophthalmic decongestant and antihistamine* [naphazoline HCl; antazoline phosphate] 0.05%●0.5%

**vasoconstrictors** *a class of cardiovascular drugs that narrow the blood vessels*

**Vasodilan** tablets ℞ *peripheral vasodilator* [isoxsuprine HCl] 10, 20 mg ⑨ Vasocidin

**vasodilators** *a class of cardiovascular drugs that dilate the blood vessels*

**Vasofem** ℞ *investigational (NDA filed) oral treatment for female sexual arousal disorder* [phentolamine mesylate]

**Vasoflux** ℞ *investigational (Phase II) anticoagulant for use in acute myocardial infarction patients* ⑨ Vasoprost; Vasosulf

**vasopressin (VP)** USP, INN *posterior pituitary hormone; antidiuretic* 20 U/mL injection

**vasopressin tannate** USP *posterior pituitary hormone; antidiuretic*

**vasopressors** *a class of posterior pituitary hormones that raise blood pressure by causing contraction of capillaries and arterioles; a class of sympathomimetic agents that raise blood pressure by increasing myocardial contractility* [also called: vasopressins]

**Vasoprost** ℞ *investigational (orphan) prostaglandin for severe peripheral arterial occlusive disease* [alprostadil] ⊡ Vasoflux

**Vasosulf** eye drops ℞ *antibiotic; ophthalmic decongestant* [sulfacetamide sodium; phenylephrine HCl] 15%• 0.125% ⊡ Velosef; Vasoflux

**Vasotate HC** ear drops ℞ *topical corticosteroidal anti-inflammatory; antibacterial; antifungal* [hydrocortisone; acetic acid] 1%•2%

**Vasotec** tablets ℞ *antihypertensive; angiotensin-converting enzyme (ACE) inhibitor; treatment for CHF* [enalapril maleate] 2.5, 5, 10, 20 mg

**Vasotec I.V.** injection (discontinued 2003) ℞ *antihypertensive; angiotensin-converting enzyme (ACE) inhibitor* [enalaprilat] 1.25 mg/mL

**Vasoxyl** IV or IM injection (discontinued 2001) ℞ *vasopressor for hypotensive shock during surgery* [methoxamine HCl] 20 mg/mL

**VAT (vinblastine, Adriamycin, thiotepa)** *chemotherapy protocol*

**vatalanib** *investigational (Phase III) tyrosine kinase inhibitor for cervical cancer*

**VATD; VAT-D (vincristine, ara-C, thioguanine, daunorubicin)** *chemotherapy protocol*

**VATH (vinblastine, Adriamycin, thiotepa, Halotestin)** *chemotherapy protocol for breast cancer*

**Vatronol** [see: Vicks Vatronol]

**VAV (VP-16-213, Adriamycin, vincristine)** *chemotherapy protocol*

**Vaxigrip** ⒸⒶⓃ IM injection ℞ *flu vaccine* [influenza split-virus vaccine] 0.5 mL/dose

**VaxSyn HIV-1** ℞ *investigational (orphan) antiviral (therapeutic, Phase II) and vaccine (preventative, Phase I) for HIV and AIDS* [gp160 antigens]

**VB (vinblastine, bleomycin)** *chemotherapy protocol*

**VBA (vincristine, BCNU, Adriamycin)** *chemotherapy protocol*

**VBAP (vincristine, BCNU, Adriamycin, prednisone)** *chemotherapy protocol for multiple myeloma*

**VBC (VePesid, BCNU, cyclophosphamide)** *chemotherapy protocol*

**VBC (vinblastine, bleomycin, cisplatin)** *chemotherapy protocol*

**VBCMP (vincristine, BCNU, cyclophosphamide, melphalan, prednisone)** *chemotherapy protocol for multiple myeloma*

**VBD (vinblastine, bleomycin, DDP)** *chemotherapy protocol*

**VBM (vincristine, bleomycin, methotrexate)** *chemotherapy protocol*

**VBMCP (vincristine, BCNU, melphalan, cyclophosphamide, prednisone)** *chemotherapy protocol*

**VBMF (vincristine, bleomycin, methotrexate, fluorouracil)** *chemotherapy protocol*

**VBP (vinblastine, bleomycin, Platinol)** *chemotherapy protocol*

**VC (VePesid, carboplatin)** *chemotherapy protocol*

**VC (vincristine)** [q.v.]

**VC (vinorelbine, cisplatin)** *chemotherapy protocol for non–small cell lung cancer (NSCLC)*

**VCAP (vincristine, cyclophosphamide, Adriamycin, prednisone)** *chemotherapy protocol for multiple myeloma*

**V-CAP III (VP-16-213, cyclophosphamide, Adriamycin, Platinol)** *chemotherapy protocol*

**VCF** (vaginal contraceptive film) OTC *spermicidal contraceptive* [nonoxynol 9] 28%

**VCF (vincristine, cyclophosphamide, fluorouracil)** *chemotherapy protocol*

**VCMP (vincristine, cyclophosphamide, melphalan, prednisone)** *chemotherapy protocol for multiple myeloma* [also: VMCP]

**VCP (vincristine, cyclophosphamide, prednisone)** *chemotherapy protocol*

**VCP 205** *investigational (Phase II) vaccine for HIV* [also: ALVAC-120TMG]

**VCR (vincristine)** [q.v.]

**VD (vinorelbine, doxorubicin)** *chemotherapy protocol for breast cancer*

**VDA (vincristine, daunorubicin, asparaginase)** *chemotherapy protocol*

**V-Dec-M** sustained-release tablets ℞ *decongestant; expectorant* [pseudoephedrine HCl; guaifenesin] 120•500 mg

**VDP (vinblastine, dacarbazine, Platinol)** *chemotherapy protocol*

**VDP (vincristine, daunorubicin, prednisone)** *chemotherapy protocol*

**Vectrin** capsules (discontinued 2003) ℞ *tetracycline antibiotic* [minocycline HCl] 50, 100 mg

**vecuronium bromide** USAN, INN, BAN *nondepolarizing neuromuscular blocker; muscle relaxant; adjunct to anesthesia* 10, 20 mg injection

**Veetids** film-coated tablets, powder for oral solution ℞ *natural penicillin antibiotic* [penicillin V potassium] 250, 500 mg; 125, 250 mg/5 mL

**vegetable oil, hydrogenated** NF *tablet and capsule lubricant*

**vegetable tallow; vegetable wax** *medicinal herb* [see: bayberry]

**VEGF (vascular endothelial growth factor)** [see: telbermin]

**Vehicle/N; Vehicle/N Mild** OTC *lotion base*

**VeIP (Velban, ifosfamide [with mesna rescue], Platinol)** *chemotherapy protocol for genitourinary and testicular cancer*

**Velban** powder for IV injection ℞ *antineoplastic for lung, breast and testicular cancers, lymphomas, sarcomas, and neuroblastoma* [vinblastine sulfate] 10 mg/vial ⊠ Valpin

**Velcade** powder for IV injection ℞ *antineoplastic for multiple myeloma (orphan)* [bortezomib] 3.5 mg/vial

**Veldona** low-dose oral lozenge ℞ *investigational (Phase II) treatment for AIDS-related xerostomia; investigational (orphan) for oral human papillo-* mavirus (HPV) warts in HIV-infected patients [interferon alfa]

**Veletri** injection ℞ *investigational (Phase III) vasoconstrictor and endothelin receptor antagonist for acute heart failure, pulmonary edema, and hepatorenal syndrome* [tezosentan]

**Velivet** tablets (in packs of 28) ℞ *triphasic oral contraceptive; emergency postcoital contraceptive* [desogestrel; ethinyl estradiol]
Phase 1 (7 days): 100•25 μg;
Phase 2 (7 days): 125•25 μg;
Phase 3 (7 days): 150•25 μg

**velnacrine** INN, BAN *cholinesterase inhibitor* [also: velnacrine maleate]

**velnacrine maleate** USAN *cholinesterase inhibitor for Alzheimer disease* [also: velnacrine]

**Velosef** capsules, oral suspension ℞ *cephalosporin antibiotic* [cephradine] 250, 500 mg; 125, 250 mg/5 mL ⊠ Vasosulf

**Velosef** powder for IV or IM injection (discontinued 2004) ℞ *cephalosporin antibiotic* [cephradine] 250, 500, 1000, 2000 mg ⊠ Vasosulf

**Velosulin BR** subcu injection OTC *antidiabetic* [human insulin (rDNA)] 100 U/mL

**Velvachol** OTC *cream base*

**Venice turpentine** *medicinal herb* [see: larch]

**venlafaxine** INN, BAN *antidepressant; anxiolytic; selective serotonin and norepinephrine reuptake inhibitor (SSNRI)* [also: venlafaxine HCl]

**venlafaxine HCl** USAN *antidepressant; anxiolytic; selective serotonin and norepinephrine reuptake inhibitor (SSNRI)* [also: venlafaxine]

**Venofer** IV injection ℞ *hematinic for iron deficiency anemia in patients undergoing chronic dialysis* [iron sucrose] 20 mg/mL

**Venoglobulin-I** powder for IV infusion (discontinued 2001; replaced by Venoglobulin-S) ℞ *passive immunizing agent for HIV and idiopathic*

thrombocytopenic purpura (ITP) [immune globulin] 50 mg/mL

**Venoglobulin-S** IV infusion ℞ *passive immunizing agent for HIV and idiopathic thrombocytopenic purpura (ITP)* [immune globulin, solvent/detergent treated] 5%, 10%

**Venomil** subcu or IM injection ℞ *venom sensitivity testing (subcu); venom desensitization therapy (IM)* [extracts of honeybee, yellow jacket, yellow hornet, white-faced hornet, mixed vespid, and wasp venom]

**Ventolin** ⒸⒶⓃ Diskus (inhalation powder device) ℞ *sympathomimetic bronchodilator* [albuterol sulfate] 200 μg/dose

**Ventolin** inhalation aerosol (discontinued 2003) ℞ *sympathomimetic bronchodilator* [albuterol] 90 μg/dose 🔃 phentolamine

**Ventolin** Rotacap (encapsulated powder for inhalation), tablets, solution for inhalation, Nebules (unit-dose solution for inhalation), syrup (discontinued 2001) ℞ *sympathomimetic bronchodilator* [albuterol sulfate] 200 μg; 2, 4 mg; 0.05%; 0.083%; 2 mg/5 mL

**Ventolin HFA** CFC-free inhalation aerosol ℞ *sympathomimetic bronchodilator* [albuterol] 90 μg/dose

**VePesid** IV injection, capsules ℞ *antineoplastic for testicular and small cell lung cancers* [etoposide] 20 mg/mL; 50 mg

**veradoline** INN *analgesic* [also: veradoline HCl]

**veradoline HCl** USAN *analgesic* [also: veradoline]

**veralipride** INN

**verapamil** USAN, INN, BAN *coronary vasodilator; calcium channel blocker*

**verapamil HCl** USAN, USP *antianginal; antiarrhythmic; antihypertensive; calcium channel blocker* 40, 80, 120, 180, 240 mg oral; 2.5 mg/mL injection

*Veratrum* **species** *medicinal herb* [see: hellebore]

**veratrylidene-isoniazid** [see: verazide]

**verazide** INN, BAN

**Verazinc** capsules OTC *zinc supplement* [zinc sulfate] 220 mg

*Verbascum nigrum; V. phlomoides; V. thapsiforme; V. thapsus* *medicinal herb* [see: mullein]

*Verbena hastata* *medicinal herb* [see: blue vervain]

**Verelan** sustained-release capsules ℞ *antihypertensive; antianginal; antiarrhythmic; calcium channel blocker* [verapamil HCl] 120, 180, 240, 360 mg

**Verelan PM** delayed-onset, extended-release capsules ℞ *antihypertensive; calcium channel blocker* [verapamil HCl] 100, 200, 300 mg

**Vergon** capsules OTC *anticholinergic; antihistamine; antivertigo agent; motion sickness preventative* [meclizine HCl] 30 mg

**Veridate** (trademarked packaging form) *patient compliance package for oral contraceptives*

**verilopam** INN *analgesic* [also: verilopam HCl]

**verilopam HCl** USAN *analgesic* [also: verilopam]

**verlukast** USAN, INN *bronchodilator; antiasthmatic*

**Verluma** technetium Tc 99 prep kit ℞ *monoclonal antibody imaging agent for small cell lung cancer* [nofetumomab merpentan]

**vermicides; vermifuges** *a class of drugs effective against parasitic infections* [also called: anthelmintics]

**Vermox** chewable tablets ℞ *anthelmintic for trichuriasis, enterobiasis, ascariasis, and uncinariasis* [mebendazole] 100 mg

**verofylline** USAN, INN *bronchodilator; antiasthmatic*

**veronal** [see: barbital]

**veronal sodium** [see: barbital sodium]

**veronica, tall** *medicinal herb* [see: Culver root]

*Veronica beccabunga* *medicinal herb* [see: brooklime]

*Veronica officinalis* *medicinal herb* [see: speedwell]

**Versacaps** sustained-release capsules ℞ *decongestant; expectorant* [pseudo-ephedrine HCl; guaifenesin] 60•300 mg

**Versed** IV or IM injection, Tel-E-Ject syringes, pediatric syrup ℞ *short-acting benzodiazepine general anesthetic adjunct for preoperative sedation* [midazolam HCl] 1, 5 mg/mL; 2 mg/mL

**versetamide** USAN *stabilizer; carrier agent for gadoversetamide*

**Versiclear** lotion ℞ *antifungal; keratolytic; antipruritic; anesthetic* [sodium thiosulfate; salicylic acid; alcohol 10%] 25%•1%

**verteporfin** USAN *light-activated treatment for subfoveal choroidal neovascularization (CNV) due to age-related macular degeneration (AMD), pathologic myopia, or ocular histoplasmosis*

**vervain** *medicinal herb* [see: blue vervain]

**Vesanoid** capsules ℞ *antineoplastic for acute promyelocytic leukemia (orphan); investigational (orphan) for other leukemias and ophthalmic squamous metaplasia* [tretinoin] 10 mg

**vesicants** *a class of agents that cause blisters*

**Vesicare** tablets ℞ *investigational (NDA filed) treatment for overactive bladder with urinary incontinence, urgency, and frequency* [solifenacin succinate] 5, 10 mg

**vesnarinone** USAN, INN *cardiotonic; inotropic for congestive heart failure*

**vesperal** [see: barbital]

**Vesprin** IV or IM injection (discontinued 2003) ℞ *conventional (typical) antipsychotic; antiemetic* [triflupromazine HCl] 10, 20 mg/mL

**Vestra** tablets ℞ *investigational (NDA filed) fast-acting selective norepinephrine reuptake inhibitor for depression* [reboxetine mesylate]

**vetrabutine** INN, BAN

**Vetuss HC** syrup (discontinued 2002) ℞ *narcotic antitussive; decongestant; antihistamine* [hydrocodone bitartrate; phenylpropanolamine HCl; phenylephrine HCl; pyrilamine maleate; pheniramine maleate; alcohol 5%] 1.7•3.3•5•3.3•3.3 mg/5 mL

**Vexol** eye drop suspension ℞ *topical ophthalmic corticosteroidal anti-inflammatory* [rimexolone] 1%

**Vfend** film-coated tablets, powder for oral suspension, powder for IV injection ℞ *triazole antifungal for invasive aspergillosis, esophageal candidiasis, and other serious fungal infections* [voriconazole] 50, 200 mg; 40 mg/mL; 200 mg/vial

**Viactiv** chewable tablets OTC *calcium supplement* [calcium carbonate; vitamin D; vitamin K] 1.25 g•100 IU•40 µg

**Viadur** DUROS (once-yearly implant) ℞ *antihormonal antineoplastic for the palliative treatment of advanced prostate cancer* [leuprolide acetate] 120 µg/day

**Viaflex** (trademarked form) *ready-to-use IV*

**Viagra** film-coated tablets ℞ *phosphodiesterase type 5 (PDE5) inhibitor; selective vasodilator for erectile dysfunction (ED)* [sildenafil citrate] 25, 50, 100 mg

**Vianain** ℞ *investigational (orphan) proteolytic enzymes for debridement of severe burns* [ananain; comosain; bromelains]

**vibesate**

**Vibramycin** capsules ℞ *tetracycline antibiotic* [doxycycline hyclate] 50, 100 mg

**Vibramycin** powder for oral suspension ℞ *tetracycline antibiotic* [doxycycline monohydrate] 25 mg/5 mL

**Vibramycin** syrup ℞ *tetracycline antibiotic* [doxycycline calcium] 50 mg/5 mL

**Vibramycin I.V.** powder for IV injection (discontinued 2003) ℞ *tetracycline antibiotic* [doxycycline hyclate] 100, 200 mg/vial

**Vibra-Tabs** film-coated tablets ℞ *tetracycline antibiotic* [doxycycline hyclate] 100 mg

**Viburnum opulus** *medicinal herb* [see: cramp bark]

**VIC (VePesid, ifosfamide [with mesna rescue], carboplatin)** *che-*

motherapy protocol for non–small cell lung cancer (NSCLC) [also: CVI]

**VIC (vinblastine, ifosfamide, CCNU)** *chemotherapy protocol*

**Vicam** injection ℞ *parenteral vitamin therapy* [multiple B vitamins; vitamin C] ≙ ● 50 mg/mL

**Vicks 44 Cough Relief** oral liquid OTC *antitussive* [dextromethorphan hydrobromide; alcohol 5%] 10 mg/5 mL

**Vicks 44 Non-Drowsy Cold & Cough** LiquiCaps (liquid-filled gelcaps) (discontinued 2002) OTC *antitussive; decongestant* [dextromethorphan hydrobromide; pseudoephedrine HCl] 30 ● 60 mg

**Vicks 44D Cough & Head Congestion Relief** oral liquid OTC *antitussive; decongestant* [dextromethorphan hydrobromide; pseudoephedrine HCl; alcohol 5%] 30 ● 60 mg/15 mL

**Vicks 44E Cough & Chest Congestion Relief** oral liquid OTC *antitussive; expectorant* [dextromethorphan hydrobromide; guaifenesin; alcohol 5%] 20 ● 200 mg/15 mL

**Vicks 44M Cold, Flu & Cough** LiquiCaps (liquid-filled gelcaps) (discontinued 2002) OTC *antitussive; decongestant; antihistamine; analgesic* [dextromethorphan hydrobromide; pseudoephedrine HCl; chlorpheniramine maleate; acetaminophen] 10 ● 30 ● 2 ● 250 mg

**Vicks 44M Cough, Cold, & Flu Relief** oral liquid OTC *antitussive; decongestant; antihistamine; analgesic* [dextromethorphan hydrobromide; pseudoephedrine HCl; chlorpheniramine maleate; acetaminophen; alcohol 10%] 30 ● 60 ● 4 ● 650 mg/20 mL

**Vicks Cough Drops; Vicks Menthol Cough Drops** OTC *topical analgesic; counterirritant; mild local anesthetic* [menthol] 10 mg; 8.4 mg

**Vicks Cough Silencers** lozenges OTC *antitussive; topical oral anesthetic* [dextromethorphan hydrobromide; benzocaine] 2.5 ● 1 mg

**Vicks DayQuil** products [see: DayQuil]

**Vicks Dry Hacking Cough** syrup (discontinued 2002) OTC *antitussive* [dextromethorphan hydrobromide; alcohol 10%] 15 mg/5 mL

**Vicks Formula 44D Cough & Decongestant; Vicks Pediatric Formula 44d Cough & Decongestant** oral liquid (discontinued 2002) OTC *antitussive; decongestant* [dextromethorphan hydrobromide; pseudoephedrine HCl] 10 ● 20 mg/5 mL; 5 ● 10 mg/5 mL

**Vicks NyQuil** products [see: NyQuil]

**Vicks Pediatric 44d Dry Hacking Cough and Head Congestion** syrup (discontinued 2002) OTC *antitussive* [dextromethorphan hydrobromide] 15 mg/15 mL

**Vicks Pediatric 44e Cough & Chest Congestion Relief** oral liquid OTC *antitussive; expectorant* [dextromethorphan hydrobromide; guaifenesin] 10 ● 100 mg/15 mL

**Vicks Pediatric 44m Cough & Cold Relief** oral liquid OTC *antitussive; decongestant; antihistamine* [dextromethorphan hydrobromide; pseudoephedrine HCl; chlorpheniramine maleate] 15 ● 30 ● 2 mg/15 mL

**Vicks Sinex** products [see: Sinex]

**Vicks Vapor** inhaler OTC *nasal decongestant* [levmetamfetamine] 50 mg

**Vicks VapoRub** vaporizing ointment, cream OTC *counterirritant; cough suppressant* [camphor; menthol; eucalyptus oil] 5.2% ● 2.8% ● 1.2%

**Vicks Vitamin C Drops** (lozenges) OTC *vitamin C supplement* [ascorbic acid and sodium ascorbate] 25 mg

**Vicodin; Vicodin ES; Vicodin HP** tablets ℞ *narcotic analgesic* [hydrocodone bitartrate; acetaminophen] 5 ● 500 mg; 7.5 ● 750 mg; 10 ● 660 mg

**Vicodin Tuss** syrup ℞ *narcotic antitussive; expectorant* [hydrocodone bitartrate; guaifenesin] 5 ● 100 mg/5 mL ⓓ Hycodan; Hycomine

**Vicon Forte** capsules ℞ *vitamin/mineral supplement* [multiple vitamins & minerals; folic acid] ≙ ● 1 mg

**Vicon Plus** capsules OTC *vitamin/mineral supplement* [multiple vitamins & minerals]

**Vicon-C** capsules OTC *vitamin/mineral supplement* [multiple B vitamins & minerals; vitamin C] ± • 300 mg

**Vicoprofen** film-coated tablets ℞ *narcotic analgesic & antitussive* [hydrocodone bitartrate; ibuprofen] 7.5 • 200 mg

**vicotrope** [see: cosyntropin]

**vidarabine** USAN, USP, INN, BAN *antiviral* ② cytarabine

**vidarabine monohydrate** [see: vidarabine]

**vidarabine phosphate** USAN *antiviral*

**vidarabine sodium phosphate** USAN *antiviral*

**Vi-Daylin** chewable tablets (discontinued 2003) OTC *vitamin supplement* [multiple vitamins; folic acid] ± • 0.3 mg

**Vi-Daylin ADC** drops OTC *vitamin supplement* [vitamins A, C, and D] 1500 IU • 35 mg • 400 IU per mL

**Vi-Daylin ADC Vitamins + Iron** drops OTC *vitamin/iron supplement* [vitamins A, C, and D; ferrous gluconate] 1500 IU • 35 mg • 400 IU • 10 mg per mL

**Vi-Daylin Multivitamin** oral liquid, drops OTC *vitamin supplement* [multiple vitamins]

**Vi-Daylin Multivitamin + Iron** chewable tablets (discontinued 2003) OTC *vitamin/iron supplement* [multiple vitamins; iron; folic acid] ± • 12 • 0.3 mg

**Vi-Daylin Multivitamin + Iron** oral liquid, drops OTC *vitamin/iron supplement* [multiple vitamins; ferrous gluconate] ± • 10 mg/5 mL; ± • 10 mg/mL

**Vi-Daylin/F ADC** drops ℞ *pediatric vitamin supplement and dental caries preventative* [vitamins A, C, and D; sodium fluoride] 1500 IU • 35 mg • 400 IU • 0.25 mg per mL

**Vi-Daylin/F ADC + Iron** drops ℞ *pediatric vitamin/iron supplement and dental caries preventative* [vitamins A, C, and D; sodium fluoride; ferrous

sulfate] 1500 IU • 35 mg • 400 IU • 0.25 mg • 10 mg per mL

**Vi-Daylin/F Multivitamin** chewable tablets (discontinued 2004) ℞ *pediatric vitamin supplement and dental caries preventative* [multiple vitamins; sodium fluoride; folic acid] ± • 1 • 0.3 mg

**Vi-Daylin/F Multivitamin** drops ℞ *pediatric vitamin supplement and dental caries preventative* [multiple vitamins; sodium fluoride] ± • 0.25 mg/mL

**Vi-Daylin/F Multivitamin + Iron** chewable tablets ℞ *pediatric vitamin/iron supplement and dental caries preventative* [multiple vitamins; sodium fluoride; ferrous sulfate; folic acid] ± • 1 • 12 • 0.3 mg

**Vi-Daylin/F Multivitamin + Iron** drops ℞ *pediatric vitamin/iron supplement and dental caries preventative* [multiple vitamins; sodium fluoride; ferrous sulfate] ± • 0.25 • 10 mg/mL

**Vidaza** suspension for subcu injection ℞ *demethylating antineoplastic for myelodysplastic syndrome (orphan)* [azacitidine] 100 mg/vial

**Videx** chewable/dispersible tablets, powder for oral solution, powder for pediatric oral solution ℞ *antiviral for advanced HIV infection* [didanosine] 25, 50, 100, 200 mg; 100, 250 mg/ pkt.; 2, 4 g/bottle

**Videx EC** delayed-release capsules with enteric-coated beads ℞ *antiviral for advanced HIV infection* [didanosine] 200, 250, 500 mg

**VIE (vincristine, ifosfamide, etoposide)** *chemotherapy protocol*

**vifilcon A** USAN *hydrophilic contact lens material*

**vifilcon B** USAN *hydrophilic contact lens material*

**Vi-Flor** [see: Poly-Vi-Flor; Tri-Vi-Flor]

**VIG (vaccinia immune globulin)** [q.v.]

**vigabatrin** USAN, INN, BAN *investigational (NDA filed) anticonvulsant*

**Vigamox** eye drops ℞ *broad-spectrum fluoroquinolone antibiotic* [moxifloxacin HCl] 0.5%

**Vigomar Forte** tablets OTC *vitamin/mineral/iron supplement* [multiple vitamins & minerals; iron] ≐•12 mg

**Vigortol** oral liquid OTC *geriatric vitamin/mineral supplement* [multiple B vitamins & minerals; alcohol 18%]

**VIL** Ṛ *investigational (orphan) for hyperphenylalaninemia* [valine; isoleucine; leucine]

**viloxazine** INN, BAN *investigational (NDA filed) bicyclic antidepressant; investigational (orphan) for cataplexy and narcolepsy* [also: viloxazine HCl]

**viloxazine HCl** USAN *bicyclic antidepressant* [also: viloxazine]

**Viminate** oral liquid OTC *geriatric vitamin/mineral supplement* [multiple B vitamins & minerals]

**viminol** INN

**vinafocon A** USAN *hydrophobic contact lens material*

**Vinate Good Start Prenatal Formula** chewable tablets Ṛ *prenatal vitamin/mineral/calcium/iron supplement* [multiple vitamins & minerals; calcium; iron; folic acid] ≐•200•29•1 mg

**Vinate GT** tablets Ṛ *prenatal vitamin/mineral/calcium/iron supplement; stool softener* [multiple vitamins & minerals; calcium; iron; folic acid; biotin; docusate sodium] ≐•200•90•1•0.03•50 mg

**vinbarbital** NF, INN [also: vinbarbitone]

**vinbarbital sodium** NF

**vinbarbitone** BAN [also: vinbarbital]

**vinblastine** INN *vinca alkaloid antineoplastic* [also: vinblastine sulfate]

**vinblastine sulfate** USAN, USP *vinca alkaloid antineoplastic* [also: vinblastine] 10 mg/vial, 1 mg/mL injection

**vinblastine sulfate & estramustine** *chemotherapy protocol for prostate cancer*

**vinburnine** INN

**vinca alkaloids** *a class of natural antineoplastics*

**Vinca major; V. minor** *medicinal herb* [see: periwinkle]

**vincaleukoblastine sulfate** [see: vinblastine sulfate]

**vincamine** INN, BAN

**vincanol** INN

**vincantenate** [see: vinconate]

**vincantril** INN

**Vincasar PFS** IV injection Ṛ *antineoplastic* [vincristine sulfate] 1 mg/mL

**vincofos** USAN, INN *anthelmintic*

**vinconate** INN

**vincristine (VC; VCR)** INN *antineoplastic* [also: vincristine sulfate]

**vincristine sulfate** USAN, USP *antineoplastic* [also: vincristine] 1 mg/mL injection

**vindeburnol** INN

**vindesine** USAN, INN, BAN *synthetic vinca alkaloid antineoplastic*

**vindesine sulfate** USAN, JAN *investigational (NDA filed) synthetic vinca alkaloid antineoplastic*

**vinegar** [see: acetic acid]

**vinepidine** INN *antineoplastic* [also: vinepidine sulfate]

**vinepidine sulfate** USAN *antineoplastic* [also: vinepidine]

**vinformide** INN

**vinglycinate** INN *antineoplastic* [also: vinglycinate sulfate]

**vinglycinate sulfate** USAN *antineoplastic* [also: vinglycinate]

**vinleurosine** INN *antineoplastic* [also: vinleurosine sulfate]

**vinleurosine sulfate** USAN *antineoplastic* [also: vinleurosine]

**vinmegallate** INN

**vinorelbine** INN *antineoplastic* [also: vinorelbine tartrate]

**vinorelbine & cisplatin** *chemotherapy protocol for cervical cancer and non–small cell lung cancer (NSCLC)*

**vinorelbine & doxorubicin** *chemotherapy protocol for breast cancer*

**vinorelbine & gemcitabine** *chemotherapy protocol for non–small cell lung cancer (NSCLC)*

**vinorelbine & paclitaxel** *chemotherapy protocol for breast cancer*

**vinorelbine tartrate** USAN *antineoplastic* [also: vinorelbine] 10 mg/mL injection

**vinpocetine** USAN, INN *natural derivative of vincamine, an extract of the periwinkle plant; increases ATP levels in the brain, which increases memory and mental function by increasing the neuronal firing rate; also increases serotonin levels in the brain*

**vinpoline** INN

**vinrosidine** INN *antineoplastic* [also: vinrosidine sulfate]

**vinrosidine sulfate** USAN *antineoplastic* [also: vinrosidine]

**vintiamol** INN

**vintoperol** INN

**vintriptol** INN

**vinyl alcohol polymer** [see: polyvinyl alcohol]

**vinyl ether** USP

**vinyl gamma-aminobutyric acid** [see: vigabatrin]

**vinylbital** INN [also: vinylbitone]

**vinylbitone** BAN [also: vinylbital]

**vinylestrenolone** [see: norgesterone]

**vinymal** [see: vinylbital]

**vinyzene** [see: bromchlorenone]

**vinzolidine** INN *antineoplastic* [also: vinzolidine sulfate]

**vinzolidine sulfate** USAN *antineoplastic* [also: vinzolidine]

**Vioform** cream, ointment (discontinued 2000) OTC *topical antifungal; antibacterial* [clioquinol] 3%

**Viogen-C** capsules OTC *vitamin/mineral supplement* [multiple B vitamins & minerals; vitamin C] ± • 300 mg

**Viokase** powder ℞ *porcine-derived digestive enzymes* [lipase; protease; amylase] 16 800 • 70 000 • 70 000 USP units/¼ tsp.

**Viokase 8; Viokase 16** tablets ℞ *porcine-derived digestive enzymes* [lipase; protease; amylase] 8000 • 30 000 • 30 000 USP units; 16 000 • 60 000 • 60 000 USP units

*Viola odorata* medicinal herb [see: violet]

*Viola tricolor* medicinal herb [see: pansy]

**violet** *(Viola odorata)* flowers and leaves *medicinal herb for asthma, bronchitis, cancer, colds, cough, sinus congestion, tumors, and ulcers*

**violet, garden** medicinal herb [see: pansy]

**violetbloom** medicinal herb [see: bittersweet nightshade]

**viomycin** INN [also: viomycin sulfate]

**viomycin sulfate** USP [also: viomycin]

**viosterol in oil** [see: ergocalciferol]

**Vioxx** tablets, oral suspension ℞ *analgesic; antiarthritic; antipyretic; COX-2 inhibitor; nonsteroidal anti-inflammatory drug (NSAID); treatment for acute migraine* [rofecoxib] 12.5, 25, 50 mg; 12.5, 25 mg/5 mL

**Viozan** ℞ *investigational treatment for chronic obstructive pulmonary disease (COPD)* [sibenadet HCl]

**VIP (VePesid, ifosfamide [with mesna rescue], Platinol)** *chemotherapy protocol for genitourinary cancers, testicular cancer, small cell lung cancer (SCLC), and non–small cell lung cancer (NSCLC)*

**VIP (vinblastine, ifosfamide [with mesna rescue], Platinol)** *chemotherapy protocol*

**VIP-B (VP-16, ifosfamide, Platinol, bleomycin)** *chemotherapy protocol*

**Viprinex** ⓒ subcu injection, IV infusion ℞ *anticoagulant for deep vein thrombosis (DVT) and severe chronic peripheral circulatory disorders; (investigational (orphan) in the U.S. for cardiopulmonary bypass in heparin-intolerant patients)* [ancrod] 70 IU/mL

**viprostol** USAN, INN, BAN *hypotensive; vasodilator*

**viprynium embonate** BAN *anthelmintic* [also: pyrvinium pamoate]

**viqualine** INN

**viquidil** INN

**Viquin Forte** cream (discontinued 2003) ℞ *hyperpigmentation bleaching agent* [hydroquinone (in a sunscreen base)] 4%

**Vira-A** ophthalmic ointment ℞ *topical antiviral for acute keratoconjunctivitis and recurrent epithelial keratitis due to herpes simplex virus infection* [vidarabine] 3%

**Viracept** film-coated tablets, powder for oral solution ℞ *antiretroviral; protease* *inhibitor for HIV-1 infection* [nelfinavir mesylate] 250, 650 mg; 50 mg/g

**Viractin** cream, gel (name changed to Cēpacol Viractin in 2001)

**Viramune** tablets, oral suspension ℞ *antiviral non-nucleoside reverse transcriptase inhibitor (NNRTI) for HIV-1 infections* [nevirapine] 200 mg; 50 mg/5 mL

**Viravan-DM** oral suspension, chewable tablets ℞ *pediatric antitussive, decongestant, and antihistamine* [dextromethorphan tannate; phenylephrine tannate; pyrilamine tannate] 25•12.5•30 mg/5 mL; 25•25•30 mg

**Viravan-S** pediatric oral suspension ℞ *decongestant antihistamine* [phenylephrine tannate; pyrilamine tannate] 12.5•30 mg/5 mL

**Viravan-T** pediatric chewable tablets ℞ *decongestant; antihistamine* [phenylephrine tannate; pyrilamine tannate] 25•30 mg

**Virazole** powder for inhalation aerosol ℞ *nucleoside antiviral for severe lower respiratory tract infections; investigational (orphan) for hemorrhagic fever with renal syndrome* [ribavirin] 6 g/vial (20 mg/mL reconstituted)

**Viread** film-coated tablets ℞ *antiviral; nucleotide reverse transcriptase inhibitor (NRTI) for HIV-1 infection* [tenofovir disoproxil fumarate] 300 mg

**Virend** ℞ *investigational (Phase II) antiviral for AIDS-related genital herpes* [crofelemer]

**Virginia mountain mint; Virginia thyme** *medicinal herb* [see: wild hyssop]

**Virginia silk** *medicinal herb* [see: milkweed]

**virginiamycin** USAN, INN *antibacterial; veterinary food additive*

**virginiamycin factor M₁** [see: virginiamycin]

**virginiamycin factor S** [see: virginiamycin]

**virgin's bower** *medicinal herb* [see: woodbine]

**viridofulvin** USAN, INN *antifungal*

**Virilon** capsules, IM injection ℞ *androgen for hypogonadism or testosterone deficiency in men, delayed puberty in boys, and metastatic breast cancer in women; also abused as a street drug* [methyltestosterone] 10 mg; 200 mg/mL

**Virogen Herpes** slide test for professional use *in vitro diagnostic aid for herpes simplex virus antigen in lesions or cell cultures* [latex agglutination test]

**Virogen Rotatest** slide test for professional use *in vitro diagnostic aid for fecal rotavirus* [latex agglutination test]

**Viroptic** Drop-Dose (eye drops) ℞ *ophthalmic antiviral for keratoconjunctivitis and epithelial keratitis due to herpes simplex virus infection* [trifluridine] 1%

**viroxime** USAN, INN *antiviral*

**viroxime component A** [see: zinviroxime]

**viroxime component B** [see: enviroxime]

**Viroxyn** oral gel OTC *germicide for cold sores/fever blisters* [benzalkonium chloride; isopropyl alcohol] 0.13%•70%

**Virulizin** *investigational (Phase III) macrophage activator for AIDS-related lymphomas, Kaposi sarcoma, and pancreatic cancer*

**Viscoat** prefilled syringes ℞ *viscoelastic agent for ophthalmic surgery* [hyaluronate sodium; chondroitin sulfate sodium] 30•40 mg/mL

**Viscum album** *medicinal herb* [see: mistletoe]

**Visicol** tablets ℞ *saline laxative; preprocedure bowel evacuant* [sodium phosphate (monobasic and dibasic)] 1.5 g (1.102•0.398 g)

**visilizumab** USAN *anti-CD3 monoclonal antibody for organ transplants, autoimmune diseases, and other T-lymphocyte disorders*

**visiluzumab** [now: visilizumab]

**Visine Allergy Relief** eye drops OTC *topical ophthalmic decongestant and astringent* [tetrahydrozoline HCl; zinc sulfate] 0.05%•0.25%

**Visine L.R.** eye drops OTC *topical ophthalmic decongestant and vasoconstrictor* [oxymetazoline HCl] 0.025%

**Visine Moisturizing** eye drops OTC *topical ophthalmic decongestant, vasoconstrictor, and lubricant* [tetrahydrozoline HCl; polyethylene glycol 400] 0.05% • 1%

**Vision** (trademarked device) OTC *needle-free insulin injection system*

**Vision Care Enzymatic Cleaner** tablets OTC *enzymatic cleaner for soft contact lenses* [pork pancreatin]

**Visipak** (trademarked packaging form) *reverse-numbered package*

**Visipaque 270; Visipaque 320** intra-arterial or IV injection ℞ *radiopaque contrast medium for CT, x-ray, and visceral digital subtraction angiography* [iodixanol (49.1% iodine)] 550 mg/mL (270 mg/mL); 652 mg/mL (320 mg/mL)

**Visken** tablets ℞ *antihypertensive; antianginal; β-blocker* [pindolol] 5, 10 mg

**visnadine** INN, BAN

**visnafylline** INN

**Vi-Sol** [see: Poly-Vi-Sol; Tri-Vi-Sol]

**Vistaril** capsules, oral suspension ℞ *anxiolytic; minor tranquilizer; antihistamine for allergic pruritus* [hydroxyzine pamoate] 25, 50, 100 mg; 25 mg/5 mL ② Restoril

**Vistaril** deep IM injection ℞ *anxiolytic; antiemetic; antihistamine for allergic pruritus; adjunct to preoperative or prepartum analgesia* [hydroxyzine HCl] 25 mg/mL ② Restoril; Zestril

**vistatolon** INN *antiviral* [also: statolon]

**Vistazine 50** IM injection (discontinued 2003) ℞ *anxiolytic; antiemetic; antihistamine for allergic pruritus* [hydroxyzine HCl] 50 mg/mL

**Vistide** IV infusion ℞ *nucleoside antiviral for AIDS-related cytomegalovirus retinitis* [cidofovir] 75 mg/mL

**Visual-Eyes** ophthalmic solution OTC *extraocular irrigating solution* [sterile isotonic solution]

**Visudyne** powder for IV infusion ℞ *treatment for subfoveal choroidal neovascularization (CNV) due to age-related macular degeneration (AMD), pathologic myopia, or ocular histoplasmosis; activated with the Opal Photoactivator laser* [verteporfin] 2 mg/mL (15 mg/vial)

**Vita-bee with C** Captabs (capsule-shaped tablets) OTC *vitamin supplement* [multiple B vitamins; vitamin C] ± • 300 mg

**Vita-Bob** softgel capsules OTC *vitamin supplement* [multiple vitamins; folic acid] ± • 0.4 mg

**Vita-C** crystals OTC *vitamin C supplement* [ascorbic acid] 4 g/tsp.

**VitaCarn** oral solution (discontinued 2001) ℞ *dietary amino acid for primary and secondary genetic carnitine deficiency (orphan) and end-stage renal disease (orphan); investigational (orphan) for pediatric cardiomyopathy* [levocarnitine]

**Vitafol** syrup ℞ *hematinic* [ferric pyrophosphate; multiple B vitamins; folic acid] 90 • ± • 0.75 mg/15 mL

**Vitafol; Vitafol-PN** film-coated caplets ℞ *hematinic; vitamin supplement* [ferrous fumarate; multiple vitamins; folic acid] 65 mg • ± • 1 mg

**Vita-Kid** chewable wafers OTC *vitamin supplement* [multiple vitamins; folic acid] ± • 0.3 mg

**Vital B-50** timed-release tablets OTC *vitamin supplement* [multiple B vitamins; folic acid; biotin] ± • 100 • 50 μg

**Vital High Nitrogen** powder OTC *enteral nutritional therapy* [lactose-free formula] 79 g

**Vitalets** chewable tablets OTC *vitamin/mineral/iron supplement* [multiple vitamins & minerals; iron; biotin] ± • 10 mg • 25 μg

**Vitalize SF** oral liquid OTC *hematinic* [ferric pyrophosphate; multiple B vitamins; lysine] 66 • ± • 300 mg/15 mL

**Vitalux** ⓐ time-release tablet OTC *vitamin/antioxidant supplement* [multiple vitamins; multiple minerals]

**vitamin A** USP *fat-soluble vitamin; antixerophthalmic; topical emollient; essen-*

tial for vision, dental development, growth, cortisone synthesis, epithelial tissue differentiation, embryonic development, reproduction, and mucous membrane maintenance 10 000, 15 000, 25 000 IU oral

**vitamin A acid** [see: tretinoin]

**vitamin A palmitate**

**vitamin A₁** [see: retinol]

**Vitamin B Complex 100** injection ℞ parenteral vitamin therapy [multiple B vitamins]

**vitamin B₁** [see: thiamine HCl]

**vitamin B₁ mononitrate** [see: thiamine mononitrate]

**vitamin B₂** [see: riboflavin]

**vitamin B₃** [see: niacin; niacinamide]

**vitamin B₅** [see: calcium pantothenate]

**vitamin B₆** [see: pyridoxine HCl]

**vitamin B₈** [see: adenosine phosphate]

**vitamin B₁₂** [now: cyanocobalamin; hydroxocobalamin]

**vitamin B_c** [see: folic acid]

**vitamin B_t** [see: carnitine]

**vitamin C** [see: ascorbic acid; calcium ascorbate; sodium ascorbate]

**vitamin D** a family of fat-soluble vitamins consisting of ergocalciferol (vitamin $D_2$) and cholecalciferol (vitamin $D_3$), which is converted to calcitriol (the active form) in the body; considered a non-endogenous hormone [see also: calcifediol; dihydrotachysterol; doxercalciferol; paricalcitol]

**vitamin D₁** [see: dihydrotachysterol]

**vitamin D₂** [see: ergocalciferol]

**vitamin D₃** [see: cholecalciferol]

**vitamin E** USP fat-soluble vitamin; antioxidant; platelet aggregation inhibitor; topical emollient [note relative potencies at alpha tocopherol, et seq.] 100, 200, 400, 500, 800, 1000 IU oral; 15 IU/30 mL oral

**Vitamin E with Mixed Tocopherols** tablets OTC vitamin supplement [vitamin E] 100, 200, 400 IU

**vitamin E-TPGS (tocopheryl polyethylene glycol succinate)** [see: tocophersolan]

**vitamin G** [see: riboflavin]

**vitamin H** [see: biotin]

**vitamin K₁** [see: phytonadione]

**vitamin K₂** [see: menaquinone]

**vitamin K₃** [see: menadione]

**vitamin K₄** [see: menadiol sodium diphosphate]

**vitamin M** [see: folic acid]

**vitamin P** [see: bioflavonoids]

**vitamin P₄** [see: troxerutin]

**Vitamin-Mineral Supplement** oral liquid OTC vitamin/mineral supplement [multiple B vitamins & minerals; alcohol 18%]

**Vitaneed** oral liquid OTC enteral nutritional therapy [lactose-free formula]

**Vita-Plus E** softgels OTC vitamin supplement [vitamin E (as d-alpha tocopheryl acetate)] 400 IU

**Vita-Plus G** softgel capsules OTC geriatric vitamin/mineral supplement [multiple vitamins & minerals]

**Vita-Plus H** softgel capsules OTC vitamin/mineral/iron supplement [multiple vitamins & minerals; iron] ± • 13.4 mg

**Vita-PMS; Vita-PMS Plus** tablets OTC vitamin/mineral supplement; digestive enzymes [multiple vitamins & minerals; folic acid; biotin; amylase; protease; lipase; betaine acid HCl] ± • 0.33 mg • 10.4 μg • 2500 U • 2500 U • 200 U • 16.7 mg

**Vitarex** tablets OTC vitamin/mineral/iron supplement [multiple vitamins & minerals; iron] ± • 15 mg

**Vite E** cream OTC emollient [vitamin E] 50 mg/g

**Vitec** cream OTC emollient [vitamin E]

**Vitelle Irospan** timed-release tablets, timed-release capsules OTC hematinic; iron supplement [iron (from ferrous sulfate, dried); ascorbic acid] 65 • 150 mg

**Vitelle Lurline PMS** tablets OTC analgesic; antipyretic; diuretic; vitamin B₆ [acetaminophen; pamabrom; pyridoxine HCl] 500 • 25 • 50 mg

**Vitelle Nesentials** tablets OTC vitamin/mineral supplement [multiple vitamins & minerals]

**Vitelle Nestabs OTC** tablets OTC *prenatal vitamin/calcium/iron supplement* [multiple vitamins; calcium; iron; folic acid] ±•200•29•0.8 mg

**Vitelle Nestrex** tablets OTC *vitamin B$_6$ supplement* [pyridoxine HCl]

**vitellin** *natural remedy* [see: lecithin]

**Vitex agnus-castus** *medicinal herb* [see: chaste tree]

**Vitinoin** ⒸⒶⓃ cream, gel (discontinued 2001) ℞ *keratolytic for acne* [tretinoin] 0.025%, 0.05%, 0.1%; 0.025%

**Vitis coigetiae; V. vinifera** *medicinal herb* [see: grape seed]

**Vitrase** ℞ *investigational (NDA filed) agent to clear vitreous hemorrhage* [hyaluronidase]

**Vitrasert** intraocular implant (5–8 months' duration) ℞ *antiviral for AIDS-related CMV retinitis (orphan)* [ganciclovir] 4.5 mg

**Vitravene** intravitreal injection ℞ *ophthalmic antiviral for AIDS-related CMV retinitis* [fomivirsen sodium] 6.6 mg/mL

**Vitron-C** chewable tablets OTC *hematinic* [iron (from ferrous fumarate); ascorbic acid] 66•125 mg ⑨ Vytone

**Vitussin** syrup ℞ *narcotic antitussive; expectorant* [hydrocodone bitartrate; guaifenesin] 5•100 mg/5 mL

**Vivactil** film-coated tablets ℞ *tricyclic antidepressant* [protriptyline HCl] 5, 10 mg

**Viva-Drops** eye drops OTC *ocular moisturizer/lubricant*

**Vivarin** tablets OTC *CNS stimulant; analeptic* [caffeine] 200 mg

**Vivelle; Vivelle-Dot** transdermal patch ℞ *estrogen replacement therapy for the treatment of postmenopausal symptoms and prevention of postmenopausal osteoporosis* [estradiol] 37.5, 50, 75, 100 μg/day

**Vivitrex** extended-release injection ℞ *investigational (Phase III) treatment for alcoholism; investigational (Phase I) treatment for opiate addiction* [naltrexone HCl]

**Vivonex T.E.N.** powder OTC *enteral nutritional therapy* [lactose-free formula]

**Vivotif Berna** enteric-coated capsules ℞ *typhoid fever vaccine* [typhoid vaccine (Ty21a), live attenuated] 2–6 × 10$^9$ viable CFU + 5–50 × 10$^9$ nonviable cells

**Vi-Zac** capsules OTC *vitamin/zinc supplement* [vitamins A, C, and E; zinc] 5000 IU•500 mg•50 mg•18 mg

**VLP (vincristine, L-asparaginase, prednisone)** *chemotherapy protocol*

**VM (vinblastine, mitomycin)** *chemotherapy protocol for breast cancer*

**VM-26** [see: teniposide]

**VM-26PP (teniposide, procarbazine, prednisone)** *chemotherapy protocol*

**VMAD (vincristine, methotrexate, Adriamycin, actinomycin D)** *chemotherapy protocol*

**VMCP (vincristine, melphalan, cyclophosphamide, prednisone)** *chemotherapy protocol for multiple myeloma* [also: VCMP]

**VMP (VePesid, mitoxantrone, prednimustine)** *chemotherapy protocol*

**VOCAP (VP-16-213, Oncovin, cyclophosphamide, Adriamycin, Platinol)** *chemotherapy protocol*

**Vofenal** ⒸⒶⓃ eye drops (discontinued 2001) ℞ *topical nonsteroidal antiinflammatory drug (NSAID)* [diclofenac sodium] 0.1%

**vofopitant dihydrochloride** USAN *tachykinin NK$_1$ receptor antagonist; antiemetic*

**voglibose** USAN *investigational α-glucosidase inhibitor; antidiabetic*

**volatile nitrites** *amyl nitrite, butyl nitrite, and isobutyl nitrite vapors that produce coronary stimulant effects, abused as street drugs* [see also: nitrous oxide; petroleum distillate inhalants]

**volazocine** USAN, INN *analgesic*

**Volmax** extended-release tablets (discontinued 2004) ℞ *sympathomimetic bronchodilator* [albuterol sulfate] 4, 8 mg

**Voltaren** delayed-release tablets ℞ *analgesic; antiarthritic; nonsteroidal anti-inflammatory drug (NSAID) for ankylosing spondylitis* [diclofenac sodium] 25, 50, 75 mg

**Voltaren** eye drops ℞ *ocular nonsteroidal anti-inflammatory drug (NSAID) for postoperative treatment following cataract extraction* [diclofenac sodium] 0.1%

**Voltaren** ⒸⒶⓃ suppositories ℞ *analgesic; antiarthritic; nonsteroidal anti-inflammatory drug (NSAID)* [diclofenac sodium] 50, 100 mg

**Voltaren Ophtha** ⒸⒶⓃ eye drops ℞ *ocular nonsteroidal anti-inflammatory drug (NSAID) for postoperative treatment following cataract extraction* [diclofenac sodium] 0.1%

**Voltaren Rapide** ⒸⒶⓃ tablets ℞ *analgesic; antiarthritic; nonsteroidal anti-inflammatory drug (NSAID)* [diclofenac potassium] 50 mg

**Voltaren SR** ⒸⒶⓃ slow-release tablets ℞ *once-daily antiarthritic; nonsteroidal anti-inflammatory drug (NSAID)* [diclofenac sodium] 75, 100 mg

**Voltaren XR** extended-release tablets ℞ *once-daily antiarthritic; nonsteroidal anti-inflammatory drug (NSAID)* [diclofenac sodium] 100 mg

**von Willebrand factor (VWF)** *antihemophilic for von Willebrand disease*

**voriconazole** *triazole antifungal for invasive aspergillosis, esophageal candidiasis, and other serious fungal infections*

**vorozole** USAN, INN, BAN *antineoplastic; aromatase inhibitor*

**vortel** [see: clorprenaline HCl]

**VōSol HC Otic** ear drops ℞ *topical corticosteroidal anti-inflammatory; antibacterial; antifungal* [hydrocortisone; acetic acid] 1% • 2%

**VōSol Otic** ear drops ℞ *antibacterial; antifungal* [acetic acid] 2%

**VoSpire ER** extended-release tablets ℞ *sympathomimetic bronchodilator* [albuterol sulfate] 4, 8 mg

**votumumab** USAN *monoclonal antibody for cancer imaging and therapy*

**Voxsuprine** tablets ℞ *peripheral vasodilator* [isoxsuprine HCl] 10, 20 mg

**VP (vasopressin)** [q.v.]

**VP (VePesid, Platinol)** *chemotherapy protocol for small cell lung cancer (SCLC)*

**VP (vincristine, prednisone)** *chemotherapy protocol*

**VP + A (vincristine, prednisone, asparaginase)** *chemotherapy protocol*

**VP-16** [see: etoposide]

**VPB (vinblastine, Platinol, bleomycin)** *chemotherapy protocol*

**VPBCPr (vincristine, prednisone, vinblastine, chlorambucil, procarbazine)** *chemotherapy protocol*

**VPCA (vincristine, prednisone, cyclophosphamide, ara-C)** *chemotherapy protocol*

**VPCMF (vincristine, prednisone, cyclophosphamide, methotrexate, fluorouracil)** *chemotherapy protocol*

**VP-L-asparaginase (vincristine, prednisone, L-asparaginase)** *chemotherapy protocol*

**VPP (VePesid, Platinol)** *chemotherapy protocol*

**VT-1** *investigational stem cell transplant adjunct for multiple myeloma and other blood-related cancers*

**V-TAD (VePesid, thioguanine, ara-C, daunorubicin)** *chemotherapy protocol for acute myelocytic leukemia (AML)*

**vulneraries** *a class of agents that promote wound healing*

**Vumon** IV infusion ℞ *antineoplastic for acute lymphocytic leukemia (orphan) and bladder cancer* [teniposide] 50 mg (10 mg/mL)

**V.V.S.** vaginal cream (discontinued 2001) ℞ *broad-spectrum antibiotic* [sulfathiazole; sulfacetamide; sulfabenzamide] 3.42% • 2.86% • 3.7%

**VWF (von Willebrand factor)** [q.v.]

**VX-175** *investigational (Phase III) protease inhibitor for HIV infections*

**Vytone** cream ℞ *topical corticosteroidal anti-inflammatory; antifungal; antibacterial* [hydrocortisone; iodoquinol] 1% • 1% ② Hytone; Vitron

**Vytorin 10/10; Vytorin 10/20; Vytorin 10/40; Vytorin 10/80** caplets ℞ *antihyperlipidemic for hypercholesterolemia; intestinal cholesterol absorption inhibitor; HMG-CoA reductase inhibitor* [ezetimibe; simvastatin] 10•10 mg; 10•20 mg; 10•40 mg; 10•80 mg

**VZIG (varicella-zoster immune globulin)** [q.v.]

patient compliance package for oral contraceptives

**wallflower; western wallflower** *medicinal herb* [see: dogbane]

**walnut (Juglans spp.)** *medicinal herb* [see: black walnut; butternut; English walnut]

**walnut, lemon; white walnut** *medicinal herb* [see: butternut]

**Walpole tea** *medicinal herb* [see: New Jersey tea]

**wandering milkweed** *medicinal herb* [see: dogbane]

**warfarin** INN, BAN *coumarin-derivative anticoagulant* [also: warfarin potassium]

**warfarin potassium** USP *coumarin-derivative anticoagulant* [also: warfarin]

**warfarin sodium** USP *coumarin-derivative anticoagulant* 1, 2, 2.5, 3, 4, 5, 6, 7.5, 10 mg oral

**Wart Remover** topical liquid OTC *keratolytic* [salicylic acid in flexible collodion] 17%

**Wartec** ⒸⒶⓃ solution ℞ *antimitotic for external genital warts* [podofilox] 0.5%

**Wart-Off** topical liquid OTC *keratolytic* [salicylic acid in flexible collodion] 17%

**water, purified** USP *solvent*

**water, tritiated** [see: tritiated water]

**water cabbage** *medicinal herb* [see: white pond lily]

**water dock (Rumex aquaticus)** *medicinal herb* [see: yellow dock]

**water eryngo (Eryngium aquaticum)** root *medicinal herb used as a diaphoretic, diuretic, emetic, expectorant, and stimulant*

**water fern** *medicinal herb* [see: buckhorn brake]

**water flag** *medicinal herb* [see: blue flag]

**water hemlock; water parsley** *medicinal herb* [see: poison hemlock]

**water lily** *medicinal herb* [see: blue flag; white pond lily]

**water lily, sweet; sweet-scented water lily; white water lily** *medicinal herb* [see: white pond lily]

**water moccasin snake antivenin** [see: antivenin (Crotalidae) polyvalent]

**water O 15** USAN *radioactive diagnostic aid for vascular disorders*

**water pepper** *medicinal herb* [see: knotweed]

**water pimpernel; water purslain** *medicinal herb* [see: brooklime]

**water shamrock** *medicinal herb* [see: buckbean]

**water smartweed** *medicinal herb* [see: knotweed]

**[¹⁵O]water** [see: water O 15]

**watercress (Nasturtium officinale)** plant *medicinal herb for anemia, cramps, kidney and liver disorders, nervousness, and rheumatism*

**water-d₂** [see: deuterium oxide]

**wax, carnauba** NF *tablet-coating agent*

**wax, emulsifying** NF *emulsifying and stiffening agent*

**wax, microcrystalline** NF *stiffening and tablet-coating agent*

**wax, white** NF *stiffening agent* [also: beeswax, white]

**wax, yellow** NF *stiffening agent* [also: beeswax, yellow]

**wax cluster** *medicinal herb* [see: wintergreen]

**wax myrtle** *medicinal herb* [see: bayberry]

**weeping spruce** *medicinal herb* [see: hemlock]

**WelChol** tablets ℞ *nonabsorbable cholesterol-lowering polymer for hyperlipidemia* [colesevelam HCl] 625 mg

**Wellbutrin** film-coated tablets ℞ *aminoketone antidepressant* [bupropion HCl] 75, 100 mg

**Wellbutrin SR** sustained-release film-coated tablets ℞ *aminoketone antidepressant* [bupropion HCl] 100, 150, 200 mg

**Wellbutrin XL** extended-release tablets ℞ *aminoketone antidepressant* [bupropion HCl] 150, 300 mg

**Wellcovorin** powder for IV infusion (discontinued 2002) ℞ *chemotherapy "rescue" agent (orphan)* [leucovorin calcium] 100 mg/vial

**Wellcovorin** tablets (discontinued 2002) ℞ *chemotherapy "rescue" agent (orphan); antidote to folic acid antagonist overdose* [leucovorin calcium] 5, 25 mg

**Wellferon** subcu or IM injection (discontinued 2000) ℞ *biological response modifier for chronic hepatitis C (orphan); investigational (Phase III) for HIV* [interferon alfa-n1] 3 MU/mL (a MU or "megaunit" is 10⁶ IU)

**Wellferon** ⒸⒶⓃ subcu or IM injection (discontinued 2001) ℞ *biological response modifier for hairy cell leukemia, laryngeal papillomatosis, condylomata acuminata, and chronic hepatitis B and C* [interferon alfa-n1] 3, 5, 10 MU/mL (a MU or "megaunit" is 10⁶ IU)

**Westcort** ointment, cream ℞ *corticosteroidal anti-inflammatory* [hydrocortisone valerate] 0.2%

**western wallflower** *medicinal herb* [see: dogbane]

**Westhroid** tablets ℞ *thyroid replacement therapy for hypothyroidism or thyroid*

*cancer* [thyroid, desiccated (porcine)] 32.4, 64.8, 129.6, 194.4 mg

**Wet-N-Soak** solution OTC *rewetting solution for rigid gas permeable contact lenses*

**Wet-N-Soak Plus** solution OTC *disinfecting/wetting/soaking solution for rigid gas permeable contact lenses* [note: RGP contact indication different from hard contact indication for same product]

**Wet-N-Soak Plus** solution OTC *wetting/soaking solution for hard contact lenses* [note: hard contact indication different from RGP contact indication for same product]

**Wetting** solution OTC *wetting solution for hard contact lenses*

**Wetting & Soaking** solution OTC *disinfecting/wetting/soaking solution for rigid gas permeable contact lenses* [note: one of two different products with the same name]

**Wetting & Soaking** solution OTC *wetting/soaking solution for hard contact lenses* [note: one of two different products with the same name]

**wheat germ oil (octacosanol)** *natural dietary supplement for increasing muscle endurance*

**WHF Lubricating Gel** OTC *vaginal antimicrobial and lubricant* [chlorhexidine gluconate; glycerin]

**white bay** *medicinal herb* [see: magnolia]

**white beeswax** [see: beeswax, white]

**White Cloverine Salve** ointment OTC *skin protectant* [white petrolatum] 97%

**White Cod Liver Oil Concentrate** capsules, chewable tablets OTC *vitamin supplement* [vitamins A, D, and E] 10 000•400• ≟ IU; 4000•200• ≟ IU

**White Cod Liver Oil Concentrate with Vitamin C** chewable tablets OTC *vitamin supplement* [vitamins A, C, and D] 4000 IU•50 mg•200 IU

**white cohosh** *(Actaea alba; A. pachypoda; A. rubra)* plant and root *medicinal herb for arthritis, bowel evacuation, colds, cough, itching, promoting labor, reviving those near death,* *rheumatism, stimulating menses, stomach disorders, and urogenital disorders*

**white endive** *medicinal herb* [see: dandelion]

**white fringe** *medicinal herb* [see: fringe tree]

**white hellebore (Veratrum album)** [see: hellebore]

**white horehound** *medicinal herb* [see: horehound]

**white lotion** USP *astringent; topical protectant*

**white mineral oil** [see: petrolatum, white]

**white mustard; white mustard seed** *medicinal herb* [see: mustard]

**white nettle** *medicinal herb* [see: blind nettle]

**white oak (Quercus alba)** bark *medicinal herb for internal and external bleeding, menstrual disorders, mouth sores, skin irritation, toothache, strep throat, ulcers, and urinary bleeding*

**white ointment** [see: ointment, white]

**white petrolatum** [see: petrolatum, white]

**white phenolphthalein** [see: phenolphthalein]

**white pine (Pinus strobus)** bark *medicinal herb for bronchitis, dysentery, laryngitis, and mucous build-up*

**white pond lily (Nymphaea odorata)** root *medicinal herb used as an antiseptic, astringent, demulcent, discutient, and vulnerary*

**white root** *medicinal herb* [see: pleurisy root]

**white sorrel** *medicinal herb* [see: wood sorrel]

**white walnut** *medicinal herb* [see: butternut]

**white water lily** *medicinal herb* [see: white pond lily]

**white wax** [see: wax, white]

**white willow (Salix alba)** *medicinal herb* [see: willow]

**whitethorn** *medicinal herb* [see: hawthorn]

**Whitfield's Ointment** OTC *antifungal; keratolytic* [benzoic acid; salicylic acid] 6%•3%

**Whitfield's ointment** [see: benzoic & salicylic acids]

**whole blood** [see: blood, whole]

**whole root rauwolfia** [see: rauwolfia serpentina]

**whole-cell pertussis vaccine** [see: diphtheria & tetanus toxoids & whole-cell pertussis (DTwP) vaccine, adsorbed]

**whorlywort** *medicinal herb* [see: Culver root]

**Wibi** lotion OTC *moisturizer; emollient*

**widow spider species antivenin** [now: antivenin (Latrodectus mactans)]

**Wigraine** suppositories ℞ *migraine-specific vasoconstrictor* [ergotamine tartrate; caffeine; tartaric acid] 2•100•21.5 mg

**Wigraine** tablets ℞ *migraine-specific vasoconstrictor* [ergotamine tartrate; caffeine] 1•100 mg

**wild bergamot (Monarda fistulosa)** leaves *medicinal herb used as a carminative and stimulant*

**wild black cherry (Prunus serotina)** bark *medicinal herb used as an astringent, pectoral, sedative, and stimulant*

**wild carrot** *medicinal herb* [see: carrot]

**wild cherry (Prunus virginiana)** bark *medicinal herb for asthma, bronchitis, cough, fever, hypertension, and mucosal inflammation with discharge; also used as an expectorant*

**wild cherry syrup** USP

**wild chicory** *medicinal herb* [see: chicory]

**wild clover** *medicinal herb* [see: red clover]

**wild cranesbill** *medicinal herb* [see: alum root]

**wild daisy (Bellis perennis)** flowers and leaves *medicinal herb used as an analgesic, antispasmodic, demulcent, digestive, expectorant, laxative, and purgative*

**wild endive** *medicinal herb* [see: dandelion]

**wild fennel** *medicinal herb* [see: fennel]

**wild geranium** *medicinal herb* [see: alum root]

**wild ginger (Asarum canadense)** root *medicinal herb used as a carminative, diaphoretic, expectorant, and irritant; sometimes used as a substitute for ginger (Zingiber)*

**wild hydrangea** *medicinal herb* [see: hydrangea]

**wild hyssop** *medicinal herb* [see: blue vervain]

**wild hyssop (Pycnanthemum virginianum)** plant *medicinal herb used as an antispasmodic, carminative, diaphoretic, and stimulant*

**wild indigo (Baptisia tinctoria)** plant *medicinal herb used as an antiseptic, astringent, emetic, purgative, and stimulant*

**wild jalap (Ipomoea pandurata)** root *medicinal herb used as a strong cathartic*

**wild lemon** *medicinal herb* [see: mandrake]

**wild lettuce (Lactuca virosa)** leaves, flowers, and seeds *medicinal herb for asthma, bronchitis, chronic pain, circulatory disorders, cramps, laryngitis, nervous disorders, stimulating lactation, swollen genitals, and urinary tract infections*

**wild marjoram** *medicinal herb* [see: marjoram]

**wild Oregon grape** *medicinal herb* [see: Oregon grape]

**wild pepper** *medicinal herb* [see: mezereon; Siberian ginseng]

**wild potato; wild scammony; wild sweet potato vine** *medicinal herb* [see: wild jalap]

**wild red raspberry** *medicinal herb* [see: red raspberry]

**wild senna** *medicinal herb* [see: senna]

**wild snowball** *medicinal herb* [see: New Jersey tea]

**wild strawberry** *medicinal herb* [see: strawberry]

**wild tobacco** *medicinal herb* [see: lobelia]

**wild turkey pea** *medicinal herb* [see: turkey corn]

**wild valerian, great** *medicinal herb* [see: valerian]

**wild woodbine** *medicinal herb* [see: American ivy]

**wild yam (Dioscorea villosa)** root *medicinal herb for arthritis, bilious colic, bowel spasms, gas, menstrual cramps, morning sickness, and spasmodic asthma*

**Willard water** *natural remedy for acne, alopecia, anxiety, arthritis, hypertension, and stomach ulcers*

**willow (Salix alba; S. caprea; S. nigra; S. purpurea)** bark and buds *medicinal herb for analgesia, diuresis, eczema, fever, inducing diaphoresis, headache, nervousness, rheumatism, and ulcerations; also used as an anaphrodisiac, antiseptic, and astringent*

**wind root** *medicinal herb* [see: pleurisy root]

**wineberry** *medicinal herb* [see: currant]

**winged elm** *medicinal herb* [see: slippery elm]

**WinRho SD** IV or IM injection (discontinued 2000; replaced by WinRho SDF) ℞ *obstetric Rh factor immunity suppressant; treatment for immune thrombocytopenic purpura (orphan)* [Rh$_O$(D) immune globulin, solvent/detergent treated] 600, 1500, 5000 IU (120, 300, 1000 μg)

**WinRho SDF** freeze-dried powder for IV or IM injection ℞ *obstetric Rh factor immunity suppressant; treatment for immune thrombocytopenic purpura (orphan)* [Rh$_O$(D) immune globulin, solvent/detergent treated] 600, 1500, 5000 IU (120, 300, 1000 μg)

**Winstrol** tablets ℞ *anabolic steroid for hereditary angioedema* [stanozolol] 2 mg

**winter bloom** *medicinal herb* [see: witch hazel]

**winter clover** *medicinal herb* [see: squaw vine]

**winter marjoram; winter sweet** *medicinal herb* [see: marjoram]

**winter savory (Calamintha montana; Satureja montana; S. obovata)** leaves and stems *medicinal herb for* diarrhea, nausea, promoting expectoration, relieving gas and flatulence, and stimulation of menstruation; also used as an aphrodisiac

**winterberry (Ilex verticillata)** bark and fruit medicinal herb used as an astringent, bitter tonic, and febrifuge

**wintergreen (Gaultheria procumbens)** leaves and oil medicinal herb for aches and pains, colds, gout, lumbago, and migraine headache; also used topically as an astringent and rubefacient

**wintergreen, bitter; false wintergreen** medicinal herb [see: pipsissewa]

**wintergreen oil** [see: methyl salicylate]

**winterlein** medicinal herb [see: flaxseed]

**Wintersteiner's compound F** [see: hydrocortisone]

**winterweed** medicinal herb [see: chickweed]

**witch hazel (Hamamelis virginiana)** bark medicinal herb for bruises, burns, colds, colitis, diarrhea, dysentery, eye irritations, hemorrhoids, internal and external bleeding, mucous membrane inflammation of mouth, gums, and throat, tuberculosis, and varicose veins

**withania (Withania somnifera)** fruit and roots medicinal herb for diuresis, inducing emesis, liver disorders, inflammation, sedation, tuberculosis, and tumors

**withe; withy** medicinal herb [see: willow]

**wobe-mugos** investigational (orphan) enzyme combination adjunct to chemotherapy for multiple myeloma

**wolf claw** medicinal herb [see: club moss]

**Women's Daily Formula** capsules OTC vitamin/calcium/iron supplement [multiple vitamins; calcium; iron; folic acid] ≟•450•25•0.4 mg

**Women's Gentle Laxative** enteric-coated tablets OTC stimulant laxative [bisacodyl] 5 mg

**Wonder Ice** gel OTC topical analgesic; counterirritant [menthol] 5.25%

**Wondra** lotion OTC moisturizer; emollient [lanolin]

**wood betony** medicinal herb [see: betony]

**wood creosote** [see: creosote carbonate]

**wood sanicle** medicinal herb [see: sanicle]

**wood sorrel (Oxalis acetosella)** plant medicinal herb used as an anodyne, diuretic, emmenagogue, irritant, and stomachic

**wood strawberry** medicinal herb [see: strawberry]

**woodbine (Clematis virginiana)** leaves medicinal herb for bowel evacuation, cancer, edema, fever, hypertension, inflammation, insomnia, itching, kidney disorders, skin cuts and sores, tuberculous cervical lymphadenitis, tumors, and venereal eruptions; not generally regarded as safe and effective

**woodbine; American woodbine; wild woodbine** medicinal herb [see: American ivy]

**woodruff** medicinal herb [see: sweet woodruff]

**woody nightshade** medicinal herb [see: bittersweet nightshade]

**Woolley's antiserotonin** [see: benanserin HCl]

**wooly parsnip** medicinal herb [see: masterwort]

**wormwood (Artemisia absinthium)** plant and leaves medicinal herb for aiding digestion, constipation, debility, fever, intestinal worms, jaundice, labor pains, menstrual cramps, and stomach and liver disorders; not generally regarded as safe and effective

**wound weed** medicinal herb [see: goldenrod]

**woundwort (Prunella vulgaris)** plant medicinal herb used as an antispasmodic, astringent, bitter tonic, diuretic, hemostatic, vermifuge, and vulnerary

**woundwort, soldier's** medicinal herb [see: yarrow]

**WOWtabs** (trademarked dosage form) quickly dissolving "without water" tablets

**WX-G250RIT** investigational (orphan) antineoplastic for renal cell carcinoma

**Wyamine Sulfate** IV or IM injection ℞ vasopressor for hypotensive shock

[mephentermine sulfate] 15, 30 mg/mL

**Wyanoids Relief Factor** rectal suppositories OTC *emollient* [cocoa butter; shark liver oil] 79%•3%

**Wycillin** IM, IV, intrapleural, or intrathecal injection, Tubex (cartridge-needle units) (discontinued 2003) ℞ *natural penicillin antibiotic* [penicillin G procaine] 600 000, 1 200 000 U/vial ② Bicillin; V-Cillin

**Wydase** IV or subcu injection, powder for injection (discontinued 2001) ℞ *adjuvant to increase absorption and dis-*

*persion of injected drugs* [hyaluronidase] 150 U/mL; 150, 1500 U/vial ② Lidex

**Wygesic** tablets (discontinued 2004) ℞ *narcotic analgesic* [propoxyphene HCl; acetaminophen] 65•650 mg

**wymote** *medicinal herb* [see: marsh mallow]

**Wymox** capsules, powder for oral suspension (discontinued 2002) ℞ *aminopenicillin antibiotic* [amoxicillin] 250, 500 mg; 125, 250 mg/5 mL

**Wyseal** (trademarked dosage form) *film-coated tablet*

**Wytensin** tablets ℞ *antihypertensive* [guanabenz acetate] 4, 8 mg

**Xalatan** eye drops ℞ *prostaglandin agonist for glaucoma and ocular hypertension* [latanoprost] 0.005% (50 µg/mL) ② Dilantin

**Xalcom** ℞ *investigational (NDA filed) combination agent for glaucoma and ocular hypertension* [latanoprost; timolol]

**xaliprodene** *investigational (Phase III) nerve growth factor–like agent for amyotrophic lateral sclerosis; investigational (Phase II) for Alzheimer disease*

**xamoterol** USAN, INN, BAN *cardiac stimulant*

**xamoterol fumarate** USAN *cardiac stimulant*

**Xanax** tablets ℞ *benzodiazepine anxiolytic; sedative; treatment for panic disorders and agoraphobia* [alprazolam] 0.25, 0.5, 1, 2 mg ② Tenex; Zantac

**Xanax XR** extended-release tablets ℞ *benzodiazepine anxiolytic for panic disorder and agoraphobia* [alprazolam] 0.5, 1, 2, 3 mg

**xanomeline** USAN *cholinergic agonist for Alzheimer disease*

**xanomeline tartrate** USAN *cholinergic agonist for Alzheimer disease*

**xanoxate sodium** USAN *bronchodilator*

**xanoxic acid** INN

**xan**

**xan** *ci*

**xan** *v*

**xanthiol** INN

**xanthiol HCl** [see: xanthiol]

**xanthocillin** BAN [also: xantocillin]

*Xanthorhiza simplicissima* *medicinal herb* [see: yellow root]

**xanthotoxin** [see: methoxsalen]

*Xanthoxylum americanum; X. fraxineum* *medicinal herb* [see: prickly ash]

**xantifibrate** INN

**xantinol nicotinate** INN *peripheral vasodilator* [also: xanthinol niacinate]

**xantocillin** INN [also: xanthocillin]

**xantofyl palmitate** INN

**Xatral** (foreign name for U.S. product Uroxatral)

**Xcytrin** injection ℞ *investigational (Phase III) radiosensitizer for brain metastases* [motexafin gadolinium]

$^{127}$**Xe** [see: xenon Xe 127]

$^{133}$**Xe** [see: xenon Xe 133]

**Xeloda** film-coated tablets ℞ *antineoplastic for metastatic breast and colorectal cancer; investigational (Phase III)* *for pancreatic cancer* [capecitabine] 150, 500 mg

**xemilofiban HCl** USAN *antianginal*

**xenalamine** [see: xenazoic acid]

**xenaldial** [see: xenygloxal]

**xenalipin** USAN, INN *hypolipidemic*

**xenazoic acid** INN

**xenbucin** USAN, INN *antihypercholesterolemic*

**xenbuficin** [see: xenbucin]

**Xenical** capsules ℞ *lipase inhibitor for weight loss; investigational (Phase III) preventative for type 2 diabetes* [orlistat] 120 mg

**xenipentone** INN

**xenon** *element (Xe)*

**xenon** ($^{133}$Xe) INN *radioactive agent* [also: xenon Xe 133]

**xenon Xe 127** USP *diagnostic aid; medicinal gas; radioactive agent*

**xenon Xe 133** USAN, USP *radioactive agent* [also: xenon ($^{133}$Xe)]

**xenthiorate** INN

**xenygloxal** INN

**xenyhexenic acid** INN

**xenysalate** INN, BAN *topical anesthetic; antibacterial; antifungal* [also: biphenamine HCl]

**xenysalate HCl** [see: biphenamine HCl]

**xenytropium bromide** INN

**Xerac AC** topical liquid ℞ *cleanser for acne* [aluminum chloride; alcohol] 6.25%•96%

**Xerecept** *investigational (Phase I/II, orphan) agent for peritumoral brain edema* [corticotropin-releasing factor]

**xibenolol** INN

**xibornol** INN, BAN

**Xifaxan** film-coated tablets ℞ *broadspectrum rifamycin antibiotic for traveler's diarrhea* [rifaximin] 200 mg

**Xigris** IV infusion ℞ *recombinant human activated protein C (rhAPC) for severe sepsis* [drotrecogin alfa] 5, 20 mg/vial

**xilobam** USAN, INN *muscle relaxant*

**ximelagatran** *investigational (NDA filed) oral anticoagulant and direct thrombin inhibitor for the prevention of* *stroke due to atrial fibrillation and the prevention and treatment of a venous thromboembolic event (VTE); prodrug of melagatran*

**ximoprofen** INN

**xinafoate** USAN, INN, BAN *combining name for radicals or groups*

**xinidamine** INN

**xinomiline** INN

**xipamide** USAN, INN *antihypertensive; diuretic*

**xipranolol** INN

**Xiral** sustained-release caplets ℞ *decongestant; antihistamine; anticholinergic to dry mucosal secretions* [pseudoephedrine HCl; chlorpheniramine maleate; methscopolamine nitrate] 120•8•2.5 mg

**Xolair** powder for subcu injection ℞ *immunoglobulin E (IgE) blocker for moderate to severe asthma* [omalizumab] 150 mg/1.2 mL dose

**XomaZyme-791** *investigational (orphan) for metastatic colorectal adenocarcinoma* [anti-TAP-72 immunotoxin]

**Xopenex** inhalation solution ℞ *sympathomimetic bronchodilator* [levalbuterol HCl] 0.31, 0.63, 1.25 mg/3 mL dose

**xorphanol** INN *analgesic* [also: xorphanol mesylate]

**xorphanol mesylate** USAN *analgesic* [also: xorphanol]

**X-Prep** oral liquid OTC *pre-procedure bowel evacuant* [senna extract] 74 mL

**X-Prep Bowel Evacuant Kit-1** oral liquid + 2 tablets + 1 suppository OTC *pre-procedure bowel evacuant* [X-Prep liquid (q.v.); Senokot-S tablets (q.v.); Rectolax suppository (q.v.)]

**X-Prep Bowel Evacuant Kit-2** oral liquid + granules + 1 suppository (discontinued 2003) OTC *pre-procedure bowel evacuant* [X-Prep liquid (q.v.); Citralax granules (q.v.); Rectolax suppository (q.v.)]

**XR-9576** *investigational (Phase III) antineoplastic*

**XRT (x-ray therapy)** *adjunct to chemotherapy* [not a pharmaceutical agent]

**X-Seb** shampoo OTC *antiseborrheic; keratolytic* [salicylic acid] 4%

**X-Seb Plus** shampoo OTC *antiseborrheic; keratolytic; antibacterial; antifungal* [salicylic acid; pyrithione zinc] 2%•1%

**X-Seb T** shampoo OTC *antiseborrheic; antipsoriatic; keratolytic* [coal tar; salicylic acid] 10%•4%

**X-Seb T Plus** shampoo OTC *antiseborrheic; antipsoriatic; keratolytic* [coal tar; salicylic acid; menthol] 10%•3%•1%

**xylamidine tosilate** INN *serotonin inhibitor* [also: xylamidine tosylate]

**xylamidine tosylate** USAN *serotonin inhibitor* [also: xylamidine tosilate]

**xylazine** INN *analgesic; veterinary muscle relaxant* [also: xylazine HCl]

**xylazine HCl** USAN *analgesic; veterinary muscle relaxant* [also: xylazine]

**xylitol** NF *sweetened vehicle*

**Xylocaine** injection ℞ *injectable local anesthetic* [lidocaine HCl] 0.5%, 1%, 2%

**Xylocaine** ointment OTC *topical local anesthetic* [lidocaine] 2.5%

**Xylocaine** topical liquid, topical solution, ointment, jelly ℞ *mucous membrane anesthetic* [lidocaine HCl] 5%; 4%; 5%; 2%

**Xylocaine 10% Oral** spray ℞ *mucous membrane anesthetic* [lidocaine HCl] 10%

**Xylocaine HCl** injection ℞ *injectable local anesthetic* [lidocaine HCl; dextrose] 1.5%•7.5%

**Xylocaine HCl** injection ℞ *injectable local anesthetic* [lidocaine HCl; epinephrine] 0.5%•1:200 000, 1%• 1:100 000, 1%•1:200 000, 2%• 1:50 000, 2%•1:100 000, 2%• 1:200 000

**Xylocaine HCl IV for Cardiac Arrhythmias** IV injection, IV admixture ℞ *antiarrhythmic* [lidocaine HCl] 1%, 2%, 4%, 20%

**Xylocaine MPF** injection ℞ *injectable local anesthetic* [lidocaine HCl] 0.5%, 1%, 1.5%, 2%, 4%

**Xylocaine MPF** injection ℞ *injectable local anesthetic* [lidocaine HCl; epinephrine] 1%•1:200 000, 1.5%• 1:200 000, 2%•1:200 000

**Xylocaine MPF** injection ℞ *injectable local anesthetic* [lidocaine HCl; glucose] 5%•7.5%

**Xylocaine Viscous** solution ℞ *mucous membrane anesthetic* [lidocaine HCl] 2%

**xylocoumarol** INN

**xylofilcon A** USAN *hydrophilic contact lens material*

**xylometazoline** INN, BAN *vasoconstrictor; nasal decongestant* [also: xylometazoline HCl]

**xylometazoline HCl** USP *vasoconstrictor; nasal decongestant* [also: xylometazoline]

**Xylo-Pfan** tablets (discontinued 2004) OTC *diagnostic aid for intestinal function* [xylose] 25 g

**xylose (D-xylose)** USP *diagnostic aid for intestinal function*

**xyloxemine** INN

**Xyotax** ℞ *investigational (Phase III) taxane for lung cancer* [polyglutamate paclitaxel]

**Xyrem** oral solution ℞ *CNS depressant for cataplexy in narcoleptic patients* [sodium oxybate] 500 mg

**Xyvion** ℞ *investigational (NDA filed) synthetic steroid for osteoporosis and other postmenopausal symptoms* [tibolone]

...ver
...ge,
...cing
...na-
tion with discharge, nosebleed, reducing
heavy menstrual bleeding and pain,
thrombosis, and topical hemostasis

**Yasmin** film-coated tablets (in packs
of 28) ℞ *monophasic oral contraceptive* [drospirenone; ethinyl estradiol]
3 mg•30 µg

**yatren** [see: chiniofon]

**[169]Yb** [see: pentetate calcium trisodium
Yb 169]

**[169]Yb** [see: ytterbium Yb 169 pentetate]

**yeast, dried** NF

**yeast cell derivative** *claimed to promote wound healing*

**Yeast-Gard** vaginal suppositories OTC
*for vaginal irritations, itching, and
burning* [pulsatilla 28x; Candida albicans 28x]

**Yeast-Gard Medicated Disposable
Douche Premix** solution OTC *antifungal; vaginal cleanser and deodorizer;
acidity modifier* [sodium benzoate;
lactic acid]

**Yeast-Gard Medicated Douche;
Yeast-Gard Medicated Disposable
Douche** solution OTC *antiseptic/germicidal; vaginal cleanser and deodorizer*
[povidone-iodine] 10%; 0.3%

**Yeast-X** vaginal suppositories OTC *for
vaginal irritations, itching, and burning*
[pulsatilla 28x]

**Yelets** tablets OTC *vitamin/mineral/iron
supplement* [multiple vitamins &
minerals; ferrous fumarate; folic
acid] ±•20•0.1 mg

**yellow bedstraw; yellow cleavers**
*medicinal herb* [see: bedstraw]

**yellow beeswax** [see: beeswax, yellow]

**yellow dock (Rumex crispus)** root
*medicinal herb for anemia, blood
cleansing, constipation, itching, liver
congestion, rheumatism, skin problems,*
and eyelid ulcerations; also used as a
dentifrice

**yellow ferric oxide** [see: ferric oxide,
yellow]

**yellow fever vaccine** USP *active
immunizing agent for yellow fever*

**yellow gentian** *medicinal herb* [see:
gentian]

**yellow ginseng** *medicinal herb* [see:
blue cohosh]

**yellow Indian paint** *medicinal herb*
[see: goldenseal]

**yellow jessamine** *medicinal herb* [see:
gelsemium]

**yellow mercuric oxide** [see: mercuric
oxide, yellow]

**yellow ointment** [see: ointment, yellow]

**yellow paint root; yellow root**
*medicinal herb* [see: goldenseal]

**yellow petrolatum** JAN *ointment base;
emollient/protectant* [also: petrolatum]

**yellow phenolphthalein** [see: phenolphthalein, yellow]

**yellow precipitate** [see: mercuric
oxide, yellow]

**yellow puccoon** *medicinal herb* [see:
goldenseal]

**yellow root (Xanthorhiza simplicissima)** *medicinal herb used for diabetes
and hypertension*

**yellow root; yellow paint root**
*medicinal herb* [see: goldenseal]

**yellow wax** [see: wax, yellow]

**yellow wood; yellow wood berries**
*medicinal herb* [see: prickly ash]

**Yentreve** (approved in Europe) ℞
*investigational (Phase II) selective serotonin and norepinephrine reuptake
inhibitor (SSNRI) for stress urinary
incontinence* [duloxetine HCl]

**yerba maté (Ilex paraguariensis)**
leaves *medicinal herb used as a CNS
stimulant, diuretic, and purifier*

**yerba santa (Eriodictyon californicum)**
leaves *medicinal herb for asthma,
bronchial congestion, colds, hay fever,*

*inducing expectoration, inflammation, rheumatic pain, and tuberculosis*

**yew (*Taxus bacatta* and other species)** leaves *medicinal herb for liver disorders, rheumatism, and urinary tract disorders*

**YF-Vax** subcu injection ℞ *yellow fever vaccine* [yellow fever vaccine] 0.5 mL

**Yocon** tablets ℞ *alpha₂-adrenergic blocker for impotence and orthostatic hypotension; sympatholytic; mydriatic; may have aphrodisiac activity; no FDA-approved indications* [yohimbine HCl] 5.4 mg

**Yodoxin** tablets, powder ℞ *amebicide* [iodoquinol] 210, 650 mg; 25 g

**yohimbe (*Corynanthe johimbe; Pausinystalia johimbe*)** bark *medicinal herb for angina, hypertension, and impotence and other sexual dysfunction; also used as an aphrodisiac*

**yohimbic acid** INN

**yohimbine HCl** *alpha₂-adrenergic blocker for impotence and orthostatic hypotension; sympatholytic; mydriatic; may have aphrodisiac activity; no FDA-sanctioned indications* 5.4 mg oral

**Yohimex** tablets (discontinued 2003) ℞ *alpha₂-adrenergic blocker for impotence; sympatholytic; mydriatic; may have aphrodisiac activity; no FDA-approved indications* [yohimbine HCl] 5.4 mg

**Yondelis** ℞ *investigational (Phase III) tetrahydroisoquinoline alkaloid for sarcoma* [ecteinascidin]

**Your Choice Non-Preserved Saline** solution OTC *rinsing/storage solution for soft contact lenses* [sodium chloride (saline solution)]

**Your Choice Sterile Preserved Saline** solution OTC *rinsing/storage solution for soft contact lenses* [sodium chloride (preserved saline solution)]

**youthwort** *medicinal herb* [see: masterwort]

**ytterbium** *element (Yb)*

**ytterbium Yb 169 pentetate** USP *radioactive agent*

**yttrium** *element (Y)*

**yttrium Y 90 ibritumomab tiuxetan** *radioimmunotherapy for non-Hodgkin B-cell lymphoma*

**yttrium Y 90 murine monoclonal antibodies (2B8-MXDTPA) & indium In 111 murine monoclonal antibodies (2B8-MXDTPA)** *investigational (orphan) for non-Hodgkin B-cell lymphoma*

**yucca (*Yucca glauca*)** root *medicinal herb for arthritis, colitis, hypertension, migraine headache, and rheumatism*

**yuma** *medicinal herb* [see: wild yam]

**Yurelax** (Spanish name for U.S. product Flexeril)

**Yutopar** IV infusion (discontinued 2003) ℞ *uterine relaxant to arrest preterm labor* [ritodrine HCl] 10, 15 mg/mL

# Z

**zabicipril** INN

**zacopride** INN *antiemetic; peristaltic stimulant* [also: zacopride HCl]

**zacopride HCl** USAN, INN *antiemetic; peristaltic stimulant* [also: zacopride]

**Zacutex** IV injection ℞ *investigational (Phase III) platelet activating factor (PAF) antagonist for acute pancreatitis* [lexipafant]

**Zadaxin** (approved in several countries) ℞ *investigational (Phase III) influenza vaccine and vaccine enhancer for lung cancer; investigational (Phase III, orphan) for chronic hepatitis B; investigational (orphan) for DiGeorge syndrome with immune defects; investigational (orphan) for hepatocellular carcinoma* [thymalfasin]

**Zaditen Ophthalmic** (foreign name for U.S. product Zaditor)

**Zaditor** eye drops ℞ *ophthalmic antihistamine and mast cell stabilizer for allergic conjunctivitis* [ketotifen fumarate] 0.025%

**zafirlukast** USAN, INN, BAN *leukotriene receptor antagonist (LTRA) for prevention and chronic treatment of asthma*

**zafuleptine** INN

**Zagam** film-coated tablets ℞ *once-daily broad-spectrum fluoroquinolone antibiotic for community-acquired respiratory infections* [sparfloxacin] 200 mg

**zalcitabine** USAN *nucleoside reverse transcriptase inhibitor; antiviral for advanced HIV infection (orphan)*

**zaleplon** USAN *pyrazolopyrimidine hypnotic for the short-term treatment of insomnia*

**zalospirone** INN *anxiolytic* [also: zalospirone HCl]

**zalospirone HCl** USAN *anxiolytic* [also: zalospirone]

**zaltidine** INN, BAN *antagonist to histamine $H_2$ receptors* [also: zaltidine HCl]

**zaltidine HCl** USAN *antagonist to histamine $H_2$ receptors* [also: zaltidine]

**zamifenacin** INN, BAN *investigational treatment for irritable bowel syndrome*

**Zanaflex** tablets, capsules ℞ *antispasmodic for multiple sclerosis and spinal cord injury (orphan)* [tizanidine HCl] 2, 4 mg; 2, 4, 6 mg

**zanamivir** USAN *influenza neuraminidase inhibitor for the treatment of acute influenza types A and B*

**Zanfel** cream, wash OTC *poison ivy treatment* [polyethylene granles]

**zankiren HCl** USAN *antihypertensive*

**Zanosar** powder for IV injection ℞ *nitrosourea-type alkylating antineoplastic for metastatic islet cell carcinoma of pancreas* [streptozocin] 1 g (100 mg/mL)

**zanoterone** USAN *antiandrogen*

**Zantac** film-coated tablets, syrup, IV or IM injection ℞ *histamine $H_2$ antagonist for gastric and duodenal ulcers* [ranitidine HCl] 150, 300 mg; 15 mg/mL; 0.5, 25 mg/mL ⑨ Xanax

**Zantac 75** tablets OTC *histamine $H_2$ antagonist for episodic heartburn* [ranitidine HCl] 75 mg

**Zantac EFFERdose** effervescent tablets, effervescent granules ℞ *histamine $H_2$ antagonist for gastric and duodenal ulcers* [ranitidine HCl] 25, 150 mg; 150 mg/pkt.

**Zantac GELdose** capsules ℞ *histamine $H_2$ antagonist for gastric and duodenal ulcers* [ranitidine HCl] 150, 300 mg

*Zanthorhiza apiifolia* medicinal herb [see: yellow root]

**Zantryl** capsules (discontinued 2001) ℞ *anorexiant; CNS stimulant* [phentermine HCl] 30 mg

*Zanzibar aloe* medicinal herb [see: aloe]

**zapizolam** INN

**zaprinast** INN, BAN

**zardaverine** INN

**Zarontin** capsules, syrup ℞ *anticonvulsant* [ethosuximide] 250 mg; 250 mg/5 mL ⑨ Zaroxolyn

**Zaroxolyn** tablets ℞ *antihypertensive; diuretic* [metolazone] 2.5, 5, 10 mg ⑨ Zarontin; Zeroxin

**zatosetron** INN, BAN *antimigraine* [also: zatosetron maleate]

**zatosetron maleate** USAN *antimigraine* [also: zatosetron]

**Zavedos** (European name for U.S. product Idamycin)

**Zavesca** capsules ℞ *treatment for type I Gaucher disease* [miglustat] 100 mg

**Z-Bec** tablets OTC *vitamin/zinc supplement* [multiple vitamins; zinc sulfate] ± •22.5 mg

**ZBT Baby** topical powder (discontinued 2003) OTC *diaper rash treatment* [talc]

**Z-Cof DM** syrup ℞ *antitussive; decongestant; expectorant* [dextromethorphan hydrobromide; pseudoephedrine HCl; guaifenesin] 30•80•400 mg/10 mL

**Z-Cof HC** syrup ℞ *narcotic antitussive; decongestant; antihistamine* [hydrocodone bitartrate; phenylephrine HCl; chlorpheniramine maleate] 3.5•10•2.5 mg/5 mL

**Z-Cof LA** sustained-release tablets ℞ *antitussive; expectorant* [dextromethorphan hydrobromide; guaifenesin] 3•650 mg

**ZDV (zidovudine)** [q.v.]

**ZE Caps** soft capsules OTC *dietary supplement* [vitamin E; zinc gluconate] 200•9.6 mg

*Zea mays medicinal herb* [see: Indian corn]

**Zeasorb AF** ⒸⒶⓃ topical solution OTC *topical antifungal* [tolnaftate] 10 mg/mL

**Zeasorb-AF** powder OTC *antifungal* [miconazole nitrate] 2%

*zeaxanthin natural carotenoid used to prevent and treat age-related macular degeneration (AMD), retinitis pigmentosa (RP), and other retinal dysfunction*

**Zebeta** film-coated tablets ℞ *antihypertensive; β-blocker* [bisoprolol fumarate] 5, 10 mg

**Zee-Seltzer** effervescent tablets OTC *antacid; analgesic* [sodium bicarbonate; citric acid; aspirin] 1916• 1000•325 mg

**Zefazone** powder or frozen premix for IV injection ℞ *cephalosporin antibiotic* [cefmetazole sodium] 1, 2 g ⑦ cefazolin

**Zegerid** powder for oral suspension ℞ *proton pump inhibitor for gastric and duodenal ulcers, erosive esophagitis, GERD, and other gastroesophageal disorders* [omeprazole] 20 mg

**zein** NF *coating agent*

**Zeldox** (European name for U.S. product Geodon)

**Zelmac** (name changed to Zelnorm upon marketing release in 2002)

**Zelnorm** tablets ℞ *selective serotonin 5-HT$_4$ receptor antagonist for irritable bowel syndrome and chronic constipation in women* [tegaserod maleate] 2, 6 mg

**Zemaira** powder for IV infusion ℞ *enzyme replacement therapy for hereditary alpha$_1$-proteinase inhibitor deficiency, which leads to progressive panacinar emphysema* [alpha$_1$-proteinase inhibitor] 50 mg/mL (1000 mg/vial)

**Zemplar** parenteral injection during dialysis ℞ *synthetic vitamin D analogue for osteodystrophy and hyperparathyroidism secondary to chronic renal failure* [paricalcitol] 5 μg/mL

**Zemuron** IV injection ℞ *nondepolarizing neuromuscular blocking agent; muscle relaxant; adjunct to general anesthesia* [rocuronium bromide] 10 mg/mL

**Zenapax** injection ℞ *immunosuppressant; monoclonal antibodies (MAb) to prevent acute rejection of organ and bone marrow transplants (orphan)* [daclizumab] 25 mg/5 mL

*zenarestat* USAN *investigational (Phase III) aldose reductase inhibitor for diabetic neuropathy*

**Zenate, Advanced Formula** film-coated tablets ℞ *vitamin/iron supplement* [multiple vitamins; iron; folic acid] ±•65•1 mg

*zenazocine mesylate* USAN *analgesic*

**Zendra** ℞ *investigational GABA (A) receptor modulator for acute ischemic stroke* [clomethiazole edisylate]

*zepastine* INN

**Zephiran Chloride** tincture, tincture spray, aqueous solution, towelettes, disinfectant concentrate OTC *topical antiseptic* [benzalkonium chloride] 1:750; 1:750; 1:750; 1:750; 17%

*zephirol* [see: benzalkonium chloride]

**Zephrex** film-coated tablets ℞ *decongestant; expectorant* [pseudoephedrine HCl; guaifenesin] 60•400 mg

**Zephrex LA** extended-release tablets ℞ *decongestant; expectorant* [pseudoephedrine HCl; guaifenesin] 120• 600 mg

*zeranol* USAN, INN *anabolic*

**Zerit** capsules, powder for oral solution ℞ *antiviral for HIV infection* [stavudine] 15, 20, 30, 40 mg; 1 mg/mL

**Zerit XR** extended-release capsules ℞ *antiviral for HIV infection* [stavudine] 37.5, 50, 75, 100 mg

**Zestoretic** tablets ℞ *antihypertensive; angiotensin-converting enzyme (ACE) inhibitor; diuretic* [hydrochlorothiazide; lisinopril] 12.5•10, 25•20 mg

**Zestril** tablets ℞ *antihypertensive; angiotensin-converting enzyme (ACE) inhibitor; adjunctive treatment for CHF* [lisinopril] 2.5, 5, 10, 20, 30, 40 mg ⑨ Restoril; Vistaril

**Zetacet** topical suspension, wash ℞ *acne treatment* [sulfacetamide sodium; sulfur] 10%•5%

**Zetar** shampoo OTC *antiseborrheic; antipsoriatic; antipruritic; antibacterial* [coal tar] 1%

**Zetar Emulsion** bath oil (discontinued 2003) ℞ *antipsoriatic; antiseborrheic; antipruritic; emollient* [coal tar] 30%

**Zetia** caplets ℞ *antihyperlipidemic; intestinal cholesterol absorption inhibitor* [ezetimibe] 10 mg

**zetidoline** INN, BAN

**Zevalin** powder for injection ℞ *radioimmunotherapy carrier; radiolabeled with indium In 111 (step 1) and yttrium Y 90 (step 2) to treat non-Hodgkin B-cell lymphoma* [ibritumomab tiuxetan]

**Zevalin therapeutic regimen** "kit" (complete package for a one-week course of treatment) ℞ *multistep treatment protocol for non-Hodgkin B-cell lymphoma* [rituximab; indium In 111 ibritumomab tiuxetan; yttrium Y 90 ibritumomab tiuxetan]

**Z-gen** tablets OTC *vitamin/zinc supplement* [multiple vitamins; zinc] ±•22.5 mg

**Zhuzishen (Panax pseudoginseng)** *medicinal herb* [see: ginseng]

**Ziac** tablets ℞ *antihypertensive; β-blocker; diuretic* [hydrochlorothiazide; bisoprolol fumarate] 6.25•2.5, 6.25•5, 6.25•10 mg

**Ziagen** film-coated caplets, oral solution ℞ *antiviral nucleoside reverse transcriptase inhibitor for HIV infection* [abacavir sulfate] 300 mg; 20 mg/mL

**ziconotide** USAN *non-narcotic analgesic; calcium channel blocker; investigational (NDA filed) intrathecal administration for intractable pain of cancer or AIDS; investigational epidural administration for spinal cord injury*

**zidapamide** INN

**zidometacin** USAN, INN *anti-inflammatory*

**zidovudine (ZDV)** USAN, INN, BAN *nucleoside antiviral for AIDS and AIDS-related complex (orphan), HIV infection, and to prevent maternal-fetal HIV transmission*

**zidovudine & amprenavir & lamivudine** *investigational (Phase III) second-generation protease inhibitor combination for AIDS*

**zidovudine & didanosine** *investigational (Phase II) heterodimer antiviral combination for AIDS*

**zidovudine & didanosine & nevirapine** *investigational (Phase III) antiviral combination for HIV infection*

**zidovudine & efavirenz & lamivudine** *investigational (Phase III) antiviral combination for HIV and AIDS*

**zidovudine & saquinavir mesylate & ritonavir** *investigational (Phase II) protease inhibitor combination for HIV infection*

**zifrosilone** USAN *acetylcholinesterase inhibitor for Alzheimer disease*

**Ziks** cream OTC *analgesic; counterirritant* [methyl salicylate; menthol; capsaicin] 12%•1%•0.025% ⑨ Vicks

**Zilactin Medicated** gel OTC *astringent for oral canker and herpes lesions* [tannic acid; alcohol 80%] 7%

**Zilactin-B Medicated** gel OTC *topical oral anesthetic* [benzocaine; alcohol 76%] 10%

**Zilactin-L** topical liquid OTC *local anesthetic* [lidocaine] 2.5%

**zilantel** USAN, INN *anthelmintic*

**zileuton** USAN, INN, BAN *5-lipoxygenase inhibitor; leukotriene receptor inhibitor; for prophylaxis and chronic treatment of asthma*

**zilpaterol** INN

**zimeldine** INN, BAN *antidepressant* [also: zimeldine HCl]

**zimeldine HCl** USAN *antidepressant* [also: zimeldine]

**zimelidine HCl** [now: zimeldine HCl]

**zimidoben** INN

**Zinacef** powder or frozen premix for IV or IM injection ℞ *cephalosporin antibiotic* [cefuroxime sodium] 0.75, 1.5, 7.5 g

**zinc** *element (Zn)*

**Zinc 15** tablets OTC *zinc supplement* [zinc sulfate] 66 mg

**zinc acetate** USP *copper blocking/complexing agent for Wilson disease (orphan)*

**zinc acetate, basic** INN

**zinc acetate dihydrate** [see: zinc acetate]

**zinc bacitracin** [see: bacitracin zinc]

**zinc caprylate** *antifungal*

**zinc carbonate** USAN *dietary zinc supplement*

**zinc chloride** USP *astringent; dentin desensitizer; dietary zinc supplement*

**zinc chloride Zn 65** USAN *radioactive agent*

**zinc citrate** *dietary zinc supplement (34% elemental zinc)*

**zinc complex bacitracins** [see: bacitracin zinc]

**zinc gelatin** USP

**zinc gluconate** USP *dietary zinc supplement* 10, 15, 50, 78 mg oral

**Zinc Lozenges** OTC *topical anti-infective to relieve sore throat* [zinc citrate and zinc gluconate] 23 mg

**zinc mesoporphyrin & hemin** *investigational (orphan) for acute porphyric syndromes*

**zinc oleate** NF

**zinc oxide** USP, JAN *astringent; topical protectant; emollient; antiseptic* 20% topical

**zinc peroxide, medicinal** USP

**zinc phenolsulfonate** NF *not generally regarded as safe and effective as an antidiarrheal*

**zinc propionate** *antifungal*

**zinc pyrithione** [see: pyrithione zinc]

**zinc stearate** USP *dusting powder; tablet and capsule lubricant; antifungal*

**zinc sulfate** USP, JAN *ophthalmic astringent; dietary zinc supplement* 200, 220, 250 mg oral; 1, 5 mg/mL injection

**zinc sulfate heptahydrate** [see: zinc sulfate]

**zinc sulfate monohydrate** [see: zinc sulfate]

**zinc sulfocarbolate** [see: zinc phenolsulfonate]

**zinc undecylenate** USP *antifungal*

**zinc valerate** USP

**Zinc-220** capsules OTC *zinc supplement* [zinc sulfate] 220 mg

**Zinca-Pak** IV injection ℞ *intravenous nutritional therapy* [zinc sulfate] 1, 5 mg/mL

**Zincate** capsules ℞ *zinc supplement* [zinc sulfate] 220 mg

**zinc-eugenol** USP

**Zincfrin** Drop-Tainers (eye drops) OTC *topical ocular decongestant and astringent* [phenylephrine HCl; zinc sulfate] 0.12%•0.25%

**Zincon** shampoo OTC *antiseborrheic; antibacterial; antifungal* [pyrithione zinc] 1%

**Zincvit** capsules ℞ *vitamin/mineral supplement* [multiple vitamins & minerals; folic acid] ±•1 mg

**zindotrine** USAN, INN *bronchodilator*

**zindoxifene** INN

**Zinecard** powder for IV drip or push ℞ *cardioprotectant for doxorubicin-induced cardiomyopathy (orphan)* [dexrazoxane] 250, 500 mg/vial

**Zingiber officinale** *medicinal herb* [see: ginger]

**zinoconazole** INN *antifungal* [also: zinoconazole HCl]

**zinoconazole HCl** USAN *antifungal* [also: zinoconazole]

**zinostatin** USAN, INN *antineoplastic* ⚠ Sandostatin; simvastatin

**zinterol** INN *bronchodilator* [also: zinterol HCl]

**zinterol HCl** USAN *bronchodilator* [also: zinterol]

**Zintevir** ℞ *investigational (Phase I/II) integrase inhibitor for HIV infection* [AR-177 (code name—generic name not yet assigned)]

**zinviroxime** USAN, INN *antiviral*

**zipeprol** INN

**ziprasidone HCl** *dihydroindolone antipsychotic; serotonin 5-HT$_2$ and dopamine D$_2$ antagonist*

**ziprasidone mesylate** *dihydroindolone antipsychotic; serotonin 5-HT$_2$ and dopamine D$_2$ antagonist*

**Ziracin** ℞ *investigational antibiotic* [evernimicin]

**Ziradryl** lotion OTC *topical antihistamine; astringent; antiseptic* [diphenhydramine HCl; zinc oxide; alcohol 2%] 1%•2%

**zirconium** *element (Zr)*

**zirconium oxide** *astringent*

**Zithromax** ⒸⒶⓃ capsules, tablets, powder for oral suspension ℞ *macrolide antibiotic* [azithromycin] 250 mg; 250 mg; 300, 600 mg/15 mL, 900 mg/22.5 mL

**Zithromax** Z-Pak (6 tablets), film-coated tablets, powder for oral suspension, powder for IV or IM injection ℞ *macrolide antibiotic* [azithromycin] 250 mg; 250, 500, 600 mg; 100, 200 mg/5 mL, 1 g/pkt.; 500 mg

**Zixoryn** ℞ *investigational (orphan) agent for neonatal hyperbilirubinemia* [flumecinol]

**⁶⁵Zn** [see: zinc chloride Zn 65]

**Zn-DTPA (zinc pentetate)** [see: pentetate zinc trisodium]

**ZNP** cleansing bar OTC *antiseborrheic; antibacterial; antifungal* [pyrithione zinc] 2%

**zocainone** INN

**Zocor** film-coated tablets ℞ *HMG-CoA reductase inhibitor for hyperlipidemia, hypertriglyceridemia, and coronary heart disease* [simvastatin] 5, 10, 20, 40, 80 mg

**Zocor Heart-Pro** film-coated tablets (available OTC in England) *HMG-CoA reductase inhibitor for hyperlipidemia, hypertriglyceridemia, and coronary heart disease* [simvastatin] 10 mg

**Zodeac-100** tablets ℞ *hematinic; vitamin/mineral supplement* [ferrous fumarate; multiple vitamins & minerals; folic acid; biotin] 60 mg• ± •1 mg•300 µg

**Zoderm** gel, cream, liquid cleanser ℞ *keratolytic for acne* [benzoyl peroxide (in a urea base)] 4.5%, 8.5%

**zofenopril** INN, BAN *angiotensin-converting enzyme (ACE) inhibitor* [also: zofenopril calcium]

**zofenopril calcium** USAN *angiotensin-converting enzyme (ACE) inhibitor* [also: zofenopril]

**zofenoprilat** INN *antihypertensive* [also: zofenoprilat arginine]

**zofenoprilat arginine** USAN *antihypertensive* [also: zofenoprilat]

**zoficonazole** INN

**Zofran** film-coated tablets, oral solution, IV infusion, IM injection ℞ *serotonin 5-HT$_3$ antagonist; antiemetic for nausea following chemotherapy, radiation, or surgery* [ondansetron HCl] 4, 8, 24 mg; 4 mg/5 mL; 32 mg/50 mL; 2 mg/mL

**Zofran ODT** (orally disintegrating tablets) ℞ *serotonin 5-HT$_3$ receptor antagonist; antiemetic for nausea following chemotherapy, radiation, or surgery* [ondansetron HCl] 4, 8 mg

**Zoladex** subcu implant in preloaded syringe ℞ *hormonal antineoplastic for palliative treatment of prostatic carcinoma, breast cancer, and endometriosis* [goserelin acetate] 3.6 mg (1-month implant), 10.8 mg (3-month implant) ⍰ sulindac

**Zoladex LA** ⒸⒶⓃ subcu implant in pre-loaded syringe ℞ *hormonal antineoplastic for palliative treatment of prostatic carcinoma; LHRH agonist for endometriosis* [goserelin acetate] 10.8 mg (3-month implant)

**zolamine** INN *antihistamine; topical anesthetic* [also: zolamine HCl]

**zolamine HCl** USAN *antihistamine; topical anesthetic* [also: zolamine]

**zolazepam** INN, BAN *sedative* [also: zolazepam HCl]

**zolazepam HCl** USAN *sedative* [also: zolazepam]

**zoledronate disodium** USAN *bone resorption inhibitor for osteoporosis*

**zoledronate trisodium** USAN *bone resorption inhibitor for osteoporosis*

**zoledronic acid** USAN *bisphosphonate bone resorption inhibitor for hypercalcemia of malignancy, multiple myeloma, and metabolic bone disorders such as Paget disease*

**zolenzepine** INN

**zolertine** INN *antiadrenergic; vasodilator* [also: zolertine HCl]

**zolertine HCl** USAN *antiadrenergic; vasodilator* [also: zolertine]

**Zolicef** powder for IV or IM injection ℞ *cephalosporin antibiotic* [cefazolin sodium] 0.5, 1 g

**zolimidine** INN

**zolimomab aritox** USAN *anti-T lymphocyte monoclonal antibody*

**zoliprofen** INN

**zoliridine** [see: zolimidine]

**zolmitriptan** USAN *vascular serotonin 5-HT$_{1B/1D}$ receptor agonist for the acute treatment of migraine*

**Zoloft** film-coated tablets, oral drops ℞ *selective serotonin reuptake inhibitor (SSRI) for depression, obsessive-compulsive disorder (OCD), panic disorder, post-traumatic stress disorder, premenstrual dysmorphic disorder (PMDD), and social anxiety disorder* [sertraline HCl] 25, 50, 100 mg; 20 mg/mL

**zoloperone** INN

**zolpidem** INN, BAN *imidazopyridine sedative/hypnotic* [also: zolpidem tartrate]

**zolpidem tartrate** USAN *imidazopyridine sedative/hypnotic* [also: zolpidem]

**Zomaril** ℞ *investigational (Phase III) selective serotonin and dopamine antagonist for schizophrenia* [iloperidone]

**zomebazam** INN

**zomepirac** INN, BAN *analgesic; anti-inflammatory* [also: zomepirac sodium]

**zomepirac sodium** USAN, USP *analgesic; anti-inflammatory* [also: zomepirac]

**Zometa** powder for IV infusion ℞ *bone resorption inhibitor for hypercalcemia of malignancy, multiple myeloma, and metabolic bone disorders such as Paget disease* [zoledronic acid] 4 mg

**zometapine** USAN *antidepressant*

**Zomig** film-coated tablets, nasal spray ℞ *vascular serotonin 5-HT$_{1B/1D}$ receptor agonist for the acute treatment of migraine* [zolmitriptan] 2.5, 5 mg; 5 mg/dose ⊘ Flomax; Slow-Mag

**Zomig Rapimelt** ⒸⒶⓃ (orally disintegrating tablets) ℞ *vascular serotonin 5-HT$_{1B/1D}$ receptor agonist for the acute treatment of migraine* [zolmitriptan] 2.5 mg

**Zomig-ZMT** orally disintegrating tablets ℞ *vascular serotonin 5-HT$_{1B/1D}$ receptor agonist for the acute treatment of migraine* [zolmitriptan] 2.5 mg ⊘ Flomax; Slow-Mag

**Zonalon** cream ℞ *antihistamine; antipruritic* [doxepin HCl] 5%

**Zone-A Forte** lotion ℞ *topical corticosteroidal anti-inflammatory; local anesthetic* [hydrocortisone acetate; pramoxine] 2.5%•1%

**Zonegran** capsules ℞ *sulfonamide anticonvulsant for partial seizures* [zonisamide] 25, 50, 100 mg

**zoniclezole** INN *anticonvulsant* [also: zoniclezole HCl]

**zoniclezole HCl** USAN *anticonvulsant* [also: zoniclezole]

**zonisamide** USAN, INN, BAN *sulfonamide anticonvulsant for partial seizures*

**Zonite Douche** solution concentrate OTC *antiseptic; antipruritic/counterirritant; vaginal cleanser and deodorizer* [benzalkonium chloride; menthol; thymol]

**Zophren** (European name for U.S. product Zofran)

**zopiclone** INN, BAN, JAN *sedative; hypnotic*

**zopolrestat** USAN *antidiabetic; aldose reductase inhibitor*

**zorbamycin** USAN *antibacterial*

**Zorbtive** powder for subcu injection ℞ *treatment for short bowel syndrome (SBS) in children* [somatropin (rDNA)] 4, 5, 6, 8.8 mg (12, 15, 18, 24.6 IU) per vial

**ZORprin** Zero Order Release tablets ℞ *analgesic; antipyretic; anti-inflammatory; antirheumatic* [aspirin] 800 mg

**zorubicin** INN *antineoplastic* [also: zorubicin HCl]

**zorubicin HCl** USAN *antineoplastic* [also: zorubicin]

**Zostrix; Zostrix-HP** cream OTC *topical analgesic* [capsaicin] 0.025%; 0.075%

**zosuquidar trihydrochloride** *investigational (Phase III) p-glycoprotein inhibitor for acute myelogenous leukemia (AML)*

**Zosyn** powder or frozen premix for IV injection R̟ *extended-spectrum penicillin antibiotic* [piperacillin sodium; tazobactam sodium] 2•0.25, 3•0.375, 4•0.5, 36•4.5 g

**zotepine** INN, JAN *investigational antipsychotic*

**Zoto-HC** ear drops R̟ *topical corticosteroidal anti-inflammatory; antibacterial; local anesthetic* [hydrocortisone; chloroxylenol; pramoxine HCl] 10%•1%•10%

**Zovant** R̟ *investigational (Phase III) recombinant human activated protein C for severe sepsis*

**Zovia 1/35E; Zovia 1/50E** tablets (in packs of 21 or 28) R̟ *monophasic oral contraceptive* [ethynodiol diacetate; ethinyl estradiol] 1 mg•35 μg; 1 mg•50 μg

**Zovirax** capsules, tablets, oral suspension R̟ *antiviral for herpes simplex, herpes zoster, and adult-onset chickenpox* [acyclovir] 200 mg; 400, 800 mg; 200 mg/5 mL

**Zovirax** cream R̟ *antiviral for recurrent herpes labialis* [acyclovir] 5%

**Zovirax** ointment R̟ *antiviral for herpes genitalis and mucocutaneous herpes simplex infections* [acyclovir] 5%

**Zovirax** powder for IV infusion R̟ *antiviral for herpes infections* [acyclovir sodium] 500, 1000 mg/vial

**zoxazolamine** NF, INN

**Z-Pak** (trademarked packaging form) *6-tablet pack of Zithromax*

**ZTuss Expectorant** oral liquid R̟ *narcotic antitussive; decongestant; antihistamine; expectorant* [hydrocodone bitartrate; pseudoephedrine HCl; chlorpheniramine maleate; guaifenesin] 5•30•4•200 mg/10 mL

**Zucapsaicin** R̟ *investigational (orphan) agent for postherpetic neuralgia of the trigeminal nerve* [civamide]

**zucapsaicin** USAN *topical analgesic*

**zuclomifene** INN

**zuclomiphene** USAN

**zuclopenthixol** INN, BAN *thioxanthene antipsychotic*

**Z-Xtra** lotion OTC *local anesthetic; antihistamine; emollient* [pyrilamine maleate; benzocaine; zinc oxide] 2.07• 2.08•41.35 mg/mL

**Zyban** sustained-release film-coated tablets R̟ *non-nicotine aid to smoking cessation* [bupropion HCl] 150 mg

**Zyderm** gel for subcu injection R̟ *dermal filler for fine-to-moderate scars and wrinkles* [collagen, purified bovine] 35, 65 mg/mL

**Zydis** (trademarked dosage form) *orally disintegrating tablets*

**Zydone** tablets, capsules R̟ *narcotic analgesic* [hydrocodone bitartrate; acetaminophen] 5•400, 7.5•400, 10•400 mg; 5•500 mg

**Zyflo** film-coated tablets R̟ *5-lipoxygenase inhibitor; leukotriene receptor inhibitor; prophylaxis and treatment for chronic asthma* [zileuton] 600 mg

**zylofuramine** INN

**Zyloprim** tablets R̟ *xanthine oxidase inhibitor for gout and hyperuricemia; antineoplastic adjunct for reducing uric acid levels following chemotherapy for leukemia, lymphoma, and solid tumor malignancies (orphan)* [allopurinol] 100, 300 mg

**Zymacap** capsules OTC *vitamin supplement* [multiple vitamins; folic acid] ±•0.4 mg

**Zymar** eye drops R̟ *broad-spectrum fluoroquinolone antibiotic* [gatifloxacin] 0.3%

**Zymase** capsules containing enteric-coated spheres (discontinued 2002) R̟ *digestive enzymes* [lipase; protease; amylase] 12 000•24 000•24 000 USP units

**Zymine** oral liquid ℞ *antihistamine* [triprolidine HCl] 1.25 mg/5 mL

**Zyplast** gel for subcu injection ℞ *dermal filler for deep scars and wrinkles* [collagen, purified bovine, cross-linked] 35 mg/mL

**Zyprexa** film-coated tablets, Zydis (orally disintegrating tablets) ℞ *novel (atypical) antipsychotic for schizophrenia and manic episodes of a bipolar disorder* [olanzapine] 2.5, 5, 7.5, 10, 15, 20 mg; 5, 10, 15, 20 mg

**Zyprexa IntraMuscular** IM injection ℞ *novel (atypical) antipsychotic for manic episodes of a bipolar disorder* [olanzapine] 5 mg/mL (10 mg/vial)

**Zyrkamine** *investigational (orphan) for non-Hodgkin lymphoma* [mitoguazone]

**Zyrtec** film-coated tablets, chewable tablets, syrup ℞ *nonsedating antihistamine for allergic rhinitis and chronic idiopathic urticaria* [cetirizine HCl] 5, 10 mg; 5, 10 mg; 5 mg/5 mL

**Zyrtec-D 12 Hour** extended-release tablets ℞ *nonsedating antihistamine and decongestant for allergic rhinitis* [cetirizine HCl; pseudoephedrine HCl] 5•120 mg

**Zyvox** film-coated tablets, powder for oral suspension, IV infusion ℞ *oxazolidinone antibiotic for gram-positive bacterial infections* [linezolid] 400, 600 mg; 100 mg/5 mL; 200, 400, 600 mg/bag

**Zyvoxam** ⒸⒶⓃ tablets, IV infusion ℞ *oxazolidinone antibiotic for gram-positive bacterial infections* [linezolid] 600 mg; 2 mg/mL

APPENDIX **A**
# Sound-Alikes

Listed below are 677 drug names that may be confused in transcription, followed by one or more possible "sound-alike" names. The list is not all-inclusive, and we would appreciate hearing of any additions the reader might suggest. These sound-alikes have also been included in the main section of the book. Look for the "ear" icon (👂).

| | |
|---|---|
| Accurbron | Accutane |
| Accutane | Accurbron |
| Aciphex | AcuTect |
| Actifed | Actidil |
| actinomycin | Achromycin; Aureomycin |
| AcuTect | Aciphex |
| adrenaline | adrenalone |
| adrenalone | adrenaline |
| Advil | Avail |
| Afrin | aspirin |
| Agoral | Argyrol |
| Akne-Mycin | Ak-Mycin |
| Alamag | Alma-Mag |
| Alco-Gel | aloe gel |
| Aldactazide | Aldactone |
| Aldactone | Aldactazide |
| Aldoril | Elavil; Eldepryl; Enovil; Equanil; Mellaril |
| Allergan | allergen; Auralgan |
| aloe | Alco-Gel |
| ALOMAD | Alomide |
| Alomide | ALOMAD |
| Alustra | Lustra |
| Ambenyl | Aventyl |
| Amicar | Amikin |
| Amikin | Amicar |
| amitriptyline | nortriptyline |
| amoxapine | amoxicillin; Amoxil |
| amoxicillin | amoxapine |
| Amoxil | amoxapine |
| Amphojel | Amphocil |
| Anacin | Unisom; Unasyn |
| Anafranil | enalapril |
| Analpram-HC | Analbalm |
| Ancobon | Oncovin |
| Ansaid | NSAID |
| Anturane | Artane |

| | |
|---|---|
| Anusol | Aplisol |
| Aplisol | Anusol; Apresoline |
| Appedrine | aprindine; ephedrine |
| aprindine | Appedrine; ephedrine |
| ara-C | ERYC |
| Aralen | Arlidin |
| Aricept | Erycette |
| Artane | Anturane |
| aspirin | Afrin |
| Atacand | Ativan |
| Atarax | Marax |
| atenolol | timolol |
| Ativan | Atacand; Adapin; Avitene |
| Ativan | Adapin; Avitene |
| Atrovent | Trovan |
| Auralgan | Allergan; allergen |
| Avail | Advil |
| Aventyl | Ambenyl; Bentyl |
| Avita | Evista |
| Avitene | Ativan |
| Axid | Biaxin |
| azolimine | Azulfidine |
| Azulfidine | Silvadene |
| Bacid | Banacid |
| bacitracin | Bacitrin; Bactrim |
| Bactocill | Pathocil |
| Bactrim | bacitracin |
| BAL | Balneol |
| Balneol | BAL in Oil |
| Banophen | Barophen |
| Banthīne | Brethine; Vantin |
| Beminal | Benemid |
| Benadryl | Bentyl; Benylin; Caladryl |
| Benemid | Beminal |
| Benoxyl | PanOxyl |
| Bentyl | Aventyl; Benadryl; Bontril |
| Benylin | Benadryl |
| Betagan | Betagen |
| Betagen | Betagan |
| Biaxin | Axid |
| Bichloracetic | dichloroacetic acid |
| Bicillin | V-Cillin; Wycillin |
| bleomycin | Cleocin |
| Bonamine | Bonine |
| Bontril | Bentyl; Vontrol |
| Boyol | boil |
| Brethine | Banthine |
| Brevital | Bretylol |
| Bromfed | Bromphen |
| Bromophen | Bromphen |

| | |
|---|---|
| Broncholate | Brondelate |
| Brondelate | Broncholate |
| butabarbital | butalbital |
| butalbital | butabarbital; Butibel |
| Butibel | butalbital |
| Butisol | Butazolidin |
| Byclomine | Hycomine |
| Caladryl | Benadryl |
| Calamox | Camalox |
| Calan | kaolin; Kaon |
| calcitonin | calcitriol |
| calcitriol | calcitonin |
| Capastat | Cepastat |
| Capitrol | captopril |
| captopril | Capitrol |
| Cardene | Cardizem |
| Cardizem | Cardene |
| Catapres | Catarase; Combipres; Ser-Ap-Es |
| Cefadyl | Cefzil |
| cefazolin | cephalothin; Zefazone |
| cefotaxime | cefoxitin |
| cefoxitin | cefotaxime |
| ceftizoxime | cefuroxime |
| cefuroxime | ceftizoxime |
| Cefzil | Cefadyl; Kefzol |
| Celebrex | Celexa; Cerebyx |
| Celexa | Celebrex |
| Cēpastat | Capastat |
| cephalexin | cefazolin; cephalothin |
| cephalothin | cefazolin |
| cephapirin | cephradine |
| cephradine | cephapirin |
| Cerebyx | Celebrex |
| chlorpheniramine | chlorphentermine |
| chlorphentermine | chlorpheniramine |
| cimetidine | dimethicone |
| Cipro | Septa; Septra |
| Citracal | Citrucel |
| Citrucel | Citracal |
| clara | Clearasil |
| claretin-12 | Claritin; Clarityne |
| clarithromycin | dirithromycin; erythromycin |
| Claritin | claretin; Clarityne |
| Clarityne | claretin; Claritin |
| Clearasil | clara cell |
| Cleocin | bleomycin; Lincocin |
| clioxanide | Clinoxide |
| clomiphene | clonidine |
| clonidine | clomiphene; Klonopin; quinidine |
| clotrimazole | co-trimoxazole |

| | |
|---|---|
| Codegest | Codehist |
| Codehist | Codegest |
| codeine | Kaodene |
| Colestid | colistin |
| colestipol | colistin |
| colistin | Colestid; colestipol |
| Combipres | Catapres |
| Cort-Dome | Cortone |
| Cortenema | quart enema |
| cortisone | Cortizone |
| Cortizone-5 | cortisone |
| Cortone | Cort-Dome |
| Cotrim | Cortin |
| co-trimoxazole | clotrimazole |
| Coumadin | Kemadrin |
| Covera-HS | Provera |
| cytarabine | vidarabine |
| dacarbazine | Dicarbosil; procarbazine |
| Dalmane | Dialume |
| danthron | Dantrium |
| Dantrium | danthron |
| Daranide | Daraprim |
| Daraprim | Daranide |
| Darvocet-N | Darvon-N |
| Darvon | Diovan |
| daunorubicin | doxorubicin |
| Decadron | Decaderm; Percodan |
| Deconsal | Deconal |
| Delcort | Dilacor |
| Demulen | Demerol; Demolin |
| Dermacort | DermiCort |
| deserpidine | desipramine |
| Desferal | Disophrol |
| desipramine | deserpidine |
| desoximetasone | dexamethasone |
| Desoxyn | digitoxin; digoxin |
| dexamethasone | desoximetasone |
| Dexedrine | dextran |
| dextran | Dexedrine; dextrin |
| dextrin | dextran |
| Dialume | Dalmane |
| dichloroacetic | Bichloracetic acid |
| dicumarol | Demerol |
| digitoxin | Desoxyn; digoxin |
| digoxin | Desoxyn; digitoxin |
| Dilacor | Delcort |
| Dilantin | Milontin; Mylanta; Xalatan |
| Dimacol | dimercaprol |
| dimenhydrinate | diphenhydramine |
| dimercaprol | Dimacol |

| | |
|---|---|
| Dimetabs | Dimetane; Dimetapp |
| Dimetapp | Dimetabs |
| dimethicone | cimetidine |
| Diovan | Darvon |
| diphenhydramine | dimenhydrinate |
| Diphenylan | Diphenylin |
| dirithromycin | clarithromycin; erythromycin |
| Disophrol | Desferal; disoprofol; Stilphostrol |
| disoprofol | Disophrol |
| Ditropan | Intropin |
| Diutensen-R | Salutensin |
| dobutamine | dopamine |
| Donnagel | Donnatal |
| Donnatal | Donnagel |
| Donnazyme | Entozyme |
| dopamine | dobutamine; Dopram |
| Dopar | Dopram |
| Dopram | dopamine; Dopar |
| doxepin | Doxidan; Loxitane |
| doxorubicin | daunorubicin |
| Dramanate | Dommanate |
| Duranest | Duratest |
| Duratest | Duranest; Duratuss |
| Duratuss | Duratest |
| Dyazide | thiazides; Tiazac |
| Dymelor | Demerol; Pamelor |
| Dyrenium | Pyridium |
| Ecotrin | Edecrin |
| Edecrin | Ecotrin; Ethaquin |
| Elavil | Aldoril; Elidel; Eldepryl; Enovil; Equanil; Mellaril |
| Eldepryl | Aldoril; Elavil; Enovil; Equanil; Mellaril |
| Elidel | Elavil |
| emetine | Emetrol |
| Emetrol | emetine |
| Enbrel | Incel |
| Endal | Intal |
| Enduron | Imuran; Inderal |
| Enduronyl | Inderal |
| ephedrine | Appedrine; aprindine |
| Epifrin | epinephrine; EpiPen |
| Epinal | Epitol |
| epinephrine | Epifrin |
| EpiPen | Epifrin |
| Epitol | Epinal |
| Epogen | "amp and gent" (ampicillin & gentamicin) |
| Equanil | Aldoril; Elavil; Eldepryl; Enovil; Mellaril |
| ERYC | ara-C |
| Erycette | Aricept |
| erythromycin | clarithromycin; dirithromycin |
| Esidrix | Lasix |

| | |
|---|---|
| Esimil | Estinyl; Isomil |
| Estinyl | Esimil |
| Estraderm | Estradurin |
| Estratab | Ethatab |
| ethacridine | ethacrynic |
| ethacrynic | ethacridine |
| ethinamate | ethionamide |
| Ethiodol | ethynodiol |
| ethionamide | ethinamate |
| ethynodiol | Ethiodol |
| Eurax | Serax; Urex |
| Evac-Q-Kwik | Evac-Q-Kit |
| Evista | Avita |
| Femiron | Remeron |
| fentanyl | Sentinel |
| Feosol | Feostat; Fer-In-Sol; Festal |
| Feostat | Feosol |
| Feverall, | Fiberall |
| Fioricet | Lorcet |
| Fiorinal | Florinef |
| Flexeril | Flaxedil |
| Flomax | Slow-Mag; Zomig |
| Florinef | Fiorinal |
| folacin | Fulvicin |
| Fostex | pHisoHex |
| Fulvicin | folacin; Furacin |
| Furacin | Fulvicin |
| Gabitril | Carbatrol |
| Garamycin | Gamastan; kanamycin; Terramycin; Theramycin |
| Gelfoam | Ger-O-Foam |
| Genatap | Genapap |
| Generet | Gentap |
| gentamicin | Jenamicin; kanamycin |
| glucose | Glutose |
| Glutose | glucose |
| Glycotuss | Glytuss |
| Glytuss | Glycotuss |
| Gonak | Gonic |
| Gonic | Gonak |
| guaifenesin | guanfacine |
| guanethidine | guanidine |
| guanfacine | guaifenesin |
| guanidine | guanethidine |
| Guiatuss | Guiatussin |
| Guiatussin | Guiatuss |
| Haldol | Halenol; Halog |
| Halog | Haldol |
| Halotestin | Halotex; Halotussin |
| Halotex | Halotestin |
| Halotussin | Halotestin |

| | |
|---|---|
| Hespan | Histatan |
| Hexadrol | Hexalol |
| Hexalen | Hexalol |
| Hycodan | Hycomine; Vicodin |
| Hycomine | Byclomine; Hycodan; Vicodin |
| Hydergine | Hydramine |
| Hydramine | Bydramine; Hydergine; Hydramyn; Hytramyn |
| Hygroton | Regroton |
| HyperHep | Hyper-Tet; Hyperstat |
| Hyperstat | Hyper-Tet; HyperHep |
| Hyper-Tet | HyperHep; Hyperstat |
| Hytone | Vytone |
| Ilosone | inosine |
| imipramine | Imferon; Norpramin; trimipramine |
| Imuran | Enduron; Imferon |
| Inderal | Enduron; Enduronyl; Inderide |
| Inderide | Inderal |
| Indocin | Lincocin; Minocin |
| InFeD | NSAID |
| inosine | Ilosone |
| insulin | inulin |
| Intal | Endal |
| Intropin | Ditropan; Isoptin |
| inulin | insulin |
| Ismelin | Ritalin |
| Isomil | Esimil |
| Isoptin | Intropin |
| Isopto | Isopto Eserine |
| Isordil | Isuprel |
| Isuprel | Isordil |
| kanamycin | Garamycin; gentamicin |
| Kaochlor | K-Lor |
| kaolin | Calan; Kaon |
| Kaon | Calan; kaolin |
| Kaopectate, | Kapectalin |
| Kapectolin | Kaopectate |
| Kay Ciel | KCl |
| KCl | Kay Ciel |
| Keflex | Keflet; Keflin |
| Kefzol | Cefzil |
| Kemadrin | Coumadin |
| Kenalog | Ketalar |
| Ketalar | Kenalog |
| Klonopin | clonidine |
| K-Lor | Kaochlor |
| Klotrix | Liotrix |
| Koromex | Komex |
| Lasix | Esidrix; Lidex |
| levallorphan | levorphanol |
| levodopa | methyldopa |

| | |
|---|---|
| levorphanol | levallorphan |
| levothyroxine | liothyronine |
| Lidex | Lasix; Lidox; Wydase |
| Lincocin | Cleocin; Indocin |
| liothyronine | levothyroxine |
| liotrix | Klotrix |
| Loniten | clonidine |
| Lonox | Lovenox |
| Lorcet | Fioricet |
| Lotrimin | Otrivin |
| Lovenox | Lonox |
| Loxitane | doxepin |
| Luminal | Tuinal |
| Lupron | Mepron; Napron |
| Lupron | Mepron; Napron |
| Maalox | Marax |
| Mandol | nadolol |
| Marax | Atarax; Maalox |
| Marcaine | Narcan |
| Maxzide | Microzide |
| mazindol | mebendazole |
| Mebaral | Medrol |
| mebendazole | mazindol |
| Meclan | Meclomen; Mezlin |
| meclizine | mescaline |
| meclozine | mescaline |
| Medrol | Mebaral |
| Mellaril | Aldoril; Elavil; Eldepryl; Enovil; Equanil; Moderil |
| meperidine | meprobamate |
| mephenytoin | Mephyton |
| Mephyton | mephenytoin; methadone |
| meprobamate | meperidine |
| Mepron | Lupron; Napron |
| Mesantoin | mephenytoin; Mestinon; Metatensin |
| mescaline | meclizine |
| Mestinon | Mesantoin; Metatensin |
| Metahydrin | Metandren |
| metaproterenol | metoprolol |
| Metatensin | Mesantoin; Mestinon |
| metaxalone | metolazone |
| metesind | medicine |
| methadone | Mephyton |
| methenamine | methionine |
| methionine | methenamine |
| methixene | methoxsalen |
| methoxsalen | methixene |
| methyldopa | levodopa |
| metolazone | metaxalone |
| Metopirone | metyrapone |
| metoprolol | metaproterenol |

| | |
|---|---|
| metyrapone | Metopirone; metyrosine |
| metyrosine | metyrapone |
| Mezlin | Meclan |
| MICRhoGAM | microgram |
| Microzide | Maxzide |
| Midrin | Mydfrin |
| Milontin | Dilantin; Miltown; Mylanta |
| Miltown | Milontin |
| Minocin | Indocin; Mithracin; niacin |
| Mithracin | Minocin |
| mithramycin | mitomycin |
| mitomycin | mithramycin; Mutamycin |
| Moban | Mobidin; Modane |
| Mobidin | Moban |
| Modane | Moban; Mudrane |
| Modicon | Mylicon |
| Moi-Stir | moisture |
| Monocaps | Monoclate; Monoket |
| Monocid | Monocete |
| Monoclate | Monocaps; Monoket |
| Monoket | Monocete |
| Mudrane | Modane |
| Mutamycin | mitomycin |
| Myambutol | Nembutal |
| Mydfrin | Midrin; Myfedrine |
| Mylanta | Dilantin; Milontin |
| Myleran | Mylicon |
| Mylicon | Modicon; Myleran |
| nadolol | Nandol |
| Naldecon | Nalfon |
| Nalfon | Naldecon |
| Napron | Lupron; Mepron |
| Naprosyn | Meprospan; Natacyn |
| Narcan | Marcaine |
| Nardil | Norinyl |
| Natacyn | Naprosyn |
| Nembutal | Myambutal |
| Neomixin | neomycin |
| neomycin | Neomixin |
| Neovastat | Novastan |
| niacin | Minocin |
| NightTime | Thera-Flur |
| Nilstat | Nitrostat; nystatin |
| Nitro-Bid | Nicobid |
| nitroglycerin | Nitroglyn |
| Nitroglyn | nitroglycerin |
| Norinyl | Nardil |
| Norpramin | imipramine |
| nortriptyline | amitriptyline |
| Novastan | Neovastat; Ovastat |

| | |
|---|---|
| NSAIDs | InFeD |
| nystatin | Nilstat; Nitrostat |
| Omnipen | Unipen |
| Oncovin | Ancobon |
| Orabase-B | Orinase |
| orarsan | Oracin; Orasone |
| Orasone | Oracin; orarsan |
| Oretic | Oreton |
| Oreton | Oretic |
| Orinase | Orabase; Ornade; Ornex; Tolinase |
| Ornade | Orinase; Ornex |
| Ornex | Orex; Orinase; Ornade |
| Orthoclone | Ortho-Creme |
| Otobiotic | Urobiotic |
| Otrivin | Lotrimin |
| OvaRex | O-Vax |
| Ovastat | Novastan |
| O-Vax | Ovarex |
| oxycodone | Roxicodone |
| oxymetazoline | oxymetholone |
| oxymetholone | oxymetazoline; oxymorphone |
| oxymorphone | oxymetholone |
| Pamelor | Dymelor; Panlor |
| Panasol-S | Panscol |
| Panlor | Pamelor |
| Panoxyl | Benoxyl |
| Panscol | Panasol |
| Parafon | Pantopon |
| paramethadione | paramethasone |
| paramethasone | paramethadione |
| Pathilon | Pathocil |
| Pathocil | Bactocill; Pathilon; Placidyl |
| Pavabid | Pavased |
| Pavulon | Paverolan |
| penicillamine | penicillin |
| penicillin | penicillamine; Polycillin |
| pentobarbital | phenobarbital |
| Pentothal | pentrinitrol |
| pentrinitrol | Pentothal |
| Percodan | Decadron |
| Perdiem | Pyridium |
| Periactin | Taractan |
| Persantine | Pertofrane |
| Phazyme | Pherazine |
| phenacetin | phenazocine |
| phenazocine | phenacetin |
| phenelzine | Phenazine; Phenylzin |
| Phenergan | Phenaphen; Theragran |
| phenobarbital | pentobarbital |
| Phenoxine | Phenazine |

| | |
|---|---|
| phentermine | phentolamine |
| phentolamine | phentermine; Ventolin |
| pHisoHex | Fostex |
| physostigmine | pyridostigmine; Prostigmin |
| piperacetazine | piperazine |
| piperazine | piperacetazine |
| piracetam | piroxicam |
| piroxicam | piracetam |
| Pitocin | Pitressin |
| Pitressin | Pitocin |
| Placidyl | Pathocil |
| Podofin | podophyllin |
| podophyllin | Podofin |
| Ponstel | Pronestyl |
| pralidoxime | pyridoxine; pramoxine |
| Pramosone | pramoxine |
| pramoxine | pralidoxime; Pramosone |
| Pravachol | Primacor |
| prazepam | prazepine; prazosin |
| prazepine | prazepam |
| prazosin | prazepam |
| prednisolone | prednisone |
| prednisone | prednisolone |
| Preven | Preveon |
| Prilosec | Prozac |
| Primacor | Pravachol |
| Priscoline | Apresoline |
| procaine | Procan |
| procarbazine | dacarbazine |
| proline | Prolene |
| promazine | Promethazine |
| Pronestyl | Ponstel |
| Proscar | Posicor |
| Prostigmin | physostigmine |
| Protopam | Protamine |
| Provera | Covera; Provir; Trovert |
| Provir | Provera; Trovert |
| Prozac | Prilosec |
| Pyridium | Dyrenium; pyridoxine; pyrithione; pyritidium |
| pyridostigmine | physostigmine |
| pyridoxine | pralidoxime; Pyridium |
| pyrithione | Pyridium |
| pyritidium | Pyridium |
| Quarzan | Questran |
| quinacrine | quinidine |
| quinidine | clonidine; quinacrine; Quinatime; quinine |
| quinine | quinidine |
| Rēgain | Rogaine |
| Reglan | Regonol |
| Regonol | Reglan |

| | |
|---|---|
| Regroton | Hygroton |
| Remeron | Femiron |
| Repan | Riopan |
| Restoril | Risperdal; Vistaril; Zestril |
| Rheumatex | Rheumatrex |
| Rheumatrex | Rheumatex |
| Rifadin | Ritalin |
| Risperdal | Restoril |
| Ritalin | Ismelin; Rifadin |
| Robaxisal | Robaxacet |
| Rogaine | Rēgain |
| Roxicodone | oxycodone |
| Salutensin | Diutensen |
| Sandostatin | simvastatin; zinostatin |
| Sentinel | fentanyl |
| Septa | Cipro; Septra |
| Septra | Cipro; Septa |
| Ser-Ap-Es | Catapres |
| Serax | Eurax; Urex; Xerac |
| Serentil | Surital |
| Silvadene | Azulfidine |
| Simplet | Singlet |
| simvastatin | Sandostatin; zinostatin |
| Singlet | Simplet |
| sirolimus | temsirolimus |
| Slow-Mag | Flomax; Zomig |
| stilbestrol | Stilphostrol |
| Stilphostrol | Disophrol; stilbestrol |
| Streptase | Streptonase |
| streptokinase | Streptonase |
| Streptonase-B | Streptase; streptokinase |
| sucrose | sucrase |
| Sulf-10 | Sulten-10 |
| sulfamethizole | sulfamethoxazole |
| sulfamethoxazole | sulfamethizole |
| sulfathiazole | sulfisoxazole |
| sulfisoxazole | sulfathiazole |
| sulindac | Zoladex |
| Supartz | sports |
| Tagamet | Tegopen |
| Targretin | Tegopen; Tegrin |
| Tegretol | Tegrin |
| Tegrin | Targretin; Tegopen; Tegretol |
| temsirolimus | sirolimus |
| Tenex | Xanax |
| Terramycin | Garamycin; Theramycin |
| testolactone | testosterone |
| testosterone | testolactone |
| thallium | Valium |
| Theoclear-80 | Theolair |

| | |
|---|---|
| Theolair | Theoclear; Thyrolar |
| TheraFlu | Thera-Flur |
| Thera-Flur | TheraFlu |
| Theragran | Theragyn |
| Theragran | Phenergan |
| Theramycin | Garamycin; Terramycin |
| Theravite | Therevac |
| Therevac-Plus | Theravite |
| Threostat | Triostat |
| Thyrolar | Theolair; Thyrar |
| Tiazac | Dyazide; thiazides |
| Ticar | Tigan |
| Tigan | Ticar; Triban |
| timolol | atenolol |
| Tinactin | Taractan |
| TobraDex | Tobrex |
| tobramycin | Trobicin |
| Tobrex | TobraDex |
| Tofranil | Tepanil |
| Tolinase | Orinase |
| Topic | Topicort |
| Topicort | Topic |
| Trasylol | Travasol |
| Travasol | Trasylol |
| triamcinolone | Triaminicin |
| Triaminic | Triaminicin; TriHemic |
| Triaminicin | triamcinolone; Triaminic |
| triamterene | trimipramine |
| Triapine | Triaprim |
| Triban | Tigan |
| TriHemic | Triaminic |
| trimeprazine | trimipramine |
| trimethaphan | trimethoprim |
| trimethoprim | trimethaphan |
| trimipramine | imipramine; triamterene; trimeprazine |
| Triostat | Threostat |
| Trobicin | tobramycin |
| Tronolane | Tronothane |
| Tronothane | Tronolane |
| Trovan | Atrovent |
| Trovert | Provir; Provera |
| Tuinal | Luminal; Tylenol |
| Tusibron | Tussigon |
| Tussafed | Tussafin |
| Tussafin | Tussafed |
| Tussex | Tussionex; Tussirex |
| Tussigon | Tusibron |
| Tussionex | Tussex; Tussirex |
| Tussirex | Tussex; Tussionex |
| Tylenol | Tuinal |

| | |
|---|---|
| Unasyn | Anacin; Unisom |
| Unipen | Omnipen |
| Unisom | Anacin; Unasyn |
| Uracid | uracil; Urised; Urocit |
| uracil | Uracel; Uracid |
| Urex | Eurax; Serax |
| Urised | Uracel; Uracid; Urispas |
| Urispas | Urised |
| Urocit | Uracid |
| Valium | thallium; Valpin |
| Vantin | Banthine; Bantron |
| Vasocidin | Vasodilan |
| Vasocine | Vaseline |
| VasoClear | VasoCare |
| Vasodilan | Vasocidin |
| Vasoflux | Vasoprost; Vasosulf |
| Vasoprost | Vasoflux |
| Vasosulf | Velosef; Vasoflux |
| Velban | Valpin |
| Velosef | Vasosulf |
| Ventolin | phentolamine |
| Vicodin | Hycodan; Hycomine |
| vidarabine | cytarabine |
| Vistaril | Restoril |
| Vistaril | Restoril; Zestril |
| Vitron | Vytone |
| Vytone | Hytone; Vitron |
| Wycillin | Bicillin; V-Cillin |
| Wydase | Lidex |
| Xalatan | Dilantin |
| Xanax | Tenex; Zantac |
| Zantac | Xanax |
| Zarontin | Zaroxolyn |
| Zaroxolyn | Zarontin; Zeroxin |
| Zefazone | cefazolin |
| Zestril | Restoril; Vistaril |
| Ziks | Vicks |
| zinostatin | Sandostatin; simvastatin |
| Zoladex | sulindac |
| Zomig | Flomax; Slow-Mag |

# Abbreviations Used with Medications and Dosages

| Abbreviation/Term | Literally | Meaning |
|---|---|---|
| a.c. | ante cibum | before meals or food |
| ad | ad | to, up to |
| A.D., AD | auris dextra | right ear |
| ad lib. | ad libitum | at pleasure |
| A.L. | auris laeva | left ear |
| a.m., A.M. | ante meridiem | morning |
| Aq. | aqua | water |
| A.S., AS | auris sinistra | left ear |
| A.U., AU* | auris uterque | each ear |
| b.i.d. | bis in die | twice daily |
| b.m. | bowel movement | |
| cc, cm$^3$ | cubic centimeter | |
| CFU | colony-forming unit(s) | |
| d. | die | day |
| EL.U. | ELISA unit(s) | |
| et | et | and |
| g | gram(s) | |
| gt. (plural gtt.) | gutta (plural guttae) | a drop (drops) |
| h. | hora | hour |
| HAU | hemagglutinating unit(s) | |
| h.s. | hora somni | at bedtime |
| IM† | intramuscular | |
| IU | international unit(s) | |
| IV† | intravenous | |
| LfU | limes flocculating unit(s) | |
| | limit of flocculation unit(s) | |
| mcg, μg | microgram(s) | |
| mg | milligram(s) | |
| mEq | milliequivalent(s) | |
| mkat | millikatal unit(s) | |
| mL, ml | milliliter(s) | |
| mU, mIU | milliunit(s) | |
| MU, MIU | megaunit(s) | one million ($10^6$) IU |
| nkat | nanokatal unit(s) | |
| O.D. | oculus dexter | right eye |
| O.L. | oculus laevus | left eye |
| O.S. | oculus sinister | left eye |
| O.U.§ | oculus uterque | each eye |
| p.c. | post cibum | after meals |

| Abbreviation/Term | Literally | Meaning |
|---|---|---|
| p.m., P.M. | post meridiem | afternoon or evening |
| p.o. | per os | by mouth |
| p.r.n. | pro re nata | as needed |
| q.d. | quaque die | every day |
| q.h. | quaque hora | every hour |
| q.i.d. | quater in die | four times a day |
| q.o.d. | | every other day |
| q.s. | quantum satis | sufficient quantity |
| q.s. ad | quantum satis ad | a sufficient quantity to make |
| ℞, Rx | recipe | take; a recipe |
| Sig. | signetur | label |
| s.o.s. | si opus sit | if there is need |
| stat | statim | at once, immediately |
| subcu, subq, SQ | subcutaneous | beneath the skin |
| t.i.d. | ter in die | three times a day |
| tsp. | teaspoonful | |
| μg, mcg | microgram(s) | |

---

\* Although some references have aures unitas (Latin, both ears), this cannot be justified by classical Latin.

† Some references suggest that IM and IV be typed with periods to distinguish from Roman numerals, but we believe context is sufficient to make this distinction.

§ Although some references have oculi unitas (Latin, both eyes), this cannot be justified by classical Latin.

# Therapeutic Drug Levels

| Drug | Class | Serum Levels<br>metric units (SI units) |
|------|-------|----------------------------------------|
| amantadine | antiviral | 300 ng/mL |
| amikacin | aminoglycoside | 16–32 μg/mL |
| amiodarone | antiarrhythmic | 0.5–2.5 μg/mL |
| amitriptyline | antidepressant | 110–250 ng/mL |
| amoxapine | antidepressant | 200–500 ng/mL |
| amrinone | cardiotonic | 3.7 μg/mL |
| bretylium | antiarrhythmic | 0.5–1.5 μg/mL |
| bupropion | antidepressant | 25–100 ng/mL |
| carbamazepine | anticonvulsant | 4–12 μg/mL<br>(17–51 μmol/L) |
| chloramphenicol | antibiotic | 10–20 μg/mL<br>(31–62 μmol/L) |
| chlorpromazine | antipsychotic | 30–500 ng/mL |
| clomipramine | antidepressant | 80–100 ng/mL |
| cyclosporine | immunosuppressive | 250–800 ng/mL<br>(whole blood, RIA*) |
|    trough values: | | 50–300 ng/mL<br>(plasma,RIA*) |
| desipramine | antidepressant | 125–300 ng/mL |
| digitoxin | antiarrhythmic | 9–25 μg/L<br>(11.8–32.8 nmol/L) |
| digoxin | antiarrhythmic | 0.5–2.2 ng/mL<br>(0.6–2.8 nmol/L) |
| disopyramide | antiarrhythmic | 2–8 μg/mL<br>(6–18 μmol/L) |
| doxepin | antidepressant | 100–200 ng/mL |
| flecainide | antiarrhythmic | 0.2–1 μg/mL |
| fluphenazine | antipsychotic | 0.13–2.8 ng/mL |
| gentamicin | aminoglycoside | 4–8 μg/mL |
| haloperidol | antipsychotic | 5–20 ng/mL |
| hydralazine | antihypertensive | 100 ng/mL |
| imipramine | antidepressant | 200–350 ng/mL |
| kanamycin | aminoglycoside | 15–40 μg/mL |
| lidocaine | antiarrhythmic | 1.5–6 μg/mL<br>(4.5–21.5 μmol/L) |
| lithium | antipsychotic | 0.5–1.5 mEq/L<br>(0.5–1.5 mmol/L) |
| maprotiline | antidepressant | 200–300 ng/mL |
| mexiletine | antiarrhythmic | 0.5–2 μg/mL |
| netilmicin | aminoglycoside | 6–10 μg/mL |

| Drug | Class | Serum Levels<br>metric units (SI units) |
|------|-------|------------------------------------------|
| nortriptyline | antidepressant | 50–150 ng/mL |
| perphenazine | antipsychotic | 0.8–1.2 ng/mL |
| phenobarbital | anticonvulsant | 15–40 μg/mL<br>(65–172 μmol/L) |
| phenytoin | anticonvulsant | 10–20 μg/mL<br>(40–80 μmol/L) |
| primidone | anticonvulsant | 5–12 μg/mL<br>(25–46 μmol/L) |
| procainamide | antiarrhythmic | 4–8 μg/mL<br>(17–34 μmol/L) |
| propranolol | antiarrhythmic | 50–200 ng/mL<br>(190–770 nmol/L) |
| protriptyline | antidepressant | 100–200 ng/mL |
| quinidine | antiarrhythmic | 2–6 μg/mL<br>(4.6–9.2 μmol/L) |
| salicylate | analgesic | 100–200 mg/L<br>(725–1448 μmol/L) |
| streptomycin | aminoglycoside | 20–30 μg/mL |
| sulfonamide | antibiotic | 5–15 mg/dL |
| terbutaline | bronchodilator | 0.5–4.1 ng/mL |
| theophylline | bronchodilator | 10–20 μg/mL<br>(55–110 μmol/L) |
| thiothixene | antipsychotic | 2–57 ng/mL |
| tobramycin | aminoglycoside | 4–8 μg/mL |
| tocainide | antiarrhythmic | 4–10 μg/mL |
| trazodone | antidepressant | 800–1600 ng/mL |
| valproic acid | anticonvulsant | 50–100 μg/mL<br>(350–700 μmol/L) |
| vancomycin | antibiotic | 30–40 ng/mL (peak) |
| verapamil | antiarrhythmic | 0.08–0.3 μg/mL |

* radioimmunoassay

# APPENDIX D
# The Most Prescribed Drugs

| Drug | Class/Indication(s) |
|------|---------------------|
| Accupril (quinapril HCl) | antihypertensive, ACE inhibitor |
| acetaminophen with codeine | analgesic, anti-inflammatory |
| Aciphex (rabeprazole sodium) | proton pump inhibitor for GERD |
| Actonel (risedronate sodium) | osteoporosis prevention and treatment |
| Actos (pioglitazone HCl) | oral antidiabetic |
| Adderall XR (mixed amphetamines) | CNS stimulant for ADHD |
| Advair Discus (salmeterol xinafoate, fluticasone propionate) | bronchodilator and corticosteroidal anti-inflammatory for asthma |
| albuterol; albuterol sulfate | bronchodilator for asthma |
| Allegra (fexofenadine HCl) | nonsedating antihistamine for allergy |
| Allegra-D (fexofenadine HCl, pseudo-ephedrine HCl) | nonsedating antihistamine and decongestant for allergy |
| allopurinol | treatment for gout and hyperuricemia |
| Alphagan P (brimonidine tartrate) | topical antiglaucoma agent |
| alprazolam | anxiolytic, sedative |
| Altace (ramipril) | antihypertensive, ACE inhibitor |
| Amaryl (glimepiride) | oral antidiabetic |
| Ambien (zolpidem tartrate) | sedative, hypnotic |
| amitriptyline HCl | tricyclic antidepressant |
| amoxicillin | aminopenicillin antibiotic |
| amoxicillin & clavulanate potassium | aminopenicillin antibiotic |
| Amoxil (amoxicillin trihydrate) | aminopenicillin antibiotic |
| Apri (desogestrel, ethinyl estradiol) | monophasic oral contraceptive |
| Aricept (donepezil HCl) | cognition aid for Alzheimer disease |
| Atacand (candesartan cilexetil) | antihypertensive, angiotensin II blocker |
| atenolol | antihypertensive, antianginal |
| Atrovent (ipratropium bromide) | bronchodilator |
| Augmentin (amoxicillin trihydrate, clavulanate potassium) | aminopenicillin antibiotic |
| Avalide (irbesartan, hydrochlorothiazide) | antihypertensive, angiotensin II blocker, diuretic |
| Avandia (rosiglitazone maleate) | antidiabetic; decreases insulin resistance |
| Avapro (irbesartan) | antihypertensive |
| Avelox (moxifloxacin HCl) | fluoroquinolone antibiotic |
| Aviane (levonorgestrel, ethinyl estradiol) | monophasic oral contraceptive |
| Bactroban (mupirocin calcium) | topical antibiotic |
| Bextra (valdecoxib) | antiarthritic, NSAID, COX-2 inhibitor |
| Biaxin; Biaxin XL (clarithromycin) | macrolide antibiotic |
| carisoprodol | skeletal muscle relaxant |
| Cartia XT (diltiazem HCl) | antihypertensive, antianginal |
| Cefzil (cefprozil) | cephalosporin antibiotic |

| Drug | Class/Indication(s) |
|------|---------------------|
| Celebrex (celecoxib) | antiarthritic, NSAID, COX-2 inhibitor |
| Celexa (citalopram hydrobromide) | SSRI antidepressant |
| cephalexin | cephalosporin antibiotic |
| Cipro (ciprofloxacin) | fluoroquinolone antibiotic |
| ciprofloxacin | fluoroquinolone antibiotic |
| clonazepam | anticonvulsant |
| clonidine | antihypertensive |
| clotrimazole & betamethasone dipropionate | broad-spectrum antifungal, corticosteroidal anti-inflammatory |
| Combivent (ipratropium bromide, albuterol sulfate) | bronchodilator for COPD |
| Concerta (methylphenidate HCl) | CNS stimulant for ADHD |
| Coreg (carvedilol) | α- and β-blocker for hypertension and congestive heart failure |
| Cotrim (trimethoprim, sulfamethoxazole) | sulfonamide antibiotic |
| Coumadin (warfarin sodium) | anticoagulant |
| Cozaar (losartan potassium) | antihypertensive, angiotensin II blocker |
| cyclobenzaprine HCl | skeletal muscle relaxant |
| Depakote (divalproex sodium) | anticonvulsant |
| Detrol LA (tolterodine tartrate) | treatment for urinary frequency |
| diazepam | anxiolytic, skeletal muscle relaxant |
| Diflucan (fluconazole) | systemic antifungal |
| Digitek (digoxin) | antiarrhythmic |
| Dilantin (phenytoin sodium) | anticonvulsant |
| diltiazem HCl | antihypertensive, antianginal |
| Diovan (valsartan) | antihypertensive, angiotensin II blocker |
| Diovan HCT (valsartan, hydrochlorothiazide) | antihypertensive, angiotensin II blocker, diuretic |
| Ditropan XL (oxybutynin chloride) | treatment for urinary frequency |
| doxycycline hyclate | tetracycline antibiotic |
| Duragesic (fentanyl) | narcotic analgesic transdermal patch |
| Effexor XR (venlafaxine) | SSNRI antidepressant, anxiolytic |
| Elidel (pimecrolimus) | topical NSAID for atopic dermatitis |
| enalapril maleate | antihypertensive, ACE inhibitor |
| Endocet (oxycodone HCl; acetaminophen) | narcotic analgesic |
| Evista (raloxifene HCl) | postmenopausal osteoporosis treatment |
| Flomax (tamsulosin HCl) | benign prostatic hypertrophy treatment |
| Flonase (fluticasone propionate) | steroidal anti-inflammatory |
| Flovent (fluticasone propionate) | steroidal anti-inflammatory |
| fluoxetine HCl | SSRI antidepressant |
| folic acid | hematopoietic, prevents birth defects |
| Fosamax (alendronate sodium) | postmenopausal osteoporosis treatment |
| furosemide | diuretic, antihypertensive |
| gemfibrozil | antihyperlipidemic |
| Glucophage XR (metformin HCl) | oral antidiabetic |
| Glucotrol XL (glipizide) | oral antidiabetic |
| Glucovance (glyburide, metformin HCl) | oral antidiabetic |

| Drug | Class/Indication(s) |
|------|---------------------|
| glyburide | oral antidiabetic |
| Humalog (insulin lispro) | parenteral antidiabetic |
| Humulin N; Humulin 70/30 (insulin) | parenteral antidiabetic |
| hydrochlorothiazide | diuretic, antihypertensive |
| hydrocodone & acetaminophen | antitussive, analgesic |
| Hyzaar (losartan potassium, hydrochlorothiazide) | antihypertensive, angiotensin II blocker, diuretic |
| ibuprofen | antiarthritic, analgesic, NSAID |
| Imitrex [oral] (sumatriptan succinate) | migraine headache treatment |
| Inderal LA (propranolol HCl) | antihypertensive, antiarrhythmic |
| isosorbide mononitrate | coronary vasodilator, antianginal |
| Kariva (desogestrel, ethinyl estradiol) | biphasic oral contraceptive |
| Klor-Con; Klor-Con M20 (potassium chloride) | potassium supplement |
| Lanoxin (digoxin) | antiarrhythmic |
| Lantus (insulin glargine) | parenteral antidiabetic |
| Lescol XL (fluvastatin sodium) | antihyperlipidemic |
| Levaquin (levofloxacin) | fluoroquinolone antibiotic |
| Levothroid (levothyroxine sodium) | thyroid hormone |
| Levoxyl (levothyroxine sodium) | thyroid hormone |
| Lexapro (escitalopram oxalate) | SSRI antidepressant |
| Lipitor (atorvastatin calcium) | antihyperlipidemic |
| lisinopril | antihypertensive, ACE inhibitor |
| lorazepam | anxiolytic, tranquilizer |
| Lotensin (benazepril HCl) | antihypertensive, ACE inhibitor |
| Lotrel (amlodipine besylate, benazepril HCl) | antihypertensive, ACE inhibitor, calcium channel blocker |
| Low-Ogestrel (norgestrel, ethinyl estradiol) | monophasic oral contraceptive |
| Macrobid (nitrofurantoin) | urinary antibiotic |
| meclizine HCl | antiemetic for motion sickness, vertigo |
| metformin HCl | oral antidiabetic |
| methylprednisolone | corticosteroidal anti-inflammatory |
| metoclopramide HCl | antiemetic for chemotherapy |
| metoprolol tartrate | antianginal, antihypertensive |
| Miacalcin (calcitonin salmon) | calcium regulator for osteoporosis |
| Microgestin Fe (norethindrone acetate, ethinyl estradiol, ferrous fumarate) | monophasic oral contraceptive, iron supplement |
| Miralax (polyethylene glycol 3350) | laxative, pre-procedure bowel evacuant |
| Mobic (meloxicam) | analgesic, antiarthritic, NSAID |
| Monopril (fosinopril sodium) | antihypertensive, ACE inhibitor |
| naproxen; naproxen sodium | analgesic, antiarthritic, NSAID |
| Nasacort AQ (triamcinolone acetonide) | nasal steroid for allergic rhinitis |
| Nasonex (mometasone furoate) | nasal steroid for allergic rhinitis |
| Necon 1/35 (norethindrone, ethinyl estradiol) | monophasic oral contraceptive |
| Neurontin (gabapentin) | anticonvulsant |
| Nexium (esomeprazole magnesium) | proton pump inhibitor for GERD |

| Drug | Class/Indication(s) |
| --- | --- |
| Niaspan (niacin) | vasodilator, antihyperlipidemic |
| Nifediac CC (nifedipine) | antianginal, antihypertensive |
| nifedipine [extended-release form] | antianginal, antihypertensive |
| Nitroquick (nitroglycerin) | antianginal, coronary vasodilator |
| Norvasc (amlodipine) | antianginal, antihypertensive |
| omeprazole | proton pump inhibitor for GERD |
| Omnicef (cefdinir) | cephalosporin antibiotic |
| Ortho Evra (norelgestromin, ethinyl estradiol) | once-weekly contraceptive patch |
| Ortho-Novum 7/7/7 (norethindrone, ethinyl estradiol) | triphasic oral contraceptive |
| Ortho Tri-Cyclen (norgestimate, ethinyl estradiol) | triphasic oral contraceptive |
| oxycodone HCl & acetaminophen | narcotic analgesic, NSAID |
| OxyContin (oxycodone HCl) | narcotic analgesic |
| Patanol (olopatadine HCl) | ophthalmic antihistamine for allergy |
| Paxil; Paxil CR (paroxetine HCl) | SSRI antidepressant |
| penicillin VK (penicillin V potassium) | natural antibiotic |
| Percocet (oxycodone HCl, acetaminophen) | narcotic analgesic, NSAID |
| phenytoin | anticonvulsant |
| Plavix (clopidogrel bisulfate) | platelet aggregation inhibitor |
| Plendil (felodipine) | antihypertensive |
| potassium chloride | potassium supplement |
| Pravachol (pravastatin sodium) | antihyperlipidemic |
| prednisone | corticosteroidal anti-inflammatory |
| Premarin (conjugated estrogens) | estrogen replacement |
| Prempro (conjugated estrogens, medroxyprogesterone acetate) | hormone replacement therapy |
| Prevacid (lansoprazole) | antisecretory, antiulcer |
| Prilosec (omeprazole) | proton pump inhibitor for GERD |
| promethazine HCl | antihistamine, antiemetic |
| promethazine with codeine | narcotic antitussive, antihistamine |
| propoxyphene napsylate/acetaminophen | narcotic analgesic, NSAID |
| propranolol HCl | antihypertensive, antiarrhythmic |
| Proscar (finasteride) | androgen inhibitor for BPH |
| Protonix (pantoprazole sodium) | proton pump inhibitor for GERD |
| Pulmicort (budesonide) | steroidal inhalant for asthma |
| ranitidine HCl | histamine antagonist for gastric ulcers |
| Remeron (mirtazapine) | tetracyclic antidepressant |
| Rhinocort Aqua (budesonide) | nasal steroid for allergic rhinitis |
| Risperdal (risperidone) | antipsychotic |
| Roxicet (oxycodone HCl, acetaminophen) | narcotic analgesic, NSAID |
| Seroquel (quetiapine fumarate) | antipsychotic |
| Singulair (montelukast sodium) | antiasthmatic |
| Skelaxin (metaxalone) | skeletal muscle relaxant |
| spironolactone | antihypertensive, diuretic |

| Drug | Class/Indication(s) |
|---|---|
| Strattera (atomoxetine HCl) | nonstimulant ADHD treatment |
| sulfamethoxazole & trimethoprim | anti-infective, antibacterial |
| Synthroid (levothyroxine sodium) | thyroid replacement |
| temazepam | tranquilizer, hypnotic |
| terazosin HCl | α-blocker for hypertension and BPH |
| timolol maleate | topical antiglaucoma agent |
| TobraDex (tobramycin, dexamethasone) | ophthalmic antibiotic and steroid |
| Topamax (topiramate) | anticonvulsant |
| Toprol XL (metoprolol succinate) | antihypertensive, antianginal |
| trazodone HCl | tetracyclic antidepressant |
| triamcinolone acetonide | topical steroidal anti-inflammatory |
| triamterene & hydrochlorothiazide | diuretic, antihypertensive |
| Tricor (fenofibrate) | antihyperlipidemic |
| trimethoprim & sulfamethoxazole | anti-infective, antibacterial |
| Trimox (amoxicillin trihydrate) | aminopenicillin antibiotic |
| Trivora (lovonorgestrel, ethinyl estradiol) | triphasic oral contraceptive |
| Tussionex (hydrocodone polistirex, chlorpheniramine polistirex) | narcotic antitussive, antihistamine |
| Ultracet (tramadol HCl, acetaminophen) | central analgesic, NSAID |
| Valtrex (valacyclovir HCl) | antiviral for herpes infections |
| verapamil HCl [sustained-release form] | antianginal, antiarrhythmic, calcium channel blocker |
| Viagra (sildenafil citrate) | vasodilator for erectile dysfunction |
| Vioxx (rofecoxib) | antiarthritic, NSAID, COX-2 inhibitor |
| warfarin sodium | anticoagulant |
| Wellbutrin SR (bupropion HCl) | aminoketone antidepressant |
| Xalatan (latanoprost) | topical antiglaucoma agent |
| Yasmin (drospirenone, ethinyl estradiol) | monophasic oral contraceptive |
| Zetia (ezetimibe) | antihyperlipidemic |
| Zithromax (azithromycin dihydrate) | macrolide antibiotic |
| Zocor (simvastatin) | antihyperlipidemic |
| Zoloft (sertraline) | SSRI antidepressant |
| Zyprexa (olanzapine) | antipsychotic, antimanic |
| Zyrtec (cetirizine HCl) | antihistamine |
| Zyrtec-D (cetirizine HCl, pseudoephedrine HCl) | antihistamine, nasal decongetant |

**Dropped from the previous year's list:**

| | |
|---|---|
| acyclovir | antiviral |
| Adalat CC (nifedipine) | antianginal, antihypertensive |
| Alesse (levonorgestrel, ethinyl estradiol) | monophasic oral contraceptive |
| aspirin | analgesic, antipyretic, NSAID |
| Azmacort (triamcinolone acetonide) | corticosteroid for asthma |
| benzonatate | antitussive |
| bisoprolol & hydrochlorothiazide | β-blocker and diuretic for hypertension |
| BuSpar (buspirone HCl) | anxiolytic |
| buspirone HCl | anxiolytic |

| Drug | Class/Indication(s) |
|---|---|
| butalbital & acetaminophen & caffeine | barbiturate sedative, analgesic |
| captopril | antihypertensive, ACE inhibitor |
| carbidopa & levodopa | antiparkinsonian |
| Cardizem CD (diltiazem HCl) | antihypertensive, antianginal |
| Cardura (doxazosin mesylate) | antihypertensive, antiadrenergic |
| Ceftin (cefuroxime axetil) | cephalosporin antibiotic |
| cimetidine | histamine antagonist for gastric ulcers |
| Clarinex (desloratadine) | nonsedating antihistamine for allergy |
| Claritin (loratadine) | nonsedating antihistamine for allergy |
| Claritin-D (loratadine, pseudoephedrine sulfate) | nonsedating antihistamine and decongestant for allergy |
| clindamycin | lincosamide antibiotic |
| Detrol (tolterodine tartrate) | treatment for urinary frequency |
| diclofenac sodium | antiarthritic, analgesic, NSAID |
| digoxin | antiarrhythmic |
| doxazosin mesylate | $\alpha$-blocker for hypertension and BPH |
| doxepin HCl | tricyclic antidepressant, anxiolytic |
| Dura-Vent (phenylpropanolamine HCl, guaifenesin) | decongestant, expectorant |
| Elocon (mometasone furoate) | topical steroidal anti-inflammatory |
| erythromycin | macrolide antibiotic |
| estradiol | oral estrogen for postmenopausal HRT |
| famotidine | histamine antagonist for gastric ulcers |
| glipizide | oral antidiabetic |
| Glucophage (metformin HCl) | oral antidiabetic |
| hydroxyzine HCl | anxiolytic, minor tranquilizer |
| hyoscyamine sulfate | gastrointestinal/urinary antispasmodic |
| K-Dur (potassium chloride) | potassium supplement |
| Loestrin Fe 1/20 (norethindrone acetate, ethinyl estradiol, ferrous fumarate) | monophasic oral contraceptive, iron supplement |
| Lo/Ovral (ethinyl estradiol, norgestrel) | monophasic oral contraceptive |
| Lotrisone (betamethasone dipropionate, clotrimazole) | topical corticosteroid, antifungal |
| medroxyprogesterone | progestin |
| methocarbamol | skeletal muscle relaxant |
| methylphenidate HCl | CNS stimulant for ADHD |
| metronidazole | oral antibiotic, antiprotozoal |
| minocycline HCl | broad-spectrum antibiotic |
| Mircette (desogestrel, ethinyl estradiol) | biphasic oral contraceptive |
| nitroglycerin | antianginal, coronary vasodilator |
| nortriptyline HCl | tricyclic antidepressant |
| nystatin | systemic antifungal |
| Ortho-Cyclen (norgestimate, ethinyl estradiol) | monophasic oral contraceptive |
| Pepcid (famotidine) | histamine antagonist for gastric ulcers |
| phenazopyridine HCl | urinary tract analgesic |
| phenobarbital | sedative, hypnotic |
| Prinivil (lisinopril) | antihypertensive, ACE inhibitor |

| Drug | Class/Indication(s) |
|------|---------------------|
| Procardia XL (nifedipine) | antianginal, antihypertensive |
| Propacet (propoxyphene napsylate, acetaminophen) | narcotic analgesic, NSAID |
| Proventil HFA (albuterol) | bronchodilator |
| Prozac (fluoxetine HCl) | SSRI antidepressant |
| Relafen (nabumetone) | antiarthritic, NSAID |
| Serevent (salmeterol xinafoate) | bronchodilator for asthma |
| Serzone (nefazodone HCl) | SSNRI antidepressant |
| tamoxifen citrate | antineoplastic for breast cancer |
| tetracycline HCl | antibiotic |
| theophylline [sustained-release form] | bronchodilator |
| Tiazac (diltiazem HCl) | antihypertensive, antianginal |
| tramadol HCl | central analgesic |
| Triphasil (levonorgestrel, ethinyl estradiol) | triphasic oral contraceptive |
| Ultram (tramadol HCl) | central analgesic |
| Vasotec (enalaprilat maleate) | antihypertensive, ACE inhibitor |
| Veetids (penicillin V potassium) | natural antibiotic |
| Vicoprofen (hydrocodone bitartrate, ibuprofen) | narcotic analgesic |
| Zestoretic (hydrochlorothiazide, lisinopril) | antihypertensive, ACE inhibitor, diuretic |
| Zestril (lisinopril) | antihypertensive |
| Ziac (hydrochlorothiazide, bisoprolol fumarate) | antihypertensive |